Fetal and Neonatal Brain Injury

Fetal and Neonatal Brain Injury

Fourth Edition

Edited by

David K. Stevenson

William E. Benitz

Philip Sunshine

Susan R. Hintz

Maurice L. Druzin

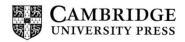

CAMBRIDGE UNIVERSITY PRESS
Cambridge, New York, Melbourne, Madrid, Cape Town, Singapore,
São Paulo, Delhi

Cambridge University Press
The Edinburgh Building, Cambridge CB2 8RU, UK

Published in the United States of America by Cambridge University Press,
New York

www.cambridge.org
Information on this title: www.cambridge.org/9780521888592

First edition published 1989 by Oxford University Press
Second edition published 1997
Third edition published 2003 by Cambridge University Press
Fourth edition published 2009

Printed in the United Kingdom at the University Press, Cambridge

A catalog record for this publication is available from the British Library

Library of Congress Cataloging-in-Publication Data

Fetal and neonatal brain injury / edited by David K. Stevenson ...
[et al.]. – 4th ed.
        p. ; cm.
    Includes bibliographical references and index.
    ISBN 978-0-521-88859-2 (hardback)
1. Fetal brain–Abnormalities. 2. Brain-damaged children. I. Stevenson,
David K. (David Kendal), 1949–
    [DNLM: 1. Brain Injuries. 2. Infant, Newborn. 3. Birth Injuries.
4. Brain Diseases. 5. Fetal Diseases. 6. Pregnancy Complications.
WS 340 F419 2009]
    RG629.B73F456 2009
    618.92'8–dc22

                                                                    2009009613

ISBN 978-0-521-88859-2 hardback

Contents

Contributors

Reinaldo Acosta
Sacred Heart Women's Health Center, Spokane,
Washington, USA

Julie M. R. Arafeh
Stanford University Medical Center, Stanford,
California, USA

Rebecca N. Baergen
New York Presbyterian Hospital, Weill Comell Medical
College, New York, USA

Patrick D. Barnes M.D.
Lucile Packard Children's Hospital at Stanford, Palo Alto,
California, USA

Robert D. Barrett
The University of Auckland, Auckland, New Zealand

William E. Benitz
Stanford University Medical Center, Stanford, California, USA

Laura Bennet
The University of Auckland, Auckland, New Zealand

Jonathan A. Bernstein
Stanford University Medical Center, Stanford,
California, USA

Yair Blumenfeld
Stanford University Medical Center, Stanford, California, USA

Theonia K. Boyd
Harvard Medical School, Boston, Massachusetts, USA

Ken Brady
Johns Hopkins School of Medicine, Baltimore, Maryland, USA

David P. Carlton
Emory University, Atlanta, Georgia, USA

Usha Chitkara
Stanford University Medical Center, Stanford, California, USA

Jane Chueh
Stanford University Medical Center, Stanford, California, USA

Ronald S. Cohen
Stanford University Medical Center, Stanford,
California, USA

Justin Collingham
Stanford University Medical Center, Stanford,
California, USA

Marvin Cornblath (deceased)
The Johns Hopkins University, Baltimore, Maryland, USA

Alexis S. Davis
Stanford University Medical Center, Stanford,
California, USA

Justin Mark Dean
The University of Auckland, Auckland, New Zealand

Maurice L. Druzin
Stanford University Medical Center, Stanford,
California, USA

Bonnie Dwyer
Stanford University Medical Center, Stanford,
California, USA

Yasser Y. El-Sayed
Stanford University Medical Center, Stanford,
California, USA

Gregory M. Enns
Stanford University Medical Center, Stanford,
California, USA

Andrea Enright
Stanford University Medical Center, Stanford,
California, USA

Heidi M. Feldman
Stanford University Medical Center, Stanford,
California, USA

Donna M. Ferriero
University of California San Francisco, San Francisco,
California, USA

Hayley A. Gans
Stanford University Medical Center, Stanford,
California, USA

Hannah C. Glass
University of San Francisco, San Francisco,
California, USA

Alistair J. Gunn
The University of Auckland, Auckland, New Zealand

Kathleen Gutierrez
Stanford University Medical Center, Stanford, California, USA

Jin S. Hahn
Stanford University Medical Center, Stanford, California, USA

Louis P. Halamek
Stanford University Medical Center, Stanford, California, USA

Rima Hanna-Wakim
Stanford University Medical Center, Stanford, California, USA

William W. Hay, Jr.
University of Colorado School of Medicine, Aurora, Colorado, USA

Israel Hendler
Sheba Medical Center, Tel Hashomer, Israel

Susan R. Hintz
Stanford University Medical Center, Stanford, California, USA

H. Eugene Hoyme
Sanford Children's Hospital, Sioux Falls, South Dakota and Stanford Medical Center, Stanford, California, USA

Louanne Hudgins
Stanford University Medical Center, Stanford, California, USA

Satish C. Kalhan
Case Reserve University, Cleveland, Ohio, USA

John A. Kerner
Stanford University Medical Center, Stanford, California, USA

Bea Latal
University of British Columbia, British Columbia, Canada

Ronald J. Lemire (deceased)
Stanford University Medical Center, Stanford, California, USA

Irene M. Loe
Stanford University Medical Center, Stanford, California, USA

Deirdre J. Lyell
Stanford University Medical Center, Stanford, California, USA

Yvonne A. Maldonado
Stanford University Medical Center, Stanford, California, USA

Melanie A. Manning
Stanford University Medical Center, Stanford, California, USA

Lee J. Martin
Johns Hopkins University School of Medicine, Baltimore, Maryland, USA

Steven P. Miller
University of British Columbia, British Columbia, Canada

Amen Ness
University of California San Francisco, San Francisco, California, USA

William Oh
Brown University, Providence, Rhode Island, USA

Donald M. Olson
Stanford University Medical Center, Stanford, California, USA

Giles J. Peek
Glenfield Hospital, Leicester, United Kingdom

Alistair G. S. Philip
Stanford University Medical Center, Stanford, California, USA

Chandra Ramamoorthy
Stanford University Medical Center, Stanford, California, USA

William D. Rhine
Stanford University Medical Center, Stanford, California, USA

Ted S. Rosenkrantz
University of Connecticut School of Medicine, Farmington, Connecticut, USA

Mark S. Scher
Rainbow Babies and Children's Hospital, Cleveland, Ohio, USA

Robert Schwartz
Brown University, Providence, Rhode Island, USA

Daniel S. Seidman
Sheba Medical Center, Tel Hashomer, Israel

Avinash K. Shetty
Wake Forest University Health Sciences, Winston-Salem, North Carolina, USA

David Sheuerman
Sheuerman, Martini & Tabari, Attorneys at Law, San Jose, California, USA

Janet Shimotake
University of California San Francisco, San Francisco, California, USA

David K. Stevenson
Stanford University Medical Center, Stanford, California, USA

Philip Sunshine
Stanford University Medical Center, Stanford, California, USA

Trenna L. Sutcliffe
Stanford University Medical Center, Stanford, California, USA

Masoud Taslimi
Stanford University Medical Center, Stanford, California, USA

Krisa P. Van Meurs
Stanford University Medical Center, Stanford, California, USA

Zinaida S. Vexler
University of California San Francisco, San Francisco, California, USA

Linda S. de Vries
Wilhelmina Children's Hospital, Utrecht, the Netherlands

Thomas E. Wiswell
Center for Neonatal Care, Orlando, Florida, USA

Ronald J. Wong
Stanford University Medical Center, Stanford, California, USA

Ernlé W. D. Young
Stanford University Medical Center, Stanford, California, USA

Foreword

Neonatal–perinatal medicine emerged as a subspecialty in the 1960s, and the first certification examination by the American Board of Pediatrics took place in 1975. Prior to the application of intensive care, neonatal–perinatal medicine could be characterized as being anecdotally based, with benign neglect and a series of disastrous interventions. Great progress has been made, and evidence-based medicine is now the order of the day. The data base has expanded exponentially and we stand on the threshold of seminal therapeutic breakthroughs. The impossible is being made possible, and we anticipate that the ability to repair organs such as the brain and spinal cord will soon be part of our armamentarium.

There has been a dizzying proliferation of scientific knowledge related to the brain that has been incorporated into the fourth edition of *Fetal and Neonatal Brain Injury*. Whereas there is a general awareness that by the time a textbook is published it typically trails current knowledge, the editors have made every effort to remedy this. The fourth edition includes new authors or topic headings for 21 of the 50 chapters, and the text *is as near to current as is humanly possible.*

Simplifying neuroscience for non-neurologists is a daunting task. Yet somehow, through their choice of contributors, the editors have successfully assembled a book that is comprehensive, up to date, understandable, and interesting to read. The sections have been somewhat rearranged but they follow a logical sequence and new chapters and contributors blend seamlessly with those that have been updated. Although the text is mainly focused on the central and peripheral nervous system, because any and all disorders in the neonate may affect the brain, the reader is subjected to an excellent refresher course on general neonatology.

When I wrote the foreword to the third edition, we could anticipate the outcomes from the hypothermia for hypoxic ischemic encephalopathy trials – the data are available and encouraging. However, additional therapy is still needed as approximately half the treated group is still significantly harmed by the perinatal insult. Furthermore, there is a suggestion that the outcomes for extremely low-birthweight infants are improving. The developing brain is slowly revealing its secrets, and we can anticipate even better outcomes in the future.

The latest advances in genetics, neurobiology, and imaging as well as the therapeutic advances in the treatment of asphyxia and seizures, to mention a few, are well described. There are also a number of journeys that can be followed from bench to bedside. I came away with an optimistic feeling that we are on the brink of major breakthroughs in neuronal repair, as well as a deep respect for the plasticity of the brain. A Canadian psychiatrist, Norman Doidge, has called neural plasticity "one of the most extraordinary discoveries of the twentieth century." Neural plasticity permits the neonatal brain to move a given function to a different location as a consequence of normal experience or brain damage/recovery. Is it really possible that thinking, learning, and acting actually change the structure and function of the brain? Certainly there is every reason, based on the accumulating evidence, to believe this to be true. Better understanding of this remarkable ability will enable the maximum recovery from insults to the brain. Also the recognition and characterization of neuromodulators and neurotrophic factors, together with a better understanding of the genetic, hormonal, and cytokine control of the neurons, should result in the successful introduction of newer and better pharmacologic agents. Ultimately we can anticipate the implantation of cells genetically modified to secrete the appropriate cytokines, hormones, or therapeutic agents to modulate the brain.

Avroy A. Fanaroff
Gertrude Lee Tucker Professor and Chair
Eliza Henry Barnes Professor of Neonatology
Department of Pediatrics
Rainbow Babies & Children's Hospital
Case Western Reserve University
Cleveland, Ohio

Preface

In preparing the fourth edition of our textbook, we have incorporated the newest data regarding the pathophysiology and cellular and molecular bases of neonatal encephalopathy. We have added the most recent data depicting the emergence of newer and promising forms of therapy, including the results of randomized clinical trials using hypothermia.

We have added two new editors for this edition, Dr. Maurice L. Druzin, who is the Chief of Maternal Fetal Medicine at Stanford University, and Susan R. Hintz, an Associate Professor of Pediatrics in the Division of Neonatal and Developmental Medicine. Dr. Druzin has reorganized the section on obstetrical factors that can contribute to fetal and neonatal brain injury and has recruited new contributors for this endeavor. Dr. Hintz, who has provided leadership in prenatal counseling and is the Director of our new Center for Comprehensive Fetal Health, has also focused on outcome studies in various disease processes in the neonate, and recruited new contributors to provide additional outcome data and recommendations.

We have added several new chapters, including ones addressing pregnancy-induced hypertension, HELLP syndrome and chronic hypertension, complications of multiple gestation, neurogenic disorders of the brain, pathogenesis of white-matter injury in the preterm infant, neonatal stroke, assessment and management of infants with cerebral palsy, the long-term outcome of neonatal events on speech, language development, and academic achievement, as well as the neurological outcome of infants with neonatal encephalopathy. We have expanded the chapters on the mechanism of brain damage in animal models of neonatal encephalopathy, the structural and functional imaging of the fetal and neonatal brain, and hemorrhagic lesion of the central nervous system.

As we noted in our previous editions, with any text that has multiple contributors, there is some overlap and repetition among the various presentations. Rather than editing these chapters to avoid such overlap entirely, we have elected to respect the authors' unique presentations and styles, as different perspectives reflect the richness of their experiences. It also allows the contributors to express their opinions freely, and the variation of opinion in similar topics can be appreciated more fully.

We thank our collaborators, especially those who met their editorial deadlines, as well as the staff of Cambridge University Press for their support and expertise in preparing the text. We thank Cele Quaintance, who helped organize the content of the text, maintained contact with our contributors, and collected and collated the chapters as they were received. We also thank Mrs. Tonya Gonzales-Clenney, who helped edit many of the chapters to fit the format of the text, and maintained communications with our publishers.

Lastly, we owe a great deal to our spouses, Joan Stevenson, Andrea Benitz, Sara Sunshine, Elizabeth Hoffman, and Henry Rosack, for their support, encouragement, and infinite patience.

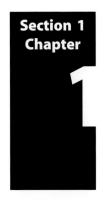

Epidemiology, pathophysiology, and pathogenesis of fetal and neonatal brain injury
Neonatal encephalopathy: epidemiology and overview

Philip Sunshine

Introduction

Since the publication of the first edition of this text in 1989, a great deal has been written regarding the issues of neonatal asphyxia and hypoxic–ischemic encephalopathy (HIE) in term and near-term infants. These manuscripts have addressed the incidence, etiology, pathophysiology, treatment, and outcome of such patients, often relating outcomes to the development of cerebral palsy (CP) and/or mental retardation in survivors [1–29]. Much of the understanding of the pathophysiology has been the result of studies carried out in laboratory animals, which have been extrapolated to the human fetus and newborn. Additional studies of complications and outcome have been population-based, comparing the injured infant to carefully selected normal controls. These studies have added a great deal to our understanding of risk factors for brain injury, and have enhanced our ability to predict and to identify patients with increasing accuracy. This has become increasingly important, as newer modalities of treatment have evolved which require more precision in the early identification of these infants so that the validity of these therapies can be ascertained. As can be seen in Chapters 39, 41, and 42, early institution of treatment becomes of paramount importance if an improved outcome is to be achieved.

While some still believe that the major injuries in these patients occur in the intrapartum period, many studies suggest otherwise, and allude to the fact that many of the problems arise antenatally, and may be exacerbated in the intrapartum period. Clearly, several important publications have defined specific criteria that must be present in order to establish that intrapartum events are the primary causes of the infant's difficulties, but not everyone agrees that such rigorous definitions are valid in each and every case [7,10].

Unfortunately, the terms birth asphyxia and HIE have been and continue to be used interchangeably to identify the depressed infant. Stanley et al. noted that "Birth asphyxia is a theoretical concept, and its existence in a patient is not easy to recognize accurately by clinical observation" [1]. Similarly, the description HIE would indicate that the cause of the condition is clearly identified. Most now refer to such infants as having neonatal encephalopathy, a term used by Nelson and Leviton to describe "a clinically defined syndrome of disturbed neurological function in the earliest days of life in the term infant, manifested by difficulty in initiating and maintaining respiration, depression of tone and reflexes, subnormal level of consciousness and often seizures" [2].

This terminology has been adopted by the International Cerebral Palsy Task Force [7] as well as by the American College of Obstetricians and Gynecologists (ACOG) and the American Academy of Pediatrics (AAP) in their text entitled *Neonatal Encephalopathy and Cerebral Palsy: Defining the Pathogenesis and Pathophysiology* [10].

Neonatal encephalopathy is a purely clinical description that avoids identification of the etiology or pathogenesis of the infant's condition. Unfortunately, neonatal encephalopathy does not exist as a distinct diagnostic category in the International Classification of Diseases, 9th Revision (ICD-9). Table 1.1 lists the categories and numerical designations used to define these infants.

Nevertheless, it is crucial that the caretakers of the injured infant have a more rigorous understanding of the factors that could possibly contribute to the infant's condition, and that they are not unduly influenced by circumstantial evidence. Many of the events leading to the infant's presentation at birth occur long before the onset of labor. With the use of sophisticated imaging, more and more infants are being recognized as having abnormalities that have already led to significant damage prior to the intrapartum period. In addition, careful examination of the placenta has been of great value in identifying lesions that are associated with infections or other anomalies that have or can lead to fetal injury (see Chapter 20).

We recognize that these infants are often unable to tolerate the stress of labor well, may have fetal heart rate abnormalities either prior to delivery or during the early stages of labor, or have abnormal contraction stress tests or non-stress testing. These infants are often difficult to resuscitate, and show neurological features that seem excessive considering the problems that occurred during labor or the birthing process. In addition, some infants may have suffered a significant intrauterine catastrophe, recover, and may even be able to

Fetal and Neonatal Brain Injury, 4th edition, ed. David K. Stevenson, William E. Benitz, Philip Sunshine, Susan R. Hintz, and Maurice L. Druzin. Published by Cambridge University Press. © Cambridge University Press 2009.

Table 1.1. International Classification of Diseases 9th Revision (ICD-9) categories used to designate neonatal encephalopathy

Unspecified birth asphyxia in newborn infants	768.9
Encephalopathy, not classified	348.3
Encephalopathy, other	348.39
Cerebral depression, coma, and other abnormal cerebral signs	779.2
Asphyxia, mild–moderate	768.6
Severe birth asphyxia	768.5
Asphyxia and hypoxemia	799.0
If seizures are present, add	779.0

Table 1.2. Acute causes of fetal brain injury (sentinel events)

Prolapsed umbilical cord
Uterine rupture
Abruptio placentae
Amniotic fluid embolism
Acute neonatal hemorrhage
Vasa previa
Acute blood loss from cord
Fetal–maternal hemorrhage
Acute maternal hemorrhage
Any condition causing an abrupt decrease in maternal cardiac output and/ or blood flow to the fetus

tolerate labor well enough not to have abnormalities noted on their fetal heart-rate tracings [23].

We also recognize that events leading to difficulties in the prematurely born infant may be different from those in infants born near or at term. Similarly, the preterm infant may have many more and vastly different difficulties in the postpartum rather than the intrapartum period, and will have different clinical features from those seen in the full-term infant. In attempts to evaluate etiology, pathogenesis, intervention, and management, one must be aware that similar events may have different consequences depending upon the patient's capacity to respond to various insults, and some of these are determined by gestational age. In addition, infants with intrauterine growth restriction (IUGR) make up a disproportionate share of infants with neonatal brain injury, suggesting that the underlying cause or causes of the growth restriction may have started in utero and continued through the intrapartum and postpartum periods.

Asphyxia

Asphyxia is defined as progressive hypoxemia and hypercapnia accompanied by the progressive development of metabolic acidosis. The definition has both clinical and biochemical components, and indicates that, unless the process is reversed, it will lead to cellular damage and ultimately to the death of the patient. We currently do not have the sophisticated technology of routinely measuring fetal cerebral activity or the neurocellular response to unfavorable conditions such as hypoxia, ischemia, or acidosis, the compensatory mechanisms that protect the brain cells, or, when such mechanisms are inadequate, the documentation of cell injury and cellular death.

In lieu of direct measurements, we have utilized indirect indicators that have been based on studies carried out in laboratory animals and extrapolated to be used in the human fetus. In a few instances direct measurements have been possible, but have not been convincingly linked to outcome. Indirect assessments include the biophysical profile, fetal heart rate measurements, evidence of severe metabolic acidosis, depressed Apgar scores, abnormal newborn neurological function, and development of seizures. As mentioned, the timing of the events is often unknown and difficult to ascertain as far as onset, duration, and severity are concerned. Based on studies in monkeys by Myers [30], and also substantiated to a great

extent in fetal lambs by the group in New Zealand [31], two major types of intrauterine asphyxial conditions have been recognized. These include acute total asphyxial events and prolonged partial asphyxia.

The causes of the acute total events are listed in Table 1.2 and have been referred to as "sentinel events" by MacLennan and the International Cerebral Palsy Task Force [7]. In the acute type of asphyxia, there is a catastrophic event: the fetus is suddenly and rapidly deprived of his or her lifeline, and usually does not have the opportunity to protect the brain by "invoking the diving reflex."

The conditions most commonly encountered include prolapse of the umbilical cord, placental abruption, fetal hemorrhage, and uterine rupture. For a period of time there was an increase in the use of vaginal birth after cesarean section (VBAC), but recently, because of the risk of uterine rupture, there has been a decrease in VBAC, with many physicians and hospitals reluctant to provide such care for patients (see Chapter 12).

Infants with acute asphyxia have damage to the deep gray matter of the brain involving the thalamus, basal ganglia, and brainstem, often with sparing of the cerebral cortex. If successfully resuscitated, these infants may not have evidence of multisystem or multiorgan dysfunction. Laboratory animals that were healthy prior to the onset of the acute asphyxial event develop evidence of neurological damage as early as 8 minutes after the acute event. Major irreversible lesions were found after 10–11 minutes, and the animals usually succumbed if not resuscitated within 18 minutes. After 20 minutes of asphyxia, some animals could be resuscitated, but usually died of cardiogenic shock within 24–48 hours even with intensive care [30].

Although data in humans are lacking, studies of infants following prolapsed cords or uterine rupture suggest similar time frames, and those infants who have occult prolapse often have a better outcome than those with overt prolapse. A study from Los Angeles County University of Southern California (LAC/USC) Medical Center noted that if it required greater than 18 minutes to deliver the fetus after spontaneous rupture of the uterus, neurological sequelae would ensue [32]. Unfortunately, the long-term follow-up of the surviving infants in this study is not available. Thus the 30-minute timing of "decision to incision," as recommended by ACOG, is not valid in these situations. The infants who have suffered this type of acute asphyxia will have varying degrees of neurological injury, often manifesting extrapyramidal types of CP and varying degrees of mental impairment depending upon the severity and extent of the injury.

The second group of infants are those that have been subjected to prolonged partial asphyxial episodes, and have involvement of the cerebral cortex in a watershed type of distribution. They often have multiorgan involvement and have pyramidal signs of CP. The incidence and severity of cognitive impairment also depend upon the extent and severity of the lesion.

An acute event may also occur in a fetus who has already been subjected to a partial prolonged asphyxial condition or a pre-existing neurological insult. That fetus may demonstrate complications of both processes and have both pyramidal and extrapyramidal neurological findings associated with varying degrees of auditory, visual, and/or cognitive abnormalities.

Incidence of neonatal encephalopathy

Haider and Bhutta noted that of the over 130 million babies born yearly worldwide, about 4 million expire in the neonatal period, primarily from complications arising during birthing [21]. Most of the infants are born in developing nations, and at least 50% of the deaths occur at home, where most of these infants are born.

In industrialized nations the incidence of neonatal encephalopathy is much lower, and it has continued to fall over the past three decades. Depending upon the criteria used to document the incidence as well as the severity of the encephalopathy, the incidence varies from 1 to 7/1000 live births. Using the Sarnat score or modifications of the score, infants are classified as having mild, moderate, or severe encephalopathy [33] (see Chapter 16). In the United Kingdom [3], France [18], and Australia [19], similar declines have been noted not only in the incidence of severe encephalopathy but also in the mortality rate of infants so affected.

In Sweden, where an Apgar score of less than 7 at 5 minutes was used to identify babies with this problem, the incidence increased from 5.7/1000 live births to 8.2/1000 over a 7-year period. The incidence of severe depression varied between 1.4 and 2.6/1000 live births. However, the incidence of stillborn infants had decreased significantly [26].

Wu et al. evaluated data from the state of California from 1991 to 2000, and included 5 364 663 live-born infants. Using ICD-9 classifications of 768.5, 768.6, and 768.9, the incidence of neonatal asphyxia fell from 14.8/1000 to 1.3/1000 live births, a 91% decrease during the study years [34]. Data from the 1996 annual summary of vital statistics also demonstrated that the infant mortality rate due to asphyxia fell 72% between 1979 and 1996 [35], and in the most recent surveys the mortality rates were 0.13/1000 in 2001 and 0.15/1000 in 2003.

The reasons for the decrease in neonatal encephalopathy have not as yet been clearly elucidated, but several factors have been suggested (Table 1.3). Perhaps one of the most important

Table 1.3. Factors that have been associated with decreased incidence and mortality due to neonatal encephalopathy in term and near-term infants

More stringent awareness and documentation of the appropriate diagnosis of neonatal encephalopathy
Early prenatal care and recognition of mothers who are at high risk of delivering an infant with neonatal encephalopathy
Pregnancy termination when severe congenital malformations are detected
Early recognition of infants with growth restriction as well as macrosomic infants and avoidance of intrapartum complications
Improved education and training of personnel who are responsible for resuscitation and stabilization of the depressed neonate
Appropriate treatment of mothers who are carriers of Group B streptococci
More liberal use of cesarean section for infants in the breech position
Improved recognition and treatment of mothers with chorioamnionitis
More appropriate induction and use of obstetrical anesthesia
Ready access to neonatal intensive care

reasons is close adherence to a more specific diagnosis of encephalopathy. Other factors playing a significant role include early prenatal care and recognition of women with high-risk pregnancies, increased recognition and appropriate treatment of mothers who are carriers of Group B *Streptococcus*, early dating of pregnancy, and avoiding post-term deliveries as well as recognizing the fetus who is over- or undergrown. There has also been early termination of pregnancy where infants with significant congenital malformation are detected. Lastly, education programs have been developed to insure that depressed infants are given appropriate resuscitation and stabilization and ready access to intensive care [34] (see Chapters 39 and 40).

Risk factors associated with neonatal encephalopathy

Most of the data regarding risk factors have been derived from data accumulated from the Western Australia case–control studies [5,19]. The infants were born at or near term and had moderate to severe neonatal encephalopathy as defined by strict criteria. The criteria included seizures alone or associated with abnormal consciousness, difficulty in maintaining respiration, difficulty in feeding, and abnormal tone and/or reflexes.

Risk factors prior to conception

These are listed in Table 1.4 and include poor socioeconomic status and advanced maternal age. The findings of a family history of seizures and/or neurological disorders are similar to those previously described by Nelson and Ellenberg [36]. The increased incidence associated with in vitro fertilization is discussed in Chapter 6.

Risk factors in the antepartum period

These are delineated in Table 1.5 and include maternal and fetal characteristics. Mothers with thyroid disease were nine times more likely to have infants with neonatal encephalopathy compared to mothers who were euthyroid. This association has also been noted in infants with CP born to mothers with various

Table 1.4. Risk factors prior to conception

Socioeconomic factors
Increased maternal age
Unemployment
Women without health insurance
Medical conditions
Family history of recurrent non-febrile seizures
Family history of other neurological disorders
Infertility treatment
Poorly controlled chronic illnesses

Table 1.5. Risk factors in the antepartum period

Maternal conditions
Thyroid disease
Severe pre-eclampsia
Moderate to severe vaginal bleeding
Viral infection requiring medical attention
Late or no prenatal care
Poorly controlled diabetes
Systemic lupus erythematosus (SLE)
Infant complications
Post-datism
Intrauterine growth restriction (IUGR)
Abnormal placenta
Congenital malformations

types of thyroid diseases. Similarly, severe pre-eclampsia, moderate to severe vaginal bleeding, and severe viral illness were other prepartum risk factors. Growth restriction and those who were post-dates were at increased risk as well.

The Australian study deliberately excluded infants with birth defects and abnormal antepartum fetal birth rate tracings, but both of these findings would indicate an at-risk infant [5].

Congenital malformations involving systems other than the nervous system were found more frequently in infants with encephalopathy, suggesting these are antepartum risk factors as well [37]. Women with chronic illnesses such as systemic lupus erythematosus (SLE) and diabetes have an increased risk of having neonates with encephalopathy.

Intrapartum risk factors

Intrapartum risk factors are often a continuum of those factors that placed the infant at risk in the antepartum period, such as growth restriction and pre-existing congenital abnormalities. Additional factors include maternal fever, a tight nucchal cord, a persistent occiput posterior position, and a persistent non-reassuring fetal heart rate pattern that develops during the intrapartum period after being normal initially [5,6]. Chorioamnionitis, a diagnosis made clinically because of maternal pyrexia, leukocytosis, and malodorous amniotic fluid, is associated with a marked increase in the incidence and severity of neonatal encephalopathy and CP [38]. In laboratory animals, the presence of various cytokines, especially interleukin 6 (IL-6), causes an increased sensitivity of the fetus to ischemia and hypoxia, as well as having a direct deleterious effect on the brain. Measurements of various cytokines in blood and cerebrospinal fluid (CSF) have been found to be significantly higher in infants with encephalopathy who were later found to have abnormal neurodevelopmental outcome [15,39]. The issue of chorioamnionitis is discussed in greater detail in Chapter 12.

Factors that are associated with sudden changes in fetal heart rate patterns leading to bradycardia that does not resolve readily have been described as sentinel events; these are listed in Table 1.2 and are highly correlative with neonatal encephalopathy.

Correlative findings associated with neonatal encephalopathy

Several findings have been correlated to some extent with the severity of encephalopathy occurring in the intrapartum period. These include a persistently low Apgar score, presence of meconium in the amniotic fluid, evidence of significant metabolic acidosis, the onset of seizures within the first 72 hours of life, the need for cardiopulmonary resuscitation, abnormal electroencephalography, evidence of multiorgan damage, corroborative findings on imaging studies, and corroborative laboratory findings.

Apgar score

The Apgar score was designed to identify infants who were depressed at birth and who required resuscitative efforts [40]. The scoring system required an "advocate" in order to evaluate the infant and provide a numerical score of the infant's condition. Dr. Virginia Apgar did not design this scoring system to evaluate neurological damage or outcome. However, a score of less than 7 at 5 minutes has been used in numerous studies to identify an infant who has suffered from intrapartum events. Unfortunately, there are many factors that influence the Apgar score including immaturity, maternal anesthesia and/or analgesia, fetal and neonatal sepsis, and neuromuscular abnormalities. Using the Apgar score as an isolated finding by itself is inappropriate to define neonatal encephalopathy.

However, the persistence of a low score for greater than 5 minutes despite intensive and appropriate resuscitation has been associated with an increase in morbidity and mortality [27]. Perlman and Risser found that an Apgar score of 5 or less at 5 minutes in combination with significant fetal acidosis and the need for cardiopulmonary resuscitation increased the risk significantly (340-fold) for the infants to develop seizures, a marker of moderate to severe encephalopathy [4,13].

Meconium

The presence of meconium in the amniotic fluid has long been thought to indicate fetal stress. Meconium is found in 8–20% of all deliveries, being uncommonly encountered in preterm gestations and more frequently in the post-term baby [41].

If meconium is recognized in amniotic fluids of infants at 34 weeks' gestation or younger, significant intrauterine stress or intrauterine infection must be suspected. In term and post-term infants, meconium staining is usually light, and the fetus and newborn are essentially symptom-free. However, heavy, thick meconium passed early in labor tends to have a more ominous significance than when it is passed more proximate to delivery. But even this finding has not been substantiated.

The presence of meconium per se in term infants is not predictive of neurological sequelae; in fact, Nelson and Ellenberg noted that fewer than 0.5% of the infants weighing more than 2500 g with meconium staining had neurological sequelae [36]. In other studies, the presence of meconium-stained amniotic fluid had no predictive value in regard to outcome, the development of neurologic symptoms in the newborn period, or acidosis measured by the pH of cord blood. Even when the presence of meconium was ascertained and used in conjunction with either Apgar scores or cord pH values or both, the finding did not alter the incidence of subsequent neurological abnormalities (see Chapters 20 and 36).

Fetal heart-rate monitoring

Fetal heart-rate monitoring has now been used for over 40 years, having been developed to decrease the rates of neonatal encephalopathy and intrauterine deaths. While it has been successful in decreasing the rate of stillbirths, its use has not significantly decreased the incidence of neurological sequelae. In one carefully controlled study comparing continuous fetal heart rate monitoring with intermittent auscultation of the fetal heart rate, the incidence of seizures was reduced in the group that was continually monitored electronically. However, the long-term neurological outcomes were the same in both groups, and most of the infants who developed CP did not have seizures in the newborn period [42]. A more complete discussion of intrapartum monitoring is found in Chapter 15.

Fetal and neonatal blood gas evaluations

Since the mid-1960s, obstetricians have utilized fetal acid–base measurements as adjuncts to fetal heart-rate monitoring to evaluate the well-being of the fetus and to identify those who were at risk to develop intrapartum difficulties. Fetal scalp blood sampling during labor has been abandoned to a great extent, and fetal heart-rate monitoring has been used exclusively. The acid–base status of the fetus has been monitored at the time of delivery by assaying the umbilical arterial and venous blood gases immediately after birth.

Initially, an arterial pH below 7.20 was considered to be abnormal, but few such infants were found to have any neonatal or subsequent neurological abnormalities. Correlative data were noted when the umbilical arterial pH was less than 7.0, and especially when it was associated with newborns who required various forms of resuscitation. The vast majority of infants with low pH and no other findings almost always have benign neonatal courses.

Chauhan et al. [43] evaluated their own data as well as several large previously published studies totaling over 43 000

infants born at term who had umbilical arterial pH levels of 7.0 or less. The prevalence of this low pH ranged from 0.2% to 1.6% of live births, with a mean of 0.6%. The incidence of neurologic injury in these infants ranged from 4.3% to 30.9%, and the mortality rate ranged from 0% to 8%.

Low [17] has noted that the threshold for significant metabolic acidosis was a base deficit between 12 and 16 mmol/L. As the degree of acidosis increased, the number of neurological abnormalities increased. In addition, the longer the acidosis persisted, the greater was the risk of neurological defects.

The finding of a low pH in itself is of little consequence unless other abnormalities are found. Perlman [23] reported on a total of 115 infants who were found to have an umbilical cord arterial pH of less that 7.0; 68 of the infants were cared for in the well-baby nursery and discharged home following an uneventful neonatal course. Over 80% of those who were admitted to the intensive care nursery also had benign courses.

Is there an arterial pH level that would predict an abnormal outcome in an infant who is depressed at birth? Goodwin et al. [44] evaluated over 120 infants born at term with a cord pH of less than 7.0. Approximately 4% died, 8% had major neurological abnormalities, 4% were suspected of having neurological problems, 6% were lost to follow-up, and 78% were normal. The same investigators, in a follow-up study of these same infants, noted that if the arteriovenous difference in PCO_2 was greater than 25 mmHg, the infants had an increased incidence of seizures, encephalopathy, and cardiac, pulmonary, and renal dysfunction, as well as abnormal neurological outcomes. The arteriovenous difference in PO_2 correlated to a much lesser extent [45].

Not all infants with neonatal encephalopathy will have abnormal umbilical arterial blood gases. Those infants with normal gases behave as if the umbilical cord had been clamped at the onset of the asphyxial episode, with little blood flow taking place from the placenta to the fetus. This would be most likely a result of cord prolapse, cord impingement, or even an asystolic event. These infants are depressed, often pale, and poorly responsive. After appropriate resuscitation has been instituted and cardiopulmonary function restored, an arterial sample of the infant's blood will be found to be markedly acidemic.

Seizures

The onset of seizures within the first 2–3 days of life has been equated with the incidence and severity of neonatal encephalopathy, as well as with the quality of intrapartum care. The incidence of seizures varies from less than 1 to 3.5/1000 live births, and has decreased significantly over the past 20 years from an incidence as high as 14/1000 live births. In a recent comprehensive study of 89 infants by Tekgul et al. [46] the major etiological factor was global encephalopathy, found in 40% of the patients. These investigators also felt that 60% of the seizures were the result of intrapartum factors, and only 25% were secondary to antepartum factors.

The second most common cause of seizures was stroke, with 18% of patients having this abnormality. Intracranial hemorrhage accounted for 17% of patients, with most due to extra-parenchymal rather than intra-parenchymal bleeding. Only 5% of the patients had developmental abnormalities and 3% had meningitis or encephalitis. Metabolic disturbances, such as hypoglycemia or hypocalcemia, were encountered infrequently, although these could accompany a severe pre- or intrapartum episode as well [46].

Neonatal stroke is being encountered more frequently as the use of imaging techniques has increased. It is found as frequently as 1/4000 live births, is probably the second most common cause of neonatal seizures, and may be associated with various types of genetic hypercoagulable states. This topic is discussed in Chapter 25.

The mortality rate associated with neonatal seizures has also fallen dramatically over the past 20 years, and has been reported to be as low as 7%. Unfortunately, the prevalence of adverse long-term outcome was 28%, with a 20% rate of later seizure recurrence. With advances and improvements in perinatal care, the incidence and mortality rate associated with seizure have decreased significantly, but the long-term damage in survivors remains unchanged [47]. The seizures themselves may contribute to the already existing brain injury by impairing energy utilization and integrity of the neurons. An aggressive approach to the treatment of neonatal seizures is warranted in order to mitigate further damage to an already compromised central nervous system (CNS) [48] (see also Chapters 17 and 43).

Multiple organ dysfunction associated with neonatal encephalopathy

The fetal response to an asphyxial episode is to preserve perfusion and oxygenation of the heart, brain, and adrenal gland at the expense of the other "non-vital" organs, such as the kidney, lungs, gastrointestinal tract, and musculoskeletal system. The incidence of single or multiple organ injury in association with neonatal encephalopathy has varied from 40% to almost 100%, and seems to correlate with the severity of the CNS injury [7,23,25,49–51]. Most often, the renal system is involved, and it is the easiest to evaluate. Findings range from mild oliguria (less than 1 mL/kg/h), proteinuria, and hematuria to renal tubular necrosis and acute renal failure.

Cardiac manifestations vary from minor arrhythmias, ST segment changes on EKG, and tricuspid insufficiency to papillary muscle necrosis, poor ventricular contractions, and cardiogenic shock. Patients with moderately severe or severe asphyxia may have a fixed, non-varying rapid heart rate of 140–160 beats/minute, which may be a prelude to impending failure and cardiogenic shock.

Pulmonary manifestations of asphyxia vary from increased pulmonary vascular resistance that responds readily to correction of acidosis and hypoxia, to persistent pulmonary hypertension of the newborn, severe pulmonary insufficiency, or pulmonary hemorrhage, all of which are difficult to manage.

Other organs that are involved, and the manifestations of their involvement, are listed in Table 1.6. One area often

Table 1.6. Effect of asphyxia on various organs in the newborn

Central nervous system injury
Hypoxic–ischemic encephalopathy (HIE)
Cerebral necrosis
Cerebral edema
Seizures
Hemorrhage
Spinal cord injury
Renal injury
Oliguria
Hematuria
Proteinuria
Acute renal failure
Pulmonary injury
Respiratory failure
Pulmonary hemorrhage
Persistent pulmonary hypertension of the newborn (PPHN)
Pulmonary edema
Meconium aspiration syndrome
Cardiovascular injury
Decreased ventricular function
Abnormalities of rate and rhythm
Tricuspid regurgitation
Papillary muscle necrosis
Hypotension
Cardiovascular shock
Gastrointestinal injury
Gastrointestinal hemorrhage
Sloughing of mucosa
Necrotizing enterocolitis (NEC)
Hepatic injury
Hyperammonemia
Elevated liver enzymes
Coagulopathies
Hematological abnormalities
Elevated nucleated red cell count
Neutropenia or neutrophilia
Thrombocytopenia
Coagulopathy
Metabolic abnormalities
Hypoglycemia
Hypocalcemia
Sodium and potassium abnormalities
Hypo- or hypermagnesemia

Source: Modified from Carter *et al.* [51].

overlooked in the patient with severe asphyxia is damage to the spinal cord. Clancy et al. [52] described 18 severely asphyxiated newborns, 12 or whom expired. On autopsy, five of the 12 demonstrated severe ischemic necrosis in the spinal cord gray matter. Electromyographic studies in the six survivors were abnormal and consistent with recent injury to the lower motor neurons above the level of the dorsal root ganglion. It is often difficult to distinguish clinically between damage to the cortical motor area and damage to the spinal cord.

Phelan et al. [53] described 57 infants with HIE, of whom 14 had no evidence of multisystem problems. Six infants were delivered following uterine rupture, one had fetal exsanguination, one had a cord prolapse, and one was delivered following maternal cardiopulmonary arrest. Five fetuses had sudden and prolonged fetal heart rate decelerations, which persisted until delivery. All of these infants would be classified as having an acute asphyxial or a sentinel episode, and would not have had the opportunity to develop the "diving reflex" necessary to protect the brain and heart at the expense of other organs.

If an infant with intrapartum asphyxia demonstrates only CNS involvement without other organ abnormalities, it may be that there was an acute hypoxic event, that the CNS damage did not occur in the intrapartum period, or that it was due to a cerebrovascular event that did not cause profound hypoxia or hypotension to affect other organs.

Laboratory correlates of neonatal encephalopathy

In addition to the abnormalities in acid–base determinations that have been described previously, various metabolic parameters have also been found to be abnormal in these patients. Some, but not all, have correlated to a certain degree with severe encephalopathy, but they often do not differentiate those infants from infants with mild to moderate encephalopathic states [29].

Urinalysis will usually detect proteinuria and hematuria. Elevations of serum and hepatic enzymes document renal and liver involvement, but may not correlate well with the degree of CNS damage. Elevation of serum ammonia is usually found when severe neurological damage has occurred. Elevations of creatine kinase (CK) in serum and CSF are often found, and both resolve quickly over a one- to two-day period. Erythropoietin, both in serum and in CSF, are excellent markers of severe encephalopathy. The level of urinary lactate/creatine ratio, measured within the first 6 hours of life, has been correlative with the severity of encephalopathy and adverse neurological sequelae at 1 year of age. Follow-up data on this measurement have not been forthcoming, and many encephalopathic infants fail to pass urine within the first 6 hours of life.

Recently, increased levels of troponin T [54] and S100B protein [55] in serum, and IL-6 in serum and CSF, have been found to correlate with the severity of the encephalopathy [15]. Troponin T has been used as a marker of myocardial

Table 1.7. Laboratory studies used to support the diagnosis and severity of neonatal encephalopathy

Study	Body fluid
Ammonia	Serum
Lactate	Serum
Creatine kinase BB (CK-BB)	Serum, CSF
Erythropoietin	Serum, CSF
Neuron-specific enolase	CSF
Myelin basic protein	CSF
Glutamate	CSF
Troponin T	Serum
S100B protein	Serum
Interleukin 6	Serum, CSF

Note:
CSF, cerebrospinal fluid.
Source: Modified from Volpe [29].

damage, and has been correlative with the degree of encephalopathy as well. Unfortunately, most of the reports have been based on a small number of patients, and their findings must be evaluated in a much larger group of encephalopathic infants.

If abnormalities are encountered, they should be re-evaluated frequently in order to assess the evolution of the injury. Table 1.7 lists the various laboratory determinations that have been used to evaluate the extent of CNS injury in affected infants. Some of these measurements are not readily available in many clinical laboratories, and samples of sera of CSF have to be sent to specialized laboratories for assay.

It is important to do a lumbar puncture in the encephalopathic individuals, in order to obtain fluid for the assays as well as to rule out meningitis and encephalitis as causes of the infant's encephalopathy [29].

The measurements and interpretations of white blood cells and nucleated red blood cell counts [56] in these infants are discussed in Chapter 21.

Clinical manifestations of neonatal encephalopathy

If significant damage has occurred to the CNS, the infant should demonstrate neurological abnormalities in the neonatal period. It is often difficult to appreciate such abnormalities in preterm infants, especially those who have cardiopulmonary abnormalities and who are being treated with assisted ventilation. Often these infants cannot be distinguished from other prematurely born infants with similar cardiopulmonary abnormalities. However, in the term or near-term infant, signs of encephalopathy are readily discernible. Sarnat and Sarnat [33] developed an infant scoring system that categorizes the patients into three stages of "postasphyxial encephalopathy," identifying mild, moderate, and severe. Although they correlated many of the findings with electroencephalographic changes, one can use their classification even if the electroencephalographic changes are not evaluated. The clinical manifestation and the gradation of severity of the encephalopathy are discussed in Chapter 16. Similarly, the electroencephalographic abnormalities found in these infants are discussed in Chapter 17.

Neuroimaging of the infant with encephalopathy

With the increased use of neuroimaging in the encephalopathic infant, investigators have been able to more clearly define the extent of the injury, and have, to some degree, determined the timing of the insult. While not being able to pinpoint timing in minutes or even hours, by following the changes that occur on imaging studies the neuroradiologist has been able to help in determining the time frames of injury in many infants. Magnetic resonance spectroscopy is also of help in evaluating the extent of damage, as well as the timing of the insult. These aspects are discussed in detail in Chapter 18.

How much of neonatal encephalopathy is due to intrapartum events?

In evaluating all of the factors that have been associated with neonatal encephalopathy, it is obvious that no one factor taken by itself can identify the infant who will have neurological injury. Using only the Apgar score, unless it is very low for a protracted period, is not a very good marker, nor is it predictive of long-term outcome.

In his excellent review of intrapartum asphyxia and its relationship to CP, Perlman noted that "a single marker of in utero stress provided little useful information regarding the asphyxial process or the fetal adaptive responses, and thus the relationship to neonatal brain injury or subsequent cerebral palsy." He noted that there had to be a "constellation of markers" in linking intrapartum events to neonatal encephalopathy and then to CP. The infants with severe encephalopathy, including seizures, could be identified by using a 5-minute Apgar score of 5 or less, the need for intubation or CPR, and an umbilical cord arterial pH of 7.0 or less [23].

For years, it was postulated that a depressed infant who developed seizures within the first 72 hours of life had suffered from an adverse intrapartum event. Currently, there is disagreement as to the correlation of intrapartum events with the development of neonatal encephalopathy. The case–control studies from Australia found that 69% of the infants with encephalopathy had only antepartum risk factors, 25% had both antepartum and evidence of intrapartum markers, 4% had evidence of intrapartum issues only, and 2% had no recognizable causes [5].

Volpe, drawing from his vast experience in evaluating encephalopathic infants, noted that 20% had insults related primarily to antepartum events, 35% had intrapartum disturbances, 35% had both intra- and antepartum events, and 10% had issues in the postpartum period. The latter was encountered primarily in prematurely born infants [29].

The International Cerebral Palsy Task Force developed a template enumerating the criteria used to define an intrapartum

Table 1.8. Criteria to define an acute intrapartum event sufficient to cause cerebral palsy

Essential criteria (must meet all four)
(1) Evidence of metabolic acidosis in fetal umbilical cord arterial blood obtained at delivery (pH < 7.00 and base deficit $\geq$ 12 mmol/L)
(2) Early onset of severe or moderate neonatal encephalopathy in infants born at 34 weeks or more of gestation
(3) Cerebral palsy of the spastic quadriplegic or dyskinetic type
(4) Exclusion of other identifiable etiologies such as trauma, coagulation disorders, infectious conditions, or genetic disorders
Criteria that collectively suggest an intrapartum timing (within close proximity to labor and delivery, e.g., 0 to 48 h), but are non-specific to asphyxial insults
(1) A sentinel (signal) hypoxic event occurring immediately before or during labor
(2) A sudden and sustained fetal bradycardia or absence of fetal heart rate variability in the presence of persistent, late, or variable decelerations, usually after a hypoxic sentinel event when the pattern was previously normal
(3) Apgar scores of 0–3 beyond 5 min
(4) Onset of multisystem involvement within 72 h of birth
(5) Early imaging study showing evidence of a non-focal cerebral abnormality

Source: Reproduced with permission of BMJ and ACOG.

event sufficient to cause CP [7]. This template was modified by the ACOG and the AAP, and published in 2003 [10]. These criteria, which are depicted in Table 1.8, include both essential criteria and criteria that collectively denote intrapartum timing. Not all investigators have agreed with these criteria, especially in regard to the issues of timing that have been advocated by the Task Force or the ACOG/AAP publications.

Cowan *et al.* [11] evaluated 351 infants with neonatal encephalopathy and/or seizures who were referred to two large intensive care units, and who were evaluated with MRIs and/or postmortem examinations. The infants were divided into two groups: 261 infants with neonatal encephalopathy and 90 who had seizures without encephalopathy. Imaging of the brain showed an acute insult in 80% of the encephalopathic infants and did not show evidence of prior injuries or atrophy. In the group with seizures only, focal damage (stroke) was found in 69% while 2% had evidence of antenatal injury. Their follow-up was disconcerting, as 66 infants in the encephalopathic group died and 85 had neurological sequelae. This study was not population-based or case-controlled, as were the studies from Australia, but was based on findings from tertiary referral centers that treated the most severely affected infants.

As noted previously, if the fetus has suffered from an acute intrapartum event, and there is not enough time to invoke the "diving reflex," the infant may not show multiorgan damage. Similarly, if the umbilical cord is acutely impinged, prolapsed, or tightly wound around the fetus's neck, the cord blood gas may be normal and may not accurately reflect the fetal condition at the time of birth.

In other situations, the fetus may have suffered an acute or subacute intrauterine asphyxial event prior to the onset of labor, followed by a period of recovery, and at the time of delivery may show no overt signs of injury. Such infants were often sent to the well-baby nursery, but within hours they developed signs of encephalopathy, often with seizures, and had the neuroimaging findings that have been associated with an acute intrapartum asphyxial episode. Perlman noted that in his experience this group of infants makes up 50% of patients with encephalopathy [23]. In addition, these same infants often may not tolerate labor well, may have poor cardiopulmonary reserve, and may develop non-reassuring fetal heart rate tracings. Even though they are delivered expeditiously, they demonstrate all of the findings that have been associated with "intrapartum asphyxia" and have neuroimaging that is compatible with an intrapartum injury.

As techniques such as hypothermia are being developed and utilized to treat encephalopathic infants, it behooves the physician to be as precise as possible in identifying the infants with intrapartum injury, in order to provide the most appropriate types of care. Treatment with hypothermia must be initiated within 6 hours after birth in order to be effective. Many infants enrolled in these trials may not have had a "true" intrapartum event, and may not respond well to treatment. These infants must be identified in a retrospective manner, if possible, and evaluated as a separate group of patients from those who had a true intrapartum injury.

Conditions causing neonatal depression that mimic or are associated with the encephalopathic infant

Nelson and Leviton were among the first to question whether all infants with neonatal encephalopathy had their insults secondary to intrapartum asphyxia [2]. One of the more common problems that can present in this fashion is the infant with neonatal sepsis. Currently, Group B *Streptococcus* is the most common organism involved. In many instances, the mother had been pretreated with antibiotics, and an organism was not able to be cultured from the newborn's blood or CSF. Indirect evidence of infection may be present, including an abnormally low or elevated white blood cell count, an elevated C-reactive protein, and/or evidence of severe chorioamnionitis. These infants have severe lactic acidosis, may have pulmonary hypertension or hemorrhage, and are very difficult to manage in the neonatal period. Even with the use of nitric oxide, high-frequency ventilation, and extracorporeal membrane oxygenation (ECMO), the mortality and morbidity rates are high.

Similarly, the infant born of a mother with chorioamnionitis may also behave like the infant with intrapartum asphyxia. Placental perfusion has been shown to be decreased in such pregnancies, further subjecting the fetus to increased risk of damage (see Chapters 12 and 20).

Although most infants with congenital infections such as cytomegalovirus, herpes, or toxoplasmosis are asymptomatic

Table 1.9. Conditions causing neonatal depression and/or neonatal encephalopathy that mimic intrapartum asphyxia

Neonatal sepsis
Chorioamnionitis without documented neonatal sepsis
Congenital infections
Viral
Toxoplasmosis
Neuronal migration disorders
Congenital myotonic disorders, including congenital and transient myasthenia gravis
Metabolic conditions causing lactic acidosis
Genetic disorders associated with thrombotic or thrombophilic abnormalities, including
Protein C and protein S deficiencies
Factor V Leiden deficiency
Anticardiolipin antibodies

at birth, and later develop clinical manifestations of their disease, a few will be symptomatic in the neonatal period and behave as if they had suffered from intrapartum asphyxia. Infants with congenital parvoviral infection are often born with generalized edema, are difficult to resuscitate, and have significant rates of morbidity and mortality. Newborns with neuronal migration disorders and those with early-onset myotonic disease have also been mislabeled as infants suffering from intrapartum encephalopathy. The infant with an intrauterine stroke may also be depressed in addition to having seizures. Too often, without substantiating evidence, it is assumed that the stroke has been caused by an adverse intrapartum hypoxic event. Lastly, infants with metabolic disorders can also present in the immediate newborn period with signs suggesting intrapartum asphyxia (see Chapters 23 and 34).

Table 1.9 lists some of these conditions, and clinicians must be aware that not all patients with encephalopathy have their insult due to an intrapartum asphyxial event.

Outcome of infants with neonatal encephalopathy

(see Chapter 48)

Although the incidence and mortality rates of infants with encephalopathy have decreased markedly, the complication rates found in the survivors have not changed appreciably in the past 20 years [11]. The infants with mild encephalopathy usually have benign courses, and have few, if any, neonatal sequelae. Those with severe encephalopathy (grade III Sarnat score) have a very high mortality rate, ranging from 25% to 100% [11]. Major handicaps are reported in as few as 42% to as high as 100% of survivors, with most studies showing that more than 80% are handicapped to a significant degree. The infants with moderate encephalopathic changes (grade II Sarnat score) have a much lower mortality rate of 5% or less, and fewer than 25% have major handicaps, with 75% or more having no discernible sequelae. Although careful follow-up of these patients to school age has shown an increased incidence of learning disabilities, similar results have been found by evaluating MRI findings in these infants and documenting the extent of the injury [57].

It is anticipated that, with the development and use of techniques such as hypothermia, growth factors, and oxygen-free-radical inhibitors, the outcome of the encephalopathic infants will improve. Early data suggest that these therapies are proving to be beneficial, especially in the moderately severe group of patients (see Chapter 42).

Cerebral palsy (CP)

(see Chapter 46)

The relationship of neonatal encephalopathy and CP with and without cognitive impairment continues to be elusive and often difficult to ascertain. The incidence of CP varies, and is dependent on the type of injury present and the cause, if it can be identified. In most developed countries the incidence is remarkably similar, varying between 1.0 and 2.5/1000 live births, and it has not changed to any significant degree over the past two decades. The rates of CP rose in the early 1970s and tended to remain constant during the early 1980s, primarily due to increased numbers of very-low-birthweight infants surviving, some of whom developed CP. Himmermann et al. [58], however, noted that the subsequent reduction in neonatal mortality has resulted in far more healthy children surviving without CP than with CP. Despite this, prematurely born infants still make up at least 25–50% of the total number of infants so afflicted, and the risk of CP increases with decreasing gestational age and birthweight. Neuroimaging has been helpful in identifying not only the area of the brain involved, but also the timing of the insult. Malformations of the brain tend to occur primarily during the first and into the second trimester of pregnancy, while lesions in the white matter occur between the 20th and the 34th weeks of gestation, and gray matter lesions and injuries to the striatum occur after the 34th week of pregnancy [59,60].

Spastic diplegia is the most frequent type of CP found in the preterm infant, and there has been an increasing incidence of hemiplegia due primarily to cerebral infarcts. In the latest study from Sweden, 30% of patients born at or near term had a prenatal cause for their CP, and 35% had perinatal causes. However, in this latter group were infants who had evidence of HIE, intracerebral hemorrhage, or infections involving the CNS. It was also noted that the maternal risk factors increased from 4.8% in term infants with CP and 8.5% in preterm infants in the period 1969–74, to 17% and 35% respectively in the years 1995–8. The most frequently encountered risk factors were maternal fever at the time of delivery and maternal diabetes. A disconcerting factor in the Swedish studies has been the increased incidence of dyskinetic CP, which is often associated with intrapartum difficulties [61].

Neonatal encephalopathy was found in 24% of the term infants with CP reported from Australia [19], 22% of those from Canada [61], and 31% of those from Norway [61].

In the large Dublin randomized trial of electronic versus intermittent auscultation, six infants who had seizures in the neonatal period were found to have CP at 4 years of age. Three were from each group of monitored patients. Interestingly, 15 additional patients with CP who were diagnosed at 4 years of age did not have neonatal seizures and were not in the high-risk group. Of the total number of patients with CP at 4 years of age, only 29% had intrapartum difficulties [42]. Thus most reports have indicated that the incidence of CP due to neonatal encephalopathy ranges between 10% and 30% in term infants.

CP found in children following neonatal encephalopathy is primarily of the spastic quadriplegic or dyskinetic types, and is associated more frequently with severe cognitive impairment and epilepsy when compared to those children with CP who were not encephalopathic. In addition, the mortality rate is almost four times greater (19% vs. 5%) in the encephalopathic patients [11,19].

Investigators have also reported an association of CP with non-cerebral birth defects, particularly cardiac defects, which has added further evidence that many of the antecedents of CP occur in the antepartum period [37].

Is it possible to decrease the incidence of CP?

The most important approach would be to decrease the incidence of preterm births, because this group contributes at least 50% of patients to the CP population [62]. This would be a formidable task and would require a multipronged attack if it were to be successful. There has been a significant increase in the number of multiple births, which has increased the number of preterm infants. In addition to being born early, these infants have an increased risk of in utero complications such as twin-to-twin transfusion and the in utero death of one of the infants. Multiple births are frequently the result of fertility-enhancing techniques, which often are used in older patients. Hopefully, improved techniques, careful counseling, and the implantation of a single rather than multiple fertilized eggs will mitigate this problem to some extent.

Early recognition and treatment of women who have or are at risk of having chorioamnionitis could be a factor in decreasing the incidence of prematurity, and it may be an important factor in decreasing the incidence of CP in the term infant as well. Similarly, careful monitoring of pregnant women with chronic illnesses, especially SLE, diabetes, and thyroid disease, would be another approach [63,64].

Electronic fetal heart rate monitoring was hailed as a method to decrease the incidence of CP. This technique has helped reduce the number of stillbirths, but has had little, if any, effect on the incidence of CP. While the rate of cesarean sections in response to abnormalities noted in fetal heart rate tracings has increased almost fivefold, the incidence of CP has remained unchanged [65].

Infants who are growth-restricted in utero contribute significantly to the number of patients with neonatal encephalopathy, seizures, and CP. Improving the early recognition and earlier intervention in these pregnancies could potentially enhance the outcome for these infants.

A question that has lingered for years is whether the increased rate of cesarean births has decreased the incidence of CP. Overall, the answer has been a resounding "no." However, if an infant is delivered by elective cesarean section, is the incidence of CP decreased? Gaffney et al. [3] studied 141 infants with CP in the UK and found seven infants delivered by elective cesarean section who did not have neonatal encephalopathy but did have CP.

Badawi et al. [5] reported that infants delivered by cesarean section without labor had an 83% reduction in the risk of having moderate or severe encephalopathy. Landon et al. [66], evaluating perinatal outcome associated with a trial of labor after a prior cesarean birth, encountered no infants with HIE in mothers who had elective repeat sections. Although elective cesarean births could decrease the incidence of neonatal encephalopathy, it may not prevent the birth of infants who would develop CP [67].

Epidemiology of mental retardation (MR)

Epidemiologists define severe mental retardation (MR) as an IQ score below 50, and mild MR as a score between 50 and 69. The prevalence of severe MR has been remarkably constant, varying between 3 and 4/1000 school-aged children. This retardation is often associated with motor handicaps, abnormal features or appearance, and seizures. These patients are generally found with equal frequency in all socioeconomic classes, and most commonly are retarded as a result of a "biologic insult to the brain" [68].

Patients with mild MR most commonly come from the most disadvantaged socioeconomic classes, have learning problems, and often require special classes or schooling in order to reach their ultimate levels of achievement. Associated neurological handicaps may be found in as many as 30% of these patients, epilepsy being the most common finding.

The incidence of mild MR has been stated to be between 23 and 30/1000 in the school-age population, and it is closely related to socioeconomic class. In Sweden, the incidence of this type of MR has fallen to only 4/1000. It appears that alterations in the socioeconomic environment may have a significant effect in lowering the incidence of mild MR.

Hagberg and Kyllerman [68] noted that patients with the fetal alcohol syndrome made up almost 10% of those with mild MR and almost 1% of the patients with severe MR. As more of these patients are being recognized in the USA, it is possible that an increased percentage will be found in both the mild and the severe MR groups in our country as well. Similarly, if the number of infants delivered of substance-abusing mothers increases, it is possible that these patients may also contribute to the number of mentally retarded infants and children encountered.

Aberrant perinatal events, including intrapartum difficulties, account for 10% of the patients with severe and mild MR, and postnatal difficulties account for another 10% with both types of MR.

In most of the patients the origin of severe MR lies in prenatal problems, including chromosomal abnormalities (40%), biochemical inborn errors of metabolism (3–5%), and intrauterine infections (5%). In approximately 30% of patients with severe MR, the cause is unknown.

For many years it has been stated that if an infant or child has severe MR without severe CP, the MR is not due to intrapartum asphyxial issues. Initially Robertson [69] challenged this premise, when she identified a group of patients with severe MR but without severe CP. Patients were found to have abnormal imaging studies that corresponded to the abnormalities seen in patients who had a severe intrapartum asphyxial event. Gonzalez and Miller [70] have reported similar findings in their review of the literature, and in evaluating patients for whom they cared. Survivors of neonatal encephalopathy were at risk of having cognitive abnormalities even in the absence of functional motor deficits, and frequently demonstrated watershed lesions of the cerebral cortex (see Chapter 48).

Conclusion

Over the past two decades, a great deal of improvement has taken place in reducing the incidence, morbidity, and mortality rates of neonatal encephalopathy. We are more cognizant of the factors that place the fetus and newborn at risk for such problems. We have improved our diagnostic capabilities so that we have become more precise in evaluating the cause and timing of the events leading to the injury, and we have increased and improved our use of neuroimaging technology to assist us in doing so. We continue to improve our ability to successfully resuscitate the depressed newborn through educational programs for pediatricians, obstetricians, nurses, and respiratory therapists. We are currently evaluating techniques such as hypothermia and various growth factors to mitigate the adverse outcomes of the encephalopathic infant.

Unfortunately, we have not decreased the incidence or the severity of CP and MR, which continue to affect a large number of children annually.

Hopefully, over the coming two decades, we will continue to make significant progress and markedly decrease the number of handicapped children, not only in the USA, but worldwide as well.

References

1. Stanley F, Blair E, Alberman E. *Cerebral Palsies: Epidemiology and Causal Pathways*. Clinics in Developmental Medicine 151. London: MacKeith Press, 2000.

2. Nelson KB, Leviton A. How much of neonatal encephalopathy is due to birth asphyxia? *Am J Dis Child* 1991; **145**: 1325–31.

3. Gaffney G, Flavell V, Johnson A, *et al.* Cerebral palsy and neonatal encephalopathy. *Arch Dis Child Fetal Neonatal Ed* 1994; **70**: F195–200.

4. Perlman JM, Risser R. Can asphyxiated infants at risk for neonatal seizures be rapidly identified by current high-risk markers? *Pediatrics* 1996; **97**: 456–62.

5. Badawi N, Kurinczuk JJ, Keogh JM, *et al.* Intrapartum risk factor for newborn encephalopathy: the Western Australian case control study. *BMJ* 1998; **317**: 1554–8.

6. Nelson KB, Grether JK. Potentially asphyxiating conditions and spastic cerebral palsy in infants of normal birth weight. *Am J Obstet Gynecol* 1998; **179**: 507–13.

7. MacLennan A. A template for defining a causal relationship between acute intrapartum events and cerebral palsy: international consensus statement International Cerebral Palsy Task Force. *BMJ* 1999; **319**: 1054–9.

8. Phelan JP, Kim JO. Fetal heart rate observations in the brain damaged infant. *Semin Perinatol* 2000; **24**: 221–9.

9. Hankins GDV, Speer M. Defining the pathogenesis and pathophysiology of neonatal encephalopathy and cerebral palsy. *Obstet Gynecol* 2003; **102**: 628–36.

10. American College of Obstetricians and Gynecologists, American Academy of Pediatrics. *Neonatal Encephalopathy and Cerebral Palsy: Defining the Pathogenesis and Pathophysiology.* Washington, DC: ACOG, 2003.

11. Cowan F, Rutherford M, Groenendaal F, *et al.* Origin and timing of brain lesions in term infants with neonatal encephalopathy. *Lancet* 2003; **361**: 736–42.

12. Shevell, MI. The "Bermuda Triangle" of neonatal neurology: cerebral palsy, neonatal encephalopathy, and intrapartum asphyxia. *Semin Pediatr Neurol* 2004; **11**: 24–30.

13. Perlman JM. Brain injury in the term infant. *Semin Perinatol* 2004; **28**: 415–24.

14. Ferriero DM. Neonatal brain injury. *N Engl J Med* 2004; **351**: 1985–95.

15. Bartha AI, Foster-Barber A, Miller SP, *et al.* Neonatal encephalopathy: association of cytokines and MR spectroscopy and outcome. *Pediatr Res* 2004; **56**: 960–6.

16. Becher JC, Bell JE, Keeling JW, *et al.* The Scottish perinatal neuropathology study: clinicopathological correlation in early neonatal deaths. *Arch Dis Child Fetal Neonatal Ed* 2004; **89**: F399–407.

17. Low JA. Determining the contribution of asphyxia to brain damage in the neonate. *J Obstet Gynaecol Res* 2004; **30**: 276–86.

18. Pierrat V, Haouari N, Liska A, *et al.* Prevalence, causes, and outcome at 2 years of age of newborn encephalopathy: population-based study. *Arch Dis Child Fetal Neonatal Ed* 2005; **90**: F257–61.

19. Badawi N, Felix JF, Kurinczuk JJ, *et al.* Cerebral palsy following term newborn encephalopathy: a population-based study. *Dev Med Child Neurol* 2005; **47**: 293–8.

20. Foley ME, Alarab M, Daly L, *et al.* Term neonatal asphyxial seizures and peripartum deaths: lack of correlation with a rising cesarean delivery rate. *Am J Obstet Gynecol* 2005; **192**: 102–8.

21. Haider BA, Bhutta ZA. Birth asphyxia in developing countries: Current status and public health implications. *Curr Probl Pediatr Adolesc Health Care* 2006; **36**: 178–88.

22. Thorngren-Jerneck K, Herbst A. Perinatal factors associated with cerebral palsy in children born in Sweden. *Obstet Gynecol* 2006; **108**: 1499–505.

23. Perlman JM. Intrapartum asphyxia and cerebral palsy: is there a link? *Clin Perinatol* 2006; **33**: 335–53.

24. Bercher JC, Stenson B, Lyon A. Is intrapartum asphyxia preventable? *BJOG* 2007; **114**: 1442–4.

25. Flidel-Rimon O, Shinwell ES. Neonatal aspects of the relationship between intrapartum events and cerebral palsy. *Clin Perinatol* 2007; **34**: 439–49.

26. Milsom I, Ladfors L, Thiringer K, *et al.* Influence of maternal, obstetric and fetal risk factors on the prevalence of birth asphyxia at term in a Swedish urban population. *Acta Obstet Gynecol Scand* 2002; **81**: 909–17.

27. Hogan L, Ingemarsson I, Thorngren-Jerneck K, *et al.* How often is a low 5-min Apgar score in term infants due to asphyxia? *Eur J Obstet Gynecol Reprod Biol* 2007; **130**: 169–75.

28. Rennie JM, Hagmann CF, Robertson NJ. Outcome after intrapartum hypoxic ischemia at term. *Semin Fetal Neonatal Med* 2007; **12**: 398–407.

29. Volpe JJ. Hypoxic–ischemic encephalopathy. In Volpe JJ, *Neurology of the Newborn,* 4th edn. Philadelphia, PA: Saunders, 2001: 217–394.

30. Myers RE. Two patterns of perinatal brain damage and their conditions of occurrence. *Am J Obstet Gynecol* 1972; **112**: 246–76.

31. Mallard EC, Williams CE, Johnston BM, *et al.* Repeated episodes of umbilical cord occlusion in fetal sheep lead to preferential damage to the striatum and sensitize the heart to further insults. *Pediatr Res* 1995; **37**: 707–13.

32. Leung AS, Leung EK, Paul RH. Uterine rupture after previous cesarean delivery: maternal and fetal consequences. *Am J Obstet Gynecol* 1993; **169**: 945–50.

33. Sarnat HB, Sarnat MS. Neonatal encephalopathy following fetal distress: a clinical and electroencephalographic study. *Arch Neurol* 1976; **33**: 696–705.

34. Wu YW, Backstrand KH, Zhao S, *et al.* Declining diagnosis of birth asphyxia in California: 1991–2000. *Pediatrics* 2004; **114**: 1584–90.

35. Martin JA, Kochanek KD, Strobino DM, *et al.* Annual summary of vital statistics: 2003. *Pediatrics* 2005; **115**: 619–34.

36. Nelson KB, Ellenberg JH. Obstetric complications as risk factors for cerebral palsy or seizure disorders. *JAMA* 1984; **251**: 1843–8.

37. Blair E, Al Asedy F, Badawi N, *et al.* Is cerebral palsy associated with birth defects other than cerebral defects? *Dev Med Child Neurol* 2007; **49**: 252–8.

38. Wu YW, Escobar GJ, Grether JK, *et al.* Chorioamnionitis and cerebral palsy in term and near-term infants. *JAMA* 2003; **290**: 2677–84.

39. Tekgul H, Yalaz M, Kutukculer N, *et al.* Value of biochemical markers for outcome in term infants with asphyxia. *Pediatr Neurol* 2004; **31**: 326–32.

40. Apgar VA. A proposal for a new method of evaluation of the newborn infant. *Curr Res Anesth Analg* 1953; **32**: 260–7.

41. Dijxhoorn MJ, Visser GHV, Touwen BC. Apgar score, meconium and acidemia at birth in small to gestational age infants born at term, and their relationship to neonatal neurological morbidity. *Br J Obstet Gynaecol* 1987; **94**: 873–9.

42. Grant A, O'Brien W, Joy MT, *et al.* Cerebral palsy among children born during the Dublin randomised trial of intrapartum monitoring. *Lancet* 1989; **2**: 1233–6.

43. Chauhan SP, Hendrix NW, Magann EF, *et al.* Neonatal organ dysfunction among newborns at gestational age ≥ 34 weeks, and umbilical arterial pH < 7.00. *J Matern Fetal Neonatal Med* 2005; **17**: 261–8.

44. Goodwin TM, Belai I, Hernandez P, *et al.* Asphyxial complications in the term newborn with severe umbilical acidemia. *Am J Obstet Gynecol* 1992; **167**: 1506–12.

45. Belai Y, Goodwin TM, Durand M, *et al.* Umbilical arteriovenous PO_2 and PCO_2 differences and neonatal morbidity in term infants with severe acidosis. *Am J Obstet Gynecol* 1998; **178**: 13–19.

46. Tekgul H, Gauvreau K, Soul J, *et al.* The current etiologic profile and neurodevelopmental outcome of seizures in term newborn infants. *Pediatrics* 2006; **117**: 1270–80.

47. Silverstein FS, Jensen FE. Neonatal seizures. *Ann Neurol* 2007; **62**: 112–20.

48. Miller SP, Weiss J, Barnwell A, *et al.* Seizure-associated brain injury in term newborns with perinatal asphyxia. *Neurology* 2002; **58**: 542–8.

49. Hankins GDV, Koen S, Gei F, *et al.* Neonatal organ system injury in acute birth asphyxia sufficient to result in neonatal encephalopathy. *Obstet Gynecol* 2002; **99**: 688–91.

50. Shah P, Riphagen S, Beyene J, *et al.* Multiorgan dysfunction in infants with post-asphyxial hypoxic–ischemic encephalopathy. *Arch Dis Child Fetal Neonatal Ed* 2004; **89**: F152–5.

51. Carter BS, Haverkamp AD, Merenstein GB. The definition of acute perinatal asphyxia. *Clin Perinatol* 1993; **20**: 287–304.

52. Clancy RR, Sladky JT, Rorke LB. Hypoxic–ischemic spinal cord injury following perinatal asphyxia. *Ann Neurol* 1989; **25**: 185–9.

53. Phelan JP, Ahn MO, Korst L, *et al.* Intrapartum fetal asphyxial brain injury with absent multi-organ system dysfunction. *J Maternal Fetal Med* 1998; **7**: 19–22.

54. Trevisanuto D, Picco G, Golin R, *et al.* Cardiac troponin I in asphyxiated neonates. *Biol Neonate* 2006; **89**: 190–3.

55. Thorngren-Jerneck K, Alling C, Herbst A, *et al.* S100 protein in serum as a prognostic marker for cerebral injury in term newborn infants with hypoxic ischemic encephalopathy. *Pediatr Res* 2004; **55**: 406–12.

56. Phelan JP, Kirkendall C, Korst LM, *et al.* Nucleated red blood cell and platelet counts in asphyxiated neonates sufficient to result in permanent neurological impairment. *J Matern Fetal Neonatal Med* 2007; **20**: 377–80.

57. Miller, SP, Ramaswamy V, Michelson D, *et al.* Patterns of brain injury in term neonatal encephalopathy. *J Pediatr* 2005; **146**: 453–60.

58. Himmelmann K, Hagberg G, Beckung E, *et al.* The changing panorama of cerebral palsy in Sweden. IX. Prevalence and origin in the birth year period 1995–1998. *Acta Paediatr* 2005; **94**: 287–94.

59. Bax M, Tydeman C, Flodmark O. Clinical and MRI correlates of cerebral palsy: the European Cerebral Palsy Study. *JAMA* 2006; **296**: 1602–8.

60. Wu YW, Croen LA, Shah SJ, *et al.* Cerebral palsy in a term population: risk factors and neuroimaging findings. *Pediatrics* 2006; **118**: 690–7.

61. Himmelmann K, Hagberg G, Wiklund LM, *et al.* Dyskinetic cerebral palsy: a population-based study of children born between 1991 and 1998. *Dev Med Child Neurol* 2007; **49**: 246–51.

62. Nelson KB. Can we prevent cerebral palsy? *N Engl J Med* 2003; **349**: 1765–9.

63. Nelson KB. The epidemiology of cerebral palsy in term infants. *Ment Retard Dev Disabil Res Rev* 2002; **8**: 146–50.

64. Blair E, Watson L. Epidemiology of cerebral palsy. *Semin Fetal Neonatal Med* 2006; **11**: 117–25.

65. Clark SL, Hankins GDV. Temporal and demographic trends in cerebral palsy: fact and fiction. *Am J Obstet Gynecol* 2003; **188**: 628–33.

66. Landon MB, Hauth JC, Leveno KJ, *et al.* Maternal and perinatal outcomes associated with a trial of labor after prior cesarean delivery. *N Engl J Med* 2004; **351**: 2581–9.

67. Hankins GDV, Clark SM, Munn MB. Cesarean section on request at 39 weeks: impact on shoulder dystocia, fetal trauma, neonatal encephalopathy, and intrauterine demise. *Semin Perinatol* 2006; **30**: 276–87.

68. Hagberg B, Kyllerman M. Epidemiology of mental retardation: a Swedish survey. *Brain Dev* 1983; **5**: 441–9.

69. Robertson CMT. Can hypoxic–ischemic encephalopathy (HIE) associated with term birth asphyxia lead to mental disability without cerebral palsy? *Can J Neurol Sci* 1999; **26**: S36.

70. Gonzalez FF, Miller SP. Does perinatal asphyxia impair cognitive function without cerebral palsy? *Arch Dis Child Fetal Neonatal Ed* 2006; **91**: F454–9.

Mechanisms of neurodegeneration and therapeutics in animal models of neonatal hypoxic–ischemic encephalopathy

Lee J. Martin

Introduction

Perinatal hypoxia–ischemia (HI) and asphyxia due to umbilical cord prolapse, delivery complications, airway obstruction, asthma, drowning, and cardiac arrest are significant causes of brain damage, mortality, and morbidity in infants and young children. The incidence of HI encephalopathy (HIE), for example, is ∼2 to 4/1000 live term births [1]. Term infants that experience episodes of asphyxia can have damage in the brainstem and forebrain, with the basal ganglia, particularly the striatum, and somatosensory systems showing selective vulnerability [2]. Infants surviving with HIE can have long-term neurological disability, including disorders in movement, visual deficits, learning and cognition impairments, and epilepsy [2]. Many of these neurological disabilities are contributors to the complex clinical syndrome of cerebral palsy [1]. Neuroimaging studies of full-term neonates [2] and experimental studies on animal models [3,4] suggest that this pattern of selective vulnerability is related to local metabolism and brain regional interconnections that instigate and propagate the damage within specific neural systems. This idea has been called the "metabolism-connectivity concept" [3,4]. The neurodegeneration is partly triggered by excitotoxic mechanisms resulting from excessive activation of excitatory glutamate receptors and oxidative stress [5–8]. The ion channel N-methyl-D-aspartate (NMDA) receptor and intracellular signaling networks involving calcium, nitric oxide synthase (NOS), mitochondria, and reactive oxygen species (ROS), such as superoxide, nitric oxide (NO), peroxynitrite, and hydrogen peroxide (H_2O_2), appear to have instrumental roles in the neuronal cell death leading to perinatal HIE [6–9].

Despite considerable progress in the epidemiological and pathophysiological understanding of perinatal HI, treatments do not exist that successfully ameliorate HIE and restore neurological function in human infants and children that are its victims. Management is limited to supportive care [1,10]. Mild hypothermia has gained American Heart Association endorsement as a neuroprotective intervention after HI caused by cardiopulmonary arrest in adult humans [11], but the use

of hypothermia on infants and children has uncertain efficacy, in part due to variations in the severity of injury and the timing of implementation [12,13]. Furthermore, it is not clear if the neurons salvaged by hypothermia are intact structurally and functionally, and the aftereffects of hypothermia on the developing brain are uncertain. Hypothermia might interfere with endogenous recovery mechanisms in the brain by reducing neurogenesis [14]. Moreover, the mechanisms of hypothermic neuroprotection are unresolved. In this chapter, I will summarize specific mechanisms of neuron degeneration and experimental therapeutics, including the application of hypothermia and neural stem cells, in animal models of HIE.

Types of cell death

Cells can die by different processes. These processes have been classified generally into two distinct categories, called necrosis and apoptosis. These forms of cellular degeneration were classified originally as different because they appeared different morphologically under a microscope (Fig. 2.1). Necrosis is a lytic destruction of individual cells or groups of cells, while apoptosis (derived from the Greek for "dropping of leaves from trees") is an orderly and compartmental dismantling of single cells or groups of cells into consumable components for nearby cells. Apoptosis is an example of programmed cell death (PCD) that is an ATP-driven (sometimes gene-transcription-requiring) form of cell suicide often committed by demolition enzymes called caspases, but other apoptotic and non-apoptotic, caspase-independent forms of PCD exist [15]. Apoptotic PCD is instrumental in developmental organogenesis and histogenesis and adult tissue homeostasis, functioning to eliminate excess cells. In normal humans, it is estimated that 50–70 billion cells in an adult and 20–30 billion cells in a child between the ages of 8 and 14 die each day due to apoptosis [16]. Another form of cell degeneration, seen first with yeast and then in metazoans, has been called autophagy [17]. Autophagy is an intracellular catabolic process that occurs by lysosomal degradation of damaged or expendable organelles. Necrosis and apoptosis both differ morphologically (Fig. 2.1) and mechanistically from autophagy [15,17].

More recently the morphological and molecular regulatory distinctions between the different forms of cell death have become blurred and uncertain due to observations made on

Fetal and Neonatal Brain Injury, 4th edition, ed. David K. Stevenson, William E. Benitz, Philip Sunshine, Susan R. Hintz, and Maurice L. Druzin. Published by Cambridge University Press. © Cambridge University Press 2009.

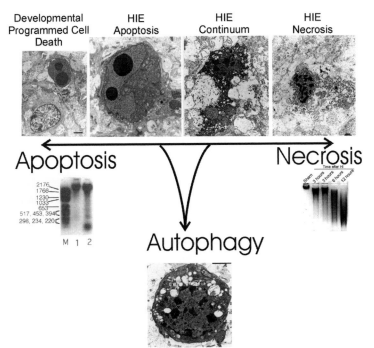

Apoptosis

Necrosis

Autophagy

Fig. 2.1. Gallery of cell death. Electron micrographs of forebrain neurons at mid- to end-stages of degeneration. Developmental programmed cell death (PCD) of neurons in the early postnatal brain is a "gold standard" for neuronal apoptosis. Neonatal HI induces the degeneration of neurons with several phenotypes. The most common forms of cell death are apoptosis, hybrids of apoptosis and necrosis (continuum cells), classical necrosis, and possibly autophagy. In some forms of apoptosis DNA endonucleases act in the nucleus to cleave DNA into internucleosomal fragments (multiples of 180–200 base pairs) to generate a DNA "ladder" (see DNA gel at left, showing molecular weight standards [M], control rat brain tissue [lane 1], and neonatal rat brain tissue undergoing apoptosis [lane 2]). During cellular necrosis (as in the piglet striatum early after HI) nuclear DNA is digested globally to generate numerous randomly sized fragments, first as high molecular weight fragments and then progressing to lower molecular weight fragments, seen as a "smear" in a DNA gel. The spectrum of cell-death morphologies that can be identified in the HI neonatal brain supports the existence of a continuum for cell death.

degenerating neurons in vivo and to a new concept that attempts to accommodate these observations. This concept, in its original form, posits that cell death exists as a continuum, with necrosis and apoptosis at opposite ends of a spectrum and hybrid forms of degeneration manifesting in between (Fig. 2.1) [18–21]. For example, the degeneration of neurons in diseased or damaged human and animal nervous systems is not always strictly necrosis or apoptosis, according to the traditional binary classification of cell death, but also occurs as intermediate or hybrid forms with co-existing morphological and biochemical characteristics that lie in a structural continuum with necrosis and apoptosis at the two extremes [18,19]. Thus, neuronal cell death can be syncretic. The different processes leading to the putative different forms of cell death can be activated concurrently, with graded contributions of the different cell-death modes to the degenerative process (Fig. 2.1).

The in vivo reality of a neuronal cell-death continuum was revealed first in neonatal and adult rat models of glutamate receptor excitoxicity [18,19] and then very nicely in rat and mouse models of neonatal HIE [22–24]. The hybrid cells can be distinguished cytopathologically by the progressive compaction of the nuclear chromatin into few, discrete, large, irregularly shaped clumps (Fig. 2.1). This morphology contrasts with the formation of few, uniformly shaped, dense, round masses in classic apoptosis, and with the formation of numerous, smaller, irregularly shaped chromatin clumps in classic necrosis. The cytoplasmic organelle pathology in hybrid cells has a basic pattern that appears more similar to necrosis than apoptosis but is lower in amplitude than in necrosis (e.g., mitochondrial swelling). Toxicological studies of cultured cells have shown that stimulus intensity influences

the mode of cell death [25–27], such that apoptosis can be induced by injurious stimuli of lesser amplitude than insults causing necrosis [28], but the cell-death modes were still considered distinct [27].

Basic research is uncloaking the molecular mechanisms of cell death [29,30] and, with this, the distinctiveness of different cell-death processes as well as the potential overlap among different cell-death mechanisms. Experimental studies on cell-death mechanisms, and particularly the cell-death continuum, are important because they could lead to the rational development of molecular-mechanism-based therapies for treating neonatal HIE. The different categories of cell death are discussed below.

Necrosis

Cell death caused by cytoplasmic swelling, nuclear dissolution (karyolysis), and lysis has been classified traditionally as necrosis [31]. Cell necrosis (sometimes termed oncosis) [32] results from rapid and severe failure to sustain cellular homeostasis, notably cell volume control [33]. The process of necrosis involves damage to the structural and functional integrity of the cell plasma membrane and associated enzymes, for example Na^+,K^+-ATPase, abrupt influx and overload of ions (e.g., Na^+ and Ca^{2+}) and H_2O, and rapid mitochondrial damage and energetic collapse [27,34–36]. Metabolic inhibition and oxidative stress from ROS are major culprits in triggering necrosis. Inhibitory crosstalk between ion pumps causes pro-necrotic effects when Na^+,K^+-ATPase "steals" ATP from the plasma-membrane Ca^{2+}-ATPase, resulting in Ca^{2+} overload [37].

The morphology and some biochemical features of classic necrosis in neurons are distinctive (Fig. 2.1). The main features

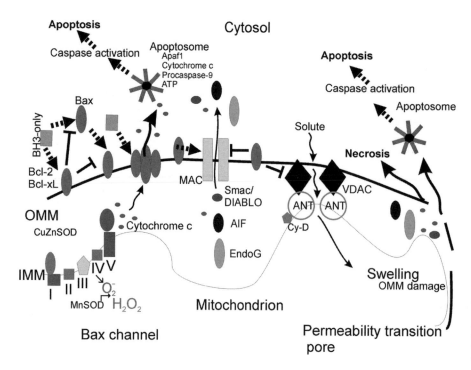

Fig. 2.2. Mitochondrial dysfunction and regulation of cell death. Mitochondria generate ROS in the respiratory chain (lower left). Complexes I, II, and III can generate O_2^-. MnSOD converts O_2^- to H_2O_2. Bcl-2 family members regulate apoptosis by modulating the release of cytochrome c from mitochondria into the cytosol. In the Bax channel model (left), Bax is a proapoptotic protein found in the cytosol that translocates to the outer mitochondrial membrane (OMM). Bax monomers physically interact and form tetrameric channels that are permeable to cytochrome c. The formation of these channels is blocked by Bcl-2 and Bcl-x_L at multiple sites. BH3-only members (Bad, Bid, Noxa, Puma) are proapoptotic and can modulate the conformation of Bax to sensitize this channel, possibly by exposing its membrane insertion domain, or by inactivating Bcl-2 and Bcl-x_L. The mitochondria apoptosis-induced channel (MAC) may be a channel similar to the Bax channel but possibly having additional components. Release of cytochrome c participates in the formation of the apoptosome in the cytosol that drives the activation of caspase-3 leading to apoptosis. Smac/DIABLO are released to inactivate the antiapoptotic actions of inhibitor of apoptosis proteins that inhibit caspases. AIF and EndoG are released and translocate to the nucleus to stimulate DNA fragmentation. Another model for cell death involves the permeability transition pore (PTP). The PTP is a transmembrane channel formed by the interaction of the ANT and the VDAC at contact sites between the inner mitochondrial membrane (IMM) and the OMM and is modulated by cyclophilin D (cy-D). Opening of the PTP induces matrix swelling and OMM rupture leading to release of apoptogenic proteins (cytochrome c, AIF, EndoG) or to cellular necrosis.

are swelling and vacuolation/vesiculation of organelles, destruction of membrane integrity, random digestion of chromatin due to activation of proteases and deoxyribonucleases (DNases), and dissolution of the cell. The overall profile of the moribund cell is maintained generally as it dissolves into the surrounding tissue parenchyma and induces an inflammatory reaction in vivo. In necrosis, dying cells do not bud to form discrete, membrane-bound fragments. The nuclear pyknosis and karyolysis appear as condensation of chromatin into many irregularly shaped small clumps, sharply contrasting with the formation of few, uniformly dense and regularly shaped chromatin aggregates that occurs in apoptosis. In cells undergoing necrosis, genomic DNA is digested globally because proteases that digest histone proteins that protect DNA and DNases are co-activated to generate many randomly sized fragments seen as a DNA "smear" (Fig. 2.1). These differences in the cytoplasmic changes and condensation and digestion of nuclear chromatin in pure apoptosis and pure necrosis are very diagnostic.

Recent work has shown that cell necrosis might not be as chaotic or random as envisioned originally but can involve the activation of specific signaling pathways to eventuate in cell death [38]. For example, DNA damage can lead to poly(ADP-ribose) polymerase activation and ATP depletion, energetic failure, and necrosis [39]. Another pathway for "programmed"

necrosis involves mitochondrial permeability transition. Mitochondrial Ca^{2+} overload, excessive oxidative stress, and decreases in the electrochemical gradient, ADP, and ATP can favor mitochondrial permeability transition [40–42].

Mitochondrial permeability transition is a mitochondrial state in which the proton-motive force is disrupted [40,41]. This disruption involves the so-called mitochondrial permeability transition pore (mPTP) which functions as a voltage, thiol, and Ca^{2+} sensor. The mPTP is a large polyprotein transmembrane channel formed at contact sites between the inner mitochondrial membrane and the outer mitochondrial membrane (Fig. 2.2). The complete components of the mPTP (Table 2.1, Fig. 2.2) are still controversial. The primary components of the mPTP are the voltage-dependent anion channel (VDAC, also called porin) in the outer mitochondrial membrane and the adenine nucleotide translocator (ANT) in the inner mitochondrial membrane [40]. The VDAC makes the inner mitochondrial membrane permeable to most small molecules ($< 5\,kDa$) for free exchange of respiratory chain substrates. The ANT mediates the exchange of ADP for ATP. During normal mitochondrial function the intermembrane space separates the outer and inner mitochondrial membranes and the VDAC and the ANT do not interact, or interact only transiently in a state described as "flicker" [42]. When the mPTP is in the open state, it permits influx of

Table 2.1. Mitochondrial associated proteins that function in cell death

Protein	Function
Bcl-2	Antiapoptotic, blocks Bax/Bak channel formation
Bcl-x_L	Antiapoptotic, blocks Bax/Bak channel formation
Boo (Diva)	Antiapoptotic, blocks cytochrome c release
Bax	Proapoptotic, forms pores for cytochrome release
Bak	Proapoptotic, forms pores for cytochrome release
Bad	Proapoptotic, decoy for Bcl-2/Bcl-x_L promoting Bax/Bak pore formation
Bid	Proapoptotic, decoy for Bcl-2/Bcl-x_L promoting Bax/Bak pore formation
Noxa	Proapoptotic, decoy for Bcl-2/Bcl-x_L promoting Bax/Bak pore formation
Puma	Proapoptotic, decoy for Bcl-2/Bcl-x_L promoting Bax/Bak pore formation
p53	Antagonizes activity of Bcl-2/Bcl-x_L, promotes Bax/Bak oligomerization
Cytochrome c	Activator of apoptosome
Smac/DIABLO	IAP inhibitor
AIF	Antioxidant flavoprotein/released from mitochondria to promote nuclear DNA fragmentation
Endonuclease G	Released from mitochondria to promote nuclear DNA fragmentation
HtrA2/Omi	Serine protease, IAP inhibitor
VDAC	PTP component in outer mitochondrial membrane
ANT	PTP component in inner mitochondrial membrane
Cyclophilin D	PTP component in mitochondrial matrix
Peripheral benzodiazepine receptor	PTP component in outer mitochondrial membrane

Notes:
IAP, inhibitor of apoptosis protein; PTP, permeability transition pore.

solutes of ~ 1500 Da and H_2O into the matrix, resulting in depolarization of mitochondria and dissipation of the proton electrochemical gradient. Consequently, the inner mitochondrial membrane loses its integrity and oxidative phosphorylation is uncoupled. When this occurs, oxidation of metabolites by O_2 proceeds with electron flux not coupled to proton pumping, resulting in further dissipation of transmembrane proton gradient and ATP production, production of ROS, and large-amplitude mitochondrial swelling, triggering necrosis or apoptosis [41]. Several proteins regulate the mPTP. Cyclophilin D is one of these proteins found in the mitochondrial matrix, and it interacts reversibly with the ANT. Inactivation of cyclophilin D can block mitochondrial swelling and cellular necrosis induced by Ca^{2+} overload and ROS [43,44]. Another protein that causes mPTP opening is BNIP3, which can integrate into the outer mitochondrial membrane and can trigger necrosis [45].

Apoptosis

Apoptosis is a form of PCD because it is carried out by active, intrinsic transcription-dependent [46] or transcription-independent mechanisms involving specific molecules (Tables 2.1 and 2.2, Fig. 2.2). Apoptosis should not be used as a synonym for PCD because non-apoptotic forms of PCD exist [47,48]. Apoptosis is only one example of PCD. It is critical for the normal growth and differentiation of organ systems in vertebrates and invertebrates (see reference 49 regarding Ernst's discovery of developmental PCD) [50–52]. The structure of apoptosis is similar to the type I form of PCD described by Clarke [53]. In physiological settings in adult tissues, apoptosis is a normal process, occurring continuously in populations of cells that undergo slow proliferation (e.g., liver and adrenal gland) or rapid proliferation (e.g., epithelium of intestinal crypts) [54,55]. Apoptosis is a normal event in the immune system when lymphocyte clones are deleted after an immune response [56]. Kerr and colleagues were the first to describe apoptosis in pathological settings [57], but many descriptions were made prior to this time in studies of developing animal systems [58].

Classical apoptosis has a distinctive structural appearance (Fig. 2.1). The cell condenses and is dismantled in an organized way into small packages that can be consumed by nearby cells. Nuclear breakdown is orderly. The DNA is digested in a specific pattern of internucleosomal fragments (Fig. 2.1), and the chromatin is packaged into sharply delineated, uniformly dense masses that appear as crescents abutting the nuclear envelope or as smooth, round masses within the nucleus (Fig. 2.1). The execution of apoptosis is linked to Ca^{2+}-activated DNases [59], one being DNA fragmentation factor 45 (DFF-45) [60], which digests genomic DNA at internucleosomal sites only (because proteases that digest histone proteins remain inactivated and the DNA at these sites is protected from DNases) to generate a DNA "ladder" (Fig. 2.1). However, the emergence of the apoptotic nuclear morphology can be independent of the degradation of chromosomal DNA [61]. Cytoplasmic breakdown is also orderly. The cytoplasm condenses (as reflected by a darkening of the cell in electron micrographs, Fig. 2.1), and subsequently the cell shrinks in size, while the plasma membrane remains intact. During the course of these events, it is believed that the mitochondria are required for ATP-dependent processes. Subsequently, the nuclear and plasma membranes become convoluted, and, then the cell undergoes a process called budding. In this process, the nucleus, containing smooth, uniform masses of condensed chromatin, undergoes fragmentation in association with the condensed cytoplasm, forming cellular debris (called apoptotic bodies) composed of pieces of nucleus surrounded by cytoplasm with closely packed and apparently intact organelles. Apoptotic cells display surface markers (e.g., phosphatidylserine or sugars) for recognition by phagocytic cells. Phagocytosis of cellular debris by adjacent cells is the final phase of apoptosis in vivo.

Variants of classical apoptosis or non-classical apoptosis can occur during nervous system development [53,62] and

Table 2.2. Some molecular regulators of apoptosis

Bcl-2 family		Caspase family	IAP family	Tumor suppressors
Antiapoptotic proteins	**Proapoptotic proteins**			
Bcl-2	Bax	Apoptosis "initiators": caspase-2, 8, 9, 10	NAIP	p53
Bcl-x_L	Bak	Apoptosis "executioners": caspase-2, 3, 6, 7	Apollon	p63
Mcl-1	Bcl-x_S	Cytokine processors: caspase-1, 4, 5, 11, 12, 14	Survivin	p73
	Bad		IAP1	
	Bid		IAP2	
	Bik		XIAP	
	Bim			
	Noxa			
	Puma			

also frequently in pathophysiological settings of nervous system injury and disease [18–20]. Axonal damage (axotomy) and target deprivation in the mature nervous system can induce apoptosis in neurons that is similar structurally, but not identical, to developmental PCD [20]. Excitotoxins can induce readily and robustly non-classical forms of apoptosis in neurons [18,19]. Types of cell death similar to those seen with excitotoxicity occur frequently in pathological cell death resulting from neonatal HI [22–24,35].

Cells can die by PCD through mechanisms that are distinct from apoptosis [47,48]. The structure of non-apoptotic PCD is similar to the type II or type III forms of cell death described by Clarke [53]. Interestingly, there is no internucleosomal fragmentation of genomic DNA in some forms of non-apoptotic PCD [47,48].

Autophagy

Autophagy is a mechanism whereby eukaryotic cells degrade their own cytoplasm and organelles [17]. The degradation of organelles and long-lived proteins is carried out by the lysosomal system. Autophagy functions as a cell-death mechanism and as a homeostatic non-lethal stress response mechanism for recycling proteins to protect cells from low supplies of nutrients. Autophagy is also called type II PCD [53]. A hallmark of autophagic cell death is accumulation of autophagic vacuoles of lysosomal origin. Autophagy has been seen in developmental and pathological conditions. For example, insect metamorphosis involves autophagy [63], and developing neurons can use autophagy as a PCD mechanism [64,65]. Degeneration of Purkinje neurons in the mouse mutant *Lurcher* appears to be a form of autophagy, thus possibly linking excitotoxic and autophagic cell deaths to constitutive activation of the GluR2 glutamate receptor [66]. Autophagy appears to have a critical role in neurodegeneration after neonatal HI in mice, because genetic deletion of the *atg7* gene results in a near-complete protection from HI [67].

The molecular controls of autophagy appear common in eukaryotic cells from yeast to human, and it is believed that autophagy evolved before apoptosis [29]. However, most of the work has been done on yeast, with detailed work on mammalian cells only beginning [68]. Double-membrane autophagosomes for sequestration of cytoplasmic components are derived from the endoplasmic reticulum (ER) or the plasma membrane. Tor kinase, phosphatidylinositol-3-kinase (PI3K), a family of cysteine proteases called autophagins, and death-associated proteins function in autophagy [69,70]. Autophagic and apoptotic cell-death pathways crosstalk. The product of the tumor suppressor gene *Beclin1* (the human homolog of the yeast autophagy gene *APG6*) interacts with the antiapoptosis regulator Bcl-2 [71]. Autophagy can block apoptosis by sequestration of mitochondria. If the capacity for autophagy is reduced, stressed cells die by apoptosis, whereas inhibition or blockade of molecules that function in apoptosis can convert the cell-death process into autophagy [72]. Thus, a continuum between autophagy and apoptosis exists (Fig. 2.1).

Molecular and cellular regulation of apoptosis

Apoptosis is a structurally and biochemically organized form of cell death. The basic machinery of apoptosis is conserved in yeast, hydra, nematode, fruitfly, zebrafish, mouse, and human [73]. Our current understanding of the molecular mechanisms of apoptosis in mammalian cells is built on studies by Horvitz and colleagues on PCD in the nematode *Caenorhabditis elegans* [74]. They pioneered the understanding of the genetic control of developmental cell death by showing that this death is regulated predominantly by three genes (*ced-3*, *ced-4*, and *ced-9*) [74]. Several families of apoptosis-regulation genes have been identified in mammals (Table 2.2), including the Bcl-2 family [74,75], the caspase family of cysteine-containing, aspartate-specific proteases [76], the p53 gene family [77], cell-surface death receptors [56], and other apoptogenic factors, including Ca^{2+}, cytochrome c, apoptosis-inducing factor (AIF), and second mitochondria-derived activator of caspases (Smac) [15,78–81]. Moreover, a family of inhibitor of apoptosis proteins (IAP) actively blocks cell death, and IAPs

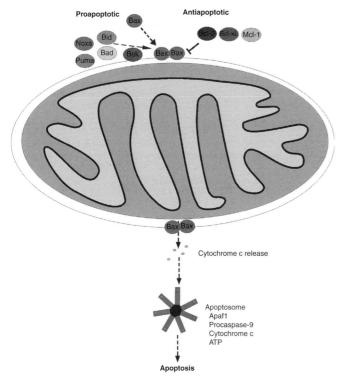

Fig. 2.3. Mitochondrial regulation of apoptosis. The intrinsic cell-death signaling pathway is regulated by mitochondria and involves Bcl-2 family members, cytochrome c release, and apoptosome formation. Bcl-2 family members regulate apoptosis by modulating the release of cytochrome c. Bax and Bak are proapoptotic; they physically interact and form channels that are permeable to cytochrome c. BH3-only members (Bad, Bid, Puma, Noxa, and others not shown) are proapoptotic, and can sequester antiapoptotic proteins to allow conformational changes in Bax or Bak. Functional antagonism of Bax and Bak could provide protection against neonatal HI brain damage. Bcl-2 and Bcl-x$_L$ are antiapoptotic, and can block the function of Bax/Bak. Mimicking the actions of negative regulators could also protect neurons. In the cytosol, cytochrome c, Apaf-1, and procaspase-9 interact to form the apoptosome that drives the activation of caspase-3. Caspases are pursued as important targets for neuroprotection in neonatal HI brain injury.

are inhibited by mitochondrial proteases [78]. Specific organelles have been identified as critical for the apoptotic process, including mitochondria and the ER (Figs. 2.2, 2.3, 2.4). In seminal work by Wang and coworkers, it was discovered that the mitochondrion integrates death signals mediated by proteins in the Bcl-2 family and releases molecules residing in the mitochondrial intermembrane space, such as cytochrome c, which complexes with cytoplasmic proteins (e.g., apoptotic peptidase activating factor-1, Apaf-1) to activate caspase proteases leading to internucleosomal cleavage of DNA [79,80]. The finding that cytochrome c has a function in apoptosis, in addition to its better-known role in oxidative phosphorylation, was astounding, although foreshadowing clues were available. The release of cytochrome c from mitochondria to the cytosol with concomitant reduced oxidative phosphorylation was described as the "cytochrome c effect" in irradiated cancer cells [82]. The ER, which regulates intracellular Ca^{2+} levels, participates in a loop with mitochondria to modulate mitochondrial permeability transition and cytochrome c release through the actions of Bcl-2 protein family members [83].

Bcl-2 family of survival and death proteins

The *bcl-2* proto-oncogene family is a large group of apoptosis-regulatory genes encoding about 25 different proteins, defined by at least one conserved B-cell lymphoma (Bcl) homology domain (BH1–BH4 can be present) in their amino acid sequence that functions in protein–protein interactions [74,75]. Some of the protein products of these genes (e.g., Bcl-2, Bcl-x$_L$, and Mcl-1) have all four BH1–BH4 domains and are antiapoptotic (Table 2.2). Other gene products, which are proapoptotic, are multidomain proteins possessing BH1–BH3 sequences (e.g., Bax and Bak) or proteins with only the BH3 domain (e.g., Bad, Bid, Bim, Bik, Noxa, and Puma) that contains the critical death domain (Table 2.2). Bcl-x$_L$ and Bax have α-helices resembling the pore-forming subunit of diphtheria toxin [84]; thus, Bcl-2 family members appear to function by conformation-induced insertion into the outer mitochondrial membrane to form channels or pores that can regulate release of apoptogenic factors (Fig. 2.2).

The expression of many of these proteins is regulated developmentally, and the proteins have differential tissue distributions and subcellular localizations. Most of these proteins are found in CNS. The subcellular distributions of Bax, Bak, and Bad in healthy adult rodent CNS tissue [85] are consistent with in vitro studies of non-neuronal cells [86,87]. Bax, Bad, and Bcl-2 reside primarily in the cytosol, whereas Bak resides primarily in mitochondria. Bcl-2 family members can form homodimers or heterodimers and higher-order multimers with other family members. Bax forms homodimers or heterodimers with Bak, Bcl-2, or Bcl-x$_L$. When Bax and Bak are present in excess, the antiapoptotic activity of Bcl-2 and Bcl-x$_L$ is antagonized. The formation of Bax homo-oligomers promotes apoptosis, whereas Bax heterodimerization with either Bcl-2 or Bcl-x$_L$ neutralizes its proapoptotic activity.

Release of cytochrome c from mitochondria may occur through mechanisms that involve the formation of membrane channels comprised of Bax or Bak [88] and Bax and the VDAC [89]. Cytochrome c triggers the assembly of the cytoplasmic apoptosome (a protein complex of Apaf-1, cytochrome c, and procaspase-9) which is the engine that drives caspase-3 activation in mammalian cells [79]. Bcl-2 and Bcl-x$_L$ block the release of cytochrome c [90,91] from mitochondria and thus the activation of caspase-3 [79,80]. The blockade of cytochrome c release from mitochondria by Bcl-2 and Bcl-x$_L$ [80,92] is caused by inhibition of Bax channel-forming activity in the outer mitochondrial membrane [88] or by modulation of mitochondrial membrane potential and volume homeostasis [92]. Bcl-x$_L$ also has antiapoptotic activity by interacting with Apaf-1 and caspase-9 and inhibiting the Apaf-1-mediated autocatalytic maturation of caspase-9 [93]. Boo (also called Bcl2L10 or Diva) can inhibit Bak- and Bik-induced apoptosis (but not Bax-induced cell death), possibly through heterodimerization and by interactions with Apaf-1 and caspase-9 (Table 2.1) [94]. Bax and Bak double-knockout cells are completely resistant to mitochondrial cytochrome c release during apoptosis [95]. BH3-only proteins such as Bim, Bid, Puma,

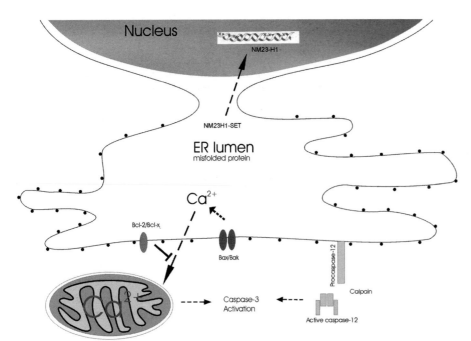

Fig. 2.4. The endoplasmic reticulum (ER) functions in apoptosis. Under conditions of ER stress, such as events resulting in protein misfolding, Bax and Bak regulate the release of Ca^{2+} from the ER into the cytosol. Increased cytosolic Ca^{2+} triggers enhanced Ca^{2+} import into mitochondria and subsequent mitochondrial dysfunction and release of apoptogenic factors that activate caspase-3. Bcl-2 and Bcl-x_L can block the release of Ca^{2+} from the ER. Procaspase-12 is localized to the ER and can be cleaved by calpain into the active form in response to prolonged stress. Activated caspase-12 can in turn activate caspase-9 and caspase-3. GrA–perforin pathway activation can lead to the translocation of ER-sequestered NM23-H1 protein and activation of DNase activity leading to DNA single-strand nicks.

and Noxa appear to induce a conformational change in Bax, or they serve as decoys for Bcl-x_L that allow Bax to form pores in the outer mitochondrial membrane [96].

Although many studies have focused on how Bcl-2 family members regulate apoptosis at mitochondria, it is now evident that ER stress can initiate apoptosis (Fig. 2.4). This finding is relevant to neonatal HIE and excitotoxicity, where ER abnormalities may be important to pathogenesis [18,19,35,97]. The ER functions to fold proteins, and when this capacity is compromised an unfolded protein response (UPR) is engaged. The UPR can lead to a return to homeostasis or to cell death. Bcl-2 localizes to the ER [98]. Overexpression of Bcl-2 and Bcl-x_L can block ER-stress-induced apoptosis [99]. Bak and Bax also operate in the ER and function in the activation of ER-specific caspase-12 [100]. Cells lacking Bax and Bak are resistant to ER-stress-induced apoptosis [95].

Protein phosphorylation regulates the functions of some Bcl-2 family members. Bcl-2 loses its antiapoptotic activity following serine phosphorylation, possibly because its antioxidant function is inactivated [101]. Bcl-2 phosphorylation at serine 24 in the BH4 domain precedes caspase-3 cleavage following cerebral HI in neonatal rats [102]. In addition to interacting with homologous proteins, Bcl-2 can associate with nonhomologous proteins, including the protein kinase Raf-1 [103]. Bcl-2 is thought to target Raf-1 to mitochondrial membranes, allowing this kinase to phosphorylate Bad at serine residues. The phosphatidylinositol-3-kinase (PI3–K)-Akt pathway also regulates the function of Bad and caspase-9 through phosphorylation [104–106]. In the presence of trophic factors, Bad is phosphorylated. Phosphorylated Bad is sequestered in the cytosol by interacting with soluble protein 14–3–3 and, when bound to protein 14–3–3, Bad is unable to interact with Bcl-2 and Bcl-x_L, thereby promoting survival [107]. Conversely, when Bad is dephosphorylated by calcineurin [108],

it dissociates from protein 14–3–3 in the cytosol and translocates to the mitochondria, where it exerts proapoptotic activity. Nonphosphorylated Bad heterodimerizes with membrane-associated Bcl-2 and Bcl-x_L, thereby displacing Bax from Bax–Bcl-2 and Bax–Bcl-x_L dimers, and promotes cell death [109]. The phosphorylation status of Bad helps regulate glucokinase activity, thereby linking glucose metabolism to apoptosis [110].

Caspase family of cell demolition proteases

Caspases (*cy*steinyl- *asp*artate-specific protein*ases*) are cysteine proteases that have a near-absolute substrate requirement for aspartate in the P_1 position of the peptide bond. Fourteen members have been identified [76]. Caspases exist as constitutively expressed inactive proenzymes (30–50 kDa) in healthy cells. The protein contains three domains, an amino-terminal prodomain, a large subunit (~20 kDa), and a small subunit (~10 kDa). Caspases are activated through regulated proteolysis of the proenzyme with "initiator" caspases activating "executioner" caspases (Table 2.2), although some caspase proenzymes (e.g., caspase-9) have low activity without processing [111]. Other caspase family members function in inflammation by processing cytokines (Table 2.2) [76]. The prodomain of initiator caspases contains amino acid sequences that are caspase recruitment domains (CARD) or death effector domains (DED) that enable the caspases to interact with other molecules that regulate their activation. Activation of caspases involves proteolytic processing between domains, and then association of large and small subunits to form a heterodimer with both subunits contributing to the catalytic site. Two heterodimers associate to form a tetramer that has two catalytic sites that function independently. Active caspases have many target proteins [112] that are cleaved during regulated and organized cell death. Caspases cleave nuclear proteins (e.g., DNases, poly(ADP) ribose polymerase, DNA-dependent protein kinase, heteronuclear ribonucleoproteins, transcription factors or lamins), cytoskeletal proteins (e.g., actin and fodrin), and cytosolic proteins (e.g., other caspases, protein kinases, Bid).

In cell models of apoptosis using human cell lines, activation of caspase-3 occurs when caspase-9 proenzyme (also known as Apaf-3) is bound by Apaf-1, which then oligomerizes in a process initiated by cytochrome c (identified as Apaf-2) and either ATP or dATP [79]. Cytosolic ATP or dATP are required cofactors for cytochrome-c-induced caspase activation. Apaf-1, a 130 kDa cytoplasmic protein, serves as a docking protein for procaspase-9 (Apaf-3) and cytochrome c [79]. Apaf-1 becomes activated when ATP is bound and hydrolyzed, with the hydrolysis of ATP and the binding of cytochrome c promoting Apaf-1 oligomerization [113]. This oligomeric complex recruits and mediates the autocatalytic activation of procaspase-9 (forming the apoptosome), which dissociates from the complex and becomes available to activate caspase-3. Once activated, caspase-3 cleaves a protein with DNase activity (i.e., DFF-45), and this cleavage activates a process leading to the internucleosomal fragmentation of genomic DNA [60].

So far three caspase-related signaling pathways have been identified that can lead to apoptosis [60,79,80,114], but crosstalk among these pathways is possible. The intrinsic mitochondria-mediated pathway is controlled by Bcl-2 family proteins. It is regulated by cytochrome c release from mitochondria, promoting the activation of caspase-9 through Apaf-1 and then caspase-3 activation. The extrinsic death receptor pathway involves the activation of cell-surface death receptors, including Fas and tumor necrosis factor receptor, leading to the formation of the death-inducible signaling complex (DISC) and the activation of caspase-8, which in turn cleaves and activates downstream caspases such as caspase-3, 6, and 7. Caspase-8 can also cleave Bid, leading to the translocation, oligomerization, and insertion of Bax or Bak into the mitochondrial membrane. Another pathway involves the activation of caspase-2 by DNA damage or ER stress as a premitochondrial signal [115]. Caspases are also critical regulators of non-death functions in cells, notably some maturation processes.

Not all forms of apoptotic cell death are caspase-dependent [116,117]. The serine protease granzyme A (GrA) mediates a caspase-independent apoptotic pathway [116]. GrA is delivered to target cells through Ca^{2+}-dependent, perforin-generated pores and activates a DNase (GrA-DNase, non-metastasis factor 23, NM23) that is sequestered in the cytoplasm. NM23 activity is inhibited by the SET complex, which is located in the ER and composed of the nucleosome assembly protein SET, an inhibitor of protein phosphatase 2A, apurinic endonuclease 1, and a high mobility group protein (a non-histone DNA-binding protein that induces alterations in DNA architecture). GrA cleaves components of the SET complex to release activated NM23, which translocates to the nucleus to induce single-strand DNA nicks and cell death, which can be apoptotic or non-apoptotic [117].

Inhibitor of apoptosis protein (IAP) family

The activity of proapoptotic proteins must be placed in check to prevent unwanted apoptosis in normal cells. Apoptosis is blocked by the IAP family in mammalian cells [118–120]. This family includes X-chromosome-linked IAP (XIAP), IAP1, IAP2, NAIP (neuronal apoptosis inhibitory protein), survivin, livin, and apollon. These proteins are characterized by 1–3 baculoviral IAP repeat domains consisting of a zinc finger domain of ∼70–80 amino acids [119]. Apollon is a huge (530 kDa) protein that also has a ubiquitin-conjugating enzyme domain. The main identified antiapoptotic function of IAPs is the suppression of caspase activity [120]. Procaspase-9 and procaspase-3 are major targets of several IAPs. IAPs reversibly interact directly with caspases to block substrate cleavage. Apollon also ubiquitylates and facilitates proteosomal degradation of active caspase-9 and second mitochondria-derived activator of caspases (Smac) [121]. However, IAPs do not prevent caspase-8-induced proteolytic activation of procaspase-3. IAPs can also block apoptosis by reciprocal interactions with the nuclear transcription factor NFκB [118]. Scant information is available on IAPs in the nervous system. Survivin is essential for nervous system development in mouse, because conditional deletion of *survivin* gene in neuronal precursor cells causes reduced brain size, severe multifocal degeneration, and death shortly after birth [122]. NAIP is expressed throughout the CNS in neurons [123]. XIAP is enriched highly in mouse spinal motor neurons [124]. The importance of the IAP gene family in pediatric neurodegeneration is underscored by the finding that NAIP is deleted partially in a significant proportion of children with spinal muscular atrophy [125].

Proteins exist that inhibit mammalian IAPs. The murine mitochondrial protein Smac and its human ortholog DIABLO (for direct IAP-binding protein with low pI) inactivate the antiapoptotic actions of IAPs and thus exert proapoptotic actions [126,127]. These IAP inhibitors are 23 kDa mitochondrial proteins (derived from 29 kDa precursor proteins processed in the mitochondria) that are released from the intermembrane space and sequester IAPs. High temperature requirement protein A2 (HtrA2), also called Omi, is another mitochondrial serine protease that exerts proapoptotic activity by inhibiting IAPs [128]. HtrA2/Omi functions as a homotrimeric protein that cleaves IAPs irreversibly and thus facilitates caspase activity. The intrinsic mitochondria-mediated cell-death pathway is regulated by Smac and HtrA2/Omi.

Apoptosis-inducing factor (AIF)

AIF is a mammalian-cell mitochondrial protein identified as a flavoprotein oxidoreductase [129]. AIF has an N-terminal mitochondrial localization signal, and after import into the intermitochondrial membrane space the mitochondrial localization signal is cleaved off to generate a mature protein of 57 kDa. Under normal physiological conditions, AIF might function as a ROS scavenger targeting H_2O_2 [81] or in redox cycling with NAD(P)H [130]. With apoptotic stimuli, AIF translocates to the nucleus [129]. Overexpression of AIF induces cardinal features of apoptosis, including chromatin condensation, high-molecular-weight DNA fragmentation, and loss of mitochondrial transmembrane potential [129].

Cell-surface death receptors

Cell death by apoptosis can also be initiated at the cell membrane by surface death receptors of the tumor necrosis factor (TNF) receptor family. Fas (CD95/Apo-1) and the 75-kDa neurotrophin receptor (p75[NTR]) are members of the TNF receptor family [56]. The signal for apoptosis is initiated at the cell surface by aggregation (trimerization) of Fas. This activation of Fas is induced by the binding of the multivalent Fas ligand (FasL), a member of the TNF-cytokine family. FasL is expressed on activated T cells and natural killer cells. Clustering of Fas on the target cell by FasL recruits Fas-associated death domain (FADD), a cytoplasmic adapter molecule that functions in the activation of the caspase-8–Bid pathway, thus forming the "death-induced signaling complex" (DISC) [114]. In this pathway, Bid (a proapoptotic family member that is a substrate for caspase-8) is cleaved in the cytosol, and then truncated Bid translocates to mitochondria, thereby functioning as a BH3-only transducer of Fas activation signal at the cell plasma membrane to mitochondria [114]. Bid translocation from the cytosol to mitochondrial membranes is associated with a conformational change in Bax (which is prevented by Bcl-2 and Bcl-x_L) and is accompanied by release of cytochrome c from mitochondria [131]. Apoptosis through Fas is independent of new RNA or protein synthesis.

Apoptosis can be mediated by p75[NTR] [132]. Activation of p75[NTR] occurs through binding of nerve growth factor. When p75[NTR] is activated without Trk receptors, neurotrophin binding induces homodimer formation and activates an apoptotic cascade. p75[NTR] activation leads to the generation of ceramide through sphingomyelin hydrolysis. Ceramide production is associated with the activation of Jun N-terminal kinase (JNK) that phosphorylates and activates c-Jun and other transcription factors. p75 mediates hippocampal neuron death in response to neurotrophin withdrawal, involving cytochrome c, Apaf-1, and caspases-9, 6, and 3 (but not caspase-8), and thus is different from Fas-mediated cell death [132].

p53/p63/p73 family of tumor suppressors

Cell death by apoptosis can be triggered by DNA damage. p53 and related DNA binding proteins identified as p73 and p63 are involved in this process [77]. p53, p73, and p63 function in apoptosis or growth arrest and repair. They can commit to death cells that have sustained DNA damage from ROS, irradiation, and other genotoxic stresses [77]. p53 and p73 have similar oligomerization and DNA sequence transactivation properties. p73 exists as a group of full-length isoforms (including p73α and p73β) and as truncated isoforms that lack the transactivation domain (ΔN-p73). p53 is the best-studied of this family of proteins.

p53 is a short-lived protein with a half-life of ~5–20 minutes in most types of cells studied. p53 rapidly accumulates several-fold in response to DNA damage. This rapid regulation is mediated by post-translational modification such as phosphorylation and acetylation as well as intracellular redox state [133]. The elevation in p53 protein levels occurs through stabilization and prevention of degradation. p53 is degraded rapidly in a ubiquitination-dependent proteosomal pathway [134,135]. Murine double minute 2 (Mdm2; the human homolog is Hdm2) has a crucial role in this degradation pathway [136]. Mdm2 functions in a feedback loop to limit the duration or magnitude of the p53 response to DNA damage. Expression of the Mdm2 gene is controlled by p53 [136]. Mdm2 binds to the N-terminal transcriptional activation domain of p53 and regulates its DNA binding activity and stability by direct association. Mdm2 has ubiquitin ligase activity for p53 through the ubiquitin-conjugating enzyme E2. Stabilization of p53 is achieved through phosphorylation of serine[15] resulting in inhibition of formation of Mdm2–p53 complexes. Activated p53 binds the promoters of several genes encoding proteins associated with growth control and cell-cycle checkpoints (e.g., p21, Gadd45, Mdm2) and apoptosis (e.g., Bax, Bcl-2, Bcl-x_L, and Fas). The BH3-only proteins Puma and Noxa are critical mediators of p53-mediated apoptosis [137].

p53 and p73 regulate neuronal cell survival. p53 has a critical apoptotic role in cultured sympathetic ganglion neurons in response to neurotrophin withdrawal [138]. p53 deficiency protects against neuronal apoptosis induced by axotomy and target deprivation in vivo [139,140]. p53-mediated neuronal apoptosis can be blocked by the ΔN-p73 isoform by direct binding and inactivation of p53 [141].

Excitotoxic cell death

Neuronal death can be induced by excitotoxicity. This observation was made originally in 1957 [142], formulated into a concept by John Olney after he showed that glutamate can kill neurons in brain [143], and then examined mechanistically by Dennis Choi [144]. This concept has fundamental importance to a variety of acute neurological insults, such as cerebral HI, epilepsy, and trauma, and possibly chronic neurodegenerative diseases [7,20,145]. This pathologic neurodegeneration is mediated by excessive activation of glutamate-gated ion channel receptors and voltage-dependent ion channels. Increased cytosolic free Ca^{2+} causes activation of Ca^{2+}-sensitive proteases, protein kinases/phosphatases, phospholipases, and NOS when glutamate receptors are stimulated. The excessive interaction of ligand with subtypes of glutamate receptors causes pathophysiological changes in intracellular ion concentrations, pH, protein phosphorylation, and energy metabolism [144,146]. The precise mechanisms of excitotoxic cell death are still being examined intensively, driven by the hope of identifying therapeutic targets for neurological/neurodegenerative disorders with putative excitotoxic components. Yet, in vitro and in vivo experimental data are discordant with regard to whether excitotoxic neuronal death is apoptotic or necrotic, or perhaps even a peculiar form of cell death that is unique to excitotoxicity.

The contribution of apoptotic mechanisms to excitotoxic death of neurons has been examined in cultured neurons. However, these studies provide conflicting results. Excitotoxicity can cause activation of endonucleases and specific internucleosomal DNA fragmentation in cultures of cortical neurons [147,148] and cerebellar granule cells [149,150]. Internucleosomal fragmentation of DNA was not seen in other studies of cerebellar granule cell cultures [151]. Excitotoxic cell death in neuronal cultures is prevented [148] or unaffected [147,150,151] by inhibitors of RNA or protein synthesis, and sensitive [148,150] or insensitive [151] to the endonuclease inhibitor aurintricarboxylic acid. In primary cultures of mouse cortical cells, the non-NMDA glutamate receptor agonist kainic acid (KA) induces increases in Bax protein, and *bax* gene deficiency significantly protects cells against KA receptor toxicity [152]. However, NMDA receptor toxicity in mouse cerebellar granule cells [153] and mouse cortical cells [154] was not Bax-related. These results support our expectation that non-NMDA glutamate receptor excitotoxicity is more likely than NMDA receptor-mediated excitotoxicity to induce apoptosis or continuum cell death [18,19]. Glutamate (100 μM) stimulation of mouse cortical cells did not cause an increase in caspase activity [155], but NMDA-treated rat cortical cells showed increased caspase activity [156]. In cerebellar granule neurons, glutamate (100 μM to 1 mM) did not activate caspase activity, and adenoviral-mediated expression of IAPs did not influence excitotoxic cell death [157]. These conflicting results can also be related to the finding that activation of different subtypes of glutamate receptors appears to activate different modes of cell death [18,19].

The morphological characteristics of excitotoxicity in many neurons in vivo include somatodendritic swelling, mitochondrial damage, and chromatin condensation into irregular clumps [18,19,143,158], features that are thought to be typical of cellular necrosis; however, in other neurons, excitotoxicity causes cytological features more like apoptosis [18,19,158]. Excitotoxic degeneration of CA3 neurons in response to KA is increased in NAIP-deleted mice, further supporting a contribution of apoptosis [159]. Excitotoxic neurodegeneration in vivo has been shown to be either sensitive [160] or insensitive [161] to protein synthesis inhibition; therefore, a role for de novo protein synthesis in the expression of a PCD cascade in excitotoxicity is uncertain.

The precise mechanisms of excitotoxic neuronal apoptosis in vivo have not been identified specifically. Neurons in the immature rodent CNS undergo massive apoptosis in response to glutamate receptor excitotoxicity [18,19]. Apoptosis is much more prominent after excitotoxic injury in the immature brain compared to the mature brain [19]. Intrastriatal administration of KA in newborn rodents causes copious apoptosis of striatal neurons [18,162], serving as an unequivocal model of apoptosis in neurons that are selectively vulnerable in HIE. This apoptosis has been verified structurally with light and electron microscopy, and by immunolocalization of cleaved caspase-3 [162]. Ubiquitous apoptosis is observed at 24 hours after the insult. DNA degradation by internucleosomal fragmentation further confirms the presence of apoptosis. Excitotoxic neuronal apoptosis is associated with rapid (within 2 hours after neurotoxin exposure) translocation of Bax and cleaved caspase-3 to mitochondria [162]. Moreover, this study revealed that the ratio of mitochondrial membrane-associated Bax to soluble Bax in normal developing striatum changes prominently with brain maturation. Newborn rat striatum has a much greater proportion of Bax in the mitochondrial fraction, with lower levels of soluble Bax. Mature rat striatum has a much larger proportion of Bax in the soluble fraction and low amounts of Bax in the mitochondrial fraction. With brain maturation there is a linear decrease in the ratio of mitochondrial Bax to soluble Bax. This developmental subcellular redistribution of Bax might be a reason why immature rodent neurons exhibit a more robust classical apoptosis response compared to adult neurons after brain damage [163].

The cell-death continuum

We discovered using animal models of neurodegeneration that cell death exists as a continuum with necrosis and apoptosis at opposite ends of a degenerative spectrum; numerous hybrid forms of degeneration manifest between necrosis and apoptosis (Fig. 2.1) [18–21]. The age or maturity of brain and the subtype of excitatory glutamate receptor that is activated influence the mode and speed of neuronal cell death [18,19,163,164]. This structural and temporal diversity of neuronal cell death is seen with a variety of brain injuries including excitotoxicity, HI, target deprivation, and axonal trauma. Hence, injury-associated neuronal death is not the same in immature and mature CNS, and can be pleiomorphic in neurons within the same brain (Fig. 2.5).

To help explain these data we formulated the concept of the cell-death continuum. A fundamental cornerstone of the continuum is thought to be gradations in the responses of cells to stress. Some specific mechanisms thought to be driving the continuum are the developmental expression of different subtypes of glutamate receptors, mitochondrial energetics, the propinquity of developing neurons to the cell cycle, neurotrophin requirements, DNA damage vulnerability, and the degree of axonal collateralization [19]. Although the molecular mechanisms that drive this cell-death continuum in the brain are uncertain currently, cell culture data hint that ATP levels [34], intracellular Ca^{2+} levels [31], and mitochondrial permeability transition [40] could be involved. Our in vivo experiments so far suggest that the relative level of Bax in the outer mitochondrial membrane could regulate the cell-death continuum in neurons [162]. We believe that the concept of the cell-death continuum is particularly pertinent to neuron degeneration, although it might be applicable to cytopathology in general.

The concept of the cell-death continuum has been challenged and deemed confusing by some investigators [165–167]. Opponents of the cell-death continuum assume that

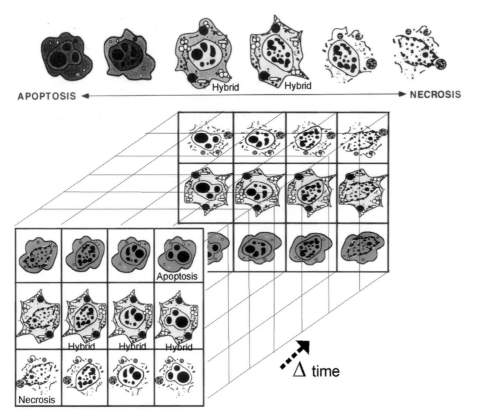

Fig. 2.5. Cell-death matrix. This diagram summarizes in linear (top) and three-dimensional matrix (bottom) formats the concept of the apoptosis–necrosis continuum of cell death. The concept as proposed in its original form organizes cell death as a linear spectrum with apoptosis and necrosis at the extremes and different syncretic hybrid forms in between (top). The front matrix of the cube (bottom) shows some of the numerous possible structures of neuronal cell death near or at the terminal stages of degeneration. Combining different nuclear morphologies and cytoplasmic morphologies generates a non-linear matrix of possible cell-death structures. In the cell at the extreme upper right corner, nuclear and cytoplasmic morphologies combine to form an apoptotic neuron that is typical of naturally occurring PCD during nervous system development. This death is classical apoptosis. In contrast, in the cell at the extreme lower left corner, the merging of necrotic nuclear and necrotic cytoplasmic morphologies forms a typical necrotic neuron resulting from NMDA receptor excitotoxicity and cerebral ischemia. Between these two extremes, hybrids of cell death can be produced with varying contributions of apoptosis and necrosis. The typical apoptosis–necrosis hybrid cell-death structure is best exemplified by neurons in the CNS dying from HI or non-NMDA GluR-mediated excitotoxicity. The death forms shown in the front matrix of the cube represent only a small number of the possible forms of cell death that we can envision to fill the empty cells of the matrix. Neuronal maturity and the subtypes of GluRs that are overactivated are known to influence where an injured/degenerating neuron falls within the matrix. The types and levels of DNA damage that are sustained by a cell might also influence the position of a degenerating cell within the death matrix. The back panel represents the possible cell-death forms occurring over a delayed period or after administration of therapeutic interventions. The matrix predicts that the cell-death patterns could change over time from apoptosis to apoptosis–necrosis variants or necrosis, and from necrosis to apoptosis–necrosis variants or apoptosis. This concept may also be relevant to cell death in general, and thus may be applicable to cancer biology and the mechanisms of action of chemotherapies and radiation therapies.

morphology and underlying biochemical processes remain binary and discrete [165]. While this is the case at the extremes of the continuum, absolute discreteness ignores the observable features of cell degeneration seen in the injured and diseased CNS. Steadfast arguments proposed by opponents of the cell-death continuum concept include (1) excitotoxic neuronal death in vivo is necrotic, regardless of age, and (2) apoptosis of neurons in the adult nervous system is extremely infrequent [165]. Experiments done by us [163,168] and others [169–172] have shown that neuronal degeneration triggered by excitoxicity and HI can be apoptotic, apoptosis–necrosis hybrids, and necrotic; furthermore, entire populations of neurons in the adult CNS can indeed undergo apoptosis after injury. Rigid conceptualization regarding cellular pathology is unrealistic and misleading and can hinder our goal of the identification of relevant molecular mechanisms in complex biological

systems, such as the injured perinatal brain, and ultimately limit the realization of therapeutic opportunities. For example, motor neuron degeneration in amyotrophic lateral sclerosis (ALS) was not considered to be a variant of apoptosis until the concept of the cell-death continuum was applied [21], and now antiapoptosis therapies are in clinical trials for the treatment of ALS [173].

The cell-death matrix

Studies show that the morphological appearance of the dying cell is a valuable tool for providing hints about the biochemical and molecular events responsible for the cell death [168]. When studying mechanisms of cell death in human disease and in animal/cell models of disease we believe that it is helpful to embrace the idea that apoptosis, necrosis, autophagy, and non-apoptotic PCD are not strictly "black and white." For the nervous system, overlay this complexity with cell-death mechanisms that are influenced by brain maturity, capacities for protein/RNA synthesis and DNA repair, antioxidant status, neurotrophin requirements, location in brain and location relative to the primary sites of injury, as well as intensity of the insult. These factors that influence nervous system damage, at least in animal models, can make the pathobiology of perinatal HIE seem to abandon strict certainty and causality, thus yielding a neuropathology that is probabilistic and uncertain.

To help organize neurodegeneration and discover laws that determine causes and effects in neurodegenerative settings, the concept of the cell-death continuum was extended to a hypothetical cell-death matrix to embrace the "fuzziness" of cell death in the injured CNS (Fig. 2.5). A matrix might be a useful modeling tool for pathology in general, and specifically for delineating the contributions of the different forms of cell death, and the possible identification of previously unrecognized forms of cell death in human neurological disorders and in their animal/cell models. A cell-death matrix could also be useful for modeling outcomes and how drugs and other treatments for human disease (e.g., cancer) will work. We need to identify better the relationships between mechanisms of cell death and the structure of dying cells in human pathology, in developing and adult CNS, as well as in animal and cell models of neurotoxicity in undifferentiated immature and terminally differentiated cells. It must be emphasized strongly that much more work needs to be done on the pathobiology of human HIE to better define its cell-death types. To help with this necessity, perinatal intensivists must encourage autopsy. The concept of a cell-death matrix could be important for understanding neuronal degeneration in a variety of pathophysiological settings, and thus may be important for mechanism-based neuroprotective treatments in neurological disorders in infants, children, and adults. If brain maturity and brain location dictate how and when neurons die relative to the insult [20,163], then the molecular mechanisms responsible for neuronal degeneration in different brain regions (and at different times after the injury) in infants and children might be different from the mechanisms of neuronal degeneration in adults; hence therapeutic targets will differ, and thus therapies will need to be customized for different brain regions, post-insult time, and age groups.

It will be extremely important to use clues from cell-death structure following different degrees and types of perinatal brain injury to better understand which injuries are most likely to respond to antinecrosis, antiapoptosis, or combination therapies, and whether these therapies actually ameliorate injury or simply delay or change the mode of cell damage. Animal studies predict that apoptosis inhibitors alone will be inadequate to ameliorate most of the early brain damage following neonatal HI, and the cell-death continuum predicts that apoptosis inhibitor drugs administered at acute and delayed time points will simply push cell degeneration from apoptosis to apoptosis-variant or necrotic cell death, as seen in vitro with caspase inhibitors applied following

chemical hypoxia [174]. Using the cell-death matrix, we predict that it will be difficult to pinpoint appropriate times for effective mechanism-based, spatially directed drug therapy. Hypothermia might be an ideal strategy, because it appears to protect against necrosis and apoptosis [175], but it has yet to be shown if these "protected" neurons are fully normal structurally and functionally, and whether there are functional benefits. More experimental and clinical work needs to be done. Nevertheless, it will be important to prepare for the possibility that pharmacological or non-drug interventions such as hypothermia might only delay, convert, or worsen the evolving brain damage associated with HIE in newborns. Alternative therapeutic approaches involving stem and progenitor cells should be considered now for the treatment of perinatal HIE.

Neurodegeneration in newborn human HIE

Detailed assessment of the cytopathological changes seen in newborn human HIE is of critical importance in order to identify the standard against which experimental animal-model observations should be compared; however, few detailed neuropathological and molecular-mechanism-based studies of cell death have been done on pediatric human HIE autopsy brains [176,177], in part because of a low frequency of autopsy [178]. Neuroimaging studies of infants at 24 hours of life after perinatal asphyxia have revealed neuronal integrity abnormalities in basal ganglia by magnetic resonance spectroscopy [179]. Most available postmortem studies of human HIE have focused on "pontosubicular necrosis" [176]. In asphyxic term humans at 1 day of life a pattern of neuronal necrosis in striatum is suggested [180]. We have begun to evaluate brain samples from a small cohort of full-term human infants ($n = 6$) that suffered from complications during delivery resulting in HIE and death between 3 days and months after the insult. Paraffin sections from cerebral cortex, striatum, and cerebellum were evaluated for cytopathology and molecular markers for cell death (p53 and cleaved caspase-3). The degeneration was seen in selective populations of neurons throughout forebrain and cerebellar cortex, with no evidence of infarct or major gliomesodermal changes. The neurodegeneration was divisible on a single-cell basis and was seen as two dominant forms: lytic, necrotic-like or condensed, traditional ischemic-like (Fig. 2.6). The necrotic-like neurons were swollen or erupted with residual cytoplasm around the nucleus. The ischemic-like neurons displayed homogenization and vacuolation of the cytoplasm, cell shrinkage (but no apparent frank lysis), and uniform nuclear condensation and collapse (pyknosis) rather than cytoplasmic or nuclear fragmentation. The absence of nuclear fragmentation is inconsistent with apoptosis and a hybrid form of cell death. There were no classically apoptotic or closely apoptotic-like neurons seen. Nevertheless, subsets of degenerating cortical neurons in human HIE were positive for cleaved caspase-3 (Fig. 2.6), but many degenerating neurons were not positive

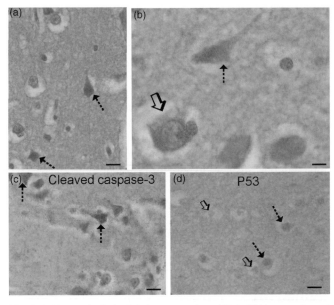

Fig. 2.6. Neuronal cell death in human newborn HIE. (a, b) Hematoxylin and eosin staining of neocortex from an infant that survived 3 days after HI due to delivery complications reveals selective degeneration of neurons (hatched arrows) in the form of typical ischemic neuronal death with eosinophilic cytoplasm, shrunken cell body, and condensed nucleus. Other damaged neurons are swollen with a vacuolated cytoplasm (open arrow in b). This pattern of neurodegeneration is much less phenotypically heterogeneous than that seen in neonatal rodent models of HI, but similar to that seen in our piglet model of HI. Scale bars = 33 μm (a), 7 μm (b). (c) Subsets of neocortical neurons (hatched arrows) in human infants with HIE display cleaved caspase-3 throughout the cell. Other cells in the field shown by the cresyl violet counterstaining have no labeling for cleaved caspase-3. Scale bar = 15 μm. (d) Subsets of neocortical neurons (hatched arrows) in human infants with HIE display active p53 within the nucleus. Other cells (open arrow) in the field have no labeling for active p53. Scale bar = 15 μm. *See color plate section.*

for cleaved caspase-3. One recent study has shown cells (of unknown identity) positive for cleaved caspase-3 in the cerebral cortex of a human neonate with HIE [177]. Many degenerating cortical neurons, surprisingly some cells with a necrotic morphology, were also positive for active (phosphorylated) p53 (Fig. 2.6). In white matter, there was no morphological evidence for oligodendrocyte apoptosis, although appreciable white-matter damage was present as evidenced by the rarefaction and vacuolation. These observations show that classic apoptosis has little contribution to the evolving neuropathology in the newborn human brain with HIE, but caspase-3- and p53-regulated cell-death mechanisms seem to be operative in driving a syncretic cell-death-continuum variant phenotype in addition to cellular necrosis.

Neurodegeneration in neonatal animal models of HIE

Relevance of animal models of HIE

Animal models are critical for identifying injury-related mechanisms of HIE and for testing preclinical efficacy of therapeutics. However, the relevance of the animal model should be understood in the context of human pathobiology

by appreciating the relative brain maturity of the model compared to that of the human term newborn, and whether the pathobiology observed in the model is similar to that seen in human neonatal HIE. Fundamental physiological, neurobiological, and pathobiological issues are very important when considering the relevance of experimental animals as models for brain injury in human newborns. Neurodegeneration in the immature brain is phenotypically heterogeneous and regionally specific, and can be dependent on model and species [20]. For example (see below for more details), the contributions of classic apoptosis to the neurodegeneration in models of neonatal HI are much more prominent in newborn rat/mouse models [22–24,181] than in piglet models [3,7,35,36]. In human newborn HIE there is very little or no evidence for involvement of classic apoptosis morphologically, but caspase-3 and p53 involvements seem operative (Fig. 2.6). Considerable experimental data on HIE mechanisms have been derived using a 7-day-old rat (and mouse) pup model of HI (modified Levine model by Rice *et al.* [182]), which is very immature and has a brain maturity much less than that of near-term humans [183]. The 7-day-old rat/mouse is a preterm model [184] and should not be considered as an animal model for HIE in the term human brain. Moreover, the small size of rat and mouse pups prohibits intensive physiological monitoring [185]. Small variations in post-ischemic temperature have a major impact on the amount of brain damage in rat pups [186]. The 7-day-old rat/mouse model of HIE is a robust model of neurodegeneration, but it displays a pattern of injury that is atypical clinically, somewhat between the pattern seen with global asphyxia and that of stroke [185]. In contrast to the newborn rat/mouse, the percentage of adult brain weight at birth in piglets is much closer to that in humans [187], and the body size of the piglet and chest and cranial geometries, as well as the cortical and basal ganglia topology, are much more similar to human infants. Thus, a piglet model of asphyxic cardiac arrest has been developed as a particularly relevant model of HIE for the full-term human newborn and young infant. The basal ganglia and somatosensory cortical injury created in this model [3,4] is strikingly similar to that seen in MR studies of full-term human neonates with perinatal asphyxia [2,188]. Neuronal integrity abnormalities in basal ganglia are seen by MR spectroscopy in 24-hour-infants after perinatal asphyxia [179]. Recent PET studies of human infants suffering for delivery-associated HI even show the transient selective brain regional hypermetabolism [189] seen in piglets after HI [3,4]. Piglet models of neonatal HIE that reveal the efficacy of hypothermic neuroprotection [190,191] are perhaps the most relevant models to identify mechanisms of neurodegeneration and to test drug and cell therapies, because of the similarities in brain anatomy and pathophysiology.

HIE in neonatal rats and mice

Despite the limitations of the rat/mouse pup model of HIE, considerable data on mechanisms of neurodegeneration continue to accrue from this model. The neuronal cell death in the rat/mouse pup model of HIE is fulminant, has acute and delayed temporal components, and occurs as several forms, including necrosis, apoptosis, and hybrids of necrosis and apoptosis [22–24]. These studies have shown that neuronal cell death early after HI is largely a form of necrosis and necrosis–apoptosis hybrids, followed by robust delayed apoptotic neurodegeneration [7,23,24]. This hybrid form of cell death is similar to the continuum cell death caused by non-NMDA glutamate receptor excitotoxins in the neonatal forebrain [7]. Based on structural and biochemical evidence, neuronal necrosis predominates in cerebral cortex, necrosis–apoptosis hybrids occur in hippocampus and striatum, and classical apoptosis is prominent in thalamus. We believe that connectivity instructed-target deprivation contributes substantially to the brain damage occurring over the longer term following perinatal HI [4,20], and this neurodegeneration is fully apoptosis. There remains, however, a fundamental question of whether or not apoptotic mechanisms are directly activated acutely by perinatal HI.

Caspases seem to be involved in the evolution of neonatal brain injury caused by HI. Caspase-3 cleavage and activation occur in brain after HI in neonatal rodents [22,24,102,193]. The extent of caspase-3 cleavage and activation following brain injury or neuronal stress is greater in developing systems compared to mature systems in vivo and in vitro [194,195]. Cerebroventricular injection of a pan-caspase inhibitor or intraperitoneal injection of a serine protease inhibitor 3 hours after neonatal HI has neuroprotective effects [181,196]. Subsequent studies have shown 30–50% decreases in neonatal HI-induced tissue loss at 15 days after the insult with non-selective inhibitors of caspase-8 and caspase-9 [197–199]. However, the lack of enzyme specificity of caspase-inhibitor drugs prevents unambiguous identification of caspases in mediating brain injury in most studies. The class of irreversible tetrapeptide caspase inhibitors covalently coupled to chloromethylketone, fluoromethylketone, or aldehydes efficiently inhibits other classes of cysteine proteases such as calpains [200,201]. Calpains, Ca^{2+}-activated, neutral, cytosolic cysteine proteases, are activated highly following neonatal HI [193,202]. MDL28170, a drug that inhibits calpains and caspase-3, exerts neuroprotective actions in the neonatal rat brain by decreasing necrosis and apoptosis [203]. Cathepsins, cysteine proteases concentrated in the lysosomal compartment, are also likely to be activated, based on electron-microscopy evidence of lysosomal and vacuolar changes found following neonatal HI [20]. More potent, selective, and reversible non-peptide caspase-3 inhibitors have been developed [204] and used to protect against brain injury following neonatal HI [199], but the protective effects were more modest compared to initial reports with non-selective pan-caspase inhibition [181].

The roles of the Bcl-2 and IAP families and AIF in regulating neonatal brain injury are being examined enthusiastically in rodent models of HIE. The level of Bax protein is increased markedly in relation to the levels of Bcl-2 or Bcl-x$_L$ protein following the injury [205]. Nevertheless, neonatal $bax^{-/-}$ mice still show caspase-3 activation in dying hippocampal neurons, despite the lack of Bax protein, though caspase-8 activation is not affected by lack of Bax protein [205]. Mice with complete homozygous deletion of *bax* genes exposed to HI at postnatal day 7 (P7) have modest neuroprotection in hippocampus and no protection in cerebral cortex at P14 [205]. In other models of neonatal CNS injury, although Bax deletion rescues neurons from axotomy-induced apoptosis, the neurons are structurally abnormal [206] (Martin *et al.*, unpublished observations), and there is no evidence that they function properly. The importance of the Bax homolog Bak needs to be investigated in neonatal HI. In addition to the multidomain Bcl-2 family mitochondrial death proteins, the roles of the BH3-only proteins in mediating neonatal HI brain damage need to be examined. Recent data seem to indicate that Bim and Bad, but not Bid, are involved in the hippocampal damage in neonatal mice with HIE [207]. Overexpression of XIAP in transgenic neonatal mice reduces brain damage after HI [208], and AIF knockdown reduces infarct volume [209]. We have found that mitochondria in the immature brain may be "primed" for apoptosis by significant amounts of Bax resident within their membranes (Figs. 2.2, 2.3). With brain maturation, Bax levels in the mitochondrial fraction of striatal tissue change from high to low [162]. We have found significant alterations in the balance of pro- and antiapoptosis Bcl-2 family protein levels following neonatal HI [210,211].

The apoptosis in thalamic neurons after HI in neonatal rat is associated with a rapid increase in the levels of Fas death receptor and caspase-8 activation [210,211], and neonatal mice with inactivated Fas are protected from some HI-related damage [210]. Concurrently, the levels of Bax in mitochondrial-enriched cell fractions increase, and cytochrome c accumulates in the soluble protein compartment. Increased levels of Fas death receptor and Bax, cytochrome c accumulation, and activation of caspase-8 precede the marked activation of caspase-3 and the occurrence of neuronal apoptosis in the thalamus in neonatal rat HI [23,210]. This thalamic neuron apoptosis in the neonatal rat brain after HI is identical structurally to the apoptosis of thalamic neurons after cortical trauma [164]. HI in the neonatal rat causes severe infarction of cerebral cortex [23], and we suspect that this thalamic neuron apoptosis is caused by target deprivation, as in our occipital cortex lesion model [212,213].

Studies have been done on the perinatal brain to determine whether apoptotic mechanisms are activated directly by injury. Biochemical evidence for the existence of an intermediate "continuum" form of cell death was verified by the co-expression of markers for both apoptosis and necrosis in neurons in the injured forebrain at 3 hours following HI in neonatal rat [202]. The significance of this finding becomes evident by the demonstration that caspase-3 inhibition provides complete blockade of caspase activation but only partial neuroprotection. Caspase-3 inhibitors fail to prevent the necrotic mode of cell death induced by HI, as revealed by the presence of necrosis markers, and thus the forebrain still sustains significant injury [199].

HIE in newborn piglets

We have developed a 7-day-old piglet model of HI that simulates the brain damage and some of the clinical deficits found in human newborns that are victims of asphyxia [3,4,214]. This injury model is most relevant to asphyxia in the full-term neonate [2,215]. Importantly, the basal ganglia are selectively vulnerable in this model. The putamen is the most vulnerable. The death of striatal neurons after HI in piglets is categorically necrosis [35], contrasting with findings in neonatal rat striatum after HI [22–24]. Nevertheless, despite the necrosis, this neurodegeneration in piglets evolves with a specific temporal pattern of subcellular organelle damage and biochemical defects [35,36]. Damage to the Golgi apparatus and rough ER occurs at 3–12 hours, while most mitochondria appear intact until 12 hours. Mitochondria undergo an early suppression of metabolic activity, then a transient burst of activity at 6 hours after the insult, followed by mitochondrial failure. Cytochrome c is depleted at 6 hours after HI, failing to accumulate in the cytosol compartment, and is not restored thereafter. Lysosomal destabilization occurs within 3–6 hours after HI, consistent with the lack of evidence for autophagy. Damage in newborn piglet striatum after cerebral HI induced by asphyxic cardiac arrest thus evolves rapidly over 24 hours, at which time ~80% of the neurons in the putamen are dead, and closely resembles excitotoxic neuronal damage caused by NMDA receptor activation [35].

A variety of biochemical mechanisms of cell injury were examined in this model. After 3 hours recovery, glutathione levels are reduced in striatum [35,36]. Peroxynitrite-mediated oxidative damage to membrane proteins occurs at 3–12 hours after HI, and the Golgi apparatus and cytoskeleton are early targets for extensive tyrosine nitration. Striatal neurons sustain hydroxyl radical damage to DNA and RNA within 6 hours after HI. The early emergence of this injury coincides with elevated NMDA receptor phosphorylation, a biochemical surrogate marker for receptor activation, and prominent oxidative damage by 5 minutes after recovery of spontaneous circulation [216]. These abnormalities are sustained through 3 hours of recovery. The early NMDA receptor phosphorylation coincides with rapid recruitment of neuronal NOS to the synaptic/plasma membrane. This work demonstrates that neuronal necrosis in the striatum after HI in piglets evolves rapidly and is possibly driven by early depletion of glutathione antioxidant capacity and oxidative stress by 3 hours after the insult. We anticipated that this brain injury would be difficult to protect against in piglets because it evolves so quickly after HI, with significant accumulation of DNA double-strand breaks (a very lethal form of genotoxicity) by 3 hours, damage to 50% of neurons by 6 hours, and degeneration of 80% of putaminal neurons by 24 hours [35]. Early implemented interventions will thus be required to protect the basal ganglia region from HI.

We have proposed that brain damage in the striatum serves as an "organizer" for the subsequent neuropathology that emerges after HI in newborns [3,4]. In this concept, damage in specific zones of striatum sets up the damage in topographically interconnected regions of cerebral cortex. This idea is supported by the progressive delayed hypermetabolism and neurodegeneration in regions of neocortex having connections that map topographically to locations of striatum with damage. Moreover, the more severe the striatal damage, the more severe the cortical damage. For example, when central putamen is damaged selectively, regions of somatosensory cortex correspondingly develop damage, and when the caudate nucleus is also damaged there is correspondingly more damage in frontal cortex. At later time points after the insult, the damage cascades into what appears to be cortically directed thalamic and brainstem damage, involving retrograde and anterograde mechanisms. Why the damage initially manifests in the central putamen in this model is still a mystery, although it seems to begin in matrix regions of the striatal mosaic that are hypermetabolic (Martin, unpublished observations). The mechanisms of topographically driven degeneration in HIE might involve changes in the sensitivities of glutamate receptors to ligand and the functioning of transporters that remove glutamate from the synaptic cleft, acute and delayed abnormalities in inhibitory interneurons, and trophic factor deprivation. A prediction based on this concept of the brain damage "organizer" of HIE is that if interventions can result in sustained neuroprotection in striatum, then protection in other brain regions will follow.

Neuroprotection and neuroregenerative strategies in the piglet model of newborn HIE

The pathophysiological mechanisms of striatal injury engage rapidly in piglets after HI. Robust ischemic cytopathology in putaminal neurons emerges between 3 and 6 hours after HI in male piglets and is associated with oxidative damage to cytosolic proteins [216]. The mechanisms for this profound degeneration of striatal neurons might involve NMDA-receptor-mediated excitotoxicity [20,35] and dopamine-receptor-mediated inactivation of Na^+,K^+-ATPase [217,218]. The NMDA receptor is a tetrameric ion channel comprising individual protein subunits designated as NR1, NR2A-D, and NR3A-B [219]. The functional channel must contain at least one NR1 subunit, of which there are several variants generated by alternate splicing of the C-terminus [219]. The physiological properties of the NMDA receptor are determined by the subunit composition of the heteromeric complex and are modulated by phosphorylation of the NR1 and NR2 subunits [219,220]. Protein kinase C (PKC) phosphorylates NR1 serine residues 890 and 896, and cyclic adenosine monophosphate (cAMP)-dependent protein kinase A (PKA) phosphorylates NR1 serine 897 [220]. NMDA receptor subunit proteins are enriched in newborn piglet striatum; moreover, the levels of the different subunits as well as the phosphorylation of NR1 change differentially in the striatum of HI piglets during the period of active cell death after HI [221], at which time there is oxidative damage and striatal neuron necrosis [35]. Recent data also suggest that striatal neuron degeneration may involve D1 dopamine-receptor-mediated toxicity involving PKA-dependent phosphorylation of NR1 and Na^+,K^+-ATPase [219]. We have also shown that 24 hours of mild, whole-body hypothermia with sedation and paralysis has profound, perhaps sustained, neuroprotective effects on the HI piglet striatum [190], consistent with other studies in newborn piglets [191] and rats [222,223]. Moreover, hypothermia blocks the apparent NMDA-receptor activation and the oxidative damage to proteins [216]. It is still uncertain if these salvaged neurons are normal. We have found that neurons can exist in damaged atrophic states with few synaptic contacts for months after injury [224].

Stem cell therapy for pediatric HIE

Regenerative medicine through novel cell-based therapies needs to be explored preclinically for treating perinatal HIE [225–227]. The possibilities for neural repair after HI include recruitment of endogenous cells and transplantation of exogenous or autologous cells. Recruitment of endogenous neural stem cells (NSCs) or neural progenitor cells (NPCs) will likely have limited benefit [228]. To date, relatively little work has been done on the transplantation of allogenic or xenogenic embryonic stem cells (SCs) or neonatal and adult SCs as a therapy in animal models of infant and childhood HIE. In a neonatal mouse model of HI, retrovirally transformed, immortalized, neonatal mouse cerebellum-derived stem-like cells (the C17.2 cell line) were transplanted into the cavitary lesion as a cell-polymer scaffold complex, and were shown to engraft and differentiate into the three primary neural cell types and to integrate structurally [225]. In a neonatal rat model of HI, multipotent astrocytic NSCs from mouse subependymal zone differentiated into neurons at locations remote from the infarcted area [227]. We used a neonatal mouse model of excitotoxicity to evaluate the behavior of transplanted human embryonic germ (EG) cell-derived NSCs in the environment of an immature host forebrain that is injured. We studied the ability of human EG-cell-derived NSCs to engraft, differentiate, and replace cells in the damaged neonatal mouse brain. We found that human NSCs can engraft successfully into injured newborn mouse forebrain, disseminate into the lesioned areas, survive, differentiate into neuronal and glial cells, and replace lost neurons [226]. Nevertheless, more data need to be collected on animal models to determine beneficial or harmful effects of this approach.

Newborn piglet olfactory bulb is a rich source of NSC/NPCs useful for transplantation after pediatric HI

The human olfactory bulb (OB) contains resident NSC/NPCs [229]. The OB of rat and mouse also contains multipotent (stem) NPCs [229,230]. The OB core is part of the anterior subventricular zone (SVZ) rostral migratory stream (RMS) system of NPCs [231]. Because the OB core is the rostral extension of the SVZ, the NPCs within this structure are more accessible than those in the SVZ, lying deep within the forebrain, for potential experimental autologous transplantation. OB-NSCs/NPCs have been used as an effective therapy in mouse ALS [232]. Thus, the OB could be of major importance to HIE neuroregenerative medicine if proof of principle is established that the OB core contains cells that are useful for transplantation in animal models of HIE.

We have begun histological and cell-culture studies on the piglet brain to identify the presence of NSC/NPCs (Fig. 2.7). Labeling of bromodeoxyuridine (BrdU), a thymidine analogue that is incorporated into DNA during its synthesis, showed that the OB core in newborn piglets accumulates numerous newly replicated cells. The piglet OB core is rich in nestin (an NSC marker), musashi (an NSC/NPC marker), polysialic acid neural cell adhesion molecule (PSA-NCAM, an NPC marker), as well as doublecortin and TUC4 (differentiating/migrating newborn neuron markers). BrdU-positive cells are immunolabeled for astrocyte and neuronal markers. Isolated and cultured OB core cells from piglets have the capacity to generate numerous neurospheres. Neurospheres are three-dimensional aggregates of viable self-adherent cells. Thus newborn OB-NSC/NPCs can be isolated and expanded in vitro. OB core neurospheres can be cryopreserved and subsequently cultured again. Single-cell clonal analysis of piglet OB neurospheres has revealed the capacity for self-renewal and multipotency. Piglet OB core cells differentiate into neurons, astrocytes, and oligodendrocytes in culture. We conclude that the newborn piglet OB core is a reservoir of multipotent NSCs/NPCs.

We have begun transplantation experiments to identify the potential use of piglet OB-NSC/NPCs for cell therapy in our newborn piglet model of HIE. Clonally derived OB-NSC/NPC neurospheres were stably transduced with a lentiviral construct to express the jellyfish green fluorescent protein (GFP) as a reporter molecule for detection of transplanted cells in the host brain (Fig. 2.7). These OB cell-derived neurospheres were transplanted by intracerebral stereotaxic microinjection into the cerebral cortex or striatum of piglets 3 days after asphyxic cardiac arrest. At 14 days after transplantation, the piglets were killed to examine the fate of the transplanted cells. The transplanted neurospheres dispersed into constituent GFP-labeled cells (Fig. 2.7). The transplanted cells were found in damaged regions (e.g., striatum) as well as in regions previously not evaluated for damage. Specifically, transplanted cells were found in cerebral cortex, corpus callosum, striatum, SVZ, globus pallidus, and basal forebrain. OB-NSC/NPCs were found to express markers for neurons and oligodendrocytes and subsets of these cells differentiated in cells appearing as neurons.

These preclinical findings are relevant to the development of novel cell-based therapies for human pediatric HIE. The OB in the human brain is a potential target for regenerative medicine using transplantation of autologous cells, with the goal of replacing neurons and oligodendrocytes in the forebrain damaged by perinatal HI. However, translating this approach into the clinic presents major hurdles. Harvesting multipotent NSCs/NPCs from the human OB is invasive, and the human

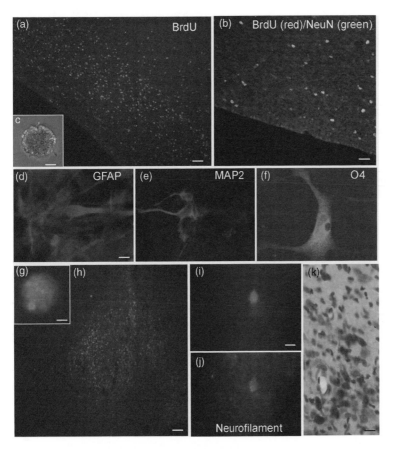

Fig. 2.7. The newborn piglet olfactory bulb (OB) is a rich source of multipotent neural progenitor cells useful for transplantation into damaged newborn brain after HI. (a) The piglet OB core (the ventricular cavity is the black area at left of image) contains numerous newly born cells (green-labeled cells) as identified by BrdU labeling of replicated DNA and antibody detection. Scale bar = 80 μm. (b) The majority of newly born cells (BrdU, red) in the newborn piglet OB core express the neuron-specific nuclear marker NeuN (green), demonstrating that they are newly born neurons. Yellow indicates overlap in two signals. Scale bar = 24 μm. (c) Newborn piglet OB-NSC/NPC neurosphere. OB core cells from newborn piglet can be harvested, cultured, and used to isolate neurosphere-forming cells. Neurospheres can be dissociated into constituent cells and shown by single-cell clonal analysis to be multipotent neural precursor cells. Scale bar = 20 μm. (d–f) Single OB core neurosphere-forming cells can be expanded in vitro to form numerous additional neurospheres with constituent cells that can differentiate into the three primary neural cell types: astrocytes positive for glial fibrillary (GFAP), neurons positive for microtubule-associated protein-2 (MAP2), and oligodendrocytes positive for the cell surface marker O4. Scale bar = 7 μm. (g) Piglet OB-NSC/NPC neurospheres can be stably transfected with a green fluorescent protein (GFP) gene using a lentiviral construct. This cell tagging serves as a reporter for transplanted cells. Scale bar = 20 μm. (h) After transplantation into the newborn piglet with HIE, GFP-OB-NSC/NPC neurospheres disperse entirely into individual green-labeled cells and migrate into damaged areas. Scale bar = 20 μm. (i, j) Subsets of transplanted GFP-labeled cells (green in i) in neocortex and basal ganglia that appear to be differentiating express neuron markers (neurofilament, red in j). Scale bar = 12 μm. (k) Immunoperoxidase detection of GFP using monoclonal antibody can be used as an alternative method to identify transplanted cells in HI piglet brain. These cells (brown-labeled cells) have engrafted, survived, and are differentiating into neurons in striatum. Scale bar = 20 μm. *See color plate section.*

OB is less accessible than the piglet OB. However, neurosurgical approaches are established for exposing the human OB and are used for olfactory grove meningiomas and OB tumors [233–235]. A unilateral biopsy of the OB to obtain a source of expandable autologous NSC/NPCs for transplantation might cause mild disability such as hemianosmia, but, when faced with the lifelong neurological consequences of perinatal HIE, such as cerebral palsy, this approach might be welcomed.

Acknowledgments

This work was supported by grants from the US Public Health Service, NIH-NINDS (NS034100, NS052098, NS020020) and NIH-NIA (AG016282). The author is grateful to Dr. Ansgar Brambrink for his original work on the development of the piglet HIE model, Dr. Dawn Mueller-Burke for her work on the piglet hypothermia intervention studies, Dr. Frances Northington for her work on the neonatal rat/mouse model of HIE, Alyssa Katzenelson for her work on the piglet OB-NSC/NPC characterization in vivo and in vitro, Dr. Zeng-Jin Yang for his help with the BrdU and transplantation experiments on piglets, and Dr. Ray Koehler for his continuous enthusiasm for the piglet model. The author dedicates this chapter to his father Joseph G. Martin (born June 10, 1926, died December 21, 2007).

References

1. Glass HC, Ferriero DM. Treatment of hypoxic–ischemic encephalopathy in newborns. *Curr Treat Options Neurol* 2007; **9**: 414–23.

2. Maller AI, Hankins LL, Yeakley JW, *et al.* Rolandic type cerebral palsy in children as a pattern of hypoxic–ischemic injury in the full-term neonate. *J Child Neurol* 1998; **13**: 313–21.

3. Martin LJ, Brambrink A, Koehler RC, *et al.* Primary sensory and forebrain motor systems in the newborn brain are preferentially damaged by hypoxia–ischemia. *J Comp Neurol* 1997; **377**: 262–85.

4. Martin LJ, Brambrink A, Koehler RC, *et al.* Neonatal asphyxic brain injury is neural system preferential and targets sensory-motor networks. In Stevenson DK, Sunshine P, eds., *Fetal and Neonatal Brain Injury: Mechanisms, Management, and the Risks of Practice*, 2nd edn. New York, NY: Oxford University Press, 1997: 374–99.

5. Volpe JJ. *Neurology of the Newborn.* Philadelphia, PA: Saunders, 2001.

6. Johnston MV, Nakajima W, Hagberg H. Mechanisms of hypoxic neurodegeneration in the developing brain. *Neuroscientist* 2002; **8**: 212–20.

7. Martin LJ. Mechanisms of brain damage in animal models of hypoxia–ischemia in newborns. In Stevenson DK, Benitz WE, Sunshine P, eds., *Fetal and Neonatal Brain Injury: Mechanisms, Management, and the Risks of Practice*, 3rd edn. Cambridge: Cambridge University Press, 2003: 30–57.

8. McQuillen PS, Ferriero DM. Selective vulnerability in the developing central nervous system. *Pediatr Neurol* 2004; **30**: 227–35.

9. Blomgren K, Hagberg H. Free radicals, mitochondria, and hypoxia–ischemia in the developing brain. *Free Rad Biol Med* 2006; **40**: 388–97.

10. Hamrick SE, Ferriero DM. The injury response in the term newborn brain: can we neuroprotect? *Curr Opin Neurol* 2003; **16**: 147–54.

11. Hypothermia after Cardiac Arrest Study Group. Mild therapeutic hypothermia to improve the neurologic outcome after cardiac arrest. *N Engl J Med* 2002; **346**: 549–56.

12. Shankaran S, Laptook AR, Ehrenkranz RA, *et al.* Whole-body hypothermia for neonates with hypoxic–ischemic encephalopathy. *N Engl J Med* 2005; **353**: 1574–84.

13. Gluckman PD, Wyatt JS, Azzopardi D, *et al.* Selective head cooling with mild systemic hypothermia after neonatal encephalopathy: multicentre randomized trial. *Lancet* 2005; **365**: 663–70.

14. Kanagawa T, Fukuda H, Tsubouchi H, *et al.* A decrease of cell proliferation by hypothermia in the hippocampus of the neonatal rat. *Brain Res* 2006; **1111**: 36–40.

15. Lockshin RA, Zakeri Z. Caspase-independent cell deaths. *Curr Opin Cell Biol* 2002; **14**: 727–33.

16. Gilbert SF. *Developmental Biology.* Sunderland, MA: Sinauer Associates, 2006.

17. Klionsky DJ, Emr SD. Autophagy as a regulated pathway of cellular degradation. *Science* 2000; **290**: 1717–21.

18. Portera-Cailliau C, Price DL, Martin LJ. Excitotoxic neuronal death in the immature brain is an apoptosis–necrosis morphological continuum. *J Comp Neurol* 1997; **378**: 70–87.

19. Portera-Cailliau C, Price DL, Martin LJ. Non-NMDA and NMDA receptor-mediated excitotoxic neuronal deaths in adult brain are morphologically distinct: further evidence for an apoptosis–necrosis continuum. *J Comp Neurol* 1997; **378**: 88–104.

20. Martin LJ, Al-Abdulla NA, Brambrink AM, *et al.* Neurodegeneration in excitotoxicity, global cerebral ischemia, and target deprivation: a perspective on the contributions of apoptosis and necrosis. *Brain Res Bull* 1998; **46**: 281–309.

21. Martin LJ. Neuronal death in amyotrophic lateral sclerosis is apoptosis: possible contribution of a programmed cell death mechanism. *J Neuropathol Exp Neurol* 1999; **58**: 459–71.

22. Nakajima W, Ishida A, Lange MS, *et al.* Apoptosis has a prolonged role in the neurodegeneration after hypoxic ischemia in the newborn rat. *J Neurosci* 2000; **20**: 7994–8004.

23. Northington FJ, Ferriero DM, Graham EM, *et al.* Early neurodegeneration after hypoxia–ischemia in neonatal rat is necrosis while delayed neuronal death is apoptosis. *Neurobiol Dis* 2001; **8**: 207–19.

24. Northington FJ, Zelaya ME, O'Riordan DP, *et al.* Failure to complete apoptosis following neonatal hypoxia–ischemia manifests as "continuum" phenotype of cell death and occurs with multiple manifestations of mitochondrial dysfunction in rodent forebrain. *Neuroscience* 2007; **149**: 822–33.

25. Lennon SV, Martin SJ, Cotter TG. Dose-dependent induction of apoptosis in human tumour cell lines by widely diverging stimuli. *Cell Prolif* 1991; **24**: 203–14.

26. Fernandes RS, Cotter TG. Apoptosis or necrosis: intracellular levels of glutathione influence mode of cell death. *Biochem Pharmacol* 1994; **48**: 675–81.

27. Bonfoco E, Krainc D, Ankarcrona M, *et al.* Apoptosis and necrosis: two distinct events induced, respectively, by mild and intense insults with N-methyl-D-aspartate or nitric oxide/superoxide in cortical cell culture. *Proc Natl Acad Sci USA* 1995; **92**: 7162–6.

28. Raffray M, Cohen GM. Apoptosis and necrosis in toxicology: a continuum or distinct modes of cell death? *Pharmacol Ther* 1997; **75**: 153–77.

29. Yuan J, Lipinski M, Degterev A. Diversity in the mechanisms of neuronal cell death. *Neuron* 2003; **40**: 401–13.

30. Orrenius S, Zhivotovsky B, Nicotera P. Regulation of cell death: the calcium–apoptosis link. *Nat Rev Mol Cell Biol* 2003; **4**: 552–65.

31. Trump BF, Berezesky IK. The role of altered $[Ca^{2+}]_i$ regulation in apoptosis, oncosis, and necrosis. *Biochim Biophys Acta* 1996; **1313**: 173–8.

32. Majno G, Joris I. Apoptosis, oncosis, and necrosis: an overview of cell death. *Am J Pathol* 1995; **146**: 3–15.

33. Trump BF, Goldblatt PJ, Stowell RE. Studies on necrosis of mouse liver *in vitro*: ultrastructural alterations in the mitochondria of hepatic parenchymal cells. *Lab Invest* 1964; **14**: 343–71.

34. Leist M, Single B, Castoldi AF, *et al.* Intracellular adenosine triphosphate (ATP) concentration: a switch in the decision between apoptosis and necrosis. *J Exp Med* 1997; **185**: 1481–6.

35. Martin LJ, Brambrink AM, Price AC, *et al.* Neuronal death in newborn striatum after hypoxia–ischemia is necrosis and evolves with oxidative stress. *Neurobiol Dis* 2000; **7**: 169–91.

36. Golden WC, Brambrink AM, Traystman RJ, *et al.* Failure to sustain recovery of Na,K-ATPase function is a possible mechanism for striatal neurodegeneration in hypoxic–ischemic newborn piglets. *Brain Res Mol Brain Res* 2001; **88**: 94–102.

37. Castro J, Ruminot I, Porras OH, *et al.* ATP steal between cation pumps: a mechanism linking Na^+ influx to the onset or necrotic Ca^{2+} overload. *Cell Death Diff* 2006; **13**: 1675–85.

38. Proskuryakov SY, Konoplyannikov AG, Gabai VL. Necrosis: a specific form of programmed cell death. *Exp Cell Res* 2003; **283**: 1–16.

39. Ha HC, Snyder SH. Poly(ADP-ribose) polymerase-1 in the nervous system. *Neurobiol Dis* 2000; **7**: 225–39.

40. Crompton M. The mitochondrial permeability transition pore and its role in cell death. *Biochem J* 1999; **341**: 233–49.

41. van Gurp M, Festjens N, van Loo G, *et al.* Mitochondrial intermembrane proteins in cell death. *Biochem Biophys Res Comm* 2003; **304**: 487–97.

42. Crompton M, Virji S, Ward JM. Cyclophilin-D binds strongly to complexes of the voltage-dependent anion channel and the adenine nucleotide translocase to form the permeability transition pore. *Eur J Biochem* 1998; **258**: 729–35.

43. Baines CP, Kaiser RA, Purcell NH, *et al.* Loss of cyclophilin D reveals a critical role for mitochondrial permeability transition in cell death. *Nature* 2005; **434**: 658–62.

44. Nakagawa T, Shimizu S, Watanabe T, *et al.* Cyclophilin D-dependent mitochondrial transition regulates some necrotic but not apoptotic cell death. *Nature* 2005; **434**: 652–8.

45. Vande Velde C, Cizeau J, Dubik D, *et al.* BNIP3 and genetic control of necrosis-like cell death through the mitochondrial

permeability transition pore. *Mol Cell Biol* 2000; **20**: 5454–68.

46. Tata JR. Requirement for RNA and protein synthesis for induced regression of tadpole tail in organ culture. *Dev Biol* 1966; **13**: 77–94.

47. Schwartz LM, Smith SW, Jones MEE, *et al.* Do all programmed cell deaths occur via apoptosis? *Proc Natl Acad Sci USA* 1993; **90**: 980–4.

48. Amin F, Bowen ID, Szegedi Z, *et al.* Apoptotic and non-apoptotic modes of programmed cell death in MCF-7 human breast carcinoma cells. *Cell Biol Intl* 2000; **24**: 253–60.

49. Jacobson M. *Developmental Neurobiology.* New York, NY: Plenum Press, 1991.

50. Glücksmann A. Cell deaths in normal vertebrate ontogeny. *Biol Rev* 1951; **26**: 59–86.

51. Lockshin RA, Williams CM. Programmed cell death: II. Endocrine potentiation of the breakdown of the intersegmental muscles of silkmoths. *J Insect Physiol* 1964; **10**: 643–9.

52. Saunders JW. Death in embryonic systems. *Science* 1966; **54**: 604–12.

53. Clarke PGH. Developmental cell death: morphological diversity and multiple mechanisms. *Anat Embryol* 1990; **181**: 195–213.

54. Bursch W, Paffe S, Putz B, *et al.* Determination of the length of the histological stages of apoptosis in normal liver and in altered hepatic foci of rats. *Carcinogenesis* 1990; **11**: 847–53.

55. Wyllie AH, Kerr JFR, Currie AR. Cell death: the significance of apoptosis. *Int Rev Cytol* 1980; **68**: 251–306.

56. Nagata S. Fas ligand-induced apoptosis. *Annu Rev Genet* 1999; **33**: 29–55.

57. Kerr JFR, Wyllie AH, Currie AR. Apoptosis: a basic biological phenomenon with wide-ranging implications in tissue kinetics. *Br J Cancer* 1972; **26**: 239–57.

58. Lockshin RA, Zakeri Z. Programmed cell death and apoptosis: origins of the theory. *Nat Rev Mol Cell Biol* 2001; **2**: 545–50.

59. Wyllie AH. Glucocorticoid-induced thymocyte apoptosis is associated with enodgenous endonuclease activation. *Nature* 1980; **284**: 555–6.

60. Liu X, Zou H, Slaughter C, *et al.* DFF, a heterodimeric protein that functions downstream of caspase-3 to trigger DNA fragmentation during apoptosis. *Cell* 1997; **89**: 175–84.

61. Sakahira H, Enari M, Ohsawa Y, *et al.* Apoptotic nuclear morphological change without DNA fragmentation. *Curr Biol* 1999; **9**: 543–6.

62. Pilar G, Landmesser L. Ultrastructural differences during embryonic cell death in normal and peripherally deprived ciliary ganglia. *J Cell Biol* 1976; **68**: 339–56.

63. Lockshin RA, Zakeri A. Programmed cell death: early changes in metamorphosing cells. *Biochem Cell Biol* 1994; **72**: 589–96.

64. Schweichel JU, Merker HJ. The morphology of various types of cell death in prenatal tissues. *Teratology* 1973; **7**: 253–66.

65. Xue LZ, Fletcher GC, Tolkovsky AM. Autophagy is activated by apoptotic signalling in sympathetic neurons: an alternative mechanism of death execution. *Mol Cell Neurosci* 1999; **14**: 180–98.

66. Yue Z, Horton A, Bravin M, *et al.* A novel protein complex linking the δ 2 glutamate receptor and autophagy: implications for neurodegeneration in Lurcher mice. *Neuron* 2002; **35**: 921–33.

67. Koike M, Shibata M, Tadakoshi M, *et al.* Inhibition of autophagy prevents hippocampal pyramidal neuron death after hypoxic–ischemic injury. *Am J Pathol* 2008; **172**: 454–69.

68. Mizushima N, Ohsumi Y, Yoshimori T. Autophagosome formation in mammalian cells. *Cell Struct Funct* 2002; **27**: 421–9.

69. Bursch W. The autophagosomal–lysosomal compartment in programmed cell death. *Cell Death Diff* 2001; **8**: 569–81.

70. Inbal B, Bialik S, Sabanay I, *et al.* DAP kinase and DRP-1 mediate membrane blebbing and the formation of autophagic vesicles during programmed cell death. *J Cell Biol* 2002; **157**: 455–68.

71. Liang XH, Kleeman LK, Jiang HH, *et al.* Protection against fatal sindbis virus encephalitis by beclin, a novel Bcl-2-interacting protein. *J Virol* 1998; **72**: 8586–96.

72. Ogier-Denis E, Codogno P. Autophagy: a barrier or an adaptive response to cancer. *Biochim Biophys Acta* 2003; **1603**: 113–28.

73. Ameisen JC. On the origin, evolution, and nature of programmed cell death: a timeline of four billion years. *Cell Death Diff* 2002; **9**: 367–93.

74. Metzstein MM, Stanfield, Horvitz NR. Genetics of programmed cell death in *C. elegans*: past, present and future. *Trends Genet* 1998; **14**: 410–16.

75. Cory S, Adams JM. The Bcl2 family: regulators of the cellular life-or-death switch. *Nat Rev Cancer* 2002; **2**: 647–56.

76. Wolf BB, Green DR. Suicidal tendencies: apoptotic cell death by caspase family proteinases. *J Biol Chem* 1999; **274**: 20049–52.

77. Levrero M, De Laurenzi V, Costanzo A, *et al.* The p53/p63/p73 family of transcription factors: overlapping and distinct functions. *J Cell Sci* 2000; **113**: 1661–70.

78. Hegde R, Srinivasula SM, Zhang Z, *et al.* Identification of Omi/HtrA2 as a mitochondrial apoptotic serine protease that disrupts inhibitor of apoptosis protein-caspase interaction. *J Biol Chem* 2002; **277**: 432–8.

79. Li P, Nijhawan D, Budihardjo I, *et al.* Cytochrome c and dATP-dependent formation of Apaf-1/caspase-9 complex initiates an apoptotic protease cascade. *Cell* 1997; **91**: 479–89.

80. Liu X, Kim CN, Yang J, *et al.* Induction of apoptotic program in cell-free extracts: Requirement for dATP and cytochrome c. *Cell* 1996; **86**: 147–57.

81. Klein JA, Longo-Guess CM, Rossmann MP, *et al.* The harlequin mouse mutation downregulates apoptosis-inducing factor. *Nature* 2002; **419**: 367–74.

82. van Bekkum DW. The effect of x-rays on phosphorylations *in vivo. Biochim Biophys Acta* 1957; **25**: 487–92.

83. Scorrano L, Oakes SA, Opferman TJ, *et al.* Bax and Bak regulation of endoplasmic reticulum Ca^{2+}: a control point for apoptosis. *Science* 2003; **300**: 135–9.

84. Muchmore SW, Sattler M, Liang H, *et al.* X-ray and NMR structure of human Bcl-xL, an inhibitor of programmed cell death. *Nature* 1999; **381**: 335–41.

85. Martin LJ, Price AC, McClendon KB. Early events of target deprivation/axotomy-induced neuronal apoptosis *in vivo*: oxidative stress, DNA damage, p53 phosphorylation and subcellular redistribution of death proteins. *J Neurochem* 2003; **85**: 234–47.

86. Wolter KG, Hsu YT, Smith CL, *et al.* Movement of Bax from the cytosol to mitochondria during apoptosis. *J Cell Biol* 1997; **139**: 1281–92.

87. Nechushtan A, Smith CL, Lamensdorf I, et al. Bax and Bak coalesce into novel mitochondria-associated clusters during apoptosis. *J Cell Biol* 2001; **153**: 1265–76.

88. Antonsson B, Conti F, Ciavatta A, et al. Inhibition of Bax channel-forming activity by bcl-2. *Science* 1997; **277**: 370–2.

89. Shimizu S, Ide T, Yanagida T, et al. Electrophysiological study of a novel large pore formed by Bax and the voltage-dependent anion channel that is permeable to cytochrome c. *J Biol Chem* 2000; **275**: 12321–5.

90. Kluck RM, Bossy-Wetzel E, Green DR, et al. The release of cytochrome c from mitochondria: a primary site for bcl-2 regulation of apoptosis. *Science* 1997; **275**: 1132–6.

91. Yang J, Liu X, Bhalla K, et al. Prevention of apoptosis by bcl-2: release of cytochrome c from mitochondria blocked. *Science* 1997; **275**: 1129–32.

92. Vander Heiden MG, Chandel NS, Williamson EK, et al. Bcl-x_L regulates the membrane potential and volume homeostasis of mitochondria. *Cell* 1997; **91**: 627–37.

93. Hu Y, Benedict MA, Wu D, et al. Bcl-x_L interacts with Apaf-1 and inhibits Apaf-1-dependent caspase-9 activation. *Proc Natl Acad Sci USA* 1998; **95**: 4386–91.

94. Song Q, Kuang Y, Dixit VM, et al. Boo, a negative regulator of cell death, interacts with Apaf-1. *EMBO J* 1999; **18**: 167–78.

95. Wei MC, Zong WX, Cheng EHY. Proapoptotic Bax and Bak: a requisite gateway to mitochondrial dysfunction and death. *Science* 2001; **292**: 727–30.

96. Letai A, Bassik MC, Walensky LD. Distinct BH3 domains either sensitize or activate mitochondrial apoptosis, serving as prototype cancer therapeutics. *Cancer Cell* 2001; **2**: 183–92.

97. Puka-Sundvall M, Gajkowska B, Cholewinski M, et al. Subcellular distribution of calcium and ultrastructural changes after cerebral hypoxia–ischemia in immature rats. *Dev Brain Res* 2000; **125**: 31–41.

98. Lithgow T, van Driel R, Bertram JF, et al. The protein product of the oncogene bcl-2 is a component of the nuclear envelope, the endoplasmic reticulum, and the outer mitochondrial membrane. *Cell Growth Differ* 1994; **5**: 411–17.

99. Murakami Y, Aizu-Yokota E, Sonoda Y, et al. Suppression of endoplasmic stress-induced caspase activation and cell death by overexpression of Bcl-xL or Bcl-2. *J Biochem* 2007; **141**: 401–10.

100. Zong WX, Li C, Hatzivassiliou G, et al. Bax and Bak can localize to the endoplasmic reticulum to initiate apoptosis. *J Cell Biol* 2003; **162**: 59–69.

101. Haldar S, Jena N, Croce CM. Inactivation of Bcl-2 by phosphorylation. *Proc Natl Acad Sci USA* 1995; **92**: 4507–11.

102. Hallin U, Kondo E, Ozaki Y, et al. Bcl-2 phosphorylation in the BH4 domain precedes caspase-3 activation and cell death after neonatal cerebral hypoxic–ischemic injury. *Neurobiol Dis* 2006; **21**: 478–86.

103. Wang HG, Rapp UR, Reed JC. Bcl-2 targets the protein kinase raf-1 to mitochondria. *Cell* 1996; **87**: 629–38.

104. Datta SR, Dudek H, Tao X. Akt phosphorylation of Bad couples survival signals to the cell-intrinsic death machinery. *Cell* 1997; **91**: 231–41.

105. del Peso L, Gonzalez-Garcia M, Page C, et al. Interleukin-3-induced phosphorylation of Bad through the protein kinase Akt. *Science* 1997; **278**: 687–9.

106. Cardone MH, Roy N, Stennicke HR. Regulation of cell death protease caspase-9 by phosphorylation. *Science* 1998; **282**: 1318–21.

107. Zha J, Harada H, Yang E, et al. Serine phosphorylation of death agonist Bad in response to survival factor results in binding to 14–3–3 not Bcl-x_L. *Cell* 1996; **87**: 619–28.

108. Wang H-G, Pathan N, Ethell IM, et al. Ca^{2+}-induced apoptosis through calcineurin dephosphorylation of Bad. *Science* 1999; **284**: 339–43.

109. Yang E, Zha J, Jockel J. Bad, a heterodimeric partner for Bcl-x_L and Bcl-2, displaces Bax and promotes cell death. *Cell* 1995; **80**: 285–91.

110. Danial NN, Gramm CF, Scorrano L. Bad and glucokinase reside in a mitochondrial complex that integrates glycolysis and apoptosis. *Nature* 2003; **424**: 952–6.

111. Stennicke HR, Deveraux QL, Humke EW. Caspase-9 can be activated without proteolytic processing. *J Biol Chem* 1999; **274**: 8359–62.

112. Schwartz LM, Milligan CE. Cold thoughts of death: the role of ICE proteases in neuronal cell death. *Trends Neurosci* 1996; **19**: 555–62.

113. Zou H, Li Y, Liu X, et al. An Apaf-1-cytochrome c multimeric complex is a functional apoptosome that activates procaspase-9. *J Biol Chem* 1999; **274**: 11549–56.

114. Li H, Zhu H, Xu CJ, et al. Cleavage of Bid by caspase 8 mediates the mitochondrial damage in the Fas pathway of apoptosis. *Cell* 1989; **94**: 491–501.

115. Robertson JD, Enoksson M, Suomela M, et al. Caspase-2 acts upstream of mitochondria to promote cytochrome c release during etoposide-induced apoptosis. *J Biol Chem* 2002; **277**: 29803–9.

116. Beresford PJ, Zhang D, Oh DY, et al. Granzyme A activates an endoplasmic reticulum-associated caspase-independent nuclease to induce single-stranded DNA nicks. *J Biol Chem* 2001; **76**: 43285–93.

117. Fan Z, Beresford PJ, Oh DY, et al. Tumor suppressor NM23-H1 is a granzyme A-activated DNase during TL-mediated apoptosis, and the nucleosome assembly protein SET is its inhibitor. *Cell* 2003; **112**: 659–72.

118. LaCasse EC, Baird S, Korneluk RG, et al. The inhibitors of apoptosis (IAPs) and their emerging role in cancer. *Oncogene* 1998; **17**: 3247–59.

119. Holcik M. The IAP proteins. *Trends Genet* 2002; **18**: 537–8.

120. Deveraux QL, Roy N, Stennicke HR, et al. IAPs block apoptotic events induced by caspase-8 and cytochrome c by direct inhibition of distinct caspases. *EMBO J* 1998; **17**: 2215–23.

121. Hao Y, Sekine K, Kawabata A, et al. Apollon ubiquitinates SMAC and caspase-9 and has essential cytoprotective function. *Nat Cell Biol* 2004; **6**: 849–60.

122. Jiang Y, de Bruin A, Caldas H, et al. Essential role for survivin in early brain development. *J Neurosci* 2005; **25**: 6962–70.

123. Xu DG, Korneluk RG, Tamai K, et al. Distribution of neuronal apoptosis inhibitory protein-like immunoreactivity in the rat central nervous system. *J Comp Neurol* 1997; **382**: 247–59.

124. Martin LJ, Liu Z, Chen K, et al. Motor neuron degeneration in amyotrophic lateral sclerosis mutant superoxide dismutase-1 transgenic mice: mechanisms of mitochondriopathy and cell death. *J Comp Neurol* 2007; **500**: 20–46.

125. Roy N, Mahadevan MS, McLean M, *et al.* The gene for neuronal apoptosis inhibitory protein is partially deleted in individuals with spinal muscular atrophy. *Cell* 1995; **80**: 167–78.

126. Du C, Fang M, Li Y, *et al.* Smac, a mitochondrial protein that promotes cytochrome c-dependent caspase activation by eliminating IAP inhibition. *Cell* 2000; **102**: 33–42.

127. Verhagen AM, Ekert PG, Pakusch M, *et al.* Identification of DIABLO, a mammalian protein that promotes apoptosis by binding to and antagonizing IAP proteins. *Cell* 2000; **102**: 43–53.

128. Suzuki Y, Takahashi-Niki K, Akagi T, *et al.* Mitochondrial protease Omi/ HtrA2 enhances caspase activation through multiple pathways. *Cell Death Diff* 2004; **11**: 208–16.

129. Susin SA, Lorenzo HK, Zamzami N, *et al.* Molecular characterization of mitochondrial apoptosis-inducing factor. *Nature* 1999; **397**: 441–6.

130. Mate MJ, Ortiz-Lombardia M, Boitel, B, *et al.* The crystal structure of the mouse apoptosis-inducing factor AIF. *Nat Struct Biol* 2002; **9**: 442–6.

131. Desagher S, Osen-Sand A, Nichols A, *et al.* Bid-induced conformational change of bax is responsible for mitochondrial cytochrome c release during apoptosis. *J Cell Biol* 1999; **144**: 891–901.

132. Troy CM, Friedman JE, Friedman WJ. Mechanisms of p75-mediated death of hippocampal neurons: role of caspases. *J Biol Chem* 2002; **277**: 34295–302.

133. Giaccia AJ, Kastan MB. The complexity of p53 modulation: emerging patterns from divergent signals. *Genes Develop* 1998; **12**: 2973–83.

134. Chang YC, Lee YS, Tejima T, *et al.* Mdm-2 and bax, downstream mediators of the p53 response, are degraded by the ubiquitin-proteasome pathway. *Cell Growth Diff* 1998; **9**: 79–84.

135. Maki CG, Huibregtse JM, Howley PM. *In vivo* ubiquitination and proteasome-mediated degradation of p53. *Cancer Res* 1996; **56**: 2649–54.

136. Shieh SY, Ikeda M, Taya Y, *et al.* DNA damage-induced phosphorylation of p53 alleviates inhibition by MDM2. *Cell* 1997; **91**: 325–34.

137. Villunger A, Michalak EM, Coultas L, *et al.* p53- and drug-induced apoptotic responses mediated by BH3-only proteins Puma and Noxa. *Science* 2003; **302**: 1036–8.

138. Aloyz RS, Bamji SX, Pozniak CD, *et al.* p53 is essential for developmental neuron death regulated by the TrkA and p75 neurotrophin receptors. *J Cell Biol* 1998; **143**: 1691–703.

139. Martin LJ, Kaiser A, Yu JW, *et al.* Injury-induced apoptosis of neurons in adult brain is mediated by p53-dependent and p53-independent pathways and requires Bax. *J Comp Neurol* 2001; **433**: 299–311.

140. Martin LJ, Liu Z. Injury-induced spinal motor neuron apoptosis is preceded by DNA single-strand breaks and is p53- and Bax-dependent. *J Neurobiol* 2002; **50**: 181–97.

141. Pozniak CD, Radinovic S, Yang A, *et al.* An anti-apoptotic role for the p53 family member, p73, during developmental neuron death. *Science* 2000; **289**: 304–6.

142. Lucas DR, Newhouse JP. The toxic effect of sodium L-glutamate on the inner layers of the retina. *Arch Ophthal* 1957; **58**: 193–201.

143. Olney JW. Glutamate-induced neuronal necrosis in the infant mouse hypothalamus: an electron microscopic study. *J Neuropathol Exp Neurol* 1971; **30**: 75–90.

144. Choi DW. Excitotoxic cell death. *J Neurobiol* 1992; **23**: 1261–76.

145. Martin LJ, Sieber FE, Traystman RJ. Apoptosis and necrosis occur in separate neuronal populations in hippocampus and cerebellum after ischemia and are associated with alterations in metabotropic glutamate receptor signaling pathways. *J Cereb Blood Flow Metab* 2000; **20**: 153–67.

146. Lipton SA, Rosenberg PA. Excitatory amino acids as a final common pathway for neurologic disorders. *N Engl J Med* 1994; **330**: 613–22.

147. Gwag BJ, Koh JY, DeMaro JA, *et al.* Slowly triggered excitotoxicity occurs by necrosis in cortical cultures. *Neuroscience* 1997; **77**: 393–401.

148. Kure S, Tominaga T, Yoshimoto T, *et al.* Glutamate triggers internucleosomal DNA cleavage in neuronal cells. *Biochem Biophys Res Commun* 1991; **179**: 39–45.

149. Ankarcrona M, Dypbukt JM, Bonfoco E, *et al.* Glutamate-induced neuronal death: a succession of necrosis or apoptosis depending on mitochondrial function. *Neuron* 1995; **15**: 961–73.

150. Simonian NA, Getz RL, Leveque JC, *et al.* Kainate induces apoptosis in neurons. *Neuroscience* 1996; **74**: 675–83.

151. Dessi F, Charriaut-Marlangue C, Khrestchatisky M, *et al.* Glutamate-induced neuronal death is not a programmed cell death in cerebellar culture. *J Neurochem* 1993; **60**: 1953–5.

152. Xiang H, Kinoshita Y, Knudson CM, *et al.* Bax involvement in p53-mediated neuronal cell death. *J Neurosci* 1998; **18**: 1363–73.

153. Miller TM, Moulder KL, Knudson CM, *et al.* Bax deletion further orders the cell death pathway in cerebellar granule cells and suggests a caspase-independent pathway to cell death. *J Cell Biol* 1997; **139**: 205–17.

154. Dargusch R, Piasecki D, Tan S, *et al.* The role of Bax in glutamate-induced nerve cell death. *J Neurochem* 2001; **76**: 295–301.

155. Johnson MD, Kinoshita Y, Xiang H, *et al.* Contribution of p53-dependent caspase activation to neuronal cell death declines with neuronal maturation. *J Neurosci* 1999; **19**: 2996–3006.

156. Tenneti L, Lipton SA. Involvement of activated caspase-3-like proteases in N-methyl-D-aspartate-induced apoptosis in cerebrocortical neurons. *J Neurochem* 2001; **74**: 134–42.

157. Simons M, Beinroth S, Gleichmann M, *et al.* Adenovirus-mediated gene transfer of inhibitors of apoptosis proteins delays apoptosis in cerebellar granule neurons. *J Neurochem* 1999; **72**: 292–301.

158. van Lookeren Campagne M, Lucassen PJ, Vermeulen JP, *et al.* NMDA and kainate induced internucleosomal DNA cleavage associated with both apoptotic and necrotic cell death in the neonatal rat brain. *Eur J Neurosci* 1995; **7**: 1627–40.

159. Holcik M, Thompson CS, Yaraghi Z, *et al.* The hippocampal neurons of neuronal apoptosis inhibitory protein 1 (NAIP1)-deleted mice display increased vulnerability to kainic acid-induced injury. *Proc Natl Acad Sci USA* 1999; **97**: 2286–90.

160. Schreiber SS, Tocco G, Najm I, *et al.* Cycloheximide prevents kainate-induced neuronal death and c-fos expression in adult rat brain. *J Mol Neurosci* 1993; **4**: 149–59.

161. Leppin C, Finiels-Marlier F, Crawley JN, *et al.* Failure of a protein synthesis inhibitor to modify glutamate receptor-mediated neurotoxicity *in vivo. Brain Res* 1992; **581**: 168–70.

162. Lok J, Martin LJ. Rapid subcellular redistribution of Bax precedes caspase-3 and endonuclease activation during excitotoxic neuronal apoptosis in rat brain. *J Neurotrauma* 2002; **19**: 815–28.

163. Martin LJ. Neuronal cell death in nervous system development, disease, and injury. *Int J Mol Med* 2001; **7**: 455–78.

164. Natale JE, Cheng Y, Martin LJ. Thalamic neuron apoptosis emerges rapidly after cortical damage in immature mice. *Neuroscience* 2002; **112**: 665–76.

165. Fujikawa DG. Confusion between neuronal apoptosis and activation of programmed cell death mechanisms in acute necrotic insults. *Trends Neurosci* 2000; **23**: 410–11.

166. Ishimaru MJ, Ikonomidou C, Tenkova TI, *et al.* Distinguishing excitotoxic from apoptotic neurodegeneration in the developing rat brain. *J Comp Neurol* 1999; **408**: 461–76.

167. Sloviter RS. Apoptosis: a guide for the perplexed. *Trends Pharmacol Sci* 2002; **23**: 19–24.

168. Northington FJ, Graham EM, Martin LJ. Apoptosis in perinatal hypoxic-ischemic brain injury: how important is it and should it be inhibited? *Brain Res Rev* 2005; **50**: 244–57.

169. Baille V, Clarke PGH, Brocher G, *et al.* Soman-induced convulsions: the neuropathology revisited. *Toxicology* 2005; **215**: 1–24.

170. Zhu C, Wang X, Xu F, *et al.* The influence of age on apoptotic and other mechanisms of cell death after cerebral hypoxia-ischemia. *Cell Death Diff* 2005; **12**: 162–76.

171. Sheldon RA, Hall JJ, Noble LJ, *et al.* Delayed cell death in neonatal mouse hippocampus from hypoxia-ischemia is neither apoptotic nor necrotic. *Neurosci Lett* 2001; **304**: 165–8.

172. Wei L, Ying D-J, Cui L, *et al.* Necrosis, apoptosis, and hybrid death in the cortex and thalamus after barrel cortex ischemia in rats. *Brain Res* 2004; **1022**: 54–61.

173. Bruijn LI. Amyotrophic lateral sclerosis: from disease mechanisms to therapies. *BioTechniques* 2002; **32**: 1112–21.

174. Formigli L, Papucci L, Tani A, *et al.* Aponecrosis: morphological and biochemical exploration of a syncretic process of cell death sharing apoptosis and necrosis. *J Cell Physiol* 2000; **182**: 41–9.

175. Ohmura A, Nakajima W, Ishida A, *et al.* Prolonged hypothermia protects neonatal rat brain against hypoxic-ischemia by reducing both apoptosis and necrosis. *Brain Dev* 2005; **27**: 517–26.

176. Takizawa Y, Takashima S, Itoh M. A histopathological study of premature and mature infants with pontosubicular neuron necrosis: neuronal cell death in perinatal brain damage. *Brain Res* 2006; **1095**: 2000–6.

177. Taniguchi H, Mohri I, Okabe-Arahori H, *et al.* Prostaglandin D2 protects neonatal mouse brain from hypoxic ischemic injury. *J Neurosci* 2007; **27**: 4303–12.

178. Squier W, Cowan FM. The value of autopsy in determining the cause of failure to respond to resuscitation at birth. *Semin Neonatol* 2004; **9**: 331–45.

179. Barkovich AJ, Westmark KD, Bedi HS, *et al.* Proton spectroscopy and diffusion imaging on the first day of life after perinatal asphyxia: preliminary report. *Am J Neuroradiol* 2001; **22**: 1786–94.

180. Meng SZ, Ohyu J, Takashima S. Changes in AMPA glutamate and dopamine D_2 receptors in hypoxic-ischemic basal ganglia necrosis. *Pediatr Neurol* 1997; **17**: 139–43.

181. Cheng Y, Deshmukh M, D'Costa A, *et al.* Caspase inhibitor affords neuroprotection with delayed adminstration in a rat model of neonatal hypoxic-ischemic brain injury. *J Clin Invest* 1998; **101**: 1992–9.

182. Rice JE, Vannucci RC, Brierley JB. The influence of immaturity on hypoxic-ischemic brain damage in the rat. *Ann Neurol* 1981; **9**: 131–41.

183. Clancy B, Darlington RB, Finlay BL. Translating developmental time across mammalian species. *Neuroscience* 2001; **105**: 7–17.

184. Romijn HJ, Hofman MA, Gramsbergen A. At what age is the developing cerebral cortex of the rat comparable to that of the full-term newborn human baby? *Early Hum Dev* 1991; **26**: 61–7.

185. Ginsberg MD, Busto R. Rodent models of cerebral ischemia. *Stroke* 1989; **20**: 1627–42.

186. Yager JY. Animal models of hypoxic-ischemic brain damage in the newborn. *Semin Pediatr Neurol* 2001; **11**: 31–46.

187. Dobbing J, Sands J. Comparative aspects of the brain growth spurt. *Early Hum Dev* 1979; **3**: 79–83.

188. Roland EH, Poskitt K, Rodriguez E, *et al.* Perinatal hypoxic-ischemic thalamic injury: clinical features and neuroimaging. *Ann Neurol* 1998; **44**: 161–6.

189. Batista CE, Chugani HT, Juhasz C, *et al.* Transient hypermetabolism of the basal ganglia following perinatal hypoxia. *Pediatr Neurol* 2007; **36**: 330–3.

190. Agnew DM, Koehler RC, Guerguerian AM, *et al.* Hypothermia for 24 hours after asphyxic cardiac arrest in piglets provides striatal neuroprotection that is sustained 10 days after rewarming. *Pediatr Res* 2003; **54**: 1–10.

191. Thoresen M, Satas S, Loberg EM, *et al.* Twenty-four hours of mild hypothermia in unsedated newborn pigs starting after a severe global hypoxic-ischemic insult is not neuroprotective. *Pediatr Res* 2001; **50**: 405–11.

192. Eicher DJ, Wagner CL, Katikaneni LP, *et al.* Moderate hypothermia in neonatal encephalopathy: efficacy outcomes. *Pediatr Neurol* 2005; **32**: 11–17.

193. Blomgren K, Zhu C, Wang X, *et al.* Synergistic activation of caspase-3 by m-calpain after neonatal hypoxia-ischemia: a mechanism of "pathological apoptosis"? *J Biol Chem* 2001; **276**: 10191–8.

194. Hu BR, Liu CL, Ouyang Y, *et al.* Involvement of caspase-3 in cell death after hypoxia-ischemia declines during brain maturation. *J Cereb Blood Flow Metab* 2000; **20**: 1294–300.

195. Lesuisse C, Martin LJ. Immature and mature cortical neurons engage different apoptotic mechanisms involving caspase-3 and the mitogen-activated protein kinase pathway. *J Cereb Blood Flow Metab* 2002; **22**: 935–50.

196. Feng Y, LeBlanc MH. Treatment of hypoxic-ischemic brain injury in newborn rats with TPCK 3 h after hypoxia decreases caspase-9 activation and improves neuropathologic outcome. *Dev Neurosci* 2003; **25**: 34–40.

197. Feng Y, Fratkin JD, LeBlanc MH. Inhibiting caspase-8 after injury reduces hypoxic-ischemic brain injury in the newborn rat. *Eur J Pharmacol* 2003; **481**: 169–73.

198. Feng Y, Fratkin JD, LeBlanc MH. Inhibiting caspase-9 after injury reduces hypoxic ischemic neuronal injury in the cortex in the newborn rat. *Neurosci Lett* 2003; **344**: 201–4.

199. Han BH, Xu D, Choi J, *et al.* Selective, reversible caspase-3 inhibitor is neuroprotective and reveals distinct pathways of cell death after neonatal hypoxic–ischemic brain injury. *J Biol Chem* 2002; **277**: 30128–36.

200. Knoblach SM, Alroy DA, Nikolaeva M, *et al.* Caspase inhibitor z-DEVD-fmk attenuates calpain and necrotic cell death in vitro and after traumatic brain injury. *J Cereb Blood Flow Metab* 2004; **24**: 1119–32.

201. Rozman-Pungercar J, Kopitar-Jerala N, Bogyo M, *et al.* Inhibition of papain-like cysteine proteases and legumain by caspase-specific inhibitors: when reaction mechanism is more important than specificity. *Cell Death Differ* 2003; **10**: 881–8.

202. Ostwald K, Hagberg H, Andine P, *et al.* Upregulation of calpain activity in neonatal rat brain after hypoxic-ischemia. *Brain Res* 1993; **630**: 289–94.

203. Kawamura M, Nakajima W, Ishida A, *et al.* Calpain inhibitor MDL 28170 protects hypoxic–ischemic brain injury in neonatal rats by inhibition of both apoptosis and necrosis. *Brain Res* 2005; **1037**: 59–69.

204. Han Y, Giroux A, Colucci J, *et al.* Novel pyrazinone mono-amides as potent and reversible caspase-3 inhibitors. *Bioorg Med Chem Lett* 2005; **15**: 1173–80.

205. Gibson ME, Han BH, Choi J, *et al.* Bax contributes to apoptotic-like death following neonatal hypoxia-ischemia: evidence for distinct apoptosis pathways. *Mol Med* 2001; **7**: 644–55.

206. Sun W, Oppenheim RW. Response of motoneurons to neonatal sciatic nerve axotomy in Bax-knockout mice. *Mol Cell Neurosci* 2003; **24**: 875–86.

207. Ness JM, Harvey CA, Strasser A, *et al.* Selective involvement of BH3-only Bcl-2 family members Bim and Bad in neonatal hypoxia-ischemia. *Brain Res* 2006; **1099**: 150–9.

208. Zhu C, Xu F, Fukuda A, *et al.* X chromosome-linked inhibitor of apoptosis protein reduces oxidative stress after cerebral irradiation or hypoxia-ischemia through up-regulation of mitochondrial antioxidants. *Eur J Neurosci* 2007; **26**: 3402–10.

209. Zhu C, Wang X, Huang Z, *et al.* Apoptosis-inducing factor is a major contributor to neuronal loss induced by neonatal cerebral hypoxia–ischemia. *Cell Death Diff* 2007; **14**: 775–84.

210. Northington FJ, Ferriero DM, Flock DL, *et al.* Delayed neurodegeneration in neonatal rat thalamus after hypoxia–ischemia is apoptosis. *J Neurosci* 2001; **21**: 1931–8.

211. Northington FJ, Ferriero DM, Martin LJ. Neurodegeneration in the thalamus following neonatal hypoxia–ischemia is programmed cell death. *Dev Neurosci* 2001; **23**: 186–91.

212. Al-Abdulla NA, Martin LJ. Apoptosis of retrogradely degenerating neurons occurs in association with the accumulation of perikaryal mitochondria and oxidative damage to the nucleus. *Am J Pathol* 1998; **153**: 447–56.

213. Al-Abdulla NA, Portera-Cailliau C, Martin LJ. Occipital cortex ablation in adult rat causes retrograde neuronal death in the lateral geniculate nucleus that resembles apoptosis. *Neuroscience* 1998; **86**: 191–209.

214. Johnston MV. Selective vulnerability in the neonatal brain. *Ann Neurol* 1998; **44**: 155–6.

215. Brambrink AM, Martin LJ, Hanley DF, *et al.* Effects of the AMPA receptor antagonist NBQX on the outcome of newborn pigs after asphyxic cardiac arrest. *J Cereb Blood Flow Metab* 1999; **19**: 927–38.

216. Yang ZJ, Torbey M, Li Z, *et al.* Dopamine receptor modulation of hypoxic–ischemic neuronal injury in striatum of newborn piglets. *J Cereb Blood Flow Metab* 2007; **27**: 1339–51.

217. Golden WC, Branbrink AM, Traystman RJ, *et al.* Nitration of the striatal Na,K-ATPaseα3 isoform occurs in normal brain development but is not increased during hypoxia–ischemia in newborn piglets. *Neurochem Res* 2003; **28**: 1883–9.

218. Mueller-Burke D, Koehler RC, Martin LJ. Rapid NMDA receptor phosphorylation and oxidative stress precede striatal neurodegeneration after hypoxic ischemia in newborn piglets and are attenuated with hypothermia. *Int J Dev Neurosci* 2008; **26**: 67–76.

219. Prybylowski K, Wenthold RJ. N-methyl-D-aspartate receptors: subunit assembly and trafficking to the synapse. *J Biol Chem* 2004; **279**: 9673–6.

220. Tingley WG, Ehlers MD, Kameyama K, *et al.* Characterization of protein kinase A and protein kinase C phosphorylation of the N-methyl-D-aspartate receptor NR1 subunit using phosphorylation site-specific antibodies. *J Biol Chem* 1997; **272**: 5157–66.

221. Guerguerian AM, Brambrink AM, Traystman RJ, *et al.* Altered expression and phosphorylation of N-methyl-D-aspartate receptors in piglet striatum after hypoxia-ischemia. *Brain Res Mol Brain Res* 2002; **104**: 66–80.

222. Trescher WH, Ishiwa S, Johnston MV. Brief post-hypoxic–ischemic hypothermia markedly delays neonatal brain injury. *Brain Dev* 1997; **19**: 326–38.

223. Bona, E, Hagberg H, Loberg EM, *et al.* Protective effects of moderate hypothermia after neonatal hypoxia-ischemia: short- and long-term outcome. *Pediatr Res* 1998; **43**: 738–45.

224. Ginsberg SD, Martin LJ. Ultrastructural analysis of the progression of neurodegeneration in the septum following fimbria–fornix transection. *Neuroscience* 1998; **86**; 1259–72.

225. Park KI, Teng YD, Snyder EY. The injured brain interacts reciprocally with neural stem cells supported by scaffolds to reconstitute lost tissue. *Nat Biotechnol* 2002; **20**: 1111–7.

226. Mueller D, Shamblott MJ, Fox HE, *et al.* Transplanted human embryonic germ cell-derived neural stem cells replace neurons and oligodendrocytes in the forebrain of neonatal mice with excitotoxic brain damage. *J Neurosci Res* 2005; **82**: 592–608.

227. Zheng T, Rossignol C, Leibovici A, *et al.* Transplantation of multipotent astrocytic stem cells into a rat model of neonatal hypoxic–ischemic encephalopathy. *Brain Res* 2006; **1112**: 99–105.

228. Ikeda T, Iwai M, Hayashi T, *et al.* Limited differentiation to neurons and astroglia from neural stem cells in the cortex and striatum after ischemia/hypoxia in the neonatal rat brain. *Am J Obstet Gynecol* 2005; **193**: 849–56.

229. Liu Z, Martin LJ. The olfactory bulb core is a rich source of neural progenitor and stem cells in adult rodent and human. *J Comp Neurol* 2003; **459**: 368–91.

230. Gritti A, Bonfanti L, Doetsch F, *et al.* Multipotent neural stem cells reside in the rostral extension and olfactory bulb of adult rodents. *J Neurosci* 2002; **22**: 437–45.

231. Alvarez-Buylla A, Garcia-Verdugo JM. Neurogenesis in adult subventricular zone. *J Neurosci* 2002; **22**: 629–34.

232. Martin LJ, Liu Z. Adult olfactory bulb neural precursor cell grafts provide temporary protection from motor neuron degeneration, improve motor function, and extend survival in amyotrophic lateral sclerosis mice. *J Neuropathol Exp Neurol* 2007; **66**: 1002–18.

233. McEvoy AW, Bartolucci M, Revesz T, *et al.* Intractable epilepsy and olfactory bulb hamartoma. *Stereotact Funct Neurosurg* 2002; **79**: 88–93.

234. Obeid F, Al-Mefty O. Recurrence of olfactory groove meningiomas. *Neurosurgery* 2003; **53**: 534–42.

235. Spektor S, Valarezo J, Fliss DM, *et al.* Olfactory groove meningiomas from neurosurgical and ear, nose, and throat perspectives: approaches, techniques, and outcomes. *Neurosurgery* 2005; **57**: 268–79.

Cellular and molecular biology of hypoxic–ischemic encephalopathy

Zinaida S. Vexler, Donna M. Ferriero, and Janet Shimotake

Introduction

The exact timing of hypoxic–ischemic brain injury and the preceding course of events are often unknown, but they play a crucial role in pathogenesis, regional susceptibility, and injury severity in humans [1,2], requiring different treatment approaches. The dynamic nature of the developing brain requires the use of age-appropriate models to advance our understanding of both the injurious mechanisms and the means to ameliorate injury.

Several aspects of injury to the immature brain caused by experimental hypoxia–ischemia (HI) or focal stroke [3–5] in animals have been recently reviewed, including the role of age [6–8], blood-flow regulation and energy metabolism [9], inflammation [7,10], intracellular injury mechanisms, and neuronal death, and these will not be covered in great detail here [10,11]. We will review recently emerging concepts, including the status of the neurovascular unit and blood–brain barrier, neuroinflammation, adaptive intracellular mechanisms, gender differences in the injury response, neuroprotection, and brain repair.

Energy failure and early intracellular injury

The role of disruption of cerebral blood flow and failure of mitochondrial ATP production in initiating injury after HI has been recently reviewed by Vannucci & Vannucci [12] and Perlman [13]. The role of elevated levels of extracellular glutamate, overactivation of excitatory amino acid (EAA) receptors, and calcium ($Ca^{2+}i$)-mediated intracellular injury, which in part depends on failure of ATP-dependent processes, have been recently reviewed as well [14]. The time course of injurious events is shown in Figure 3.1. Recent studies have demonstrated the importance of the link between the N-methyl-D-aspartate (NMDA) receptor, postsynaptic density (PSD)-93 and PSD-95 membrane-associated guanylate kinases (MAGUKs), and neuronal nitric oxide synthase (nNOS) in HI injury and the role of activation of Src family kinases in neuronal injury [15]. Further studies confirming that reactive oxygen species play a major role in HI injury have been

conducted in mice with manipulated CuZn-superoxide dismutase (SOD) and glutathione peroxidase (Gpx) activities [16].

Neurovascular unit and blood–brain barrier (BBB) permeability

It has become apparent that neuronal survival depends on the microenvironment and cellular interactions, leading to the concept of the "neurovascular unit." The neurovascular unit includes brain microvascular endothelium, and the BBB as a whole: glia, neurons, and extracellular matrix, along with the complexities of cell–cell communication within the brain and the crosstalk between the systemic circulation and the brain.

In adults, the BBB is disrupted after stroke, with the temporal-spatial extent dependent on both the systemic and the local inflammatory reaction [17]. Peripheral leukocytes contribute to the opening of the BBB [17], release of toxic mediators [18], and basal lamina degradation [19]. Leukocyte extravasation occurs through several discrete steps and depends on a number of integrins, adhesion molecules, and chemokine gradients in the brain [10]. Microglia, locally and systemically produced cytokines, and matrix metalloprotease activation also potentiate damage to BBB constituents [19–21].

The early postnatal BBB is not as permeable as once thought. Entrance of proteins is restricted by tight junctions early in embryonic development [22]. By birth the BBB is functional, with no fenestrations [23]. Regulation of the BBB is age-dependent but does not change linearly with brain maturation. BBB is more permeable in 21-day-old (P21) than in P1 pups following intrastriatal injections of the inflammatory cytokines IL-1β or TNF-α [24]. The mechanisms that keep the BBB relatively preserved are not well understood but may be related to the very limited transmigration of neutrophils and monocytes in the injured parenchyma during the neonatal period [25–27]. Extracellular matrix degradation and MMP-9 activation are injurious acutely after HI in P9 but so far there are no data on this process in immature rodents of other ages [28].

Neuroinflammation
Microglial cells and astrocytes

Microglial cells are the resident macrophages of the CNS, primarily responsible for maintenance of the microenvironment, production of cytokines, chemokines and growth

Fetal and Neonatal Brain Injury, 4th edition, ed. David K. Stevenson, William E. Benitz, Philip Sunshine, Susan R. Hintz, and Maurice L. Druzin. Published by Cambridge University Press. © Cambridge University Press 2009.

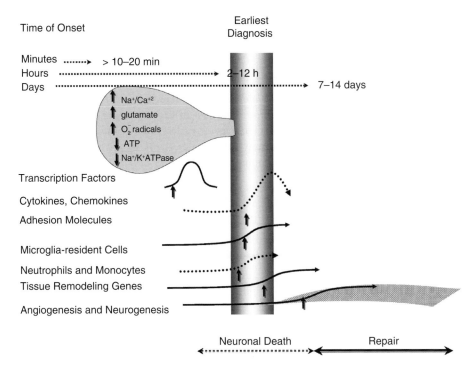

Fig. 3.1. Mechanisms of ischemia-induced injury in the neonate.

factors, and removal of debris. For a long time, activated microglial cells were viewed as uniformly injurious in acute and chronic neurodegenerative conditions [29]. They were also believed to adversely affect repair in adult stroke [30]. This view is being reconsidered, based on accumulating data regarding the ability of these cells to support neurogenesis in vitro and in vivo and minimize (rather than enhance) neurodegeneration [31,32].

Microglia, which populate the developing brain by birth, can provoke the death of neurons during the period of synaptogenesis rather than clear the debris of neurons dying by caspase-3-dependent mechanisms [33]. Microglial activation is rapid in neonates and is seen after transient focal ischemia [27,34], hypoxia–ischemia, and excitotoxic injury [26,35,36]. A broad range of anti-inflammatory drugs that target various intracellular inflammatory pathways in the microglial cells, such as minocycline [37], iminobiotin [38], chloroquine [36], and aminoguanidine [39], show varying degrees of protection against acute injury in neonates.

Astrocytes contribute to neuronal homeostasis and function, play an immune modulating role in the brain, and are an important part of the BBB [40]. As a major source of inflammatory mediators such as cytokines, chemokines, and inducible nitric oxide synthase (iNOS), activated astrocytes have the potential to harm the ischemic brain. At the same time, astrocytes may be beneficial following cerebral ischemia, as is evidenced by larger cortical infarct volumes in glial fibrillary acidic protein (GFAP)-null mice [41]. While mechanisms of astrocytic death in the immature post-ischemic brain are not well understood, at least a subpopulation of these cells is dying in a caspase-3-dependent way [42]. Increased cytochrome c release from mitochondria, DNA fragmentation,

and poly (ADP-ribose) polymerase (PARP-1) cleavage contribute to their death [43].

Other inflammatory cells

Infiltration of T and B cells following neonatal HI and focal stroke may be less profound or more transient than in adult stroke [26,42]. There is, however, increasing evidence for the injurious role of mast cells after neonatal HI and focal stroke [44,45]. Agents that inhibit histamine release and degranulation of mast cells in mast-cell-deficient neonatal mice reduce injury size [44,46]. The injurious effects of mast cells have been shown to depend on TGF-β and IL-9 [47].

Cytokines and chemokines

Cytokines are polypeptides that affect long-term developmental events such as proliferation, differentiation, and cell survival, as well as short-term events such as modulation of synaptic activity and inflammatory responses. They are expressed by cells in the immune system and also by resident brain cells, including glia and neurons. Cytokines are upregulated rapidly in the neonatal brain after HI and focal stroke. IL-1β, IL-6, and TNF-α exacerbate local inflammation by activating astrocytes and microglia and inducing a number of other cytokines and chemokines in neonatal models of HI [48] and focal ischemia [49]. Pretreatment with inflammatory Th1 cytokines IL-1β, IL-6, or TNF-α or the Th2 cytokine IL-9 prior to an excitotoxic stimulus in P5 rats significantly exacerbates injury severity and increases density of activated microglia [50,51]. The pleotrophic Th2 cytokine IL-10, in turn, can reverse injury caused by IL-1β and IL-6 if administered after HI [52]. Our study using minocycline suggested that attenuation of the elevated levels of circulating cytokines without reduction in the elevated cytokine levels in ischemic–reperfused brain provides only short-term protection [49].

Chemoattractant cytokines, chemokines, and their receptors exert a variety of physiological functions, including control of cell migration, proliferation, differentiation, and angiogenesis in normal and disease states [53]. The breakdown of inflammatory genes by functional category in a microarray analysis has shown that chemokines are the first family of molecules to increase following HI in P7 rats [54]. The injurious role of CC-chemokines MCP-1 and MIP-1α, and complement activation, has been demonstrated after excitotoxic and HI injury [55–57].

Mechanisms of ischemic neuronal death and gender differences

Several concepts have emerged regarding the complexity of the apoptotic machinery. First, expression of many of the key components of apoptosis declines with age in normal brain [58–60]. Therefore it is not surprising that apoptotic pathways are more readily activated in immature brain after injury, resulting in increases in caspase-3-dependent apoptosis up to 100-fold after HI [59,60] and focal ischemia–reperfusion [61]. While pharmacological inhibition of caspase-3 protects the neonatal brain against HI [59,62], a lack of caspase-3 exacerbates injury via amplification of necrosis and caspase-3-independent injury pathways [63], suggesting that complete abolition of caspase-3 activity can be injurious rather than purely beneficial. Second, data on the central role of mitochondria in apoptosis after HI and the ability to attenuate mitochondrial response by counteracting oxidative stress via modulation of expression of proteins within the apoptotic pathways continue to accumulate [64,65]. Finally, failure to complete apoptosis may result in the "continuum" or hybrid cell death, an intermediate form of cell death that exhibits features of both necrosis and apoptosis [11,66]. The insufficient clearance of apoptotic cells also enhances necrosis and inflammation, exacerbating injury [14,63,67].

Many CNS diseases display sexual dimorphism, specifically affecting one gender. Cerebral palsy (CP) and related developmental disorders are more common in males than in females [68], but the reasons for this disparity are uncertain. Sex hormones can provide protection against ischemic injury, but the neonatal brain may not be as influenced by these hormones as the adult brain. Recent experimental data demonstrate gender predominance in the mechanisms of apoptotic death and the ability of antiapoptotic drugs to protect immature brain from ischemia [69–71]. Inhibition or lack of the gene for PARP-1 protected male but not female mouse pups from HI [69]. The existence of intrinsic gender-specific differences in cell-death pathways in the fetal or neonatal period seems likely.

Data are emerging that the effects of therapeutics can be gender-specific. As an example, 2-iminobiotin (2-IB), an inhibitor of iNOS, can reduce long-term brain damage (6 weeks) in female but not male P7 rats, likely through inhibition of the HI-induced increase in cytosolic cytochrome c and caspase-3 activation. Activation of apoptosis-inducing factor (AIF), observed in males only, is not affected by 2-IB [72]. Similarly, in P3 rats, neuroprotection after HI is observed only in female rats [73]. Protection is associated with reversal of HI-induced elevated HSP70 protein expression and cytochrome c release from the mitochondria in female but not male rats [72]. Therefore, gender-specific effects of therapeutics are important for the design of future clinical trials of potential neuroprotective strategies.

Adaptive response of cells to injury

In addition to injurious responses to hypoxia–ischemia, the cell also exhibits protective mechanisms. Innate responses to HI include upregulation of the hypoxia-inducible factor 1 (HIF-1) cascade and many downstream targets, including erythropoietin (EPO) and vascular endothelial growth factor (VEGF).

Hypoxia-inducible factor 1 (HIF-1)

HIF-1 is a heterodimeric transcription factor that consists of an inducible α subunit and a constitutive β subunit [74]. It is found in neurons, glia, and endothelial cells [75,76]. Under normoxic conditions, HIF-1α is expressed but rapidly hydroxylated and ultimately degraded via the ubiquitin pathway by the oxygen-dependent EGLN family of HIF prolyl hydroxylases [77]. Following hypoxia, HIF-1α is stabilized and upregulated by inhibition of these prolyl hydroxylases. The phosphorylated form of HIF-1α dimerizes with the constitutive β subunit, forming the active complex that binds to the transcriptional co-activator p300/CBP and to the hypoxia response element (HRE) in the promotor region of a variety of genes, including EPO, glucose transporters, glycolytic enzymes, VEGF and other growth factors (Fig. 3.2) [78]. These HIF-1 target genes, which maintain energy metabolism, angiogenesis, and possibly neurogenesis, contribute to protection and recovery after stroke in adults, as is demonstrated by exacerbation of injury in neuron-specific HIF-1α conditional knockouts and reduction of ischemic injury in animals treated with HIF-1α stimulators [75,79,80]. Although HIF-1α is generally considered neuroprotective, it is also shown to induce various pro-death proteins (such as bNIP3) and caspase-3 activation [81,82], interfering with protective responses in the hippocampus in a model of global hypoxia [83]. The exact mechanisms of these opposing effects of HIF-1α on ischemic injury are not clear, but the extent of temporal–spatial HIF-1α-dependent induction of genes like EPO and VEGF after ischemic injury, and the balance between pro-survival and pro-death proteins, seem to play a major role in HIF-1α-dependent outcomes [75,79,83].

In neonatal models, HIF-1α is induced by HI, focal ischemia–reperfusion, and desferoxamine (DFO), which acts in both a HIF-dependent and independent manner [84–86]. Increased HIF-1α expression occurs as early as 4 hours, peaks at 8 hours, and returns to baseline by about 24 hours following

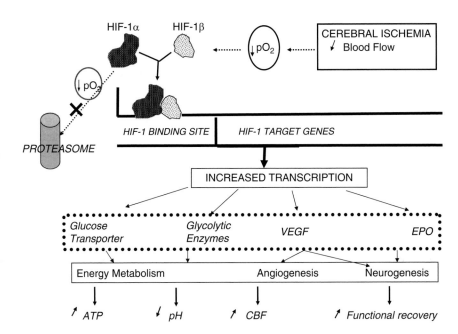

Fig. 3.2. HIF-1-mediated protection and repair following HI.

a transient middle cerebral artery occlusion (MCAO) in P10 rats, and is followed by increases in both VEGF and EPO expression [85,86]. HIF-1α upregulation is mediated in part by the PI3K–Akt and ERK1–2 pathways, as evidenced by attenuation of HIF-1α upregulation by inhibitors of proteins in these pathways [87,88]. HIF-1 is also believed to contribute to hypoxic preconditioning in neonatal rat brain, likely through induction of a variety of HIF-1-inducible genes, including VEGF, EPO, GLUT-1, adrenomedullin, and propyl 4-hydroxylase α [89,90].

Erythropoietin (EPO)

EPO is a pleotrophic growth factor and a member of the type I superfamily of cytokines. While EPO was identified for its role in erythropoiesis [91], biological activity of EPO extends far beyond erythropoiesis. It contributes directly to brain development, by supporting neural cell progenitor cells and promoting survival and proliferation of these cells [92,93]. EPO knockout is embryonic-lethal by E13, with fetuses exhibiting severe anemia and a paucity of neural progenitor cells and neurogenesis [92,94].

EPO receptor (EPOR) binding results in phosphorylation of Janus-tyrosine kinase 2 (JAK-2) that activates several pathways, including Ras- and phosphatidylinositol-3-kinase (PI3K) pathways. In neurons, EPO activates the nuclear factor κB (NFκB) [95] and reduces glutamate release [96]. EPO administration protects against focal and global ischemia, glutamate toxicity, and kainate-induced seizures by reducing neuronal apoptosis [97–99], stimulating neuronal precursors, and stimulating angiogenesis [92,93,100]. EPO also contributes to neuroprotection via attenuation of inflammation [101].

In neonatal rodents, EPO treatment reduces brain injury, apoptosis, and gliosis days after the HI insult [102], in part by rapid EPOR upregulation [103]. It preserves auditory processing and learning/memory after HI even when administered in low doses, 0.3–1 U/g [104], and improves sensorimotor, memory, and behavioral outcomes [105,106]. However, a U-shaped dose response to the range of EPO concentrations is reported [102]. In a focal ischemia–reperfusion model in neonatal rats, we showed that EPO (5 U/g) markedly preserved hemispheric volume, decreased the expansion of the subventricular zone (SVZ) unilaterally, and significantly improved sensorimotor and memory function up to 6 weeks after MCAO [107]. The effect on tissue preservation is in part due to increased percentage of newly generated neurons versus decreased newly generated astrocytes following brain injury, suggesting that in neonatal stroke EPO may redirect cell fate toward neurogenesis and away from gliogenesis, allowing for repair and replacement of damaged tissue [108].

Vascular endothelial growth factor (VEGF)

VEGF is a family of growth factors involved in vasculogenesis, neurogenesis, and angiogenesis. There are three VEGF isoforms, which signal by binding to two endothelial tyrosine kinase receptors: VEGFR1 (Flt-1) and VEGFR2 (Flk-1) [109]. VEGFR2 has higher affinity to VEGF-A (i.e., VEGF) and is thought to be responsible for most biological signaling by VEGF in the CNS. Loss of a single VEGF allele is embryonic-lethal [110].

VEGF-induced VEGFR2 autophosphorylation leads to binding of several SH2-containing molecules and activation of several downstream signaling pathways including the MAPK [111], ERK1–2, and PI3K–Akt pathways [112,113]. VEGFR1, in turn, mediates monocyte and macrophage migration [114] and can affect integrity of BBB via the PI3K–Akt pathway [115]. VEGFR1 can also modulate VEGR2 activity [116,117]. In vitro, VEGF stabilizes and promotes survival of neurons after hypoxia, nutrient deprivation, or glutamate administration [118].

In stroke, VEGF expression is robustly upregulated [119]. VEGF administration or overexpression results in decreased infarct volume, increased angiogenesis and neurogenesis, and improved functional outcomes 4–8 weeks post-injury [120,121]. However, a rush to use VEGF as a salvage treatment following CNS injury must be tempered with caution, as early administration of VEGF after stroke actually can increase BBB leakage and infarct size [122]. A U-shaped curve – protection after low, non-angiogenic doses of VEGF, and increased damage and hemorrhagic transformation associated with doses high enough to stimulate angiogenesis – is reported after adult stroke [123]. Delayed administration of VEGF shows enhanced microvascular perfusion and no increase in BBB leakage [122], reinforcing the importance of the timing for VEGF biological effects for long-term outcomes.

VEGF and VEGFR2 expression is high in the developing brain, in concert with developmental cerebral angiogenesis, and is further upregulated following HI and focal stroke in neonatal animals [85,87,88,124]. The increase in VEGF (and HIF-1α) expression is blocked by the PI3K–Akt and ERK inhibitors [88]. Endogenous VEGF is a necessary piece of the neuroprotection offered by hypoxic preconditioning, with exogenous VEGF augmenting the benefits of hypoxic preconditioning [125]. In an ongoing study using the VEGFR2 antagonist SU5416, we showed injury exacerbation and increased gliosis after neonatal focal ischemia [126].

New trends in neuroprotection: hypothermia and natural ingredients

Two recent large multicenter randomized studies of newborn infants with hypoxic–ischemic encephalopathy demonstrate the neuroprotective potential of hypothermia, using head cooling or whole-body cooling [127,128]. The benefits may be limited to infants with moderate injury [127], and these studies, while indicating great promise, show the need to better understand optimal depth, timing, and duration of hypothermia to maximize beneficial effects [129].

Several studies in immature rats showed that hypothermia during HI insult is protective and significantly attenuates spatial learning deficits [130,131]. When induced immediately after HI in P7 rats, hypothermia provides protection and inhibition of caspase activation via the intrinsic pathway in the neonatal brain, thereby preventing apoptotic cell death [132]. Delayed cooling of P7 rats is shown to reduce cerebral infarction and behavioral deficits at 6 weeks after the insult [133]. Yet other studies show that hypothermia alone did not improve long-term outcomes but is beneficial as a part of combined treatment [134]. In larger species, e.g., piglets, mild hypothermia reduces HI injury and neuronal apoptosis, and preserves sensorimotor and behavioral function [135,136]. The timing of hypothermia is critical for protection. Deep cooling is needed to protect between 6 and 12 hours after HI in rodents [137]. In fetal lambs, cooling protects against HI when delayed up to 5 hours [138] but not to 8 hours post-insult [139]. Combinatory strategies show further benefits.

The long-term benefits of hypothermia can be augmented by co-administering topiramate, N-acetylcysteine, or xenon [134,140,141].

Two recent studies show that pomegranate juice protects against neonatal HI when given as maternal dietary supplementation prior to subjecting newborn pups to HI, and when pups are drinking pomegranate juice after HI [142,143]. Polyphenols, which are believed to be active ingredients in the juice, and resveratrol in particular, can reduce caspase-3 activation and calpain activation following neonatal HI [143], presumably via the SIRT signaling pathway. Pretreatment with grape-seed extract protects against HI, possibly due to its antioxidant characteristics and ability to restore regulation within the prostaglandin pathways [144].

Repair: neurogenesis and angiogenesis

Generation of new neurons – neurogenesis – is a critical element of repair following neurodegenerative conditions, including stroke and HI. Ischemic focal stroke gives rise to cell proliferation in the SVZ in both adult and neonatal brains [107,145–147]. The newly formed neuroblasts migrate from the SVZ into the damaged striatum and differentiate to become mature neurons of appropriate phenotypes [145,148,149]. This suggests a potential for self-repair strategies after stroke [146]. However, endogenous neurogenesis is short-lived and ineffective, as shown by several laboratories including ours [107,145,150,151].

Some studies show that neonatal HI depletes the SVZ of progenitors, while other studies have demonstrated expansion of the SVZ after HI [147] and focal stroke [107]. Activated calpains and caspase-3 co-localized to regions with progenitor cell death, whereas neither enzyme was activated in the medial SVZ, which harbors the neural stem cells that are resilient to this insult [152]. Increased neocortical production was associated with increases in insulin-like growth factor 1 and MCP-1, but statistically insignificant production of EPO, brain-derived neurotrophic factor, glial-derived neurotrophic factor, and transforming growth factor α, suggesting that HI injury in the neonatal brain initiates a regenerative response from the SVZ [153]. HIF-1α modulates neurogenesis through increased expression of genes like VEGF and EPO, and EPO by itself is a major inducer of neurogenesis after neonatal ischemic insults.

The formation of new blood vessels – angiogenesis – is a limiting factor in post-ischemic repair [154]. Angiogenesis is a complex multistep process, with numerous soluble factors strictly controlling this process [155]. The presence of newly formed blood vessels is critical in several aspects of repair, including not only ensuring the blood supply but also providing an angiogenic–neurogenic niche in the brain, as neurogenesis appears to be intimately associated with active vascular recruitment and remodeling [154].

Evidence continues to accumulate that angiogenesis is coupled with neurogenesis [154]. The VEGFR2 receptor mediates antiapoptotic effects and supports survival of the endothelial cells that have been induced by VEGF [118].

Future directions

Considerable progress has been made in delineating the complexity of cellular injury, including better understanding of the network of intracellular signaling pathways and the rationale for identification of therapeutic targets and development of effective therapies. Two new aspects of thinking in the field have been acknowledgement of the integrative nature of brain injury, which evolves via communication between different cell types, and the dynamic nature of changes during brain maturation. Recent studies have begun targeting repair as the way of improving long-term recovery following HI injury during the newborn period. Currently, promising clinical studies are being conducted on the effects of hypothermia and erythropoietin following perinatal HIE, but much needs to be learned about the optimal conditions for these interventions and ways of targeting severely injured brains. Therefore, future work should address the optimal timing for modulating effects of interventions. Elucidating how to enhance the repair process, by supporting angiogenesis, neurogenesis, and preservation of function, will be the major markers of success. Emerging evidence suggests that different interventions may be necessary to accomplish improvement in males and females. Studies are also needed to determine whether proposed interventions adversely affect long-term brain development.

References

1. Volpe JJ. Brain injury in the premature infant: overview of clinical aspects, neuropathology, and pathogenesis. *Semin Pediatr Neurol* 1998; **5**: 135–51.

2. Ferriero DM. Neonatal brain injury. *N Engl J Med* 2004; **351**: 1985–95.

3. Vannucci RC, Vannucci SJ. A model of perinatal hypoxic–ischemic brain damage. *Ann N Y Acad Sci* 1997; **835**: 234–49.

4. Derugin N, Ferriero DM, Vexler ZS. Neonatal reversible focal cerebral ischemia: a new model. *Neurosci Res* 1998; **32**: 349–53.

5. Ashwal S, Tone B, Tian HR, et al. Core and penumbral nitric oxide synthase activity during cerebral ischemia and reperfusion. *Stroke* 1998; **29**: 1037–47.

6. McQuillen PS, Ferriero DM. Selective vulnerability in the developing central nervous system. *Pediatr Neurol* 2004; **30**: 227–35.

7. Hagberg H, Mallard C. Effect of inflammation on central nervous system development and vulnerability. *Curr Opin Neurol* 2005; **18**: 117–23.

8. Vexler ZS. Hypoxic ischemic insults and inflammation in the developing brain. In Yenari MA, Giffard RG, eds., *Glia and Inflammation in Neurodegenerative Disease*. New York, NY: Nova Science, 2006: 197–220.

9. Vannucci SJ, Hagberg H. Hypoxia–ischemia in the immature brain. *J Exp Biol* 2004; **207**: 3149–54.

10. Vexler ZS, Tang D, Yenari M. Inflammation in adult and neonatal stroke. *Clin Neurosci Res* 2006; **6**: 293–313.

11. Northington FJ, Zelaya ME, O'Riordan DP, et al. Failure to complete apoptosis following neonatal hypoxia–ischemia manifests as "continuum" phenotype of cell death and occurs with multiple manifestations of mitochondrial dysfunction in rodent forebrain. *Neuroscience* 2007; **149**: 822–33.

12. Vannucci RC, Vannucci SJ. Glucose metabolism in the developing brain. *Semin Perinatol* 2000; **24**: 107–15.

13. Perlman JM. Intervention strategies for neonatal hypoxic–ischemic cerebral injury. *Clin Ther* 2006; **28**: 1353–65.

14. Vexler ZS, Ferriero DM. Mechanisms of ischemic cell death in the developing brain. In Chan P, Lajtha A, eds., *Handbook of Neurochemistry and Molecular Neurobiology*. New York, NY: Springer, 2007: 209–34.

15. Jiang X, Mu D, Biran V, et al. Activated Src kinases interact with N-methyl-D-aspartate receptor after neonatal brain ischemia. *Ann Neurol* 2008; **63**: 632–41.

16. Sheldon RA, Christen S, Ferriero DM. Genetic and pharmacologic manipulation of oxidative stress after neonatal hypoxia–ischemia. *Int J Dev Neurosci* 2008; **26**: 87–92.

17. Garcia JH, Liu KF, Yoshida Y, et al. Influx of leukocytes and platelets in an evolving brain infarct (Wistar rat). *Am J Pathol* 1994; **144**: 188–99.

18. Hallenbeck JM. Significance of the inflammatory response in brain ischemia. *Acta Neurochir Suppl* 1996; **66**: 27–31.

19. Rosenberg GA. Matrix metalloproteinases in neuroinflammation. *Glia* 2002; **39**: 279–91.

20. Allan SM, Tyrrell PJ, Rothwell NJ. Interleukin-1 and neuronal injury. *Nat Rev Immunol* 2005; **5**: 629–40.

21. Pan W, Ding Y, Yu Y, et al. Stroke upregulates TNFα transport across the blood–brain barrier. *Exp Neurol* 2006; **198**: 222–33.

22. Kniesel U, Risau W, Wolburg H. Development of blood–brain barrier tight junctions in the rat cortex. *Brain Res Dev Brain Res* 1996; **96**: 229–40.

23. Engelhardt B. Development of the blood–brain barrier. *Cell Tissue Res* 2003; **314**: 119–29.

24. Blamire AM, Anthony DC, Rajagopalan B, et al. Interleukin-1β-induced changes in blood–brain barrier permeability, apparent diffusion coefficient, and cerebral blood volume in the rat brain: a magnetic resonance study. *J Neurosci* 2000; **20**: 8153–9.

25. Palmer C, Roberts RL, Young PI. Timing of neutrophil depletion influences long-term neuroprotection in neonatal rat hypoxic–ischemic brain injury. *Pediatr Res* 2004; **55**: 549–56.

26. Bona E, Andersson AL, Blomgren K, et al. Chemokine and inflammatory cell response to hypoxia–ischemia in immature rats. *Pediatr Res* 1999; **45**: 500–9.

27. Denker SP, Ji S, Dingman A, et al. Macrophages are comprised of resident brain microglia not infiltrating peripheral monocytes acutely after neonatal stroke. *J Neurochem* 2007; **100**: 893–904.

28. Svedin P, Hagberg H, Savman K, et al. Matrix metalloproteinase-9 gene knock-out protects the immature brain after cerebral hypoxia–ischemia. *J Neurosci* 2007; **27**: 1511–8.

29. Raivich G, Bohatschek M, Kloss CU, et al. Neuroglial activation repertoire in the injured brain: graded response, molecular mechanisms and cues to physiological function. *Brain Res Brain Res Rev* 1999; **30**: 77–105.

30. Monje ML, Toda H, Palmer TD. Inflammatory blockade restores adult hippocampal neurogenesis. *Science* 2003; **302**: 1760–5.

31. Walton NM, Sutter BM, Laywell ED, et al. Microglia instruct subventricular

zone neurogenesis. *Glia* 2006; **54**: 815–25.

32. Britschgi M, Wyss-Coray T. Immune cells may fend off Alzheimer disease. *Nat Med* 2007; **13**: 408–9.

33. Marin-Teva JL, Dusart I, Colin C, *et al.* Microglia promote the death of developing Purkinje cells. *Neuron* 2004; **41**: 535–47.

34. Derugin N, Wendland M, Muramatsu K, *et al.* Evolution of brain injury after transient middle cerebral artery occlusion in neonatal rat. *Stroke* 2000; **31**: 1752–61.

35. McRae A, Gilland E, Bona E, *et al.* Microglia activation after neonatal hypoxic-ischemia. *Brain Res Dev Brain Res* 1995; **84**: 245–52.

36. Dommergues MA, Plaisant F, Verney C, *et al.* Early microglial activation following neonatal excitotoxic brain damage in mice: a potential target for neuroprotection. *Neuroscience* 2003; **121**: 619–28.

37. Tikka T, Fiebich BL, Goldsteins G, *et al.* Minocycline, a tetracycline derivative, is neuroprotective against excitotoxicity by inhibiting activation and proliferation of microglia. *J Neurosci* 2001; **21**: 2580–8.

38. van den Tweel ER, van Bel F, Kavelaars A, *et al.* Long-term neuroprotection with 2-iminobiotin, an inhibitor of neuronal and inducible nitric oxide synthase, after cerebral hypoxia-ischemia in neonatal rats. *J Cereb Blood Flow Metab* 2005; **25**: 67–74.

39. Dingman A, Lee SY, Derugin N, *et al.* Aminoguanidine inhibits caspase-3 and calpain activation without affecting microglial activation following neonatal transient ischemia. *J Neurochem* 2006; **96**: 1467–79.

40. Dong Y, Benveniste EN. Immune function of astrocytes. *Glia* 2001; **36**: 180–90.

41. Nawashiro H, Brenner M, Fukui S, *et al.* High susceptibility to cerebral ischemia in GFAP-null mice. *J Cereb Blood Flow Metab* 2000; **20**: 1040–4.

42. Benjelloun N, Renolleau S, Represa A, *et al.* Inflammatory responses in the cerebral cortex after ischemia in the P7 neonatal rat. *Stroke* 1999; **30**: 1916–1923.

43. Ducrocq S, Benjelloun N, Plotkine M, *et al.* Poly(ADP-ribose) synthase inhibition reduces ischemic injury and inflammation in neonatal rat brain. *J Neurochem* 2000; **74**: 2504–11.

44. Jin Y, Silverman AJ, Vannucci SJ. Mast cell stabilization limits hypoxic–ischemic brain damage in the immature rat. *Dev Neurosci* 2007; **29**: 373–84.

45. Biran V, Cochois V, Karroubi A, *et al.* Stroke induces histamine accumulation and mast cell degranulation in the neonatal rat brain. *Brain Pathol* 2008; **18**: 1–9.

46. Mesples B, Fontaine RH, Lelievre V, *et al.* Neuronal TGF-β1 mediates IL-9/ mast cell interaction and exacerbates excitotoxicity in newborn mice. *Neurobiol Dis* 2005; **18**: 193–205.

47. Hedtjarn M, Mallard C, Hagberg H. Inflammatory gene profiling in the developing mouse brain after hypoxia-ischemia. *J Cereb Blood Flow Metab* 2004; **24**: 1333–51.

48. Szaflarski J, Burtrum D, Silverstein FS. Cerebral hypoxia-ischemia stimulates cytokine gene expression in perinatal rats. *Stroke* 1995; **26**: 1093–100.

49. Fox C, Dingman A, Derugin N, *et al.* Minocycline confers early but transient protection in the immature brain following focal cerebral ischemia-reperfusion. *J Cereb Blood Flow Metab* 2005; **25**: 1138–49.

50. Dommergues MA, Patkai J, Renauld JC, *et al.* Proinflammatory cytokines and interleukin-9 exacerbate excitotoxic lesions of the newborn murine neopallium. *Ann Neurol* 2000; **47**: 54–63.

51. Patkai J, Mesples B, Dommergues MA, *et al.* Deleterious effects of IL-9-activated mast cells and neuroprotection by antihistamine drugs in the developing mouse brain. *Pediatr Res* 2001; **50**: 222–30.

52. Mesples B, Plaisant F, Gressens P. Effects of interleukin-10 on neonatal excitotoxic brain lesions in mice. *Brain Res Dev Brain Res* 2003; **141**: 25–32.

53. Gerard C, Rollins BJ. Chemokines and disease. *Nat Immunol* 2001; **2**: 108–15.

54. Hedtjarn M, Mallard C, Eklind S, *et al.* Global gene expression in the immature brain after hypoxia-ischemia. *J Cereb Blood Flow Metab* 2004; **24**: 1317–32.

55. Galasso JM, Miller MJ, Cowell RM, *et al.* Acute excitotoxic injury induces expression of monocyte chemoattractant protein-1 and its receptor, CCR2, in neonatal rat brain. *Exp Neurol* 2000; **165**: 295–305.

56. Cowell RM, Xu H, Galasso JM, *et al.* Hypoxic–ischemic injury induces macrophage inflammatory protein-1α expression in immature rat brain. *Stroke* 2002; **33**: 795–801.

57. Cowell RM, Plane JM, Silverstein FS. Complement activation contributes to hypoxic–ischemic brain injury in neonatal rats. *J Neurosci* 2003; **23**: 9459–68.

58. Hu BR, Liu XL, Ouyang Y, *et al.* Involvement of caspase-3 in cell death after hypoxia–ischemia declines during brain maturation. *J Cereb Blood Flow Metab* 2000; **20**: 1294–1300.

59. Han BH, Xu D, Choi J, *et al.* Selective, reversible caspase-3 inhibitor is neuroprotective and reveals distinct pathways of cell death following neonatal hypoxic–ischemic brain injury. *J Biol Chem* 2002; **277**: 30128–36.

60. Zhu C, Wang X, Xu F, *et al.* The influence of age on apoptotic and other mechanisms of cell death after cerebral hypoxia-ischemia. *Cell Death Differ* 2005; **12**: 162–76.

61. Manabat C, Han BH, Wendland M, *et al.* Reperfusion differentially induces caspase-3 activation in ischemic core and penumbra after stroke in immature brain. *Stroke* 2003; **34**: 207–13.

62. Cheng Y, Deshmukh M, D'Costa A, *et al.* Caspase inhibitor affords neuroprotection with delayed administration in a rat model of neonatal hypoxic–ischemic brain injury. *J Clin Invest* 1998; **101**: 1992–9.

63. West T, Atzeva M, Holtzman DM. Caspase-3 deficiency during development increases vulnerability to hypoxic–ischemic injury through caspase-3-independent pathways. *Neurobiol Dis* 2006; **22**: 523–37.

64. Zhu C, Xu F, Fukuda A, *et al.* X chromosome-linked inhibitor of apoptosis protein reduces oxidative stress after cerebral irradiation or hypoxia–ischemia through up-regulation of mitochondrial antioxidants. *Eur J Neurosci* 2007; **26**: 3402–10.

65. Matsumori Y, Hong SM, Aoyama K, *et al.* Hsp70 overexpression sequesters AIF and reduces neonatal hypoxic/ ischemic brain injury. *J Cereb Blood Flow Metab* 2005; **25**: 899–910.

66. Blomgren K, Leist M, Groc L. Pathological apoptosis in the developing brain. *Apoptosis* 2007; **12**: 993–1010.

67. Carloni S, Carnevali A, Cimino M, *et al.* Extended role of necrotic cell death after hypoxia–ischemia-induced neurodegeneration in the neonatal rat. *Neurobiol Dis* 2007; **27**: 354–61.

68. Johnston MV, Hagberg H. Sex and the pathogenesis of cerebral palsy. *Dev Med Child Neurol* 2007; **49**: 74–8.

69. Hagberg H, Wilson MA, Matsushita H, *et al.* PARP-1 gene disruption in mice preferentially protects males from perinatal brain injury. *J Neurochem* 2004; **90**: 1068–75.

70. Renolleau S, Fau S, Charriaut-Marlangue C. Gender-related differences in apoptotic pathways after neonatal cerebral ischemia. *Neuroscientist* 2008; **14**: 46–52.

71. Renolleau S, Fau S, Goyenvalle C, *et al.* Sex, neuroprotection, and neonatal ischemia. *Dev Med Child Neurol* 2007; **49**: 477–8.

72. Nijboer CH, Groendendaal F, Kavelaars A, *et al.* Gender-specific neuroprotection by 2-iminobiotin after hypoxia–ischemia in the neonatal rat via a nitric oxide independent pathway. *J Cereb Blood Flow Metab* 2007; **27**: 282–92.

73. Nijboer CH, Kavelaars A, van Bel F, *et al.* Gender-dependent pathways of hypoxia–ischemia-induced cell death and neuroprotection in the immature P3 rat. *Dev Neurosci* 2007; **29**: 385–92.

74. Wang GL, Semenza GL. Characterization of hypoxia-inducible factor 1 and regulation of DNA binding activity by hypoxia. *J Biol Chem* 1993; **268**: 21513–18.

75. Bergeron M, Yu AY, Solway KE, *et al.* Induction of hypoxia-inducible factor-1 (HIF-1) and its target genes following focal ischaemia in rat brain. *Eur J Neurosci* 1999; **11**: 4159–70.

76. Chavez JC, LaManna JC. Activation of hypoxia-inducible factor-1 in the rat cerebral cortex after transient global ischemia: potential role of insulin-like growth factor-1. *J Neurosci* 2002; **22**: 8922–31.

77. Bruick RK, McKnight SL. A conserved family of prolyl-4-hydroxylases that modify HIF. *Science* 2001; **294**: 1337–40.

78. Semenza GL. Hypoxia-inducible factor 1: master regulator of O2 homeostasis. *Curr Opin Genet Dev* 1998; **8**: 588–94.

79. Baranova O, Miranda LF, Pichiule P, *et al.* Neuron-specific inactivation of the hypoxia inducible factor 1 alpha increases brain injury in a mouse model of transient focal cerebral ischemia. *J Neurosci* 2007; **27**: 6320–32.

80. Zaman K, Ryu H, Hall D, *et al.* Protection from oxidative stress-induced apoptosis in cortical neuronal cultures by iron chelators is associated with enhanced DNA binding of hypoxia-inducible factor-1 and ATF-1/CREB and increased expression of glycolytic enzymes, p21(waf1/cip1), and erythropoietin. *J Neurosci* 1999; **19**: 9821–30.

81. Bruick RK. Expression of the gene encoding the proapoptotic Nip3 protein is induced by hypoxia. *Proc Natl Acad Sci USA* 2000; **97**: 9082–7.

82. Van Hoecke M, Prigent-Tessier AS, Garnier PE, *et al.* Evidence of HIF-1 functional binding activity to caspase-3 promoter after photothrombotic cerebral ischemia. *Mol Cell Neurosci* 2007; **34**: 40–7.

83. Helton R, Cui J, Scheel JR, *et al.* Brain-specific knock-out of hypoxia-inducible factor-1α reduces rather than increases hypoxic–ischemic damage. *J Neurosci* 2005; **25**: 4099–107.

84. Bergeron M, Gidday JM, Yu AY, *et al.* Role of hypoxia-inducible factor-1 in hypoxia-induced ischemic tolerance in neonatal rat brain. *Ann Neurol* 2000; **48**: 285–96.

85. Mu D, Jiang X, Sheldon RA, *et al.* Regulation of hypoxia-inducible factor 1α and induction of vascular endothelial growth factor in a rat neonatal stroke model. *Neurobiol Dis* 2003; **14**: 524–34.

86. Mu D, Chang YS, Vexler ZS, *et al.* Hypoxia-inducible factor 1α and erythropoietin upregulation with deferoxamine salvage after neonatal stroke. *Exp Neurol* 2005; **195**: 407–15.

87. Li L, Qu Y, Mao M, *et al.* The involvement of phosphoinositid 3-kinase/Akt pathway in the activation of hypoxia-inducible factor-1α in the developing rat brain after hypoxia–ischemia. *Brain Res* 2008; **1197**: 152–8.

88. Li L, Xiong Y, Qu Y, *et al.* The requirement of extracellular signal-related protein kinase pathway in the activation of hypoxia inducible factor 1α in the developing rat brain after hypoxia–ischemia. *Acta Neuropathol* 2008; **115**: 297–303.

89. Jones NM, Bergeron M. Hypoxic preconditioning induces changes in HIF-1 target genes in neonatal rat brain. *J Cereb Blood Flow Metab* 2001; **21**: 1105–14.

90. Bernaudin M, Tang Y, Reilly M, *et al.* Brain genomic response following hypoxia and re-oxygenation in the neonatal rat. Identification of genes that might contribute to hypoxia-induced ischemic tolerance. *J Biol Chem* 2002; **277**: 39728–38.

91. Jelkmann W. Erythropoietin: structure, control of production, and function. *Physiol Rev* 1992; **72**: 449–89.

92. Chen ZY, Asavaritikrai P, Prchal J, *et al.* Endogenous erythropoietin signaling is required for normal neural progenitor cell proliferation. *J Biol Chem* 2007; **282**: 25875–83.

93. Shingo T, Sorokan ST, Shimazaki T, *et al.* Erythropoietin regulates the in vitro and in vivo production of neuronal progenitors by mammalian forebrain neural stem cells. *J Neurosci* 2001; **21**: 9733–43.

94. Wu H, Liu X, Jaenisch R, *et al.* Generation of committed erythroid BFU-E and CFU-E progenitors does not require erythropoietin or the erythropoietin receptor. *Cell* 1995; **83**: 59–67.

95. Digicaylioglu M, Lipton SA. Erythropoietin-mediated neuroprotection involves cross-talk between Jak2 and NF-κB signalling cascades. *Nature* 2001; **412**: 641–7.

96. Kawakami M, Sekiguchi M, Sato K, *et al.* Erythropoietin receptor-mediated inhibition of exocytotic glutamate release confers neuroprotection during chemical ischemia. *J Biol Chem* 2001; **276**: 39469–75.

97. Marti HH, Bernaudin M, Petit E, *et al.* Neuroprotection and angiogenesis: dual role of erythropoietin in brain ischemia. *News Physiol Sci* 2000; **15**: 225–9.

98. Solaroglu I, Solaroglu A, Kaptanoglu E, *et al.* Erythropoietin prevents ischemia–reperfusion from inducing oxidative damage in fetal rat brain. *Childs Nerv Syst* 2003; **19**: 19–22.

99. Sola A, Wen C, Hamrick SE, *et al.* Potential for protection and repair following injury to the developing brain: a role for erythropoietin? *Pediatr Res* 2005; **57**: 110R–117R.

100. Wang L, Zhang Z, Wang Y, *et al.* Treatment of stroke with erythropoietin enhances neurogenesis and angiogenesis and improves neurological function in rats. *Stroke* 2004; **35**: 1732–7.

101. Sun Y, Calvert JW, Zhang JH. Neonatal hypoxia/ischemia is associated with decreased inflammatory mediators after erythropoietin administration. *Stroke* 2005; **36**: 1672–8.

102. Kellert BA, McPherson RJ, Juul SE. A comparison of high-dose recombinant erythropoietin treatment regimens in brain-injured neonatal rats. *Pediatr Res* 2007; **61**: 451–5.

103. Spandou E, Papousopoulou S, Soubasi V, *et al.* Hypoxia–ischemia affects erythropoietin and erythropoietin

receptor expression pattern in the neonatal rat brain. *Brain Res* 2004; **1021**: 167–72.

104. McClure MM, Threlkeld SW, Fitch RH. Auditory processing and learning/ memory following erythropoietin administration in neonatally hypoxic–ischemic injured rats. *Brain Res* 2007; **1132**: 203–9.

105. Iwai M, Cao G, Yin W, et al. Erythropoietin promotes neuronal replacement through revascularization and neurogenesis after neonatal hypoxia/ischemia in rats. *Stroke* 2007; **38**: 2795–803.

106. Kumral A, Uysal N, Tugyan K, et al. Erythropoietin improves long-term spatial memory deficits and brain injury following neonatal hypoxia–ischemia in rats. *Behav Brain Res* 2004; **153**: 77–86.

107. Chang YS, Mu D, Wendland M, et al. Erythropoietin improves functional and histological outcome in neonatal stroke. *Pediatr Res* 2005; **58**: 106–11.

108. Gonzalez F, McQuillen P, Mu D, et al. Erythropoietin enhances long-term neuroprotection and neurogenesis in neonatal stroke. *Dev Neurosci* 2007; **29**: 321–30.

109. Ferrara N, Gerber HP. The role of vascular endothelial growth factor in angiogenesis. *Acta Haematol* 2001; **106**: 148–56.

110. Carmeliet P, Ferreira V, Brier G, et al. Abnormal blood vessel development and lethality in embryos lacking a single VEGF allele. *Nature* 1996; **380**: 435–9.

111. Dougher M, Terman BI. Autophosphorylation of KDR in the kinase domain is required for maximal VEGF-stimulated kinase activity and receptor internalization. *Oncogene* 1999; **18**: 1619–27.

112. Takahashi T, Yamaguchi S, Chida K, et al. A single autophosphorylation site on KDR/Flk-1 is essential for VEGF-A-dependent activation of PLC-gamma and DNA synthesis in vascular endothelial cells. *EMBO J* 2001; **20**: 2768–78.

113. Fujio Y, Walsh K. Akt mediates cytoprotection of endothelial cells by vascular endothelial growth factor in an anchorage-dependent manner. *J Biol Chem* 1999; **274**: 16349–54.

114. Shibuya M. Structure and dual function of vascular endothelial growth factor receptor-1 (Flt-1). *Int J Biochem Cell Biol* 2001; **33**: 409–20.

115. Vogel C, Bauer A, Wiesnet M, et al. Flt-1, but not Flk-1 mediates hyperpermeability through activation of the PI3-K/Akt pathway. *J Cell Physiol* 2007; **212**: 236–43.

116. Rahimi N, Dayanir V, Lashkari K. Receptor chimeras indicate that the vascular endothelial growth factor receptor-1 (VEGFR-1) modulates mitogenic activity of VEGFR-2 in endothelial cells. *J Biol Chem* 2000; **275**: 16986–92.

117. Autiero M, Waltenberger J, Communi D, et al. Role of PlGF in the intra- and intermolecular cross talk between the VEGF receptors Flt1 and Flk1. *Nat Med* 2003; **9**: 936–43.

118. Jin KL, Mao XO, Greenberg DA. Vascular endothelial growth factor: direct neuroprotective effect in in vitro ischemia. *Proc Natl Acad Sci USA* 2000; **97**: 10242–7.

119. Shweiki D, Itin A, Soffer D, et al. Vascular endothelial growth factor induced by hypoxia may mediate hypoxia-initiated angiogenesis. *Nature* 1992; **359**: 843–5.

120. Sun Y, Jin K, Xie L, et al. VEGF-induced neuroprotection, neurogenesis, and angiogenesis after focal cerebral ischemia. *J Clin Invest* 2003; **111**: 1843–51.

121. Wang Y, Jin K, Mao XO, et al. VEGF-overexpressing transgenic mice show enhanced post-ischemic neurogenesis and neuromigration. *J Neurosci Res* 2007; **85**: 740–7.

122. Zhang ZG, Zhang L, Jiang O, et al. VEGF enhances angiogenesis and promotes blood–brain barrier leakage in the ischemic brain. *J Clin Invest* 2000; **106**: 829–38.

123. Manoonkitiwongsa PS, Schultz RL, McCreery DB, et al. Neuroprotection of ischemic brain by vascular endothelial growth factor is critically dependent on proper dosage and may be compromised by angiogenesis. *J Cereb Blood Flow Metab* 2004; **24**: 693–702.

124. Ogunshola OO, Stewart WB, Mihalcik V, et al. Neuronal VEGF expression correlates with angiogenesis in postnatal developing rat brain. *Brain Res Dev Brain Res* 2000; **119**: 139–53.

125. Laudenbach V, Fontaine RH, Medja F, et al. Neonatal hypoxic preconditioning involves vascular endothelial growth factor. *Neurobiol Dis* 2007; **26**: 243–52.

126. Shimotake J, et al. Effect of a VEGF receptor inhibitor SU5416 on short-term outcome in neonatal rodent stroke. Pediatric Academic Societies meeting, 2008.

127. Gluckman PD, Wyatt JS, Azzopardi D, et al. Selective head cooling with mild systemic hypothermia after neonatal encephalopathy: multicentre randomised trial. *Lancet* 2005; **365**: 663–70.

128. Shankaran S, Laptook AR, Ehrenkranz RA, et al. Whole-body hypothermia for neonates with hypoxic–ischemic encephalopathy. *N Engl J Med* 2005; **353**: 1574–84.

129. Wyatt JS, Gluckman PD, Liu PY, et al. Determinants of outcomes after head cooling for neonatal encephalopathy. *Pediatrics* 2007; **119**: 912–21.

130. Yager JY, Armstrong EA, Jaharus C, et al. Preventing hyperthermia decreases brain damage following neonatal hypoxic–ischemic seizures. *Brain Res* 2004; **1011**: 48–57.

131. Mishima K, Ikeda, Yoshikawa T, et al. Effects of hypothermia and hyperthermia on attentional and spatial learning deficits following neonatal hypoxia-ischemic insult in rats. *Behav Brain Res* 2004; **151**: 209–17.

132. Zhu C, Wang X, Cheng X, et al. Post-ischemic hypothermia-induced tissue protection and diminished apoptosis after neonatal cerebral hypoxia–ischemia. *Brain Res* 2004; **996**: 67–75.

133. Wagner BP, Nedelcu J, Martin E. Delayed postischemic hypothermia improves long-term behavioral outcome after cerebral hypoxia-ischemia in neonatal rats. *Pediatr Res* 2002; **51**: 354–60.

134. Liu Y, Barks JD, Xu G, et al. Topiramate extends the therapeutic window for hypothermia-mediated neuroprotection after stroke in neonatal rats. *Stroke* 2004; **35**: 1460–5.

135. Thoresen M, Haaland K, Loberg EM, et al. A piglet survival model of posthypoxic encephalopathy. *Pediatr Res* 1996; **40**: 738–48.

136. Bona E, Hagberg H, Loberg EM, et al. Protective effects of moderate hypothermia after neonatal hypoxia–ischemia: short- and long-term outcome. *Pediatr Res* 1998; **43**: 738–45.

137. Taylor DL, Mehmet H, Cady EB, et al. Improved neuroprotection with hypothermia delayed by 6 hours following cerebral hypoxia–ischemia in the 14-day-old rat. *Pediatr Res* 2002; **51**: 13–19.

138. Gunn AJ, Gunn TR, de Haan HH, *et al.* Dramatic neuronal rescue with prolonged selective head cooling after ischemia in fetal lambs. *J Clin Invest* 1997; **99**: 248–56.

139. Gunn AJ, Bennet L, Gunning MI, *et al.* Cerebral hypothermia is not neuroprotective when started after postischemic seizures in fetal sheep. *Pediatr Res* 1999; **46**: 274–80.

140. Jatan M, Singh I, Singh AK, *et al.* Combination of systemic hypothermia and N-acetylcysteine attenuates hypoxic–ischemic brain injury in neonatal rats. *Pediatr Res* 2006; **59**: 684–9.

141. Hobbs CT, Tucker M, Aquilina A, *et al.* Xenon and hypothermia combine additively, offering long-term functional and histopathologic neuroprotection after neonatal hypoxia/ischemia. *Stroke* 2008; **39**: 1307–13.

142. Loren DJ, Seeram NP, Schulman RN, *et al.* Maternal dietary supplementation with pomegranate juice is neuroprotective in an animal model of neonatal hypoxic–ischemic brain injury. *Pediatr Res* 2005; **57**: 858–64.

143. West T, Atzeva M, Holtzman DM. Pomegranate polyphenols and resveratrol protect the neonatal brain against hypoxic–ischemic injury. *Dev Neurosci* 2007; **29**: 363–72.

144. Feng Y, Liu YM, Leblanc MH, *et al.* Grape seed extract given three hours after injury suppresses lipid peroxidation and reduces hypoxic–ischemic brain injury in neonatal rats. *Pediatr Res* 2007; **61**: 295–300.

145. Parent JM, Vexler ZS, Gong C, *et al.* Rat forebrain neurogenesis and striatal neuron replacement after focal stroke. *Ann Neurol* 2002; **52**: 802–13.

146. Lindvall O, Kokaia Z. Recovery and rehabilitation in stroke: stem cells. *Stroke* 2004; **35**: 2691–4.

147. Plane JM, Liu R, Wang TW, *et al.* Neonatal hypoxic–ischemic injury increases forebrain subventricular zone neurogenesis in the mouse. *Neurobiol Dis* 2004; **16**: 585–95.

148. Arvidsson A, Collin T, Kirik D, *et al.* Neuronal replacement from endogenous precursors in the adult brain after stroke. *Nat Med* 2002; **8**: 963–70.

149. Zhang R, Zhang Z, Wang L, *et al.* Activated neural stem cells contribute to stroke-induced neurogenesis and neuroblast migration toward the infarct boundary in adult rats. *J Cereb Blood Flow Metab* 2004; **24**: 441–8.

150. Zhang R, Zhang Z, Zhang C, *et al.* Stroke transiently increases subventricular zone cell division from asymmetric to symmetric and increases neuronal differentiation in the adult rat. *J Neurosci* 2004; **24**: 5810–15.

151. Ohab JJ, Fleming S, Blesch A, *et al.* A neurovascular niche for neurogenesis after stroke. *J Neurosci* 2006; **26**: 13007–16.

152. Romanko MJ, Zhu C, Bahr BA, *et al.* Death effector activation in the subventricular zone subsequent to perinatal hypoxia/ischemia. *J Neurochem* 2007; **103**: 1121–31.

153. Yang Z, Covey MV, Bitel CL, *et al.* Sustained neocortical neurogenesis after neonatal hypoxic/ischemic injury. *Ann Neurol* 2007; **61**: 199–208.

154. Greenberg DA, Jin K. From angiogenesis to neuropathology. *Nature* 2005; **438**: 954–9.

155. Distler JH, Hirth A, Kurowska-Stolarska M, *et al.* Angiogenic and angiostatic factors in the molecular control of angiogenesis. *Q J Nucl Med* 2003; **47**: 149–61.

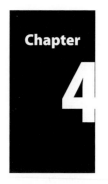

Chapter 4

The pathogenesis of preterm brain injury

Laura Bennet, Justin Mark Dean, and Alistair J. Gunn

Introduction

Neurodevelopmental disability in prematurely born infants remains a very significant problem worldwide, for which there is no specific treatment. While there have been significant improvements in the survival of preterm infants [1], this has not been matched by improvements in morbidity; indeed there is some evidence that disability has increased [1], with a moderate rise in the childhood prevalence of cerebral palsy [2]. The high incidence of neurological morbidity within this group of babies poses a considerable burden on families and the health system. We need to considerably increase our understanding of when and how this injury occurs to develop effective ways of alleviating the burden.

Traditionally, brain injury in preterm infants has been thought to reflect a fundamental vulnerability of the developing periventricular white matter to damage. However, recent evidence suggests a much more complex picture. In the present review, we will critically dissect the neuropathology of hypoxic preterm brain injury, including the underappreciated importance of acute gray-matter as well as white-matter damage, and the timing and mechanisms of injury, and highlight key unresolved issues.

The long-term problem: neurodevelopmental handicap

Children born preterm (< 37 weeks) have high rates of disability including visual damage, mental retardation, epileptic seizures, and cerebral palsy [3,4]. The incidence of these deficits increases steeply with decreasing gestational age and birthweight [4]. Even in those children who survive without apparent motor disability, there is substantial reduction in mean intelligence quotient and more frequent cognitive and educational difficulties [4].

Preterm neuropathology

The most distinctive pathological feature of prematurely born infants is white-matter injury, predominantly in the periventricular tracts (periventricular leukomalacia; PVL) [5]. The incidence of severe cystic PVL has steadily fallen to very low levels with modern intensive care, so that the great majority of cases now involve milder, diffuse cell loss without cystic changes [6,7]. Injury to white matter is highly visible on ultrasound and magnetic resonance imaging (MRI), and thus this feature has been the primary focus of most clinical and experimental investigations.

However, the consistent link between preterm white-matter damage and neurodevelopmental impairment [8,9] seems to be contradictory, since we think with our neurons not with white matter [10]. Indeed, there has been no apparent improvement in neurodevelopmental outcomes of premature infants despite the progressive reduction in the incidence of the severe cystic form of PVL over the last 10 years [11]. A recent key insight comes from quantitative MRI studies, which have shown that preterm birth is also associated with regionally specific long-term reductions in brain gray-matter volumes, in both cortical and subcortical regions, in addition to reduced white-matter volumes [8,12,13]. In turn, neurodevelopmental outcomes are correlated with reduced gray-matter volume, even after adjustment for the presence of PVL [8,13]. White-matter injury was associated with greater reduction in gray-matter volume [8]; however, a quantitative reduction in cortical surface area and complexity of cortical folding was observed at term-equivalent in premature infants without overt parenchymal lesions [14], and in ex-preterm infants at older ages [13,15,16], which correlated with reduced IQ [13,17]. A similar correlation is seen between reduced volume of subcortical gray matter and long-term functional problems in ex-preterm children, including cognitive ability and memory problems in later childhood and adolescence [18,19].

A role for acute neural injury?

There is increasing evidence that these *chronic* anatomical deficits partly reflect *acute* neuronal damage sustained during the peripartum period. In a population-based postmortem survey there was a 32% incidence of neuronal loss, particularly in the pons [20]. Consistent with this, a subsequent series of 41 premature infants found that PVL was associated with neuronal loss in over a third of infants, particularly in the basal ganglia and cerebellum [10], and that more than half had gray-matter astrogliosis that is highly suggestive of milder, selective injury.

Fetal and Neonatal Brain Injury, 4th edition, ed. David K. Stevenson, William E. Benitz, Philip Sunshine, Susan R. Hintz, and Maurice L. Druzin. Published by Cambridge University Press. © Cambridge University Press 2009.

Further, MR imaging of preterm infants exposed to known severe perinatal hypoxia has demonstrated a consistent pattern of acute subcortical damage involving the thalamus and basal ganglia, and cerebellar infarction combined with diffuse periventricular white-matter injury, but sparing of the cortex [21–24]. These studies suggest that acute gray-matter injury is probably confined to a subset of infants; this may be an underestimate, since MRI is not sensitive to selective neuronal loss [25,26].

Can acute injury really account for the marked chronic deficits?

The data reviewed above provide compelling evidence that acute subcortical neuronal injury does accompany white-matter injury in a substantial subset of preterm infants. However, this does not seem to be sufficient to explain long-term impairment of brain growth in a majority of premature infants. Indeed, since the preterm cortex is consistently spared both on neuroimaging and histologically [10,22,25], a chronic reduction in cortical volumes must involve additional mechanisms.

Potential mechanisms include loss of the key population of dividing cells that contribute to brain growth such as stem and progenitor cells, and chronic upregulation of programmed cell death. Both are likely to be contributory. Premature birth, before 32 weeks' gestation, corresponds with a phase when large numbers of proliferating immature oligodendrocytes and precursors are present in cerebral white matter [27,28]. In part, then, adverse events may result in a larger long-term impact on brain growth in premature infants than in later life because of loss of progenitor cells that provide the substrate for brain growth [29,30].

In addition, there is increasing evidence that clinical brain injury evolves progressively. Over half of premature infants who go on to develop cerebral palsy do not show white-matter lesions during the first few days to weeks after birth, but have marked white-matter loss on longer-term MRI and evidence of delayed myelination [8]. This is consistent with an experimental study in the postnatal-day-seven rat (broadly equivalent to the preterm infant of around 32 weeks gestation), in which no significant damage was seen during the initial 2 weeks of recovery from moderate hypoxia–ischemia, followed by the development of delayed infarction by 8 weeks [31], in contrast with rapid but non-progressive infarction after a severe insult. Thus, a mild to moderate ischemic insult to the perinatal brain may establish a vulnerable region in which cell death develops over time. This is likely mediated by enhanced physiological apoptosis (programmed cell death).

During normal neural development, cells which are surplus to requirement are eliminated by apoptosis [32]. Cell survival is tightly linked to extrinsic signals from neighboring cells and synaptic activity [33], and thus apoptosis is triggered when cells lose essential input from other cells, for example due to injury elsewhere in the brain or to damage to the interconnecting axons. This ensures matching between the number of myelinating cells and the axonal surface area requiring myelination, and between the number of neurons and the size of their target fields [33].

Thus, loss of input from other cells can trigger secondary cell death. There is evidence of axonal injury within and around periventricular white-matter necrosis [34–36], which may then lead to target deprivation in the cortex. For example, in a recent postmortem study there was diffuse axonal injury both around and distant from areas of white-matter necrosis, while 31% of infants with white-matter injury had thalamic damage and 15% had neuronal injury in the cerebral cortex overlying areas of PVL [36]. These data support the hypothesis that chronic neuronal loss is partly related to acute primary neural injury, and partly to target degeneration secondary to damage to the corticothalamic tracts.

Timing and etiology of preterm brain injury

Although the precise etiology of acute neural injury in preterm infants is still poorly defined, there is increasing evidence that key events include exposure to hypoxia around the time of birth and preceding (in utero) exposure to infection/inflammation. Early imaging, postmortem, and electroencephalogram (EEG) data suggest that neural injury occurs in the immediate perinatal period in approximately two-thirds of cases, while an appreciable number of cases occur before the onset of labor, and cases in the chronic postnatal period are the least common [37–39]. The presence of EEG abnormalities in the perinatal period is highly predictive of long-term outcome [38,40]. In turn, adverse neonatal and long-term outcomes of premature birth are strongly associated with evidence of exposure to perinatal hypoxia, as shown by metabolic acidosis, active labor, abnormal heart rate traces in labor, and subsequent low Apgar scores [37,41,42]. Although severe perinatal hypoxia occurs in only a minority of premature infants, the incidence is much higher (73/1000 live births, of whom 50% are moderate or severe) than at term (25/1000 live births, of whom 15% are moderate or severe) [43]. While clinical encephalopathy is difficult to assess in very premature infants, larger premature infants, from 31 to 36 weeks' gestation, with moderate to severe metabolic acidosis on cord blood, have a high rate of evolving clinical encephalopathy after birth, which in turn is associated with adverse neurological outcome [44].

Mechanisms of hypoxia and ischemic injury

Experimentally, prolonged complete umbilical cord occlusion in preterm fetal sheep at 0.6 and 0.7 of gestation is associated with severe neuronal loss in subcortical gray-matter regions such as the basal ganglia and hippocampus, and diffuse loss of oligodendrocytes in the periventricular white matter, but sparing of the cortex [45–48]. As noted above, this pattern is highly consistent with that seen after clinical asphyxia in preterm infants [22]. These data highlight the observation that preterm fetuses and newborns can consistently survive far longer periods of such profound hypoxia than at term before brain injury occurs [49]. Potentially, this remarkable ability to survive may paradoxically allow the preterm fetus to survive longer periods of severe hypoperfusion than is possible at term, as discussed further in Chapter 14.

Potentially, the localization of white-matter injury to the periventricular region may reflect either anatomical vulnerability or relative vulnerability of different populations of oligodendroglia. Thus, older data suggest that there is a transient watershed zone between the short and long penetrating arteries arising from the pia in premature infants [5], which resolves after 32 weeks' gestation. However, there are recent data from preterm fetal sheep suggesting that the distribution of white-matter damage after cerebral ischemia was not explained by differences in local blood flow [50], and so supporting the hypothesis that it is the presence of a population of relatively susceptible oligodendrocyte progenitors that underlies periventricular white-matter injury.

Postnatal hypotension/hypoperfusion may also contribute to injury. Pathologically low upper-body blood flow was found in one-third of infants born before 30 weeks' gestation [51]. In 80% of cases it was lowest at 5–12 hours of age, and progressively resolved with time; less than 5% of infants had low flows by 48 hours [51,52]. These indirect estimates of cerebral perfusion are supported by evidence of cerebral hypoperfusion on near-infrared spectroscopy [53], and the finding that hypoperfusion is strongly and independently associated with mortality and adverse neurodevelopmental outcome [54].

The mechanisms of this early hypoperfusion are widely debated. It has been suggested that this is potentiated by immaturity of the cerebrovascular autoregulatory response, leading to a pressure-passive circulation whereby cerebral blood flow is reduced in response to even mild systemic hypotension [55]. Some support for this hypothesis is seen in the finding that many premature infants show a temporal association between changes in mean arterial pressure and intravascular cerebral oxygenation consistent with reduced autoregulation [56]. Further, systemic hypotension after preterm birth has been associated with neurological deficits in some studies [57–59]. In contrast, many studies in preterm infants have *not* found an association between hypotension during the early neonatal period and PVL or cerebral palsy [60–64]. Curiously, one study found an association only with one definition of hypotension but not with others, and even then only for "larger" preterm infants $\geq 27/40$ and those with less severe illness [64]. This may be because blood pressure is a poor marker of impaired cardiac output, and thus of reduced cerebral perfusion [51], and many infants who later develop PVL had impaired superior vena cava flow despite normal blood pressure [51]. Some have speculated that, in part, systemic hypoperfusion may be a secondary consequence of preceding exposure to hypoxia [65]. Clearly it is essential to better understand the underlying etiology of hypotension or hypoperfusion before we can understand what to treat. It is striking, for example, that there is still no systematic evidence that treating blood pressure with volume or inotropic agents improves outcome for the majority of babies [66].

Glutamate excitotoxicity and preterm white-matter injury

It is widely hypothesized that exposure of the immature white matter to excitatory amino acids such as glutamate ("excitotoxicity") during or after exposure to hypoxia–ischemia plays a pivotal role in preterm periventricular white-matter injury [5]. It is well established that extracellular glutamate increases dramatically in gray matter during severe hypoxia–ischemia in the term-equivalent and older fetus and newborn [67], and that glutamate is highly toxic in vitro [68]. However, even in gray matter there is no clear correlation between the regional increase in glutamate levels during hypoxia–ischemia and ultimate cell death [69], pointing towards differential glutamate receptor distribution and composition as central to in vivo cellular vulnerability [70].

Since white matter lacks synapses it may seem counterintuitive to implicate glutamate in oligodendrocyte injury. Exposure to high-dose glutaminergic agonists causes severe loss of immature oligodendrocytes both in vivo and in vitro [71,72], and there is in vitro evidence that the major excitatory amino acid, glutamate, can be released from developing oligodendrocytes and axons during hypoxia–ischemia [73,74], for example, through reversal of the glutamate transporter [73,74]. Oligodendrocytes express high levels of the α-amino-3-hydroxy-5-methyl-4-isoxazolepropionic acid (AMPA) subtype of glutamate receptor [75], and there is some evidence for transient overexpression of Ca^{2+}-permeable AMPA receptors that could contribute to selective vulnerability of premyelinating oligodendrocytes to hypoxia compared with mature cells [76]. However, against this, in the fetal sheep analysis of receptor subunit expression suggested a high expression of calcium-permeable AMPA receptors in subcortical white matter from near-mid-gestation to term [75]. Finally, there are limited data in the neonatal rat that AMPA receptor blockade after hypoxia–ischemia can reduce loss of oligodendrocytes [77].

Despite these data, it remains unclear whether excitatory amino acids are released by oligodendrocytes or astrocytes at meaningful levels during ischemia in vivo. Although hypoxia–ischemia was associated with a reduction in intracellular glutamate-like reactivity in axons and oligodendrocytes in the white matter of the neonatal rat, extracellular levels of glutamate were not measured [78]. In contrast, a recent study in preterm (0.65 gestation) fetal sheep, an age closely equivalent to the 26- to 28-week human fetus [50], used microdialysis to demonstrate that there was no significant change in extracellular glutamate levels during or shortly after severe cerebral ischemia in periventricular white matter [79]. Although a subset of fetuses that were exposed to severe cerebral ischemia showed a delayed increase in extracellular accumulation of most excitatory amino acids, this occurred many days after ischemia, at a time when secondary cytotoxic edema was present [80], strongly suggesting that these changes are mainly an epiphenomenon of failure of release–reuptake mechanisms during evolving cell death, and cell lysis.

These findings are consistent with data from more mature animals that suggest that there is either no or a minimal increase in extracellular glutamate levels in the white-matter tracts during ischemia or asphyxia, despite a considerable rise in gray matter [81–83]. Indeed, in adult cats, whereas extracellular calcium levels rapidly fell after the start of ischemia in gray matter, they actually increased in white matter during the first 20–30 minutes of ischemia, and then gradually declined [84], consistent with a lack of acute synaptic activation in white matter during ischemia.

Oxygen free radicals

Alternatively, immature oligodendroglia are also more vulnerable to oxygen free radicals (OFRs) in vitro than mature cells [85]. Such oxidative stress can be mediated by increased extracellular glutamate levels via non-receptor-mediated toxicity in vitro [86], but other pathways may be involved. Consistent with a significant role for OFRs, elevated cerebrospinal-fluid (CSF) levels of the lipid peroxidation products, malondialdehyde (MDA) and 8-isoprostane, in the human premature infant are associated with adverse outcomes [87], and protein nitration and lipid peroxidation of premyelinating oligodendrocytes occurs in the diffuse component of PVL [88]. Experimentally, there was a marked increase in cerebral ascorbyl radical production in preterm fetal sheep following umbilical-cord occlusion, a model that led to subsequent white-matter injury [89].

In contrast, Fraser *et al.* found that there was no overall evidence of increased lipid peroxidation in periventricular white matter after cerebral ischemia in preterm fetal sheep [79]. There was only a trend to increased 8-isoprostane after ischemia, while MDA increased during the secondary phase of cytotoxic edema, suggesting that lipid peroxidation is also primarily linked with cell death in developing white matter [79]. Further, the finding that excitatory amino acid levels were not raised during even severe ischemia also strongly suggests that non-receptor-mediated glutamate toxicity (Fig. 4.1) [86] is unlikely to make a material contribution to PVL. However, it remains possible that there may be aberrantly enhanced activation of Ca^{2+}-permeable AMPA/kainate receptors in response to physiological extracellular levels of glutamate in the first few hours after cerebral ischemia [90]. Such a mechanism would be consistent with the apparent beneficial effects of AMPA/kainate receptor blockade after hypoxia–ischemia [77], and should be explored further.

Infection/inflammation and preterm brain injury

In addition to exposure to hypoxia–ischemia, there is increasing evidence of a link between exposure to infection and inflammation and brain damage in preterm infants. Exposure to bacteria and their products such as endotoxin can trigger an inflammatory reaction in the mother or child. This self-defense reaction helps to eliminate or neutralize injurious

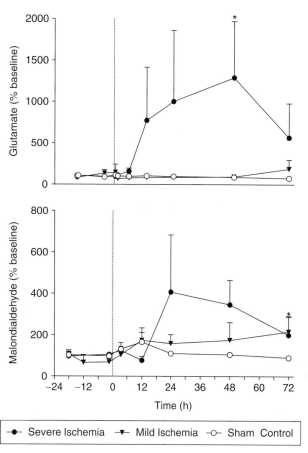

Fig. 4.1. Time course of the percentage change in extracellular levels of glutamate (top panel) and the lipid peroxidation product malondialdehyde (bottom panel) as measured by microdialysis in periventricular white matter in preterm fetal sheep before, during, and after 30 minutes of cerebral ischemia (starting at time zero, shown by the dashed line). Note that malondialdehyde was not measured during ischemia because of sample volume limitations. *$p < 0.05$, severe vs. sham-occlusion group by ANCOVA. There was no significant accumulation of either excitatory amino acids such as glutamate or lipid peroxidation products during or shortly after severe cerebral ischemia that was associated with PVL, whereas there was a marked rise well after ischemia [79]. Data are mean ± SEM.

stimuli and restore tissue integrity [91]. However, excessive neural inflammation may contribute to neural injury [92].

Chorioamnionitis (low-grade infection of the chorionic and amniotic membranes) complicates more than 25% of preterm pregnancies and is strongly associated with preterm labor [93]. In turn, fetal vasculitis (inflammation of blood vessels) in the chorionic plate of the placenta and/or umbilical cord, and high levels of proinflammatory cytokines in amniotic and umbilical blood, are all highly associated with risk of periventricular white-matter injury in premature babies and with later cerebral palsy, as recently reviewed [93].

It is striking that cerebral palsy is much more strongly associated with fetal vasculitis than with chorioamnionitis [92,93]. This suggests that it is the fetal inflammatory response that mediates white-matter injury. These data lead to the hypothesis that inflammatory cytokines released during intra-uterine infection both promote preterm delivery and trigger or exacerbate the development of neural injury in premature infants, and later cerebral palsy [93,94].

Cytokines and preterm brain injury

Increased levels of proinflammatory cytokines such as IL-6 and TNF-α in cord blood or amniotic fluid have been associated with abnormal cranial ultrasound appearances consistent with white-matter injury and later impaired neurodevelopmental outcome [92]. Preterm infants with cerebral white-matter injury on MRI had higher levels of IL-6, IL-10, and TNF-α in the CSF than infants without white-matter injury [95]. Similarly, elevated cytokine levels in umbilical-cord blood predicted cerebral lesions on MRI soon after delivery [96]. In autopsy studies, increased expression of TNF-α, IL-1β, and IL-6 are observed in white-matter lesions, mainly in hypertrophic astrocytes and microglial cells around the area of injury [93,97].

Experimental evidence for a pathological role for infection and cytokines

There is increasing direct experimental evidence that these clinical associations are causal. For example, intrauterine infection with Gram-negative bacteria in the rabbit leads to fetal white-matter lesions [93]. In order to investigate the mechanisms of this link, most studies have used the Gram-negative endotoxin lipopolysaccharide (LPS), a potent inflammatory agent that initiates most components of an inflammatory response [98]. LPS given to the mother intra-amniotically, and to the fetus in a variety of species including the fetal rat, mouse, and sheep, is associated with white-matter damage [92].

The cytokines upregulated following LPS administration include IL-6, IL-8, and TNF-α [98–100]. Their levels typically increase within 2–6 hours after LPS administration and then resolve [98], and there is marked attenuation of response with repeated exposure [98]. In fetal sheep, plasma IL-6 and IL-8 concentrations were undetectable 28 days after LPS exposure [99].

In turn, there is evidence that exogenous administration or overexpression of cytokines increases hypoxic or excitotoxic injury in white and gray matter [101], whereas inhibition or downregulation of cytokines can reduce ischemic injury [102,103]. Further, in adult mice, neural inflammation precedes the progressive enlargement of brain infarction after hypoxia–ischemia, suggesting that the inflammation is causal rather than a consequence of damage [102].

It is important to appreciate that some cytokines have anti-inflammatory [104] and neuroprotective properties [105]. For example, exogenous transforming growth factor β (TGF-β) or IL-10 can reduce post-ischemic injury [106,107]. Thus, it is likely that the balance between pro- and anti-inflammatory mediators helps to determine whether the inflammatory response causes injury. The potential mechanisms of inflammatory injury include direct toxicity to neurons and white-matter cells; immature oligodendrocytes at the stage found in premature infants when they are at greatest risk of PVL [27] seem to be particularly vulnerable [108].

Cytokines can induce apoptosis in many cell types, and promote stimulation of capillary endothelial cell proinflammatory responses and leukocyte adhesion and infiltration into the ischemic brain [109]. Further, intracerebral injection of cytokines induces a marked local astrogliosis [110], and cytokines trigger microglial activation with subsequent release of nitric oxide, superoxides, and other inflammatory mediators [111]. Combined neuronal and inducible nitric oxide synthase inhibition in the newborn rat is neuroprotective after hypoxia–ischemia, without altering cytokine responses [112], strongly suggesting that much of the toxicity associated with cytokine induction is mediated through release of inducible nitric oxide from microglia.

The role of microglia

Microglia form a network of endogenous immunocompetent cells whose primary function is to provide continuous surveillance of the parenchyma and protect the brain during injury and disease [113]. In parallel with the evidence that inflammation has both protective and damaging effects, activated microglia seem to be a "double-edged sword" in the central nervous system [114]. In vitro, for example, microglia promote viability and differentiation of oligodendrocyte progenitor cells under physiological conditions, whereas they mediate cytotoxic effects after activation by LPS [115]. Activated microglia produce a range of potentially toxic mediators, including cytokines, which in turn increase the permeability of the blood–brain barrier [116], and may increase entry of macrophages and leukocytes into the brain. High levels of TNF-α, IL-6, and IFN-γ are expressed in macrophages and/or astrocytes in regions of white-matter damage in the developing brain [93,117].

Consistent with these data, LPS exposure in fetal sheep was associated with microgliosis rather than astrogliosis in regions of subcortical white-matter injury [100]. There was a significant correlation between the intensity of microglial/macrophage invasion and the severity of white-matter injury, supporting a role for microglial activation in the manifestation of and/or response to injury [100]. A similar link has been reported after excitotoxin damage in mice [118] and in neonatal human neuropathology [119]. It is still unclear whether these cells mainly originate from populations of microglia resident in the brain, or may be macrophages invading from the circulation [100].

Conversely, suppression of microglial activation with the tetracycline antibiotic minocycline reduced neural cell loss after LPS infusion in neonatal rats [120]. Similarly, reduced white-matter injury with IL-10 injections in fetal rat pups that had been exposed to E. coli infection was associated with suppression of microglial activation, supporting a central role for activated microglia in the genesis of antenatal PVL [121].

Potential confounding factors

Potential confounding factors associated with exposure to bacterial products, and the inflammatory response in general, include pyrexia and secondary tissue hypoxia. For example, maternal pyrexia is associated with adverse neurological outcome in newborn infants, and hyperthermia greatly exacerbates neurological injury after hypoxia–ischemia [122]. However, fetal infusions of LPS do not cause pyrexia [123], and thus LPS can cause white-matter injury independently of pyrexia [98,124]. Infection/inflammation may also be associated with secondary hypoxemia and transient hypotension that could compromise cerebral perfusion [98,125]. However, in practice, in preterm fetal sheep carotid blood flow was increased despite the fall in blood pressure [125]. Further, others found mild cerebral injury despite no change in mean arterial blood pressure following a single intra-amniotic dose of LPS in near-term fetal sheep [126].

Exposure to infection can sensitize to hypoxia–ischemia

It is important to appreciate that direct injury is not the only possible adverse effect of exposure to inflammatory agents. There is increasing evidence that exposure to LPS modifies responses to subsequent hypoxia–ischemia [127,128]. A low dose of LPS given either shortly (4 or 6 hours) or well before (72 hours or more) hypoxia–ischemia in rat pups was associated with increased injury ("sensitization") [127,129]. Curiously, when given at an intermediate time (24 hours) before hypoxia–ischemia, LPS actually reduced injury [129]. Further, in mice fetal exposure to endotoxin affected the responses to hypoxia–ischemia even in adulthood, with both reduced and increased injury, in different regions [130]. The mechanisms for this complex sensitization are unclear. One study implicated changes in blood glucose levels [131]; however, normalization of blood glucose levels did not prevent sensitization, and so other factors are likely to be involved, such as chronic changes in glial responses [132].

Conclusion

In conclusion, the most striking concept to emerge from recent clinical and experimental studies of the very immature brain has been that perinatal white-matter injury is associated with both acute subcortical gray-matter injury and a long-term reduction in cortical complexity and cortical and subcortical volume, and with cognitive impairment. The emerging concept which underpins these observations is that acute early white- and gray-matter cell loss is associated with exposure to hypoxia and to infection/inflammation, and that this acute injury initiates a phase of chronic programmed cell death that underlies

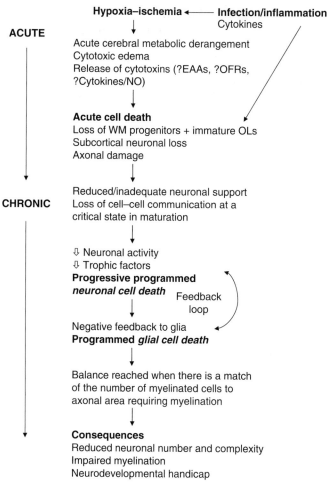

Fig. 4.2. Flow diagram outlining the hypothesized relationship between acute hypoxic injury in the developing brain, exposure to infection/inflammation, and long-term reductions in regional brain growth. OFR, oxygen free radicals; EAA, excitatory amino acids; WM, white matter; NO, nitric oxide; OLs, oligodendrocytes.

impaired neurodevelopment (Fig. 4.2). The widely hypothesized roles for free-radical-mediated injury and excitotoxicity on the one hand, and of hypotension/hypoperfusion on the other, remain surprising unclear, and require further research.

Acknowledgments

The authors' work reported in this review has been supported by the Health Research Council of New Zealand, the Lottery Health Board of New Zealand, the Auckland Medical Research Foundation, and the March of Dimes Birth Defects Foundation.

References

1. Wilson-Costello D, Friedman H, Minich N, *et al.* Improved survival rates with increased neurodevelopmental disability for extremely low birth weight infants in the 1990s. *Pediatrics* 2005; **115**: 997–1003.

2. Bhushan V, Paneth N, Kiely JL. Impact of improved survival of very low birth weight infants on recent secular trends in the prevalence of cerebral palsy. *Pediatrics* 1993; **91**: 1094–100.

3. Wilson-Costello D, Friedman H, Minich N, *et al.* Improved neurodevelopmental outcomes for extremely low birth weight infants in 2000–2002. *Pediatrics* 2007; **119**: 37–45.

4. Hack M. Young adult outcomes of very-low-birth-weight children. *Semin Fetal Neonatal Med* 2006; **11**: 127–37.

5. Volpe JJ. Neurobiology of periventricular leukomalacia in the premature infant. *Pediatr Res* 2001; **50**: 553–62.

6. Inder TE, Anderson NJ, Spencer C, *et al.* White matter injury in the premature infant: a comparison between serial cranial sonographic and MR findings at term. *AJNR Am J Neuroradiol* 2003; **24**: 805–9.

7. Maalouf EF, Duggan PJ, Rutherford MA, *et al.* Magnetic resonance imaging of the brain in a cohort of extremely preterm infants. *J Pediatr* 1999; **135**: 351–7.

8. Woodward LJ, Anderson PJ, Austin NC, *et al.* Neonatal MRI to predict neurodevelopmental outcomes in preterm infants. *N Engl J Med* 2006; **355**: 685–94.

9. Miller SP, Ferriero DM, Leonard C, *et al.* Early brain injury in premature newborns detected with magnetic resonance imaging is associated with adverse early neurodevelopmental outcome. *J Pediatr* 2005; **147**: 609–16.

10. Pierson CR, Folkerth RD, Billiards SS, *et al.* Gray matter injury associated with periventricular leukomalacia in the premature infant. *Acta Neuropathol (Berl)* 2007; **114**: 619–31.

11. Hamrick SE, Miller SP, Leonard C, *et al.* Trends in severe brain injury and neurodevelopmental outcome in premature newborn infants: the role of cystic periventricular leukomalacia. *J Pediatr* 2004; **145**: 593–9.

12. Lin Y, Okumura A, Hayakawa F, *et al.* Quantitative evaluation of thalami and basal ganglia in infants with periventricular leukomalacia. *Dev Med Child Neurol* 2001; **43**: 481–5.

13. Peterson BS, Vohr B, Staib LH, *et al.* Regional brain volume abnormalities and long-term cognitive outcome in preterm infants. *JAMA* 2000; **284**: 1939–47.

14. Ajayi-Obe M, Saeed N, Cowan FM, *et al.* Reduced development of cerebral cortex in extremely preterm infants. *Lancet* 2000; **356**: 1162–3.

15. Nosarti C, Al-Asady MH, Frangou S, *et al.* Adolescents who were born very preterm have decreased brain volumes. *Brain* 2002; **125**: 1616–23.

16. Martinussen M, Fischl B, Larsson HB, *et al.* Cerebral cortex thickness in 15-year-old adolescents with low birth weight measured by an automated MRI-based method. *Brain* 2005; **128**: 2588–96.

17. Isaacs EB, Edmonds CJ, Chong WK, *et al.* Brain morphometry and IQ measurements in preterm children. *Brain* 2004; **127**: 2595–607.

18. Abernethy LJ, Cooke RW, Foulder-Hughes L. Caudate and hippocampal volumes, intelligence, and motor impairment in 7-year-old children who were born preterm. *Pediatr Res* 2004; **55**: 884–93.

19. Gimenez M, Junque C, Narberhaus A, *et al.* Hippocampal gray matter reduction associates with memory deficits in adolescents with history of prematurity. *Neuroimage* 2004; **23**: 869–77.

20. Bell JE, Becher JC, Wyatt B, *et al.* Brain damage and axonal injury in a Scottish cohort of neonatal deaths. *Brain* 2005; **128**: 1070–81.

21. Johnsen SD, Tarby TJ, Lewis KS, *et al.* Cerebellar infarction: an unrecognized complication of very low birthweight. *J Child Neurol* 2002; **17**: 320–4.

22. Barkovich AJ, Sargent SK. Profound asphyxia in the premature infant: imaging findings. *AJNR Am J Neuroradiol* 1995; **16**: 1837–46.

23. de Vries LS, Smet M, Goemans N, *et al.* Unilateral thalamic haemorrhage in the pre-term and full-term newborn. *Neuropediatrics* 1992; **23**: 153–6.

24. Leijser LM, Klein RH, Veen S, *et al.* Hyperechogenicity of the thalamus and basal ganglia in very preterm infants: radiological findings and short-term neurological outcome. *Neuropediatrics* 2004; **35**: 283–9.

25. Felderhoff-Mueser U, Rutherford MA, Squier WV, *et al.* Relationship between MR imaging and histopathologic findings of the brain in extremely sick preterm infants. *AJNR Am J Neuroradiol* 1999; **20**: 1349–57.

26. Fraser M, Bennet L, Helliwell R, *et al.* Regional specificity of magnetic resonance imaging for cerebral ischemic changes in preterm fetal sheep. *Reprod Sci* 2007; **14**: 182–91.

27. Back SA, Luo NL, Borenstein NS, *et al.* Late oligodendrocyte progenitors coincide with the developmental window of vulnerability for human perinatal white matter injury. *J Neurosci* 2001; **21**: 1302–12.

28. de Graaf-Peters VB, Hadders-Algra M. Ontogeny of the human central nervous system: what is happening when? *Early Hum Dev* 2006; **82**: 257–66.

29. Romanko MJ, Rothstein RP, Levison SW. Neural stem cells in the subventricular zone are resilient to hypoxia/ischemia whereas progenitors are vulnerable. *J Cereb Blood Flow Metab* 2004; **24**: 814–25.

30. Barrett RD, Bennet L, Davidson J, *et al.* Destruction and reconstruction: hypoxia and the developing brain. *Birth Defects Res C Embryo Today* 2007; **81**: 163–76.

31. Geddes R, Vannucci RC, Vannucci SJ. Delayed cerebral atrophy following moderate hypoxia–ischemia in the immature rat. *Dev Neurosci* 2001; **23**: 180–5.

32. Goldberg JL, Barres BA. The relationship between neuronal survival and regeneration. *Annu Rev Neurosci* 2000; **23**: 579–612.

33. Jacobson MD, Weil M, Raff MC. Programmed cell death in animal development. *Cell* 1997; **88**: 347–54.

34. Meng SZ, Arai Y, Deguchi K, *et al.* Early detection of axonal and neuronal lesions in prenatal-onset periventricular leukomalacia. *Brain Dev* 1997; **19**: 480–4.

35. Hirayama A, Okoshi Y, Hachiya Y, *et al.* Early immunohistochemical detection of axonal damage and glial activation in extremely immature brains with periventricular leukomalacia. *Clin Neuropathol* 2001; **20**: 87–91.

36. Haynes RL, Billiards SS, Borenstein NS, *et al.* Diffuse axonal injury in periventricular leukomalacia as determined by apoptotic marker fractin. *Pediatr Res* 2008; **63**: 656–61.

37. de Vries LS, Eken P, Groenendaal F, *et al.* Antenatal onset of haemorrhagic and/or ischaemic lesions in preterm infants: prevalence and associated obstetric variables. *Arch Dis Child Fetal Neonatal Ed* 1998; **78**: F51–6.

38. Hayakawa F, Okumura A, Kato T, *et al.* Determination of timing of brain injury in preterm infants with periventricular leukomalacia with serial neonatal electroencephalography. *Pediatrics* 1999; **104**: 1077–81.

39. Becher JC, Bell JE, Keeling JW, *et al.* The Scottish perinatal neuropathology study: clinicopathological correlation in early neonatal deaths. *Arch Dis Child Fetal Neonatal Ed* 2004; **89**: F399–407.

40. Kubota T, Okumura A, Hayakawa F, *et al.* Combination of neonatal electroencephalography and ultrasonography: sensitive means of early diagnosis of periventricular leukomalacia. *Brain Dev* 2002; **24**: 698–702.

41. Weinberger B, Anwar M, Hegyi T, *et al.* Antecedents and neonatal consequences of low Apgar scores in preterm newborns: a population study. *Arch Pediatr Adolesc Med* 2000; **154**: 294–300.

42. Osborn DA, Evans N, Kluckow M. Hemodynamic and antecedent risk factors of early and late periventricular/intraventricular hemorrhage in premature infants. *Pediatrics* 2003; **112**: 33–9.

43. Low JA. Determining the contribution of asphyxia to brain damage in the neonate. *J Obstet Gynaecol Res* 2004; **30**: 276–86.

44. Salhab WA, Perlman JM. Severe fetal acidemia and subsequent neonatal encephalopathy in the larger premature infant. *Pediatr Neurol* 2005; **32**: 25–9.

45. George S, Gunn AJ, Westgate JA, *et al.* Fetal heart rate variability and brainstem injury after asphyxia in preterm fetal sheep. *Am J Physiol Regul Integr Comp Physiol* 2004; **287**: R925–33.

46. Dean JM, George SA, Wassink G, *et al.* Suppression of post hypoxic–ischemic EEG transients with dizocilpine is associated with partial striatal protection in the preterm fetal sheep. *Neuropharmacology* 2006; **50**: 491–503.

47. Dean JM, Gunn AJ, Wassink G, *et al.* Endogenous α_2-adrenergic receptor-mediated neuroprotection after severe hypoxia in preterm fetal sheep. *Neuroscience* 2006; **142**: 615–28.

48. Bennet L, Roelfsema V, George S, *et al.* The effect of cerebral hypothermia on white and grey matter injury induced by severe hypoxia in preterm fetal sheep. *J Physiol* 2007; **578**: 491–506.

49. Gunn AJ, Quaedackers JS, Guan J, *et al.* The premature fetus: not as defenseless as we thought, but still paradoxically vulnerable? *Dev Neurosci* 2001; **23**: 175–9.

50. Riddle A, Luo NL, Manese M, *et al.* Spatial heterogeneity in oligodendrocyte lineage maturation and not cerebral blood flow predicts fetal ovine periventricular white matter injury. *J Neurosci* 2006; **26**: 3045–55.

51. Osborn DA, Evans N, Kluckow M. Clinical detection of low upper body blood flow in very premature infants using blood pressure, capillary refill time, and central–peripheral temperature difference. *Arch Dis Child Fetal Neonatal Ed* 2004; **89**: F168–73.

52. Kluckow M, Evans N. Superior vena cava flow in newborn infants: a novel marker of systemic blood flow. *Arch Dis Child Fetal Neonatal Ed* 2000; **82**: F182–7.

53. Meek JH, Elwell CE, McCormick DC, *et al.* Abnormal cerebral haemodynamics in perinatally asphyxiated neonates related to outcome. *Arch Dis Child Fetal Neonatal Ed* 1999; **81**: F110–15.

54. Hunt RW, Evans N, Rieger I, *et al.* Low superior vena cava flow and neurodevelopment at 3 years in very preterm infants. *J Pediatr* 2004; **145**: 588–92.

55. Lou HC, Lassen NA, Tweed WA, *et al.* Pressure passive cerebral blood flow and breakdown of the blood–brain barrier in experimental fetal asphyxia. *Acta Paediatr Scand* 1979; **68**: 57–63.

56. Soul JS, Hammer PE, Tsuji M, *et al.* Fluctuating pressure-passivity is common in the cerebral circulation of sick premature infants. *Pediatr Res* 2007; **61**: 467–73.

57. Martens SE, Rijken M, Stoelhorst GM, *et al.* Is hypotension a major risk factor for neurological morbidity at term age in very preterm infants? *Early Hum Dev* 2003; **75**: 79–89.

58. Murphy DJ, Hope PL, Johnson A. Neonatal risk factors for cerebral palsy in very preterm babies: case–control study. *BMJ* 1997; **314**: 404–8.

59. Low JA, Froese AB, Galbraith RS, *et al.* The association between preterm newborn hypotension and hypoxemia and outcome during the first year. *Acta Paediatr* 1993; **82**: 433–7.

60. Trounce JQ, Shaw DE, Levene MI, *et al.* Clinical risk factors and periventricular leucomalacia. *Arch Dis Child* 1988; **63**: 17–22.

61. Perlman JM, Risser R, Broyles RS. Bilateral cystic periventricular leukomalacia in the premature infant: associated risk factors. *Pediatrics* 1996; **97**: 822–7.

62. Dammann O, Allred EN, Kuban KC, *et al.* Systemic hypotension and white-matter damage in preterm infants. *Dev Med Child Neurol* 2002; **44**: 82–90.

63. Cunningham S, Symon AG, Elton RA, *et al.* Intra-arterial blood pressure reference ranges, death and morbidity in very low birthweight infants during the first seven days of life. *Early Hum Dev* 1999; **56**: 151–65.

64. Limperopoulos C, Bassan H, Kalish LA, *et al.* Current definitions of hypotension do not predict abnormal cranial ultrasound findings in preterm infants. *Pediatrics* 2007; **120**: 966–77.

65. Bennet L, Booth L, Malpas SC, *et al.* Acute systemic complications in the preterm fetus after asphyxia: The role of cardiovascular and blood flow responses. *Clin Exp Pharmacol Physiol* 2006; **33**: 291–9.

66. Osborn DA. Diagnosis and treatment of preterm transitional circulatory compromise. *Early Hum Dev* 2005; **81**: 413–22.

67. Tan WK, Williams CE, During MJ, *et al.* Accumulation of cytotoxins during the development of seizures and edema after hypoxic–ischemic injury in late gestation fetal sheep. *Pediatr Res* 1996; **39**: 791–7.

68. Choi DW. Excitotoxic cell death. *J Neurobiol* 1992; **23**: 1261–76.

69. Mitani A, Andou Y, Kataoka K. Selective vulnerability of hippocampal CA1 neurons cannot be explained in terms of an increase in glutamate concentration during ischemia in the gerbil: brain microdialysis study. *Neuroscience* 1992; **48**: 307–13.

70. McDonald JW, Johnston MV, Young AB. Differential ontogenic development of three receptors comprising the NMDA receptor/channel complex in the rat hippocampus. *Exp Neurol* 1990; **110**: 237–47.

71. Fern R, Moller T. Rapid ischemic cell death in immature oligodendrocytes: a fatal glutamate release feedback loop. *J Neurosci* 2000; **20**: 34–42.

72. Follett PL, Rosenberg PA, Volpe JJ, *et al.* NBQX attenuates excitotoxic injury in developing white matter. *J Neurosci* 2000; **20**: 9235–41.

73. Rossi DJ, Oshima T, Attwell D. Glutamate release in severe brain ischaemia is mainly by reversed uptake. *Nature* 2000; **403**: 316–21.

74. Desilva TM, Kinney HC, Borenstein NS, *et al.* The glutamate transporter EAAT2 is transiently expressed in developing human cerebral white matter. *J Comp Neurol* 2007; **501**: 879–90.

75. Dean JM, Fraser M, Shelling AN, *et al.* Ontogeny of AMPA and NMDA receptor gene expression in the developing sheep white matter and cerebral cortex. *Mol Brain Res* 2005; **139**: 242–50.

76. Itoh T, Beesley J, Itoh A, *et al.* AMPA glutamate receptor-mediated calcium signaling is transiently enhanced during development of oligodendrocytes. *J Neurochem* 2002; **81**: 390–402.

77. Follett PL, Deng W, Dai W, *et al.* Glutamate receptor-mediated oligodendrocyte toxicity in periventricular leukomalacia: a protective role for topiramate. *J Neurosci* 2004; **24**: 4412–20.

78. Back SA, Riddle A, McClure MM. Maturation-dependent vulnerability of

perinatal white matter in premature birth. *Stroke* 2007; **38**: 724–30.

79. Fraser M, Bennet L, van Zijl PL, *et al.* Extracellular amino acids and peroxidation products in the periventricular white matter during and after cerebral ischemia in preterm fetal sheep. *J Neurochem* 2008; **105**: 2214–23.

80. Fraser M, Bennet L, Gunning M, *et al.* Cortical electroencephalogram suppression is associated with post-ischemic cortical injury in 0.65 gestation fetal sheep. *Dev Brain Res* 2005; **154**: 45–55.

81. Dohmen C, Kumura E, Rosner G, *et al.* Extracellular correlates of glutamate toxicity in short-term cerebral ischemia and reperfusion: a direct *in vivo* comparison between white and gray matter. *Brain Res* 2005; **1037**: 43–51.

82. Henderson JL, Reynolds JD, Dexter F, *et al.* Chronic hypoxemia causes extracellular glutamate concentration to increase in the cerebral cortex of the near-term fetal sheep. *Dev Brain Res* 1998; **105**: 287–93.

83. Loeliger M, Watson CS, Reynolds JD, *et al.* Extracellular glutamate levels and neuropathology in cerebral white matter following repeated umbilical cord occlusion in the near term fetal sheep. *Neuroscience* 2003; **116**: 705–14.

84. Kumura E, Graf R, Dohmen C, *et al.* Breakdown of calcium homeostasis in relation to tissue depolarization: comparison between gray and white matter ischemia. *J Cereb Blood Flow Metab* 1999; **19**: 788–93.

85. Back SA, Gan X, Li Y, *et al.* Maturation-dependent vulnerability of oligodendrocytes to oxidative stress-induced death caused by glutathione depletion. *J Neurosci* 1998; **18**: 6241–53.

86. Rosin C, Bates TE, Skaper SD. Excitatory amino acid induced oligodendrocyte cell death *in vitro*: receptor-dependent and -independent mechanisms. *J Neurochem* 2004; **90**: 1173–85.

87. Inder T, Mocatta T, Darlow B, *et al.* Elevated free radical products in the cerebrospinal fluid of VLBW infants with cerebral white matter injury. *Pediatr Res* 2002; **52**: 213–18.

88. Haynes RL, Folkerth RD, Keefe RJ, *et al.* Nitrosative and oxidative injury to premyelinating oligodendrocytes in periventricular leukomalacia. *J Neuropathol Exp Neurol* 2003; **62**: 441–50.

89. Welin AK, Sandberg M, Lindblom A, *et al.* White matter injury following prolonged free radical formation in the 0.65 gestation fetal sheep brain. *Pediatr Res* 2005; **58**: 100–5.

90. Deng W, Rosenberg PA, Volpe JJ, *et al.* Calcium-permeable AMPA/kainate receptors mediate toxicity and preconditioning by oxygen-glucose deprivation in oligodendrocyte precursors. *Proc Natl Acad Sci USA* 2003; **100**: 6801–6.

91. Willoughby RE, Nelson KB. Chorioamnionitis and brain injury. *Clin Perinatol* 2002; **29**: 603–21.

92. Wang X, Rousset CI, Hagberg H, *et al.* Lipopolysaccharide-induced inflammation and perinatal brain injury. *Semin Fetal Neonatal Med* 2006; **11**: 343–53.

93. Yoon BH, Park CW, Chaiworapongsa T. Intrauterine infection and the development of cerebral palsy. *BJOG* 2003; **110** (Suppl 20): 124–7.

94. Holcroft CJ, Blakemore KJ, Allen M, *et al.* Association of prematurity and neonatal infection with neurologic morbidity in very low birth weight infants. *Obstet Gynecol* 2003; **101**: 1249–53.

95. Ellison VJ, Mocatta TJ, Winterbourn CC, *et al.* The relationship of CSF and plasma cytokine levels to cerebral white matter injury in the premature newborn. *Pediatr Res* 2005; **57**: 282–6.

96. Duggan PJ, Maalouf EF, Watts TL, *et al.* Intrauterine T-cell activation and increased proinflammatory cytokine concentrations in preterm infants with cerebral lesions. *Lancet* 2001; **358**: 1699–700.

97. Kadhim H, Tabarki B, Verellen G, *et al.* Inflammatory cytokines in the pathogenesis of periventricular leukomalacia. *Neurology* 2001; **56**: 1278–84.

98. Duncan JR, Cock ML, Scheerlinck JP, *et al.* White matter injury after repeated endotoxin exposure in the preterm ovine fetus. *Pediatr Res* 2002; **52**: 941–9.

99. Nitsos I, Rees SM, Duncan J, *et al.* Chronic exposure to intra-amniotic lipopolysaccharide affects the ovine fetal brain. *J Soc Gynecol Investig* 2006; **13**: 239–47.

100. Duncan JR, Cock ML, Suzuki K, *et al.* Chronic endotoxin exposure causes brain injury in the ovine fetus in the absence of hypoxemia. *J Soc Gynecol Investig* 2006; **13**: 87–96.

101. Dommergues MA, Patkai J, Renauld JC, *et al.* Proinflammatory cytokines and interleukin-9 exacerbate excitotoxic lesions of the newborn murine neopallium. *Ann Neurol* 2000; **47**: 54–63.

102. Basu A, Lazovic J, Krady JK, *et al.* Interleukin-1 and the interleukin-1 type 1 receptor are essential for the progressive neurodegeneration that ensues subsequent to a mild hypoxic/ischemic injury. *J Cereb Blood Flow Metab* 2005; **25**: 17–29.

103. Loddick SA, Wong ML, Bongiorno PB, *et al.* Endogenous interleukin-1 receptor antagonist is neuroprotective. *Biochem Biophys Res Commun* 1997; **234**: 211–15.

104. Kremlev SG, Palmer C. Interleukin-10 inhibits endotoxin-induced pro-inflammatory cytokines in microglial cell cultures. *J Neuroimmunol* 2005; **162**: 71–80.

105. Loddick SA, Turnbull AV, Rothwell NJ. Cerebral interleukin-6 is neuroprotective during permanent focal cerebral ischemia in the rat. *J Cereb Blood Flow Metab* 1998; **18**: 176–9.

106. Guan J, Miller OT, Waugh KM, *et al.* TGFβ-1 and neurological function after hypoxia–ischemia in adult rats. *Neuroreport* 2004; **15**: 961–4.

107. Spera PA, Ellison JA, Feuerstein GZ, *et al.* IL-10 reduces rat brain injury following focal stroke. *Neurosci Lett* 1998; **251**: 189–92.

108. Cai Z, Lin S, Pang Y, *et al.* Brain injury induced by intracerebral injection of interleukin-1β and tumor necrosis factor-α in the neonatal rat. *Pediatr Res* 2004; **56**: 377–84.

109. Allan SM, Rothwell NJ. Inflammation in central nervous system injury. *Philos Trans R Soc Lond B Biol Sci* 2003; **358**: 1669–77.

110. Woiciechowsky C, Schoning B, Stoltenburg-Didinger G, *et al.* Brain-IL-1 beta triggers astrogliosis through induction of IL-6: inhibition by propranolol and IL-10. *Med Sci Monit* 2004; **10**: BR325–30.

111. Bal-Price A, Brown GC. Inflammatory neurodegeneration mediated by nitric oxide from activated glia-inhibiting neuronal respiration, causing glutamate release and excitotoxicity. *J Neurosci* 2001; **21**: 6480–91.

112. van den Tweel ER, Nijboer C, Kavelaars A, *et al.* Expression of nitric oxide synthase isoforms and nitrotyrosine formation after hypoxia–ischemia in the neonatal rat brain. *J Neuroimmunol* 2005; **167**: 64–71.

113. Raivich G, Bohatschek M, Kloss CU, *et al.* Neuroglial activation repertoire in the injured brain: graded response, molecular mechanisms and cues to physiological function. *Brain Res Brain Res Rev* 1999; **30**: 77–105.

114. Rock RB, Gekker G, Hu S, *et al.* Role of microglia in central nervous system infections. *Clin Microbiol Rev* 2004; **17**: 942–64.

115. Pang Y, Cai Z, Rhodes PG. Effects of lipopolysaccharide on oligodendrocyte progenitor cells are mediated by astrocytes and microglia. *J Neurosci Res* 2000; **62**: 510–20.

116. Yan E, Castillo-Melendez M, Nicholls T, *et al.* Cerebrovascular responses in the fetal sheep brain to low-dose endotoxin. *Pediatr Res* 2004; **55**: 855–63.

117. Folkerth RD, Keefe RJ, Haynes RL, *et al.* Interferon-gamma expression in periventricular leukomalacia in the human brain. *Brain Pathol* 2004; **14**: 265–74.

118. Tahraoui SL, Marret S, Bodenant C, *et al.* Central role of microglia in neonatal excitotoxic lesions of the murine periventricular white matter. *Brain Pathol* 2001; **11**: 56–71.

119. Kinney HC. Human myelination and perinatal white matter disorders. *J Neurol Sci* 2005; **228**: 190–2.

120. Fan LW, Pang Y, Lin S, *et al.* Minocycline attenuates lipopolysaccharide-induced white matter injury in the neonatal rat brain. *Neuroscience* 2005; **133**: 159–68.

121. Pang Y, Rodts-Palenik S, Cai Z, *et al.* Suppression of glial activation is involved in the protection of IL-10 on maternal *E. coli* induced neonatal white matter injury. *Dev Brain Res* 2005; **157**: 141–9.

122. Gunn AJ, Bennet L. Is temperature important in delivery room resuscitation? *Semin Neonatol* 2001; **6**: 241–9.

123. Yoneyama Y, Sawa R, Kubonoya K, *et al.* Evidence for mechanisms of the acute-phase response to endotoxin in late-gestation fetal goats. *Am J Obstet Gynecol* 1998; **179**: 750–5.

124. Mallard C, Welin AK, Peebles D, *et al.* White matter injury following systemic endotoxemia or asphyxia in the fetal sheep. *Neurochem Res* 2003; **28**: 215–23.

125. Peebles DM, Miller S, Newman JP, *et al.* The effect of systemic administration of lipopolysaccharide on cerebral haemodynamics and oxygenation in the 0.65 gestation ovine fetus in utero. *BJOG* 2003; **110**: 735–43.

126. Nitsos I, Moss TJ, Cock ML, *et al.* Fetal responses to intra-amniotic endotoxin in sheep. *J Soc Gynecol Investig* 2002; **9**: 80–5.

127. Eklind S, Mallard C, Leverin AL, *et al.* Bacterial endotoxin sensitizes the immature brain to hypoxic–ischaemic injury. *Eur J Neurosci* 2001; **13**: 1101–6.

128. Larouche A, Roy M, Kadhim H, *et al.* Neuronal injuries induced by perinatal hypoxic-ischemic insults are potentiated by prenatal exposure to lipopolysaccharide: animal model for perinatally acquired encephalopathy. *Dev Neurosci* 2005; **27**: 134–42.

129. Eklind S, Mallard C, Arvidsson P, *et al.* Lipopolysaccharide induces both a primary and a secondary phase of sensitization in the developing rat brain. *Pediatr Res* 2005; **58**: 112–16.

130. Wang X, Hagberg H, Nie C, *et al.* Dual role of intrauterine immune challenge on neonatal and adult brain vulnerability to hypoxia–ischemia. *J Neuropathol Exp Neurol* 2007; **66**: 552–61.

131. Eklind S, Arvidsson P, Hagberg H, *et al.* The role of glucose in brain injury following the combination of lipopolysaccharide or lipoteichoic acid and hypoxia–ischemia in neonatal rats. *Dev Neurosci* 2004; **26**: 61–7.

132. Kramer BW, Joshi SN, Moss TJ, *et al.* Endotoxin-induced maturation of monocytes in preterm fetal sheep lung. *Am J Physiol Lung Cell Mol Physiol* 2007; **293**: L345–53.

Pregnancy, labor, and delivery complications causing brain injury
Prematurity and complications of labor and delivery

Yasser Y. El-Sayed, Maurice L. Druzin, Justin Collingham, and Amen Ness

Introduction

Prematurity is a major contributor to perinatal morbidity and mortality in the USA and around the world. Preterm birth is officially defined as delivery occurring prior to 37 completed weeks from the first day of the last menstrual period [1]. The term "low birthweight" is used to describe infants weighing less than 2500 g at birth. This includes neonates who are born after 37 weeks gestational age, of which approximately one-third are in the category of "growth restriction." This group of neonates is distinct from the group of premature infants, and is the subject of another chapter (see Chapter 7). The discussion in this chapter will be confined to the preterm fetus, that which is delivered between viability (23–24 weeks) and 37 completed weeks of gestation.

Complications of labor and delivery in both preterm and term gestations have been implicated in adverse neonatal outcomes. Traditionally, cerebral palsy and "brain damage" have been linked to intrapartum events that resulted in "birth asphyxia" and subsequent neurologic damage. This association has continued to be proposed despite the fact that current evidence suggests that only about 10% of patients with cerebral palsy, about 1–2 per 10 000 births, experience serious birth asphyxia [2]. Most studies in this field refer to the term fetus. The preterm neonate has its own unique complications and resultant sequelae.

The problem of preterm birth

In the United States, one out of eight infants is born preterm. The incidence of preterm birth has increased by 30% over the past 20 years, reaching 12.7% in 2005 [3]. Although preterm deliveries occur in only about 13% of all pregnancies, they account for one in five children with mental retardation, and one in three children with vision impairment, and almost half of children with cerebral palsy [4].

Two-thirds of preterm births follow preterm labor or premature rupture of membranes, while one-third are due to indicated preterm deliveries for maternal or fetal indications. The incidence of preterm birth among African-Americans is twice that of whites, and it is the leading cause of death among African-American infants [1]. Preterm births also account for the majority of perinatal deaths around the world [4]. Birthweight is the best predictor of survival after 30 weeks gestation, while gestational age predicts survival prior to 30 weeks. The lower limits of viability are changing, and recent studies have demonstrated survival and improved short-term outcome at gestational ages as early as 23–24 weeks [5]. However, delivery prior to 27 weeks has a high incidence of serious long-term impairment [6]. Major improvements in survival occur with each completed week of gestation from 24 to 33 weeks, after which time minimal increases in survival occur, although morbidity may be decreased.

Yet, despite the significant improvements in the survival of preterm infants over the last 10–20 years, there has been little if any improvement in neonatal morbidity; in fact there is some evidence that rates of disability have increased [7]. The neurological morbidity suffered by these infants imposes a considerable burden on families and the health system.

Traditionally, brain injury in preterm infants has been thought to reflect a fundamental vulnerability to damage of immature oligodendrocytes in periventricular white matter. Cerebral white-matter injury is the most common form of brain injury in preterm infants. This lesion occurs predominantly in neonates less than 34 weeks, and in this group 60–100% of survivors develop cerebral palsy [8].

However, recent evidence suggests a much more complex picture. Experimental studies have consistently shown that premature animals can survive far longer periods of profound hypoxia or ischemia before injury occurs than at term or postnatally [9]. The mechanisms that mediate this remarkable tolerance to hypoxia of the preterm brain are not fully understood. Yet it is precisely this tolerance that, although allowing for survival, may increase the risk for neurologic injury [10].

This chapter will review the etiologies, management, and complications of preterm birth which impact the risks for neurologic injury related to prematurity.

Etiology of preterm birth

A history of preterm birth is associated with a 20–40% recurrence risk [11]. Preterm delivery may result from preterm labor, preterm premature rupture of membranes (PPROM), or maternal or fetal conditions requiring intervention for

Fetal and Neonatal Brain Injury, 4th edition, ed. David K. Stevenson, William E. Benitz, Philip Sunshine, Susan R. Hintz, and Maurice L. Druzin. Published by Cambridge University Press. © Cambridge University Press 2009.

maternal or fetal reasons. Fetal indications for delivery include non-reassuring fetal status, placental insufficiency, chorioamnionitis, and abruption placentae, while maternal factors include hypertensive disorders and other maternal illness. The short- and long-term outcomes for these infants has continued to improve as a result of the widespread use of antenatal corticosteroids, liberal use of cesarean delivery for fetal indications, and improvements in neonatal resuscitation with the use of surfactant therapy.

The majority of preterm births result from preterm labor and PPROM, with approximately 20% resulting from maternal/fetal indications for delivery. The cause of premature birth may vary according to socioeconomic status, with the incidence of PPROM being higher in lower socioeconomic groups [12].

The pathogenesis of spontaneous preterm labor with intact membranes has been categorized into four general pathogenic pathways. These are (1) maternal and/or fetal stress with premature activation of the placental–fetal hypothalamic–pituitary–adrenal axis, (2) inflammation resulting from either systemic inflammation or local infection, (3) abruption/decidual hemorrhage, and (4) mechanical stretching from either multiple gestation or polyhydramnios. Intra-amniotic infection/inflammation may be unrecognized, as these patients often do not have overt evidence of chorioamnionitis [17, 18]. They may have preterm labor that is refractory to tocolysis [13–16]. In addition, there is evidence to suggest that maternal and fetal genotypes may play a role in the genesis of preterm birth.

Demographic factors

Lower socioeconomic status, ethnicity, and maternal age all have been associated with increased incidence of preterm birth [19]. African-American women have an incidence of preterm birth that is about double that of Caucasian women. Even if socioeconomic status is accounted for, this disparity remains apparent [20]. The incidence of preterm birth is higher in women under the age of 20 years irrespective of whether they have their first or subsequent pregnancies before age 20 years. First pregnancies after age 35 years are also at increased risk for preterm birth [21]. Poor nutritional status and inadequate weight gain during pregnancy are associated with an increased incidence of preterm birth [22].

A body mass index (BMI) less than 19.8 kg/m^2, a large interpregnancy weight loss (decrease in one BMI category or more than 5 kg/m^2), or a short interpregnancy interval (less than 18 months) have all been shown to increase the risk for a preterm birth [4].

Substance abuse

Cocaine abuse [23], alcohol use, and cigarette smoking [24] have all been associated with increased rates of preterm birth. The confounding variables of poor nutrition, inadequate weight gain, and associated medical problems seen commonly in patients suffering substance abuse make it difficult to pinpoint the exact etiology of preterm delivery in such cases.

Obstetrical risk factors

As noted, a history of preterm birth is one of the most important risk factors for subsequent preterm delivery. The risk increases with the number of preterm births, and is higher the earlier in gestation they occurred, and it decreases with the number of term deliveries [25]. There is some debate over whether induced abortions in the first trimester increase the rate of preterm delivery [26,27]. There seems to be an increased incidence in women who have had second-trimester terminations [21].

Multiple gestations account for about 10% of all preterm births in the USA, where the incidence of multiple births increased from 2.4% of all births in 1992 to 3.3% in 2002 (38% increase) [28]. Between 30% and 50% of multiple gestations deliver prior to 37 weeks, with higher-order multiple gestations delivering the earliest [29,30]. Approximately 94% of multiple gestations are twins, which deliver preterm about 55% of the time. Thus the majority of the increase in premature delivery noted from 1992 to 2002 is due to the increase in multiple gestations [28]. Assisted reproductive technologies (ART) lead to multiple gestation in about 20% of cases, but the incidence of preterm delivery in singleton pregnancies resulting from ART is also higher – about 15%. The overall incidence of preterm delivery from ART is approximately 27% [31].

Fetal anomalies especially those leading to polyhydramnios, may precipitate preterm labor. First-trimester bleeding [32] and third-trimester bleeding from placental abnormalities also increase the risk of preterm delivery, either by precipitating preterm labor or because of maternal–fetal compromise [21,33].

Uterine abnormalities increase the risk of preterm delivery. These abnormalities are often congenital, or may be related to in utero exposure to diethylstilbestrol (DES). Preterm birth rates of 15–30% have been reported in these cases. The greatest incidence is noted in patients with demonstrable abnormalities of the genital tract, such as T-shaped uterus or cervical abnormalities [34,35].

Cervical incompetence is a clinical diagnosis made following a history of recurrent rapid painless cervical dilation in the second or early third trimester, or repetitive extremely premature deliveries with minimal uterine activity. It has been associated with DES exposure, cervical trauma from a prior delivery or surgery such as a cone biopsy, and subclinical intrauterine infection/inflammation. The gold standard is the documentation of cervical effacement, shortening, or dilation in the absence of obvious premature contractions [36]. Ultrasonographic evaluation of the length of the cervix has been proposed as a method of diagnosing cervical incompetence and/or risk of preterm labor [37]. Traditionally, cervical competence was thought to be an all-or-nothing phenomenon, but a more recent understanding is that it functions along a continuum and appears to be the result of an interplay between various factors including prior cervical trauma, innate cervical weakness, and premature ripening of an otherwise normal cervix. Although the original reports of the use of cerclage in the management of women with an underlying mechanical defect of the cervix and a history of recurrent loss showed success rates of 75–90% compared to pre-cerclage survival of 10–50%, these were simply case series using historical cohorts and with poorly defined diagnoses and endpoints [25,38]. There have been only four randomized trials of cerclage for sonographically diagnosed short cervix, none of which has shown benefit of this procedure [39–42]. In women presenting with a dilated cervix in the mid trimester a single small randomized trial showed some benefit [43].

About 20% of preterm deliveries are due to medical and surgical complications of pregnancy that lead to iatrogenic preterm delivery. These include conditions such as hypertensive disorders of pregnancy, renal disease, systemic lupus erythematosus, cardiac disease, acute infections, acute appendicitis, and other surgical and medical conditions.

Preterm premature rupture of membranes (PPROM) is defined as rupture of the amniotic membranes prior to term (less than 37 weeks' gestation). The interval between PPROM and onset of labor is the latency period, and it is inversely related to gestational age. Pediatricians are concerned about the latency period in term gestations and often refer to "prolonged" rupture of membranes when the latency period exceeds 18–24 hours. PPROM accounts for up to 30% of all preterm deliveries and thus is a major concern in perinatal medicine [44]. The causes of PPROM are not clearly understood, but weakening of the chorioamniotic membrane has been demonstrated as the pregnancy progresses [45,46]. Local infection from vaginal flora ascending through the cervix has been implicated as the etiology in a substantial number of cases [47]. Carriers of certain sexually transmitted organisms such as Group B β-hemolytic *Streptococcus* (GBS), *Chlamydia*, *Trichomonas*, *Gonococcus*, and bacterial vaginosis have a higher incidence of PPROM than those who are not carriers [48].

Some bacteria release proteases, which cause membrane weakening and probably early rupture [49]. There are host factors and immune activation mechanisms that probably account for the great variation in incidence of PPROM between populations. Polyhydramnios, cervical cerclage procedures, amniocentesis, smoking, and multiple gestation have all been implicated as etiological factors in PPROM [50]. However, in the majority of cases the etiology is unknown. The major complications of PPROM are premature labor and preterm delivery. The latency period is inversely related to gestational age, with 50% of patients with PPROM prior to 26 weeks being in labor within 1 week [51]. When PPROM occurs between 28 and 34 weeks, 50% are in labor within 24 hours and 80–90% within 1 week [52,53]. The other significant risk factor for PPROM is maternal/fetal/neonatal sepsis.

Chorioamnionitis occurs in 15–25% of PROM cases [54]. Incidence of neonatal sepsis at term is in the range of 1/500 deliveries. This incidence increases dramatically with PPROM, and even more significantly in the presence of chorioamnionitis

[55–57]. Umbilical-cord compression occurs more often in cases of PROM, with the associated complications of hypoxia and even asphyxia leading to fetal death or neonatal compromise [58–61]. Umbilical-cord prolapse may also complicate pregnancies with PPROM when the fetal presentation is other than vertex. Fetal deformation syndrome from PROM prior to 26 weeks is seen in approximately 3–4% of cases. This syndrome includes compression malformations and lethal pulmonary hypoplasia [62,63].

Diagnosis of preterm labor

The diagnosis of preterm labor is important in order to initiate appropriate tocolytic therapy to prolong gestation and thus decrease the incidence of neonatal complications. The criteria for the diagnosis of preterm labor seem deceptively simple, i.e., gestational age of 20–37 weeks and documented uterine contractions of $\geq 4/20$ minutes or $\geq 8/60$ minutes. In addition, in the presence of intact membranes there should be documented cervical change in either dilation or effacement or an initial cervical effacement of at least 80% and/or dilation of ≥ 2 cm [64]. Unfortunately, the diagnosis of cervical change based on a manual exam is subjective, and overtreatment is common. In fact, the majority of women diagnosed with preterm labor do not deliver preterm. In order to improve the diagnosis of preterm labor, two predictive tests, fetal fibronectin and transvaginal ultrasound measurement of cervical length, are now being used to help triage women in suspected preterm labor. Fetal fibronectin may help rule out preterm labor, by virtue of its high negative predictive value [65].

Initial assessments of the patient in suspected preterm labor include confirming the diagnosis and careful fetal evaluation by both sonography and continuous electronic fetal monitoring (EFM). Conditions which would contraindicate tocolysis, such as fetal anomalies incompatible with life, evidence of fetal compromise, significant intrauterine growth restriction (IUGR), chorioamnionitis, or severe maternal medical or surgical disorders, should be ruled out prior to initiation.

With PPROM in the absence of clinical chorioamnionitis, antibiotic prophylaxis helps prolong latency, and should be administered for a period of 7–10 days [66,67].

Preparation for delivery of the preterm fetus
Maternal transport

The most important factor to consider in cases in which preterm delivery may occur is availability of resources to deliver optimal care to both the neonate and the mother. Preterm neonates delivered in a perinatal center specializing in providing care for these patients have a much improved prognosis compared to neonates who are transported after birth [68–70]. Prior to arranging for maternal transport the gestational age and birthweight need to be determined. The use of real-time sonography will reliably estimate fetal weight and gestational age, with a small margin of error, in the preterm fetus [71,72]. The clinical estimation of gestational age and birthweight is subject to many errors, including inaccurate menstrual history, oligo- or polyhydramnios, fetal presentation, maternal body habitus, and other pathology such as myomata uteri. The tendency is often to underestimate fetal weight [73]. In most circumstances the gestational age at which maternal transfer would not be indicated will vary according to the level of neonatal care available. At gestational ages of 36 weeks or greater, and birthweights of > 2500 g, most obstetrical/pediatric facilities would have the resources to care for these neonates. If the gestation is previable, then transport may not confer an advantage in terms of neonatal survival. In practical terms, many community hospitals are uncomfortable with the possibility that a supposedly previable gestation may turn out to be larger than anticipated and delivery will have occurred without adequate facilities. The philosophy of "When in doubt, ship them out" is often the most prudent approach. Most maternal transports will be made for gestational ages of 24–36 weeks. However, diagnosis of fetal anomalies or serious maternal illness may require transfer at any gestational age.

Close communication between referring physicians, accepting maternal–fetal physicians, neonatologists, and other appropriate pediatric staff is essential. The patient and her family need to be given a realistic and consistent evaluation of the situation, including risks, benefits, alternatives, and ultimately prognosis. Survival rates and follow-up data need to be known for the institution, and counseling should be initiated by both obstetrics and neonatology staff as soon as is feasible. The type of transportation used will be quite region-specific but, as a general rule, transports from less than 100 miles (160 km) can be accomplished by ground ambulance while air transport is often used for greater distances. Mountains, road conditions, and weather will all influence the choice of method of transport. Once the decision to transport is made it is advantageous to have a transport team available. At many institutions, physicians and nurse teams are specially trained to transport either the pregnant mother or the neonate. These are two distinctly different types of health professionals: maternal–fetal transport is done by personnel trained in obstetrics, while neonatal transports are done by persons trained in care of the sick neonate.

Communication is vital between all the parties involved in caring for maternal–fetal and neonatal transports. There must be an efficient mechanism of initiating a request for transport. One phone call to the referring center or regional dispatch center should set in motion a chain of events leading to appropriate transportation. Medical staff at the referring hospital will need to contact the accepting institution's staff without difficulty in order to provide appropriate information concerning the patient. The obstetricians accepting a maternal–fetal transport will need to contact their neonatology group to inform them of the impending transport and confirm availability of a neonatal bed. If there is a problem with this, alternative strategies need to be devised.

The referring institution needs to provide as much information as possible, so that adequate resources can be mobilized to deal with specific problems. Examples would be availability of pediatric surgical specialties or availability of blood for transfusion. There are cases in which a maternal–fetal transport team may arrive after an unexpected delivery, or find that transport would be inadvisable and delivery preparations should be undertaken. In this type of situation, close communication between the maternal–fetal and neonatal teams is vital.

Discussion needs to be instituted concerning the use of medications or other interventions prior to initiation of transport. When there is a maternal–fetal transport, discussion usually centers around the use of tocolytic agents, antihypertensive and antiseizure medications in cases of hypertensive disorders of pregnancy, and sometimes the use of antibiotics in cases of preterm labor and/or PPROM.

Antenatal steroids for fetal lung maturity

The use of pharmacologic agents given to the pregnant patient in order to improve neonatal outcome is an extremely important consideration. The most effective and well-studied therapy is antenatal corticosteroid administration. The most commonly used regimens are either dexamethasone 5 mg intramuscularly every 12 hours for four doses or betamethasone 12 mg intramuscularly repeated in 24 hours.

Currently, the consensus conference of the National Institutes of Health [74] recommends that all women between 24 and 34 weeks of pregnancy at risk for preterm delivery be considered candidates for antenatal corticosteroid therapy. Optimal therapeutic benefits begin 24 hours after initiation of therapy and last 7 days. Because there is evidence suggesting that mortality, respiratory distress syndrome, and intraventricular hemorrhage are reduced even when treatment lasts for less than 24 hours, steroids should be given unless delivery is imminent.

Management of labor and delivery

Once delivery is imminent, optimal management of the delivery process is important. Pain relief is an essential element in the management of patients in preterm labor. It should be accepted that all analgesic medications commonly used in obstetrics cross the placenta. The long-held misconception about neonatal depression secondary to analgesic medication continues to prevent physicians from administering adequate pain relief in labor. Some medications may indeed lead to temporary respiratory depression of the neonate, but other causes for the problem must be sought. There is evidence that central nervous system depressants may in fact protect the central nervous system of the fetus from the effects of hypoxia [75].

Continuous epidural anesthesia is a safe and effective method of pain relief in preterm labor. Avoidance of maternal hypotension is important to prevent in utero placental insufficiency. General anesthesia for emergency operative delivery poses no threat to the fetus provided maternal oxygenation is maintained and hypotension avoided.

Route of delivery

Vertex presentation

There has been some controversy over the method of delivery of the premature fetus. Enthusiasm for liberal use of cesarean delivery has been tempered by the findings of several retrospective studies showing no difference in mortality between cesarean and vaginal delivery [76–78]. The current accepted approach is to allow labor with intensive fetal monitoring. Indication for cesarean section is very similar to that for the term fetus. The difference is that the preterm fetus probably tolerates hypoxia less effectively than the term fetus, and prompt atraumatic delivery should be considered early in the process. Delivery *en caul* (membranes intact) has been advocated to decrease risk of trauma and fluctuations of cerebral blood flow in response to cord compression [79].

Of historical interest is the practice of prophylactic forceps-assisted vaginal delivery of the premature fetus, with the rationale that decreasing the length of the second stage with forceps may reduce neonatal morbidity and mortality. Neonatal outcomes of low-birthweight infants delivered by prophylactic forceps have not been shown to be different, however, than outcomes of those born spontaneously, and this practice has been largely abandoned [21]. In some studies the use of "prophylactic forceps" for preterm delivery has been proven to be potentially hazardous [80,81].

Breech presentation

Criteria for singleton breech delivery have traditionally been a gestational age greater than 37 weeks and an estimated fetal weight of 2500–4000 g. The recommended mode of delivery for the preterm non-vertex singleton, therefore, in the absence of much data, has been cesarean section. A recent population-based study concluded that vaginal breech delivery of the preterm low-birthweight singleton fetus is associated with a 6–16-fold increase in risk of neonatal mortality, and that cesarean delivery is protective [82]. With an incidence of breech presentation of around 20% at 25–26 weeks of gestation, some authors have advocated *en caul* vaginal breech delivery of the extremely premature breech singleton. In a recent series, there was no difference in perinatal morbidity or mortality in nine infants under 26 weeks of gestation delivered breech and *en caul* vaginally when compared to six infants matched for gestational age and delivered via cesarean section [83]. Proponents of *en caul* vaginal delivery of the extremely premature breech fetus note reduced risk of head entrapment of the aftercoming head by an incompletely dilated cervix and a reduced risk of cord prolapse requiring emergent cesarean delivery, as well as avoidance of a likely classical cesarean delivery and its attendant risks (see below).

Malpresentation, multiple gestations

Malpresentations are common in the preterm fetus. The incidence of breech presentation at 28 weeks' gestation approaches 25%. The incidence of fetal abnormalities is increased with breech presentation, including neuromuscular deficits. The risk of the lower extremities, abdomen, and thorax delivering through an incompletely dilated cervix, leaving the relatively larger fetal head trapped behind the cervix prior to 32 weeks has led to a liberal policy of cesarean delivery for the premature fetus. The increased risk of cord prolapse also supports this approach. There have been conflicting reports in the literature regarding cesarean section for breech [84–86]. The very-low-birthweight fetus (less than 1500 g) is at greatest risk for head entrapment, and thus may benefit most from a cesarean section. However, even with term breech, a study did show greater morbidity with the vaginal approach [84].

Atraumatic cesarean delivery must be accomplished, and this will often require a vertical uterine incision in a poorly developed lower uterine segment. A wide transverse incision is preferable, but an adequate incision must be employed. The splint technique is often helpful in assisting with atraumatic delivery of a malpresentation [87].

Multiple gestations of a higher order (greater than two) are generally delivered by cesarean section. In twin gestations, with the leading twin presenting as a breech, cesarean delivery is indicated. If the lead twin is vertex and twin B is either concordant with or smaller than twin A, vaginal delivery of twin A and either external version or breech delivery of twin B may be undertaken. Clinical judgment is important, and there should be no hesitation in abandoning difficult vaginal delivery and performing cesarean section if indicated. Real-time sonography should be used to help determine the position and route of delivery. Availability of both obstetric and neonatal expertise is important in decisions on the location of delivery. Obstetrical management is often not a problem, but expertise in resuscitation and stabilization of the preterm fetus is crucial in optimizing subsequent outcome [88,89]. This will often require maternal–fetal transportation.

Fetal monitoring

Intrapartum hypoxia and acidosis in the preterm fetus may be a significant factor in subsequent complications of prematurity [90]. Continuous EFM appears to predict fetal hypoxia in the preterm fetus with some degree of accuracy [91,92]. Skilled auscultation may also be used [93]. However, this is often not practical because of the more labor-intensive nature of surveillance by auscultation. Amnioinfusion has been demonstrated to reduce the incidence of cord compression and cesarean delivery in patients with PPROM [94].

Progressive intrapartum hypoxemia and acidosis (asphyxia) in the preterm fetus contributes to CNS and other organ-system complications. Depending on its degree and duration, the asphyxial insult may cause brain damage, which accounts for major handicaps in surviving children, and fetal and early neonatal death [95]. Studies by Low *et al.* have observed that preterm pregnancies have three times the frequency of moderate and severe asphyxia compared to term pregnancies [95–97]. Yet recent studies have demonstrated that mid-trimester fetal sheep are neurologically more tolerant of cord occlusion than mature fetal sheep. This means that the immature fetus will tolerate a longer exposure to asphyxia than the term fetus, but this survival eventually results in sudden profound cardiovascular decompensation with resultant systemic hypotension and cerebral hypoperfusion [97].

In a study of 40 preterm pregnancies with biochemically confirmed fetal acidosis (base deficit > 12 mmol/L) EFM was predictive in 71% (60% of those with mild acidosis and 83% of those with moderate or severe acidosis) [95]. Unfortunately, some of the pregnancies with moderate to severe asphyxia are difficult to prevent, either because the fetal asphyxial exposure began before fetal surveillance was initiated or because of the acute and sudden onset of a profound fetal insult. Nevertheless, the use of EFM may help to identify the preterm fetus with mild intrapartum asphyxia and allow for intervention prior to the development of moderate or severe asphyxia, and possibly reduce the morbidity and death caused by more severe asphyxia.

The influence of events of labor and delivery on perinatal "brain damage" has been the focus of both obstetricians and pediatricians since the early nineteenth century. Little [98] and Freud [99] stated that the major cause of cerebral palsy (CP) and mental retardation (MR) was intrapartum "brain damage." Prolonged labors and traumatic deliveries supported this impression, and it has only recently been proved that only about 10% of cases of CP and MR can be attributed to events of labor and delivery [100–102]. However, this group of patients is one in which some type of intervention may have a meaningful impact on perinatal outcome. Fetal heart rate (FHR) patterns, determined by continuous EFM, may be of value in predicting hypoxemia and acidosis during labor, thus allowing potentially beneficial therapy. FHR patterns may be obtained through EFM or by auscultation. Continuous EFM may be a less labor-intensive and more practical method of monitoring than auscultation. FHR monitoring is only one parameter of fetal condition, and it must be evaluated along with the total clinical picture. Transient and repetitive episodes of fetal hypoxemia are extremely common during normal labor. These episodes are usually well tolerated by the fetus. Only when hypoxia and resultant metabolic acidemia reach extreme levels is the fetus at risk for long-term neurologic damage [103]. It should be noted that umbilical cord blood gases, particularly arterial, are more accurate in assessing fetal condition in the preterm neonate than are Apgar scores, which are quite unreliable at early gestational ages [104].

Terminology must be appropriately used, and the following definitions reflect current thinking [105]:

Hypoxemia: Decreased oxygen content in blood

Hypoxia: Decreased level of oxygen in tissue

Acidemia: Increased concentration of hydrogen ions in the blood

Acidosis: Increased concentration of hydrogen ions in tissue

Asphyxia: Hypoxia with metabolic acidosis

The fetus is well adapted to tolerating the intermittent episodes of decreased oxygen delivery that occur with contractions in labor. However, numerous factors can lead to significant hypoxemia and eventually to metabolic acidemia. Decreased uterine blood flow will influence the level of fetal oxygenation. Contractions, maternal position, and blood pressure will all have an effect on uterine blood flow. The umbilical cord is also vulnerable during labor. Intermittent cord compression is common and normally well tolerated by the fetus, but prolonged compression may lead to hypoxemia, acidosis, and asphyxia. The premature fetus and those with growth disorders are more susceptible to the effects of hypoxemia in the intrapartum period, and the onset of metabolic acidosis may occur more rapidly. This may lead to fetal or neonatal death or poor long-term outcome [106,107]. Alterations in the FHR are under CNS control and may be sensitive indicators of fetal hypoxia [108,109]. A normal FHR is reassuring and is almost always associated with a healthy newborn. The term "reassuring" thus implies normal oxygenation and acid–base status. On the other hand, non-reassuring patterns have a wider range of predictability. In many cases non-reassuring patterns are a result of early gestational age, fetal rest cycles, and medications. These patterns may be difficult to distinguish from patterns resulting from hypoxia and early acidosis. The term "fetal distress" should be abandoned, and the type of heart-rate pattern should be described.

The FHR should be evaluated systematically, a mechanism for changes in FHR proposed, and the clinical situation assessed. Judgment concerning further management of labor should be made with all relevant information (see Chapter 15).

Management of FHR patterns

If the sequential approach is strongly suggestive of fetal acidosis, further fetal evaluation and assessment of the clinical situation are necessary. If there is an impression of significant acidosis, delivery by the most expedient method may be indicated. If there are conflicting data and evidence of acidosis is not overwhelming, further evaluation of the fetus and strategies to improve uterine blood flow, fetal oxygenation, and acid–base status must be undertaken.

Standard measures to improve fetal status include maintenance of normal maternal cardiac output, maximizing maternal and fetal oxygenation, and control of uterine activity. Fluid administration and occasionally medication may be required to correct maternal hypotension. Avoidance of the supine position will prevent aortocaval compression. Maternal position change may alleviate cord compression. Discontinuation of oxytocin administration will treat uterine hyperstimulation.

Another potentially valuable tool in the management of intrapartum events is the use of tocolytic agents to decrease uterine activity. Terbutaline [110], magnesium sulfate [111], and nitroglycerin [112] have all been used. Use of these agents is usually temporary, while preparing for expeditious delivery.

It should be emphasized that individual circumstances in each case must be considered. Decisions on whether to continue labor or expedite delivery will be dictated by the complete clinical picture, and not by isolated pieces of information. The overriding principle must be optimal outcome for both the mother and the fetus. Giving the fetus the benefit of the doubt in confusing situations is often the most prudent approach.

Operative vaginal delivery

Normal spontaneous vaginal delivery is considered a physiological process, and complications with spontaneous delivery are relatively uncommon. Acute events in the late second stage of labor, prior to anticipated delivery, may cause fetal and neonatal complications. These include abruptio placentae, umbilical cord prolapse, ruptured uterus, ruptured vasa previa, and shoulder dystocia. Diagnosis of these complications may lead to operative vaginal delivery. Instruments for operative vaginal delivery include forceps and vacuum extraction. Cesarean section is classified as operative abdominal delivery.

Maternal indications

There are certain medical conditions in which the mother needs to avoid or cannot perform voluntary expulsive efforts, such as certain cardiovascular, cerebral, gastrointestinal, or neuromuscular diseases. Maternal exhaustion, lack of cooperation, and excessive analgesia may affect the patient's ability to assist adequately in the expulsion of the fetus.

Fetal indications

Non-reassuring FHR pattern is a major indication for operative delivery. Second-stage FHR monitoring patterns are frequently misinterpreted as non-reassuring, with subsequent intervention. These patterns are often confusing, and they need to be evaluated carefully to determine whether there is fetal intolerance of labor [113]. Failure of spontaneous vaginal delivery following an appropriately managed second stage is another major indication for operative vaginal delivery. The use of "prophylactic" forceps for the delivery of a preterm fetus is generally discouraged, and standard obstetrical indications should be used in making decisions on whether forceps should be used in these circumstances.

When operative vaginal delivery of the preterm fetus is indicated, whether for non-reassuring fetal status or for a prolonged second stage, the gestational age of the fetus should be considered when choosing between vacuum-assisted and forceps-assisted vaginal deliveries. The American College of Obstetricians and Gynecologists notes that most authorities consider vacuum extraction inappropriate before 34 weeks of gestation because of concerns for intraventricular hemorrhage [114]. Although there are case reports of serious intracranial hemorrhage with vacuum extraction of the preterm fetus [115], two retrospective case–control studies of low-birth-weight infants delivered by vacuum-assisted vaginal delivery compared to spontaneously delivered low-birthweight infants have not confirmed this concern for increased morbidity with vacuum extraction in the preterm neonate [116,117].

Cesarean delivery

When abdominal delivery of the preterm fetus is indicated, whether secondary to malpresentation or to non-reassuring fetal status or other routine obstetric indications, a lack of development of the lower uterine segment may preclude a low transverse incision. A vertical uterine incision that extends into the more muscular upper uterine segment and/or uterine fundus may therefore be required, often termed a classical incision. Classical cesarean deliveries are associated with an increased risk of maternal postoperative morbidity [118] and impart an increased risk of uterine rupture with labor in a subsequent pregnancy of 4–9% [119]; this increased risk of rupture over incisions in the lower uterine segment therefore increases the risk of perinatal morbidity and mortality for the fetus in a subsequent pregnancy.

Miscellaneous obstetric interventions for the preterm fetus

Delayed cord clamping in the premature infant has been advocated by some experts to increase blood volume and potentially decrease neonatal morbidity. A trial in which singleton fetuses of less than 32 weeks gestation were randomly assigned to either immediate cord clamping or delayed cord clamping (30–45 seconds) showed no increase in hematocrit in those with delayed cord clamping but showed a reduction in intraventricular hemorrhage and late-onset sepsis in these patients [120]. There may therefore be a potential benefit in delaying cord clamping after delivery of the premature infant.

The Maternal–Fetal Medicine Units Network has demonstrated a potential benefit of magnesium sulfate before delivery of the premature infant. This multicenter randomized controlled trial involved administration of magnesium sulfate to women with advanced preterm labor, preterm premature rupture of membranes, or indicated delivery from 24–31 weeks of gestation, compared to administration of placebo, and noted a reduction by 50% of moderate to severe cerebral palsy of surviving infants at age 2 years [121].

Conclusion

The premature fetus and neonate are at increased risk for brain injury compared to term infants. This is due both to prenatal factors that may have brought about the preterm delivery and to neonatal complications. In addition, it is now clear that, despite improvements in obstetric and neonatal care that have decreased the incidence of intrapartum and neonatal deaths, there has been no corresponding decrease in the incidence of cerebral palsy. This finding has served to highlight the issue of how much cerebral palsy is related to intrapartum as opposed to antepartum events. Recent studies have demonstrated that at least 40% of asphyxia in the preterm fetus occurs before the onset of labor [97]. If we are to reduce brain injury in preterm infants we must not only improve our intrapartum and neonatal care but must also focus our research efforts on early detection of antenatal precursors for brain injury.

References

1. World Health Organization. Prevention of Perinatal Morbidity. *Public Health Papers 42*. Geneva: WHO, 1969.

2. Nelson KB, Ellenberg JH. Antecedents of cerebral palsy: multivariate analysis of risk. *N Engl J Med* 1986; **315**: 81–6.

3. Martin JA, Hamilton BE, Sutton PD, *et al.* Births: final data for 2004. *Natl Vital Stat Rep* 2006; **55**: 1–101.

4. Spong CY. Prediction and prevention of recurrent spontaneous preterm birth. *Am J Obstet Gynecol* 2007; **110**: 404–15.

5. Cooper RK, Goldenberg RL, Creasy RK, *et al.* A multicenter study of preterm birth weight and gestational age specific mortality. *Am J Obstet Gynecol* 1993; **168**: 78–84.

6. Ferrara TB, Hoekstra RE, Couser RS, *et al.* Survival and follow-up of infants born at 23–26 weeks gestational age: effects of surfactant therapy. *J Pediatr* 1994; **124**: 119–24.

7. Wilson-Costello D, Friedman H, Minich N, *et al.* Improved survival rates with increased neurodevelopmental disability for extremely low birth weight infants in the 1990s. *Pediatrics* 2005; **115**: 997–1003.

8. Leviton A, Paneth N. White matter damage in preterm newborns: an epidemiologic perspective. *Early Hum Dev* 1990; **24**: 1–22.

9. Gunn AJ, Quaedackers JS, Guan J, *et al.* The premature fetus: not as defenseless as we thought, but still paradoxically vulnerable? *Dev Neurosci* 2001; **23**: 175–9.

10. Barrett RD, Bennet L, Davidson J, *et al.* Destruction and reconstruction: hypoxia and the developing brain. *Birth Defects Res C Embryo Today* 2007; **81**: 163–76.

11. Papiernik E, Kaminski M. Multifactorial study of the risk of prematurity at 32 weeks of gestation. *J Perinat Med* 1974; **2**: 30–6.

12. Meis PJ, MacErnest J, Moore ML. Causes of low birth weight births in public and private patients. *Am J Obstet Gynecol* 1987; **156**: 1165–8.

13. Leigh J, Garite TJM. Amnionitis and the management of premature labor. *Obstet Gynecol* 1986; **67**: 500–6.

14. Gravett MG, Hummel D, Eschenbach DA, *et al.* Preterm labor associated with subclinical amniotic infection and with bacterial vaginosis. *Obstet Gynecol* 1986; **67**: 229–37.

15. Hameed C, Teiane N, Verma UL, *et al.* Silent chorioamnionitis as a cause of preterm labor refractory to tocolytic therapy. *Am J Obstet Gynecol* 1984; **149**: 726–30.

16. Duff P, Kopelman JN. Subclinical intraamniotic infection in asymptomatic patients with refractory preterm labor. *Obstet Gynecol* 1987; **69**: 756–69.

17. Bobbitt JR, Ledger WJ. Unrecognized amnionitis and prematurity: a preliminary report. *J Reprod Med* 1977; **19**: 8–12.

18. Bobbitt JR, Ledger WJ. Amniotic fluid analysis: its role in maternal and neonatal infection. *Obstet Gynecol* 1978; **51**: 56–62.

19. Fedrick J, Anderson ABM. Factors associated with spontaneous preterm birth. *Br J Obstet Gynaecol* 1976; **83**: 342–50.

20. US Department of Health and Human Services. Report of the Secretary's Task Force on Black and Minority Health, publication 0–487–637 (QL3). Vol. 6. *Infant Mortality and Low Birth Weight.* Hyattsville, MD: National Center for Health Statistics, 1985.

21. Bakketeig LS, Hoffman HJ. Epidemiology of preterm birth: results from longitudinal study of births in Norway. In Elder MG, Dendricks CH, eds., *Preterm Labour*. London: Butterworths, 1981: 17–46.

22. Abrams B, Newman V, Key T, *et al.* Maternal weight gain and preterm delivery. *Obstet Gynecol* 1989; **74**: 577–83.

23. MacGregor SW, Keith LG, Chasnoff IJ, *et al.* Cocaine use during pregnancy: adverse perinatal outcome. *Am J Obstet Gynecol* 1987; **57**: 686–90.

24. Shiono PH, Klebanoff MA, Rhoads GG. Smoking and drinking during pregnancy. *JAMA* 1986; **255**: 82–4.

25. Keirse M, Rush R, Anderson A, *et al.* Risk of pre-term delivery in patients with previous preterm delivery and/or abortion. *Br J Obstet Gynaecol* 1978; **85**: 81–5.

26. Linn S, Schoenbaum S, Monson R, *et al.* The relationship between induced abortion and outcome of subsequent pregnancies. *Am J Obstet Gynecol* 1983; **146**: 136–40.

27. Chung C, Smith R, Steinhoff P, *et al.* Induced abortion and spontaneous fetal loss in subsequent pregnancies. *Am J Public Health* 1982; **72**: 548–54.

28. Elliot JP. High order multiple gestations. *Semin Perinatol* 2005; **5**: 305–11.

29. US Department of Health and Human Services. Public Health Service. *Vital Statistics of the United States, 1982. Vol. 1. Natality.* Hyattsville, MD: Department of Health, 1986.

30. Neilson JP, Verkuyl DAA, Crowther CA, *et al.* Preterm labor in twin pregnancies: prediction by cervical assessment. *Obstet Gynecol* 1988; **72**: 719–23.

31. Australian Institute of Health and Welfare National Perinatal Statistics Unit. *Assisted Conception in Australia and New Zealand.* Sydney: AIHW, 1992.

32. Williams MA, Millendorf R, Liererman E, *et al.* Adverse infant outcomes associated with first trimester vaginal bleeding. *Obstet Gynecol* 1991; **78**: 14–8.

33. Roberts G. Unclassified antepartum haemorrhage incidence and perinatal mortality in a community. *J Obstet Gynaecol Br Commonwlth* 1970; **77**: 492–5.

34. Herbst AL, Hubby MM, Blough RR, *et al.* A comparison of pregnancy experiment in DES-exposed and DES-unexposed daughters. *J Reprod Med* 1980; **24**: 62–9.

35. Kaufman RH, Noller K, Adam E, *et al.* Upper genital tract abnormalities and pregnancy outcome in diethylstilbestrol-exposed progeny. *Am J Obstet Gynecol* 1985; **148**: 973–84.

36. Harger JH. Cervical cerclage: patient selection, morbidity and success rates. *Clin Perinatol* 1983; **10**: 321–41.

37. Zemlyn S. The length of the uterine cervix and its significance. *J Clin Ultrasound* 1981; **9**: 267–9.

38. Rush RLO. Incidence of preterm delivery in patients with previous preterm delivery and/or abortion. *S Afr Med J* 1979; **56**: 1085–7.

39. Rust OA, Atlas RO, Jones KJ, *et al.* A randomized trial of cerclage versus no cerclage among patients with ultrasonographically detected second-trimester preterm dilatation of the internal os. *Am J Obstet Gynecol* 2000; **183**: 830–5.

40. Berghella V, Odibo AO, Tolosa JE. Cerclage for prevention of preterm birth in women with a short cervix found on transvaginal ultrasound examination: a randomized trial. *Am J Obstet Gynecol* 2004; **191**: 1311–17.

41. To MS, Alfirevic Z, Heath VCF, *et al.* Cervical cerclage for prevention of preterm delivery in women with short cervix: randomized controlled trial. *Lancet* 2004; **363**: 1849–53.

42. Althuisius SM, Dekker GA, Hummel P, *et al.* Final results of the cervical

incompetence prevention randomized cerclage trial (CIPRACT): therapeutic cerclage with bed rest versus bed rest alone. *Am J Obstet Gynecol* 2001; **185**: 1106–12.

43. Althuisius SM, Dekker GA, Hummel P, *et al.* Cervical incompetence prevention randomized cerclage trial: emergency cerclage with bed rest versus bed rest alone. *Am J Obstet Gynecol* 2003; **189**: 907–10.

44. Kaltreider DF, Kohl S. Epidemiology of preterm delivery. *Clin Obstet Gynecol* 1980; **23**: 17–31.

45. Artal JP, Sokol RJ, Newman M, *et al.* The mechanical properties of prematurely and non-prematurely ruptured membranes. *Am J Obstet Gynecol* 1976; **125**: 655–9.

46. Lavery JP, Miller CE, Knight RD. The effect of labor on the rheologic response of chorioamniotic membranes. *Obstet Gynecol* 1982; **60**: 87–91.

47. Lonky NN, Hayashi RH. A proposed mechanism for premature rupture of membranes. *Obstet Gynecol Surv* 1988; **43**: 22–8.

48. Minkoff H, Grunebaum AN, Schwarz RH, *et al.* Risk factors for prematurity and premature rupture of membranes; a prospective study of vaginal flora in pregnancy. *Am J Obstet Gynecol* 1984; **150**: 965–72.

49. Iams JD, McGregor JA. Cervicovaginal microflora and pregnancy outcome: results of a double blind, placebo-controlled trial of erythromycin treatment. *Am J Obstet Gynecol* 1990; **163**: 1580–91.

50. Naeye RL. Factors that predispose to premature rupture of the fetal membranes. *Obstet Gynecol* 1982; **60**: 93–8.

51. Taylor J, Garite TJ. Premature rupture of membranes before fetal viability. *Obstet Gynecol* 1984; **64**: 615–20.

52. Mead PB. Management of the patient with premature rupture of the membranes. *Clin Perinatol* 1980; **7**: 243–55.

53. Kennedy KA, Clark SL. Premature rupture of the membranes: management controversies. *Clin Perinatol* 1992; **19**: 385–97.

54. Garite TJ, Freeman RK, Linzy EM, *et al.* Prospective randomized study of corticosteroids in the management of premature rupture of membranes and the premature gestation. *Am J Obstet Gynecol* 1981; **141**: 508–15.

55. Gibbs RS, Blanco JD, St Clair PJ, *et al.* Quantitative bacteriology of amniotic fluid from patients with clinical intra-amniotic infection at term. *J Infect Dis* 1982; **145**: 1–8.

56. Yoder PR, Gibbs RS, Blanco JD, *et al.* A prospective controlled study of maternal and perinatal outcome after intra-amniotic infection at term. *Am J Obstet Gynecol* 1983; **145**: 695–701.

57. Garite TJ. Premature rupture of the membranes. In Creasy RK, Resnick R, eds., *Maternal–Fetal Medicine: Principles and Practices*. Philadelphia, PA: Saunders, 1994: 625–38.

58. Garite TJ, Freeman RK. Chorioamnionitis in the preterm gestation. *Obstet Gynecol* 1982; **54**: 539–45.

59. Gabbe SG, Ettinger BB, Freeman RK, *et al.* Umbilical cord compression associated with amniotomy: laboratory observations. *Am J Obstet Gynecol* 1976; **126**: 353–6.

60. Wilson JC, Levy DC, Wilds PL. Premature rupture of membranes prior to term: consequences of non-intervention. *Obstet Gynecol* 1982; **60**: 601–6.

61. Moberg LJ, Garite TJ. Antepartum fetal heart rate testing in PROM. *Seventh Annual Meeting of the Society of Perinatal Obstetricians*, 1987.

62. Morretti M, Sibai BM. Maternal and perinatal outcome of expectant management of premature rupture of membranes in the mid-trimester. *Am J Obstet Gynecol* 1988; **159**: 390–6.

63. Major CA, Kitzmiller JL. Perinatal survival with expectant management of mid-trimester rupture of membranes. *Am J Obstet Gynecol* 1990; **163**: 838–44.

64. Creasy RK. Preterm labor and delivery. In Moberg LJ, Garite TJ, eds. *Disorders of Parturition*, Part III. 1985: 494–520.

65. Peaceman AM, Andrews WW, Thorp JM, *et al.* Fetal fibronectin as a predictor of preterm birth in patients with symptoms: a multicenter trial. *Am J Obstet Gynecol* 1997; **177**: 13–18.

66. Mercer BM, Arheart KL. Antimicrobial therapy in expectant management of preterm premature rupture of the membranes. *Lancet* 1995; **346**: 1271–9.

67. Mercer BM, Miodovnik M, Thurnau GR, *et al.* Antibiotic therapy for reduction of infant morbidity after preterm premature rupture of the membranes: a randomized controlled trial. *JAMA* 1997; **278**: 989–95.

68. Usher R. Changing mortality rates with perinatal intensive care and regionalization. *Semin Perinatol* 1977; **1**: 309–19.

69. Gortmaker S, Sobol A, Clark C, *et al.* The survival of very low-birth weight infants by level of hospital of birth: a population study of perinatal systems in four states. *Am J Obstet Gynecol* 1985; **152**: 517–24.

70. Kitchen W, Ford G, Orgill A, *et al.* Outcome in infants with birth weight 500–999 grams: a regional study of 1979 and 1980 births. *J Pediatr* 1984; **104**: 921–7.

71. Hadlock FP, Harrist RB, Carpenter RJ, *et al.* Sonographic estimation of fetal weight: the value of fetal length in addition to head and abdominal measurements. *Radiology* 1984; **152**: 497–501.

72. Seeds JW, Cefalo RL, Bowes WA. Femur lengths in the estimation of fetal weight less than 1500 grams. *Am J Obstet Gynecol* 1984; **149**: 233–5.

73. Paul RH, Hon EH. Clinical fetal monitoring. V. Effect on perinatal outcome. *Am J Obstet Gynecol* 1974; **118**: 529–33.

74. National Institutes of Health Consensus Statement. Effect of antenatal steroids for fetal maturation on perinatal outcomes. *NIH Consensus Statement* 1994; **12** (2): 1–24.

75. Myers RE, Myers SE. Use of sedative, analgesic and anesthetic drugs during labor and delivery: bane or boon? *Am J Obstet Gynecol* 1979; **133**: 83–108.

76. Olshan AF, Shy KK, Luthy DA. Cesarean birth and neonatal mortality in very low birth weight infants. *Obstet Gynecol* 1984; **64**: 267–70.

77. Yu VYH, Bajak B, Cutting D, *et al.* Effect of mode of delivery on outcome of very low birthweight infants. *Br J Obstet Gynaecol* 1984; **91**: 633–9.

78. Kithen W, Ford GW, Doyle LW, *et al.* Cesarean section or vaginal delivery at 24 to 28 weeks' gestation: comparison of survival and neonatal and two year morbidity. *Obstet Gynecol* 1985; **66**: 149–57.

79. Goldenberg RL, Davis RO. In caul delivery of the very premature infant. *Am J Obstet Gynecol* 1983; **145**: 645–6.

80. Schwarz DB, Miodovnik MK, Lavin JP Jr. Neonatal outcome among low birth weight infants delivered spontaneously or by low forceps. *Obstet Gynecol* 1983; **62**: 283–6.

81. Kriewall TJ. Structural, mechanical, and material properties of fetal cranial bone. *Am J Obstet Gynecol* 1982; **143**: 707–14.

82. Robilio PA, Boe NM, Danielsen B, *et al.* Vaginal vs. cesarean delivery for preterm

breech presentation of singleton infants in California. *J Reprod Med* 2007; **52**: 473–9.

83. Richmond JR, Morin L, Benjamin A. Extremely preterm vaginal breech delivery en caul. *Obstet Gynecol* 2002; **99**: 1025–30.

84. Bowes WA, Taylor ES, O'Brien M, *et al.* Breech delivery: evaluation of the method of delivery on perinatal results and maternal morbidity. *Am J Obstet Gynecol* 1979; **135**: 965–73.

85. Bodmer B, Benjamin A, McLean FH, *et al.* Has use of cesarean section reduced the risk of delivery in the preterm breech presentation? *Am J Obstet Gynecol* 1986; **154**: 244–50.

86. Rosen G, Chick L. The effect of delivery route on outcome in breech presentation. *Am J Obstet Gynecol* 1984; **148**: 909–14.

87. Druzin ML. Atraumatic delivery in cases of malpresentation of the very low birth weight fetus at cesarean section: the splint technique. *Am J Obstet Gynecol* 1986; **154**: 941–2.

88. Harris TR, Isman J, Giles HR. Improved neonatal survival through maternal transport. *Obstet Gynecol* 1978; **52**: 294–300.

89. Paneth N, Kiely JL, Wallenstein S, *et al.* The choice of place of delivery: effect of hospital level on mortality in all singleton births in New York City. *Am J Dis Child* 1987; **141**: 60–4.

90. Low JA, Gallbraith RS, Muir DW, *et al.* Factors associated with motor and cognitive deficits in children after intrapartum fetal hypoxia. *Am J Obstet Gynecol* 1984; **148**: 533–9.

91. Bowes WA, Gabbe S, Bowes C. Fetal heart rate monitoring in premature infants weighing 1500 grams or less. *Am J Obstet Gynecol* 1980; **137**: 791–6.

92. Westgren LMR, Malcus P, Sveningsen NW. Intrauterine asphyxia and longterm outcome in preterm fetuses. *Obstet Gynecol* 1986; **67**: 512–16.

93. Luthy DA, Kirkwood KS, van Belle G, *et al.* A randomized trial of electronic fetal monitoring in preterm labor. *Obstet Gynecol* 1987; **69**: 637–95.

94. Nageotte MP, Freeman RK, Garite TJ, *et al.* Prophylactic intrapartum amnioinfusion in patients with preterm premature rupture of membranes. *Am J Obstet Gynecol* 1985; **153**: 557–62.

95. Low JA, Killen, H, Derrick J. The prediction of asphyxia in preterm pregnancies. *Am J Obstet Gynecol* 2001; **186**: 279–82.

96. Low JA, Killen H, Derrick J. Antepartum fetal asphyxia in the preterm pregnancy. *Am J Obstet Gynecol* 2002; **188**: 461–5.

97. Low JA. Determining the contribution of asphyxia to brain damage in the neonate. *J Obstet Gynaecol Res* 2004; **30**: 276–86.

98. Little WJ. On the influence of abnormal parturition, difficult labors, premature birth, and asphyxia neonatorum on the mental and physical condition of the child, especially in relation to deformities. *Trans Obstet Soc Lond* 1862; **2**: 293–344.

99. Freud S. *Die infantile Cerebrallähmung.* Vienna: Hölder, 1897.

100. Blair E, Stanley FJ. Intrapartum asphyxia: a rare cause of cerebral palsy. *J Pediatr* 1988; **112**: 515–19.

101. Committee on Obstetrics, Maternal and Fetal Medicine. Fetal and Neonatal Neurologic Injury. *ACOG Technical Bulletin 163.* Washington, DC: ACOG, 1992.

102. Naeye RL, Peters EC, Bartholomew M, *et al.* Origins of cerebral palsy. *Am J Dis Child* 1989; **143**: 1154–6.

103. Stanley FJ, Blair E. Why have we failed to reduce the frequency of cerebral palsy? *Med J Aust* 1991; **154**: 623–6.

104. Goldenberg RL, Huddlestone JF, Nelson KG. Apgar scores and umbilical arterial pH in preterm newborn infants. *Am J Obstet Gynecol* 1984; **149**: 651–4.

105. American College of Obstetricians and Gynecologists. Fetal Heart Rate Patterns: Monitoring, Interpretation, and Management. *ACOG Technical Bulletin 207.* Washington, DC: ACOG, 1995.

106. Low JA, Boston RW, Pancham FR. Fetal asphyxia during the intrapartum period in intrauterine growth retarded infants. *Am J Obstet Gynecol* 1972; **113**: 351–7.

107. Westgran LMR, Malcus P, Svenningsen NW. Intrauterine asphyxia and longterm outcome in preterm fetuses. *Obstet Gynecol* 1986; **67**: 512–16.

108. Myers RE, Mueller-Huebach E, Adamson K. Predictability of the state of fetal oxygenation from quantitative analysis of the components of late decelerations. *Am J Obstet Gynecol* 1992; **115**: 1083–94.

109. Watasuki A, Murata Y, Ninomiya Y, *et al.* Autonomic nervous system regulation of baseline heart rate in the fetal lamb. *Am J Obstet Gynecol* 1992; **167**: 519–23.

110. Arias F. Intrauterine resuscitation with terbutaline: a method for the management of acute intrapartum fetal distress. *Am J Obstet Gynecol* 1978; **131**: 139–13.

111. Reece EA, Chervenak FA, Romero R, *et al.* Magnesium sulfate in the management of acute intrapartum fetal distress. *Am J Obstet Gynecol* 1984; **148**: 104–7.

112. Riley ET, Flanagan B, Cohen SE, *et al.* Intravenous nitroglycerin: a potent uterine relaxant for emergency obstetric procedures. Review of the literature and report of three cases. *Int J Obstet Anesth* 1996; **5**: 264–8.

113. Clark SL, Gimovsky ML, Miller FC. Fetal heart rate response to scalp blood sampling. *Am J Obstet Gynecol* 1982; **44**: 706–8.

114. Tejani N, Verma U, Hameed C, *et al.* Method and route of delivery in the low birth weight vertex presentation correlated with early periventricular/intraventricular hemorrhage. *Obstet Gynecol* 1987; **69**: 1–4.

115. Riskin A, Riskin-Mashiah S, Lusky A, *et al.* The relationship between delivery mode and mortality in very low birthweight singleton vertex-presenting infants. *BJOG* 2004; **111**: 1365–71.

116. Qiu H, Paneth N, Lorenz JM, *et al.* Labor and delivery factors in brain damage, disabling cerebral palsy, and neonatal death in low-birth-weight infants. *Am J Obstet Gynecol* 2003; **189**: 1143–9.

117. Grant A, Glazener CM. Elective caesarean section versus expectant management for delivery of the small baby. *Cochrane Database Syst Rev* 2001; **2**: CD000078.

118. Lee HC, Gould JB. Survival advantage associated with cesarean delivery in very low birth weight vertex neonates. *Obstet Gynecol* 2006; **107**: 97–105.

119. Lee HC, Gould JB. Survival rates and mode of delivery for vertex preterm neonates according to small- or appropriate-for-gestational-age status. *Pediatrics* 2007; **1118**: e1836–44.

120. Mercer JS, Vohr BR, McGrath MM, *et al.* Delayed cord clamping in very preterm infants reduces the incidence of intraventricular hemorrhage and late-onset sepsis: a randomized, controlled trial. *Pediatrics* 2006; **117**: 1235–42.

121. Rouse D, Hirtz DG, Thom E, *et al.* A randomized controlled trial of magnesium sulfate for the prevention of cerebral palsy. *N Engl J Med* 2008; **359**: 895–905.

Chapter 6

Risks and complications of multiple gestations

Yair Blumenfeld and Usha Chitkara

Introduction

In the United States in 2004, 3.4% of all births were multiple births [1]. Between 1994 and 2004, the multiple birth ratio in the United States increased by 32% (from 2.6% to 3.4%), largely due to increased use of assisted reproductive technology. This increase in multiple birth rates has had a tremendous impact on prematurity. In 2004, one in eight babies (12.5% of live births) was born prematurely; and of multiple gestations, 61.4% were born preterm, 58.5% were low birthweight (less than 2500 g), and 11.5% were very low birthweight (less than 1500 g) [1]. Infants from multiple gestations thus carry a tremendous economic burden, in 2005 the annual cost of prematurity in the United States was well over $26 billion [1].

Among multiple gestations, the highest incidence is contributed by twins. Besides prematurity, twins, regardless of type, are at higher risk for neurological injury. Over the years, several studies have correlated cerebral palsy with multiple gestations [2–6]. A recently published large case–control study based on the Swedish Medical Birth Registry between 1984 and 1998 showed a 1.4 odds ratio (95% CI 1.1–1.6) of cerebral palsy in twin gestations relative to their singleton counterparts [7].

Besides their effect on society, twins pose interesting and challenging diagnostic and management dilemmas. From conception to delivery, and even beyond, twin gestations behave remarkably differently from their singleton counterparts, and have a myriad of unique physiologic changes and pathologic conditions that one must consider when caring for these special pregnancies.

Embryology

Approximately two-thirds of twins are dizygotic, with an incidence of 7–11/1000 births [8]. The incidence of dizygotic twinning is influenced by race, heredity, maternal age, parity, and especially fertility drugs [8]. Dizygotic twins result from fertilization of two oocytes by different spermatozoa, and thus each zygote has a different genetic makeup. Each twin implants separately in the uterus and has a separate chorionic sac and amniotic cavity. Monozygotic twins, on the other hand, occur at a relatively constant rate, approximately

one per 250 births, and result from splitting of the zygote at various stages of development. When splitting occurs at the two-cell stage (within 3 days post fertilization), each resulting embryo will have its own placenta, amniotic sac, and chorionic cavity [9]. If splitting occurs later, at the early bastocyst stage (between 4 and 8 days post fertilization), the resulting embryos will have a common placenta and chorionic sac, but separate amniotic cavities [9]. Rarely, the separation occurs at the bilaminar germ disc stage (between 8 and 12 days post fertilization), resulting in two embryos that share a single placenta, as well as a common chorionic and amniotic sac [9]. Even rarer are conjoined twins, resulting from a split during development of the primitive node and streak (after day 13 post fertilization).

Zygosity can be determined prenatally by ultrasound only if the fetuses are monoamnionic or monochorionic. Dichorionic, diamnionic twins may be either dizygotic or monozygotic. Obstetrically, clarifying the chorionicity of twin gestations as early as possible is of vital importance, since antenatal, intrapartum, and postnatal risks vary by chorionic type.

Diagnosis

Until the use of real-time ultrasound in the 1970s, twin gestations were largely diagnosed at the time of delivery. The treating obstetrician may have been suspicious clinically of the possibility of multiple gestations by a larger than expected abdominal size or by multiple moving fetal parts. Advances in ultrasound imaging, and more recently the shift towards increased first-trimester imaging, have had a tremendous impact on the antenatal diagnosis and care of multiple gestations.

Probably no parameter on ultrasound evaluation is more important than determining the chorionicity of multiple gestations. Imaging parameters such as determining the sex of the fetuses, placental location and origin, thickness (less than or greater than 2 mm) and number of layers of the membranes are often utilized to achieve this goal [10]. Sometimes, in pregnancies in which there is a single placental mass, it may be difficult to distinguish one large placenta from two placentas that are "fused." In these situations, the presence of a triangular projection of placental tissue extending beyond the chorionic surface, termed the "twin peak" sign, indicates two fused placentas [8]. A prospective study comparing ultrasound criteria with placental pathology found that the combination

Fetal and Neonatal Brain Injury, 4th edition, ed. David K. Stevenson, William E. Benitz, Philip Sunshine, Susan R. Hintz, and Maurice L. Druzin. Published by Cambridge University Press. © Cambridge University Press 2009.

of placental location, dividing membrane thickness, presence or absence of the twin peak sign, and fetal gender had 91% specificity and sensitivity for determining the chorionicity, amnionicity, and zygosity of 110 twins at mid-gestation [11].

Prematurity

The mean gestational age of delivery for twin pregnancies is 35.3 weeks, more than 4 weeks earlier than for singletons [12]. Multiple gestations are also six times more likely to be born preterm (less than 37 weeks) and eight times more likely to be born very preterm (less than 32 weeks) [1]. In a large cohort study of more than 33 800 neonates, twins represented only 2.6% of newborns but 12.2% of all preterm births, 15.4% of neonatal deaths and 9.5% of all fetal deaths [13]. Spontaneous labor accounted for 54% of all preterm twin pregnancies, premature rupture of membranes accounted for 22%, and indicated deliveries for 23% (including maternal hypertension, fetal distress, and fetal growth abnormalities) [13].

The pathophysiologic mechanisms leading to preterm labor and delivery in twins may be quite different from those in singletons. Stretching alone can induce increased myometrial contractility, prostaglandin release, expression of gap junction protein or connexin 43, and increased oxytocin receptors in pregnant and non-pregnant myometrium [14,15]. Compared with spontaneous twins, IVF twins are at an increased risk for preterm delivery and have been reported to deliver at earlier gestational ages [16].

Prediction

Currently, the most validated predictive markers of preterm labor are cervical length and fetal fibronectin measurements. A short cervix, often defined as less than 2.5 cm in the second trimester (normal cervix is approximately 3.5–4 cm), is associated with a 25% risk of preterm labor in singletons but up to 70% in twins [17]. Similarly, the presence of fetal fibronectin (FFN), a protein released by the decidual membrane, has a positive predictive value of 83.1% in singletons and up to 100% in twins [17,18]. Studies comparing the utility of combining both have shown that the presence of short cervix and positive FFN at 24 weeks carries a 25% risk of delivery within 2–4 weeks for singleton gestations but up to 50% in twins [17]. Today, both are utilized in assessing the risk of preterm labor in twin gestations [19–21].

Prevention

Cervical cerclage in the setting of a history of cervical incompetence or for short cervix remains controversial in singleton pregnancies [22], and it is even more controversial for twin gestations. In the 1980s two prospective studies evaluating the role of prophylactic cerclage in multiple gestations did not show a definitive benefit from the procedure [23,24]. More recently, in their study of prophylactic cerclage in twins, Eskandar et al. also showed no benefit to cerclage over expectant management [25]. Furthermore, two recent retrospective studies of ultrasound-indicated cerclage due to a short cervix also demonstrated no benefit to cerclage [26,27].

Progesterone supplementation has recently been introduced as a possible means of preventing the recurrence of preterm labor in singleton gestations [28]. When the same study group evaluated the role of progesterone for multiple gestations, equal benefit was not found [29]. There is still debate regarding the role of progesterone in twin pregnancies, including the optimal dose and route of administration. There is currently no consensus, nor enough data to support the routine use of progesterone supplementation for preterm labor prevention in twins [30].

Treatment

There are limited data regarding the benefit of acute tocolysis for preterm labor in twin pregnancies. Most of the information available has come from the few retrospective and prospective trials that mostly included singletons but also some twin sets. Hales et al. reported magnesium sulfate to be as efficacious in twins as it is in singletons [31]. O'Leary in 1986 described prophylactic oral terbutaline to increase the mean gestational age of delivery in 28 twin pairs [32]. More recently, in the largest randomized prospective trial comparing magnesium sulfate to nifedipine, which included 37 twin pregnancies out of 192 participants, no difference was observed in delay of delivery, gestational age of delivery, or major neonatal outcomes between the two study drugs [33]. Overall, there is limited information regarding the benefit of tocolytics in twin pregnancies, especially their efficacy and effects on birthweight and neonatal mortality [12]. On the other hand, corticosteroids for improvement of neonatal outcomes in the setting of preterm labor are recommended by the National Institutes of Health despite a lack of studies assessing the optimal dose in twin gestations [12].

Twin-to-twin transfusion syndrome

Twin-to-twin transfusion syndrome (TTTS) is a pathological condition in which placental arterial and venous anastamoses lead to unequal sharing of fetal blood supply and discordant growth in monozygotic twins. Studies conducted on placentas of TTTS twins suggest that it is the deep arteriovenous connections that lead to this phenomenon [34]. Classically, the condition will result in a "donor twin," characterized by intrauterine growth restriction, anemia, and oligohydramnios; and a "recipient twin," in which the blood volume overload will ultimately lead to hydropic changes, polycythemia, polyhydramnios, and heart failure. TTTS is seen in approximately 5–15% of monochorionic twins [35].

Clinical presentation and diagnosis

In 1999, a staging system for TTTS was introduced that incorporated discordant amniotic fluid volumes between gestational sacs, absent bladder in the donor twin, arterial Doppler abnormalities, presence of fetal hydrops, and neonatal demise [36]. The staging system, designated from class 1 to 5 in severity, has not only prognostic implications for neonatal morbidity and mortality, but also has since been used to triage patients for prenatal invasive surgical treatment modalities [36].

In cases of severe oligohydramnios, the donor twin may have a "stuck twin" appearance due to its proximity to the uterine wall and limited ability to move freely within its amniotic cavity.

Management

Early studies of TTTS reported perinatal mortality rates as high as 100% when the disease was diagnosed mid-trimester [37]. Today, the management and outcome of these twins will vary by center depending upon the gestational age and severity of disease at the time of diagnosis. The natural course of TTTS is relatively unpredictable. In a limited study of 18 TTTS twins followed for 90 "week-to-week changes," a progression of disease was seen in 14.5%, downstaging was present in 12.2%, and no change was seen in 72.2% [38].

Over the years, multiple treatment modalities have been attempted aimed at resolving the unequal sharing of blood supply. Amnioreduction via serial amniocentesis, amniotic septostomy, and selective fetocide via cord occlusion of one of the co-twins have all been described. Serial amniocentesis remains the most widely available and practiced therapy for TTTS. A large review of neonatal outcomes from 223 sets of twins undergoing amnioreduction for TTTS showed a 78% live birth rate, 60% alive at 4 weeks of life, and 48% of sets with both neonates alive at 4 weeks of life. Neurological scans in survivors revealed abnormalities in 24% of recipients and 25% of donors [39].

Endoscopic laser photocoagulation was introduced in the late 1980s and early 1990s as a treatment for early and severe TTTS. A recent European multicenter prospective randomized study comparing serial amnioreduction with endoscopic laser surgery was stopped early due to the observation of increased neonatal survival and decreased incidence of periventricular leukomalacia and other fetal neurological complications in the laser photocoagulation group [40]. A similar multicenter prospective clinical trial conducted in the United States did not show a difference in the overall fetal and neonatal survival between amnioreduction and laser surgery [41].

Neonatal outcomes

Progressive TTTS is often associated with severe neonatal morbidity and mortality, including severe adverse neurological outcomes. Overall, neonatal outcomes will depend largely on the gestational age at diagnosis, severity of disease, treatment modality, and presence of co-twin demise [42]. In a large cohort study of monochorionic twins, those with TTTS had higher rates of respiratory distress syndrome (RDS), intraventricular hemorrhage (IVH), periventricular leukomalacia (PVL), renal failure, persistent pulmonary hypertension of the newborn (PPHN), and fetal demise, and lower 1-year survival [35]. Intracranial Doppler flow abnormalities have also been reported in monochorionic twins with TTTS, and these have been correlated with worse outcomes [43]. In a retrospective study of 29 TTTS cases, 18 treated with serial amnioreduction and 11 with conservative management, perinatal mortality was 50%, with a mean gestational age of delivery of 28 weeks. Abnormal cranial ultrasounds were seen

in 41% of neonates and the incidence of cerebral palsy was 21% (50% in cases of a single twin survivor and 14.3% in cases of double survivors) [44]. A recent prospective long-term study of 167 surviving neonates of second-trimester TTTS treated with laser photocoagulation from a single center reported 86% intact neurodevelopmental outcomes in survivors, 7% mild neurological abnormalities, and 6% major neurodevelopmental abnormalities [45]. Another report of 82 TTTS pregnancies treated with fetoscopic laser surgery reported a 70% perinatal survival and 17% (19/115) neurodevelopmental impairment at 2 years of life, including cerebral palsy (eight cases), mental developmental delay (nine cases), psychomotor developmental delay (12 cases), and deafness (one case) [46].

Abnormal growth

Aside from twin-to-twin transfusion syndrome, abnormal growth is present in approximately 15–25% of twin gestations [12]. Abnormal growth may be either *discordant growth*, classified as 15–25% weight difference between the co-twins, or *small for gestational age (SGA)/intrauterine growth restriction (IUGR)*, classified as estimated weight less than 10% for either one or both twins. Abnormal growth in twin gestations may be a result of abnormal placentation as well as increased fetal metabolic demand. In a study of 1318 twin pairs (926 with twins of appropriate weight for gestational age and 392 with twins small for gestational age), discordant growth was an independent risk factor for cesarean delivery and adverse neonatal outcomes [47]. Other studies have also shown similar increased risk of neonatal morbidity and mortality with discordant growth [48,49]. A prospective cohort study of 42 expectantly managed monochorionic twins with selective intrauterine growth restriction, compared with 29 dichorionic and 32 monochorionic appropriately grown twin controls, showed higher rates of parenchymal brain damage in the monochorionic growth-restricted group (12% vs. 1.7% and 0% respectively) [50].

Because of the adverse neonatal risks with abnormal growth, twins are routinely monitored with serial growth ultrasounds in the second and third trimesters. Management of growth abnormalities will depend upon the gestational age and severity at the time of diagnosis. Bed rest and hospitalization, though often recommended, have not been proven to correct or prevent progressive fetal growth abnormalities [51].

Monochorionic twins

Monochorionic twins, twins resulting from division of the fertilized egg at various stages, have a relatively stable prevalence of approximately 1/250 births. All monochorionic twins are monozygotic, but not all monozygotic twins are monochorionic. Though originally thought to arise independently of assisted reproductive technology, recent studies from a single academic IVF center describe lower rates of monozygotic twins after 2002, and higher rates of monozygotic twins with blastocyst transfer compared to day-three embryo transfers, thus suggesting an effect on the rates of monochorionic twins by assisted reproduction [52,53].

Besides twin-to-twin transfusion syndrome, monochorionic twins are at a higher risk for single twin demise, twin growth abnormalities, preterm labor and delivery, and adverse neonatal outcomes including neurological deficits [42]. A retrospective study of day-three cranial ultrasounds performed on 101 multiple-gestation neonates delivered prior to 36 weeks, including 89 twins and 12 triplets, revealed a 13.8% antenatal necrosis of the cerebral white matter [54]. The incidence of antenatal necrosis of the cerebral white matter was much higher in monochorionic than in dichorionic twins (30% vs 3.3%; $p < 0.001$) [54]. Interestingly, a recent meta-analysis has even shown monochorionic twins to be at increased risk for congenital cardiac defects [55].

The death of one twin in a monochorionic pair is associated with significant risk of brain hypoxic–ischemic damage in the survivor [42,56,57]. This neurological injury likely happens instantaneously following the demise of the co-twin, and it is thought to be caused either by acute vascular flow changes or by embolization of fetal material through vascular anastomoses. Antenatal MRI has been performed on surviving co-twins, and various lesion types and locations have been reported [58].

The management, counseling, and neonatal risk stratification for monochorionic twins will depend largely on whether the twins are monoamnionic or diamnionic. Monochorionic, monoamnionic twins are at extremely high risk for cord entanglement, single twin demise, and preterm delivery. These twins are often admitted to the hospital at 24–28 weeks gestation and delivered by 32 weeks gestation [59]. Monochorionic, diamnionic twins are often managed on an outpatient basis as long as adequate fetal growth and neonatal well-being are reassuring. There is a debate regarding the optimal timing of delivery in monochorionic, diamnionic twins due to the risk of single co-twin demise with progressive gestation. Large cohort studies addressing perinatal mortality rates and gestational age in twins have shown the lowest perinatal mortality at 37–38 weeks (compared with 39–40 weeks for singletons) [60,61]. A recent large retrospective Dutch cohort study showed higher rates of fetal mortality in monochorionic than dichorionic twins after 32 weeks gestation, and suggested that the optimal time to deliver monochorionic twins is at or before 37 weeks gestation [62].

Peripartum management

Although delivery by cesarean section is a well-accepted practice for multiple gestations of triplets and greater, the mode of delivery for twin gestations remains controversial. Though often delivered via cesarean section, most physicians will determine the optimal route of delivery based on fetal presentation and clinical experience. Most obstetricians are comfortable delivering twin gestations vaginally if the twins are of concordant weight and in the vertex–vertex presentation. Fewer obstetricians feel comfortable performing a vertex–breech delivery, and even fewer would perform an internal podalic version and breech extraction for a vertex–transverse presentation.

Vertex–vertex twins are present in 38% of twins at the time of delivery, vertex–breech in 42% and non-vertex presenting twins in 20% [63]. The data regarding the safety of vertex delivery, followed by a breech extraction, is mixed for vertex–breech presentation. The American College of Obstetricians and Gynecologists (ACOG) states that "the route of delivery for twins should be determined by the position of the fetuses, the ease of fetal heart rate monitoring, and maternal and fetal status. Data are insufficient to determine the best route of delivery for higher order multiple gestations" [12]. A large retrospective study of 15 185 second non-vertex twins reported increased neonatal morbidity and mortality with vaginal delivery versus elective cesarean section, even when excluding those twins who were delivered via a combined vaginal–cesarean section [64]. Morbidity included infant injury, low Apgar scores, ventilation use, and seizures.

There is also some controversy regarding the vertex–breech delivery of fetuses weighing less than 1500 grams. Most experts refrain from doing so despite multiple retrospective studies showing no benefit to cesarean section in this situation [65–67]. Also, most clinicians will not attempt a vertex–breech delivery if the estimated weight of the second twin is 20% more than that of the presenting fetus.

There are some data regarding vaginal birth after cesarean (VBAC) delivery in twin gestations. Most studies, including a large cohort study of over 1600 twin pregnancies, report uterine rupture rates similar to those in singleton VBAC deliveries [68–70].

Conclusion

The rates of multiple gestations are rising and will undoubtedly continue to do so over the coming years. With this increase, the high incidence of complications in multiple gestations, namely prematurity and growth abnormalities, will continue to occupy future obstetricians and neonatologists. It is our hope that advances in our understanding of pathophysiologic mechanisms leading to these adverse outcomes will result in improved preventive, diagnostic, prophylactic, and therapeutic modalities, thereby reducing the risks and complications associated with these special pregnancies.

References

1. March of Dimes. *Peri Stats*. www.marchofdimes.com/peristats. Accessed February, 2008.

2. Alberman ED. Cerebral palsy in twins. *Guys Hosp Rep* 1964; **113**: 285–95.

3. Goodman R. Cerebral palsy in twins. *Dev Med Child Neurol* 1993; **35**: 370.

4. Livinec F, Ancel PY, Marret S, *et al.* Prenatal risk factors for cerebral palsy in very preterm singletons and twins. *Obstet Gynecol* 2005; **105**: 1341–7.

5. Petterson B, Nelson KB, Watson L, *et al.* Twins, triplets, and cerebral palsy in births in Western Australia in the 1980s. *BMJ* 1993; **307**: 1239–43.

6. Pharoah PO. Twins and cerebral palsy. *Acta Paediatr Suppl* 2001; **90**: 6–10.

7. Thorngren-Jerneck K, Herbst A. Perinatal factors associated with cerebral palsy in children born in Sweden. *Obstet Gynecol* 2006; **108**: 1499–505.

8. Cunningham FG, Williams JW, eds. *Williams Obstetrics*, 21st edn. New York, NY: McGraw-Hill, 2001.

9. Sadler TW, Langman J, eds. *Langman's Medical Embryology*, 10th edn. Philadelphia, PA: Lippincott Williams & Wilkins, 2006.

10. Monteagudo A, Timor-Tritsch IE, Sharma S. Early and simple determination of chorionic and amniotic type in multifetal gestations in the first fourteen weeks by high-frequency transvaginal ultrasonography. *Am J Obstet Gynecol* 1994; **170**: 824–9.

11. Scardo JA, Ellings JM, Newman RB. Prospective determination of chorionicity, amnionicity, and zygosity in twin gestations. *Am J Obstet Gynecol* 1995; **173**: 1376–80.

12. ACOG Practice Bulletin #56: Multiple gestation: complicated twin, triplet, and high-order multifetal pregnancy. *Obstet Gynecol* 2004; **104**: 869–83.

13. Gardner MO, Goldenberg RL, Cliver SP, *et al.* The origin and outcome of preterm twin pregnancies. *Obstet Gynecol* 1995; **85**: 553–7.

14. Newman RB, Iams JD, Das A, *et al.* A prospective masked observational study of uterine contraction frequency in twins. *Am J Obstet Gynecol* 2006; **195**: 1564–70.

15. Romero R, Espinoza J, Kusanovic JP, *et al.* The preterm parturition syndrome. *BJOG* 2006; **113**: 17–42.

16. Nassar AH, Usta IM, Rechdan JB, *et al.* Pregnancy outcome in spontaneous twins versus twins who were conceived through in vitro fertilization. *Am J Obstet Gynecol* 2003; **189**: 513–18.

17. Goldenberg RL, Iams JD, Das A, *et al.* The Preterm Prediction Study: sequential cervical length and fetal fibronectin testing for the prediction of spontaneous preterm birth. National Institute of Child Health and Human Development Maternal–Fetal Medicine Units Network. *Am J Obstet Gynecol* 2000; **182**: 636–43.

18. Lockwood CJ, Senyei AE, Dische MR, *et al.* Fetal fibronectin in cervical and vaginal secretions as a predictor of preterm delivery. *N Engl J Med* 1991; **325**: 669–74.

19. Gibson JL, Macara LM, Owen P, *et al.* Prediction of preterm delivery in twin pregnancy: a prospective, observational study of cervical length and fetal fibronectin testing. *Ultrasound Obstet Gynecol* 2004; **23**: 561–6.

20. Goldenberg RL, Iams JD, Miodovnik M, *et al.* The preterm prediction study: risk factors in twin gestations. National Institute of Child Health and Human Development Maternal–Fetal Medicine Units Network. *Am J Obstet Gynecol* 1996; **175**: 1047–53.

21. Ruiz RJ, Fullerton J, Brown CE. The utility of fFN for the prediction of preterm birth in twin gestations. *J Obstet Gynecol Neonatal Nurs* 2004; **33**: 446–54.

22. Berghella V, Odibo AO, To MS, *et al.* Cerclage for short cervix on ultrasonography: meta-analysis of trials using individual patient-level data. *Obstet Gynecol* 2005; **106**: 181–9.

23. Dor J, Shalev J, Mashiach S, *et al.* Elective cervical suture of twin pregnancies diagnosed ultrasonically in the first trimester following induced ovulation. *Gynecol Obstet Invest* 1982; **13**: 55–60.

24. Interim report of the Medical Research Council/Royal College of Obstetricians and Gynaecologists multicentre randomized trial of cervical cerclage. MRC/RCOG Working Party on Cervical Cerclage. *Br J Obstet Gynaecol* 1988; **95**: 437–45.

25. Eskandar M, Shafiq H, Almushait MA, *et al.* Cervical cerclage for prevention of preterm birth in women with twin pregnancy. *Int J Gynaecol Obstet* 2007; **99**: 110–12.

26. Roman AS, Rebarber A, Pereira L, *et al.* The efficacy of sonographically indicated cerclage in multiple gestations. *J Ultrasound Med* 2005; **24**: 763–71.

27. Newman RB, Krombach RS, Myers MC, *et al.* Effect of cerclage on obstetrical outcome in twin gestations with a shortened cervical length. *Am J Obstet Gynecol* 2002; **186**: 634–40.

28. Meis PJ, Klebanoff M, Thom E, *et al.* Prevention of recurrent preterm delivery by 17 alpha-hydroxyprogesterone caproate. *N Engl J Med* 2003; **348**: 2379–85.

29. Rouse DJ, Caritis SN, Peaceman AM, *et al.* A trial of 17 alpha-hydroxyprogesterone caproate to prevent prematurity in twins. *N Engl J Med* 2007; **357**: 454–61.

30. ACOG Committee Opinion. Use of progesterone to reduce preterm birth. *Obstet Gynecol* 2003; **102**: 1115–16.

31. Hales KA, Matthews JP, Rayburn WF, *et al.* Intravenous magnesium sulfate for premature labor: comparison between twin and singleton gestations. *Am J Perinatol* 1995; **12**: 7–10.

32. O'Leary JA. Prophylactic tocolysis of twins. *Am J Obstet Gynecol* 1986; **154**: 904–5.

33. Lyell DJ, Pullen K, Campbell L, *et al.* Magnesium sulfate compared with nifedipine for acute tocolysis of preterm labor: a randomized controlled trial. *Obstet Gynecol* 2007; **110**: 61–7.

34. Bajoria R, Wigglesworth J, Fisk NM. Angioarchitecture of monochorionic placentas in relation to the twin–twin transfusion syndrome. *Am J Obstet Gynecol* 1995; **172**: 856–63.

35. Lutfi S, Allen VM, Fahey J, *et al.* Twin–twin transfusion syndrome: a population-based study. *Obstet Gynecol* 2004; **104**: 1289–97.

36. Quintero RA, Morales WJ, Allen MH, *et al.* Staging of twin–twin transfusion syndrome. *J Perinatol* 1999; **19**: 550–5.

37. Chescheir NC, Seeds JW. Polyhydramnios and oligohydramnios in twin gestations. *Obstet Gynecol* 1988; **71**: 882–4.

38. Luks FI, Carr SR, Plevyak M, *et al.* Limited prognostic value of a staging system for twin-to-twin transfusion syndrome. *Fetal Diagn Ther* 2004; **19**: 301–4.

39. Mari G, Roberts A, Detti L, *et al.* Perinatal morbidity and mortality rates in severe twin–twin transfusion syndrome: results of the International Amnioreduction Registry. *Am J Obstet Gynecol* 2001; **185**: 708–15.

40. Senat MV, Deprest J, Boulvain M, *et al.* Endoscopic laser surgery versus serial amnioreduction for severe twin-to-twin transfusion syndrome. *N Engl J Med* 2004; **351**: 136–44.

41. Crombleholme TM, Shera D, Lee H, *et al.* A prospective, randomized, multicenter trial of amnioreduction vs. selective fetoscopic laser photocoagulation for the treatment of severe twin–twin transfusion syndrome. *Am J Obstet Gynecol* 2007; **197**: 396.e1–9.

42. Adegbite AL, Castille S, Ward S, *et al.* Neuromorbidity in preterm twins in relation to chorionicity and discordant birth weight. *Am J Obstet Gynecol* 2004; **190**: 156–63.

43. Degani S, Leibovitz Z, Shapiro I, *et al.* Instability of Doppler cerebral blood flow in monochorionic twins. *J Ultrasound Med* 2006; **25**: 449–54.

44. Lopriore E, Nagel HT, Vandenbussche FP, *et al.* Long-term neurodevelopmental outcome in twin-to-twin transfusion syndrome. *Am J Obstet Gynecol* 2003; **189**: 1314–19.

45. Graef C, Ellenrieder B, Hecher K, *et al.* Long-term neurodevelopmental outcome of 167 children after intrauterine laser treatment for severe twin–twin transfusion syndrome. *Am J Obstet Gynecol* 2006; **194**: 303–8.

46. Lopriore E, Middeldorp JM, Sueters M, *et al.* Long-term neurodevelopmental outcome in twin-to-twin transfusion syndrome treated with fetoscopic laser surgery. *Am J Obstet Gynecol* 2007; **196**: 231.e1–4.

47. Amaru RC, Bush MC, Berkowitz RL, *et al.* Is discordant growth in twins an independent risk factor for adverse neonatal outcome? *Obstet Gynecol* 2004; **103**: 71–6.

48. Branum AM, Schoendorf KC. The effect of birth weight discordance on twin neonatal mortality. *Obstet Gynecol* 2003; **101**: 570–4.

49. Demissie K, Ananth CV, Martin J, *et al.* Fetal and neonatal mortality among twin gestations in the United States: the role of intrapair birth weight discordance. *Obstet Gynecol* 2002; **100**: 474–80.

50. Gratacos E, Carreras E, Becker J, *et al.* Prevalence of neurological damage in monochorionic twins with selective intrauterine growth restriction and intermittent absent or reversed end-diastolic umbilical artery flow. *Ultrasound Obstet Gynecol* 2004; **24**: 159–63.

51. Gulmezoglu AM, Hofmeyr GJ. Bed rest in hospital for suspected impaired fetal growth. *Cochrane Database Syst Rev* 2000; **2**: CD000034.

52. Milki AA, Jun SH, Hinckley MD, *et al.* Incidence of monozygotic twinning with blastocyst transfer compared to cleavage-stage transfer. *Fertil Steril* 2003; **79**: 503–6.

53. Moayeri SE, Behr B, Lathi RB, *et al.* Risk of monozygotic twinning with blastocyst transfer decreases over time: an 8-year experience. *Fertil Steril* 2007; **87**: 1028–32.

54. Bejar R, Vigliocco G, Gramajo H, *et al.* Antenatal origin of neurologic damage in newborn infants. II. Multiple gestations. *Am J Obstet Gynecol* 1990; **162**: 1230–6.

55. Bahtiyar MO, Dulay AT, Weeks BP, *et al.* Prevalence of congenital heart defects in monochorionic/diamniotic twin gestations: a systematic literature review. *J Ultrasound Med* 2007; **26**: 1491–8.

56. Okumura A, Hayakawa F, Kato T, *et al.* Brain malformation of the surviving twin of intrauterine co-twin demise. *J Child Neurol* 2007; **22**: 85–8.

57. Morokuma S, Tsukimori K, Anami A, *et al.* Brain injury of the survivor diagnosed at 18 weeks of gestation after intrauterine demise of the co-twin: a case report. *Fetal Diagn Ther* 2007; **23**: 138–40.

58. Righini A, Salmona S, Bianchini E, *et al.* Prenatal magnetic resonance imaging evaluation of ischemic brain lesions in the survivors of monochorionic twin pregnancies: report of 3 cases. *J Comput Assist Tomogr* 2004; **28**: 87–92.

59. Ezra Y, Shveiky D, Ophir E, *et al.* Intensive management and early delivery reduce antenatal mortality in monoamniotic twin pregnancies. *Acta Obstet Gynecol Scand* 2005; **84**: 432–5.

60. Minakami H, Sato I. Reestimating date of delivery in multifetal pregnancies. *JAMA* 1996; **275**: 1432–4.

61. Kahn B, Lumey LH, Zybert PA, *et al.* Prospective risk of fetal death in singleton, twin, and triplet gestations: implications for practice. *Obstet Gynecol* 2003; **102**: 685–92.

62. Hack KE, Derks JB, Elias SG, *et al.* Increased perinatal mortality and morbidity in monochorionic versus dichorionic twin pregnancies: clinical implications of a large Dutch cohort study. *BJOG* 2008; **115**: 58–67.

63. Chasen ST, Spiro SJ, Kalish RB, *et al.* Changes in fetal presentation in twin pregnancies. *J Matern Fetal Neonatal Med* 2005; **17**: 45–8.

64. Yang Q, Wen SW, Chen Y, *et al.* Neonatal death and morbidity in vertex–nonvertex second twins according to mode of delivery and birth weight. *Am J Obstet Gynecol* 2005; **192**: 840–7.

65. Chasen ST, Chervenak FA. Delivery of twin gestations. *UpToDate*; 2007.

66. Davison L, Easterling TR, Jackson JC, *et al.* Breech extraction of low-birth-weight second twins: can cesarean section be justified? *Am J Obstet Gynecol* 1992; **166**: 497–502.

67. Morales WJ, O'Brien WF, Knuppel RA, *et al.* The effect of mode of delivery on the risk of intraventricular hemorrhage in nondiscordant twin gestations under 1500 g. *Obstet Gynecol* 1989; **73**: 107–10.

68. Ford AA, Bateman BT, Simpson LL. Vaginal birth after cesarean delivery in twin gestations: a large, nationwide sample of deliveries. *Am J Obstet Gynecol* 2006; **195**: 1138–42.

69. Miller DA, Mullin P, Hou D, *et al.* Vaginal birth after cesarean section in twin gestation. *Am J Obstet Gynecol* 1996; **175**: 194–8.

70. Sansregret A, Bujold E, Gauthier RJ. Twin delivery after a previous caesarean: a twelve-year experience. *J Obstet Gynaecol Can* 2003; **25**: 294–8.

Intrauterine growth restriction

Alistair G. S. Philip, David K. Stevenson, and William W. Hay Jr.

Introduction

Fetuses that grow at rates less than their inherent growth potential have intrauterine growth restriction or IUGR. Such infants, particularly when the IUGR is severe, tend to have significant problems later in life, with structural and functional neurodevelopmental disorders. Animal models confirm that decreased brain neuronal number and dendritic arborization, cognitive capacity, and behavioral function are common when growth at critical early stages of development is restricted. Understanding the basic problems that contribute to IUGR and the characteristics of such infants, therefore, is important to complement other discussions in this textbook about fetal and neonatal brain injury.

Terminology and definitions

IUGR refers to a slower than normal rate of fetal growth. Several terms have been used, often interchangeably, for IUGR. These include fetal growth retardation, fetal mal- or undernutrition, small for gestational age (SGA), small or light for dates, dysmature, placental insufficiency syndrome, "runting" syndrome, and hypotrophy. The term "restriction" is preferred to "retardation," because parents tend to link "retardation" with mental retardation [1]. Unfortunately, these terms do not all mean the same [2], which has led to some confusion, both with regard to etiologic classification and to follow-up and outcome. In interpreting studies dealing with IUGR, it is important to know how the term has been defined for the particular study. Most importantly, birthweight does not always determine fetal growth rate. See Table 7.1 for a classification schema of fetal growth that now is standard.

Even for studies dealing with infants who are called SGA, it is important to know the normative data used for comparison. For years, the growth curves developed in Denver, Colorado [3], were used as the basis for comparison by many authors. These data were gathered from infants born at an altitude of 5000 ft (1525 m), and altitude independently reduces birthweight for gestational age, largely an effect of reduced oxygen supply combined with a failure of the fetus to produce enough additional hemoglobin to maintain blood oxygen content [4,5]. Thus, infants classified as below the 10th percentile by birthweight for gestational age in Colorado probably represent infants below the 3rd percentile at sea level if using Montreal curves [6]. Data from Sweden, also at sea level, indicate that birthweights in recent years may be even higher than noted in an earlier era [7]. This may be partially related to the extreme limitation on weight gain during pregnancy that was imposed by most obstetricians in North America during the 1950s and 1960s, when these data were being gathered, as well as more recent trends toward larger infants from the now worldwide epidemic of maternal obesity.

While the majority of SGA infants will have some degree of IUGR, some are predestined to fall below the 10th percentile on a genetic or racial basis. On the other hand, some infants who have a birthweight that is appropriate for gestational age (AGA, between the 10th and 90th percentiles) may be suffering from the effects of IUGR. These infants will usually display some evidence of wasting or appear scrawny. The ponderal index or weight/length ratio helps to quantify the degree of "wasting" or "scrawniness" that some of these infants have. The ponderal index is derived as the weight (g) divided by the length (cm) cubed times 100 [3,8,9]. Different authors have used the ponderal index to classify infant growth, mostly for research purposes [8,10]. Unfortunately, this may lead to multiple subgroups within the total population of IUGR infants [11]. While this may reflect the great heterogeneity of this group of infants, it can also lead to confusion.

The simplest classification is to consider infants with IUGR as either proportionally (symmetrically) or disproportionally (asymmetrically) grown. Most proportionally grown infants will have a normal ponderal index, whereas the disproportionally grown infants will have a decreased ponderal index. However, such clear-cut distinctions are not always possible [11]. Proportionally grown infants are likely to have had a chronic insult (e.g., a chromosomal problem such as trisomy 18), whereas the disproportionally grown infants are likely to have suffered a subacute or acute insult (e.g., decreased uteroplacental blood flow with maternal preeclampsia). For many years it was believed that a chronic insult resulted in a decrease in cell number, but a subacute or acute insult produced a decrease in cell size [12]. Both proportional and disproportional growth patterns begin in the second trimester [13]. The principal distinction of

Fetal and Neonatal Brain Injury, 4th edition, ed. David K. Stevenson, William E. Benitz, Philip Sunshine, Susan R. Hintz, and Maurice L. Druzin. Published by Cambridge University Press. © Cambridge University Press 2009.

Table 7.1. Classification of fetal growth

Small for gestational age (SGA)	Birthweight < 10th percentile for gestational age
Appropriate for gestational age (AGA)	Birthweight between 10th and 90th percentile for gestational age
Large for gestational age (LGA)	Birthweight > 90th percentile for gestational age
Intrauterine growth restriction (IUGR)	Slower than normal rate of fetal growth
Normal birthweight	> 2500 g at term gestation
Low birthweight (LBW)	< 2500 g
Very low birthweight (VLBW)	< 1500 g
Extremely low birthweight (ELBW)	< 1000 g

Table 7.2. Maternal conditions associated with intrauterine growth restriction (IUGR)

Both very young and advanced maternal age
Maternal pre-pregnancy short stature and thinness
Poor maternal weight gain during the latter third of pregnancy
Maternal illness during pregnancy
Failure to obtain normal medical care during pregnancy
Lower socioeconomic status
African-American race (in the United States)
Multiple gestation
Uterine and placental anomalies
Polyhydramnios
Pre-eclampsia
Hypertension, both chronic and pregnancy-induced
Chronic, severe diabetes
Intrauterine infections
Cigarette smoking, cocaine use, and other substance abuse

disproportionally or asymmetrically grown infants is their apparently greater head/weight ratio but more normal head/length ratio, implying greater reduction in growth of soft tissue compared with brain growth, leading to the concept of "brain sparing." This is misleading, because the brain also is growth-restricted in such infants, although not as much as the soft tissues. Thus the head circumference may appear to be relatively large, but it is frequently below the 10th percentile for gestational age [14]. Furthermore, a study could not support evidence of "brain sparing" when asymmetric SGA infants were compared to symmetric SGA infants [13]. Although redistribution of blood flow may favor brain growth, this "adaptation" may be incomplete and result in deficient growth of the brain. Supporting evidence comes from studies using magnetic resonance imaging that showed decreases in brain volume, although this was less affected than body weight [15]. Although the overall growth of the brain in IUGR infants may be deficient, there may be acceleration of brain maturation, with neurobehavioral development at birth [16]. However, this may not result in long-term benefit (see later).

In many instances of IUGR, decrease in size may represent an appropriate adaptive response to the availability of nutrients, but extreme IUGR may represent pathology [17]. This adaptation to adverse nutrient transfer may also result in long-term sequelae (see later) [18]. Mild IUGR may allow for "catch-up growth," whereas severe IUGR is more likely to result in permanent growth restriction. Work by Sands *et al.* indicated that cell size increased much earlier than originally believed, and that cell multiplication continues unabated throughout tissue growth [19]. They stated that "The hypothesized early circumscribed phase of cell division, which is said to be particularly vulnerable to permanent stunting, does not appear to exist" [19]. This helps to explain the difficulty in predicting subsequent growth based on birthweight [20].

Factors affecting fetal growth

The maternal phenotype exerts a major influence on fetal size at birth, primarily by regulating the growth, size, and functional capacity of the placenta, which is the primary determinant of fetal growth [21]. The maternal influence on placental and fetal size was demonstrated in the classic studies of Walton and Hammond in 1938, when they bred the Shetland pony with the Shire horse [22]. If the mother was the pony, the offspring was smaller by far than if the mother was the Shire. This discrepancy in size persisted for at least the first 3 years and probably throughout the lives of the animals. The principle involved is known as maternal constraint, and it represents the capacity of the uterus, particularly the endometrial surface area, to support growth of the placenta and thus the fetus. Nutritional deficiencies in the mother also reduce fetal growth, but even severe maternal fasting to the point of chronic starvation seldom reduces fetal weight at term by more than 10%. Table 7.2 identifies a large variety of maternal factors that affect the rate of fetal growth.

Placental growth factors

The primary regulator of fetal growth is the placenta, both its size and its functional capacity to transport nutrients to the fetus. Thus growth and maturation of the placenta are key to determining growth of the fetus. Placental growth disorders that can restrict fetal growth are noted in Table 7.3.

The placenta also elaborates various hormones that maintain the fetoplacental unit, including chorionic gonadotropins, placental growth hormone, and placental somatotropins. Placental growth hormone and placental lactogen are important in maintaining increased concentrations of glucose and amino acids in the mother, which are then available for transplacental passage to the fetus [23]. The placenta also produces leptin, although the contributions of the fetus and placenta have not yet been clearly delineated. Leptin may also be linked to the transfer of glucose and amino acids [24].

Fetal growth factors

The major growth factor elaborated by the fetus is insulin. Overproduction of insulin leads to macrosomia [25], while

Table 7.3. Placental growth disorders that lead to or are associated with IUGR

Abnormal umbilical vascular insertions (circumvallate, velamentous)
Abruption (chronic, partial)
Avascular villi
Decidual arteritis
Fibrinosis, atheromatous changes
Cytotrophoblast hyperplasia, basement membrane thickening
Infectious villitis
Ischemic villous necrosis and umbilical vascular thromboses; multiple infarcts
Multiple gestation (limited endometrial surface area, vascular anastomoses)
Partial molar pregnancy
Placenta previa
Single umbilical artery
Spiral artery vasculitis, failed or limited erosion into intervillous space
Syncytial knots
Tumors, including chorioangioma and hemangiomas

underproduction, as found in congenital agenesis of the pancreas [26], or in transient or persistent neonatal diabetes mellitus, is associated with growth restriction [25]. All growth-restricted fetuses, in animal models, naturally growth-restricted animals, and humans, have low insulin concentrations. The principal disorder involves reduced pancreatic β-cell replication from cell-cycle arrest, although reduced angiogenesis is seen commonly in such pancreases [27]. As a result, the number of β cells is reduced, which limits overall capacity to produce insulin.

Insulin-like growth factors, IGF-1 and IGF-2, especially IGF-1, are also important growth factors in the fetus, and circulating levels of IGF-1 in fetal and cord blood correlate well with fetal size [28]. The mechanisms involved are beginning to be better understood [29], and there is evidence for genetic control, which may go awry [30]. Additionally, IGF-1 seems to play an important role in brain development [30].

Maternal IGF-1 and IGF-2 and insulin do not cross the placenta and have little direct effect on the fetus. They interact with the placenta and are instrumental in maintaining an intact fetoplacental unit. Similarly, the IGF-binding proteins and proteases that affect the binding proteins function to modulate the delivery of IGF to the placenta.

For years it was thought that fetal growth hormone (GH) had little effect on the intrauterine growth of the fetus, but recent data demonstrate that fetuses with GH deficiency tend to be short at birth [31]. Some infants with IUGR have hypersecretion of GH, but there may be a reduction or delayed development of receptor sites for GH or in the amount of GH-binding protein [32]. Most infants with IUGR will not respond to GH soon after birth [33], although some children demonstrate linear growth in response to GH at a later age [34]. Thyroid hormones have little effect on fetal growth, and the absence or abundance of the various sex hormones also

does not affect fetal growth. However, the male fetus is usually 100–150 g heavier than the female.

Recently there has been considerable interest in the hormone leptin, which has been linked to fetal growth. Although early results were somewhat confusing, it appears that leptin concentrations are significantly lower in IUGR than in AGA fetuses after 34 weeks' gestation [24,35]. However, significantly higher levels of leptin per kilogram fetal weight were found in IUGR fetuses with more severe signs of fetal distress [24].

Incidence of IUGR

The true incidence of IUGR on a worldwide basis is difficult to ascertain. While a close approximation can be made in developed countries, it is not known in many developing nations because many women in these countries give birth at home and often the weight, gestational age, and follow-up evaluations of the infants are not known. Using the World Health Organization classification of low birthweight as newborns weighing less than 2500 g, 16% of the infants born worldwide in 1982 were of low birthweight [36]. Many of these infants were most likely growth-retarded. These data were similar to those reported by Villar and Belizan for 1979 [37].

Chiswick noted that up to 10% of all live-born infants and at least 30% of low-birthweight (LBW) infants suffered from IUGR [38]. He also noted that the perinatal mortality rate in these infants was 4–10 times that of appropriately grown infants.

Villar and Belizan noted that 90% of LBW infants were born in developing countries, where the incidence of LBW infants could be as great as 45%. They also stated that when the incidence of low birthweight exceeds 10%, it is almost always due to the increase in the number of infants with IUGR, since the rate of preterm births tends to remain between 5% and 7% [37]. It has been proposed that chest circumference could be used as a proxy for birthweight in developing countries. At term gestation, a chest circumference ≤ 29 cm indicates IUGR [39].

Etiology of IUGR

Gluckman and Harding stated that IUGR is a result of one of three general mechanisms: (1) chromosomal/genetic abnormalities, (2) fetal infection/toxicity, or (3) compromised substrate delivery to the fetus [21]. The last group accounts for the majority of infants with IUGR. However, the etiology is clearly multifactorial [40], and in this section factors are classified as fetal, placental, maternal, and environmental.

Fetal factors

Fetal factors leading to low birthweight include genetic errors, chromosomal abnormalities, non-chromosomal syndromes, congenital malformations, and intrauterine infections.

Infectious agents causing or associated with IUGR are listed in Table 7.4. Klein *et al.* state that there is evidence to establish a causal relationship with IUGR only for rubella, cytomegaloviral infection, and toxoplasmosis [41]. These

Table 7.4. Infectious agents causing or associated with IUGR

Viral	Cytomegalovirus
	Rubella
	Varicella-zoster
	Human immunodeficiency virus
Bacterial	Syphilis
Protozoal	*Toxoplasma gondii*
	Plasmodium malariae
	Trypanosoma cruzi

Table 7.5. Placental factors associated with IUGR

Decreased placental mass
Absorption
Infarction
Partial separation
Multiple gestation
Intrinsic placental disorders
Poor implantation
Placental malformation
Vascular disease
Villitis
Decreased placental blood flow
Maternal vascular disease
Hypertension
Hyperviscosity

Source: Modified from Gabbe [48].

agents directly inhibit cell division, which may lead to cellular death and a decreased number of fetal cells. However, intra-uterine infections with other organisms, including syphilis, varicella-zoster, human immunodeficiency virus (HIV), *Trypanosoma*, and malaria have also been associated with IUGR. It has been difficult in most of these cases to differentiate between infection-specific causes and those related to poor maternal health and nutrition. Placental infection without affecting the neonate directly has been demonstrated in tuberculosis, syphilis, malaria, and coccidiomycosis. Congenital infection is implicated in less than 10% of patients with IUGR, and the incidence may be as low as 3%.

Chromosomal abnormalities include infants with trisomy 21, 13, and 18. In addition, infants with triploidy, various deletion syndromes, and super X syndromes (XXY, XXXY, XXXX) tend to be of low birthweight [42]. Another association with IUGR is maternal uniparental disomy 7 (where both chromosomes come from the same parent – in this case, the mother) [43]. Only 2–5% of infants with IUGR have chromosomal abnormalities, but the incidence may be much greater if both IUGR and mental retardation are present [44].

As many as 5–15% of fetuses with growth restriction have congenital malformation and/or dysmorphic syndromes such as thanatophoric dwarfing, leprechaunism, or Potter's, Cornelia de Lange, Smith–Lemli–Opitz, Seckel, Silver, or Williams syndromes, and VATER or VACTERL (vertebral, anal, cardiovascular, tracheoesophageal, renal, radial, and limb) associations [45].

Infants with varying types of congenital heart disease, those with single umbilical arteries, and monozygotic twins also frequently suffer from IUGR. Donors of twin-to-twin transfusions tend to be growth-restricted, while the recipient twin is often normally grown. These factors account for less than 2% of infants with IUGR [38].

Certain metabolic and endocrine disorders are associated with low birthweight and growth restriction. These include infants with transient neonatal diabetes mellitus, neonatal thyrotoxicosis, Menkes syndrome, hypophosphatasia, and I-cell disease [44]. Recently, a form of iron-overload disease associated with fetal growth restriction has been reported [46].

The role of race also cannot be ignored, with consistent increases in the number of LBW infants born to African-American women in the USA, which is not all explained by increased rates of preterm delivery [47]. However, environmental factors (see later) may be more important than genetic factors in this regard [47]. "Race very often serves as a proxy for poverty," so that undernutrition, malnutrition, poor prenatal care, and other factors may be important etiologic considerations [47].

Placental factors

Abnormalities of placental function leading to IUGR are listed in Table 7.5 [48]. The placenta has a great reserve capacity and may lose up to 30% of its function without affecting fetal growth [38]. Placental abnormalities such as hemangiomas, circumvallate placentas, or infarctions account for less than 1% of infants with IUGR [38]. It has also been stated that no single lesion of the placenta accounts for IUGR, but rather that it is an accumulation (or total burden) of placental injury and secondary growth failure that produces growth restriction [48]. The most common maternal condition that reduces placental growth, pre-eclampsia, involves decreased growth of terminal villi in the placenta, which will primarily reduce oxygen and glucose transport to the fetus. Reduced glucose supply alone decreases fetal growth rate and oxygen consumption rate (metabolic rate) proportionally, showing the tight linkage of energy supply and growth during periods of rapid growth such as occurs in the fetus [49].

With multiple gestation, there is an increased incidence of IUGR due to the inability of the placentas to grow large enough to meet the growth needs of the fetuses. As many as 15–25% of twins suffer from IUGR, and the incidence increases with triplets and quadruplets. Monochorionic twinning contributes disproportionately to IUGR [50]. Increasing discordance in size also contributes to an increase in preterm delivery before 32 weeks' gestation, with the discordance attributable to IUGR (most often in the second-born twin) [51].

Table 7.6. Maternal factors associated with IUGR

Maternal malnutrition
Disordered eating prior to pregnancy
Decreased maternal pre-pregnancy weight and height
Decreased weight gain during pregnancy
Labor-intensive occupation
Decreased plasma volume
Prior poor obstetrical history
Previous stillbirth
Previous infant with IUGR
Low socioeconomic status
Maternal illness
Maternal drug use and abuse

Maternal factors

Maternal factors are the most common causes of IUGR, and many of them are listed in Table 7.6. The state of maternal nutrition is a major factor in determining fetal growth and size at birth. Significant maternal malnutrition will make conception less likely, as demonstrated in the siege of Leningrad during World War II [52]. If the malnourished woman does conceive, the adequacy of maternal nutrition tends to affect the fetus primarily during the last trimester of pregnancy. This was clearly delineated in the studies of women during the Dutch famine in 1944–5, when food intake was severely curtailed. This reduction resulted in a 10% decrease in birthweights of their infants and a 15% reduction in the weights of the placentas [53,54]. Interestingly, data from the Netherlands also demonstrate that female fetuses exposed to starvation in the first trimester of pregnancy subsequently gave birth to growth-restricted infants themselves [55].

Dietary supplementation of malnourished pregnant women, especially if the supplementation is provided for more than 13 weeks during gestation, can increase the birthweight of their infants significantly [56], but Prentice and coworkers, working with Gambian women, reported that this only occurs when women were in negative energy balance before the supplements and also had a high energy workload. In these women, dietary supplementation reduced the incidence of LBW infants from 28.2% to 4.7% [57]. However, when the women were in positive energy balance, dietary supplementation had little effect on birthweight. There also are conflicting data regarding the effect of supplemental nutrition in various populations, and not all have shown beneficial effects. In fact, most studies have shown worse IUGR and increased fetal and neonatal morbidity and even mortality, particularly with protein supplementation [56]. To date, there has been no research that defines why in such cases supplementation has produced such adverse effects. This is a major limitation to any potential for prenatal prevention or amelioration of IUGR and all of its many adverse outcomes.

Specific deficiencies of micronutrients also can contribute to reduced fetal growth even if the mother's diet appears to be adequate as far as caloric and protein intake is concerned. Deficiency of zinc in pregnant women has been associated with increased rates of prematurity, perinatal death, and growth retardation of the fetus [58]. Zinc supplementation in such women has improved perinatal outcome. Thiamine deficiency in pregnancy has also been associated with the growth-retarded newborn, and has been found in mothers with inadequate nutritional intake, hyperemesis, alcohol abuse, and various infections, including HIV [59].

Although severe maternal malnutrition is uncommon in developed countries, it still exists in population areas where appropriate nutrition, nutritional supplementation, or nutritional consultation is lacking. It also is seen in pregnant women with severe gastrointestinal disease, such as Crohn's disease or ulcerative colitis, women with hyperemesis, or in women who use excessive energy in labor-intensive occupations. It has been documented that among women delivering SGA infants at term, there was a much higher incidence (32%) of disordered eating in the 3 months prior to pregnancy, compared to controls (5%) or those delivering prematurely (9%) [60].

Maternal illness, especially pre-eclampsia, not only has an adverse effect on the growth of the fetus, but it also predisposes the infant to preterm birth, especially if the mother's or infant's condition necessitates early delivery. The presence of IUGR adversely affects survival in these preterm infants [61]. It is of interest to note that multiparous women with pre-eclampsia have a greater risk of having an infant with IUGR than does a nulliparous mother [62]. During gestation, the mother's plasma volume and cardiac output increase primarily because of increased uterine blood flow. Studies by Rosso and coworkers [63] showed that women who had infants with IUGR had much lower plasma volumes and decreased cardiac outputs compared to women who had normally grown fetuses. Hypertensive women with growth-restricted fetuses have decreased plasma volumes compared to hypertensive women whose fetuses are normally grown [64].

Chronic illnesses in the mother, including those listed in Table 7.7, are associated with the birth of growth-restricted infants. The more common of these are women with chronic hypertension and chronic anemias, such as sickle-cell disease, sickle-C disease, and thalassemia. Women who have antiphospholipid antibodies, even if they are not diagnosed as having systemic lupus erythematosus (SLE), have an increased risk of giving birth to infants with IUGR [44]. When studying subgroups, it is important to evaluate carefully the total population, because some controls will have high rates of SGA infants. A recent study documented that 21% of infants born to mothers with antiphospholipid antibodies were SGA, while control mothers had an incidence of 13% SGA infants [65].

Wolfe and coworkers have reported that women with a history of poor outcome in pregnancy have an increased risk of having a subsequent birth of a growth-restricted infant [66]. A woman who has had a growth-restricted infant doubles her risk of having a second infant with IUGR. After two such outcomes, the risk of having a fetus with IUGR is quadrupled.

Table 7.7. Maternal illness associated with IUGR

Acute illness
Pre-eclampsia
Eclampsia
HELLP syndrome
Chronic illness
Chronic hypertension
Chronic renal disease
Collagen vascular disease
Cyanotic heart disease
Chronic pulmonary disease
Diabetes mellitus (classes B–F)
Thyrotoxicosis
Chronic anemia
Maternal phenylketonuria

Note:
HELLP, hemolysis, elevated liver enzymes, and low platelet count.

Table 7.8. Drugs taken by mothers that are associated with IUGR

Tobacco
Alcohol
Marijuana
Heroin
Methadone
Cocaine
LSD
Coumadin
Hydantoin
Trimethadone

These authors urged that women who have growth-restricted infants should have a thorough search for an underlying maternal disorder if the reason for the IUGR is otherwise not apparent. Ounsted and Ounsted also noted that mothers of infants with IUGR were often growth-restricted at birth themselves [67].

Environmental factors

It is difficult to separate maternal factors from some factors that might be considered to be environmental, such as tobacco usage. Therefore, these are discussed together in the ensuing section.

Medications and drugs taken by mothers can not only lead to various congenital malformations, but can also be associated with the birth of growth-retarded newborns [68]. Maternal smoking is one of the most prevalent causes of IUGR in their offspring. Birthweight may be reduced by a significant amount as compared to infants of non-smoking mothers [69]. Haddow and coworkers assayed serum cotinine, the major metabolite of nicotine, in smoking and non-smoking women, and correlated the concentration of the metabolite with the birthweight of their offspring [70]. The infants of women with the highest concentrations of serum cotinine were over 440 g lighter at birth than the infants of women who did not smoke. The mechanism by which smoking affects the fetus is not completely understood, but factors such as decreased maternal nutrition, decreased uterine blood flow, increased production of carbon monoxide (CO), and impaired fetal oxygenation have all been implicated. If the mother stops smoking before she enters the second trimester of pregnancy, her fetus tends to have normal intrauterine growth [69]. Of particular concern is a report from Sweden which showed a highly significant association between smoking and a small head circumference (and thus brain size) for gestational age [71].

Other drugs taken by the mother that have been implicated in causing growth retardation are shown in Table 7.8. Alcohol not only causes fetal growth impairment, but may lead to permanent damage to the fetus and newborn. The quantity of alcohol ingested, maternal size, and the ability of the mother to metabolize alcohol all determine how much alcohol is transported to the fetus [72]. Although the incidence of fetal alcohol effects is not known in the USA, the incidence in Sweden is 1 in 300 births, and 1 in 600 have recognizable features of the fetal alcohol syndrome [73]. (See also Chapter 10).

The incidence of illicit drug use by pregnant women in the USA can only be surmised, and accurate follow-up data are not available for the infants delivered from such women. The consensus is that 15–40% of infants of drug-abusing mothers are growth-restricted, and in some infants of cocaine-abusing mothers, the decrease in head circumference (and thus brain size) is more pronounced than is the decrease in length and weight [74]. Similar data indicate that the same outcome occurs in pregnant women who regularly smoke marijuana [75].

Caffeine, especially if taken in quantities greater than 300 mg/day, has been associated with decreased fetal growth [76]. Lesser intakes of caffeine do not seem to have an adverse effect on fetal growth, but high caffeine intake may be related to smoking, and this has not always been considered [77]. Specific syndromes such as fetal hydantoin, fetal warfarin, and fetal trimethadione syndromes are associated with an increased incidence of growth retardation [68].

Maternal hypoxia that produces fetal hypoxia also significantly reduces fetal growth [78]. Infants born to mothers who live at 10 000 ft (3000 m) or more above sea level weigh approximately 250 g less at birth than infants born to mothers who live at sea level [4]. Kruger and Arias-Stella reported that women who live in the Peruvian Andes at levels of over 15 000 ft (4500 m) had infants whose birthweights were 15% less than those who live in Lima, Peru (elevation 500 ft or 150 m), but the placentas of these infants weighed 15% more than those near sea level [79]. This would suggest that the placentas were consuming relatively large amounts of oxygen and nutrients in order to provide adequate nutrients and oxygen to the fetus. More recently, Moore's group has shown that long-term adaptation to higher altitude has led to improved birthweight relative to recent immigrants to high-altitude regions, who more commonly produce smaller infants. A principal multigenerational adaptation that has improved fetal growth involves relatively increased uteroplacental blood flow [80]. Indigenous high-altitude ancestry also protects against hypoxia-associated fetal growth reduction in a dose-dependent fashion consistent with the involvement of genetic factors. Further, some of the genes involved appear to be influenced by parent-of-origin effects, given that maternal transmission restricts and paternal transmission enhances fetal growth [81].

Maternal stress from excessive workload also may restrict fetal growth. In a recent study from Thailand, the risk of delivering an SGA infant was increased for women working more than 50 hours per week, for those whose work involved protracted squatting, and for those having high psychological job demands [82].

Mercury toxicity in pregnant women and their fetuses was highlighted during the 1950s to 1970s when three separate epidemics of mercury poisoning occurred in Minamoto and Niigata, Japan, and in Iraq. Koos and Longo reviewed the problem in depth and noted that, while all mercury compounds can cause harm to the fetus, methyl mercury has the greatest toxicity [83]. These compounds cross the placenta readily and have teratogenic and adverse growth effects in the fetus.

Mothers exposed to radiation, other pollutants, and contaminated food or water over a period of time appear to be at risk for delivery of infants with IUGR. The incidence of these factors, and the severity of their possible effects, are not known at present.

Detection of the fetus with IUGR

Currently, ultrasound is the preferred method of evaluating fetal growth and, in many instances, fetal well-being as well [84,85]. In populations where routine ultrasound is not available, careful review of risk factors, physical examination, and measurements of symphysis–fundus height (SFH) must be used to screen for IUGR. In populations where ultrasound is readily available, initial studies are often performed at 8–10 weeks' gestation. This examination documents fetal viability, the presence of multiple gestation, and gross fetal malformation, and confirms the gestational age of the fetus. This early examination is not used to determine abnormalities of intrauterine growth [85]. The biparietal diameter (BPD), the abdominal circumference (AC), and the femur length (FL) are the usual biometric measurements taken during the ultrasonographic examination [84]. Measurements of the BPD between 12 and 18 weeks' gestation are accurate in detecting gestational age within 5–6 days. However, measurements of individual parameters are not very good predictors of IUGR. To predict appropriateness of intrauterine growth more accurately, the ultrasound examination should be performed serially in the second and third trimester, but at least early in the third trimester. The estimated fetal weight (EFW) at such times relies on multiple measurements, including the abdominal

Table 7.9. Techniques to evaluate fetal growth and well-being

Measurements of symphysis-to-fundus height
Ultrasound examination
Endocrine measurements of maternal serum or urine
Estriol
Placental lactogen
Pregnanediol
Biophysical profile (including measurements of amniotic fluid index)
Contraction and non-contraction stress tests
Vibroacoustic stimulation
Doppler flow velocity waveforms
Cordocentesis

circumference and ratios of head circumference (HC)/AC or FL/AC. The optimal time to perform the examination is not clear, but it is estimated that over 50% of infants with IUGR will be detected by 32 weeks' gestation. Thus, several ultrasounds may have to be performed in order to monitor the growth of the fetus and to determine the optimal time of delivery of these infants. In pregnancies with multiple gestations, more frequent serial ultrasonographic examinations should be carried out during the last trimester.

Other studies to evaluate fetal well-being, especially in growth-restricted infants, are shown in Table 7.9. Few, if any, centers are currently using endocrine measurements of estrogens, pregnanediol, or placental lactogen in maternal serum or urine. Decreased amounts of amniotic fluid were found to correlate well with IUGR, but subsequent studies have not confirmed this observation [84].

Assessment of fetal well-being with the biophysical profile (BPP), while not used to detect IUGR, has been found to be more useful in predicting an abnormal fetal outcome than either the contraction stress test (CST) or the non-stress test (NST) alone [84,86,87]. Vibroacoustic stimulation may also help in evaluation.

Doppler flow velocity waveforms of the fetal circulation have also been used as adjuncts in evaluating fetal well-being and appropriate growth. The fetal umbilical artery, aorta, and cerebral arteries have been studied, and varying indices have been evaluated, including the resistance index (RI), the pulsatility index (PI), and the systolic/diastolic ratio (S/D) of these vessels. Abnormalities of these indices have been evaluated as to their capabilities in detecting the growth-retarded fetus and in evaluating the state of well-being of the fetus. The most accurate predictor of poor neonatal outcome was shown to be umbilical-cord Doppler waveform abnormalities [88], which have been associated with abnormal blood flow in the fetal middle cerebral artery in IUGR [89]. However, Doppler assessment of the middle cerebral artery may reveal blood flow redistribution even when umbilical-artery Doppler is normal, especially when the HC/AC ratio is elevated [90]. Lastly, cordocentesis, which has an increased risk-to-benefit ratio, can be utilized to document hypoxemia, lactic acidemia, and increased numbers of nucleated red blood cells (NRBCs) in the fetal circulation, and to identify those infants who are in need of immediate delivery [91].

These improved techniques of diagnosing and evaluating the status of the infant with IUGR have also resulted in improved management of the fetus and newborn [92]. Specific interventions, such as maternal hyperoxygenation [93], have been undertaken on a more rational basis, and decisions about delivery are based on what is optimal for the fetus. At times it is difficult to decide on what the best management may be; in many cases it may be "better out than in" for the fetus [86]. These decisions should involve a combined obstetrical–pediatric approach.

Associated problems and complications
(Table 7.10)

Fetal and neonatal asphyxia

The infant with IUGR is much more likely to experience difficulties during labor and delivery, although this is primarily related to the etiology of IUGR. Since many cases result from uteroplacental insufficiency, it is hardly surprising that a partially compromised fetus becomes a severely compromised fetus during labor. Recent experiments in pregnant sheep with IUGR placenta and fetus suggest that the association of severe IUGR with hypoxia is related to an imbalance in the development of placental structure and oxidative metabolism, which leads to a progressive decrease in oxygen transfer to the fetus and a reduction in net umbilical O_2 uptake (fetal oxygen consumption rate) [94]. Whatever the cause of the fetal hypoxia in IUGR, understanding its consequences for the fetus as labor approaches is useful. For example, Salihagić-Kadić et al. have suggested that a parameter that could take into account the degree and duration of hypoxia might be predictive of neurological outcome [95]. The Doppler cerebral/umbilical ratio (cerebral resistance index/umbilical resistance index) is a way of assessing adaptive response of the fetus to the hypoxic stress. As variability (vasoconstriction and vasodilation) is lost over time, reflected in the daily % ratio reduction from the cutoff value of one over time, the vulnerability of the fetus is exposed. Such a fetus facing labor and delivery is at high risk. A study by Figueras et al. has questioned the reliability of Doppler measurements to distinguish between SGA fetuses who are normal and those who have IUGR and are compromised metabolically [96]. Particularly as labor progresses, the frequency and strength of contractions increase, minimizing blood flow to the fetus and not allowing the fetus to recover between contractions. Lack of blood flow leads to decreased oxygen delivery and development of metabolic acidosis. The ability to remove carbon dioxide is also compromised, and the combination results in fetal hypoxia–ischemia, frequently manifest by late decelerations on fetal heart-rate monitoring. In addition, there may be variable decelerations (or cord-compression patterns) because decreased blood flow to the fetus may have produced a decrease in the quantity of amniotic fluid surrounding the fetus. This increases the probability that uterine contractions will be transmitted to the umbilical cord (especially the umbilical vein), further compromising

Table 7.10. Clinical problems commonly encountered with IUGR

Fetal and neonatal asphyxia
Fetal heart-rate abnormalities
Require resuscitation in delivery room
Persistent pulmonary hypertension
Glucose disorders
Hypoglycemia
Hyperglycemia
Hypocalcemia
Hypothermia
Hematologic problems
Neutropenia
Thrombocytopenia
Increased nucleated red blood cells
High hematocrit/hyperviscosity
Susceptibility to infection
Necrotizing enterocolitis
Pulmonary hemorrhage
Large anterior fontanel

blood flow to the fetus. An additional factor that may contribute to compromise is that, in fetuses with IUGR, the umbilical cord is frequently very thin, so that the umbilical vessels lack the protection of Wharton's jelly.

At the time of delivery, the hypoxic–ischemic, acidotic fetus becomes a hypoxic–ischemic, acidotic neonate, and prompt attention is required in the delivery room and early neonatal period to prevent further compromise. Those infants with a low ponderal index are more likely to have such problems [97]. If the fetus has been subjected to chronic intrauterine hypoxia there is the potential for change in the pulmonary vasculature, with changes in vascular tone that reduce vascular compliance and elasticity [98]. In most milder cases, nitric oxide and oxygen can reduce the contractile portion of the pulmonary vascular resistance, but when the fetal hypoxia is chronic and more severe, structural overgrowth of myocytes and other perivascular adventitial cells of arterioles and capillaries occurs, leading to irreversible narrowing of the vessel lumen and persistently increased and nitric-oxide non-responsive pulmonary vascular resistance. Particularly when combined with neonatal hypoxia, the potential for developing persistent pulmonary hypertension is great.

Hypoglycemia and other metabolic disturbances
(see Chapter 26)

The majority of infants who are born with IUGR demonstrate a lack of subcutaneous fat, and those with asymmetric IUGR usually have a decreased abdominal circumference documented before and after delivery [99]. For many years it has been recognized that preterm infants and SGA infants are prone to develop hypoglycemia, with the highest risk occurring in those infants born preterm and SGA with IUGR [25].

It is generally believed that the predisposition to develop hypoglycemia results from depletion of the glycogen stores; however, infants with IUGR and hypoglycemia are able to respond to the administration of glucagon and increase their concentrations of glucose in serum [100]. Infants with IUGR also have limited capabilities to utilize 3-carbon precursors to make glucose via the gluconeogenic pathways [25]. Additionally, hyperinsulinemia has been documented in some infants with IUGR, with hypoglycemia developing after 48 hours or so [101]. Moreover, increased insulin action, glucose production, shunting of glucose utilization to glycogen production, and maintenance of glucose transporter concentrations all contribute to the likelihood of hypoglycemia after birth [102]. In such cases, it appears that an increase in peripheral-tissue glucose transporter abundance allows increased glucose uptake at normal to low glucose and insulin concentrations, which could aggravate the relative hypoglycemia [102,103].

Since the supply of nutrients to IUGR infants has been less than optimal prior to delivery, their glucose levels at delivery are comparatively low [104] and may not be maintained because of the altered homeostatic mechanisms noted above. The brain is relatively large in many infants with IUGR (especially when it is asymmetric) and since the brain relies heavily on glucose metabolism, it is necessary to calculate glucose requirements (oral or intravenous) based on what the weight should have been (e.g., choose a weight consistent with the size of the head rather than the actual weight).

Somewhat paradoxically, treatment of hypoglycemia with "normal" amounts of glucose may lead to hyperglycemia in some infants [105]. This may be because the IUGR fetus is exposed to relative hypoglycemia in utero, which suppresses the production of insulin (the major hormone involved in growth) before delivery [106], and this cannot be "turned on" after delivery. Such infants have reduced maximal capacity for glucose utilization at high glucose and insulin concentrations. This may help to explain how hyperglycemia occurs when glucose delivery from aggressive intravenous infusions (above 7–8 mg/min/kg) is provided.

Further support for this idea comes from the condition of transient diabetes mellitus of the newborn, which seems to be the result of hypoinsulinism, or insulin dependence. Although this is a relatively uncommon condition, neonates with this problem may have hyperglycemia lasting from days to weeks, or even months [25]. Almost always, infants with this condition are born SGA [25], as they are with congenital agenesis of the pancreas [26,107]. On the other hand, as previously mentioned, some infants with IUGR have been shown to have hyperinsulinism and to develop later-onset (at approximately 48 hours) hypoglycemia [101].

Many infants prone to develop hypoglycemia are also prone to develop hypocalcemia. This is certainly true for those infants with IUGR [108]. Hypocalcemia may be due to transient hypoparathyroidism or possibly to an overproduction of calcitonin, which is increased in stressed neonates. With modern-day neonatal intensive care, it would be unusual to encounter the more severe clinical manifestations of hypocalcemia such as seizure activity. The problem is anticipated, evaluated, and treated [109].

Another problem of IUGR SGA infants is hypothermia. The increased surface-area-to-body-weight ratio of the IUGR infant promotes heat loss more rapidly than in the appropriately grown infant [110]. The ability to produce heat may be compromised in IUGR infants [110] for three reasons: (1) there is decreased insulation from adipose tissue (white fat); (2) the stores of brown fat, used for non-shivering thermogenesis, are markedly depleted; and (3) the tendency to develop hypoglycemia means that oxidative metabolism of glucose to produce heat is deficient. For all these reasons, it is more likely that IUGR infants will not be able to maintain their body temperature and will develop hypothermia [110]. In the most extreme cases, when appropriate management is not provided, one may encounter neonatal cold injury syndrome [111].

The end result of cooling is metabolic acidosis, because peripheral vasoconstriction decreases the delivery of oxygen to the tissues and increases anaerobic metabolism, with the accumulation of lactic acid. In extreme circumstances, the resultant decrease in pH may have wide-reaching effects, including altered metabolism of the brain.

Hematologic problems

Infants with IUGR are more likely to be born with a high hematocrit, an erythropoietic response to hypoxia from placental insufficiency. More recently, particularly in infants born to hypertensive mothers, thrombocytopenia and neutropenia have been observed [112]. It is believed that the pluripotent stem cell is stimulated to produce the erythroid series at the expense of neutrophils and platelets [112]. These same authors have demonstrated that there is an inhibitor of neutrophil production which is elaborated by the placenta and which is present in the infant's serum [113]. Such conditions are noted particularly in IUGR infants born to mothers with HELLP syndrome secondary to advanced pre-eclampsia.

Overproduction of erythropoietin has been noted in both term and preterm SGA infants [114,115], and studies in the fetus using cordocentesis have documented hypoxic–ischemic conditions and lactic acidemia [116]. The number of erythroblasts (NRBCs) is markedly increased in some of these fetuses [116]. Cordocentesis also has demonstrated that levels of erythropoietin are increased in those IUGR fetuses displaying erythroblastosis [117], and it may be possible to distinguish IUGR from the small but healthy fetus on this basis [118]. Thus, in the neonate with a marked increase in the number of NRBCs and a normal to high hematocrit, the most likely explanation is chronic intrauterine hypoxemia (although infection may also stimulate NRBC production). It is not clear what the duration of the hypoxemic insult needs to be to produce a significant elevation of NRBCs [119], although the duration of insult can be estimated based on numbers of NRBCs, which are more elevated with persistent fetal heart-rate abnormalities [120].

High hematocrits, especially a venous hematocrit over 65%, may lead to hyperviscosity syndrome [121], which includes several clinical manifestations involving the central nervous system, including lethargy alternating with jitteriness or even seizures. While partial exchange transfusion with saline has been used to lower the hematocrit to prevent sequelae of the hyperviscosity syndrome, this intervention does not prevent such sequelae, and exchange with protein-containing solutions actually can produce worse outcomes, probably due to clumping of red blood cells with the added protein [121].

At the opposite end of the spectrum, some infants with IUGR are anemic. This occurs most notably in the twin-to-twin transfusion syndrome, where the donor twin is inadequately perfused and has compromise of intrauterine growth in association with anemia [50,122]. The combination of anemia and reduced circulation may decrease oxygen supply to the brain and cause brain injury [50].

Susceptibility to infection

IUGR fetuses and newborns are more likely to develop hypoxic–ischemic conditions, which may predispose to bacterial infection [123]. Total T cells, helper and inducer T lymphocytes, and B cells all are deficient in number in infants who are SGA [124]. Such immunologic handicap seems to predispose to severe infection, including meningitis. This problem may be more severe in SGA infants who were stressed with recent nutritional deficiency as indicated by a low ponderal index. In one study [125], infection was four times more common in IUGR infants with low ponderal index than in those with appropriate ponderal index. Hypothermia (see earlier) also has been associated with a predisposition to develop bacterial infection, as SGA infants may not respond to infectious agents as do normally grown infants [112,113].

Necrotizing enterocolitis (NEC)

Because IUGR infants often have increased incidence of hypoxia–ischemia, acidosis, and hyperviscosity, their intestinal blood flow might be compromised. The increased susceptibility to infection adds an additional risk. It is therefore not surprising that an increased incidence of NEC has been seen in IUGR infants [126], which may be predictable based on absent end-diastolic frequencies in fetal Doppler studies [127].

Neurobehavioral abnormalities
Accelerated neurological development

Historically, it was considered that preterm infants with documented IUGR or who were born SGA were more likely to have accelerated lung maturity, and that some of these infants might have accelerated neurological development as well. The link between these developmental changes was first described in 25 infants by Gould et al. [128]. However, the concept of accelerated lung maturation has been challenged by Tyson et al. [129], who carefully compared infants who were SGA and those who were AGA and evaluated the outcome of the infants of similar gestational ages, race, and sex. Their studies documented that the SGA infants actually had increased rates of respiratory distress syndrome, respiratory failure, and death compared to the AGA preterm infants.

Acceleration of neurological maturation was confirmed by Amiel-Tison [130] in other high-risk pregnancies, some of which (but not all) resulted in infants with growth restriction. This acceleration of maturation was at least 4 weeks in 16 infants, and may relate to the severity of placental insufficiency, with the benefits being lost in the most severe cases. Maternal hypertension was implicated in approximately half of the cases.

Further observations have confirmed the acceleration of neurological maturation in stressed pregnancies. Although many of these infants are born SGA, this is not always the case, suggesting that the effects on the nervous system may precede the effects on overall growth [16]. The exact mechanism for accelerated maturation remains to be elucidated. Additional support comes from neurophysiological studies in which brainstem auditory evoked responses were more rapid in SGA infants than in AGA infants [131]. Further documentation has been provided in growth-restricted fetal lambs [132]. In contrast, development of visual evoked potentials in IUGR and SGA infants may be delayed [133]. Whether the accelerated maturational effects are documented when infants are evaluated by methods similar to those used by Tyson et al. [129] remains to be seen.

Furthermore, although accelerated neurological maturation would seem to provide an unanticipated benefit, when infants with IUGR are followed for longer periods of time they do not sustain this advantage. Indeed, by school age, they may be at a disadvantage [134].

Altered behavior

Despite accelerated neurological development in some IUGR/SGA infants, this is not always the case. With increasing severity of insult, it is likely that the behavior of the infant will be compromised by more injurious conditions, such as hypoxia. Data from the 1980s indicated that fetal behavioral states may be delayed in IUGR fetuses, with fetal movements being particularly involved [135], but, with increasing experience, the assessment of fetal behavioral organization is not considered to be of great clinical value [136].

Increasing severity of fetal hypoxia and ischemia will have a marked effect on the biophysical profile [137], one aspect of which is fetal movement. In uncomplicated IUGR cases, there is no clear effect on the quality of general movements [136]. However, it is commonly observed that infants with IUGR behave differently soon after delivery. In particular, they may feed poorly. Inevitably, this will affect parental perceptions of the baby. Low et al. [138] documented lower activity scores in IUGR infants compared to controls, with a trend to less visual fixation and visual pursuit. Studies using the Brazelton Behavioral Assessment Scale have documented less muscle tone, decreased activity, less responsiveness, and more difficulty in modulating state [139]. A high-pitched cry tends to take longer to be stimulated [140]. Most behavioral studies have been performed in term IUGR infants. Little is known about differences in preterm IUGR infants.

Parental interaction

Many infants with IUGR appear scrawny (especially those with low ponderal index) and are less attractive to parents than the expectation of what their baby "should" look like [139]. In addition, as noted above, the infant's behavior may be distorted and provide less interaction between infant and parents. The cry may be particularly aversive to adults [140]. This lack of "positive reinforcement" was believed to place these infants at particular risk for child abuse or neglect, but more recently this idea seems to have been disproved [141].

There are quite limited data available on subsequent parent–infant interaction. Although there may be some differences early in the first year [142] these differences in interaction seem to resolve by 6 months [143].

Outcome
Historical perspective

After the recognition that not all small infants were born preterm, but could be growth-restricted [144], interest shifted to focus on the etiologic heterogeneity of IUGR and more appropriate definitions and standards [10]. Improved study designs eliminated infants with chronic intrauterine infection and congenital abnormalities, which probably skewed the follow-up in one study [145].

One group of infants that could be evaluated was twins with markedly discordant birthweights. These follow-up studies (few in number) were largely performed on preterm twin infants, but continued growth restriction was usually the case in the smaller of discordant twins [146]. This was accompanied by a disadvantage in intellect, persisting into adulthood [147]. However, it was observed that head circumference was less affected than other measures [146]. Some years later, in a small sample of discordant twins, continued weight deficit in the smaller twin was noted, but without height or IQ deficit at 6 years of age [148].

The ability to have "catch-up" growth in the smaller twin also was reported [149]. In a remarkable report, Buckler and Robinson described a female twin pair with marked disparity in birthweights (2.99 vs. 1.35 kg), where the smaller twin had very rapid "catch-up" after birth. By 1 year of age there was essentially no difference in physical measurements, and evaluation at 10 years of age showed no difference in intelligence quotients [150].

In contrast to the twin studies, singleton IUGR infants show considerable variability in catch-up growth [11], leading to the conclusion that appropriate classification at birth is needed, together with categorization by etiology of IUGR. Some of the older studies may have been complicated by problems such as hypoglycemia. Nevertheless, despite the tendency to remain smaller than average in physical dimensions, the intellectual deficits of infants with IUGR described in the 1970s were not always striking, and major neurological deficits were considered to be uncommon. For example, Fitzhardinge and Steven followed 95 full-term SGA infants and noted cerebral palsy (CP) in only 1% and seizures in 6% [151]. However, although the average IQ was normal, a large percentage

(50% of boys and 36% of girls) had poor school performance [151]. In other studies, the IQ did not seem to be impaired, although it was somewhat higher in those with normal head circumference, as described by Babson and Henderson, who concluded that "severe fetal undergrowth, not complicated by severe asphyxia at birth, or congenital disease, may not severely impair later mental development, even in those whose head size remained at the 3rd percentile" [152].

Although it is now less common to see infants with IUGR born at term, Strauss has provided follow-up on two large national cohorts born many years ago [153,154]. The first group were those followed in the US National Collaborative Perinatal Project (1959–76), with a 7-year follow-up. IUGR had little impact on intelligence and motor development, except when associated with large deficits in head circumference at birth [154]. The second group included those enrolled in the 1970 British Birth Cohort Study, where follow-up was available until 1996 [153]. Although 93% had been followed at 5 years of age, only 53% were seen at 26 years of age. Among 489 SGA infants (of the original 1064) born at term and assessed as adults, academic achievement and professional attainment were significantly lower than among the adults who had normal birthweight ($n = 6981$). However, there appeared to be no long-term social or emotional consequences of being born SGA [153].

One study of preterm SGA infants indicated that approximately 50% had a developmental handicap, with 20% having major neurologic sequelae [155]. Handicap could not be related to the degree of IUGR or the rate of postnatal head or linear growth. However, it did seem to be related to perinatal "asphyxia." These infants all were born in outlying hospitals and referred to a center [155]. When more aggressive obstetrical intervention was undertaken, the outlook appeared to improve (in a different setting). Cesarean section at 28–33 weeks' gestation for suspected growth restriction and abnormal unstressed cardiotocograms resulted in 17 survivors among 25 infants. Only two survivors were neurologically abnormal [156].

As obstetrical evaluation and intervention changed, more infants with IUGR were delivered at earlier stages of gestation. The Oxford group demonstrated that attempting to prolong gestation beyond about 36 weeks may not benefit the fetus, but earlier delivery seemed to enhance the chances of compromised fetuses, with IUGR infants achieving their full developmental potential later [157]. More recently, IUGR fetuses are delivered at even earlier gestations. It seems likely that some of these fetuses would have died in utero and others might have suffered severe neurological injury. Several recent studies have provided reasonably encouraging data about long-term outcome (see section on follow-up of VLBW infants born SGA).

Mortality and morbidity

Short-term outcome involves both mortality and morbidity. The morbidity in these infants has been described in the section on associated problems and complications. The frequency of problems is in large measure dependent upon the etiology. The same holds true for mortality. It is clear that if there are many infants with chromosomal abnormalities (e.g., trisomy 18) or chronic intrauterine infections (e.g., congenital rubella syndrome) in the population being evaluated, mortality rates are likely to be high. Classically, Lubchenco *et al.* showed that the more severe the degree of growth restriction, the higher the mortality risk [158]. In a separate analysis, morbidity was found to increase progressively as birthweight fell below the 10th percentile at each gestational age [159].

In contrast, more recent studies have found that SGA infants have a lower risk for neonatal death than AGA infants, but have a higher risk of problems manifest during the first year after birth [160]. Other studies confirm the original findings that both mortality and morbidity are increased in term infants born SGA (< 3rd percentile) [161].

Physical growth

The literature shows considerable variability and many contradictions regarding physical growth of IUGR infants. Probably this reflects variable inclusion of confounders such as preterm birth, variability in anthropometric measurements, postnatal nutrition, and inclusion of infants with different underlying disorders. Most studies have shown considerable catch-up growth in some infants, with significantly lower weights, heights, and head circumferences at 3 years compared to control infants [162]. Large variations in measurements of SGA infants at follow-up are common when parents make the measurements [163]. Also, some reports of the subsequent growth of infants with IUGR have included modifiers that might influence the outcome, such as asymmetric IUGR (with a low ponderal index), which seems to persist as underweight-for-length at 3 years of age despite catch-up growth in the first 6 months [164]. Furthermore, term infants with a low ponderal index were taller than those with adequate ponderal index when evaluated at age 24 months in one study [165], while in another study of preterm infants there appeared to be no effect of the degree of IUGR on later growth [165]. Decreased ossification also may predispose to catch-up in linear growth [11], although most studies have shown that SGA infants are shorter even into adolescence [166]. Catch-up growth in the first 6 months has been noted by others [167], and adequate ponderal index at birth predicts reduced size at 12 months of age compared with those with low ponderal index [168]. SGA infants with high head-to-chest ratios at birth appear to grow faster during the first 6 months, with a sustained effect to 7 years in girls [169]. Another factor that likely produces variation in growth outcomes in IUGR infants is the variability of response to insulin [170]. At 6 months of age, those SGA infants that had increased incremental linear growth demonstrated greater insulin secretion [170]. Growth variation also might be linked to later evidence of glucose intolerance [18]. Given the variability of insulin levels in IUGR infants noted earlier, this is an area that deserves further study.

Development and intelligence quotient

While limited physical growth may have some practical implications, and many parents are concerned about short stature, neurobehavioral and intellectual development are of more concern. Allen noted that prior to 1984 most term SGA infants developed normal IQs [171]. Another study documented that in non-"asphyxiated" SGA newborns, despite residual physical deficits at age 13–19 years, neurologic and cognitive testing demonstrated scores well within the normal range, although somewhat lower than controls [172]. Additional studies also show variation in neurodevelopmental outcomes. SGA infants born to hypertensive mothers performed better on developmental tests at 4–7 years of age, but had more major neurological problems compared with those whose mothers were normotensive [173]. In another 7-year follow-up study, neurological problems were detected in 9.5% of growth-restricted infants and in 8.5% of control infants [174]. Others have described surprisingly little difference in developmental status at 4 years of age between small- and average-for-dates infants [157]. More recent evidence tends to confirm these findings, although lower IQ scores and poorer neurodevelopmental outcome were noted in IUGR infants with neonatal complications [162]. Nevertheless, these neurodevelopmental problems might be characterized as minor, with no CP and no severe hearing or visual impairment [162].

Using a slightly different approach, when ponderal index at birth was taken into consideration, one study showed that term IUGR infants with adequate ponderal index (symmetric IUGR) had lower developmental scores than those with low ponderal index (asymmetric IUGR), which in turn were lower than those with normal birthweight [175]. Preterm infants with asymmetric or symmetric IUGR also have been compared to AGA infants. In the asymmetric SGA group there were more children with low visuoauditory perception scores and social abilities scores at 18 months than in the control group. The symmetric SGA group had deficits in all developmental areas except visuoauditory perception [176]. There also were more neurological abnormalities in both SGA groups [176].

Follow-up of VLBW infants born SGA

When VLBW (< 1500 g) infants were initially evaluated, SGA infants had significantly lower developmental performance at 9 months through 3 years of age, but differences were not observed at 4 and 5 years [177]. A decade later, results from the same authors showed similar outcomes among VLBW and SGA infants [178]. At 3 years of age, development of SGA infants was significantly less than that of gestation-matched controls, but did not differ from that of weight-matched controls [178].

Amin *et al.* evaluated 52 IUGR infants (with birthweight < 1250 g) at 3 years of age. They were compared with groups of birthweight and gestational age-matched controls and had no significant differences in neurodevelopmental outcome, although all three groups had major disabilities of approximately 15%. Head sparing correlated with a good outcome (35 of 37 were normal) [1]. Similarly, in a large cohort of even smaller infants followed for 4–18 years, the majority of SGA infants with birthweight < 1000 g had catch-up of head circumference, although this was more likely in the asymmetric

SGA group (85%) than in the symmetric group (73%) [179]. Although developmental outcome was not completely addressed in this report, normal head circumference was usually associated with a good outcome.

It is important to note that there are difficulties in extrapolating results of follow-up to current VLBW populations, since management of such neonates continues to change and improve. Exogenous surfactant has only been commercially available since 1990, and prenatal use of corticosteroids to accelerate fetal lung maturity increased considerably after the National Institutes of Health consensus conference in 1994. As a result, certain complications of the VLBW infant (e.g., pneumothorax and intraventricular hemorrhage) have decreased, which could influence neurodevelopmental outcome. Finally, neonatal death or CP has decreased more in IUGR infants than in VLBW infants, and there is less neurodevelopmental impairment among the survivors [180].

Cerebral palsy (CP)

Most of the early follow-up studies of IUGR/SGA infants did not specifically address the issue of CP, although a low incidence was mentioned earlier [151]. However, in Sweden, trends in the incidence of CP have been followed over several years. Uvebrant and Hagberg followed numerous infants with CP, and noted that the rate of CP in SGA infants was increased significantly compared to control infants born during the same years [181]. Similar data have been reported from Western Australia by Blair and Stanley in growth-retarded infants of $\geq$ 34 weeks' gestation [182].

In a large cohort of preterm singletons with CP born in 1971–82 ($n = 191$) in Denmark, the association of SGA with CP was observed only in preterm infants born at more than 33 weeks' gestation [183]. The comparison group consisted of all preterm live-born singletons born in 1982 ($n = 2203$). Cerebral palsy risk was highest at 28–30 weeks' gestation, but lower in the SGA group at this gestation [183].

Learning deficits

As with CP, until recently most follow-up studies of IUGR infants did not extend into the school years. In 1984, however, a study of term infants with intrauterine malnutrition (not all were SGA) followed from birth to 12–14 years reported lower IQ scores and a greater need for special education in malnourished infants compared to well-nourished infants [184]. A study from England showed no differences in IQ or school achievement between boys weighing below the 2nd percentile at birth and controls at age 10–11 years [185]. In another study, from Canada, outcome at 9–11 years of age was measured [186]. A wide range of learning deficits was evaluated in 216 high-risk newborns, 77 of whom had IUGR. Learning deficits were encountered in 35% of the total, but 50% of preterm SGA and 46% of term SGA infants were affected [186].

Another study from England evaluated infants born in 1980–81 with a gestational age of less than 32 weeks or birthweight < 2 kg, at 8–9 years of age [187]. The authors concluded that those with fetal growth restriction in the first two trimesters did less well than normally grown infants. Both cognitive ability (measured by IQ testing and reading comprehension) and motor ability were negatively associated with the degree of fetal growth restriction.

Still another study from the Netherlands looked at a 1983 cohort born with gestational age < 32 weeks or birthweight < 1500 g, at both 5 and 9 years of age [188]. Of an original cohort of 134 SGA infants, 85 were seen at 5 years and 73 at 9 years, compared to 410 AGA infants of whom 274 and 249 were seen at 5 and 9 years respectively. Cognitive outcome was worse in the SGA group. When neurological disorders were excluded, 16.4% of the SGA children needed special education at 9 years, compared to 11.9% of AGA. When no exclusions were made, only 31.5% of SGA children were in mainstream education, compared to 43.2% of AGA [188].

On a more encouraging note, data from the Jerusalem Perinatal Study showed that long-term follow-up (at age 17) produced minimal differences in IQ tests and no differences in academic achievement, when term SGA and AGA were evaluated [189]. Longer-term studies, however, affirm the association between IUGR and worse neurodevelopmental outcome. Using a comprehensive neuropsychological evaluation at 9 years of age, Geva et al. reported a lower IQ and relatively greater difficulties in creative problem solving, attention, and executive functions, as well as visuomotor organization and higher-order verbal skills in children with a history of IUGR [190]. They further suggest that restricted head circumference was a harbinger of frontal-lobe-related suboptimal development. A 10-year population cohort of children in Western Australia affirmed the association of IUGR and poor head growth with severe intellectual disability [191]. Another 10-year prospective study by Leitner et al. pointed out the importance of perinatal complications as contributors to the worse neurocognitive outcome among IUGR children [192]. The association of severe IUGR and reduced head circumference with poor neurodevelopmental outcomes, long-term neuropsychological problems, and difficulties in school is better understood in the context of severe reduction in cortical growth and a significant decrease in cell number in the future cortex of affected individuals, as well as discrete injuries to particular regions of the brain, such as the hippocampus.

Some of these studies are summarized in Table 7.11.

Effect of fetal malnutrition on disease in adult life

Several studies in the past two decades have alluded to the relationship of IUGR with the subsequent increased incidence of cardiovascular disease when these patients reach adult life [18,193,194]. Both hypertension [195] and ischemic heart disease are increased in IUGR infants [18], and the risk of stroke is also increased [195]. Such infants also grow up to have increased incidence of obesity and diabetes. Barker and coworkers [194] suggested that undernutrition during fetal life alters the relationships between nutrient substrates and

Table 7.11. Neurodevelopmental and cognitive outcome in infants with IUGR

Authors	Category	Age at evaluation	Method of evaluation	Number evaluated	Outcome		
					Impaired	*Disabled*	
Roth et al. 1999 [210]	Term infants	1 year	Neurological exam	49 SGA	37%	6%	
	Fetal abdominal circumference		Developmental assessment	18 IUGR	33%	6%	
					CP	*Major disability*	
Amin et al. 1997 [1]	BW < 1250 g	3 years	Neurodevelopmental assessment	52 IUGR	7.7%	15.4%	
				55 BW-matched	9.1%	16.4%	
				56 GA-matched	12.5%	16.1%	
					Neuro-developmental	*IQ*	
Fattal-Valevski et al. 1999 [162]	< 34 weeks GA U/C ratio	3 years	Neurodevelopmental assessment and IQ test	85 IUGR	89.0	94.9	
				42 Controls	93.2	94.9	
Scherjon et al. 2000 [134]	< 34 weeks GA U/C ratio	5 years	IQ test	73 IUGR	Lower IQ with raised U/C ratio (87 vs. 96)		
					Special education	*CP*	*Normal development*
Kok et al. 1998 [188]	< 32 weeks GA and BW < 1500 g	9 years	Speech-language development Need for special education	73 SGA	16.4%	7%	48%
				149 AGA	11.9%	15%	63%
			Neurological exam		Cognitive outcome worse in SGA		
				Males	*IQ*		
Paz et al. 2001 [189]	Term	17 years	IQ test, academic achievement	154 severe SGA	100.7		
				431 moderate SGA	102.8		
				5928 AGA	105.1		
				Females			
				86 severe SGA	102.6		
				273 moderate SGA	102.4		
				3664 AGA	103.9		
				No difference in academic achievements			

Notes:
U/C ratio, umbilical artery to middle cerebral artery pulsatility index ratio; GA, gestational age; BW, birthweight; CP, cerebral palsy; SGA, small for gestational age; AGA, appropriate for gestational age; IUGR, intrauterine growth restriction; IQ, intelligence quotient.

hormones, such as between glucose and insulin and between growth hormone and IGF. Since IGF-1 is decreased in many growth-restricted fetuses, and since fetal undernutrition may predispose to insulin resistance in various tissues and organs later in life, these infants also appear to become insulin-resistant, glucose-intolerant, and diabetic as adults [196]. Reduced concentrations of IGF also have been associated with arterial wall thickening, in particular abdominal aortic intima-media thickness, a marker for atherosclerosis [35,197]. While the fetus may adapt to nutritional deprivation in utero, such adaptation may lead to an increased incidence of cardiovascular disease and related metabolic problems in adulthood [198].

Prevention

Although outcome in the non-"asphyxiated", normally grown fetus appears to be good, the potential for developing fetal hypoxia–ischemia in the growth-restricted fetus is high [116]. Indeed, the risk of intrauterine demise drives many obstetrical decisions. For this reason, a number of techniques have been used with the intent to improve placental perfusion.

The first of these, which was originally reported from South Africa to produce "superbabies," was intermittent abdominal decompression. The technique was evaluated in a controlled trial reported in 1973 [199]. Negative pressure is applied to the abdomen to encourage blood flow in the uterus and hence the placenta. In 70 treated versus 70 controls there were some striking differences, with improved growth of fetal biparietal diameter in the treated group and only 26% "light-for-dates" babies in the treated group compared to 83% in the controls [199]. Rates of fetal distress, low 1-minute Apgar scores, and perinatal deaths also were lower in the treated group [199]. Further support for the technique was provided in 64 pregnant women with identified placental insufficiency [200]. Abdominal decompression applied over 4 weeks or so improved placental perfusion measurements and serum unconjugated estriol and human placental lactogen levels [200]. To date, this approach has not gained widespread support, although a review provided considerable support for the method [201].

As mentioned earlier, another approach to the fetus with IUGR is to evaluate fetal oxygenation using cordocentesis. Several attempts have been made in situations where fetal hypoxia has been documented to use maternal oxygen therapy to produce maternal hyperoxygenation and secondarily improved fetal oxygenation [93]. However, a recent meta-analysis revealed only two studies using randomized controls, which involved only 62 women and did not provide enough evidence to evaluate adequately the benefits and risks of maternal oxygen therapy [202].

Another approach, which has been tested in a randomized, placebo-controlled, double-blind trial, is the use of low-dose aspirin [203]. Women were chosen on the basis of previous fetal growth restriction and/or fetal death or abruptio placentae. The frequency of fetal growth restriction in the placebo group was twice (26% vs. 13%) that in the treated group [203]. The benefits of low-dose aspirin were greater in patients with two or more previous poor outcomes. More recent evaluation of low-dose aspirin showed no evidence of improved uteroplacental or fetoplacental hemodynamics [203], although another study supported the use of a combination of aspirin and glyceryl trinitrate [204]. This too has not been adequately evaluated.

A specific cause of IUGR is severe maternal nutritional deprivation. The role of dietary supplementation and specific deficiencies has been discussed previously [56–59,205]. It is possible, under certain adverse circumstances, to support adequate fetal growth using maternal intravenous nutrition [206]. Extending this approach to other situations of less severe nutritional deprivation might allow supplemental parenteral nutrition to prevent fetal growth restriction [206]. However, a recent meta-analysis revealed only three studies involving 121 women, which did not provide enough evidence to allow an adequate evaluation of nutrient supplementation [207].

Two other analyses from the Cochrane Database of Systematic Reviews also showed insufficient evidence to demonstrate a conclusive effect of either plasma volume expansion [208] or bed rest in hospital on fetal growth [209].

Prevention remains an area for careful evaluation with randomized trials, and it is hoped that many cases of IUGR will be prevented in the future [210]. Determining the cause of IUGR is difficult, but, if possible, is important in assessing the risk for IUGR in future pregnancies [211]. A good example in this regard would be the identification of thrombophilia, which may occur in 15–25% of Caucasian populations. Thrombophilia is exacerbated by pregnancy (an acquired hypercoagulable state) and can lead to vascular complications associated with IUGR [212].

Conclusion

Major advances have been made in our understanding of infants who are growth-restricted in utero. Many of the factors that lead to IUGR have been recognized, and many of the women who are at risk of giving birth to such infants can be identified. In many cases, problems can be avoided by improving the intrauterine environment, maternal nutrition, care of chronic illness in the mother, maternal immunization, and improved counseling of pregnant women regarding smoking, alcohol, and drug abuse.

Infants also can be classified according to the types of growth restriction that are present, and it is recognized that many of these infants do not thrive in a hostile intrauterine environment, do not tolerate the stresses of labor well, and do not have an appropriate transitional period from the fetal to the newborn state.

These infants also have markedly different problems in the neonatal period than do prematurely born infants of the same size or normally grown infants of the same gestational age. Unfortunately, many of these IUGR fetuses are not being identified early enough to alter these environments, and we are still late in responding to their problems in the neonatal period rather than anticipating and preventing them from developing.

Although significant strides have been made in our understanding of the problems of IUGR infants, we need to focus attention on prevention, early detection, and appropriate management of their problems in order to produce the best outcome possible.

References

1. Amin H, Singhal N, Sauve RS. Impact of intrauterine growth restriction on neurodevelopmental and growth outcomes in very low birthweight infants. *Acta Paediatr* 1997; **86**: 306–14.

2. Metcoff J. Clinical assessment of nutritional status at birth: fetal malnutrition and SGA are not synonymous. *Pediatr Clin North Am* 1994; **41**: 875–91.

3. Lubchenco LO, Hansman C, Boyd E. Intrauterine growth in length and head circumference as estimated from live births at gestational ages from 26 to 42 weeks. *Pediatrics* 1966; **37**: 403–8.

4. Unger C, Weiser JK, McCullough RE, *et al.* Altitude, low birth weight, and infant mortality in Colorado. *JAMA* 1988; **259**: 3427–32.

5. Kitanaka T, Alonso JG, Gilbert RD, *et al.* Fetal responses to long-term hypoxemia in sheep. *Am J Physiol* 1989; **256**: R1348–54.

6. Usher R, McLean F. Intrauterine growth of live-born Caucasian infants at sea level: standards obtained from measurements in 7 dimensions of infants born between

25 and 44 weeks of gestation. *J Pediatr* 1969; **74**: 901–10.

7. Niklasson A, Ericson A, Fryer JG, *et al.* An update of the Swedish reference standards for weight, length and head circumference at birth for given gestational age (1977–1981). *Acta Paediatr Scand* 1991; **80**: 756–62.

8. Miller HC, Hassanein K. Diagnosis of impaired fetal growth in newborn infants. *Pediatrics* 1971; **48**: 511–22.

9. Röhrer R. Der Index der Körperfülle als Mass des Ernährungszustandes. *Münchener Medizinische Wochenschrift* 1921; **68**: 580–95.

10. Lubchenco LO. Assessment of gestational age and development of birth. *Pediatr Clin North Am* 1970; **17**: 125–45.

11. Philip AG. Fetal growth retardation: femurs, fontanels, and follow-up. *Pediatrics* 1978; **62**: 446–53.

12. Winick M. Cellular growth in intrauterine malnutrition. *Pediatr Clin North Am* 1970; **17**: 69–78.

13. Vik T, Vatten L, Jacobsen G, *et al.* Prenatal growth in symmetric and asymmetric small-for-gestational-age infants. *Early Hum Dev* 1997; **48**: 167–76.

14. Kramer MS, McLean FH, Olivier M, *et al.* Body proportionality and head and length "sparing" in growth-retarded neonates: a critical reappraisal. *Pediatrics* 1989; **84**: 717–23.

15. Toft PB, Leth H, Ring PB, *et al.* Volumetric analysis of the normal infant brain and in intrauterine growth retardation. *Early Hum Dev* 1995; **43**: 15–29.

16. Amiel-Tison C, Pettigrew AG. Adaptive changes in the developing brain during intrauterine stress. *Brain Dev* 1991; **13**: 67–76.

17. Warshaw JB. Intrauterine growth retardation: adaptation or pathology? *Pediatrics* 1985; **76**: 998–9.

18. Barker DJ. *In utero* programming of chronic disease. *Clin Sci (Lond)* 1998; **95**: 115–28.

19. Sands J, Dobbing J, Gratrix CA. Cell number and cell size: organ growth and development and the control of catch-up growth in rats. *Lancet* 1979; **2**: 503–5.

20. Ounsted M, Ounsted C. *On Fetal Growth Rate.* Clinics in Developmental Medicine. London: Spastics International Publications, 1973.

21. Gluckman PD, Harding JE. Nutritional and hormonal regulation of fetal growth:

evolving concepts. *Acta Paediatr Suppl* 1994; **399**: 60–3.

22. Walton A, Hammond J. The maternal effects on growth and conformation in Shire horse – Shetland pony crosses. *Proc R Soc Lond Biol* 1938; **125**: 311–35.

23. Stein ZA, Susser M. Intrauterine growth retardation: epidemiological issues and public health significance. *Semin Perinatol* 1984; **8**: 5–14.

24. Cetin I, Morpurgo PS, Radaelli T, *et al.* Fetal plasma leptin concentrations: relationship with different intrauterine growth patterns from 19 weeks to term. *Pediatr Res* 2000; **48**: 646–51.

25. Cornblath M, Schwartz R. *Disorders of Carbohydrate Metabolism in Infancy,* 3rd edn. Boston, MA: Blackwell, 1991.

26. Lemons JA, Ridenour R, Orsini EN. Congenital absence of the pancreas and intrauterine growth retardation. *Pediatrics* 1979; **64**: 255–7.

27. Limesand SW, Jensen J, Hutton JC, *et al.* Diminished beta-cell replication contributes to reduced beta-cell mass in fetal sheep with intrauterine growth restriction. *Am J Physiol Regul Integr Comp Physiol* 2005; **288**: R1297–305.

28. Evain-Brion D. Hormonal regulation of fetal growth. *Horm Res* 1994; **42**: 207–14.

29. Guevara-Aguirre J. Insulin-like growth factor I: an important intrauterine growth factor. *N Engl J Med* 1996; **335**: 1389–91.

30. Woods KA, Camacho-Hubner C, Savage MO, *et al.* Intrauterine growth retardation and postnatal growth failure associated with deletion of the insulin-like growth factor I gene. *N Engl J Med* 1996; **335**: 1363–7.

31. Gluckman PD, Gunn AJ, Wray A, *et al.* Congenital idiopathic growth hormone deficiency associated with prenatal and early postnatal growth failure. The International Board of the Kabi Pharmacia International Growth Study. *J Pediatr* 1992; **121**: 920–3.

32. Fisher DA. Intrauterine growth retardation: endocrine and receptor aspects. *Semin Perinatol* 1984; **8**: 37–41.

33. Lafeber HN. Nutritional management and growth hormone treatment of preterm infants born small for gestational age. *Acta Paediatr Suppl* 1997; **423**: 202–5.

34. Chernausek SD, Breen TJ, Frank GR. Linear growth in response to growth hormone treatment in children with short stature associated with intrauterine growth retardation: the National

Cooperative Growth Study experience. *J Pediatr* 1996; **128**: S22–7.

35. Koklu E, Ozturk MA, Kurtoglu S, *et al.* Aortic intima-media thickness, serum IGF-I, IGFBP-3, and leptin levels in intrauterine growth-restricted newborns of healthy mothers. *Pediatr Res* 2007; **62**: 704–9.

36. Kramer MS. Determinants of low birth weight: methodological assessment and meta-analysis. *Bull World Health Organ* 1987; **65**: 663–737.

37. Villar J, Belizan JM. The relative contribution of prematurity and fetal growth retardation to low birth weight in developing and developed societies. *Am J Obstet Gynecol* 1982; **143**: 793–8.

38. Chiswick ML. Intrauterine growth retardation. *Br Med J* 1985; **291**: 845–8.

39. Rondo PH, Tomkins AM. Chest circumference as an indicator of intrauterine growth retardation. *Early Hum Dev* 1996; **44**: 161–7.

40. O'Callaghan MJ, Harvey JM, Tudehope DI, *et al.* Aetiology and classification of small for gestational age infants. *J Paediatr Child Health* 1997; **33**: 213–8.

41. Klein JO, Baker CJ, Remington JS, *et al.* Current concepts of infection of the fetus and newborn infants. In Remington JS, Klein JO, Wilson CB, Baker CJ, eds., *Infectious Diseases of the Fetus and Newborn Infant,* 6th edn. Philadelphia, PA: Elsevier Saunders, 2006: 1–25.

42. Droste S. Fetal growth in aneuploid conditions. *Clin Obstet Gynecol* 1992; **35**: 119–25.

43. Kalousek DK, Harrison K. Uniparental disomy and unexplained intrauterine growth retardation. *Contemp Ob/Gyn* 1995; September: 41–52.

44. Creasy RK, Resnick R. Intrauterine growth restriction. In Creasy RK, Resnick R, eds., *Maternal Fetal Medicine,* 5th edn. Philadelphia, PA: Saunders, 2003: 495–512.

45. Kleigman RM. Intrauterine growth restriction. In Fanaroff AA, Martin RJ, Walsh MC, eds., *Neonatal–Perinatal Medicine: Diseases of the Fetus and Infant,* 5th edn. Philadelphia, PA: Mosby Elsevier, 2006: 221–306.

46. Fellman V, Rapola J, Pihko H, *et al.* Iron-overload disease in infants involving fetal growth retardation, lactic acidosis, liver haemosiderosis, and aminoaciduria. *Lancet* 1998; **351**: 490–3.

47. Foster HW. The enigma of low birth weight and race. *N Engl J Med* 1997; **337**: 1232–3.

48. Gabbe SG. Intrauterine growth retardation. In Gabbe SG, Niebyl JR, Simpson JL, eds., *Obstetrics: Normal and Problem Pregnancies*, 2nd edn. New York, NY: Churchill Livingstone, 1991: 923–44.

49. DiGiacomo JE, Hay WW. Fetal glucose metabolism and oxygen consumption during sustained hypoglycemia. *Metabolism* 1990; **39**: 193–202.

50. Gaziano EP, De Lia JE, Kuhlmann RS. Diamnionic monochorionic twin gestations: an overview. *J Matern Fetal Med* 2000; **9**: 89–96.

51. Cooperstock MS, Tummaru R, Bakewell J, *et al.* Twin birth weight discordance and risk of preterm birth. *Am J Obstet Gynecol* 2000; **183**: 63–7.

52. Antonov AN. Children born during the siege of Leningrad in 1942. *J Pediatr* 1947; **30**: 250–9.

53. Stein Z, Susser M. The Dutch famine, 1944–1945, and the reproductive process. I. Effects of six indices at birth. *Pediatr Res* 1975; **9**: 70–6.

54. Stein Z, Susser M. The Dutch famine, 1944–1945, and the reproductive process. II. Interrelations of caloric rations and six indices at birth. *Pediatr Res* 1975; **9**: 76–83.

55. Lumey LH. Decreased birthweights in infants after maternal *in utero* exposure to the Dutch famine of 1944–1945. *Paediatr Perinat Epidemiol* 1992; **6**: 240–53.

56. Suescun J, Mora JO. Food supplements during pregnancy: intrauterine growth retardation. In Senterre J, ed. *Nestle Nutrition Workshop Series*. New York, NY: Vevey/Raven, 1989.

57. Prentice AM, Whitehead RG, Watkinson M, *et al.* Prenatal dietary supplementation of African women and birth-weight. *Lancet* 1983; **1**: 489–92.

58. Jameson S. Zinc status in pregnancy: the effect of zinc therapy on perinatal mortality, prematurity, and placental ablation. *Ann NY Acad Sci* 1993; **678**: 178–92.

59. Butterworth RF. Maternal thiamine deficiency: a factor in intrauterine growth retardation. *Ann NY Acad Sci* 1993; **678**: 325–9.

60. Conti J, Abraham S, Taylor A. Eating behavior and pregnancy outcome. *J Psychosom Res* 1998; **44**: 465–77.

61. Witlin AG, Saade GR, Mattar F, *et al.* Predictors of neonatal outcome in women with severe preeclampsia or eclampsia between 24 and 33 weeks'

62. Eskenazi B, Fenster L, Sidney S, *et al.* Fetal growth retardation in infants of multiparous and nulliparous women with preeclampsia. *Am J Obstet Gynecol* 1993; **169**: 1112–18.

63. Rosso P, Donoso E, Braun S, *et al.* Maternal hemodynamic adjustments in idiopathic fetal growth retardation. *Gynecol Obstet Invest* 1993; **35**: 162–5.

64. Hays PM, Cruikshank DP, Dunn LJ. Plasma volume determination in normal and preeclamptic pregnancies. *Am J Obstet Gynecol* 1985; **151**: 958–66.

65. Brewster JA, Shaw NJ, Farquharson RG. Neonatal and pediatric outcome of infants born to mothers with antiphospholipid syndrome. *J Perinat Med* 1999; **27**: 183–7.

66. Wolfe HM, Gross TL, Sokol RJ. Recurrent small for gestational age birth: perinatal risks and outcomes. *Am J Obstet Gynecol* 1987; **157**: 288–93.

67. Ounsted M, Ounsted C. Maternal regulation of intrauterine growth. *Nature* 1966; **212**: 995–7.

68. Anderson MS, Hay WW, Jr. Intrauterine growth restriction and the small-for-gestational age infant. In MacDonald MG, Seskice MMK, Mullett MD, eds., *Neonatology: Pathophysiology and Management of the Newborn*, 6th edn. Philadelphia, PA: Lippincott Williams & Wilkins, 2005: 490–522.

69. Butler NR, Goldstein H, Ross EM. Cigarette smoking in pregnancy: its influence on birth weight and perinatal mortality. *Br Med J* 1972; **2**: 127–30.

70. Haddow JE, Knight GJ, Palomaki GE, *et al.* Cigarette consumption and serum cotinine in relation to birthweight. *Br J Obstet Gynaecol* 1987; **94**: 678–81.

71. Kallen K. Maternal smoking during pregnancy and infant head circumference at birth. *Early Hum Dev* 2000; **58**: 197–204.

72. Mills JL, Graubard BI, Harley EE, *et al.* Maternal alcohol consumption and birth weight: how much drinking during pregnancy is safe? *JAMA* 1984; **252**: 1875–9.

73. Olegard R, Sabel KG, Aronsson M, *et al.* Effects on the child of alcohol abuse during pregnancy: retrospective and prospective studies. *Acta Paediatr Scand Suppl* 1979; **275**: 112–21.

74. Little BB, Snell LM. Brain growth among fetuses exposed to cocaine *in utero*:

asymmetrical growth retardation. *Obstet Gynecol* 1991; **77**: 361–4.

75. Frank DA, Bauchner H, Parker S, *et al.* Neonatal body proportionality and body composition after *in utero* exposure to cocaine and marijuana. *J Pediatr* 1990; **117**: 622–6.

76. Fortier I, Marcoux S, Beaulac-Baillargeon L. Relation of caffeine intake during pregnancy to intrauterine growth retardation and preterm birth. *Am J Epidemiol* 1993; **137**: 931–40.

77. Golding J. Reproduction and caffeine consumption: a literature review. *Early Hum Dev* 1995; **43**: 1–14.

78. Giussani DA, Salinas CE, Villena M, *et al.* The role of oxygen in prenatal growth: studies in the chick embryo. *J Physiol* 2007; **585**: 911–17.

79. Kruger H, Arias-Stella J. The placenta and the newborn infant at high altitudes. *Am J Obstet Gynecol* 1970; **106**: 586–91.

80. Wilson MJ, Lopez M, Vargas M, *et al.* Greater uterine artery blood flow during pregnancy in multigenerational (Andean) than shorter-term (European) high-altitude residents. *Am J Physiol Regul Integr Comp Physiol* 2007; **293**: R1313–24.

81. Bennett A, Sain SR, Vargas E, *et al.* Evidence that parent-of-origin affects birth-weight reductions at high altitude. *Am J Hum Biol* 2008; **20**: 592–7.

82. Tuntiseranee P, Geater A, Chongsuvivatwong V, *et al.* The effect of heavy maternal workload on fetal growth retardation and preterm delivery: a study among southern Thai women. *J Occup Environ Med* 1998; **40**: 1013–21.

83. Koos BJ, Longo LD. Mercury toxicity in the pregnant woman, fetus, and newborn infant: a review. *Am J Obstet Gynecol* 1976; **126**: 390–409.

84. Craigo SD. The role of ultrasound in the diagnosis and management of intrauterine growth retardation. *Semin Perinatol* 1994; **18**: 292–304.

85. Kennedy A. Fetal ultrasound. *Curr Probl Diagn Radiol* 2000; **29**: 109–40.

86. Peleg D, Kennedy CM, Hunter SK. Intrauterine growth restriction: identification and management. *Am Fam Physician* 1998; **58**: 453–60, 466–7.

87. Weiner Z, Peer E, Zimmer EZ. Fetal testing in growth restriction. *Clin Obstet Gynecol* 1997; **40**: 804–13.

88. Dubinsky T, Lau M, Powell F, *et al.* Predicting poor neonatal outcome: a comparative study of noninvasive

antenatal testing methods. *AJR Am J Roentgenol* 1997; **168**: 827–31.

89. Forouzan I, Tian ZY. Fetal middle cerebral artery blood flow velocities in pregnancies complicated by intrauterine growth restriction and extreme abnormality in umbilical artery Doppler velocity. *Am J Perinatol* 1996; **13**: 139–42.

90. Hershkovitz R, Kingdom JC, Geary M, *et al.* Fetal cerebral blood flow redistribution in late gestation: identification of compromise in small fetuses with normal umbilical artery Doppler. *Ultrasound Obstet Gynecol* 2000; **15**: 209–12.

91. Shalev E, Blondheim O, Peleg D. Use of cordocentesis in the management of preterm or growth-restricted fetuses with abnormal monitoring. *Obstet Gynecol Surv* 1995; **50**: 839–44.

92. Lin CC, Santolaya-Forgas J. Current concepts of fetal growth restriction: Part II. Diagnosis and management. *Obstet Gynecol* 1999; **93**: 140–6.

93. Nicolaides KH, Campbell S, Bradley RJ, *et al.* Maternal oxygen therapy for intrauterine growth retardation. *Lancet* 1987; **1**: 942–5.

94. Regnault TR, de Vrijer B, Galan HL, *et al.* Development and mechanisms of fetal hypoxia in severe fetal growth restriction. *Placenta* 2007; **28**: 714–23.

95. Salihagić-Kadić A, Medić M, Jugović D, *et al.* Fetal cerebrovascular response to chronic hypoxia: implications for the prevention of brain damage. *J Matern Fetal Neonatal Med* 2006; **19**: 387–96.

96. Figueras F, Eixarch E, Meler E, *et al.* Small-for-gestational-age fetuses with normal umbilical artery Doppler have suboptimal perinatal and neurodevelopmental outcome. *Eur J Obstet Gynecol Reprod Biol* 2008; **136**: 34–8.

97. Walther FJ, Ramaekers LH. Neonatal morbidity of SGA infants in relation to their nutritional status at birth. *Acta Paediatr Scand* 1982; **71**: 437–40.

98. Murphy JD, Rabinovitch M, Goldstein JD, *et al.* The structural basis of persistent pulmonary hypertension of the newborn infant. *J Pediatr* 1981; **98**: 962–7.

99. Warsof SL, Cooper DJ, Little D, *et al.* Routine ultrasound screening for antenatal detection of intrauterine growth retardation. *Obstet Gynecol* 1986; **67**: 33–9.

100. Hawdon JM, Aynsley-Green A, Ward Platt MP. Neonatal blood glucose concentrations: metabolic effects of intravenous glucagon and intragastric medium chain triglyceride. *Arch Dis Child* 1993; **68**: 255–61.

101. Collins JE, Leonard JV, Teale D, *et al.* Hyperinsulinaemic hypoglycaemia in small for dates babies. *Arch Dis Child* 1990; **65**: 1118–20.

102. Limesand SW, Rozance PJ, Smith D, *et al.* Increased insulin sensitivity and maintenance of glucose utilization rates in fetal sheep with placental insufficiency and intrauterine growth restriction. *Am J Physiol Endocrinol Metab* 2007; **293**: E1716–25.

103. Wallace JM, Milne JS, Aitken RP, *et al.* Sensitivity to metabolic signals in late-gestation growth-restricted fetuses from rapidly growing adolescent sheep. *Am J Physiol Endocrinol Metab* 2007; **293**: E1233–41.

104. Hawdon JM, Ward Platt MP. Metabolic adaptation in small for gestational age infants. *Arch Dis Child* 1993; **68**: 262–8.

105. Chance GW, Bower BD. Hypoglycaemia and temporary hyperglycaemia in infants of low birth weight for maturity. *Arch Dis Child* 1966; **41**: 279–85.

106. Economides DL, Proudler A, Nicolaides KH. Plasma insulin in appropriate- and small-for-gestational-age fetuses. *Am J Obstet Gynecol* 1989; **160**: 1091–4.

107. Howard CP, Go VL, Infante AJ, *et al.* Long-term survival in a case of functional pancreatic agenesis. *J Pediatr* 1980; **97**: 786–9.

108. Tsang RC, Gigger M, Oh W, *et al.* Studies in calcium metabolism in infants with intrauterine growth retardation. *J Pediatr* 1975; **86**: 936–41.

109. Kramer MS, Olivier M, McLean FH, *et al.* Impact of intrauterine growth retardation and body proportionality on fetal and neonatal outcome. *Pediatrics* 1990; **86**: 707–13.

110. Sinclair JC. Heat production and thermoregulation in the small-for-date infant. *Pediatr Clin North Am* 1970; **17**: 147–58.

111. Jackson R, Yu JS. Cold injury of the newborn in Australia: a study of 31 cases. *Med J Aust* 1973; **2**: 630–3.

112. Koenig JM, Christensen RD. Incidence, neutrophil kinetics, and natural history of neonatal neutropenia associated with maternal hypertension. *N Engl J Med* 1989; **321**: 557–62.

113. Koenig JM, Christensen RD. The mechanism responsible for diminished neutrophil production in neonates delivered of women with pregnancy-induced hypertension. *Am J Obstet Gynecol* 1991; **165**: 467–73.

114. Philip AG, Tito AM. Increased nucleated red blood cell counts in small for gestational age infants with very low birth weight. *Am J Dis Child* 1989; **143**: 164–9.

115. Meberg A, Jakobsen E, Halvorsen K. Humoral regulation of erythropoiesis and thrombopoiesis in appropriate and small for gestational age infants. *Acta Paediatr Scand* 1982; **71**: 769–73.

116. Soothill PW, Nicolaides KH, Campbell S. Prenatal asphyxia, hyperlacticaemia, hypoglycaemia, and erythroblastosis in growth retarded fetuses. *Br Med J* 1987; **294**: 1051–3.

117. Snijders RJ, Abbas A, Melby O, *et al.* Fetal plasma erythropoietin concentration in severe growth retardation. *Am J Obstet Gynecol* 1993; **168**: 615–9.

118. Minior VK, Shatzkin E, Divon MY. Nucleated red blood cell count in the differentiation of fetuses with pathologic growth restriction from healthy small-for-gestational-age fetuses. *Am J Obstet Gynecol* 2000; **182**: 1107–9.

119. Benirschke K. Placenta pathology questions to the perinatologist. *J Perinatol* 1994; **14**: 371–5.

120. Korst LM, Phelan JP, Ahn MO, *et al.* Nucleated red blood cells: an update on the marker for fetal asphyxia. *Am J Obstet Gynecol* 1996; **175**: 843–6.

121. Black VD. Neonatal hyperviscosity syndromes. *Curr Probl Pediatr* 1987; **17**: 73–130.

122. Elliott JP, Urig MA, Clewell WH. Aggressive therapeutic amniocentesis for treatment of twin–twin transfusion syndrome. *Obstet Gynecol* 1991; **77**: 537–40.

123. Töllner U, Pohlandt F. Septicemia in the newborn due to gram-negative bacilli: risk factors, clinical symptoms, and hematologic changes. *Eur J Pediatr* 1976; **123**: 243–54.

124. Thomas RM, Linch DC. Identification of lymphocyte subsets in the newborn using a variety of monoclonal antibodies. *Arch Dis Child* 1983; **58**: 34–8.

125. Villar J, de Onis M, Kestler E, *et al.* The differential neonatal morbidity of the intrauterine growth retardation syndrome. *Am J Obstet Gynecol* 1990; **163**: 151–7.

126. Wiswell TE, Robertson CF, Jones TA, *et al.* Necrotizing enterocolitis in full-term infants: a case–control study. *Am J Dis Child* 1988; **142**: 532–5.

127. Hackett GA, Campbell S, Gamsu H, *et al.* Doppler studies in the growth retarded fetus and prediction of neonatal necrotising enterocolitis, haemorrhage, and neonatal morbidity. *Br Med J* 1987; **294**: 13–16.

128. Gould JB, Gluck L, Kulovich MV. The relationship between accelerated pulmonary maturity and accelerated neurological maturity in certain chronically stressed pregnancies. *Am J Obstet Gynecol* 1977; **127**: 181–6.

129. Tyson JE, Kennedy K, Broyles S, *et al.* The small for gestational age infant: accelerated or delayed pulmonary maturation? Increased or decreased survival? *Pediatrics* 1995; **95**: 534–8.

130. Amiel-Tison C. Possible acceleration of neurological maturation following high-risk pregnancy. *Am J Obstet Gynecol* 1980; **138**: 303–6.

131. Pettigrew AG, Edwards DA, Henderson-Smart DJ. The influence of intra-uterine growth retardation on brainstem development of preterm infants. *Dev Med Child Neurol* 1985; **27**: 467–72.

132. Cook CJ, Gluckman PD, Williams C, *et al.* Precocial neural function in the growth-retarded fetal lamb. *Pediatr Res* 1988; **24**: 600–4.

133. Stanley OH, Fleming PJ, Morgan MH. Development of visual evoked potentials following intrauterine growth retardation. *Early Hum Dev* 1991; **27**: 79–91.

134. Scherjon S, Briet J, Oosting H, *et al.* The discrepancy between maturation of visual-evoked potentials and cognitive outcome at five years in very preterm infants with and without hemodynamic signs of fetal brain-sparing. *Pediatrics* 2000; **105**: 385–91.

135. van Vliet MA, Martin CB, Jr., Nijhuis JG, *et al.* Behavioural states in growth-retarded human fetuses. *Early Hum Dev* 1985; **12**: 183–97.

136. Nijhuis IJ, ten Hof J, Nijhuis JG, *et al.* Temporal organization of fetal behavior from 24-weeks gestation onwards in normal and complicated pregnancies. *Dev Psychobiol* 1999; **34**: 257–68.

137. Vintzileos AM, Fleming AD, Scorza WE, *et al.* Relationship between fetal biophysical activities and umbilical cord blood gas values. *Am J Obstet Gynecol* 1991; **165**: 707–13.

138. Low JA, Galbraith RS, Muir D, *et al.* Intrauterine growth retardation: a preliminary report of long-term morbidity. *Am J Obstet Gynecol* 1978; **130**: 534–45.

139. Als H, Tronick E, Adamson L, *et al.* The behavior of the full-term but underweight newborn infant. *Dev Med Child Neurol* 1976; **18**: 590–602.

140. Zeskind PS, Lester BM. Analysis of cry features in newborns with differential fetal growth. *Child Dev* 1981; **52**: 207–12.

141. Leventhal JM, Berg A, Egerter SA. Is intrauterine growth retardation a risk factor for child abuse? *Pediatrics* 1987; **79**: 515–19.

142. Watt J, Strongman KT. Mother–infant interactions at 2 and 3 months in preterm, small-for-gestational-age, and full-term infants: their relationship with cognitive development at 4 months. *Early Hum Dev* 1985; **11**: 231–46.

143. Watt J. Interaction and development in the first year. II. The effects of intrauterine growth retardation. *Early Hum Dev* 1986; **13**: 211–23.

144. Warkany J, Monroe BB, Sutherland BS. Intrauterine growth retardation. *Am J Dis Child* 1961; **102**: 249–79.

145. Goldenberg RL, Cliver SP. Small for gestational age and intrauterine growth restriction: definitions and standards. *Clin Obstet Gynecol* 1997; **40**: 704–14.

146. Babson SG, Kangas J, Young N, *et al.* Growth and development of twins of dissimilar size at birth. *Pediatrics* 1964; **33**: 327–33.

147. Babson SG, Phillips DS. Growth and development of twins dissimilar in size at birth. *N Engl J Med* 1973; **289**: 937–40.

148. Wilson RS. Twin growth: initial deficit, recovery, and trends in concordance from birth to nine years. *Ann Hum Biol* 1979; **6**: 205–20.

149. Philip AGS. Term twins with discordant birth weights: observations at birth and one year. *Acta Genet Med Gemellol (Roma)* 1981; **30**: 203–12.

150. Buckler JM, Robinson A. Matched development of a pair of monozygous twins of grossly different size at birth. *Arch Dis Child* 1974; **49**: 472–6.

151. Fitzhardinge PM, Steven EM. The small-for-date infant. II. Neurological and intellectual sequelae. *Pediatrics* 1972; **50**: 50–7.

152. Babson SG, Henderson NB. Fetal undergrowth: relation of head growth to later intellectual performance. *Pediatrics* 1974; **53**: 890–4.

153. Strauss RS. Adult functional outcome of those born small for gestational age: twenty-six-year follow-up of the 1970 British Birth Cohort. *JAMA* 2000; **283**: 625–32.

154. Strauss RS, Dietz WH. Growth and development of term children born with low birth weight: effects of genetic and environmental factors. *J Pediatr* 1998; **133**: 67–72.

155. Commey JO, Fitzhardinge PM. Handicap in the preterm small-for-gestational age infant. *J Pediatr* 1979; **94**: 779–86.

156. Huisjes HJ, Baarsma R, Hadders-Algra M, *et al.* Follow-up of growth-retarded children born by elective cesarean section before 33 weeks. *Gynecol Obstet Invest* 1985; **19**: 169–73.

157. Ounsted M, Moar VA, Scott A. Small-for-dates babies, gestational age, and developmental ability at 7 years. *Early Hum Dev* 1989; **19**: 77–86.

158. Lubchenco LO, Searls DT, Brazie JV. Neonatal mortality rate: relationship to birth weight and gestational age. *J Pediatr* 1972; **81**: 814–22.

159. Lubchenco LO. Intrauterine growth and neonatal morbidity and mortality. In Lubchenco LO, ed., *The High Risk Infant.* Philadelphia, PA: Saunders, 1976: 99–124.

160. Starfield B, Shapiro S, McCormick M, *et al.* Mortality and morbidity in infants with intrauterine growth retardation. *J Pediatr* 1982; **101**: 978–83.

161. McIntire DD, Bloom SL, Casey BM, *et al.* Birth weight in relation to morbidity and mortality among newborn infants. *N Engl J Med* 1999; **340**: 1234–8.

162. Fattal-Valevski A, Leitner Y, Kutai M, *et al.* Neurodevelopmental outcome in children with intrauterine growth retardation: a 3-year follow-up. *J Child Neurol* 1999; **14**: 724–7.

163. Ounsted MK, Moar VA, Scott A. Children of deviant birthweight at the age of seven years: health, handicap, size and developmental status. *Early Hum Dev* 1984; **9**: 323–40.

164. Walther FJ, Ramaekers LH. Growth in early childhood of newborns affected by disproportionate intrauterine growth retardation. *Acta Paediatr Scand* 1982; **71**: 651–6.

165. Tenovuo A, Kero P, Piekkala P, *et al.* Growth of 519 small for gestational age infants during the first two years of life. *Acta Paediatr Scand* 1987; **76**: 636–46.

166. Paz I, Seidman DS, Danon YL, *et al.* Are children born small for gestational age at increased risk of short stature? *Am J Dis Child* 1993; **147**: 337–9.

167. Fitzhardinge PM, Inwood S. Long-term growth in small-for-date children. *Acta Paediatr Scand Suppl* 1989; **349**: 27–33.

168. Adair LS. Low birth weight and intrauterine growth retardation in Filipino infants. *Pediatrics* 1989; **84**: 613–22.

169. Ounsted M, Moar VA, Scott A. Proportionality of small-for-gestational age babies at birth: perinatal associations and postnatal sequelae. *Early Hum Dev* 1986; **14**: 77–88.

170. Colle E, Schiff D, Andrew G, *et al.* Insulin responses during catch-up growth of infants who were small for gestational age. *Pediatrics* 1976; **57**: 363–71.

171. Allen MC. Developmental outcome and followup of the small for gestational age infant. *Semin Perinatol* 1984; **8**: 123–56.

172. Westwood M, Kramer MS, Munz D, *et al.* Growth and development of full-term nonasphyxiated small-for-gestational-age newborns: follow-up through adolescence. *Pediatrics* 1983; **71**: 376–82.

173. Winer EK, Tejani NA, Atluru V, *et al.* Four- to seven-year evaluation in two groups of small-for-gestational age infants. *Am J Obstet Gynecol* 1982; **143**: 425–9.

174. Drew JH, Bayly J, Beischer NA. Prospective follow-up of growth retarded infants and of those from pregnancies complicated by low oestriol excretion: 7 years. *Aust NZ J Obstet Gynaecol* 1983; **23**: 150–4.

175. Villar J, Smeriglio V, Martorell R, *et al.* Heterogeneous growth and mental development of intrauterine growth-retarded infants during the first 3 years of life. *Pediatrics* 1984; **74**: 783–91.

176. Martikainen MA. Effects of intrauterine growth retardation and its subtypes on the development of the preterm infant. *Early Hum Dev* 1992; **28**: 7–17.

177. Vohr BR, Oh W. Growth and development in preterm infants small for gestational age. *J Pediatr* 1983; **103**: 941–5.

178. Sung IK, Vohr B, Oh W. Growth and neurodevelopmental outcome of very low birth weight infants with intrauterine growth retardation: comparison with control subjects matched by birth weight and gestational age. *J Pediatr* 1993; **123**: 618–24.

179. Monset-Couchard M, de Bethmann O. Catch-up growth in 166 small-for-gestational age premature infants weighing less than 1,000 g at birth. *Biol Neonate* 2000; **78**: 161–7.

180. Spinillo A, Gardella B, Preti E, *et al.* Rates of neonatal death and cerebral palsy associated with fetal growth restriction among very low birthweight infants: a temporal analysis. *BJOG* 2006; **113**: 775–80.

181. Uvebrant P, Hagberg G. Intrauterine growth in children with cerebral palsy. *Acta Paediatr* 1992; **81**: 407–12.

182. Blair E, Stanley F. Intrauterine growth and spastic cerebral palsy. I. Association with birth weight for gestational age. *Am J Obstet Gynecol* 1990; **162**: 229–37.

183. Topp M, Langhoff-Roos J, Uldall P, *et al.* Intrauterine growth and gestational age in preterm infants with cerebral palsy. *Early Hum Dev* 1996; **44**: 27–36.

184. Hill RM, Verniaud WM, Deter RL, *et al.* The effect of intrauterine malnutrition on the term infant: a 14-year progressive study. *Acta Paediatr Scand* 1984; **73**: 482–7.

185. Hawdon JM, Hey E, Kolvin I, *et al.* Born too small: is outcome still affected? *Dev Med Child Neurol* 1990; **32**: 943–53.

186. Low JA, Handley-Derry MH, Burke SO, *et al.* Association of intrauterine fetal growth retardation and learning deficits at age 9 to 11 years. *Am J Obstet Gynecol* 1992; **167**: 1499–505.

187. Hutton JL, Pharoah PO, Cooke RW, *et al.* Differential effects of preterm birth and small for gestational age on cognitive and motor development. *Arch Dis Child Fetal Neonatal Ed* 1997; **76**: F75–81.

188. Kok JH, den Ouden AL, Verloove-Vanhorick SP, *et al.* Outcome of very preterm small for gestational age infants: the first nine years of life. *Br J Obstet Gynaecol* 1998; **105**: 162–8.

189. Paz I, Laor A, Gale R, *et al.* Term infants with fetal growth restriction are not at increased risk for low intelligence scores at age 17 years. *J Pediatr* 2001; **138**: 87–91.

190. Geva R, Eshel R, Leitner Y, *et al.* Neuropsychological outcome of children with intrauterine growth restriction: a 9-year prospective study. *Pediatrics* 2006; **118**: 91–100.

191. Leonard H, Nassar N, Bourke J, *et al.* Relation between intrauterine growth and subsequent intellectual disability in a ten-year population cohort of children in Western Australia. *Am J Epidemiol* 2008; **167**: 103–11.

192. Leitner Y, Fattal-Valevski A, Geva R, *et al.* Neurodevelopmental outcome of children with intrauterine growth retardation: a longitudinal, 10-year prospective study. *J Child Neurol* 2007; **22**: 580–7.

193. Barker DJ, Bull AR, Osmond C, *et al.* Fetal and placental size and risk of hypertension in adult life. *Br Med J* 1990; **301**: 259–62.

194. Barker DJ, Gluckman PD, Godfrey KM, *et al.* Fetal nutrition and cardiovascular disease in adult life. *Lancet* 1993; **341**: 938–41.

195. Gortner L. Intrauterine growth restriction and risk for arterial hypertension: a causal relationship? *J Perinat Med* 2007; **35**: 361–5.

196. Forsen T, Eriksson J, Tuomilehto J, *et al.* The fetal and childhood growth of persons who develop type 2 diabetes. *Ann Intern Med* 2000; **133**: 176–82.

197. Skilton MR, Evans N, Griffiths KA, *et al.* Aortic wall thickness in newborns with intrauterine growth restriction. *Lancet* 2005; **365**: 1484–6.

198. Bloomfield FH, Oliver MH, Harding JE. The late effects of fetal growth patterns. *Arch Dis Child Fetal Neonatal Ed* 2006; **91**: F299–304.

199. Varma TR, Curzen P. The effects of abdominal decompression on pregnancy complicated by the small-for-dates fetus. *J Obstet Gynaecol Br Commonw* 1973; **80**: 1086–94.

200. Pavelka R, Salzer H. Abdominal decompression: an approach towards treating placental insufficiency. *Gynecol Obstet Invest* 1981; **12**: 317–24.

201. Pollack RN, Yaffe H, Divon MY. Therapy for intrauterine growth restriction: current options and future directions. *Clin Obstet Gynecol* 1997; **40**: 824–42.

202. Gulmezoglu AM, Hofmeyr GJ. Maternal oxygen administration for suspected impaired fetal growth. *Cochrane Database Syst Rev* 2000; (2): CD000137.

203. Grab D, Paulus WE, Erdmann M, *et al.* Effects of low-dose aspirin on uterine and fetal blood flow during pregnancy: results of a randomized, placebo-controlled, double-blind trial. *Ultrasound Obstet Gynecol* 2000; **15**: 19–27.

204. Oyelese KO, Black RS, Lees CC, *et al.* A novel approach to the management of pregnancies complicated by uteroplacental insufficiency and previous stillbirth. *Aust NZ J Obstet Gynaecol* 1998; **38**: 391–5.

205. Rush D, Stein Z, Susser M. A randomized controlled trial of prenatal nutritional supplementation in New York City. *Pediatrics* 1980; **65**: 683–97.

206. Rivera-Alsina ME, Saldana LR, Stringer CA. Fetal growth sustained by parenteral nutrition in pregnancy. *Obstet Gynecol* 1984; **64**: 138–41.

207. Gulmezoglu AM, Hofmeyr GJ. Maternal nutrient supplementation for suspected impaired fetal growth. *Cochrane Database Syst Rev* 2000; (2): CD000148.

208. Gulmezoglu AM, Hofmeyr GJ. Plasma volume expansion for suspected impaired fetal growth. *Cochrane Database Syst Rev* 2000; (2): CD000167.

209. Gulmezoglu AM, Hofmeyr GJ. Bed rest in hospital for suspected impaired fetal growth. *Cochrane Database Syst Rev* 2000; (2): CD000034.

210. Roth S, Chang TC, Robson S, *et al.* The neurodevelopmental outcome of term infants with different intrauterine growth characteristics. *Early Hum Dev* 1999; **55**: 39–50.

211. Kinzler WL, Kaminsky L. Fetal growth restriction and subsequent pregnancy risks. *Semin Perinatol* 2007; **31**: 126–34.

212. Brenner B, Aharon A. Thrombophilia and adverse pregnancy outcome. *Clin Perinatol* 2007; **34**: 527–41.

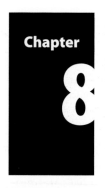

Chapter

8

Maternal diseases that affect fetal development

Bonnie Dwyer and Maurice L. Druzin

Introduction

Most maternal diseases that affect fetal development probably do so by multiple mechanisms. However, for the purpose of study, it is useful to categorize diseases by mechanism of teratogenesis. Maternal disease can effect fetal development in the following ways: (1) specific effects of metabolic end products or antibodies, (2) placental insufficiency, (3) maternal medications or toxic exposures, (4) infection, and (5) genetic disease. The main focus of this chapter is to discuss maternal disease that has primary effects on fetal development. Placental insufficiency, medication/toxic exposures, infection, and genetic disease are mentioned for the sake of completeness and will be discussed briefly. All maternal illnesses, whether they directly affect the fetus or not, can cause iatrogenic premature delivery in the case of an unstable mother.

Specific fetal effects of over- or underproduced metabolic end products or antibodies

Maternal diseases that cause specific fetal disease can do so by transplacental passage of a toxic maternal metabolic end product (e.g., high glucose or high androgen), by lack of transplacental passage of an essential maternal metabolic end product (e.g., thyroxine), or by transplacental passage of a maternal antibody. Well-studied maternal diseases that are prototypes for the above-described mechanisms of fetal disease include (1) diabetes mellitus, congenital adrenal hyperplasia, and phenylketonuria (toxic metabolic end product), (2) hypothyroidism (maternal underproduction of an essential metabolic end product), and (3) Grave's disease, systemic lupus erythematosus, and rhesus alloimmunization (maternal antibody transfer). There are many other examples of maternal diseases which affect fetal development. However, the above-mentioned prototypic diseases will be discussed below.

Toxic metabolic end product

Maternal disease can cause overproduction of normal metabolic end products. High levels of these are toxic to both the mother and the fetus. Well-studied examples include hyperglycemia in diabetes mellitus, high levels of androgens in congenital adrenal hyperplasia, and high levels of phenylalanine in phenylketonuria.

Diabetes Mellitus

In maternal diabetes mellitus, hyperglycemia has been shown to be the primary teratogen with regard to congenital malformation, pregnancy loss, and macrosomia. This is supported by studies showing that these risks are minimized with good glucose control before and during pregnancy [1–5]. However, attributing all embryopathy and fetopathy to high maternal glucose levels may be an oversimplification. Some studies have also linked the high levels of maternal ketonemia, specifically high levels of β-hydroxybutyrate, to lower scores on neurodevelopmental and behavioral tests in offspring [1,5–7]. Placental insufficiency in patients with long-standing diabetes and vascular disease likely also plays a role.

Distinguishing pregestational diabetes from gestational diabetes is important. Pregestational diabetes is associated with more preconceptual hyperglycemia, more placental vascular disease, and more difficulty controlling hyperglycemia and hypoglycemia in pregnancy. An early elevated hemoglobin A1c is highly associated with congenital malformations and early miscarriage. Gestational diabetes, on the other hand, usually starts in the third trimester and is not associated with an elevated hemoglobin A1c, congenital malformations, or early miscarriage [2]. Fetal consequences common to pregestational diabetes and gestational diabetes are macrosomia, birth trauma, and neonatal metabolic complications.

Management of diabetes in pregnancy includes diet and medical therapy (insulin or oral hypoglycemic) in order to approximate euglycemia [1,8]. Fetal ultrasound, antepartum testing, intrapartum glucose monitoring, and appropriate timing and mode of delivery make contemporary morbidity and mortality rates similar to those of the normal population [1].

Embryonic effects

Infants of insulin-dependent diabetic mothers have a two- to eightfold increased risk of congenital malformations [1,5]. The most common malformations are in the central nervous system (spina bifida/anencephaly), heart, kidney, and skeleton (caudal regression) [1,2,5]. Pregestational diabetics also have an increased risk of spontaneous miscarriage, likely related to lethal malformations or direct glucose toxicity [1].

The higher the extent of the hyperglycemia and hemoglobin A1c, the higher the risk of major malformation and

Fetal and Neonatal Brain Injury, 4th edition, ed. David K. Stevenson, William E. Benitz, Philip Sunshine, Susan R. Hintz, and Maurice L. Druzin. Published by Cambridge University Press. © Cambridge University Press 2009.

early miscarriage [1,5]. A classic study by Miller *et al.* in 1981 showed that in patients with a hemoglobin A1c of < 8.5%, the malformation rate was 3.4%, similar to the normal population. However, when the hemoglobin A1c was > 8.5%, the malformation rate was 22.4%. Lucas *et al.* in 1989 demonstrated a linear correlation between hemoglobin A1c and malformation rate [1,5,9,10].

Fetal effects

The most common effect of diabetes is fetal macrosomia. Fetal macrosomia, that is birthweight above the 90th percentile, is present in 25–42% of diabetic pregnancies [1,3]. It is directly correlated to postprandial glucose control. The fetal skeleton is not affected, and macrosomia is largely a result of increased adipose deposition in the shoulder and abdominal regions [5]. Macrosomia is related to an increased rate of cesarean delivery and an increased rate of birth injury due to shoulder dystocia and fetal compromise [1,5]. The risk of birth injury is also directly related to glucose control [5]. Insulin therapy decreases the rate of macrosomia, birth injury, and perinatal morbidity [4].

In addition to macrosomia, pregestational diabetes can be associated with intrauterine growth restriction. This may be due to maternal hypoglycemia and/or vascular abnormalities in the placenta [2,5,8].

Neonatal effects

In addition to macrosomia at birth, neonatal complications include metabolic derangements such as hypoglycemia, polycythemia, hypocalcemia, and hyperbilirubinemia. The incidence and severity of neonatal hypoglycemia is directly correlated with the extent of maternal hyperglycemia immediately antepartum and during labor. Polycythemia is also a direct consequence of hyperglycemia, as hyperglycemia is a stimulus for erythropoietin production [5]. Other complications such as delayed lung maturation and hypertrophic cardiomyopathy have been associated with chronically poor glycemic control [1,3,5].

Childhood/adulthood effects

An infant born to a diabetic mother has a higher risk of developing obesity, impaired glucose intolerance, and diabetes at an early age [3,5]. These infants are at higher risk for diabetes than infants born to diabetic fathers. This implies that the intrauterine environment, in addition to genetics, plays a role in childhood and adult disease. Whether childhood and adulthood obesity and glucose intolerance are directly associated with maternal and fetal hyperglycemia remains to be seen [3,5].

Maternal congenital adrenal hyperplasia (CAH)

Congenital adrenal hyperplasia is another example of a maternal disease in which a toxic maternal metabolite is teratogenic. Congenital adrenal hyperplasia is a group of inherited enzyme deficiencies in the adrenal steroid biosynthesis pathway, which result in elevated levels of maternal androgens [1,11].

21-hydroxylase deficiency is the most common enzyme deficiency. It causes a bottleneck, resulting in low levels of glucocorticoids and elevated levels of steroid precursors, which are shunted to the androgen pathway. Low levels of glucocorticoids stimulate elevated levels of ACTH, further stimulating production of steroid precursors and further stimulating androgen production. In an affected mother, high levels of maternal androgens can cross the placenta, virilize a female fetus, and cause ambiguous genitalia [1,11,12].

In non-pregnant states, exogenous glucocorticoids, like dexamethasone, are used to suppress steroid precursor production and decrease androgen production in order to decrease maternal virilization and allow menstruation. The steroid precursor 17-hydroxyprogesterone, androstenedione, and free testosterone are followed to adjust glucocorticoid dosing. Treatment with dexamethasone is also effective to avoid virilization of a female fetus. In pregnancy, free testosterone may be the most reliable marker for glucocorticoid dose adjustment, because 17-hydroxyprogesterone and androstenedione levels can be altered. Stress-dose steroids should be given at delivery [11,12]. Excessive glucocorticoid treatment can cause transient adrenal suppression in the neonate, so the neonate should be evaluated and monitored [12].

Congenital adrenal hyperplasia is autosomal recessive in inheritance, and therefore the disease can be present in the fetus of an unaffected mother. High androgen production by the fetus herself can also virilize a female fetus. In cases of an affected female fetus, high-dose dexamethasone can be given to the mother to suppress the fetal pituitary–adrenal axis. Prenatal diagnosis for the most common forms of CAH is available [12].

Phenylketonuria (PKU)

Phenylketonuria (PKU) is another example of a maternal disease in which toxic maternal metabolic products are teratogenic. It is an autosomal recessive disorder that is caused by a defect in phenylalanine metabolism. Elevated levels of phenylalanine cause mental retardation in the affected individual and also in a fetus of an affected mother. A diet low in phenylalanine will prevent mental retardation in both individuals [1,13].

In an affected mother, high levels of phenylalanine in maternal blood cross the placenta, causing high levels in the fetal blood. High levels of phenylalanine are teratogenic to the fetus [14]. With untreated maternal PKU, children have a 92% risk of mental retardation, a 73% risk of microcephaly, a 40% risk of low birthweight, and a 12% risk of congenital heart disease. The extent of fetal damage correlates with maternal blood levels of phenylalanine [1,13,14]. The Maternal PKU Collaborative Study in 1984–2002 reported on 572 children of 382 affected women. Mothers with metabolic control (120–360 μmol/L) prior to conception or up to 10 weeks' gestation had children who scored the highest on cognitive function and behavioral tests [1,13]. In fact, these infants had normal cognitive function and only 1/109 had congenital heart disease. Even late treatment (after 20 weeks) showed better cognitive function in offspring compared with untreated pregnancies [1,13].

Breastfeeding should be avoided due to high levels of phenylalanine in the breast milk [14]. Because women who are affected by PKU are often themselves cognitively impaired, metabolic control during pregnancy often requires intensive medical support.

PKU is autosomal recessive in inheritance, so the neonate of an affected mother should be screened for the disease. In fact, PKU screening is routine in all neonates. Affected infants should have diets low in phenylalanine to avoid cognitive impairment [1,14].

Underproduction of essential metabolic product

A maternal disease that underproduces a maternal metabolic product that is essential for fetal development can also cause abnormal development in a fetus. Hypothyroidism is likely one of these diseases, as low maternal thyroxine and related low fetal thyroxine early in pregnancy are associated with poor neurologic outcome. More data are needed to clarify if low maternal thyroxine early in pregnancy is truly the only teratogenic mechanism in this disease.

Hypothyroidism

Maternal hypothyroidism is common, present in 1–3/1000 pregnancies. It has long been associated with decreased intellectual functioning in offspring, independent of etiology (primary hypothyroidism related to iodine deficiency or Hashimoto's thyroiditis) [15,16].

Human and animal studies support the hypothesis that maternal hypothyroidism causes abnormal fetal brain development by lack of maternal T_4 and thus subsequent lack of fetal T_4 [15–21]. Pop and coworkers directly associated low maternal T_4 levels in early pregnancy (12 weeks' gestation) with neurologic impairment in offspring at 3 weeks, 1 year, and 2 years of age [17,18]. Even before fetal thyroid hormone is produced, T_3 receptors, with local conversion of T_4 to T_3, are found in early fetal brain tissue, suggesting a role for maternal T_4 in early fetal neurologic development [19]. Thyroid hormone is also likely important later in fetal life when neuronal organization associated with higher cognitive functioning occurs [1].

A landmark study by Haddow *et al.* in 1999 demonstrated that compared to women without hypothyroidism, women with hypothyroidism had offspring who scored less well on neuropsychological tests between ages 7 and 9 years. Among the offspring of women with hypothyroidism, offspring of untreated mothers had larger deficits. Furthermore, offspring of treated mothers did not have deficits compared to controls [15]. This study suggests that treatment of hypothyroidism with levothyroxine may prevent intellectual deficits in offspring [15–17].

Maternal hypothyroidism is also associated with early pregnancy loss, pre-eclampsia, placental abruption, poor fetal growth, and stillbirth. Treatment of overt hypothyroidism has been associated with improved perinatal outcomes [16,20].

In pregnancy, maternal hypothyroidism should be managed early and aggressively with levothyroxine, with the goal of normalizing TSH and free T_4. An empiric increase by one-third of the pre-pregnancy dose is recommended upon confirmation of pregnancy. On average a woman will need a 50% increase in levothyroxine dose by 20 weeks' gestation. Frequent testing to guide levothyroxine dosing should be instituted throughout pregnancy [22].

Antibody-related fetal disease

Transplacental passage of maternal antibodies can cause fetal disease. Although there are many examples of this type of teratogenesis, Grave's disease, systemic lupus erythematosus, and rhesus alloimmunization with hemolytic disease of the newborn will be discussed below.

Grave's disease

Grave's disease is the most common form of hyperthyroidism, and it is an example of a maternal disease that can cause fetal disease via transplacental passage of maternal autoantibodies. Grave's disease is an autoimmune disorder that is mediated by antibodies that bind to the TSH receptor called thyroid-stimulating immunoglobulins (TSI). TSI can be present in women with Grave's disease even after thyroid ablation, or in patients with Hashimoto's thyroiditis. TSI, which can be stimulating or blocking, can cross the placenta, bind to fetal thyroid receptors, and cause fetal hyper- or hypothyroidism. The fetal thyroid becomes sensitive to these antibodies around 20–24 weeks [1,19].

One percent of pregnancies with elevated TSI levels are affected by fetal/neonatal hyperthyroidism. Typically, TSI levels > 300% of control values are predictive of fetal disease [1,19]. Fetal hyperthyroidism is associated with fetal tachycardia, growth restriction, advanced bone age, and craniosynostosis. Hydrops fetalis and fetal death can occur. It can be treated with maternal administration of propylthiouracil (PTU). Neonatal thyrotoxicosis is associated with poor weight gain, hyperkinesis, ophthalmopathy, arrhythmias, heart failure, pulmonary and systemic hypertension, hepatosplenomegaly, thrombocytopenia, and craniosynostosis [1,19].

Less commonly, placental transfer of maternal TSI can block fetal thyroid activity (thyroid-stimulating blocking antibodies) and cause transient fetal or neonatal congenital hypothyroidism [19]. Transient hypothyroidism can also be due to maternal medications or high levels of maternal thyroxine in the fetus suppressing the fetal hypothalamic–pituitary axis. Untreated congenital hypothyroidism, even if transient, can lead to irreversible neurologic damage. Newborn thyroid screening is, therefore, routine [1,19,23].

Systemic lupus erythematosus (SLE)

Systemic lupus erythematosus (SLE) is a common autoimmune disease seen in pregnancy. Fetal effects of SLE can be secondary to maternal autoantibody transfer, placental insufficiency, prematurity, or maternal drug therapy. However, the purpose of this discussion is to highlight a unique fetal and neonatal syndrome associated with lupus, which is caused by transplacental passage of maternal autoantibodies. This syndrome is called "neonatal lupus syndrome" [24,25]. Neonatal lupus syndrome can also be associated with other autoimmune diseases such as rheumatoid arthritis, undifferentiated connective tissue disease, mixed connective tissue disease, Sjögren's syndrome, juvenile rheumatoid arthritis, and systemic sclerosis [1,24].

Neonatal lupus syndrome is a rare, passively acquired autoimmune disorder that affects offspring of women with SSA (anti-Ro) or SSB (anti-La) antibodies. Antibodies against U1 RNP are also associated with the cutaneous manifestations of the illness [24]. Fetal and neonatal manifestations include congenital heart block, which may be complete or incomplete, myocarditis, cutaneous rash, hepatitis, thrombocytopenia, leukopenia and hemolytic anemia [24,26]. Of women with SSA or SSB antibodies, approximately 2% have fetuses with congenital heart block and 1% have fetuses with cutaneous manifestations [24,25,27]. The incidence of the other manifestations is unknown. Of 360 children in a neonatal lupus registry, 50% had congenital heart block, 26% had rash, 8% had both cardiac disease and rash, and 2% had hematologic disease. These proportions, however, may reflect reporting bias [25]. Mothers with an infant previously affected by any neonatal lupus manifestation have a 25% risk of recurrence in a subsequent pregnancy [24,25,27]. It is not clear why there is only a 25% recurrence rate, or why only 2% of fetuses of antibody-positive mothers are affected. Individual fetuses may have more or less vulnerability [24,25].

Fetal and neonatal heart block/myocarditis is the most serious manifestation of neonatal lupus syndrome, associated with a 20–30% mortality rate. Sixty-seven percent of surviving children require pacemaker placement. Incomplete heart block that occurs prenatally can progress postnatally to complete heart block. Congenital heart block is thought to occur due to time-limited expression of SSA and SSB antigens in the fetal myocardium. Maternal SSA or SSB antibodies attack these fetal antigens, causing transient myocarditis and subsequent AV-node fibrosis [24,25].

Dexamethasone suppression of maternal autoimmune activity has been used to treat affected fetuses. A retrospective study showed that steroid treatment improved incomplete heart block and hydropic changes associated with heart block, but did not reverse complete heart block [24]. Fetal echocardiography with measurement of prolonged PR intervals, myocardial dysfunction, or effusion may provide an opportunity for early intervention with steroid treatment. However, therapy has not been proven. Many experts recommend serial fetal echocardiography in pregnancies complicated by the presence of maternal SSA or SSB antibodies, with maternal steroid treatment if abnormalities are identified. Prophylactic steroid treatment in high-risk pregnancies is not warranted [24–27]. The cutaneous rash, mild hepatitis, and hematologic manifestations of the disease are transient. The rash is an erythematous skin rash that often involves the scalp and periorbital region and can be exacerbated by ultraviolet light exposure. It often occurs several weeks after birth and can last until 6–8 months of life. Resolution of the skin rash is coincident with clearance of maternal antibodies from the infant's circulation. There is no long-term morbidity for infants with cutaneous disease. However, a mother with a previously affected infant should have careful fetal cardiac screening in a subsequent pregnancy [24–27].

Rhesus (Rh) alloimmunization

Rhesus (Rh) alloimmunization with hemolytic disease of the fetus/neonate, although not technically a maternal disease, is another example of transplacental passage of maternal antibodies that causes fetal/neonatal disease. The pathophysiology of this disease has been well characterized. Maternal alloimmunization occurs when maternal B cells from an RhD-negative (D-antigen-negative) woman are sensitized to D-antigen on fetal red blood cells after a significant fetomaternal hemorrhage. The fetomaternal hemorrhage usually occurs at the delivery of a previous pregnancy, but can occur in an affected pregnancy. Spontaneous fetomaternal hemorrhage occurs with increasing frequency and increasing volume as pregnancy progresses. Once a significant hemorrhage occurs, maternal anti-D antibody is produced quickly. IgM production quickly changes to IgG production [28]. Anti-D IgG can then cross the placenta, bind to D-antigen on fetal red cells, and cause hemolysis of the fetal red blood cells. In subsequent pregnancies, repeat maternal exposure to D-antigen generates quick production of higher titer anti-D IgG antibodies. Depending on the degree of the fetal anemia, hepatosplenomegaly, hydrops fetalis, and fetal death can occur.

Administration of Rh immune globulin (anti-D antibody) to RhD-negative, anti-D antibody-negative women at 28 weeks and after delivery decreases the incidence of maternal sensitization from 2% to 0.1% [28]. Currently, only 1–6/1000 newborns are affected [28]. However, administration of Rh immune globulin after a woman has been sensitized is not effective for preventing fetal/neonatal disease.

A mother with anti-D antibody should have serial titers every 4 weeks until 24 weeks and then every 2 weeks. If the mother has an anti-D titer $\geq 1/16$ or has had a prior affected infant, an attempt should be made to determine if the fetus is RhD-positive and therefore at risk for hemolytic disease. First, the RhD phenotype and genotype of the father should be determined. Paternal zygosity can now be determined by quantitative PCR. If the father is RhD-negative, the fetus will not be affected. If the father is RhD-positive, but found to be a heterozygote, there is a 50% chance the fetus will be affected. Chorionic villi sampling or amniocentesis can be done to determine the fetal genotype [28]. Increasingly, a newer technology, cell-free fetal DNA extraction, can determine fetal genotype from maternal blood. The fetus is at risk for hemolysis if it is RhD-positive [28,29].

The fetus at risk should have serial monitoring. Fetal anemia can be detected by serial amniocentesis measuring the amount of bilirubin (a red-cell breakdown product) or by serial Doppler ultrasound of the middle cerebral artery.

Doppler ultrasound of the middle cerebral artery is a relatively new technology, which is based on the fact that a fetus with anemia has a higher cardiac output and lower blood viscosity than a fetus without anemia. This results in a higher middle cerebral artery peak systolic blood-flow velocity. In a recent prospective international study [30], Doppler ultrasound of the middle cerebral artery was found to be more accurate than serial amniocentesis for diagnosis of severe fetal anemia [28–31].

If a fetus is determined to have significant anemia based on antenatal testing, anemia can be confirmed by percutaneous umbilical blood sampling (PUBS). Intrauterine transfusion can be performed at the same time. Often, serial intrauterine transfusion with neonatal exchange transfusion is needed to protect the fetus/neonate from life-threatening complications of anemia [28–31].

Other fetal red-cell antigens such as Kell, Duffy, c, and E, in the case of maternal–fetal incompatibility, can cause maternal alloimmunization and fetal/neonatal anemia as described above. Management of these diseases is similar to that of Rh alloimmunization [1].

Neonatal alloimmune thrombocytopenia (NAIT) is a platelet analog for Rh alloimmunization. In this disease, maternal platelet alloimmunization to fetal platelet antigens can cause fetal thrombocytopenia and in utero intracranial hemorrhage. The maternal antibody is directed against the HPA-1a fetal platelet antigen 80% of the time in Caucasians. Unlike red-cell alloimmunization, a first pregnancy is commonly affected [31–33].

Placental insufficiency

Placental insufficiency is probably the most common way that maternal disease affects fetal development. It is a general effect associated with any disease that causes uteroplacental hypoperfusion (due to macrovascular or microvascular disease) or hypoxemia. Placental insufficiency syndromes include intrauterine growth restriction, oligohydramnios, placental abruption, and pre-eclampsia. Any manifestation of placental insufficiency can cause iatrogenic premature delivery in the setting of an unstable mother or fetus. Diseases commonly associated with placental insufficiency include chronic hypertension, cardiac disease associated with low cardiac output or hypoxemia, respiratory disease, renal disease, autoimmune disease, and thrombophilias.

In general, management of pregnancies at risk for placental insufficiency includes treating maternal disease to minimize the effect of the disease on the pregnancy, i.e., increased cardiac output/oxygen delivery in a cardiac patient, frequent dialysis in a renal patient, suppression of autoimmune flares in a lupus patient, or anticoagulation in a thrombophilic patient. Many of these therapies, while proven to help the mother, are not necessarily proven to decrease the incidence or extent of placental insufficiency. The mother should also have frequent blood-pressure monitoring in the third trimester to screen for pre-eclampsia. Fetal monitoring includes monthly ultrasounds

to monitor fetal growth after 28 weeks and early weekly/twice-weekly antenatal testing. Timing of delivery is also important to minimize maternal and perinatal morbidity. Placental insufficiency is discussed more thoroughly in Chapter 11.

Medications and toxins

Maternal medications and toxins can affect fetal development, usually by crossing into the placental circulation. Although the effects of most medications and toxins have not been well studied, specific medications such as antiepileptics are well known to specifically affect fetal development and are associated with malformations. Other medications, including chemotherapeutic agents, can directly affect the functioning of fetal organ systems such as bone marrow. Toxic exposures, like illicit drugs, are also known to affect fetal development and can cause withdrawal syndromes. Such toxic exposures will be discussed elsewhere (Chapter 10), and a full discussion of the teratogenic effects of medications and toxins is beyond the scope of this chapter. However, as an example, we will highlight teratogenic effects of antiepileptic medications.

Antiepileptic medications

Maternal seizure disorders affect 2–7/1000 pregnant women. An increased rate of fetal malformation is found in the offspring of women with seizure disorders. It is felt, based on observational studies, that antiepileptic medications are the primary teratogens. In addition to the treatment of seizure disorders, many antiepileptic medications are now being used to treat psychiatric illness and neuropathic pain. Thus this discussion relates to all women being treated with these medications, not only to women with seizure disorders [34].

The risk of congenital malformation is increased threefold in women taking older-generation epileptic drugs such as phenytoin, phenobarbital, carbamazepine, and valproic acid. The risk is dose-dependent and also increases with the number of antiepileptic drugs. Risk of fetal malformation is 3% with one drug, 5% with two drugs, 10% with three drugs, and 20% with four drugs. The most common fetal malformations associated with antiepileptic drugs are neural tube defects, cardiac malformations, and urogenital malformations. A syndrome initially ascribed to phenytoin – fetal hydantoin syndrome, consisting of dysmorphic facial features, cleft lip and palate, digital hypoplasia, and nail dysplasia – has now been associated with phenytoin, carbamazepine, and valproic acid. Up to 10% of exposed fetuses may have some features of this syndrome. Newer antiepileptic drugs have been less well studied. There has been one report associating lamotrigine with an increased risk of cleft palate. Other studies show similar malformation rates in offspring of patients on lamotrigine monotherapy to that in controls [34,35].

Specific fetal syndromes have been associated with specific drugs. With monotherapy, observational studies have demonstrated that valproic acid is associated with the highest rate of fetal malformation, 6–11% [34,35]. Valproic acid has a specifically increased risk of neural tube defects, 1–2% of those exposed. It has also been associated with impaired cognitive function. One study has shown dose-dependent cognitive impairment in offspring of mothers treated with valproic acid compared to offspring of mothers treated with carbamazepine or phenytoin, and to unexposed controls [34]. Carbamazepine is also specifically associated with an increased risk of neural tube defects [14,34]. Folate supplementation pre-pregnancy and during pregnancy with 4–5 mg a day is recommended for all women taking antiepileptic medications to avoid neural tube defects. However, the efficacy of this has not been proven [14,34].

In general, monotherapy with the lowest effective dose is recommended for pregnant women with epilepsy. The medication should be tailored to the specific type of seizure disorder. However, if valproic acid can be avoided, it should be. Ideally, any changes in drug therapy should occur prior to conception. In patients whose last seizure was remote, preconception discontinuation of antiepileptic medication may be appropriate, and should be carefully considered by a neurologist. Drug levels during pregnancy should be monitored. Screening for fetal malformations with ultrasound and fetal echocardiography is appropriate [14,34,35].

Infection

Fetal effects of maternal infection are beyond the scope of this chapter, but are mentioned as a category for completeness.

Genetic disease

Maternal genetic disease that can affect fetal development deserves attention for completeness and because of our increasing ability to provide prenatal diagnosis for couples who are affected by or are carriers of a genetic disease. Maternal genetic disease can be passed to the fetus in an autosomal dominant, autosomal recessive, X-linked, or polygenetic fashion. The list of disorders for which prenatal diagnosis is available by chorionic villi sampling or amniocentesis is rapidly expanding. Preimplantation genetic diagnosis, a technique in which one or two cells from an embryo at the 6–8-cell stage are tested for genetic disease prior to intrauterine implantation, is also available for some genetic diseases. The practical and ethical issues surrounding prenatal diagnosis of genetic disease is complex. A full discussion of genetic disease is beyond the scope of this chapter [1,36].

Summary

Maternal disease and treatment of maternal disease can profoundly alter embryonic and fetal development and cause neonatal disease. This chapter has highlighted well-studied maternal illness which due to alterations in maternal metabolism or the maternal immune system cause specific fetal disease. For women with chronic diseases, preconception counseling is crucial. Goals of preconception counseling include (1) maximizing medical control of chronic disease pre-pregnancy, (2) avoiding medications associated with teratogenesis when appropriate, (3) offering preimplantation genetic diagnosis when available in the case of known parental genetic disease, and (4) controlling maternal expectations with regard to pregnancy outcome. Most medical disease can be managed in pregnancy. Rarely, women should be counseled to avoid pregnancy, if the physiologic changes in pregnancy could threaten their life or organ function. In this setting alternatives to pregnancy, such as surrogacy or adoption, should be discussed. Communication between the obstetrician and the pediatrician at the time of delivery is important, so that the neonate can be screened for expected sequelae of maternal illness or medications.

References

1. Sorem KA, Druzin ML. Maternal diseases that affect fetal development. In Stevenson DK, Benitz WE, Sunshine P, eds., *Fetal and Neonatal Brain Injury: Mechanisms, Management, and Risks of Practice*, 3rd edn. Cambridge: Cambridge University Press, 2003: 191–211.

2. Jovanovic L. Prepregnancy counseling and evaluation of women with diabetes mellitus, version 15.3. In Rose B, Rush JM, eds., *UpToDate*. Waltham, MA: UpToDate, 2007.

3. Jovanovic L, Pettitt DJ. Gestational diabetes mellitus. *JAMA* 2001; **286**: 2516–18.

4. Kjos SL, Buchanan TA. Gestational diabetes mellitus. *NEJM* 1999; **341**: 1749–56.

5. Moore TR. Diabetes in pregnancy. In Creasy RK, Resnik R, Iams JD, eds., *Maternal–Fetal Medicine: Principles and Practice*, 5th edn. Philadelphia, PA: Saunders, 2004: 1023–61.

6. Rizzo TA, Metzger BE, Burns WJ, *et al.* Correlations between antepartum maternal metabolism and intelligence of offspring. *NEJM* 1991; **325**: 911–16.

7. Rizzo TA, Silverman BL, Metzger BE, *et al.* Behavioral adjustment in children of diabetic mothers. *Acta Paediatr* 1997; **86**: 969–74.

8. Langer O, Conway DL, Berkus MD, *et al.* A comparison of glyburide and insulin in women with gestational diabetes mellitus. *NEJM* 2000; **343**: 1134–8.

9. Miller E, Hare JW, Cloherty JP, *et al.* Elevated maternal hemoglobin A1c in early pregnancy and major congenital anomalies in infants of diabetic mothers. *NEJM* 1981; **304**: 1331–4.

10. Lucas MJ, Leveno KJ, Williams ML, *et al.* Early pregnancy glycosylated hemoglobin, severity of diabetes, and fetal malformations. *Am J Obstet Gynecol* 1989; **161**: 426–31.

11. Garner PR. Congenital adrenal hyperplasia in pregnancy. *Semin Perinatol* 1998; **22**: 446–56.

12. Nader S. Other endocrine disorders of pregnancy. In Creasy RK, Resnik R, Iams JD, eds., *Maternal–Fetal Medicine: Principles and Practice*, 5th edn. Philadelphia, PA: Saunders, 2004: 1083–107.

13. Koch R, Hanley W, Levy H, *et al.* The maternal phenylketonuria international study: 1984–2002. *Pediatrics* 2003; **112**: 1523–9.

14. Aminoff MJ. Neurologic disorders. In Creasy RK, Resnik R, Iams JD, eds., *Maternal–Fetal Medicine: Principles and Practice*, 5th edn. Philadelphia, PA: Saunders, 2004: 1165–91.

15. Haddow JE, Palomaki GE, Allan WC, *et al.* Maternal thyroid deficiency during

pregnancy and subsequent neuropsychological development in the child. *NEJM* 1999; **341**: 549–55.

16. Casey BM, Leveno KJ. Thyroid disease in pregnancy. *Obstet Gynecol* 2006; **108**: 1283–92.

17. Pop VJ, Brouwers EP, Vader HL, *et al.* Maternal hypothyroxinemia during early pregnancy and subsequent child development: a 3-year follow-up study. *Clin Endocrinol* 2003; **59**: 282–8.

18. Kooistra L, Crawford S, van Baar AL, *et al.* Neonatal effects of maternal hypothyroxinemia during early pregnancy. *Pediatrics* 2006; **117**: 161–7.

19. Nader S. Thyroid disease and pregnancy. In Creasy RK, Resnik R, Iams JD, eds., *Maternal–Fetal Medicine: Principles and Practice*, 5th edn. Philadelphia, PA: Saunders, 2004: 1063–81.

20. Casey BM, Dashe JS, Spong CY, *et al.* Perinatal significance of isolated maternal hypothyroxinemia identified in the first half of pregnancy. *Obstet Gynecol* 2007; **109**: 1129–35.

21. Morreale de Escobar G, Obregon MJ, Ecobar del Rey F. Is neuropsychological development related to maternal hypothyroidism or to maternal hypothyroxinemia? *J Clin Endocrinol Metab* 2000; **85**: 3975–87.

22. Alexander EK, Marqusee E, Lawrence J, *et al.* Timing and magnitude of increases in levothyroxine requirements during pregnancy in women with hypothyroidism. *NEJM* 2004; **351**: 241–9.

23. Dallas JS. Autoimmune thyroid disease and pregnancy: relevance for the child. *Autoimmunity* 2003; **36**: 339–50.

24. Buyon JP, Rupel A, Clancy RM. Neonatal lupus syndromes. *Lupus* 2004; **13**: 705–12.

25. Buyon JP, Clancy RM. Neonatal lupus: review of proposed pathogenesis and clinical data from the US-based research registry for neonatal lupus. *Autoimmunity* 2003; **36**: 41–50.

26. Hankins GD, Suarez VR. Rheumatologic and connective tissue disorders. In Creasy RK, Resnik R, Iams JD, eds., *Maternal–Fetal Medicine: Principles and Practice*, 5th edn. Philadelphia, PA: Saunders, 2004: 1147–63.

27. Boh EE. Neonatal lupus erythematosus. *Clin Dermatol* 2004; **22**: 125–8.

28. Moise KJ. Management of rhesus alloimmunization in pregnancy. *Obstet Gynecol* 2002; **100**: 600–11.

29. Bianchi DW, Avent ND, Costa JM, *et al.* Noninvasive prenatal diagnosis of fetal rhesus D: Ready for prime(r) time. *Obstet Gynecol* 2005; **106**: 841–4.

30. Oepkes D, Seaward G, Vandenbussche FP, *et al.* Doppler ultrasonography versus amniocentesis to predict fetal anemia. *NEJM* 2006; **355**: 156–64.

31. Moise KJ. Hemolytic disease of the fetus and newborn. In Creasy RK, Resnik R, Iams JD, eds., *Maternal–Fetal Medicine: Principles and Practice*, 5th edn. Philadelphia, PA: Saunders, 2004: 537–61.

32. Kilpatrick SJ, Laros RK. Maternal hematologic disorders. In Creasy RK, Resnik R, Iams JD, eds., *Maternal–Fetal Medicine: Principles and Practice*, 5th edn. Philadelphia, PA: Saunders, 2004: 975–1004.

33. Paidas M. Prenatal management of neonatal alloimmune thrombocytopenia, version 15.3. In Rose B, Rush JM, eds., *UpToDate*. Waltham, MA: UpToDate, 2007.

34. Tomson T, Hiilesmaa V. Epilepsy in pregnancy. *BMJ* 2007; **335**: 769–73.

35. Brodie MJ, Dichter MA. Antiepileptic drugs. *NEJM* 1996; **334**: 168–75.

36. Schulman LP. Preimplantation genetic diagnosis, version 15.3. In Rose B, Rush JM, eds., *UpToDate*. Waltham, MA: UpToDate, 2007.

Obstetrical conditions and practices that affect the fetus and newborn

Justin Collingham, Jane Chueh, and Reinaldo Acosta

Placenta previa

The implantation of the placenta over the cervical os or very near to it is known as placenta previa. It may be total, when the internal cervical os is completely covered by placenta; partial, when the internal os is partially covered by placenta; marginal, when the edge of the placenta is at the margin of the internal os; or low-lying, when the placental edge does not reach the internal os but is in close proximity to it [1].

Incidence

The incidence of placenta previa is about 3–6/1000 singleton pregnancies [2,3]. In an unscarred uterus it has been reported to be 0.26%, and it increases almost linearly with the number of prior cesarean deliveries, up to 10% in patients with four or more prior cesareans [4]. In a study from the state of New Jersey evaluating almost 550 000 deliveries where the diagnosis of placenta previa was confirmed only in pregnancies delivered by cesarean, the incidence was 5/1000 births [5].

Etiology and risk factors

The likelihood of placenta previa rises with multiparity [6], advancing maternal age, especially in women older than 35 years old [7], and a history of prior cesarean deliveries [8]. Smoking during pregnancy can double the risk of this condition [9,10], and women of Asian origin have been reported to have an increased risk of a delivery complicated by placenta previa compared to Caucasian women [11].

Clinical presentation and diagnosis

The classic symptom of placenta previa is painless bright red vaginal bleeding in the second or third trimester. In fact, almost three-quarters of all women with placenta previa experience at least one episode of painless antepartum bleeding, which usually presents without warning. In most situations, the initial episode resolves spontaneously [12]. The antepartum diagnosis of placenta previa is primarily based on the ultrasonographic visualization of the placental location and its relationship to the internal cervical os. Transvaginal sonography is more accurate than transabdominal sonography in making the diagnosis [13,14]. Transperineal [15] and translabial

ultrasonography [16] may also provide good resolution of the internal os. Placenta previa has been diagnosed in 5% of patients undergoing ultrasound examination between 16 and 18 weeks; 90% of these placentas are no longer identified as previas in the third trimester, however. This phenomenon has been called placental migration. In these patients extra care is not required unless the diagnosis persists beyond 30 weeks of gestation or if the patient becomes symptomatic before that time. In general, the earlier in pregnancy the initial episode of bleeding occurs, the worse the outcome of the pregnancy [17].

Management

Management of placenta previa varies according to the clinical situation. In preterm pregnancies with no active bleeding, expectant management is the general rule. Strict bed rest, blood transfusions as required, administration of corticosteroids to reduce the rate and severity of fetal respiratory distress syndrome, as well as the occasional use of tocolytic agents for inhibition of premature labor in the presence of vaginal bleeding are appropriate in the conservative aggressive management of this condition [18–20]. One of the most controversial issues is whether the mother should be kept hospitalized after she has been stabilized. D'Angelo and Irwin reported an improved outcome in neonatal morbidity in these patients maintained in hospital [21], but Wing and coworkers noted that, in selected patients, outpatient management may be safe and appropriate [22]. Anti-D immunoglobulin should be given after a bleeding episode if the patient is Rh-negative. It is advisable to perform a scheduled cesarean delivery after determination of fetal pulmonary maturity: this approach significantly reduces overall neonatal morbidity and mortality [18]. Emergent and expeditious cesarean delivery, however, may be warranted in cases of persistent hemorrhage, failed tocolysis, fetal distress, or coagulopathy.

Complications

Major maternal complications of placenta previa are related to massive bleeding leading to hemorrhagic shock. Following placental removal, hemorrhage at the site of implantation may occur. Almost 7% of placenta previas have an abnormal placental attachment to the myometrium (see section below on placenta accreta) [3]. If uterotonic medication, hemostatic sutures, and other conservative methods fail to control the hemorrhage, hysterectomy may be necessary.

Fetal and Neonatal Brain Injury, 4th edition, ed. David K. Stevenson, William E. Benitz, Philip Sunshine, Susan R. Hintz, and Maurice L. Druzin. Published by Cambridge University Press. © Cambridge University Press 2009.

Some investigators have reported a high incidence of fetal growth restriction with previa [23]. Others have not found this association after controlling for gestational age [2,5,24]. Despite tocolysis and transfusions to delay delivery, nearly two-thirds of the patients are delivered before 36 weeks, and they account for at least 10–15% of all premature births [5]. The perinatal mortality due to placenta previa decreased significantly from 37% in the early 1970s [25] to as low as 4–8% in the 1980s [26]. Crane *et al.*, in a population-based retrospective cohort study of over 92 000 births in Nova Scotia, Canada, identified 305 cases of placenta previa [2]. The perinatal mortality rate in their patients was 2.3%, compared to 0.78% in controls. These investigators also noted no differences in birthweights after controlling for gestational age in the patients and controls. After controlling for potential confounders, neonatal complications associated with placenta previa included major congenital anomalies, respiratory distress syndrome, and anemia [2]. There is a significant correlation between antepartum maternal hemorrhage and the need for neonatal transfusion, and between neonatal anemia and the amount of intrapartum maternal blood loss [17].

Summary

Placenta previa is a life-threatening condition for the mother and the fetus. Prompt diagnosis by ultrasound, and treatment with strict bed rest, tocolysis, and blood transfusions are mainstays of care. A planned cesarean delivery as close to term as feasible and with documented fetal maturity is optimal. Emergent preterm delivery is frequently necessary, however.

Placental abruption

The premature separation of the normally implanted placenta is known as placental abruption. Usually this phenomenon is accompanied by painful uterine contractions and a variable amount of vaginal bleeding. Bleeding may also be concealed behind the detached placenta.

Incidence

The incidence of placental abruption is between 5 and 7/1000 births [27,28]. Ananth and Wilcox, evaluating 7 508 655 singleton births in the USA in the years 1995 and 1996, found that abruption was encountered in 6.5/1000 live births [29]. A perinatal mortality rate of 119/1000 live births has been reported [29], and up to 14% of the fetuses that survive may have significant neurological deficits [30].

Etiology and risk factors

Although the precise cause of placental abruption remains unknown, various risk factors have been identified. Many reports suggest that the incidence increases with advancing maternal age and parity [31,32], although other studies have been unable to confirm this association [33,34]. It has also been reported to be more common in African-American women than Caucasians and less frequent in Hispanic women [31]. There is a strong association of this condition with hypertension, either pre-existing or pregnancy-associated [28,35–37], with a threefold increased incidence of abruption with chronic hypertension and a fourfold increase with severe pre-eclampsia [38]. Women who smoke during their pregnancies also have an increased risk of abruption [39]. If one adds the effects of smoking and hypertension during pregnancy, the risk is increased even greater [28]. There is also an increased incidence of abruption with premature rupture of membranes [36], especially in patients who have recurrent bleeding episodes during the period of expectant management [40,41]. Studies have consistently documented placental abruption as a maternal reproductive risk associated with cocaine use [42–44]. Recent reports have also found an increased frequency of genetic thrombophilias in patients with placental abruption [45,46]. Placental abruption may also be present even in cases of minor trauma, and may not be a clinically immediately evident condition [47,48]. Uterine leiomyomas may predispose to abruption, especially if they are located behind the placental implantation site [49]. A history of placental abruption may increase the risk of occurrence up to 10-fold in subsequent pregnancies [27]. Other risk factors that have been associated with this condition include severe fetal growth restriction, chorioamnionitis, polyhydramnios, a short umbilical cord, sudden uterine decompression, external version and diabetes [32,33,50].

Clinical presentation and diagnosis

Because of the wide variety of signs and symptoms associated with placental abruption, it is necessary to have a high index of suspicion in order to make an accurate diagnosis. The clinical spectrum ranges from asymptomatic states in which the diagnosis is made only after delivery upon the evaluation of the placenta, to cases with fetal demise, maternal hypovolemic shock, and severe coagulopathy. The most common presentation, however, is an acute onset of vaginal bleeding accompanied by intermittent cramping or constant abdominal pain. Other findings that may be present are non-reassuring fetal status, frequent and intense contractions, preterm labor, and intrauterine fetal demise [51]. Ultrasound visualization of a clot occurs in only about 25% of the cases and appears to have little or no impact on course or management. The absence of these findings should not preclude the diagnosis. Ultrasound assessment and clinical inspection are both essential in order to rule out placenta previa and other causes of bleeding, however. In assessing a woman with placental abruption, the possibility of physical abuse or the use of cocaine must not be disregarded. Unless specific questions about these issues are asked, the precipitating cause of the abruption may not be identified [50].

Management

Once the diagnosis of placental abruption has been made, intravenous access, blood-product availability, and maternal hemodynamic stability must be secured. The next step in management will depend upon gestational age and maternal and fetal statuses.

In preterm pregnancies without evidence of maternal or fetal compromise, expectant management may be considered. Tocolysis in this clinical situation is a matter of controversy [51–53]. Administration of steroids should be considered, in the hope of reducing the risk of fetal respiratory distress syndrome.

Expectant management generally is not a choice for the majority of patients, and delivery is indicated because of maternal or fetal deterioration or both. Delivery is also indicated in viable, mature fetuses. If vaginal delivery is not imminent, cesarean section is the best approach. However, if the fetus has died or if the mother is anticipated to deliver vaginally in the immediate future, labor can be pursued provided that the mother does not continue to have deterioration of her clinical status. Cesarean delivery in the case of fetal demise should be reserved for maternal indications alone [20]. Rh-negative mothers with placental abruption require anti-D immunoglobulin to avoid Rh isoimmunization.

Complications

Most of the serious maternal complications of placental abruption are related to hypovolemia secondary to maternal hemorrhage, which may lead to acute renal and other organ failure. Almost 40% of cases of renal failure in pregnancy are secondary to placental abruption [54]. Abruption is also the most frequent cause of disseminated intravascular coagulation (DIC) in pregnancy. DIC may aggravate hemorrhagic problems, is found in about 30% of women with abruption, and may be severe enough to cause fetal demise [55]. With respect to the fetus, most of the complications result from prematurity and hypoxia. Low-birthweight infants delivered after placental abruption tend to have low Apgar scores and are at increased risk of neonatal death and the development of intraventricular hemorrhage and cerebral palsy [56].

Summary

Placental abruption is an extremely dangerous condition for both the mother and the fetus, carrying significant morbidity and mortality for both. The diagnosis requires a high index of suspicion as well as prompt assessment of the fetal and maternal statuses. Whether expectant management or expeditious delivery is warranted depends upon the severity of the condition and the gestational age at the time of diagnosis. The route of delivery is dictated by the severity of the condition and the viability of the fetus.

Vasa previa

Vasa previa is a rare condition in which the fetal blood vessels, unsupported by either the umbilical cord or placental tissue, traverse the fetal membranes of the lower segment of the uterus below the presenting part and directly over the cervix. This condition typically arises when the umbilical cord inserts into the placental membranes (velamentous cord insertion) near the cervix. It can also arise when a placenta previa or low-lying placenta "migrates" away from the lower uterine segment, leaving the cord insertion behind, attached only to membranes (velamentous insertion). If the fetal vessels between the umbilical cord and the main placental disc happen to traverse close to the cervix, a vasa previa would result. A vasa previa can also result from fetal vessels traversing over the cervix in their journey from the succenturiate lobe of a placenta to the main placenta disc, or between two lobes of a bilobed placenta.

Incidence

It is difficult to estimate the true incidence of this condition, as vasa previa is likely to be under-reported. It has been estimated to occur in about 1/2000 to 1/3000 deliveries. Thus, a relatively active obstetric service may expect one case per year [57].

Etiology and risk factors

Vasa previa has been associated with in vitro fertilization, multiple pregnancies, low-lying placentas, and multilobed or succenturiate placentas [58–60]. It is not clear why IVF appears to be associated with vasa previa [11,14,18]. A study of 100 placentas from IVF pregnancies revealed 14 cases of velamentous insertion among them [18]. This prevalence was higher than the prevalence of velamentous cord insertion in the general population, even after correcting for the higher prevalence of velamentous insertion in multiple pregnancies [18]. Similarly, in a recent study, Schachter and colleagues [11] found an incidence of vasa previa at their institution of 1 in 293 IVF deliveries compared with a vasa previa rate of 1 in 6068 total deliveries.

Clinical presentation and diagnosis

The usual clinical presentation of this condition is vaginal bleeding after either spontaneous or artificial rupture of membranes, leading to the rupture of the velamentous vessels, and fetal death from exsanguination. However, vessel rupture may occur independently of membrane rupture; therefore, this condition should be suspected in any patient with antepartum or intrapartum hemorrhage [61]. Occasionally, fetal heart-rate abnormalities such as progressive severe variable decelerations, fetal bradycardia, or a sinusoidal pattern due to fetal anemia may be the only manifestations of vasa previa [62,63].

Transabdominal and transvaginal ultrasound with color Doppler is the current method used for the antenatal diagnosis of vasa previa [64–68]. Pulsed wave Doppler placed directly over vessels can help distinguish between maternal and fetal pulsations. Three-dimensional ultrasound has also been reported as a useful diagnostic tool for this condition [69]. In situations where the source of vaginal bleeding is uncertain and maternal and fetal status are stable, hemoglobin denaturing tests such as the bedside Apt test may help distinguish between fetal and maternal blood, thereby establishing the origin, and therefore the acuity, of the bleed.

Management

If the diagnosis of vasa previa has been made antenatally, and there is no evidence of fetal compromise, the safest form of delivery would be by planned cesarean at around 35 weeks' gestation, or earlier if fetal lung maturity is documented. This is earlier than the 39 weeks that is generally recommended for elective cesarean delivery, but it mitigates the risk of membrane rupture and fetal exsanguination prior to delivery. One study showed a perinatal mortality rate of 56% for neonates delivered at 38 weeks without prenatal diagnosis.

Immediate delivery is mandatory in a viable pregnancy in the setting of bleeding from a vasa previa. The infant has a total blood volume of approximately 250 ml at term and is therefore very intolerant to blood loss. If the cervix is fully dilated and vaginal delivery can be accomplished rapidly, this becomes the route of choice [57]. Vaginal delivery is also indicated when the fetus is too immature to survive or when fetal demise has already occurred. An emergency cesarean delivery provides the most favorable outcome if performed immediately upon recognition of the condition. Optimizing neonatal outcome requires rapid and aggressive neonatal resuscitative techniques. These include immediate basic and advanced life support measures, and establishment of vascular access for fluids, blood, and blood-component therapy [70]. Rh-negative patients should receive anti-D immunoglobulin when indicated. Because of the risk of unexpected and catastrophic hemorrhage from fetal vessels, admission to the hospital early in the third trimester may be reasonable. An alternative approach is to follow the pregnancies with serial transvaginal cervical length determinations, along with hospitalization should the patient experience contractions or spotting. It is unknown whether either plan would be successful in averting bad outcomes associated with unexpected premature rupture of membranes or preterm labor, but hospitalized patients might theoretically have a better chance. Elective cesarean delivery at about 35 weeks of gestation is reasonable when considering benefits and risks. Because of the potential for emergency preterm delivery, consideration should be given to administering steroids to promote fetal lung maturation.

Complications

Vasa previa is mainly a risk to the fetus. The fetal mortality rate ranges from 33% to 100% [64]. Complications are associated with bleeding from fetal vessels prior to and during labor, and after rupture of membranes. In a recent review of 155 cases of vasa previa [57], the overall perinatal mortality was 36%. The only significant predictors of neonatal survival were prenatal diagnosis and gestational age at delivery. Of the patients who did not have prenatal diagnosis, intrapartum bleeding occurred in 41 of 94 (44%) [57]. The most striking finding was that, when the diagnosis was made prenatally, more than 96% of infants survived, whereas more than half of all fetuses/infants died when there was no prenatal diagnosis. Among survivors when the diagnosis had not been made prenatally, 1- and 5-minute Apgar scores were very low (median 1 and 4, respectively). In addition, more than half of surviving neonates required blood transfusions when the diagnosis was not made prenatally.

Summary

Vasa previa is an obstetric condition that may have catastrophic consequences for the fetus. If unsuspected hemorrhage occurs from a vasa previa, immediate delivery and aggressive resuscitation of the newborn are mandatory, but this carries a high neonatal morbidity and mortality. Prenatal diagnosis by transabdominal and transvaginal ultrasound, with cesarean delivery before rupture of membranes, appears to dramatically improve the neonatal outcome. In women at increased risk (those with second-trimester low-lying placentas, pregnancies resulting from IVF, and accessory placental lobes), transvaginal color Doppler sonography of the region over the cervix should be considered if vasa previa cannot be excluded by transabdominal sonography. Neonates delivered after vasa previa diagnosed prenatally have a significantly higher chance of survival, higher Apgar scores, and lower incidence of blood transfusions, compared with cases not diagnosed prenatally.

Placenta accreta

Placenta accreta is an abnormality in placental implantation in which the placental chorionic villi are attached to the myometrium instead of to the decidua basalis and the stratum spongiosum. Placenta accreta can be further specified as placenta increta, where the villi invade into the myometrium, and placenta percreta, where the villi reach the uterine serosa and may invade surrounding structures such as the bladder or rectum.

Incidence

Once a rare occurrence in obstetrics with an incidence of less than one in 30 000 deliveries in the 1930s to 1950s, placenta accreta now occurs in approximately 1/500 deliveries, largely as a result of an increase in rates of cesarean delivery [71].

Etiology and risk factors

The mechanism behind the abnormal placentation of placenta accreta is hypothesized to be a dysfunctional or absent decidua basalis, particularly in the scarred uterus. Risk factors identified for placenta accreta include advanced maternal age and previous uterine surgery such as cesarean delivery, especially when accompanied by a placenta previa. The risk of accreta with prior cesarean delivery and the existence of a placenta previa has been shown to be 3%, 11%, 40%, 61%, and 67% for first, second, third, fourth, and fifth or more repeat cesarean deliveries, respectively [72].

Clinical presentation and diagnosis

The first clinical sign of placenta accreta is often the failure of placental separation to occur, usually at the time of repeat cesarean delivery, with attendant profuse hemorrhage. The intraoperative diagnosis of placenta percreta may be made by visualization of placental invasion through the uterine wall and/or into adjacent structures, with invasion of the bladder the most common. Prenatal diagnosis of placenta accreta has gained much attention recently. Ultrasound with color Doppler to assist in identifying abnormal placental vasculature, either abdominally or transvaginally, has been determined to be useful in identifying those patients with a high likelihood of placenta accreta; magnetic resonance imaging (MRI) has also proven useful. A recent cohort study reported a sensitivity of 0.77 and a specificity of 0.96 for ultrasound in detecting placenta accreta in patients at risk for accreta, and a similar sensitivity of 0.88 and specificity of 1.0 for MRI performed in those patients with equivocal or inconclusive ultrasound findings [73].

Management

The mainstays of management include a planned cesarean delivery, usually at approximately 35–36 weeks of gestation, or earlier if fetal lung maturity is established. A lower threshold for delivery is often employed, as specialty anesthesia and surgery teams, as well as blood products, may be required for intraoperative management of expected hemorrhage. Hysterectomy is the definitive treatment, although uterine preservation in rare circumstances has been described [74].

Complications

Fetal and neonatal effects of placenta accreta have not been well documented, but as most cases of placenta accreta occur in the setting of placenta previa, the attendant perinatal risks of placenta previa can be presumed to occur with placenta accreta. Although limited by its format as a questionnaire of practicing perinatologists, one review showed a 9% perinatal mortality rate, largely due to previable iatrogenic deliveries. The rising rate of cesarean delivery has prompted investigators to examine the potential increased maternal and fetal risks of repeat cesarean delivery, particularly in the setting of placenta previa. A recent large study of patients undergoing cesarean delivery for placenta previa showed an increase in adverse maternal outcome as the number of prior cesarean deliveries rose; adverse perinatal outcomes and gestational age at delivery, however, remained unrelated to the number of prior cesarean deliveries [75].

Summary

Placenta accreta is a maternally life-threatening condition of abnormal placentation growing in incidence, largely related to an increased rate of cesarean delivery. Although prenatal imaging techniques such as ultrasound and MRI do not have perfect sensitivity and specificity for predicting placenta accreta, these tests, when coupled with a high index of suspicion in those patients most at risk, can provide invaluable information and therefore allow the practitioner to prepare adequately for massive hemorrhage and surgical intervention at the time of delivery.

Miscellaneous cord and placental abnormalities

The presence of a short umbilical cord at delivery has historically been associated with increasing the predictive value of low Apgar scores for subsequent low IQ scores and neurologic abnormalities [76]. A recent large retrospective review of short cord diagnosed after delivery showed an association between short cord in non-anomalous singleton pregnancies and maternal labor and delivery complications, as well as death within the first year among term infants [77]. Variation exists, however, in the reference standards for diagnosis of short cord, and the inability to reliably diagnose the entity in the antenatal period limits the utility of the predictive power of the diagnosis. The diagnosis has utility mainly in postnatal life, where there is a suggestion that neonates born with short umbilical cords may benefit from increased monitoring.

Postnatally diagnosed marginal cord insertion, often defined as a placental cord insertion within 1–2 cm from the placental edge, has classically been associated with reduced birthweight [78]. Recent advances in Doppler ultrasound have allowed the diagnosis to be made in the antenatal period; a recent retrospective review, however, failed to show an association between marginal cord insertion and increased risks of growth restriction or preterm delivery [79].

Postnatally diagnosed velamentous cord insertion has also been associated with low birthweight, preterm delivery, low Apgar scores, and abnormal fetal heart rate patterns [80]. Doppler ultrasound has also allowed for the antenatal diagnosis of velamentous cord insertion, with recent data suggesting an association between antenatally diagnosed velamentous insertions into the lower third of the uterus and intrapartum heart-rate abnormalities [81].

References

1. Cunningham FG, Gant NF, Leveno KJ, et al. Williams Obstetrics, 21st edn. New York, NY: McGraw-Hill, 2001: 630–635.

2. Crane JM, van den Hof MC, Dodds L, et al. Neonatal outcomes with placenta previa. Obstet Gynecol 1999; 93: 541–4.

3. Frederiksen MC, Glassenberg R, Stika CS. Placenta previa: a 22-year analysis. Am J Obstet Gynecol 1999; 180: 1432–7.

4. Clark SL, Koonings PP, Phelan JP. Placenta previa/accreta and prior cesarean sections. Obstet Gynecol 1985; 66: 89–92.

5. Ananth CV, Demissie K, Smulian JC, et al. Relationship among placenta previa, fetal growth restriction and preterm delivery: a population-based study. Obstet Gynecol 2001; 98: 299–306.

6. Babinszki A, Kerenyi T, Torok O, et al. Perinatal outcome in grand and great grand multiparity: effects of parity on obstetric risk factors. Am J Obstet Gynecol 1999; 181: 669–74.

7. Iyasu S, Saftlas AK, Rowley DL, et al. The epidemiology of placenta previa in the United States, 1979 through 1987. Am J Obstet Gynecol 1993; 168: 1424–9.

8. Ananth CV, Smulian JC, Vintzileos AM. The association of placenta previa with history of cesarean delivery and abortion: a metaanalysis. Am J Obstet Gynecol 1997; 177: 1071–8.

9. Williams MA, Mittendorf R, Lieberman E, et al. Cigarette smoking during pregnancy in relation to placenta previa. Am J Obstet Gynecol 1991; 165: 28–32.

10. Handler AS, Mason ED, Rosenberg DL, *et al.* The relationship between exposure during pregnancy to cigarette smoking and cocaine use and placenta previa. *Am J Obstet Gynecol* 1994; **170**: 884–9.

11. Schachter M, Torbin Y, Arieli S, *et al.* In vitro fertilization is a risk factor for vasa previa. *Fertil Steril* 2002; **78**: 642–3.

12. Love CD, Wallace EM. Pregnancies complicated by placenta previa: what is appropriate management? *Br J Obstet Gynaecol* 1996; **103**: 864–7.

13. Farine D, Fox HE, Jakobson S, *et al.* Is it really a placenta previa? *Eur J Obstet Gynecol Reprod Biol* 1989; **31**: 103–8.

14. Smith RS, Lauria MR, Comstock CH, *et al.* Transvaginal ultrasonography for all placentas that appear to be low lying or over the internal cervical os. *Ultrasound Obstet Gynecol* 1997; **9**: 22–4.

15. Hertzberg BS, Bowie JD, Carroll BA, *et al.* Diagnosis of placenta previa during the third trimester: role of transperineal sonography. *AJR Am J Roetgenol* 1992; **159**: 83–7.

16. Dawson WB, Dumas MD, Romano WM, *et al.* Translabial ultrasonography and placenta previa: does measurement of the os–placenta distance predict outcome? *Ultrasound Med* 1996; **15**: 441–6.

17. McShane PM, Heyl PS, Epstein MF. Maternal and perinatal morbidity resulting from placenta previa. *Obstet Gynecol* 1985; **65**: 176–82.

18. Cotton DB, Read JA, Paul RH, *et al.* The conservative aggressive management of placenta previa. *Am J Obstet Gynecol* 1980; **137**: 687–95.

19. Besinger RE, Moniak CW, Paskiweicz LS, *et al.* The effect of tocolytic use in the management of symptomatic placenta previa. *Am J Obstet Gynecol* 1995; **172**: 1770–5.

20. Chamberlain G, Steer P. ABC of labour care: obstetric emergencies. *BMJ* 1999; **318**: 1342–5.

21. D'Angelo LJ, Irwin LF. Conservation management of placenta previa: a cost benefit analysis. *Am J Obstet Gynecol* 1984; **149**: 320–6.

22. Wing DA, Paul RH, Millar LK. Management of the symptomatic placenta previa: a randomized, controlled trial of inpatient versus outpatient expectant management. *Am J Obstet Gynecol* 1996; **175**: 806–11.

23. Brar HS, Platt LD, De Vore GR, *et al.* Fetal umbilical velocimetry for the surveillance of pregnancies complicated by placenta previa. *Reprod Med* 1988; **33**: 741–4.

24. Wolf EJ, Mallozi A, Rodis JF, *et al.* Placenta previa is not an independent risk factor for a small for gestational age infant. *Obstet Gynecol* 1991; **77**: 707–9.

25. Crenshaw C, Jones DED, Parker RT. Placenta previa: a survey of twenty years experience with improved perinatal survival by expectant therapy and cesarean delivery. *Obstet Gynecol Surv* 1973; **28**: 461–70.

26. Silver R, Depp R, Sabbagha RE, *et al.* Placenta previa: aggressive expectant management. *Am J Obstet Gynecol* 1984; **150**: 15–22.

27. Kåregård M, Gennser G. Incidence and recurrence rate of abruptio placentae in Sweden. *Obstet Gynecol* 1986; **67**: 523–8.

28. Ananth CV, Smulian JC, Vintzileos AM. Incidence of placental abruption in relation to cigarette smoking and hypertensive disorders during pregnancy: a meta-analysis of observational studies. *Obstet Gynecol* 1999; **93**: 622–8.

29. Ananth CV, Wilcox AJ. Placental abruption and perinatal mortality in the United States. *Am J Epidemiol* 2001; **153**: 332–7.

30. Abdella TN, Sibai BM, Hays JM, *et al.* Perinatal outcome in abruptio placentae. *Obstet Gynecol* 1984; **63**: 365–70.

31. Pritchard JA, Cunningham FG, Pritchard SA, *et al.* On reducing the frequency of severe abruptio placentae. *Am J Obstet Gynecol* 1991; **165**: 1345–51.

32. Kramer MS, Usher RH, Pollack R, *et al.* Etiologic determinants of abruptio placentae. *Obstet Gynecol* 1997; **89**: 221–6.

33. Krohn M, Voig L, McKnight B, *et al.* Correlates of placental abruption. *Br J Obstet Gynaecol* 1987; **94**: 333–40.

34. Toohey JS, Keegan KA, Morgan MA, *et al.* The "dangerous multipara": fact or fiction? *Am J Obstet Gynecol* 1995; **172**: 683–6.

35. Ananth CV, Savitz DA, Williams MA. Placental abruption and its association with hypertension and prolonged rupture of membranes: a methodologic review and meta-analysis. *Obstet Gynecol* 1996; **88**: 309–18.

36. Ananth CV, Savitz DA, Bowes WA, *et al.* Influence of hypertensive disorders and cigarette smoking on placental abruption and uterine bleeding during pregnancy. *Br J Obstet Gynaecol* 1997; **104**: 572–8.

37. Sibai BM, Lindheimer M, Hauth J, *et al.* Risk factors for preeclampsia, abruptio placentae and adverse neonatal outcomes among women with chronic hypertension. National Institute of Child Health and Human Development network of maternal–fetal medicine units. *N Engl J Med* 1998; **339**: 667–71.

38. Ananth CV, Berkowitz GS, Savitz DA, *et al.* Placental abruption and adverse perinatal outcomes. *JAMA* 1999; **282**: 1646–51.

39. Misra DP, Ananth CV. Risk factor profiles of placental abruption in first and second pregnancies: heterogeneous etiologies. *J Clin Epidemiol* 1999; **52**: 453–61.

40. Gonen R, Hannah ME, Milligan JE. Does prolonged premature rupture of the membranes predispose to abruptio placentae? *Obstet Gynecol* 1989; **74**: 347–50.

41. Major CA, de Veciana M, Lewis DF, *et al.* Preterm premature rupture of membranes and abruptio placentae: is there an association between these pregnancy complications? *Am J Obstet Gynecol* 1995; **172**: 672–6.

42. Bingol N, Fuchs M, Diaz V, *et al.* Teratogenicity of cocaine in humans. *J Pediatr* 1987; **110**: 93–6.

43. Hoskins IA, Friedman DM, Frieden FJ, *et al.* Relationship between antepartum cocaine abuse, abnormal umbilical artery Doppler velocimetry, and placental abruption. *Obstet Gynecol* 1991; **78**: 279–82.

44. Slutsker L. Risks associated with cocaine use during pregnancy. *Obstet Gynecol* 1992; **79**: 778–89.

45. Kupferminc MJ, Eldor A, Steinman N, *et al.* Increased frequency of genetic thrombophilia in women with complications of pregnancy. *N Engl J Med* 1999; **340**: 50–2.

46. Gherman RB, Goodwin TM. Obstetric implications of activated protein C resistance and factor V Leiden mutation. *Obstet Gynecol Surv* 2000; **55**: 117–22.

47. Kettel LM, Branch DW, Scott JR. Occult placental abruption after maternal trauma. *Obstet Gynecol* 1988; **71**: 449–53.

48. Stafford PA, Biddinger PW, Zumwalt RE. Lethal intrauterine fetal trauma. *Am J Obstet Gynecol* 1988; **159**: 485–9.

49. Rice JP, Kay HH, Mahony BS. The clinical significance of uterine leiomyomas in pregnancy. *Am J Obstet Gynecol* 1989; **160**: 1212–16.

50. Nimrod CA, Oppenheimer LW. *Medicine of the Fetus and Mother,*

2nd edn. Philadelphia, PA: Lippincott–Raven, 1999: 1498–501.

51. Hurd WW, Miodovnik M, Hertzberg V, *et al.* Selective management of abruptio placentae: a prospective study. *Obstet Gynecol* 1983; **61**: 467–73.

52. Combs CA, Nyberg DA, Mack LA, *et al.* Expectant management after sonographic diagnosis of placental abruption. *Am J Perinatol* 1992; **9**: 170–4.

53. Towers CV, Pircon RA, Heppard M. Is tocolysis safe in the management of third trimester bleeding? *Am J Obstet Gynecol* 1999; **180**: 1572–8.

54. Grunfeld JP, Pertuiset N. Acute renal failure in pregnancy: 1987. *Am J Kidney Dis* 1987; **9**: 359–62.

55. Shaw KJ. Abruptio placentae. In Mishell DR, Brenner DR, eds., *Management of Common Problems in Obstetrics and Gynecology*, 3rd edn. Boston, MA: Blackwell, 1994: 211–15.

56. Spinillo A, Fazzi E, Stronati I, *et al.* Early morbidity and neurodevelopmental outcome in low birth weight infants born after third trimester bleeding. *Am J Perinatol* 1994; **11**: 85–90.

57. Oyelese Y, Catanzarite V, Prefumo F, *et al.* Vasa previa: the impact of prenatal diagnosis on outcomes. *Obstet Gynecol* 2004; **103**: 937–42.

58. Englert Y, Imbert MC, Van Rosendael E, *et al.* Morphological anomalies in the placentae of IVF pregnancies: preliminary report of a multicentric study. *Hum Reprod* 1987; **2**: 155–7.

59. Burton G, Saunders DM. Vasa praevia: another cause of concern in in vitro fertilization pregnancies. *Aust NZ J Obstet Gynaecol* 1988; **28**: 180–1.

60. Oyelese KO, Schwarzler P, Coates S, *et al.* A strategy for reducing the mortality rate from vasa previa using transvaginal sonography with color Doppler. *Ultrasound Obstet Gynecol* 1998; **12**: 377–9.

61. Carp HJ, Mashiach S, Serr DM. Vasa previa: a major complication and its management. *Obstet Gynecol* 1979; **53**: 273–5.

62. Cordero DR, Helfgofft AW, Landy HJ, *et al.* A non-hemorrhagic manifestation of vasa previa: a clinico-pathologic case report. *Obstet Gynecol* 1993; **82**: 698–700.

63. Antoine C, Young BK, Silverma F, *et al.* Sinusoidal fetal heart rate pattern with vasa previa in twin pregnancy. *J Reprod Med* 1982; **27**: 295–300.

64. Oyelese KO, Turner M, Lees C, *et al.* Vasa previa: an avoidable obstetric tragedy. *Obstet Gynecol Surv* 1999; **54**: 138–45.

65. Harding JA, Lewis DF, Major CA, *et al.* Color flow Doppler: a useful instrument in the diagnosis of vasa previa. *Am J Obstet Gynecol* 1990; **163**: 1566–8.

66. Meyer WJ, Blumenthal L, Cadkin A, *et al.* Vasa previa: prenatal diagnosis with transvaginal color Doppler flow imaging. *Am J Obstet Gynecol* 1993; **169**: 1627–9.

67. Hata K, Hata T, Fujiwaki R, *et al.* An accurate antenatal diagnosis of vasa previa with transvaginal color Doppler ultrasonography. *Am J Obstet Gynecol* 1994; **171**: 265–7.

68. Clerici G, Burnelli L, Lauro V, *et al.* Prenatal diagnosis of vasa previa presenting as amniotic band: "a not so innocent amniotic band." *Ultrasound Obstet Gynecol* 1996; **7**: 61–3.

69. Lee W, Kirk JS, Comstock CH, *et al.* Vasa previa: prenatal detection by three-dimensional ultrasonography. *Ultrasound Obstet Gynecol* 2000; **16**: 384–7.

70. Schellpfeffer MA. Improved neonatal outcome of vasa previa with aggressive intrapartum management: a report of two cases. *J Reprod Med* 1995; **40**: 327–32.

71. Wu S, Kocherginsky M, Hibbard JU. Abnormal placentation: twenty-year analysis. *Am J Obstet Gynecol* 2005; **192**: 1458–62.

72. Silver RM, Landon MB, Rouse DJ, *et al.* Maternal morbidity associated with multiple repeat cesarean deliveries. *Obstet Gynecol* 2006; **107**: 1226–32.

73. Warshak CR, Eskander R, Hull AD, *et al.* Accuracy of ultrasonography and magnetic resonance imaging in the diagnosis of placenta accreta. *Obstet Gynecol* 2006; **108**: 573–81.

74. Riggs JC, Jahshan A, Schiavello HJ. Alternative conservative management of placenta accreta: a case report. *J Reprod Med* 2000; **45**: 595–8.

75. Grobman WA, Gersnoviez R, Landon MB, *et al.* Pregnancy outcomes for women with placenta previa in relation to the number of prior cesarean deliveries. *Obstet Gynecol* 2007; **110**: 1249–55.

76. Naeye RL. Umbilical cord length: clinical significance. *J Pediatr* 1985; **107**: 278–81.

77. Krakowiak P, Smith EN, de Bruyn G, *et al.* Risk factors and outcomes associated with a short umbilical cord. *Obstet Gynecol* 2004; **103**: 119–27.

78. Rolschau J. The relationship between some disorders of the umbilical cord and intrauterine growth retardation. *Acta Obstet Gynecol Scand Suppl* 1978; **72**: 15–21.

79. Liu CC, Pretorious DH, Scioscia AL, *et al.* Sonographic prenatal diagnosis of marginal placental cord insertion: clinical importance. *J Ultrasound Med* 2002; **21**: 627–32.

80. Heinonen S, Ryynaenen M, Kirkinen P, *et al.* Perinatal diagnostic evaluation of velamentous and umbilical cord insertion: clinical, Doppler, and ultrasonic findings. *Obstet Gynecol* 1996; **87**: 112–17.

81. Hasegawa J, Matsuoka R, Ichizuka K, *et al.* Velamentous cord insertion into the lower third of the uterus is associated with intrapartum fetal heart rate abnormalities. *Ultrasound Obstet Gynecol* 2006; **27**: 425–9.

Fetal and neonatal injury
as a consequence of maternal substance abuse

H. Eugene Hoyme, Melanie A. Manning, and Louis P. Halamek

Introduction

Substance abuse is widely prevalent in our society, and women in their child-bearing years are not immune to this epidemic. In addition to the many problems substance abuse causes for these women, it may also place the children they are carrying at risk for lifelong sequelae. Despite the paucity of information on the safety of drugs in pregnancy and lactation, virtually all pregnant women are exposed to prescription and/or non-prescription drugs in some form. The 1991 World Health Organization (WHO) International Survey on Drug Utilization in Pregnancy observed that 86% of women surveyed took medication in pregnancy, with an average of 2.9 prescriptions per woman, excluding over-the-counter and herbal preparations [1]. It is estimated that approximately 10% of pregnant women are exposed to illicit substances [2]. The purpose of this chapter is to describe the fetal and neonatal effects of various legal and illegal sensorium-altering substances ingested by pregnant women.

Drug distribution in pregnancy

It is important to first understand general principles of drug distribution during pregnancy, including the roles of the placenta and breast in biotransformation and secretion. The characteristics that favor transport of a drug across the lipo-protein barriers between the circulation and the central and peripheral nervous systems include high lipid solubility, minimal ionization at physiologic pH, low protein-binding, and low molecular weight. High lipid solubility may result in storage of such substances in maternal body fat with subsequent release and transfer into fetal lipid stores during pregnancy. These same characteristics also enable drugs to cross the placenta readily and enter the fetal circulation. Drugs with a lower molecular weight (< 500 g/mol) cross the placenta readily, while drugs with a molecular weight between 600 and 1000 cross at a slower rate. A few drugs with a high molecular weight (> 1000 g/mol), such as heparin and insulin, do not cross the placenta in any appreciable amount [3]. Deposition and retention of drugs in placental tissue, while limiting acute fetal exposure during maternal binges, may

result in chronic long-term exposure to low levels of the same substance or its metabolites. Because the activity levels of certain fetal hepatic enzyme systems critical to drug metabolism are suboptimal, concentrations of such substances may be higher in the fetus than in the mother. Fetal organs such as the kidney may also be relatively inefficient in drug excretion, producing higher serum levels. Fetal swallowing of amniotic fluid contaminated with active drugs and metabolites results in continued exposure. The umbilical cord and its vessels, along with the vessels present on the surface of the placenta, provide yet another potential route of absorption of drugs and metabolites present in amniotic fluid [4]. Cutting the umbilical cord at birth does not fully protect the newborn from maternal substance abuse. Drugs stored in fetal fat can be released over time, resulting in continued exposure of the neonate over the first hours, days, weeks, or months of life. High lipophilicity enables these same substances to pass into breast milk, resulting in continued neonatal exposure and potential overdose.

General effects of substance abuse during pregnancy

Substance-abusing women often do not seek access to prenatal care, or lack access to health care, and are therefore at high risk for serious adverse health effects, including withdrawal, malnutrition, iron- and/or folate-deficiency anemia, and parenterally transmitted diseases such as bacterial endocarditis, human immunodeficiency virus, and hepatitis B virus. Pregnancy further increases the health risks faced by these women.

Fetal effects of maternal substance abuse depend on many variables. Most agents to which the mother and the fetus are exposed during gestation are not harmful; however, many substances are known human teratogens (drugs, chemicals, infectious agents, and other physical and environmental agents that cause structural and/or neurobehavioral disabilities postnatally). The specific substance used by the mother may have profound effects on the fetus that are readily apparent during pregnancy or shortly after birth, subtle influences manifested during school-age years, or no detectable consequences. The dose of the substance ingested and the duration of exposure during pregnancy also play an important role. Heavy use of any drug over a long period of time places the fetus at greater risk than light use over a similar time frame. Binge use (high intake of a drug over a relatively short period

Fetal and Neonatal Brain Injury, 4th edition, ed. David K. Stevenson, William E. Benitz, Philip Sunshine, Susan R. Hintz, and Maurice L. Druzin. Published by Cambridge University Press. © Cambridge University Press 2009.

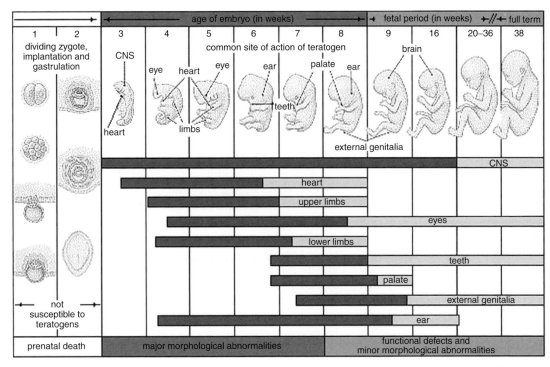

Fig. 10.1. Malformations by organ system as a function of gestational timing. Note that the embryo is not susceptible to teratogenic damage during days 0–10 post-conception. Adapted from: Moore KL, *Before We Were Born: Basic Embryology and Birth Defects*, 2nd edn. Philadelphia, PA: Saunders, 1993. With permission. *See color plate section.*

of time) is also potentially toxic to the fetus. Similarly, the timing of ingestion during pregnancy helps determine fetal and neonatal effects (Fig. 10.1). Use during the first trimester, a period critical for organogenesis, may result in malformations of organs rapidly undergoing morphogenesis. The exception is the first 10–14 days of gestation, prior to implantation of the embryo, during which no recognizable teratogenic effects are observed. This is likely due to an "all or none" phenomenon, in which if an embryo undergoes significant damage implantation (and recognizable pregnancy) will not occur; conversely, if implantation does occur following the exposure, it implies absence of significant adverse effects. Use in later trimesters may unduly influence processes such as synapse formation in the central nervous system, which may produce neurobehavioral abnormalities or result in the neonatal abstinence syndrome. The genetic constitution of both mother and fetus is likewise important, in that drug metabolism by enzyme systems is under genetic control and inherited enzymatic defects may greatly potentiate the deleterious effects of various ingested substances [5].

Exposure to substances of abuse in utero may be associated with lifelong consequences. The effects of fetal exposure to human teratogens can present in the neonatal period and may be incompatible with long-term survival. Other more subtle alterations in morphogenesis may present months or even years after birth, as neurodevelopmental delay or similar abnormalities. Clamping of the umbilical cord produces an abrupt cessation of drug administration, and may result in withdrawal as newborn blood levels fall. Continuing exposure

of the neonate to substances of abuse, as through breastfeeding, may produce a state of prolonged intoxication.

Methodological limitations

Many methodological problems exist with studies performed on substance-abusing women and their children. Because many women abuse more than a single substance during pregnancy, identification of a population of women and neonates exposed to a single substance is difficult at best. Small selective sample sizes and the lack of suitable control groups are problems which plague many clinical investigations; such studies tend to focus on those with the most intense exposures, who are most likely to exhibit detectable effects. Concomitant use of multiple drugs may produce an additive harmful effect when compared to use of a single substance. Investigators are also faced with an inherent inability to document the frequency and dose of drug exposure. Illicit drugs are not regulated for purity and are often adulterated or "cut" with other substances, making dose ascertainment problematic, even in those who apparently have limited their exposure to a single drug. While elicitation of a drug-use history is a vital component of any obstetric or neonatal evaluation, it has been shown in multiple studies that patient historical recall alone grossly underestimates prenatal substance abuse. Therefore, historical data must be accompanied by analysis of maternal and neonatal body fluids or tissues. Analysis of urine is capable of detecting only relatively recent (hours to days) exposure. Neonatal meconium analysis, while more sensitive than urine analysis, is useless in the detection of drug exposure very early in gestation, since meconium is formed beginning at approximately 16 weeks' gestation. Maternal hair analysis may provide the best information regarding timing of exposure, dose ingested, and duration of exposure, but it requires the cooperation of the mother. Neonatal hair may be lacking in sufficient quantity to allow study, and also is not present early in gestation (fetal hair begins to appear at approximately 9 weeks' gestation). Selection of only the most severely affected cases for presentation in the literature and ignorance of negative studies are common. The presence of numerous confounding variables such as poor nutrition, poverty, previous obstetric history, and lack of access to prenatal and pediatric care greatly complicates any study of the effects of maternal substance abuse. In utero exposure and subsequent biologic predisposition are complicated by environmental influences, which is reflected in the multi-hit model of neurological handicap [6]. Follow-up studies are hampered by high attrition rates and bias toward better-performing outcomes. Thus, while many of these substances are associated with adverse maternal, fetal, and neonatal outcome, it is impossible to state that a cause-and-effect relationship exists for most of the drugs ingested by pregnant women.

Substances of abuse
Ethanol

Of all the potential substances that women might abuse during pregnancy, ethanol poses the greatest risk to the embryo and fetus. Fetal alcohol syndrome is the most common identifiable cause of mental retardation, affecting 0.1–0.5% of all live births, and more subtle forms of teratogenic damage from prenatal alcohol exposure may affect 1% of all children born in the USA [7]. The societal burden of the teratogenic effects of alcohol is immense, in terms of suffering, lost productivity, and excess medical and educational expenses [8]. It was estimated that the annual costs of the damage caused by maternal alcohol abuse in the USA reached $4 billion by 1998 [9].

Ethanol consumption is common in the population at large, and various studies indicate that approximately one-half of women in their child-bearing years drink. The incidence of ethanol ingestion by pregnant women steadily declines as pregnancy advances: by the third month only 10–15% of women continue to ingest alcohol [10]. Many women are unaware they are pregnant until they reach the second or third month; therefore their fetuses are exposed to ethanol and its metabolites during the critical period of organogenesis.

The level of glucuronyl transferase and alcohol dehydrogenase activity is decreased in the fetus as compared to maternal levels [11]. Catabolism is delayed, resulting in higher fetal than maternal ethanol concentrations, thereby potentiating teratogenic risk.

It has long been recognized that maternal ethanol consumption during pregnancy produces a range of adverse effects in the fetus and neonate: such effects may be subtle, expressing themselves in mild neurodevelopmental abnormalities, or profound,

with characteristic phenotypic manifestations and mental retardation [12]. This continuum of structural anomalies and behavioral and neurocognitive disabilities is most accurately termed fetal alcohol spectrum disorders (FASD) [13].

In 1996, the Institute of Medicine set forth four specific diagnostic categories within FASD, thereby defining the clinical spectrum: fetal alcohol syndrome (FAS), partial fetal alcohol syndrome (PFAS), alcohol-related birth defects (ARBD), and alcohol-related neurodevelopmental disorder (ARND) [14]. Fetal alcohol syndrome (FAS) denotes a specific pattern of malformations, with a confirmed history of maternal alcohol abuse during pregnancy, prenatal onset of growth deficiency (length and/or weight) that persists postnatally, a specific pattern of minor anomalies of the face, and neurocognitive deficits. Children with PFAS display the facial characteristics of FAS, but demonstrate only some of the growth and/or neurocognitive deficits. ARBD represents a specific pattern of structural birth defects in affected individuals with the characteristic facies, but who demonstrate normal behavior and cognitive development. Finally, ARND represents a group of affected children with the typical neurodevelopmental profile of FAS, but who exhibit normal structural development and normal growth. It is perhaps this last group of children who represent the most difficult diagnostic challenge. Specific diagnostic criteria within each of these categories were published in 2005 (Table 10.1) [15]. A typically affected child with FAS is depicted in Figure 10.2.

Just as the intoxicating effects of ethanol on adults vary directly with blood levels, the effects seen in the newborn undoubtedly reflect the variability in dose, timing of exposure during gestation, frequency of exposure, and the genotype of mother and fetus.

Both ethanol and its primary metabolite acetaldehyde are teratogenic to numerous organ systems; however, the primary target of ethanol teratogenesis is the developing brain. Central nervous system abnormalities, especially involving midline structures, are a prominent component of fetal alcohol syndrome [16]. Structural malformations include microcephaly, cerebellar dysplasia, heterotopias, agenesis of the corpus callosum, and anomalies secondary to the interruption of neuronal and glial migration [17]. Neuroimaging studies have also documented that, in addition to an overall reduction of brain size and specific structural malformations, prominent brain shape abnormalities have been observed, with narrowing in the parietal region and reduced brain growth in portions of the frontal lobe [18].

Multiple mechanisms by which ethanol and its metabolites impair normal development have been implicated. Events such as neuronal migration depend upon the developmentally regulated expression and function of cell adhesion molecules (CAMs); CAMs are also expressed in osteoblasts, and appear to play a role in bone formation. Ethanol has been shown to alter the migration of neurons into the cortex in animal models and suppress the expression of CAMs in tissue culture in a dose-dependent fashion [19]. Ethanol also alters the levels of endogenous retinoids and the expression of retinoic acid

Table 10.1. Revised Institute of Medicine criteria for diagnoses within the fetal alcohol spectrum disorders (FASD) continuum [15]

(I) Diagnostic criteria for FAS or PFAS (with or without confirmed maternal alcohol exposure) (FAS requires all features A–C; PFAS requires A and: B or C or evidence of a complex pattern of behavioral or cognitive abnormalities inconsistent with developmental level and that cannot be explained by genetic predisposition, family background, or environment alone [see ARND])
(A) Evidence of a characteristic pattern of minor facial anomalies, including at least two of the following:
Short palpebral fissures ($\leq$ 10th percentile)
Thin vermilion border of the upper lip (score 4 or 5 on the lip/philtrum guide)
Smooth philtrum (score 4 or 5 on the lip/philtrum guide)
(B) Evidence of prenatal and/or postnatal growth retardation: height or weight $\leq$ 10th percentile
(C) Evidence of deficient brain growth or abnormal morphogenesis, including one or more of the following:
Structural brain abnormalities
Head circumference $\leq$ 10th percentile
(II) Diagnostic criteria for alcohol-related effects (ARBD and ARND) (A diagnosis in these categories requires a confirmed history of prenatal alcohol exposure)
ARBD requires the characteristic facies as above plus specific congenital structural defects (including malformations and dysplasias) in at least one organ system (if the patient displays minor anomalies only, at least two must be present). This category assumes the subject to have normal growth and intellectual/behavioral characteristics
ARND assumes the subject to have normal growth and structure and at least one of the following (A or B):
(A) Evidence of deficient brain growth or abnormal morphogenesis, including one or more of the following:
Structural brain abnormalities
Head circumference $\leq$ 10th percentile
(B) Evidence of a complex pattern of behavioral or cognitive abnormalities inconsistent with developmental level and that cannot be explained by genetic predisposition, family background, or environment alone
This pattern includes: marked impairment in the performance of complex tasks (complex problem solving, planning, judgment, abstraction, metacognition, and arithmetic tasks); higher-level receptive and expressive language deficits; and disordered behavior (difficulties in personal manner, emotional lability, motor dysfunction, poor academic performance, and deficient social interaction)

Notes:
FAS, fetal alcohol syndrome; PFAS, partial fetal alcohol syndrome; ARBD, alcohol-related birth defects; ARND, alcohol-related neurodevelopmental disorder.

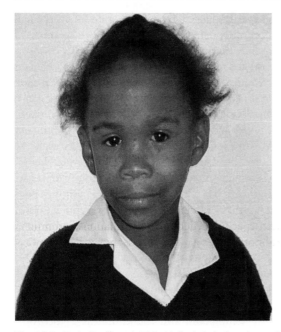

Fig. 10.2. Typically affected child with fetal alcohol syndrome. Short palpebral fissures, a smooth philtrum and a thin vermilion border of the upper lip are evident.

receptors in rats, producing cardiac anomalies similar to those seen in vitamin A teratogenesis [20].

Some studies have revealed that ethanol inhibits cell division and protein synthesis. Quantitative decreases in brain DNA and delays in the appearance of messenger RNA for various developmentally regulated central nervous system proteins have been detected in rat pups [21]. Delayed neuronal migration and proliferation have been documented in rats exposed to ethanol in utero [22]. The incidence of germinal matrix and intraventricular hemorrhage is increased in ethanol-exposed premature human neonates [23]. This may be indicative of an ethanol-induced alteration in the developmental biology of the germinal matrix, the site of both neuroblastogenesis and glioblastogenesis. Ethanol may also stimulate cell proliferation and thereby inhibit terminal neuronal differentiation and synapse formation [24]. Studies indicate that ethanol can impair gene expression at the transcriptional level, disrupting the temporal and spatial patterns of differential gene expression, potentially having a profound impact on eventual structure and function. Recent studies in experimental animals have also documented that alcohol downregulates many early developmental genetic pathways in the embryo (e.g., *Shh*, *Pax6*, and *Fgf8*), thus leading to many of the observed changes in structure and function [25–27].

Functional abnormalities such as mental retardation, hypotonia, irritability, and poor coordination are observed in patients with fetal alcohol syndrome. Exposure to ethanol in utero has been shown quantitatively and temporally to alter the development of numerous neurotransmitters, including the serotonergic, cholinergic, dopaminergic, and glutamatergic systems, as well as to alter the activity of membrane-bound receptors for various neurotransmitters [28].

Prenatal ethanol exposure is associated with amblyopia, astigmatism, and other visual defects in humans. Animal studies in rats indicate that ethanol produces both macroscopic and microscopic changes in the optic nerves, including a gross decrease in cross-sectional diameter, cytostructural maldevelopment of glial cells, neurons, and myelin, and abnormalities in various organelles [29]. External ear anomalies and sensorineural hearing loss have also been described [30].

Associated cardiovascular abnormalities include atrial septal defect, ventricular septal defect, and anomalies of the great vessels. Myocardial ultrastructural changes, including decreased myofibrillar density and dysplasia, have been produced in rats exposed to ethanol prenatally [31]. The genitourinary system may also be involved, and hydronephrosis is a common finding. Murine embryos exposed to ethanol show excessive cell death in the region of the mesonephric duct proximal to the cloaca and in neural crest cells proximal to the posterior neuropore [32]. This is followed by abnormalities in the location of the ureterovesicle junction, leading to ureteral obstruction and hydronephrosis. Other common anomalies include hirsutism, cleft lip and palate, nail hypoplasia, pectus excavatum, diastasis recti, hypospadius, and camptodactyly, among other anomalies [33].

Prenatal and postnatal growth deficiency are manifested as decreased weight, length, and head circumference [34]. Animal data indicate that prenatal ethanol exposure reduces fetal concentrations of insulin-like growth factor 1 (IGF-1) as well as the concentration of IGF-binding proteins later in life [35]. Ethanol has also been shown to reduce the secretion of IGF-2 from explanted fetal rat organs [36]. Such studies indicate that this may be but one mechanism by which prenatal ethanol exposure results in both short- and long-term alterations in growth and development. Lactase activity in the small intestine of rat pups exposed to transplacental ethanol is decreased in comparison to controls, and this may represent another factor contributing to the growth retardation seen in this syndrome [37].

Women giving birth to infants with fetal alcohol syndrome typically use more ethanol and use it earlier in gestation. While it is clear that daily consumption of more than approximately 1.5 oz (42 g) of absolute ethanol (the equivalent of three beers) greatly increases the risk of alcohol-induced teratogenicity, there is no uniform fetal response to a particular dose of ethanol: therefore there is no amount of alcohol that can be considered entirely safe for the pregnant woman to consume. The American Medical Association, the American Academy of Pediatrics, the American College of Obstetricians and Gynecologists, and the Surgeon General recommend that women who are attempting to conceive or who are already pregnant should not drink ethanol in any amount.

Ethanol withdrawal has been described in neonates born to chronically intoxicated mothers. Given the potent teratogenic effects of ethanol, it may be difficult to determine whether such manifestations represent true withdrawal or are manifestations of the central nervous system effects of fetal alcohol syndrome.

Maternal ethanol abuse complicates breastfeeding in several ways [38]. Lactation is impaired and the let-down reflex is inhibited by ethanol. Ethanol is readily secreted in breast milk, and acute neonatal intoxication can result. The motor capabilities of infants at 1 year of age regularly exposed to ethanol in breast milk have been shown to be significantly impaired [39]. Investigators have shown that the facial characteristics and other stigmata of fetal alcohol syndrome persist beyond the neonatal and infancy periods. It has also become apparent that children with a history of prenatal exposure but lacking the typical stigmata at birth may develop signs and symptoms over time. Longitudinal follow-up of neonates with prenatal ethanol exposure is necessary [40].

The neurodevelopmental deficits seen in the fetal alcohol syndrome persist into adulthood. Affected individuals manifest an inability to stay on task and poor memory, and they are at increased risk for attention-deficit disorder with hyperactivity [41]. Their comprehension, judgment, and reasoning are also impaired, making it difficult for them to anticipate the consequences of their actions. Because of mood lability, social interaction is impaired; this may accentuate feelings of withdrawal and depression [42].

Tobacco

Tobacco leaves when burned liberate thousands of compounds including toxins (such as carbon monoxide and hydrogen cyanide), trace elements (lead, nickel, and cadmium), and carcinogens. While the prevalence of smoking has declined in the general population, it remains a significant problem among women of child-bearing age. In fact, most smokers do not quit when they become pregnant. A Canadian study reported that 1/3 of women smoked before pregnancy, and, of those, over 2/3 still smoked at the time of delivery [43]. Similarly, less than 31% of women in the United States who smoke abstain from smoking during pregnancy [44].

Carbon monoxide avidly binds to hemoglobin, competitively inhibiting oxygen from being taken up in the pulmonary capillaries. At atmospheric partial pressures this results in essentially irreversible displacement of oxygen. Carboxyhemoglobin levels in pregnant women who smoke are many times those of non-smokers [45]. Increased maternal carboxyhemoglobin implies increased fetal carboxyhemoglobin, impaired oxygen content and delivery, and fetal hypoxemia [46]. Neonates born to mothers who smoke tobacco have elevated levels of erythropoietin in umbilical cord blood and increased numbers of nucleated red blood cells in peripheral circulation; both of these results indicate a response to hypoxemia [47]. Cyanide acts in a similar manner by binding to the iron moiety of both hemoglobin and mitochondrial cytochrome oxidase, inhibiting oxygen uptake and delivery as well as cellular respiration. Cyanide is also capable of inhibiting carbonic anhydrase, resulting in decreased carbon dioxide excretion. Chronic fetal hypoxemia results in intrauterine growth restriction and a small-for-gestational-age neonate. Newborns so affected are at risk for sequelae such as hypoxic–ischemic encephalopathy, polycythemia, and pulmonary hypertension.

Nicotine is primarily excreted by the kidneys, although the lungs and liver are also sites of metabolism. Nicotine crosses the placenta and accumulates in the amniotic fluid and fetus to the extent that fetal levels exceed those seen in the mother [48].

It is a common belief among pregnant adolescents that smoking will allow for an easier (quicker and less painful) vaginal delivery. Indeed, studies have shown that mothers who smoke deliver neonates weighing 200–300 g less than gestational-age-matched controls; this appears to be due to a difference in fat-free mass [49]. Some studies have indicated a dose–response relationship between weight and length at birth and prenatal exposure to tobacco [50]. Another series revealed less severe growth restriction in neonates born to mothers who quit smoking during pregnancy compared with women who continued to smoke [51]. The pathophysiology of the intrauterine growth restriction seen in offspring of smoking mothers is multifactorial. Uterine artery vasoconstriction and decreased substrate delivery to the fetus may play a role [52]. Cigarette smoking may also alter the bioavailability of certain nutrients such as folate, zinc, and vitamins, producing relative maternal and fetal deficiencies. While gross placental size is not affected by smoking, structural changes in the cytoarchitecture at the placental–lacunar interface have been described [53]. Epidermal growth factor plays an important role in implantation, placental growth and endocrine function, and other aspects of fetoplacental development. Alterations in epidermal growth factor receptor autophosphorylation have been described and may represent another mechanism by which smoking may impair fetal growth [54]. It is also possible that embryonic and fetal cell number and size are diminished by premature termination of cell division, abnormal differentiation, alterations in neuronal synapse formation, or an as yet undetermined mechanism [55].

The existence of a tobacco embryopathy is unclear. The association of smoking with cleft lip and cleft lip/palate remains controversial [56].

Most of the studies assessing the risk of placenta previa associated with maternal smoking have reported a positive association, with odds ratios ranging from 1.28 to 7.42 [57]. The evidence for an association between smoking during pregnancy and placental abruption is more compelling than in the case of placenta previa. A consensus opinion now exists that prenatal smoking is a major factor in the causation of placental abruption. The odds ratios for the association between prenatal smoking and placental abruption range from 1.4 to 4.0 [58]. A causal relationship between smoking and abruption is also supported by the observed impact of interventions. In the Collaborative Perinatal Project of the National Institute of Neurological and Communicative Disorders and Stroke, women who stopped smoking early in the pregnancy showed a risk of abruption that was similar to that of those women who never smoked [59]. The causative mechanism may involve a chronic inflammatory process that triggers a chain of responses (increased oxidative stress, vascular reactivity, etc.) leading finally to increased necrosis, apoptosis, and destruction of the extracellular matrix at the maternal–fetal interface [60].

Other adverse perinatal outcomes proven by epidemiological studies to be associated with maternal smoking include placenta accreta, preterm birth, and stillbirth [61–63].

Intrauterine exposure to tobacco may have serious consequences for the fetus and neonate extending beyond the immediate newborn period. Alterations in cerebral blood flow have been documented in animal models [64]. Prenatal tobacco exposure decreases arousal to auditory stimuli and may increase the risk of obstructive sleep apnea [65]. Maternal smoking during pregnancy is also a risk factor for sudden infant death syndrome (SIDS) [66]. Brainstem gliosis has been found in a number of autopsies of victims of SIDS; this histologic finding is consistent with repetitive hypoxemia, possibly secondary to abnormalities in the control of respiration [67]. In addition, maternal smoking appears to have an adverse effect on early intellectual function [68,69].

Nicotine, cotinine, and other substances found in tobacco are secreted in breast milk. Levels in the neonate correlate with those seen in the mother. Nicotine has been shown to impair lactation and decrease the supply of breast milk. Nicotine has been associated with neonatal emesis, respiratory problems such as frequent upper respiratory tract infections, and reactive airway disease, and a potential increased risk of childhood cancer [70]. The effects on the newborn of the many other substances found in tobacco and secreted in breast milk are currently unknown. This is especially concerning, as many women who quit smoking during pregnancy are likely to start again after delivery, feeling that the danger to their newborn no longer exists. All mothers should be counseled as to the potential risks presented by tobacco products secreted in breast milk and those found in environmental smoke [71].

The consumption of smokeless tobacco ("chew," "chaw," "dip"), while primarily a male activity in the population at large, is more common in females in certain ethnic groups, such as native Americans. Animal studies indicate that ingestion of this form of tobacco increases the risk of intrauterine growth restriction, decreased bone ossification, and embryonic demise [72].

The dangers of environmental tobacco smoke exposure ("second-hand smoke," "passive" or "involuntary" smoking) are now also coming to light. As much as 50% of non-smoking pregnant women may be exposed to "second-hand" smoke, and fetal exposure to nicotine and its metabolites may remain significant even in these cases [73]. Fetal exposure to environmental smoke appears to increase the risk of poor developmental outcome. In one study, children between the ages of 6 and 9 years exposed to environmental smoke in utero were found to perform at a level inferior to those born to nonsmoking mothers but superior to those born to smoking mothers [74]. Paternal smoking with subsequent maternal passive inhalation of "sidestream" smoke has also been associated with intrauterine growth restriction [75,76]. An increased risk of respiratory tract disease (recurrent infection, reactive airway disease), impaired pulmonary development, otitis media, and lung cancer in later life has been associated with the inhalation of environmental tobacco smoke; however, most of these studies are retrospective in nature, and prospective, well-controlled analyses are lacking. One of the most alarming findings to date is that smoking in the same room as the infant increases the risk of SIDS in a dose-dependent fashion [77].

Marijuana

D-9-tetrahydrocannabinol (D-9-THC) is the major active metabolite derived from the plant *Cannabis sativa* (over 60 similar cannabinoid compounds are present). Marijuana is the term applied to the dried leaves, stems, and seeds of this plant. It is the most frequently abused of all illicit drugs in the USA, and its use by women in their child-bearing years is extremely common. Other derivatives of marijuana include hashish and hashish oil. While oral consumption is possible, smoking is the usual route of ingestion, and this results in the absorption of a much greater proportion of active drug [78]. Burning or heating marijuana, hashish, and hashish oil allows for the inhalation of smoke containing D-9-THC and rapid absorption across the pulmonary epithelium. Marijuana smoke contains more carcinogens, irritants, and particulates than tobacco smoke [79]. Marijuana cigarettes ("joints") may be adulterated with other substances such as cocaine and phencyclidine (PCP) to produce a more intense high. Intoxication may also be seen in those exposed to second-hand smoke.

Prolonged, arrested labor has been reported with acute marijuana intoxication. While no teratogenic effects have been directly linked to prenatal marijuana, the adulteration of cigarettes with other drugs of abuse may raise the potential risk. Frequent marijuana use during pregnancy has been shown to be associated with a small decrease in birthweight, although this decrease does not reach statistical significance in all studies and in and of itself probably carries little clinical significance [80]. A 1997 meta-analysis of 10 studies concluded that there was inadequate evidence to suggest that marijuana reduces birthweight at the amount typically consumed by pregnant women [81]. However, frequent use (>4 times/week) was associated with a 131 g decrease in birthweight. The effect of prenatal marijuana exposure on long-term growth remains unclear [82].

Reported effects on neonatal behavior of in utero marijuana exposure include prolongation of the startle response, tremors, irritability, poor state regulation, and altered visual and auditory responses [83]. Reports of the effects of prenatal exposure to marijuana on neurobehavioral development during childhood are contradictory [84–86]. Continued exposure of the neonate to marijuana after birth is experienced by breastfeeding newborns because D-9-THC is excreted in breast milk.

Cocaine

Cocaine or benzoylmethylecgonine is one of several alkaloids found in the leaves of *Erythroxylon coca*, which grows primarily in Peru, Ecuador, and Bolivia; raw leaves contain approximately 0.5–2% cocaine [87]. The major metabolite of cocaine is benzoylecgonine. In addition to its local anesthetic and vasoconstrictor properties, it blocks presynaptic catecholamine reuptake, resulting in catecholamine accumulation at postsynaptic receptors and pronounced central nervous system stimulation. Benzoylmethylecgonine hydrochloride ("coke," "snow," "lady," "gold dust") is produced in the form of crystals, granules, and powder. Cocaine base ("freebase") is formed by the extraction of cocaine from the hydrochloride salt with the use of alkaline solutions and subsequent recrystallization employing highly flammable solvents. Cocaine hydrochloride mixed with water and sodium bicarbonate, then hardened in a microwave oven, results in a free alkaloid form ("crack," "rock"). Smoking crack allows for rapid diffusion and entry into the blood and central nervous system, producing high serum levels and short, very intense highs. Because cholinesterase activity is low in pregnancy as well as in the fetal and neonatal periods, pregnant women who abuse cocaine and their newborns may be exposed to high levels for protracted periods of time. The placenta binds cocaine and its metabolites and thus may effectively serve as a depot for drug release during pregnancy [88].

The perinatal literature is replete with case reports of fetal and neonatal problems attributed to prenatal cocaine exposure. The biologically plausible pathogenetic mechanism underlying these many and varied effects is suspected to be a disruption of blood flow, either globally to the uteroplacental unit or locally within specific fetal organs [89]. Thus cocaine exerts its teratogenic potential primarily through its vasoconstrictive effects, producing disruptions of normally formed tissues, rather than inducing primary malformations.

Cocaine primarily exerts its negative effects on the fetoplacental unit by global rather than focal disruption of blood flow. Uterine arterial vasospasm as a result of cocaine ingestion impairs fetal substrate delivery, predisposing the fetus to intrauterine growth restriction [90]. Prostaglandin production is altered in placental explants incubated in the presence of cocaine: thromboxane A2 synthesis is increased and prostacyclin production decreased. Thromboxane A2 induces vasoconstriction and platelet aggregation and may represent one mechanism whereby uteroplacental blood flow is impaired [91]. Although the duration of action of cocaine in producing uterine arterial vasoconstriction is relatively short-lived, even women who are relatively infrequent users of the drug remain at risk for fetal growth abnormalities [92]. Therefore it is probable that mechanisms other than vasoconstriction play a role in the increased risk of intrauterine growth restriction [93]. Even though vasoconstriction may be intermittent, other processes such as inhibition of placental uptake of substrates such as alanine may be altered in a more chronic fashion.

Several epidemiologic studies have confirmed the negative effects of maternal cocaine use on birthweight, length, and head circumference, even after adjustment for tobacco, alcohol, or other drug use, nutritional indicators, and various sociodemographic factors [94,95]. Studies also have confirmed dose–response effects of cocaine exposure on fetal growth. For example, a retrospective cohort study in a New York City hospital found a 27 g decrement in birthweight with each log unit increase in cocaine concentration in maternal hair at delivery, adjusted for gestation, smoking, and alcohol consumption [96].

Focal impairment of blood flow to specific organs in the embryo and fetus accompanying maternal cocaine use has been suggested to cause a myriad of disruptive events leading to structural defects, including: limb–body wall complex [97], limb reduction defects, intestinal atresia, cranial defects (e.g., encephalocele and exencephaly) [98,99], genitourinary tract abnormalities [100], and congenital heart defects [101]. Despite the number of such case reports, a "fetal cocaine syndrome" has not been delineated.

Cocaine use is associated with premature labor, premature rupture of membranes, advanced cervical dilation at admission, and a shortened latency period to labor and delivery [102,103]. In addition, maternal cocaine ingestion appears to carry an increased risk of placenta previa, abruptio placentae, uterine rupture, and precipitous delivery [104,105]. The incidence of spontaneous abortion and fetal demise is also higher in the cocaine-exposed population.

Neonatal effects of prenatal cocaine exposure primarily reflect focal disruption of vascular flow. Prenatal cocaine exposure is associated with an increased risk of necrotizing enterocolitis in both premature and term newborns [106]. Pregnant rats injected with cocaine delivered newborns with mesenteric vascular thrombosis and focal areas of inflammation, hemorrhage, and necrosis in their gastrointestinal tract [107].

Various central nervous system manifestations have been described in neonates, infants, and children born to cocaine-abusing women. Discrete anatomic lesions such as cerebral artery infarction have been detected in exposed neonates [108]. An increased incidence of intracranial hemorrhage has been described; this is felt to be due at least in part to an increase in mean arterial blood pressure and cerebral blood flow velocity [109]. Periventricular leukomalacia, thought to be secondary to in utero cerebral ischemia, has also been associated with prenatal cocaine exposure [110]. However, not all studies reveal an association between prenatal cocaine exposure and structural brain abnormalities [111]. Seizures have also been described in neonates after receiving a transplacental cocaine bolus shortly before birth and after passive inhalation of environmental "crack" smoke [112]. Alterations in both respiratory control and sleep regulation in the fetus and neonate have been described in human and animal studies. Cocaine-exposed term newborns have been shown to have increased apnea and periodic breathing in comparison with controls [113]. Abnormal sleep and awake state transition has been found in infants exposed to cocaine [114]. Direct intravascular administration of cocaine to fetal sheep suppresses low-voltage electrocortical activity and increases catecholamine levels [115]. Fetal sleep state regulation is in part controlled by norepinephrine, which normally decreases in active fetal sleep. Transplacentally acquired cocaine elevates norepinephrine levels and decreases active sleep. Tryptophan and serotonin also function as regulators of the sleep–wake cycle; cocaine has been found to interfere with tryptophan uptake and serotonin biosynthesis [116]. The effects of these

alterations upon the developmental biology of the central nervous system are unknown. Abnormalities in respiratory control and sleep state regulation increase the risk of SIDS. However, it is not clear that cocaine-exposed neonates are at an increased risk of SIDS, as studies have produced conflicting results [117,118].

Numerous developmental studies have been performed on children exposed to cocaine prenatally. Studies have shown poor on-task performance, fine motor deficits, impaired habituation, low threshold for overstimulation, inability to self-regulate, and cognitive and motor developmental delay at 1.5–2 years [119,120]. Other studies indicate a dose-response effect of prenatal cocaine exposure upon assessments of growth and behavior [121,122].

The lay press was quick to sensationalize the cocaine epidemic and the purported effects of this drug on the unborn. Despite limited evidence generated by studies complicated by all of the problems outlined earlier, "crack babies" were labeled as irrevocably damaged and a burden to society. A more scientific analysis of the available data fails to substantiate the universality and inevitability of these early claims. A meta-analysis published in 2001 stated that there was no convincing evidence that in utero exposure to cocaine and its metabolites results in developmental defects in children aged 6 and younger [123].

No definitive withdrawal syndrome from in utero cocaine exposure has been described in neonates; it is uncertain whether the signs observed in some neonates prenatally exposed to cocaine represent true withdrawal or are secondary to the direct effects of the drug still present in the newborn. These signs typically appear in the first 24–48 hours after birth and peak in intensity by 72 hours [124]. The most frequently observed findings include tachycardia, tachypnea, hypertension, irritability, exaggerated Moro response, impaired visual tracking, increased tremulousness, abnormal sleep patterns, increased generalized motor tone, and feeding abnormalities, including poor suck and emesis [125].

Cocaine is excreted in breast milk up to 36 hours after the last dose, representing another potential route of neonatal exposure. Cases of neonatal intoxication marked by irritability, vomiting, diarrhea, tachycardia, tachypnea, hypertension, and tremulousness in breastfed newborns have been described [126]. One case described an 11-day-old breastfeeding neonate who developed apnea and seizures after ingesting cocaine used as a topical anesthetic for maternal nipple soreness [127].

Opioids

Opiate refers to a drug derived from opium, the dried milky exudate of the opium poppy, *Papaver somniferum*. An opioid is a natural or synthetic substance which produces opium- or morphine-like effects when ingested. Narcotic is the non-specific term applied to any drug derived from opium or similar compounds capable of inducing analgesia, sedation, and sleep, and which will cause dependence with repeated use. Opioids may be ingested orally or inhaled; they may also be injected intravenously, intramuscularly, and subcutaneously.

One opioid is heroin; its lipid solubility is greater than that of morphine, allowing it to enter the central nervous system more rapidly and producing a quicker, more intense "high."

Despite the frequency of fetal exposure to opioids, no consistent teratogenic effects have been observed. Most studies of prenatal opioid, heroin, or methadone use show higher rates of low birthweight (LBW), preterm birth, and intrauterine growth restriction, although few have controlled for associated risk factors. A meta-analysis estimated a 483 g reduction in birthweight and a relative risk for LBW of 3.81 associated with any opiate use during pregnancy [128].

Endogenous opioid peptides and opioid receptors are expressed transiently in the developing mammalian brain [129]. The significance of this developmentally regulated process and the effects that fetal opioid exposure have on this phenomenon are unknown at this time. Methadone delays pulmonary surfactant synthesis by an unknown mechanism and places the newborn at higher risk of respiratory distress syndrome and the need for assisted ventilation [130]. Unlike methadone, heroin accelerates pulmonary surfactant synthesis; exposed neonates have a decreased risk of respiratory distress.

Maternal withdrawal implies fetal withdrawal. While the addicted mother manifests the typical signs and symptoms of opioid withdrawal, the fetus experiences hypoxia and in response may pass meconium. Chronic fetal hypoxia produces pulmonary vascular remodeling and increased vascular reactivity, predisposing the newborn to pulmonary hypertension after birth. Both meconium aspiration and pulmonary hypertension increase neonatal morbidity and mortality. Chronic intrauterine hypoxia also increases the risk of hypoxic–ischemic encephalopathy and fetal demise. Because of the significant maternal, fetal, and neonatal sequelae, withdrawal in pregnancy should be treated promptly and appropriately.

A neonate exposed to opioids in utero is at risk of respiratory depression in the hours after birth. Naloxone (Narcan), an opioid antagonist, may be used to reverse respiratory depression in the newborn secondary to maternal opioid administration within 4 hours of delivery in the absence of a maternal history of opioid abuse. However, acute opioid reversal in a newborn chronically exposed in utero may produce withdrawal, thus naloxone should be used very judiciously on a case-by-case basis. It is preferable to support the neonate's respirations with positive-pressure ventilation and achieve a heart rate above 100 beats per minute prior to establishing the need for and administration of naloxone. Any neonate receiving naloxone should be monitored carefully in the hours to days after birth, as the duration of action of many opioids is longer than that of naloxone.

Opioids appear to have effects that extend beyond the immediate newborn period. Neonates born to methadone-using mothers have been shown to have a decreased sensitivity to carbon dioxide during the first days of life in comparison to controls [131]. The risk of SIDS in babies born to opioid-abusing mothers is 5–10 times that of unexposed newborns

(approximately 20–30/1000 live births versus 2–3/1000 in the general population) [132].

Once the umbilical cord is clamped, the newborn is disengaged from all that was once supplied by the mother and placenta. Neonates born to opioid-addicted mothers are at risk for withdrawal. Withdrawal in the newborn is characterized by central nervous system signs such as yawning, lacrimation, mydriasis, irritability, and seizures. While these effects are transitory, some may produce permanent nervous system injury if not treated appropriately (e.g., seizures). Heroin and methadone are the most commonly used opioids by pregnant women. Heroin has a relatively short half-life and exposed newborns typically experience withdrawal soon after birth. Methadone is a synthetic opioid used in the treatment of maternal addiction and prevention of withdrawal signs and symptoms. The majority of neonates exposed to methadone in utero undergo withdrawal, usually showing signs within 1–2 days of birth. Withdrawal from methadone is typically more severe and longer in duration in comparison with other prenatally acquired opioids. Given the long half-life of this drug and the fact that methadone is present in low concentrations in breast milk, some neonates may not experience withdrawal until several weeks of age. While the presence of methadone in breast milk in levels approximating those found in serum may prevent or delay neonatal withdrawal, it may also result in intoxication, respiratory depression, and death in the breastfeeding newborn [133]. The American Academy of Pediatrics states that breastfeeding is contraindicated if the maternal dose of methadone exceeds 20 mg/day [134].

Sedative-hypnotics

The group of drugs known as the sedative-hypnotics includes the benzodiazepines, barbiturates, and others, including methaqualone, meprobamate, and ethchlorvynol. Ethanol potentiates the absorption of these drugs and therefore may lead to overdose if used simultaneously. Because they can be ingested orally they are common substances of abuse; they can also be administered intravenously or intramuscularly. As a class of drugs, these substances typically have long half-lives, and their effects may persist for days. They are metabolized by hepatic glucuronidases and excreted by the kidneys.

Benzodiazepine levels in fetal blood exceed those in maternal blood [135]. Fetal effects have included decreased beat-to-beat variability in heart-rate pattern. Although minor facial anomalies and cleft lip and palate have been described in exposed infants [136], no significant teratogenic effects have been observed in benzodiazepine-exposed pregnancies in large population-based studies [137]. Reduced head circumference and cognitive deficits have been associated with in utero exposure to anticonvulsant barbiturates [138]. However, no definitive evidence of a "sedative-hypnotic syndrome" exists.

Withdrawal in the neonate is similar to that seen with opioids: at its most severe, hypothermia, hypotonia, and respiratory depression ensue [139]. Sedative-hypnotics are secreted in breast milk, and this route affords another possible route of intoxication.

Sympathomimetics

Sympathomimetics produce physiologic responses similar to endogenous catecholamines, stimulating neurotransmitter release at alpha, beta, dopaminergic, and serotonergic receptors [123]. Unlike catecholamines, these drugs retain their efficacy when ingested orally, readily enter the central nervous system, and are metabolized much more slowly than the endogenous catecholamines, with large proportions excreted unchanged in urine. Many sympathomimetics can be obtained in over-the-counter medications, including phenylephrine, ephedrine, pseudoephedrine, and phenylpropanolamine. The most commonly abused sympathomimetics include amphetamine, methamphetamine ("crystal"), and methylphenidate. The amphetamines are collectively known as "speed." Some users ingest "speedballs," combinations of amphetamine with barbiturates (to calm the agitated feelings associated with amphetamine use) or heroin (to enhance the "rush" associated with heroin). Routes of ingestion include oral consumption, nasal insufflation, inhalation of smoke (smokable methamphetamine hydrochloride is known as "ice"), as well as intravenous and subcutaneous injection ("skin popping"). Metabolism occurs in the liver, and excretion is via the kidney.

As with cocaine, the sympathomimetics may produce potent vasoconstriction and limit blood flow to various organs. Uterine artery constriction results in relative placental insufficiency, decreased substrate delivery to the fetus, and risk of intrauterine growth restriction [140]. A slight reduction in birthweight but no differences in length or head circumference have been reported in studies of antepartum methamphetamine use [141,142].

Animal studies reveal that prenatal amphetamine exposure is associated with structural and functional alterations in brain development [143–145]. In a study of CNS structure and neurocognitive function, methamphetamine-exposed children scored lower on measures of visual motor integration, attention, verbal memory, and long-term spatial memory. There were no differences among the groups in motor skills, short-delay spatial memory, or measures of non-verbal intelligence. Despite comparable whole-brain volumes in each group, the meth-exposed children had smaller putamen bilaterally, smaller globus pallidus, smaller hippocampus, and a smaller caudate bilaterally. The reduction in these brain structures correlated with poorer performance on sustained attention and delayed verbal memory. No group differences in volumes were noted in the thalamus, midbrain, or cerebellum [146]. Methamphetamine use in late gestation has been associated with neonatal intracranial lesions, including white-matter cavitary lesions and intraventricular, subarachnoid, and subependymal hemorrhage [147]. Because the fetus has little central nervous system blood-flow autoregulatory capacity, it is possible that the sympathomimetic-induced alterations in uterine and placental blood flow produce both uncompensated hypertensive spikes and hypotensive nadirs in the fetal circulation, predisposing the fetus to ischemic damage and reperfusion injury.

Sympathomimetic use during pregnancy has also been associated with premature labor, preterm delivery, abruptio placentae, and postpartum hemorrhage [148].

Tremors, feeding difficulties, and irritability followed by prolonged periods of lethargy have been described in the first days of life in neonates exposed to methamphetamine in utero. Since methamphetamine persists for days in the neonate after clamping of the umbilical cord, it is possible that these signs represent drug toxicity rather than withdrawal [149].

PCP

PCP (1-(1-phenylcyclohexyl)piperidene hydrochloride) was formerly used as an anesthetic agent until a high incidence of side effects, including hallucinations and violent behavior, resulted in its removal from legal use in humans [150]. It exists in a liquid and a powder form (PCP, "angel dust") and can be smoked as an additive to tobacco or marijuana cigarettes. It may also be insufflated, injected intravenously, ingested orally, or absorbed percutaneously. Hepatic metabolism and renal excretion account for elimination of the drug.

PCP readily crosses the placenta and enters the fetal circulation. While reports of microcephaly and dysmorphic facies associated with maternal PCP ingestion are found in the literature, no conclusive evidence of a PCP embryopathy exists [151]. Studies using human cerebral cortical tissue culture indicate that PCP has the potential to suppress axonal outgrowth and induce neuronal necrosis, possibly via an inhibitory effect on potassium channels [152]. However, no in vivo correlation of these findings has been made.

Neonates exposed to PCP in utero may display jitteriness, irritability, and rapid swings in levels of consciousness [153]. As with many other substances of abuse, signs manifested in the neonatal period most likely reflect continued exposure to the active drug rather than true withdrawal [154]. PCP is secreted in breast milk, and breastfeeding carries the potential risk of neonatal chronic exposure and intoxication [155].

LSD

LSD ("acid") is a synthetic diethylamide derivative of lysergic acid. It is classified as a psychedelic (a substance capable of producing a distorted perception of reality) rather than a hallucinogen (a substance which produces a vision with no basis in reality). While LSD may be insufflated, inhaled, injected intravenously or subcutaneously, and instilled into the conjunctival sac, it is most commonly taken orally. Metabolism is primarily hepatic, and excretion is both renal and hepatic.

LSD has been associated with chromosomal breakage in offspring of mothers abusing the drug; however, this finding has no clinical correlate. While several case reports of cardiac, ophthalmologic, and other malformations exist, no causal link has been shown [156–159]. Withdrawal has not been reported. The extent of excretion into breast milk is also unknown.

Volatile substances of abuse

Volatile substances of abuse are primarily hydrocarbon derivatives: aromatic and aliphatic hydrocarbons such as those found in paint solvents, adhesives, and fuels; alkyl halides and nitrites present in aerosol propellants, refrigerants, cleaning fluids, and fuels; and ether and ketone components of fuels, solvents, oils, sealants, and plastics. Such substances are ubiquitous in society, found in products such as lighter fluids, nail-polish remover, and typewriter correction fluid. Because they may be obtained so readily (and legally) they are common substances of abuse, especially among those unable to afford the more expensive illicit drugs [160].

Metabolism is primarily carried out in the liver, and metabolites are excreted in bile, urine, and exhaled gas.

The teratogenic potential of many of these chemicals is significant, especially in view of the fact that it is impossible to control the amount ingested [161]. Teratogenicity is dependent upon the particular substance abused. Toluene embryopathy serves as an example. Toluene, an aromatic hydrocarbon found in paints and adhesives, readily crosses the placenta; however, the fetus appears unable to metabolize toluene adequately [162]. Animal studies indicate that prenatal exposure to toluene results in intrauterine growth restriction and neurological, cardiovascular, skeletal, and craniofacial abnormalities [163–165]. Reports in humans describe microcephaly, narrow bifrontal diameter, midface hypoplasia, developmental delay, and craniofacial abnormalities, including micrognathia, short palpebral fissures, ear anomalies, unusual scalp hair patterning, smooth philtrum, and thin upper lip. Much phenotypic similarity exists in patients exposed in utero to toluene and those diagnosed with fetal alcohol spectrum disorders [166]. This has raised the possibility of a common mechanism of craniofacial teratogenesis.

Adulterants, substitutes, and contaminants

In order to increase the bulk quantity of illicit drug and maximize profits, drugs are commonly diluted with other substances before being sold [167]. Adulterants are substances that appear similar to the illicit drug in color, structure, and consistency. Common adulterants include talc, sugar, starch, and cellulose. Adulterants are inert and do not possess psychotropic potential; the major complication associated with their incorporation into illicit drugs lies in their ability to embolize. Substitutes, like adulterants, increase the apparent volume of illicit drug by dilution. Substitutes, however, do possess intrinsic psychotropic activity similar to that of the illicit drug. Ephedrine, phenylpropanolamine, and caffeine produce a stimulant effect when added to illicit drugs. Procaine, lidocaine, and other local anesthetics are difficult to distinguish from cocaine. Contaminants are substances used in the preparation of illicit drugs that are not completely removed in the production and purification processes and therefore remain in the final formulation. Contaminants may or may not possess psychotropic or other potentially harmful effects in the user. The presence of adulterants, substitutes, and contaminants in the manufacture of illicit drugs adds further complexity to the determination of potential maternal, fetal, and neonatal toxicities.

Screening

A maternal drug history is a mandatory part of any obstetric or neonatal history and physical. The history should be obtained in a non-threatening manner and should review the use of over-the-counter medications, prescription drugs, tobacco, ethanol, and illicit drugs. When the concern of substance abuse is raised by the history or the examination of the mother, fetus, or neonate, the mother should be informed in a non-judgmental manner. The physician should always be cognizant of the potential for spousal abuse when contemplating the manner in which this information is communicated to the father. Ideally this is accomplished after obtaining maternal permission and with the support of social workers trained in substance abuse. Maternal self-reporting of substance abuse uniformly underestimates the actual frequency of in utero exposure [168]. In addition, it is recognized that drug use cuts across racial and socioeconomic boundaries [169]. Suspected substance abuse should be confirmed not only by elicitation on history but also by appropriate screening of selected maternal, fetal, and neonatal body fluids or tissues. Hospital policies vary, although permission of the mother is generally required for maternal screening, whereas neonatal testing is often considered implied when general consent to treat is provided upon newborn admission.

Urine is the body fluid most frequently tested for substances of abuse. The kidney acts to concentrate drugs and their metabolites, producing higher concentrations in urine than in serum. Because of the lack of proteins and other cellular constituents which can interfere with the equipment used in assays, urine is relatively easy to analyze. Finally, urine offers the benefit of long-term stability if specimens are frozen. Screening tests commonly used include the fluorescence polarization immunoassay and the enzyme multiplication immunoassay technique. False-positive results depend on the extent of cross-reactivity with other substances. Positive results should be confirmed by more definitive methods such as gas chromatography/mass spectrometry. The most serious drawback in using urine to screen for intrauterine substance exposure lies in the fact that drugs and their metabolites are excreted quite quickly, usually within hours to several days after maternal ingestion. Therefore the ability of a urine drug screen to detect any exposure occurring more than 48–72 hours preceding sampling is minimal. Other reasons for false-negative results include concentrations below the detectable limits of the assay and alterations in urinary pH affecting drug solubility [170].

Meconium is the first stool passed by the newborn. It is composed of swallowed amniotic fluid and secretions such as bile, vernix caseosa, epithelial cells, and other debris shed into the lumen of the fetal gastrointestinal tract starting early in the second trimester. Because of its appearance early in gestation, it functions as a reservoir for drugs delivered to the fetus via the umbilical cord and amniotic fluid, and therefore provides a much better chronologic record of intrauterine drug exposure than does urine. Large quantities can easily be obtained in a non-invasive manner. However, it is a tenaciously thick fluid with abundant particulate matter that requires extensive processing before conventional screening methods can be employed. Whereas most hospitals in the USA offer urine toxicological testing, fewer centers are currently testing meconium on a routine basis. In addition, the number of drugs capable of being detected in meconium is limited in comparison with urine. Nevertheless, its utility in increasing the yield of positive exposures for cocaine and other selected drugs is well documented [171].

Fetal hair appears at approximately 8–9 weeks of gestation. As epidermal cells surrounding the dermal papillae divide, the hair shaft grows, and drugs and metabolites in the intrauterine environment are incorporated into the developing hair shafts. Like meconium, hair acts as a depot for drugs of abuse and provides a source for detection of drugs used early in gestation. The timing of exposure during gestation can be approximated by measuring the length of the hairs in the sample, incorporating the average rate of hair growth and preserving the proximal–distal orientation of the hair strands [172]. Obviously, the longer the strands of hair obtained, the better the historical assessment of substance exposure will be: therefore it is best to obtain full-length hair. A core of hair approximately 5 mm in diameter is required. Because of the quantity of hair required the mother is usually a much better source than the neonate. The hair is then washed and any drugs extracted [173]. Quantitative analysis is carried out by radioimmunoassay with a specific antibody or gas chromatography/mass spectrometry. While it is an extremely useful tool in the determination of prenatal drug exposure, hair analysis is not completely foolproof, as various hair treatments may limit the amount of drug which can be extracted [174].

Serum may also be used for drug screening, although its use entails all of the limitations of urine testing, including the inability to establish distant or chronic exposures.

Summary

With the exception of ethanol (fetal alcohol spectrum disorders), tobacco, and toluene (toluene embryopathy), little is definitively known about the potential fetal and neonatal consequences of intrauterine drug exposure. While the many case reports and abundant anecdotal experience allow for the listing of numerous associations of the substances of abuse with various malformations, disruptions, and neurodevelopmental disabilities, few well-designed, controlled, prospective clinical studies with appropriate follow-up have been carried out. The further elucidation of embryopathic effects will require expansion of the concept of teratogenesis beyond gross morphologic abnormalities, to include postnatal development (behavioral teratology). A lack of gross structural anomalies implies neither normal molecular structure nor normal physiologic function. Direct damage to DNA is but one mechanism by which drugs may affect the fetus. The cytoplasm is truly "where the action is," and it is in this dynamic milieu that drugs may exert their effects on transcription, mRNA stability, and other processes vital to normal cellular function. This is an especially important concept in view of the many neurobehavioral problems purportedly associated with prenatal substance abuse that occur in the absence of gross nervous system malformations. Further clinical studies, coupled with bench research at the molecular level, should provide a better understanding of the impact of prenatal drug use on the fetus.

The fetal and neonatal brain exhibits remarkable resilience. Although prenatal drug exposure may create vulnerability, it is clear that the majority of children, given appropriate care, stimulation, and follow-up can overcome such potential insults. It is also clear that the quality of the postnatal environment may be just as important as, if not more important than, the intrauterine environment in determining long-term outcome. Although children with prenatal drug exposure have been shown to attain a performance level equal to non-exposed peer groups, it is also true that such peer groups may function at levels below the national norm. This illustrates the profound effect other factors such as poverty and malnutrition can have on child development. It also illustrates how elimination of these other factors can positively impact the development of our youth.

The transition to an extrauterine existence is a difficult task. A baby must learn what actions elicit the desired responses from its parents. Caring for a newborn is a tremendous challenge, and parents must learn to interpret their baby's wants and needs and be able to respond appropriately. A neonate exposed to drugs in utero may be lethargic or irritable and thus unable to process stimuli from the outside world. Substance-abusing parents may be unable to care for themselves adequately, let alone their newborn. The potential for frustration, under- or overstimulation, neglect, and abuse is great. The importance of family support, beyond that provided by substance abuse programs, cannot be underestimated. Multidisciplinary assessment and intervention programs must be easily accessible to those most in need of their services. Intrauterine drug exposure, unlike many other hazards faced by the fetus and neonate, is potentially a preventable problem.

Finally, criminalization of drug use and legitimization of the concept of "fetal abuse" in regard to prenatal drug use is not the means to achieve adequate care for a mother and her unborn child. For physicians who have not experienced, either personally or professionally, a dependency disorder, it is difficult to understand how a woman can knowingly risk potential harm to her unborn child. We can only understand when we realize that these women, plagued by a society that not only reinforces their feelings of inadequacy but also convinces them that inadequacy is their fault, are ridden with guilt and self-deprecation and therefore easily succumb to the temporary but nevertheless real reprieve offered by illicit drugs.

References

1. Yaffe SJ. Introduction. In *Drugs in Pregnancy and Lactation*, 6th edn. Philadelphia, PA: Lippincott, Williams & Wilkins, 2002: xv–xxii.

2. Committee on Substance Abuse, American Academy of Pediatrics. Drug-exposed infants. *Pediatrics* 1995; 96: 364–7.

3. Kraemer K. Placental transfer of drugs. *Neonatal Netw* 1997; 16: 65–7.

4. Mahone PR, Scott K, Sleggs G, et al. Cocaine and metabolites in amniotic fluid may prolong fetal drug exposure. *Am J Obstet Gynecol* 1994; 171: 465–9.

5. Brent RL. Environmental causes of human congenital malformations: the pediatrician's role in dealing with these complex clinical problems caused by a multiplicity of environmental and genetic factors. *Pediatrics* 2004; 113: 957–68.

6. Snodgrass SR. Cocaine babies: a result of multiple teratogenic influences. *J Child Neurol* 1994; 9: 227–33.

7. Sampson PD, Streissguth AP, Bookstein FL, et al. Incidence of fetal alcohol syndrome and prevalence of alcohol-related neurodevelopmental disorder. *Teratology* 1997; 56: 317–26.

8. Lupton C, Burd L, Harwood R. Cost of fetal alcohol spectrum disorders. *Am J Med Genet* 2004; 127C: 42–50.

9. Harwood H. Updating estimates of the economic costs of alcohol abuse in the United States: estimates, updated methods, and data. *Report Prepared by the Lewin Group*. Bethesda, MD, National Institute on Alcohol Abuse and Alcoholism, 2000.

10. Day NL, Richardson GA. Prenatal alcohol exposure: a continuum of effects. *Semin Perinatol* 1991; 15: 271–9.

11. Jacobson JL, Jacobson SW, Sokol RJ, et al. Effects of alcohol use, smoking, and illicit drug use on fetal growth in black infants. *J Pediatr* 1994; 124: 757–64.

12. Jones KL, Smith DW, Ulleland CW, et al. Pattern of malformation in offspring of alcoholic mothers. *Lancet* 1973; 1: 1267–71.

13. Barr HM, Streissguth AP. Identifying maternal self-reported alcohol use associated with fetal alcohol spectrum disorders. *Alcohol Clin Exp Res* 2001; 25: 283–7.

14. Stratton KR, Howe CJ, Battaglia FC, eds. *Fetal Alcohol Syndrome: Diagnosis, Epidemiology, Prevention, and Treatment*. Washington, DC: National Academy Press, 1996.

15. Hoyme HE, May PA, Kalberg WO, et al. A practical clinical approach to diagnosis of fetal alcohol spectrum disorders: clarification of the 1996 Institute of Medicine criteria. *Pediatrics* 2005; 115: 39–47.

16. Swayze VW, Johnson VP, Hanson JW, et al. Magnetic resonance imaging of brain anomalies in fetal alcohol syndrome. *Pediatrics* 1997; 99: 232–40.

17. Clarren SK, Alvord EC, Sumi SM, et al. Brain malformations related to prenatal exposure to ethanol. *J Pediatr* 1978; 92: 64–7.

18. Spadoni AD, McGee CL, Fryer SL, et al. Neuroimaging and fetal alcohol spectrum disorders. *Neurosci Biobehav Rev* 2007; 31: 231–45.

19. Charness ME, Safran RM, Perides G. Ethanol inhibits neural cell–cell adhesion. *J Biol Chem* 1994; 269: 9304–9.

20. DeJonge MH, Zachman RD. The effect of maternal ethanol ingestion on fetal rat heart vitamin A: a model for fetal alcohol syndrome. *Pediatr Res* 1995; 37: 418–23.

21. Naus CCG, Bechberger JF. Effect of prenatal ethanol exposure on postnatal neural gene expression in the rat. *Dev Genet* 1991; 12: 293–8.

22. Miller MW. Prenatal exposure to ethanol delays the schedule and rate of migration of neurons to rat somatosensory cortex. Fifth Congress of the International Society for Biomedical Research on Alcoholism, Toronto, Canada, 1990.

23. Holzman C, Paneth N, Little R, et al. Perinatal brain injury in premature infants born to mothers using alcohol in pregnancy. *Pediatrics* 1995; 95: 66–73.

24. Armant DR, Saunders DE. Exposure of embryonic cells to alcohol: contrasting effects during preimplantation and postimplantation development. *Semin Perinatol* 1996; 20: 127–39.

25. Ahlgren SC, Thakur V, Bronner-Fraser M. Sonic hedgehog rescues cranial neural crest from cell death induced by ethanol exposure. *Proc Natl Acad Sci USA* 2002; 99: 10476–81.

26. Peng Y, Yang PH, Ng SSM, et al. A critical role of *Pax6* in alcohol induced fetal microcephaly. *Neurobiol Dis* 2004; 16: 370–6.

27. Chrisman K, Kenney R, Comin J, et al. Gestational ethanol exposure disrupts the expression of *Fgf8* and Sonic hedgehog during limb patterning. *Birth Defects Res A Clin Mol Teratol* 2004; 70: 163–71.

28. Druse MJ, Kuo A, Tajuddin N. Effects of *in utero* ethanol exposure on the developing serotonergic system. *Alcohol Clin Exp Res* 1991; 15: 678–84.

29. Pinazo-Duran MD, Renau-Piqueras J, Guerri C. Developmental changes in the optic nerve related to ethanol consumption in pregnant rats: analysis of the ethanol-exposed optic nerve. *Teratology* 1993; 48: 305–22.

30. Church MW, Gerkin KP. Hearing disorders in children with fetal alcohol syndrome: findings from case reports. *Pediatrics* 1988; 82: 147–54.

31. Syslak PH, Nathaniel EJH, Novak C, et al. Fetal alcohol effects on the postnatal development of the rat myocardium: an ultrastructural and morphometric analysis. *Exp Mol Pathol* 1994; 60: 158–72.

32. Gage JC, Sulik KK. Pathogenesis of ethanol-induced hydronephrosis and hydroureter as demonstrated following in vivo exposure of mouse embryos. *Teratology* 1991; 44: 299–312.

33. Autti-Rämö I, Fagerlund A, Ervalahti N, et al. Fetal alcohol spectrum disorders in Finland: clinical delineation of 77 older children and adolescents. *Am J Med Genet A* 2006; 140: 137–43.

34. Day NL, Richardson G, Robles N, et al. Effect of prenatal alcohol exposure on growth and morphology of offspring at 8 months of age. *Pediatrics* 1990; 85: 748–52.

35. Breese CR, D'Costa A, Ingram RL, et al. Long-term suppression of insulin-like growth factor-1 in rats after *in utero* ethanol exposure: relationship to somatic growth. *J Pharmacol Exp Ther* 1993; 264: 448–57.

36. Mauceri HJ, Lee W, Conway S. Effect of ethanol on insulin-like growth factor-II release from fetal organs. *Alcohol Clin Exp Res* 1994; 18: 35–41.

37. Guo W, Gregg JP, Fonkalsrud EW. Effect of maternal ethanol intake on fetal rabbit gastrointestinal development. *J Pediatr Surg* 1994; 29: 1030–4.

38. American College of Obstetricians and Gynecologists. Breastfeeding: maternal and infant aspects. *Educational Bulletin Number 258*. Washington, DC: ACOG, 2000.

39. Little RE, Anderson KW, Ervin CH, et al. Maternal alcohol use during breast-feeding and infant mental and motor development at one year. *N Engl J Med* 1989; 321: 425–30.

40. Graham JM, Hanson JW, Darby BL, et al. Independent dysmorphology evaluations at birth and 4 years of age for children exposed to varying amounts of alcohol in utero. Pediatrics 1988; 81: 772–8.

41. Streissguth AP. The behavioral teratology of alcohol: performance, behavioral, and intellectual deficits in prenatally exposed children. In West JR, ed., Alcohol and Brain Development. New York, NY: Oxford University Press, 1986: 3–44.

42. Streissguth AP, Aase JM, Clarren SK, et al. Fetal alcohol syndrome in adolescents and adults. JAMA 1991; 265: 1961–7.

43. Kirkland SA, Dodds LA, Brosky G. The natural history of smoking during pregnancy among women in Nova Scotia. CMAJ 2000; 163: 281–2.

44. Kendrick JS, Merritt RK. Women and smoking: an update for the 1990s. Am J Obstet Gynecol 1996; 175: 528–35.

45. Secker-Walker RH, Vacek PM, Flynn BS, et al. Smoking in pregnancy, exhaled carbon monoxide, and birth weight. Obstet Gynecol 1997; 89: 648–53.

46. Visnjevac V, Mikov M. Smoking and carboxyhemoglobin concentrations in mothers and their newborn infants. Toxicology 1986; 5: 175–7.

47. Jazayeri A, Tsibris JCM, Spellacy WN. Umbilical cord plasma erythropoietin levels in pregnancies complicated by maternal smoking. Am J Obstet Gynecol 1998; 178: 433–5.

48. Jordanov JS. Cotinine concentrations in amniotic fluid and urine of smoking, passive smoking and non-smoking pregnant women at term and in the urine of their neonates on the 1st day of life. Eur J Pediatr 1990; 149: 734–7.

49. Bernstein IM, Plociennik K, Stahle S, et al. Impact of maternal cigarette smoking on fetal growth and body composition. Am J Obstet Gynecol 2000; 183: 883–6.

50. Bardy AH, Seppälä T, Lillsunde P, et al. Objectively measured tobacco exposure during pregnancy: neonatal effects and relation to maternal smoking. Br J Obstet Gynaecol 1993; 100: 721–6.

51. Cliver SP, Goldenberg RL, Cutter GR, et al. The effect of cigarette smoking on neonatal anthropometric measurements. Obstet Gynecol 1995; 85: 625–30.

52. Resnik R, Brink GW, Wilkes M. Catecholamine-mediated reduction in uterine blood flow after nicotine infusion in the pregnant ewe. J Clin Invest 1979; 63: 1133–6.

53. Burton GJ, Palmer ME, Dalton KJ. Morphometric differences between the placental vasculature of non-smokers, smokers and ex-smokers. Br J Obstet Gynaecol 1989; 96: 907–15.

54. Gabrial R, Alsat E, Evain-Brion D. Alteration of epidermal growth factor receptor in placental membranes of smokers: relationship with intrauterine growth retardation. Am J Obstet Gynecol 1994; 170: 1238–43.

55. Slotkin TA, McCook EC, Lappi SE, et al. Altered development of basal and forskolin-stimulated adenylate cyclase activity in brain regions of rats exposed to nicotine prenatally. Dev Brain Res 1992; 68: 233–9.

56. Khoury MJ, Gomez-Frias M, Mulinare J. Does maternal cigarette smoking during pregnancy cause cleft lip and palate in offspring? Am J Dis Child 1989; 143: 333–7.

57. Ananth CV, Savitz DA, Luther ER. Maternal cigarette smoking as a risk factor for placental abruption, placenta previa, and uterine bleeding in pregnancy. Am J Epidemiol 1996; 144: 881–9.

58. Castles A, Adams K, Melvin CL, et al. Effects of smoking during pregnancy: five meta-analyses. Am J Prev Med 1999; 16: 208–15.

59. Naeye RL. Abruptio placentae and placenta previa: frequency, perinatal mortality, and cigarette smoking. Obstet Gynecol 1980; 55: 701–4.

60. Ananth CV, Getahun D, Peltier MR, et al. Placental abruption in term and preterm gestations: evidence for heterogeneity in clinical pathways. Obstet Gynecol 2006; 107: 785–92.

61. Usta IM, Hobeika EM, Musa AA, et al. Placenta previa–accreta: risk factors and complications. Am J Obstet Gynecol 2005; 193: 1045–49.

62. Nabet C, Ancel PY, Burguet A, et al. Smoking during pregnancy and preterm birth according to obstetric history: French national perinatal surveys. Paediatr Perinat Epidemiol 2005; 19: 88–96.

63. Salihu HM, Sharma PP, Getahun G. Prenatal tobacco use and risk of stillbirth: a case–control and bi-directional case–crossover study. Nicotine Tob Res 2008; 10: 159–66.

64. Arbeille P, Bosc M, Vaillant MC, et al. Nicotine-induced changes in the cerebral circulation in ovine fetuses. Am J Perinatol 1992; 79: 645–8.

65. Franco P, Groswasser J, Hassid S, et al. Prenatal exposure to cigarette smoking is associated with a decrease in arousal in infants. J Pediatr 1999; 135: 34–8.

66. Hoffman HJ, Hillman LS. Epidemiology of the sudden infant death syndrome: maternal, neonatal, and postneonatal risk factors. Clin Perinatol 1992; 19: 717–37.

67. Takashima S, Armstrong D, Becker LE, et al. Cerebral hypoperfusion in the sudden infant death syndrome, brainstem gliosis and vasculature. Ann Neurol 1978; 4: 257–62.

68. Drews CD, Murphy CC, Yeargin-Allsop M, et al. The relationship between idiopathic mental retardation and maternal smoking during pregnancy. Pediatrics 1996; 97: 547–53.

69. Olds DL, Henderson CR, Tatelbaum R. Intellectual impairment in children of women who smoke cigarettes during pregnancy. Pediatrics 1994; 93: 221–7.

70. John EM, Savitz DA, Sandler DP. Prenatal exposure to parents' smoking and childhood cancer. Am J Epidemiol 1991; 133: 123–32.

71. Charlton A. Children and passive smoking: a review. J Fam Pract 1994; 38: 267–77.

72. Paulson RB, Shanfeld J, Mullet D, et al. Prenatal smokeless tobacco effects on the rat fetus. J Craniofac Genet Dev Biol 1994; 14: 16–25.

73. Ostrea EM, Knapp DK, Romera A, et al. Meconium analysis to assess fetal exposure to nicotine by active and passive maternal smoking. J Pediatr 1994; 124: 471–6.

74. Makin J, Fried PA, Watkinson B. A comparison of active and passive smoking during pregnancy: long-term effects. Neurotoxicol Teratol 1991; 13: 5–12.

75. Witschi H, Lundgaard SM, Rajini P, et al. Effects of exposure to nicotine and to sidestream smoke on pregnancy outcome in rats. Toxicol Lett 1994; 71: 279–86.

76. Davis DL. Paternal smoking and fetal health. Lancet 1991; 337: 123.

77. Klonoff-Cohen HS, Edelstein SL, Lefkowitz ES, et al. The effect of passive smoking and tobacco exposure through breast milk on sudden infant death syndrome. JAMA 1995; 273: 795–8.

78. Selden BS, Clark RF, Curry SC. Marijuana. Emerg Med Clin North Am 1990; 8: 8527–39.

79. Wu TC, Tashkin DP, Djahed B, *et al.* Pulmonary hazards of smoking marijuana as compared with tobacco. *N Engl J Med* 1988; **318**: 347–51.

80. Cornelius MD, Taylor PM, Geva D, *et al.* Prenatal tobacco and marijuana use among adolescents: effects on offspring gestational age, growth, and morphology. *Pediatrics* 1995; **95**: 738–43.

81. English DR, Hulse GK, Milne E, *et al.* Maternal cannabis use and birth weight: a meta-analysis. *Addiction* 1997; **92**: 1553–60.

82. Fried PA, Watkinson B, Gray R. Growth from birth to early adolescence in offspring prenatally exposed to cigarettes and marijuana. *Neurotoxicol Teratol* 1999; **21**: 513–25.

83. Fried PA, Makin JE. Neonatal behavioral correlates of prenatal exposure to marijuana, cigarettes and alcohol in a low risk population. *Neurotoxicol Teratol* 1987; **9**: 1–7.

84. Dahl RE, Scher MS, Williamson DE, *et al.* A longitudinal study of prenatal marijuana use: effects on sleep and arousal at age 3 years. *Arch Pediatr Adolesc Med* 1995; **149**: 145–50.

85. Fried PA. Prenatal exposure to marijuana and tobacco during infancy, early and middle childhood: effects and an attempt at synthesis. *Arch Toxicol Suppl* 1995; **17**: 233–60.

86. Fried PA. The Ottawa Prenatal Prospective Study (OPPS): methodologic issues and findings. It's easy to throw the baby out with the bathwater. *Life Sci* 1995; **56**: 2159–68.

87. Farrar HC, Kearns GL. Cocaine: clinical pharmacology and toxicology. *J Pediatr* 1989; **115**: 665–75.

88. Bailey DN. Cocaine and cocaethylene binding to human placenta in vitro. *Am J Obstet Gynecol* 1997; **177**: 527–31.

89. Jones KL. Developmental pathogenesis of defects associated with prenatal cocaine exposure: fetal vascular disruption. *Clin Perinatol* 1991; **18**: 139–46.

90. Arbeille P, Maulik D, Salihagic A, *et al.* Effect of long-term cocaine administration to pregnant ewes on fetal hemodynamics, oxygenation, and growth. *Obstet Gynecol* 1997; **90**: 795–802.

91. Monga M, Chmielowiec S, Andres RL, *et al.* Cocaine alters placental production of thromboxane and prostacyclin. *Am J Obstet Gynecol* 1994; **171**: 965–9.

92. Burkett G, Yasin SY, Palow D, *et al.* Patterns of cocaine binging: effect on pregnancy. *Am J Obstet Gynecol* 1994; **171**: 372–9.

93. Dicke JM, Verges DK, Polakoski KL. The effects of cocaine on neutral amino acid uptake by human placental basal membrane vesicles. *Am J Obstet Gynecol* 1994; **171**: 485–91.

94. Bandstra ES, Morrow CE, Anthony JC, *et al.* Intrauterine growth of full-term infants: impact of prenatal cocaine exposure. *Pediatrics* 2001; **108**: 1309–19.

95. Bateman DA, Chiriboga CA. Dose-response effect of cocaine on newborn head circumference. *Pediatrics* 2000; **106**: e33.

96. Kuhn L, Kline J, Ng S, *et al.* Cocaine use during pregnancy and intrauterine growth retardation: new insights based on maternal hair tests. *Am J Epidemiol* 2000; **152**: 112–19.

97. Viscarello RR, Ferguson DD, Nores J, *et al.* Limb–body wall complex associated with cocaine abuse: further evidence of cocaine's teratogenicity. *Obstet Gynecol* 1992; **80**: 523–6.

98. Hoyme HE, Jones KL, Dixon SD, *et al.* Prenatal cocaine exposure and fetal vascular disruption. *Pediatrics* 1990; **85**: 743–7.

99. Dominguez R, Vila-Coro AA, Slopis JM, *et al.* Brain and ocular abnormalities in infants with *in utero* exposure to cocaine and other street drugs. *Am J Dis Child* 1991; **145**: 688–95.

100. Chavez GF, Mulinare J, Cordero JF. Maternal cocaine use during early pregnancy as a risk factor for congenital urogenital anomalies. *JAMA* 1989; **262**: 795–8.

101. Kain ZN, Kain TS, Scarpelli EM. Cocaine exposure *in utero*: perinatal development and neonatal manifestations: review. *Clin Toxicol* 1992; **30**: 607–36.

102. Dinsmoor MJ, Irons SJ, Christmas JT. Preterm rupture of the membranes associated with recent cocaine use. *Am J Obstet Gynecol* 1994; **171**: 305–9.

103. Kliegman RM, Madura D, Kiwi R, *et al.* Relation of maternal cocaine use to the risks of prematurity and low birth weight. *J Pediatr* 1994; **124**: 751–6.

104. Iriye BK, Bristow RE, Hsu CD, *et al.* Uterine rupture associated with recent antepartum cocaine abuse. *Obstet Gynecol* 1994; **83**: 840–1.

105. Macones GA, Sehdev HM, Parry S, *et al.* The association between maternal cocaine use and placenta previa. *Am J Obstet Gynecol* 1997; **177**: 1097–100.

106. Czyrko C, Del Pin CA, O'Neill JA, *et al.* Maternal cocaine abuse and necrotizing enterocolitis: outcome and survival. *J Pediatr Surg* 1991; **26**: 414–18.

107. Büyükünal C, Kiliç N, Dervisoglu S, *et al.* Maternal cocaine abuse resulting in necrotizing enterocolitis: an experimental study in a rat model. *Acta Paediatr* 1994; **396**: 91–3.

108. Chasnoff IJ, Bussey ME, Savich R, *et al.* Perinatal cerebral infarction and maternal cocaine use. *J Pediatr* 1986; **108**: 456–9.

109. Singer LT, Yamashita TS, Hawkins S, *et al.* Increased incidence of intraventricular hemorrhage and developmental delay in cocaine-exposed, very low birth weight infants. *J Pediatr* 1994; **124**: 765–71.

110. Sims ME, Walther FJ. Antenatal brain injury and maternal cocaine use. *J Perinatol* 1989; **9**: 349–50.

111. Behnke M, Eyler FD, Conlon M, *et al.* Incidence and description of structural brain abnormalities in newborns exposed to cocaine. *J Pediatr* 1998; **132**: 291–4.

112. Mott SH, Packer RJ, Soldin SJ. Neurologic manifestations of cocaine exposure in childhood. *Pediatrics* 1994; **93**: 557–60.

113. Chen C, Duara S, Neto GS, *et al.* Respiratory instability in neonates with *in utero* exposure to cocaine. *J Pediatr* 1991; **119**: 111–13.

114. Tronick EZ, Frank DA, Cabral H, *et al.* Late dose–response effects of prenatal cocaine exposure on newborn neurobehavioral performance. *Pediatrics* 1996; **98**: 76–83.

115. Chan K, Dodd PA, Day L, *et al.* Fetal catecholamine, cardiovascular, and neurobehavioral responses to cocaine. *Am J Obstet Gynecol* 1992; **167**: 1616–23.

116. Knapp S, Mandell AJ. Narcotic drugs: effect on the serotonin biosynthetic systems of the brain. *Science* 1972; **177**: 1209–11.

117. Durand DJ, Espinoza AM, Nickerson BG. Association between prenatal cocaine exposure and sudden infant death syndrome. *J Pediatr* 1990; **117**: 909–11.

118. Bauchner H, Zuckerman B, McClain M, *et al.* Risk of sudden infant death syndrome among infants with *in utero* exposure to cocaine. *J Pediatr* 1988; **113**: 831–4.

119. Mayes LC, Granger RH, Frank MA, *et al.* Neurobehavioral profiles of neonates exposed to cocaine prenatally. *Pediatrics* 1993; **91**: 778–83.

120. Eisen LN, Field TM, Bandstra ES, *et al.* Perinatal cocaine effects on neonatal stress behavior and performance on the Brazelton scale. *Pediatrics* 1991; **88**: 477–80.

121. Eyler FD, Behnke M, Conlon M, *et al.* Birth outcome from a prospective, matched study of prenatal crack/ cocaine use. I. Interactive and dose effects on health and growth. *Pediatrics* 1998; **101**: 229–37.

122. Eyler FD, Behnke M, Conlon M, *et al.* Birth outcome from a prospective, matched study of prenatal crack/ cocaine use. II. Interactive and dose effects on neurobehavioral assessment. *Pediatrics* 1998; **101**: 237–41.

123. Frank DA, Augustyn M, Knight WG, *et al.* Growth, development, and behavior in early childhood following prenatal cocaine exposure: a systematic review. *JAMA* 2001; **285**: 1613–25.

124. Roland EH, Volpe JJ. Effect of maternal cocaine use on the fetus and newborn: review of the literature. *Pediatr Neurosci* 1989; **15**: 88–94.

125. Oro A, Dixon S. Perinatal cocaine and methamphetamine exposure: maternal and neonatal correlates. *J Pediatr* 1987; **111**: 571–8.

126. Chasnoff IJ, Lewis DE, Squires L. Cocaine intoxication in a breast-fed infant. *Pediatrics* 1987; **80**: 836–8.

127. Chaney NE, Franke J, Waddington WB. Cocaine convulsions in a breast-feeding baby. *J Pediatr* 1988; **112**: 134–5.

128. Hulse GK, Milne E, English DR, *et al.* The relationship between maternal use of heroin and methadone and infant birth weight. *Addiction* 1997; **92**: 1571–9.

129. Barg J, Rius A, Bem WT, *et al.* Differential development of beta-endorphin and mu-opioid binding sites in mouse brain. *Dev Brain Res* 1992; **66**: 71–6.

130. Suguihara C, Bancalari E. Substance abuse during pregnancy: effects on respiratory function in the infant. *Semin Perinatol* 1991; **15**: 302–9.

131. Olson GD, Lees MH. Ventilatory response to carbon dioxide of infants following chronic prenatal methadone exposure. *J Pediatr* 1980; **96**: 983–9.

132. Bunikowski R, Grimmer I, Heiser A, *et al.* Neurodevelopmental outcome after prenatal exposure to opiates. *Eur J Pediatr* 1998; **157**: 724–30.

133. Smialek JE, Monforte JR, Aronow R, *et al.* Methadone deaths in children: a continuing problem. *JAMA* 1977; **238**: 2516–17.

134. Committee on Drugs, American Academy of Pediatrics. Transfer of drugs and other chemicals into human milk. *Pediatrics* 1989; **84**: 924–36.

135. Idänpään-Heikkilä JE, Jouppila PI, Puolakka JO, *et al.* Placental transfer and fetal metabolism of diazepam in early pregnancy. *Am J Obstet Gynecol* 1971; **109**: 1011–16.

136. Laegreid L, Olegärd R, Walström J, *et al.* Teratogenic effects of benzodiazepine use during pregnancy. *J Pediatr* 1989; **114**: 126–31.

137. Eros E, Czeizel AE, Rockenbauer M, *et al.* A population-based case control teratologic study of nitrazepam, medazepam, tofisopam, alprazolum and clonazepam treatment during pregnancy. *Eur J Obstet Gynecol Reprod Biol* 2002; **101**: 147–54.

138. Dessens AB, Cohen-Kettenis PT, Mellenbergh GJ, *et al.* Association of prenatal phenobarbital and phenytoin exposure with small head size at birth and with learning problems. *Acta Paediatr* 2000; **89**: 533–41.

139. Rementeria JL, Bhatt K. Withdrawal symptoms in neonates from intrauterine exposure to diazepam. *J Pediatr* 1977; **90**: 123–6.

140. Stek AM, Baker RS, Fisher BK, *et al.* Fetal responses to maternal and fetal methamphetamine administration in sheep. *Am J Obstet Gynecol* 1995; **173**: 1592–8.

141. Little BB, Snell LM, Gilstrap LC. Methamphetamine abuse during pregnancy: outcome and fetal effects. *Obstet Gynecol* 1988; **72**: 541–4.

142. Ramin SM, Little BB, Trimmer KJ, *et al.* Peripartum methamphetamine use in a large urban population. *J Maternal Fetal Med* 1994; **3**: 101–3.

143. Nasif FJ, Cuadra GR, Ramirez OA. Permanent alteration of cerebral noradrenergic system by prenatally administered amphetamine. *Brain Res Dev Brain Res* 1999; **112**: 181–8.

144. Tavares MA, Silva MC. Differential effects of prenatal exposure to cocaine and amphetamine on growth parameters and morphometry of the prefrontal cortex in the rat. *Ann NY Acad Sci* 1996; **801**: 256–73.

145. Tavares MA, Silva MC, Silva-Araujo A, *et al.* Effects of prenatal exposure to amphetamine in the medial prefrontal cortex of the rat. *Int J Dev Neurosci* 1996; **14**: 585–96.

146. Chang L, Smith LM, LoPresti C, *et al.* Smaller subcortical volumes and cognitive deficits in children with prenatal methamphetamine exposure. *Psychiatry Res* 2004; **132**: 95–106.

147. Dixon SD, Bejar R. Echoencephalographic findings in neonates associated with maternal cocaine and methamphetamine use: incidence and clinical correlates. *J Pediatr* 1989; **115**: 770–8.

148. Eriksson M, Larsson C, Zetterström R. Amphetamine addiction and pregnancy. *Acta Obstet Gynecol Scand* 1981; **60**: 253–9.

149. Oro AS, Dixon SP. Perinatal cocaine and methamphetamine exposure: maternal and neonatal correlates. *J Pediatr* 1987; **111**: 571–8.

150. Baldridge EB, Bessen HA. Phencyclidine. *Emerg Med Clin North Am* 1990; **8**: 541–50.

151. Strauss AA, Modanlou HD, Bosu SK. Neonatal manifestations of maternal phencyclidene (PCP) abuse. *Pediatrics* 1981; **68**: 550–2.

152. Mattson MP, Rychlik B, Cheng B. Degenerative and axon outgrowth-altering effects of phencyclidine in human fetal cerebral cortical cells. *J Pharmacol* 1992; **31**: 279–91.

153. Golden NL, Kuhnert BR, Sokol RJ, *et al.* Neonatal manifestations of maternal phencyclidene exposure. *J Perinat Med* 1987; **15**: 185–91.

154. Rahbar F, Fomufod A, White D, *et al.* Impact of intrauterine exposure to phencyclidene (PCP) and cocaine on neonates. *J Natl Med Assoc* 1993; **85**: 349–52.

155. Kaufman KR, Petrucha RA, Pitts FN, *et al.* PCP in amniotic fluid and breast milk: case report. *J Clin Psychiatry* 1983; **44**: 269–70.

156. Eller JL, Morton JA. Bizarre deformities in offspring of users of lysergic acid diethylamide. *N Engl J Med* 1970; **283**: 395–7.

157. Hecht F, Beals RK, Lees MH, *et al.* Lysergic-acid-diethylamide and

cannabis as possible teratogens in man. *Lancet* 1968; **2**: 1087.

158. Carakushansky G, Neu RL, Gardner LI. Lysergide and cannabis as possible teratogens in man. *Lancet* 1969; **1**: 150–1.

159. Jacobson CB, Berlin CM. Possible reproductive detriments in LSD users. *JAMA* 1972; **222**: 1367–73.

160. Linden CH. Volatile substances of abuse. *Emerg Med Clin North Am* 1990; **8**: 559–78.

161. Jones HE, Balster RL. Inhalant abuse in pregnancy. *Obstet Gynecol Clin North Am* 1998; **25**: 153–67.

162. Ghantous H, Danielsson BRG. Placental transfer and distribution of toluene, xylene, and benzene and their metabolites during gestation in mice. *Biol Res Pregnancy* 1986; **7**: 98–105.

163. Stoltenbeurg-Didinger G, Altenkirch H, Wagner M. Neurotoxicity of organic solvent mixtures: embryotoxicity and fetotoxicity. *Neurotoxicol Teratol* 1990; **12**: 585–9.

164. Gospe SM, Zhou SS. Prenatal exposure to toluene results in abnormal neurogenesis and migration in rat somatosensory cortex. *Pediatr Res* 2000; **47**: 362–8.

165. Gospe SM, Zhou SS. Toluene abuse embryopathy: longitudinal neurodevelopmental effects of prenatal exposure to toluene in rats. *Reprod Toxicol* 1998; **12**: 119–26.

166. Pearson MA, Hoyme HE, Seaver LH, *et al.* Toluene embryopathy: delineation of the phenotype and comparison with fetal alcohol syndrome. *Pediatrics* 1994; **93**: 211–15.

167. Schauben JL. Adulterants and substitutes. *Emerg Med Clin North Am* 1990; **8**: 595–611.

168. Schutzman DL, Frankenfield-Chernicoff M, Clatterbaugh HE, *et al.* Incidence of intrauterine cocaine exposure in a suburban setting. *Pediatrics* 1991; **88**: 825–7.

169. Chasnoff IJ, Landres HJ, Barrett ME. The prevalence of illicit-drug or alcohol use during pregnancy and discrepancies in mandatory reporting in Pinellas County, Florida. *N Engl J Med* 1990; **322**: 1202–6.

170. Farrar HC, Kearns GL. Cocaine: clinical pharmacology and toxicology. *J Pediatr* 1989; **115**: 665–75.

171. Ryan RM, Wagner CL, Schultz JM, *et al.* Meconium analysis for improved identification of infants exposed to cocaine *in utero. J Pediatr* 1994; **125**: 435–40.

172. Saitoh M, Uzuka M, Sakamoto M. Rate of hair growth. *Adv Biol Skin* 1969; **9**: 183–201.

173. Baumgartner WA, Hill VA, Bland WH. Hair analysis for drug abuse. *J Forensic Sci* 1989; **34**: 1433–53.

174. Marques PR, Tippetts AS, Branch DG. Cocaine in the hair of mother–infant pairs: quantitative analysis and correlations with urine measurements and self report. *Am J Drug Alcohol Abuse* 1993; **19**: 159–75.

Hypertensive disorders of pregnancy

Bonnie Dwyer and Deirdre J. Lyell

Introduction

Hypertensive disorders in pregnancy complicate up to 12–22% of all pregnancies and are the second leading cause of maternal deaths [1]. They also contribute significantly to neonatal morbidity and mortality.

The National High Blood Pressure Education Program Working Group on High Blood Pressure in Pregnancy separates hypertensive disease in pregnancy into four categories: (1) *chronic hypertension*, (2) *gestational hypertension*, (3) *pre-eclampsia*, and (4) *superimposed pre-eclampsia* [2]. This classification is an effort to create uniformity in diagnosis for diagnostic and research purposes. It is designed to describe distinct diseases with distinct pathophysiologies, and therefore distinct associated maternal and neonatal morbidity and mortality. However, hypertensive disease in pregnancy may represent a spectrum of disease, and thus the distinctions between these classifications can be blurred. This chapter will separately discuss chronic hypertension, gestational hypertension, and pre-eclampsia/superimposed pre-eclampsia and their known fetal effects. Treatment and intervention will also be discussed.

Fetal and neonatal effects of hypertension and pre-eclampsia are mainly due to alterations in placental perfusion, iatrogenic prematurity, and effects of maternal medications. In addition, there has been widespread interest in a controversial theory called the "Barker hypothesis." This postulates that the intrauterine environment may program fetal physiology to be predisposed to specific adult diseases. Data used to support this theory include multiple retrospective studies which have correlated low birthweight (intrauterine growth restriction, IUGR) to multiple diverse adult diseases ranging from hypertension, coronary artery disease, and type 2 diabetes to depression and schizophrenia [3]. Whether these correlations imply that adult diseases are specifically a result of intrauterine environment, or whether they rather reflect the multiple causes of IUGR and are markers for genetic heredity and/or childhood environment, is unclear.

Hypertension in pregnancy

Integral to understanding hypertension in pregnancy is the fact that in normal pregnancy maternal blood pressure decreases early and nadirs between 16 and 20 weeks. Subsequently, blood pressure gradually increases, returning to near baseline by the end of the third trimester [4]. Thus if a patient presents with hypertension in the second or third trimester without documented blood pressure measurements from pre-pregnancy or the first trimester, it may be impossible to know whether these elevated blood pressures represent a chronic condition or a pregnancy-related one. Distinguishing chronic hypertension, gestational hypertension, and pre-eclampsia is important because the diagnosis correlates strongly with the disease course and with maternal, fetal, and neonatal outcomes. Diagnosis, therefore, informs clinical management.

Chronic hypertension

Chronic hypertension is defined as hypertension (systolic blood pressure ≥ 140 mmHg or diastolic blood pressure ≥ 90) that is diagnosed pre-pregnancy or at < 20 weeks' gestation (Table 11.1). If hypertension is diagnosed after 20 weeks' gestation, but does not resolve postpartum, it is also classified as chronic hypertension [1,2].

Chronic hypertension affects both maternal and fetal physiology. Ideally a woman with chronic hypertension should be evaluated prior to pregnancy or early in pregnancy. First, she should be classified as having primary or secondary hypertension. Secondary causes of hypertension should be suspected if blood pressure is particularly high or particularly difficult to control (high doses of a single antihypertensive or multiple antihypertensives are needed). Secondary causes of hypertension include coarctation of the aorta, underlying renal disease, renal artery stenosis, pheochromocytoma, Cushing's disease, hyperthyroidism, malignant hypertension, and drug-induced hypertension. They are important to identify because they necessitate treatment of an underlying cause as well as control of the blood pressure itself. Effects of maternal hypertension, such as left ventricular hypertrophy or renal dysfunction, are also important to identify in order to further risk-stratify the pregnancy and to prevent further end-organ damage [2]. A baseline assessment of 24 hour urine proteinuria is key to helping distinguish between worsening hypertension in the third trimester and superimposed pre-eclampsia.

Fetal and Neonatal Brain Injury, 4th edition, ed. David K. Stevenson, William E. Benitz, Philip Sunshine, Susan R. Hintz, and Maurice L. Druzin. Published by Cambridge University Press. © Cambridge University Press 2009.

Table 11.1. Definitions of chronic hypertension, gestational hypertension, pre-eclampsia, and superimposed pre-eclampsia

Chronic hypertension
Systolic blood pressure ≥ 140 mmHg or diastolic blood pressure ≥ 90 that is diagnosed pre-pregnancy or at < 20 weeks' gestation, or hypertension diagnosed after 20 weeks' gestation which does not resolve postpartum [1,2]

Gestational hypertension
Systolic blood pressure ≥ 140 or diastolic blood pressure ≥ 90 that is diagnosed after 20 weeks' gestation and is *not* associated with significant proteinuria (≥ 300 mg/24 hours). The blood pressure must be elevated at least two times, 6 hours apart [2]

Pre-eclampsia
Systolic blood pressure ≥ 140 or diastolic blood pressure ≥ 90 that occurs after 20 weeks' gestation in a previously normotensive patient *and* significant proteinuria (≥ 300 mg/24 hours). The blood pressure must be elevated at least two times, 6 hours apart [5]

Superimposed pre-eclampsia
The development of pre-eclampsia in a woman with underlying chronic hypertension. This is characterized by new-onset proteinuria, worsening proteinuria in a woman with pre-existing proteinuria, or the development of severe signs or symptoms of pre-eclampsia [5]

Chronic hypertension affects the fetus primarily by altering placental vessels and placental perfusion. Decidual vessels of women with chronic hypertension demonstrate microvascular changes similar to those seen in renal arterioles in women with long-standing hypertension [4]. These changes are thought to explain increased risks for placental abruption (twofold increased risk) and IUGR (30–50%). Early abnormal placental vasculature/implantation may also be related to the pathogenesis of superimposed pre-eclampsia [1,4] (see section on pre-eclampsia). Up to one-third of women with chronic hypertension will have a small-for-gestational-age infant (< 10th percentile) and two-thirds will have a preterm delivery. Approximately 20–25% of women with chronic hypertension will develop superimposed pre-eclampsia [2,4]. Women with chronic hypertension are more likely to have earlier and more severe pre-eclampsia. Most of the fetal morbidity associated with chronic hypertension is probably due to IUGR and superimposed pre-eclampsia [1,4].

In a pregnancy complicated by chronic hypertension, there is no consensus on fetal monitoring. Most recommend a baseline ultrasound at 18–20 weeks to confirm gestational age, and subsequent growth scans thereafter. Some recommend routine non-stress testing or biophysical profiles only if growth restriction is detected, whereas others perform routine testing [2]. Early delivery due to chronic hypertension alone is not indicated. Timing of delivery should be dictated by the presence or absence of non-reassuring fetal status, including intrauterine growth restriction, or the presence or absence of superimposed pre-eclampsia. The route of delivery should be decided by usual obstetric indications.

Treatment of chronic hypertension in pregnancy is controversial. Women with blood pressure 140–179/90–109 and normal renal function are generally considered to be at low risk for maternal cardiovascular complications in the relatively short time frame of pregnancy [2]. However, very little data exist to support this. Furthermore, treatment of hypertension in pregnancy may be beneficial to the mother in the long term,

especially when the patient has renal disease or left ventricular hypertrophy. However, there are no data to show that treatment of chronic hypertension improves fetal outcome or that it prevents pre-eclampsia [1,2]. Further, there is theoretic concern that decreasing the maternal blood pressure will decrease uterine–placental perfusion and impair fetal growth/development. Studies comparing neonatal outcomes with and without treatment of chronic hypertension have conflicting outcomes [1]. Thus the decision to treat chronic hypertension in pregnancy should weigh the risks and benefits to the mother and the fetus.

The Working Group recommends that hypertension be treated to maintain systolic blood pressures < 150 and diastolic blood pressures < 100 [2]. Many experts, however, prefer keeping blood pressure < 140/90. In the presence of end-organ dysfunction, such as left ventricular hypertrophy or renal insufficiency, the treatment threshold should be lower [4].

Antihypertensive medications used to treat chronic hypertension in pregnancy generally include α-methyldopa, labetalol, hydralazine, and long-acting calcium channel blockers, such as nifedipine XL. None of these medications has been associated with teratogenesis [4].

Gestational hypertension

Gestational hypertension is a less well-defined diagnosis and likely represents a heterogeneous group which includes patients with true transient hypertension, patients with undiagnosed chronic hypertension, and patients with early/incompletely manifested pre-eclampsia. Up to 25% of women with gestational hypertension will develop pre-eclampsia [5].

Gestational hypertension is defined as hypertension (systolic blood pressure ≥ 140 or diastolic blood pressure ≥ 90) first diagnosed after 20 weeks' gestation that is *not* associated with significant proteinuria (≥ 300mg/24 hour period). The blood pressure must be elevated in at least two measurements, taken 6 hours apart [2]. Severe gestational hypertension is defined as systolic blood pressure ≥ 160 or diastolic blood pressure ≥ 110 [6]. Gestational hypertension is a temporary diagnosis. If hypertension does not resolve in the first 12 weeks postpartum, then the diagnosis of chronic hypertension is given. A woman with gestational hypertension who does not become pre-eclamptic and whose hypertension resolves postpartum is considered to have had "transient hypertension of pregnancy" [2,7].

Because patients with gestational hypertension likely represent a heterogeneous group, it is hard to characterize gestational hypertension as a benign or malignant pregnancy condition. The course of the disease likely reflects underlying pathophysiology. That 15–25% of patients with gestational hypertension will develop pre-eclampsia [5,8] suggests that a significant subset of gestational hypertension represents undiagnosed chronic hypertension or an early/incomplete manifestation of pre-eclampsia. In fact, one study reports that up to 19% of patients with eclampsia had gestational hypertension only, without proteinuria, at the time of the seizure [9].

Distinguishing which patients with gestational hypertension will have a benign or morbid clinical course is a significant clinical problem. Because gestational hypertension is distinguished from pre-eclampsia based on the absence of proteinuria, many incorrectly assume that the absence or presence of proteinuria distinguishes perinatal risk. Some studies do support the idea that the presence of proteinuria increases perinatal risk. North *et al.* reported that compared to women with gestational hypertension alone, women with pre-eclampsia were more likely to develop severe maternal hypertension (63.4% vs. 26.5%, $p < 0.001$), deliver small-for-gestational-age infants < 10th percentile (25.4% vs. 20.5%, $p < 0.01$), and deliver at < 37 weeks (35.2% vs. 6%, $p < 0.0001$) [10]. However, it is clear from the above study that gestational hypertension without proteinuria also confers increased risk of maternal and perinatal complications compared to normotensive patients. Buchbinder *et al.* showed that women with severe gestational hypertension had higher rates of preterm delivery < 35 weeks (25% vs. 8.4%) and small-for-gestational-age infants < 10th percentile (20.8% vs. 6.5%) compared to women who were normotensive or had mild gestational hypertension. In this study, multivariate analysis showed that severe hypertension was strongly associated with poor perinatal outcome, whereas proteinuria was not [6]. Thus both the degree of proteinuria and the degree of hypertension likely confers perinatal risk.

Until more is understood about the pathophysiology of pre-eclampsia and superimposed pre-eclampsia, we are unlikely to be able to better distinguish between gestational hypertension which is benign and that which goes on to be associated with maternal and perinatal morbidity. Gestational hypertension should be viewed as a sign that identifies a heterogeneous group. It is possibly benign, but also possibly a harbinger of severe maternal or perinatal disease. Patients with earlier gestational age of onset of hypertension and patients with severe hypertension are more likely to have poorer outcomes [6,8]. Careful monitoring and evaluation of all women with gestational hypertension should be performed. This includes frequent evaluation of maternal blood pressure, maternal symptoms, proteinuria, and fetal well-being. It may also include assessment of maternal renal function, hepatic function, and platelets. An evaluation of fetal well-being should include an evaluation of growth, amniotic fluid, and a non-stress test or biophysical profile.

Pre-eclampsia and superimposed pre-eclampsia

Pre-eclampsia differs from chronic hypertension in that it is a *syndrome* specific to pregnancy. Pre-eclampsia is defined as hypertension (systolic blood pressure ≥ 140 or diastolic blood pressure ≥ 90, two times 6 hours apart) occurring after 20 weeks in a previously normotensive patient *and* significant proteinuria (≥ 300 mg/24 hour urine collection) [5]. Superimposed pre-eclampsia is the development of pre-eclampsia in a

Table 11.2. Criteria for severe pre-eclampsia [5]

(1) Systolic blood pressure ≥ 160 on two occasions at least 6 hours apart
(2) Diastolic blood pressure ≥ 110 on two occasions at least 6 hours apart
(3) Proteinuria of ≥ 5000 mg/24 hours or $\geq 3+$ on two random protein dipsticks at least 4 hours apart
(4) Oliguria (< 500 ml/24 hours) or acute renal failure
(5) Cerebral or visual disturbances including seizures (eclampsia)
(6) Pulmonary edema or cyanosis
(7) Epigastric or right upper quadrant pain
(8) Elevated liver enzymes
(9) Thrombocytopenia
(10) Fetal growth restriction

woman with chronic hypertension. Superimposed pre-eclampsia can be difficult to diagnose due to the similarity of signs between chronic hypertension and pre-eclampsia, but is characterized by new onset of proteinuria in a woman with chronic hypertension, a sudden increase in pre-existing proteinuria, or the development of severe signs/symptoms of pre-eclampsia in a woman with chronic hypertension (Table 11.1) [5].

The incidence of pre-eclampsia is approximately 5–8% [5,11]. The incidence of severe pre-eclampsia is 0.9% [12]. Risk factors include nulliparity, African-American race, chronic hypertension, renal disease, autoimmune disease, pregestational diabetes, maternal age > 35, and obesity [5].

The clinical features of pre-eclampsia are caused by vasospasm (increased systemic vascular resistance) and endothelial cell dysfunction (increased vascular permeability and platelet aggregation). Most often, the disease course is mild, with mild hypertension and proteinuria. However, severe cases are marked by uncontrollable hypertension, thrombotic microangiopathy (small-vessel thrombosis), and tissue edema, leading to end-organ damage. End-organ damage can involve seizures (< 1%), stroke (< 1%), pulmonary edema (2–5%), renal insufficiency, hepatic failure (< 1%), and thrombocytopenia/hemolytic anemia (10–20%) [11]. The syndrome also can affect the fetus, manifesting as intrauterine growth restriction (10–25%), oligohydramnios, and/or abruption (1–4%) [11]. Table 11.2 lists criteria for the diagnosis of severe pre-eclampsia.

Women with underlying medical disease, such as chronic hypertension, renal disease, or autoimmune disease, are at increased risk to develop pre-eclampsia earlier and more severely [11]. The severity of illness in the mother and fetus are not always concordant.

Multiple theories for the pathogenesis of pre-eclampsia exist. Historically the most prevalent theories have implicated (1) abnormal placental implantation or (2) abnormal maternal immunologic response to the placenta. A recent, literature-substantiated hypothesis marries these theories and implicates maternal–fetal immune maladaptation as causing superficial placentation. Subsequent placental events may trigger a systemic inflammatory response in the mother, which causes endothelial cell dysfunction and vasospasm [11,13]. Key players likely include the placental-derived antiangiogenic proteins soluble fms-like tyrosine kinase 1 (sFlt1) and soluble endoglin, which diffuse into the maternal sera. sFlt1 likely acts by inhibiting placental growth factor (PlGF) and vascular endothelial growth factor (VEGF), causing direct endothelial cell dysfunction and inhibiting vasodilation. Soluble endoglin likely acts as a soluble inhibitor of TGF-β1, blocking its activation of endothelial nitric oxide synthase and increasing local intravascular tone [11,13–18].

Why one pregnancy complicated by immune maladaptation and poor placentation manifests as maternal disease, another manifests as fetal disease, and still another manifests as both is unclear. Placental pathology in pregnancies complicated by pre-eclampsia reveals changes similar to those seen with intrauterine growth restriction. The difference in clinical presentation may result from the degree of placental damage, the extent of inflammatory reaction, and/or the maternal response to molecular mediators [13].

Treatment

The only known treatment for pre-eclampsia is delivery of the placenta. Key elements of treatment involve timing of delivery, seizure prophylaxis, treatment of stroke-level blood pressure, and glucocorticoids for fetal maturation.

Timing of delivery

Controlling the timing of delivery is the best tool for limiting maternal and perinatal mortality [2]. In cases of pre-eclampsia at term ($\geq$ 37 weeks), a decision for delivery is easy. A decision to deliver a preterm infant is more difficult, and thus the extent of disease in the mother and the degree of prematurity of the fetus must be carefully weighed. Guidelines for timing of delivery are based on observational studies, randomized trials, and expert opinion [11,12].

In general, mild pre-eclampsia can be managed with close observation as long as maternal disease remains mild and fetal status remains reassuring. Delivery is indicated when neonatal complications from prematurity are minimal. This gestational age is generally 37–38 weeks [11].

Severe pre-eclampsia is characterized by progressive deterioration in both the mother and fetus. Delivery should always be considered. However, expectant management may be considered in pregnancies $\leq$ 32 weeks, as it can decrease perinatal mortality and significantly increases gestational age at delivery. Expectant management necessitates intensive maternal and fetal monitoring [7,11,12].

Pre-eclampsia which develops prior to viability is most often severe. Attempts to prolong gestation when pre-eclampsia develops prior to viability risk severe maternal morbidity and even mortality. Neonatal morbidity and mortality are also high. Termination prior to viability is recommended.

Between 24 and 32 weeks, severe pre-eclampsia can be managed expectantly with careful blood pressure control. However, signs or symptoms of severe pre-eclampsia that imply end-organ dysfunction are indications for delivery. These include the inability to control blood pressure below the stroke range despite maximal antihypertensive medications, headache, seizures/neurologic symptoms, right upper quadrant/epigastric pain with elevated liver enzymes, significantly elevated liver enzymes, pulmonary edema, acute renal failure/oliguria, thrombocytopenia < 100 000, and/or a non-reassuring fetal status. Patients with severe pre-eclampsia that is stable are generally delivered by 32–34 weeks due to the ongoing maternal and fetal risks. If severe pre-eclampsia occurs with a non-reassuring fetal status such as growth restriction or a non-reassuring fetal heart tracing, delivery is almost always indicated [11,12].

Vaginal delivery is generally preferred. However, cesarean delivery is appropriate for the usual obstetrical indications, in cases of severe maternal disease where an expedient induction and vaginal delivery appear unlikely, or when vaginal delivery has not been achieved within 24 hours after initiating an induction of labor.

Seizure prophylaxis

The incidence of seizures (eclampsia) with mild and severe pre-eclampsia informs treatment patterns for seizure prophylaxis. Fewer than 1% of patients with mild pre-eclampsia develop seizures, and approximately 2–3% of patients with severe pre-eclampsia develop seizures [19].

Magnesium is the preferred antiepileptic, and is generally recommended for severe pre-eclampsia at least during labor and immediately postpartum. Randomized controlled trials have demonstrated that magnesium is superior to phenytoin, diazepam, and placebo for seizure prophylaxis in severe pre-eclampsia [5]. There is no consensus on the use of magnesium for mild pre-eclampsia [5,11,19].

Antihypertensive medications

Antihypertensive medication is used in patients with severe hypertension to prevent cerebral vascular and cardiovascular complications. However, antihypertensive therapy given to patients with pre-eclampsia does not alter rates of maternal disease progression, perinatal death, IUGR, or prematurity. Controlling severe hypertension, however, may prolong gestation, providing time for fetal steroid effect and decreasing the degree of prematurity. Treatment is usually recommended for acute elevations in systolic blood pressure $\geq$ 150–160 or diastolic blood pressure $\geq$ 105 [5,11]. The most commonly used antihypertensive medications are parenteral hydralazine, parenteral labetalol, or short-acting oral nifedipine. Nitroprusside is used when hypertension is otherwise refractory.

Glucocorticoids for fetal lung maturity

Administration of corticosteroids to women at risk for preterm delivery between 24 and 34 weeks has been shown to reduce the incidence and severity of neonatal respiratory distress syndrome, intraventricular hemorrhage, and necrotizing enterocolitis. It has also been shown to decrease perinatal mortality [20]. Glucocorticoids in the form of betamethasone or dexamethasone should be given to a woman with pre-eclampsia at less than 34 weeks, as preterm delivery is likely.

Fetal and neonatal effects of hypertensive disease in pregnancy

Neonatal effects of hypertensive disease in pregnancy are due primarily to placental insufficiency, iatrogenic prematurity, and drug effects of medications.

Placental insufficiency

Hypertension and pre-eclampsia are associated with a vasculopathy in the placenta, which may or may not be the same. Similar features of the vasculopathy include shallow placental implantation and maternal spiral arteries which fail to become low-resistance [13]. Cytotrophoblastic hyperplasia, thickening of the basement membrane, placental infarction, and chorionic villitis are also seen. These changes are associated with increased vascular resistance and decreased diffusion capacity in the placenta [21]. Fetal consequences of placental vasculopathy include increased placental vascular resistance, IUGR (< 10th percentile), increased cerebral blood flow (centralization), oligohydramnios, and placental abruption. Approximately 1/3 of IUGR is caused by uteroplacental insufficiency [21].

IUGR is associated with neonatal polycythemia, hyperbilirubinemia, hypoglycemia, hypothermia, and apneic episodes. Long-term follow-up suggests that small-for-gestational-age infants may have increased risks of adult hypertension and cardiovascular complications (Barker hypothesis) [22].

Iatrogenic prematurity

Anywhere from 15% to 67% of pregnancies complicated by hypertensive diseases of pregnancy result in preterm delivery [11]. Most poor perinatal outcome is related to the usual complications of prematurity, including neonatal death, respiratory distress syndrome, intraventricular hemorrhage, necrotizing enterocolitis, and sepsis. Although there is a common belief that in utero "stress" associated with pre-eclampsia causes accelerated fetal maturation, this was not supported in a study by Freidman *et al.* The authors found no difference in the incidence of the above complications of prematurity at ≤ 32 weeks and at ≤ 35 weeks when infants born to pre-eclamptic mothers were compared to infants born to normotensive controls. This was also true when infants of mothers with severe pre-eclampsia or severe pre-eclampsia with IUGR were compared to infants of normotensive controls [23].

Fetal effects of maternal medications

Magnesium

Magnesium sulfate crosses the placenta, enters the fetal circulation, and may cause neonatal respiratory depression before toxicity is seen in the mother. It may also decrease neonatal intestinal motility, resulting in early feeding problems [7]. There are conflicting reports regarding the effect of magnesium on neonatal neurologic outcome. One randomized controlled trial of 194 women using magnesium for tocolysis versus "other tocolytic" demonstrated a trend toward more intraventricular hemorrhage, cerebral palsy, and neonatal death in the magnesium-treated group (combined adverse outcome, 32% vs. 19%, $p = 0.07$). In this study, infants who had adverse outcomes had 25% higher levels of umbilical cord magnesium ($p = 0.03$) [24]. However, another randomized controlled trial of 1062 women comparing magnesium versus placebo for neonatal neuroprotection showed magnesium had no deleterious effect on the neonate and possibly reduced the incidence of gross motor dysfunction at 2-year follow-up [25]. Most recently, outcomes of 6922 children at 18 months of age whose mothers had been randomized to magnesium versus placebo for pre-eclampsia were published. There was no difference between groups with regard to death or neurosensory disability [26]. Taken together, it is unlikely that magnesium given for seizure prophylaxis will adversely affect the fetus/neonate in the long term.

Antihypertensive medications

Antihypertensive medications used to treat chronic hypertension or to treat severe hypertension in expectantly managed severe pre-eclampsia (chronic management) include α-methyldopa, labetalol, hydralazine, and long-acting calcium channel blockers such as nifedipine. Antihypertensive medications used to treat acute hypertension related to severe gestational hypertension, pre-eclampsia, or superimposed pre-eclampsia include parenteral hydralazine, parenteral labetalol, and short-acting nifedipine. A complete discussion regarding indications for treatment is found above.

Chronic management

Oral α-methyldopa, labetolol, and long-acting calcium channel blockers are used for chronic management of hypertension in pregnancy. α-Methyldopa was historically the drug of choice. Longitudinal data show no decrease in uteroplacental blood flow and no adverse neonatal effects in the long term with its use. However, because α-methyldopa can cause maternal lethargy and elevated liver enzymes, many practitioners favor other classes of drugs. Labetalol is commonly used, despite concerns regarding associated growth restriction. Although beta-blockers have been associated with growth restriction in meta-analysis, one study comparing α-methyldopa to labetalol showed no difference in fetal outcome [1]. Hydralazine is also commonly used, but can be limited by maternal rebound tachycardia. Long-acting calcium channel blockers, such as nifedipine, are used with minimal side effects [1,2]. Diuretics are controversial in pregnancy because of concerns that reduction in maternal blood volume will reduce uterine blood flow. However, a meta-analysis revealed no detrimental effects [1,2]. Angiotensin-converting enzyme inhibitors (ACE inhibitors) and angiotensin II receptor blockers (ARBs) are contraindicated in pregnancy because of teratogenic concerns. Although ACE inhibitors have traditionally been thought to be teratogenic only in the second and third trimesters, recent data suggest that even first-trimester exposure to ACE inhibitors can cause teratogenesis. Specific related anomalies are cardiac anomalies (risk ratio 3.72, 95% CI 1.89–7.30) and central nervous system anomalies (risk ratio 4.39, 95% CI 1.37–14.02) [27].

Acute management

Parenteral hydralazine and labetalol are the most commonly use antihypertensive agents. Short-acting oral nifedipine is less commonly used [5]. There has been some concern in meta-analysis that hydralazine may be more associated with fetal distress and lower Apgar scores than other antihypertensive agents. However, major perinatal morbidity, including admission to intensive care, neonatal hypotension, and complications from prematurity has not been shown to be different between hydralazine and other antihypertensive agents [11,28]. Oral short-acting nifedipine, though commonly used and accepted by experts, has never been FDA approved for the treatment of hypertension or hypertensive emergencies in pregnant or non-pregnant patients. Specific concern exists because it has been associated with untoward fatal and non-fatal cardiovascular events in non-pregnant patients [2,12]. No randomized trials have been done comparing neonatal effects of antihypertensives used for acute management of severe hypertension.

Summary

Hypertensive disease in pregnancy is common, and it is responsible for significant maternal and neonatal morbidity. Distinguishing between chronic hypertension, gestational hypertension, and pre-eclampsia/superimposed pre-eclampsia is important, because the diagnosis predicts associated morbidity and directs care. However, at times, distinguishing between these entities is impossible.

Management of all hypertensive disease in pregnancy includes close surveillance of both maternal and fetal health. Once pre-eclampsia develops, particularly in the preterm setting, its course is usually progressive and can accelerate. Appropriate timing of delivery, seizure prophylaxis, treatment of severe hypertension, and glucocorticoids for fetal maturation are the mainstays of pre-eclampsia care. Expectant management of severe pre-eclampsia between 24 and 32 weeks can significantly reduce perinatal morbidity and significantly extend gestation. Delivery is indicated when end-organ dysfunction is notable in the mother or the fetus. Hypertensive disease in pregnancy causes morbidity for the fetus/neonate via placental insufficiency, prematurity, and magnesium toxicity.

When more is understood about the pathophysiology of pre-eclampsia and its interaction with chronic hypertension, biochemical markers may become available to better predict which mothers, and which fetuses, have the highest risk for morbidity.

References

1. American College of Obstetricians and Gynecologists. Practice Bulletin Number 29, July 2001. Chronic hypertension in pregnancy. In *2007 Compendium of Selected Publications, Volume II: Practice Bulletins*. Washington, DC: ACOG, 2007: 609–17.

2. Report of the National High Blood Pressure Education Program Working Group on High Blood Pressure in Pregnancy. *Am J Obstet Gynecol* 2000; **183**: S1–22.

3. De Boo HA, Harding JE. The developmental origins of adult disease (Barker) hypothesis. *Aust NZ J Obstet Gynaecol* 2006; **46**: 4–14.

4. Roberts JM. Pregnancy-related hypertension. In Creasy RK, Resnik R, Iams JD, eds., *Maternal–Fetal Medicine: Principles and Practice*, 5th edn. Philadelphia, PA: Saunders, 2004: 859–99.

5. American College of Obstetricians and Gynecologists. Practice Bulletin Number 33, January 2002. Diagnosis and management of preeclampsia and eclampsia. In *2007 Compendium of Selected Publications, Volume II: Practice Bulletins*. Washington DC: ACOG, 2007: 640–8.

6. Buchbinder A, Sibai BM, Caritis S, *et al.* Adverse perinatal outcomes are significantly higher in severe gestational hypertension than in mild preeclampsia. *Am J Obstet Gynecol* 2002; **186**: 66–71.

7. Lyell, DJ. Hypertensive disorders of pregnancy: relevance for the neonatologist. *NeoReviews* 2004; **5**; e1–7.

8. Saudan P, Brown MA, Buddle ML, *et al.* Does gestational hypertension become pre-eclampsia. *Br J Obstet Gynaecol* 1998; **105**: 1177–84.

9. Sibai BM. Eclampsia. VI. Maternal–perinatal outcome in 254 consecutive cases. *Am J Obstet Gynecol* 1990; **163**: 1049–54.

10. North RA, Taylor RS, Schellenberg JC. Evaluation of a definition of pre-eclampsia. *Br J Obstet Gynaecol* 1999; **106**: 767–73.

11. Sibai BM. Pre-eclampsia. *Lancet* 2005; **365**: 785–99.

12. Sibai BM, Barton JR. Expectant management of severe preeclampsia remote from term: patient selection, treatment, and delivery indications. *Am J Obstet Gynecol* 2007; **196**: 514.e1–9.

13. Ness RB, Sibai BM. Shared and disparate components of the pathophysiologies of fetal growth restriction and preeclampsia. *Am J Obstet Gyncol* 2006; **195**: 40–9.

14. Maynard SE, Min JY, Merchan J, *et al.* Excess placental soluble fms-like tyrosine kinase 1 (sFlt1) may contribute to endothelial dysfunction, hypertension, and proteinuria in preeclampsia. *J Clin Invest* 2003; **111**: 649–58.

15. Venkatesha S, Toporsian M, Lam C, *et al.* Soluble endoglin contributes to the pathogenesis of preeclampsia. *Nat Med* 2006; **12**: 642–9.

16. Thadhani R, Mutter WP, Wolf M, *et al.* First trimester placental growth factor and soluble fms-like tyrosine kinase 1 and risk for preeclampsia. *J Clin Endocrinol Metab* 2004; **89**: 770–5.

17. Levine RJ, Maynard S, Qian C, *et al.* Circulating angiogenic factors and the risk of preeclampsia. *N Engl J Med* 2004; **350**: 672–83.

18. Levine RJ, Lam C, Qian C, *et al.* Soluble endoglin and other circulating antiangiogenic factors in preeclampsia. *N Engl J Med* 2006; **335**: 992–1005.

19. Sibai, BM. Magnesium sulfate prophylaxis in preeclampsia: lessons learned from recent trials. *Am J Obstet Gynecol* 2004; **190**: 1520–6.

20. American College of Obstetricians and Gynecologists. Practice Bulletin Number 43, May 2003. Management of preterm labor. In *2007 Compendium of Selected Publications, Volume II: Practice Bulletins*. Washington, DC: ACOG, 2007: 688–96.

21. Resnik R, Creasy RK. Intrauterine growth restriction. In Creasy RK, Resnik R, Iams JD, eds., *Maternal–Fetal Medicine: Principles and Practice*,

5th edn. Philadelphia, PA: Saunders, 2004: 495–512.

22. American College of Obstetricians and Gynecologists. Practice Bulletin Number 12, January 2000. Intrauterine growth restriction. In *2007 Compendium of Selected Publications, Volume II: Practice Bulletins*. Washington, DC: ACOG, 2007: 524–35.

23. Friedman SA, Schiff E, Kao L, *et al.* Neonatal outcome after preterm delivery for preeclampsia. *Am J Obstet Gynecol* 1995; **172**: 1785–92.

24. Mittendorf R, Dambrosia J, Pryde P, *et al.* Association between the use of antenatal magnesium sulfate in preterm labor and adverse health outcomes in infants. *Am J Obstet Gynecol* 2002; **186**: 1111–18.

25. Crowther CA, Hiller JE, Doyle LW, *et al.* Effect of magnesium sulfate given for neuroprotection before preterm birth: a randomized controlled trial. *JAMA* 2003; **290**: 2669–76.

26. Magpie Trial Follow-up Study Collaborative Group. The Magpie Trial: a randomised trial comparing magnesium sulphate with placebo for pre-eclampsia. Outcome for children at 18 months. *BJOG* 2007; **114**: 289–99.

27. Cooper WO, Hernandez-Diaz S, Arbogast PG, *et al.* Major congenital malformations after first-trimester exposure to ACE inhibitors. *N Engl J Med* 2006; **354**: 2443–51.

28. Magee LA, Cham C, Waterman EJ, *et al.* Hydralazine for treatment of severe hypertension in pregnancy: meta-analysis. *BMJ* 2003; **327**: 955–64.

Chapter 12

Complications of labor and delivery

Yair Blumenfeld and Masoud Taslimi

Introduction

Despite a common misconception among the general public, intrapartum events rarely lead to fetal injury. Approximately 70% of cases of neonatal encephalopathy are secondary to events arising prior to the onset of labor [1]. Moreover, the overall incidence of neonatal encephalopathy attributable to intrapartum hypoxia, in the absence of any other potential preconceptional or antepartum causes, is estimated to be approximately 1.6/10 000 [1]. Despite this, the practice of obstetrics is rapidly evolving as a reaction to both extrinsic and intrinsic factors. Today, cesarean section rates are at all-time highs, operative vaginal delivery rates are decreasing, and evidence-based obstetrics is threatened to be replaced by defensive, anecdotally based medicine.

In this chapter, we shall review the available evidence regarding complications of labor and delivery and their potential effects on adverse neonatal injury in general and neurological morbidity in particular. We hope this information will enable physicians to make educated, informed, and rational obstetrical decisions, thereby improving overall patient care.

Cesarean section

In the United States in 2004, 29.1% of live births were via cesarean section [2]. The rate of primary cesarean section in 2004 was 20.6%, compared with 14.6% in 1996 [2]. On the other hand, in 2004 the rate of vaginal delivery after previous cesarean (VBAC) was only 9.2%, while in 1996 the rate was 28.3% [2]. The current rise in cesarean section rates is driven by multiple factors including increasing multiple gestations, obstetrical litigation, rising elective cesarean section on maternal demand, advanced maternal age, and decreasing operative vaginal delivery. The old adage of "once a cesarean, always a cesarean" is slowly making its way back into obstetrical practice after a 30-year hiatus.

Until very recently, there were minimal data regarding the potential harmful effects of cesarean section on the fetus and neonate. To illustrate this, in 2006 the National Institutes of Health convened a State of the Science Conference to evaluate the available data regarding cesarean delivery on maternal

request. Following its review, the panel concluded that there were insufficient data to compare the safety of cesarean section on maternal request with planned vaginal delivery [3]. They further stated that "any decision to perform cesarean delivery . . . should be carefully individualized."

Since that time, a large prospective cohort study of over 94 000 deliveries in South America compared vaginal delivery to elective and intrapartum cesarean section. In this multicenter cohort, cesarean delivery reduced the risk of intrapartum fetal death, but increased the risk of severe neonatal morbidity and mortality. Also, lack of labor was a risk factor for prolonged stay in the neonatal intensive care unit, and neonatal mortality was higher for neonates delivered by elective cesarean when compared with vaginal delivery [4]. In the same study, maternal morbidity and mortality, including admission to the ICU, blood transfusion, hysterectomy, and prolonged hospital stay were higher in both the elective and intrapartum cesarean groups when compared with the vaginal delivery group [4].

Multiple studies have recently addressed maternal complications following one or more cesarean sections. Minor morbidities including difficult delivery, adhesions, and longer operative times, as well as significant morbidities including hysterectomy, blood transfusion, placenta accreta, and ICU admissions have all been shown to increase with increasing cesarean deliveries [5,6]. Moreover a recently published large case-controlled Australian study of over 35 000 women linked adverse neonatal outcomes including preterm birth, low birthweight, small for gestational age, and unexplained stillbirth in subsequent pregnancies to primary cesarean delivery [7].

As we continue to analyze these drastic changes in practice in the years to come, we must ask ourselves whether neonatal morbidity and mortality is improving, whether maternal safety is compromised, and what if any effects these trends will have on future pregnancies.

Vaginal births after cesarean (VBAC) and uterine rupture

The practice of vaginal birth after cesarean (VBAC) was introduced and rapidly endorsed by obstetricians in the 1980s and 1990s. It was initially intended to counteract what were then perceived as high cesarean section rates resulting largely from the discontinued practice of mid-forceps and vaginal breech deliveries. As the practice grew, reports of maternal and

Fetal and Neonatal Brain Injury, 4th edition, ed. David K. Stevenson, William E. Benitz, Philip Sunshine, Susan R. Hintz, and Maurice L. Druzin. Published by Cambridge University Press. © Cambridge University Press 2009.

neonatal morbidity and mortality were published, leading to a rapid decline in VBAC rates. Today, most labor units require 24-hour in-hospital obstetrical and anesthesia staff if VBAC is to be attempted. Though the risk of rupture is less than 1% for most cases of spontaneous laboring patients, the potential for severe neonatal and maternal morbidity is causing many hospitals and physician groups to avoid the practice altogether.

Data published over the last 10 years have focused on identifying the optimal VBAC candidate based on prior cesarean section scar, as well as other fetal and maternal characteristics [8–10]. In 2004 the American College of Obstetricians and Gynecologists (ACOG) published guidelines for VBAC candidates. In this chapter, the following selection criteria were deemed most useful: one previous low-transverse cesarean delivery, clinically adequate pelvis, no other uterine scars or previous rupture, and physicians and anesthesia immediately available for emergency delivery [11]. Other studies have attempted to stratify the risk of rupture based on primary surgical technique (mainly single- vs. double-layer uterine closure), as well as labor management of the VBAC, including the use of cervical induction agents and labor augmentation [12,13].

In a review comparing elective cesarean section and VBAC in over 33 000 patients, those attempting a vaginal trial of labor had statistically significant higher rates of transfusion, endometritis, and neonatal hypoxic–ischemic encephalopathy (HIE) [14]. A recently published large cohort study from the USA of over 39 000 patients at term with a history of a prior cesarean section reported 0.27% risk of adverse perinatal outcomes including stillbirth, HIE, and neonatal death [15]. The overall rate of uterine rupture was 0.32%, while the rate among those attempting a vaginal delivery was 0.74%.

Because the majority of morbidity related to VBAC trials is associated with failure to delivery vaginally, identifying the proportion of patients who are more likely to successfully deliver vaginally is important [16]. Two large studies, one retrospective and one prospective observational, reported similar overall VBAC success rates of 75.5% and 73.6% respectively [17,18]. Prior successful vaginal delivery and spontaneous labor have been reported in multiple studies to be strong predictors of successful VBAC [18,19]. Also, multiple studies have shown that the cost-effectiveness of VBAC depends on the a priori chance of success [20,21].

Counseling a woman with a prior cesarean is complex, and requires consideration not only of her likely success, risk factors for uterine rupture, and risk of maternal and neonatal morbidity, but also of the long-term consequences of delivery mode should she desire a large family. Though most studies on VBAC safety have focused on short-term maternal and neonatal outcomes, multiple cesarean deliveries may have longer reproductive consequences for women. In a large observational study of over 30 000 patients undergoing cesarean delivery, the risks of placenta accreta, cystotomy, bowel injury, ureteral injury, and ileus, the need for postoperative ventilation, intensive care unit admission, hysterectomy, and blood transfusion requiring four or more units, and the duration of operative time and hospital stay significantly increased with increasing number of cesarean deliveries [6]. A recent decision analysis suggested that allowing women with a single prior cesarean delivery a VBAC attempt will result in fewer cumulative hysterectomies compared with elective repeat cesareans if the woman desires two or more additional children [22].

Once a VBAC is attempted, close maternal and fetal monitoring is crucial. Certain clinical parameters including increased maternal abdominal pain, vaginal bleeding or hypotension, loss of fetal station, and non-reassuring fetal heart rates (FHRs) may be indicative of uterine rupture. In a case-controlled study of 48 uterine ruptures and 100 controls, fetal bradycardia in the first and second stage was the only finding to differentiate uterine ruptures from successful VBAC patients [23]. Some have previously raised concerns of regional anesthesia masking the pain associated with uterine rupture. These concerns have not been confirmed in any observational studies, and ACOG also states that VBAC is not a contraindication to epidural anesthesia [11].

Spontaneous uterine rupture

Rupture of the unscarred uterus is a rare obstetric complication, with an estimated incidence of between 1/8000 and 1/15 000 deliveries [24,25]. In a recent review of 36 reported primigravid uterine rupture cases in the English literature, only 20 cases presented with a live, viable infant, and among those there was evidence of fetal compromise in 80% [26]. Most of the cases, 89%, presented in the third trimester, and only 11% had vaginal bleeding. Risk factors for the cases included previous uterine surgery, adherent placenta, congenital uterine anomaly, adenomyosis, connective tissue disorders, oxytocin and prostaglandin induction, and labor. Twenty-six percent of the cases resulted in a hysterectomy, and maternal mortality was reported in one case.

Operative vaginal delivery

A significant reason for the rise in cesarean section rates is the decrease in operative vaginal delivery rates. Forceps deliveries are slowly becoming obsolete as the negative public perception of these instruments is increasing and resident experience and training is decreasing. This is in sharp contrast to the practice of elective forceps that permeated labor and delivery units only 30–40 years ago. Because of the experience necessary to acquire skill in performing forceps deliveries, and the decrease in available cases in teaching institutions, vacuum deliveries have recently gained relative popularity, though still in smaller numbers than previously.

The indications for operative vaginal delivery, via forceps or vacuum, have not changed over the years. These include prolonged second stage, suspicion of immediate or potential fetal compromise, and shortening of the second stage for maternal benefit [27]. Peripartum considerations, namely fetal position, presentation, lie, engagement, and clinical pelvimetry are of vital importance when attempting an operative vaginal delivery.

Mostly, the decision to proceed with either forceps or vacuum is based on operator experience and comfort.

Complications

Two randomized trials comparing elective low-forceps delivery with spontaneous vaginal delivery in 50 and 333 patients respectively failed to show any differences in neonatal outcomes between the two modalities [28,29]. Studies addressing the use of forceps in the setting of fetal macrosomia illustrated higher rates of significant injury, including neurologic abnormalities, when compared to spontaneous delivery or cesarean section [30]. Multiple studies comparing vacuum to forceps illustrated greater neonatal injury, including scalp lacerations, cephalohematomas, subgaleal hematomas, and intracranial hemorrhage, with vacuum delivery [31,32]. In a study comparing 308 vacuum-assisted deliveries with 200 forceps-assisted deliveries, cephalohematomas were seen in 20.5% of vacuum compared with 12.5% of forceps, and caput and molding were seen in 28.2% of vacuum compared with 13.5% of forceps [31]. Despite these, the overall incidence of serious complications with vacuum extraction is approximately 5%.

When considering an operative vaginal delivery, risks related to forceps-assisted delivery should also be considered and relayed to the patient prior to their use. Corneal abrasions and external ocular trauma are more common with forceps delivery. In one study, 36.5% of forceps-assisted deliveries resulted in instrument bruising [31]. Greater maternal morbidity, including perineal lacerations, is also seen with forceps. A large cohort study from a California database compared over 83 000 deliveries between 1992 and 1994 [33]. The lowest morbidity and mortality was seen with spontaneous vaginal delivery, an intermediate risk was seen with vacuum, forceps, or cesarean section during labor, while the highest risk was seen in those who delivered with combined forceps and vacuum extraction or who were delivered by cesarean section following failed operative vaginal delivery.

Long-term infant consequences

A few randomized studies have addressed the long-term consequences of operative vaginal delivery. One randomized study comparing vacuum to forceps failed to show a statistical difference in head circumference, weight, hearing, or vision at 9 months of age [34]. A separate large cohort study of 3413 children failed to show cognitive differences between those delivered by forceps and those delivered spontaneously [35]. Finally, a 10-year follow-up of 295 children delivered by vacuum and 302 controls delivered spontaneously revealed no difference in scholastic performance, speech, ability of self-care, or neurologic abnormality between the groups [36].

Shoulder dystocia

Shoulder dystocia is most often defined as a delivery that requires additional obstetric maneuvers following failure of gentle downward traction on the fetal head to effect delivery of the shoulders [37]. The most common mechanism is impaction of the anterior fetal shoulder behind the maternal pubic symphysis, and rarely impaction of the posterior fetal shoulder on the sacral promontory. It is thought to complicate less than 1% of vaginal deliveries, and is a significant contributor of maternal and neonatal injury, including brachial plexus injuries. Of note, approximately 4% of brachial plexus injuries are as a result of cesarean delivery.

Despite aggressive treatment of gestational diabetes, decreased operative vaginal delivery rates, and strict management guidelines for elective cesarean section to prevent shoulder dystocia published by ACOG, the incidence of shoulder dystocia has not decreased. In fact, a recent large UK cohort study of over 79 000 deliveries reported increased incidence of shoulder dystocia, brachial plexus injury, and neonatal asphyxia between 1991 and 2005 [38].

Risk factors for shoulder dystocia include gestational diabetes, macrosomia (fetal weight greater than 5000 g in non-diabetics and 4500 g in diabetics) [39], operative vaginal delivery, prior history of shoulder dystocia, protracted labor, pitocin use, and prolonged second stage. In only 10% of the cases a risk factor can be identified; the majority of cases are surprise presentations.

More than 95% of shoulder dystocias are uncomplicated, yet severe cases of shoulder dystocia may result in hypoxic–ischemic encephalopathy and even death [37]. Of the 5% of shoulder dystocias associated with fetal injury, less than 10% lead to permanent neurological morbidity, mostly brachial plexus injury. Other neonatal morbidity includes bone fractures, low Apgar scores, acidosis, and NICU admissions [38]. Maternal complications of shoulder dystocia include postpartum hemorrhage and perineal injury.

Amniotic fluid embolism

Amniotic fluid embolism (AFE) is a rare but catastrophic event. It arises when small amounts of amniotic fluid, rich in thromboplastin and thrombin, enter the maternal circulation via the exposed uterine spiral arterioles at the placental bed. Suggested risk factors for AFE include advanced maternal age, medical induction of labor, polyhydramnios, amnioinfusion, multiple gestations, cesarean section, operative vaginal delivery, placenta previa or abruption, eclampsia, and uterine rupture [40]. Maternal morbidity includes emergency delivery, cardiopulmonary arrest, pulmonary embolus, disseminated intravascular coagulopathy (DIC), and death. Fetal morbidity includes neonatal hypoxia, low Apgar scores, NICU admissions, and demise.

A large population-based retrospective cohort study reported the incidence of AFE to be about 1/17 000 singleton pregnancies [40]. A review of 46 suspected cases of AFE revealed that approximately 70% occurred during labor, 11% following vaginal delivery, and 19% during cesarean section following delivery of the infant. Maternal mortality was 61%, with neurologically intact survival seen in only 15% of women. Of the fetuses in utero at the time of the event, only 39% survived [41]. Other large cohort studies have described maternal mortality rates as low as 13% [40].

Clark *et al.* postulated that a biphasic hemodynamic response exists in the setting of amniotic fluid embolism [42]. First, an initial transient period of intense pulmonary vasospasm leads to acute right ventricular failure and hypoxemia. This may explain the 50% occurrence of maternal deaths during the acute episode. Subsequently, however, the predominant feature is one of left ventricular heart failure. The National Amniotic Fluid Registry revealed marked similarities between the hemodynamic, clinical, and hematologic manifestations of amniotic fluid embolism and both anaphylactic and septic shock [41]. Therefore, some authors recommend that the term "amniotic fluid embolism" be discarded altogether and replaced by "anaphylactoid syndrome of pregnancy" [41,43]. Reports of "atypical amniotic fluid embolisms" have recently described clinical hemorrhage and coagulopathy as the initial presentation rather than the classical pattern of cardiopulmonary collapse [44–46].

Early diagnosis of AFE is an integral step in the delivery of timely and appropriate care [47]. Despite efforts to identify a gold-standard diagnostic test, AFE remains a clinical diagnosis dependent on bedside judgment and exclusion of other diseases in the broad differential diagnosis [47]. Patients with AFE are best managed using a multidisciplinary approach. There are no pharmacologic or other therapies that prevent or treat the AFE, and supportive care typically involves aggressive treatment of multiple types of shock simultaneously [48]. Invasive monitoring, and aggressive treatment of hypoxia, hypotension, coagulopathy, hemorrhage, and left ventricular dysfunction are paramount [48]. The difficulty in managing AFE is the rapidity with which progression of signs and symptoms occurs, most often including considerations of both mother and fetus. In the cases in which AFE occurs during labor, immediate delivery of the fetus is mandated to prevent further hypoxic damage to the fetus and to facilitate cardiopulmonary resuscitative efforts [48].

Intra-amniotic infection

Intra-amniotic infection refers to infection of any fetal compartment including fetal membranes. It includes infection of the chorion (*chorioamnionitis* or *villitis*), amniotic fluid (*amnionitis*), umbilical cord (*funisitis*), and fetal circulation [49]. Clinically evident intra-amniotic infection occurs in approximately 0.5–10% of pregnancies [50].

Intra-amniotic infection is a major risk factor for preterm labor and delivery [51]. Risk factors for intrapartum chorioamnionitis at term include preterm rupture of membranes (rupture of membranes prior to uterine contractions), prolonged labor, performing multiple vaginal exams, intrauterine fetal surveillance monitors such as intrauterine pressure catheters and scalp electrodes, and maternal infections. The most common pathway for development of chorioamnionitis is via the ascent of lower genital tract organisms into the amniotic cavity. Less frequently, hematogenous or transplacental passage of bacteria may be the culprit.

Clinical chorioamnionitis at term is the leading risk factor for neonatal sepsis. Multiple studies have linked chorioamnionitis with NICU admissions, pneumonia, cerebral palsy (CP), respiratory distress syndrome (RDS), and periventricular leukomalacia (PVL) [52,53]. Despite this, among term infants born after intra-amniotic infection, perinatal mortality is less than 1% [43].

However, many infants born to mothers with chorioamnionitis have features of neonatal encephalopathy such as low Apgar scores, metabolic acidosis, and FHR abnormalities. These infants are at increased risk of developing CP, and studies have documented a four- to ninefold increase in the incidence of CP in term and near-term infants of mothers with chorioamnionitis [52,53]. As noted by Wu and Colford, maternal infection leads to an elevation of fetal cytokines that can damage the fetal central nervous system and impair placental blood flow and gas exchange [53]. Maternal fever may also raise the core temperature of the fetus, which may be harmful to the developing fetus.

The pathophysiology involved in chorioamnionitis is clearly delineated in preterm infants in Chapter 4, and similar processes can be seen in the term infant as well.

Chorioamnionitis is usually a polymicrobial disorder, arising from *Bacteroides* species, *Gardnerella vaginalis*, Group B *Streptococcus*, *Escherichia coli*, *Mycoplasma*, and other aerobic streptococci as well as aerobic Gram-negative rods. Diagnosis is typically made clinically, by the presence of maternal fever, fetal tachycardia, uterine tenderness, and/or foul-smelling odor of the amniotic fluid. Several treatment regimens have been studied in the setting of chorioamnionitis, including combinations of ampicillin, gentamycin, clindamycin, vancomycin, cephalosporins, macrolides, and others [54]. Despite the lack of a clear standard, the goal of treatment regardless of regimen is to provide broad-spectrum antibiotic coverage in order to reduce neonatal morbidity and mortality.

Post-term and meconium staining

Post-term pregnancy is defined as any pregnancy extending beyond 42 weeks' gestation. The reported incidence of post-term pregnancy is approximately 7% [55]. An important task when confronting a post-term pregnancy is to adequately assess the gestational age, as poor dating is the most common cause of apparently prolonged gestation. Data now indicate that any pregnancy lasting beyond term is associated with increased neonatal morbidity and mortality, and these risks should be discussed with the patients in order to develop a delivery plan based on individual obstetrical history, cervical Bishop score, and likelihood of spontaneous labor.

Pregnancy beyond term is associated with increased neonatal demise. The nadir of neonatal mortality is at 39–40 weeks for singletons and rises exponentially following 42 weeks. Moreover, meconium staining, labor induction, cesarean section, macrosomia, shoulder dystocia, and operative vaginal delivery all increase in pregnancies beyond term. Low umbilical artery pH and low 5-minute Apgar scores have also been linked to post-term pregnancies.

Twenty percent of post-term fetuses have dysmaturity syndrome, which refers to infants with characteristics similar to intrauterine growth restriction and placental insufficiency [55]. The syndrome is also associated with cord compression, oligohydramnios, meconium aspiration and short-term neonatal complications such as hypoglycemia, seizures, and respiratory insufficiency [55].

Meconium-stained amniotic fluid results from the passing of fetal stool prior to delivery and occurs in approximately 12–22% of women in labor [56]. Though often linked to fetal stress, meconium at term, without other signs of fetal compromise, does not result in adverse neonatal outcomes. Meconium aspiration syndrome comprises a combination of airway obstruction, inflammation, atelectasis, lung overexpansion, inhibition of surfactant, and secondary surfactant deficiency, hypoxia, and pulmonary hypertension [57,58]. The syndrome occurs in up to 10% of infants exposed to meconium-stained amniotic fluid and is associated with significant morbidity and mortality [56]. Initial small cohort studies of amnioinfusion as a treatment for meconium-stained fluid suggested a benefit. Larger follow-up studies including a large multicenter trial showed no benefit to amnioinfusion in terms of moderate or severe meconium aspiration, perinatal mortality, or cesarean delivery [59].

Malpresentation

Determining fetal presentation is an important step in the evaluation of the laboring patient. Most fetuses at term will align along the longitudinal axis of the uterus. Transverse and oblique lies are less common at term, seen most often in the setting of multiple gestations and grand multiparity. The most common fetal presentation is vertex (sometimes referred to as occiput), occurring in 96% of fetuses at term. Less common non-vertex presentations include breech (further defined as frank, footling, complete), face, brow, and compound. Non-vertex presentations may complicate the labor process by compromising the ability of the fetus to either enter the pelvic inlet (engagement) or flex its neck as it traverses the maternal pelvis. Flexion and fetal descent occur most often in the mid-pelvis, the narrowest portion of the pelvis bordered by the ischial spines. Inability to enter or maneuver through the pelvis leads to protracted labor and may even lead to severe maternal and neonatal morbidity. Though mostly a clinical diagnosis, ultrasound confirmation of fetal presentation and position may assist with the diagnosis of malpresentation in labor [60].

Face presentation

Fetal face presentation is caused by sharp extension of the fetal neck during the process of labor. Face presentation is often associated with fetal anencephaly, anterior neck masses, or hydrocephalus. Also, cephalopelvic disproportion, macrosomia, abnormal pelvic structures, and factors leading to laxity of the anterior abdominal tone such as multiparity and connective tissue disorders may lead to abnormal presentation.

Face presentation is often diagnosed in the second stage of labor on digital exam. The position of the face relative to the pelvis will determine the likelihood of a successful vaginal delivery. Sixty percent of face presentations occur in the mentum anterior position, 15% in the mentum transverse, and 26% in the mentum posterior [61]. Up to 50% of fetuses in the mentum transverse and mentum posterior positions will spontaneously convert to mentum anterior during the course of labor. Knowing the fetal position is crucial, since most mentum anterior positions are likely to deliver vaginally. FHR abnormalities and low 5-minute Apgar scores are also associated with face presentation.

In the mentum anterior presentation, as the face descends onto the perineum, the fetal chin passes under the maternal pubic symphysis. Flexion of the head follows as the baby is delivered. On the other hand, in the mentum posterior position, the fetal neck must extend the length of the maternal sacrum in order to reach the perineum, a difficult task given its short length. Vaginal delivery is therefore usually not possible unless spontaneous rotation occurs or the fetus is very small. Manual rotation of the mentum posterior to the vertex or mentum anterior position should only be attempted with extreme caution. Case reports of uterine rupture, neonatal asphyxia due to cord prolapse, and neonatal neurologic injury from spine trauma have been described.

Breech presentation

Delivery of a breech presentation has been described as early as the first century AD. For over 1000 years obstructed labor was treated by converting the presentation to a footling breech and delivering the baby by traction. Different techniques have been described to deliver a breech singleton, including assisted vaginal delivery, spontaneous vaginal delivery, and total breech extraction. The assisted vaginal breech delivery includes spontaneous delivery of the fetus to the umbilicus followed by the Pinard (flexion of the leg at the knee in order to facilitate its delivery out of the vagina), Loveset (rotation of the body and sweeping of the fetal arms), and Mauriceau (delivery of the aftercoming head) maneuvers. In the eighteenth century William Smellie applied forceps to the aftercoming head, and in 1924 Edmund Piper designed forceps specifically for the aftercoming head.

In the 1900s, concerns over vaginal breech delivery grew as reports of birth trauma, including intraventricular hemorrhage, spinal cord and brachial plexus injury, fractures, genital injury, birth asphyxia, and perinatal mortality, surfaced. In 2000, Hanah *et al.* published their results from a multicenter randomized trial of planned cesarean section versus planned vaginal birth trial [62]. The study had planned to enroll 2800 participants in 26 countries, with a primary outcome of perinatal or neonatal mortality. The study was halted early when an interim analysis showed 5% perinatal mortality or serious neonatal morbidity in the planned vaginal group versus 1.6% in the planned cesarean section group. Moreover, the authors concluded that "for every additional 14 cesarean sections done, one baby will avoid death or serious morbidity." Following the study, ACOG released a committee opinion stating that a "planned vaginal delivery of a singleton term breech may no longer be appropriate," and that "patients with persistent breech presentation at term in singleton gestation should undergo a planned cesarean section" [63]. Over the last seven years, criticisms of the Term Breech Trial have surfaced, including a study failing to show a significant difference in long-term neurologic sequelae between neonates delivered by cesarean or breech delivery, which resulted in ACOG rescinding its original statement and replacing it with the following in 2006: "In light of recent studies that further clarify the long-term risks of vaginal breech delivery, ACOG recommends that the decision regarding mode of delivery should depend on the experience of the health care provider . . . Cesarean delivery will be the preferred mode for most physicians because of the diminishing expertise in vaginal breech delivery" [64,65].

External cephalic version

External cephalic version (ECV), or the manual rotation of a malpositioned fetus by the application of external pressure to the maternal abdomen, has been described as early as 400 BC by Hippocrates. In 1997 ACOG published guidelines for ECV, including gestational age greater than 36 completed weeks [66]. Success rates for ECV have ranged from approximately 30% to 80%, with greater success reported in multiparous patients and those with oblique or transverse lie. Greater success has also been reported with the use of uterine relaxants, including terbutaline and ritodrine [67]. Data are limited and conflicting regarding the use of spinal or epidural [67]. Reported complications of ECV include intrauterine fetal demise, antepartum hemorrhage, premature labor, and preterm premature rupture of membranes (PPROM). Controversy regarding ECV still exists regarding patients with prior cesarean section, decreased amniotic fluid volume, or uterine malformations. Contraindications to ECV include PPROM, placenta previa, suspected placental abruption, and non-reassuring FHR.

Prolonged second stage

ACOG defines labor as the presence of uterine contractions of sufficient intensity, frequency, and duration to bring about demonstrable effacement and dilation of the cervix [68]. Normal labor is divided into three stages. The first stage, including both the latent and active phases, begins with cervical change and concludes with full cervical dilation. The second stage is the time from full cervical dilation to delivery of the neonate, and the third stage is the time interval from delivery of the neonate to delivery of the placenta.

The term "cephalopelvic disproportion" has been used to describe a disparity between the size of the maternal pelvis and the fetal head that precludes vaginal delivery [68]. Protracted and arrested disorders can occur throughout the course of labor, and their management depends on evaluation of maternal uterine contractions, the size, presentation, and position of the fetus, and maternal pelvic characteristics, assessed most commonly using clinical pelvimetry. Labor dystocia accounts for the majority of cesarean deliveries performed.

The median duration for the second stage of labor is 20 minutes for multiparous women and 50 minutes for nulliparous women [69]. Prolonged second stage should be considered in nulliparous women if the second stage lasts beyond 2 hours, or 3 hours with regional anesthesia [68]. Prolonged second stage in multiparous women should be considered if the second stage lasts longer than 1 hour, or 2 hours with regional anesthesia [68]. Management of prolonged second stage will vary depending upon reassessment of the woman, fetus, and expulsive forces. Once a second-stage arrest disorder is diagnosed, the obstetrician has three options: (1) continued observation, (2) operative vaginal delivery, or (3) cesarean delivery.

Risk factors for prolonged labor include nulliparity, diabetes, macrosomia, epidural anesthesia, oxytocin usage, and chorioamnionitis [70]. Arrested and prolonged labor, particularly in the second stage, may lead to severe neonatal and maternal morbidity. Chorioamnionitis, particularly in the setting of prolonged ruptured membranes, has been linked to protracted labor. Fetal infection and bacteremia, including pneumonia caused by aspiration of infected amniotic fluid, has also been linked to prolonged labor [68]. From a maternal perspective, increased cesarean operative times, greater extensions at the time of cesarean section, increased operative vaginal delivery rates, and increased third- and fourth-degree lacerations have all been linked to prolonged second stage [71,72]. Prolonged second stage may also result in injuries of the pelvic floor, and in developing nations very prolonged second stages of labor have resulted in severe necrosis and development of vesico- and rectovaginal fistulas [73].

Recently, despite historical concerns for fetal asphyxia, evidence has emerged suggesting improved vaginal delivery rates with expectant management of prolonged second stage [70]. In a large retrospective cohort study of over 6000 patients in the second stage of labor, there were no perinatal deaths unrelated to anomaly in the prolonged second stage group [74]. Also, there was no significant relationship between second-stage duration and low 5-minute Apgar score, neonatal seizures, or admission to the neonatal intensive care unit. ACOG thus states that the decision to perform an operative delivery in the second stage versus continued observation should be made on the basis of clinical assessment of the woman and the fetus, and the skill and training of the obstetrician [68].

Fetal heart-rate monitoring

FHR monitors are ubiquitous on labor and delivery units across the United States and other developed countries. In 2002, approximately 85% of all live births were assessed with electronic fetal heart-rate monitoring (EFM) [75]. Despite widespread use, major limitations to EFM remain, including poor inter- and intra-observer reliability, uncertain efficacy, and a high false-positive rate [76].

A large meta-analysis comparing EFM with intermittent auscultation showed higher rates of cesarean section and operative vaginal deliveries in the EFM group [77]. Also, despite a lower rate of perinatal mortality caused by fetal hypoxia in the EFM group, the overall perinatal mortality was equal [77]. Most studies comparing the two modalities exclude high-risk pregnancies such as suspected fetal growth restriction, pre-eclampsia, and type 1 diabetes mellitus; ACOG still recommends continuous monitoring of such pregnancies [76].

Marked inter- and intra-observer variability in EFM has been described in multiple studies [78–80]. For example, when four obstetricians examined 50 tracings, agreement was reached in only 22% of cases. Moreover, 2 months later, the same clinicians interpreted 21% of the tracings differently than they did during the first evaluation [78].

The greatest limitation of EFM is its high false-positive rate. The positive predictive value of a non-reassuring FHR pattern to predict CP among singletons with a birthweight of 2500 g or more is only 0.14% [81]. Thus, for 1000 fetuses with a non-reassuring FHR pattern, only one or two will develop CP [76]. Despite increasing prevalence, the widespread use of EFM has not led to the reduction of CP over time [82,83]. This is also consistent with the fact that only 4% of encephalopathies can be attributed solely to intrapartum events [1].

References

1. American College of Obstetricians and Gynecologists. *Neonatal Encephalopathy and Cerebral Palsy*. Executive summary. www.acog.org. Accessed October, 2008.

2. March of Dimes. Peri Stats. Births by method of delivery, 1994–2004. http://www.marchofdimes.com/peristats/. Accessed January, 2008.

3. NIH State-of-the-Science Conference Statement on Cesarean Delivery on Maternal Request. *NIH Consensus Statements* 2006; **23**: 1–29.

4. Villar J, Carroli G, Zavaleta N, *et al.* Maternal and neonatal individual risks and benefits associated with caesarean delivery: multicentre prospective study. *BMJ* 2007; **335**: 1025–35.

5. Nisenblat V, Barak S, Griness OB, *et al.* Maternal complications associated with multiple cesarean deliveries. *Obstet Gynecol* 2006; **108**: 21–6.

6. Silver RM, Landon MB, Rouse DJ, *et al.* Maternal morbidity associated with multiple repeat cesarean deliveries. *Obstet Gynecol* 2006; **107**: 1226–32.

7. Kennare R, Tucker G, Heard A, *et al.* Risks of adverse outcomes in the next birth after a first cesarean delivery. *Obstet Gynecol* 2007; **109**: 270–6.

8. Grobman WA, Lai Y, Landon MB, *et al.* Development of a nomogram for prediction of vaginal birth after cesarean delivery. *Obstet Gynecol* 2007; **109**: 806–12.

9. Peaceman AM, Gersnoviez R, Landon MB, *et al.* The MFMU Cesarean Registry: impact of fetal size on trial of labor success for patients with previous cesarean for dystocia. *Am J Obstet Gynecol* 2006; **195**: 1127–31.

10. Landon MB, Spong CY, Thom E, *et al.* Risk of uterine rupture with a trial of labor in women with multiple and single prior cesarean delivery. *Obstet Gynecol* 2006; **108**: 12–20.

11. ACOG Practice Bulletin #54: vaginal birth after previous cesarean. *Obstet Gynecol* 2004; **104**: 203–12.

12. Gyamfi C, Juhasz G, Gyamfi P, *et al.* Single- versus double-layer uterine incision closure and uterine rupture. *J Matern Fetal Neonatal Med* 2006; **19**: 639–43.

13. Cahill AG, Stamilio DM, Odibo AO, *et al.* Does a maximum dose of oxytocin affect risk for uterine rupture in candidates for vaginal birth after cesarean delivery? *Am J Obstet Gynecol* 2007; **197**: 495.e1–5.

14. Landon MB, Hauth JC, Leveno KJ, *et al.* Maternal and perinatal outcomes associated with a trial of labor after prior cesarean delivery. *N Engl J Med* 2004; **351**: 2581–9.

15. Spong CY, Landon MB, Gilbert S, *et al.* Risk of uterine rupture and adverse perinatal outcome at term after cesarean delivery. *Obstet Gynecol* 2007; **110**: 801–7.

16. Cahill AG, Macones GA. Vaginal birth after cesarean delivery: evidence-based practice. *Clin Obstet Gynecol* 2007; **50**: 518–25.

17. Macones GA, Peipert J, Nelson DB, *et al.* Maternal complications with vaginal birth after cesarean delivery: a multicenter study. *Am J Obstet Gynecol* 2005; **193**: 1656–62.

18. Landon MB, Leindecker S, Spong CY, *et al.* The MFMU Cesarean Registry: factors affecting the success of trial of labor after previous cesarean delivery. *Am J Obstet Gynecol* 2005; **193**: 1016–23.

19. Cahill AG, Stamilio DM, Odibo AO, *et al.* Is vaginal birth after cesarean (VBAC) or elective repeat cesarean safer in women with a prior vaginal delivery? *Am J Obstet Gynecol* 2006; **195**: 1143–7.

20. Macario A, El-Sayed YY, Druzin ML. Cost-effectiveness of a trial of labor after previous cesarean delivery depends on the a priori chance of success. *Clin Obstet Gynecol* 2004; **47**: 378–85.

21. Chung A, Macario A, El-Sayed YY, *et al.* Cost-effectiveness of a trial of labor after previous cesarean. *Obstet Gynecol* 2001; **97**: 932–41.

22. Pare E, Quinones JN, Macones GA. Vaginal birth after caesarean section versus elective repeat caesarean section: assessment of maternal downstream health outcomes. *BJOG* 2006; **113**: 75–85.

23. Ridgeway JJ, Weyrich DL, Benedetti TJ. Fetal heart rate changes associated with uterine rupture. *Obstet Gynecol* 2004; **103**: 506–12.

24. Miller DA, Goodwin TM, Gherman RB, *et al.* Intrapartum rupture of the unscarred uterus. *Obstet Gynecol* 1997; **89**: 671–3.

25. Sweeten KM, Graves WK, Athanassiou A. Spontaneous rupture of the unscarred uterus. *Am J Obstet Gynecol* 1995; **172**: 1851–5.

26. Walsh CA, Baxi LV. Rupture of the primigravid uterus: a review of the literature. *Obstet Gynecol Surv* 2007; **62**: 327–34.

27. American College of Obstetricians and Gynecologists. Operative vaginal delivery: clinical management guidelines for obstetrician–gynecologists. *Int J Gynaecol Obstet* 2001; **74**: 69–76.

28. Carmona F, Martinez-Roman S, Manau D, *et al.* Immediate maternal and neonatal effects of low-forceps delivery according to the new criteria of the American College of Obstetricians and Gynecologists compared with spontaneous vaginal delivery in term pregnancies. *Am J Obstet Gynecol* 1995; **173**: 55–9.

29. Yancey MK, Herpolsheimer A, Jordan GD, *et al.* Maternal and neonatal effects of outlet forceps delivery compared with spontaneous vaginal delivery in term pregnancies. *Obstet Gynecol* 1991; **78**: 646–50.

30. Kolderup LB, Laros RK, Musci TJ. Incidence of persistent birth injury in macrosomic infants: association with mode of delivery. *Am J Obstet Gynecol* 1997; **177**: 37–41.

31. Johnson JH, Figueroa R, Garry D, *et al.* Immediate maternal and neonatal effects of forceps and vacuum-assisted deliveries. *Obstet Gynecol* 2004; **103**: 513–18.

32. Caughey AB, Sandberg PL, Zlatnik MG, *et al.* Forceps compared with vacuum: rates of neonatal and maternal morbidity. *Obstet Gynecol* 2005; **106**: 908–12.

33. Towner D, Castro MA, Eby-Wilkens E, *et al.* Effect of mode of delivery in nulliparous women on neonatal intracranial injury. *N Engl J Med* 1999; **341**: 1709–14.

34. Carmody F, Grant A, Mutch L, *et al.* Follow up of babies delivered in a randomized controlled comparison of vacuum extraction and forceps delivery. *Acta Obstet Gynecol Scand* 1986; **65**: 763–6.

35. Wesley BD, van den Berg BJ, Reece EA. The effect of forceps delivery on cognitive development. *Am J Obstet Gynecol* 1993; **169**: 1091–5.

36. Ngan HY, Miu P, Ko L, *et al.* Long-term neurological sequelae following vacuum extractor delivery. *Aust NZ J Obstet Gynaecol* 1990; **30**: 111–14.

37. Sokol RJ, Blackwell SC. ACOG practice bulletin: shoulder dystocia. Number 40, November 2002. *Int J Gynaecol Obstet* 2003; **80**: 87–92.

38. MacKenzie IZ, Shah M, Lean K, *et al.* Management of shoulder dystocia: trends in incidence and maternal and neonatal morbidity. *Obstet Gynecol* 2007; **110**: 1059–68.

39. Fetal macrosomia. ACOG Technical Bulletin Number 159, September 1991. *Int J Gynaecol Obstet* 1992; **39**: 341–5.

40. Kramer MS, Rouleau J, Baskett TF, *et al.* Amniotic-fluid embolism and medical induction of labour: a retrospective, population-based cohort study. *Lancet* 2006; **368**: 1444–8.

41. Clark SL, Hankins GD, Dudley DA, *et al.* Amniotic fluid embolism: analysis of the national registry. *Am J Obstet Gynecol* 1995; **172**: 1158–67.

42. Clark SL, Montz FJ, Phelan JP. Hemodynamic alterations associated with amniotic fluid embolism: a reappraisal. *Am J Obstet Gynecol* 1985; **151**: 617–21.

43. Creasy RK, Resnik R, Iams JD. *Maternal–Fetal Medicine*, 5th edn. Philadelphia, PA: Saunders, 2004.

44. Yang JI, Kim HS, Chang KH, *et al.* Amniotic fluid embolism with isolated coagulopathy: a case report. *J Reprod Med* 2006; **51**: 64–6.

45. Levy G. [Amniotic fluid embolism]. *Ann Fr Anesth Reanim* 2004; **23**: 861.

46. Awad IT, Shorten GD. Amniotic fluid embolism and isolated coagulopathy: atypical presentation of amniotic fluid embolism. *Eur J Anaesthesiol* 2001; **18**: 410–13.

47. Moore J. Amniotic fluid embolism: on the trail of an elusive diagnosis. *Lancet* 2006; **368**: 1399–401.

48. Moore J, Baldisseri MR. Amniotic fluid embolism. *Crit Care Med* 2005; **33**: S279–85.

49. Cunningham FG, Williams JW. *Williams Obstetrics*, 21st edn. New York, NY: McGraw-Hill, 2001.

50. Gibbs RS, Duff P. Progress in pathogenesis and management of clinical intraamniotic infection. *Am J Obstet Gynecol* 1991; **164**: 1317–26.

51. Romero R, Espinoza J, Kusanovic JP, *et al.* The preterm parturition syndrome. *BJOG* 2006; **113**: 17–42.

52. Grether JK, Nelson KB. Maternal infection and cerebral palsy in infants of normal birth weight. *JAMA* 1997; **278**: 207–11.

53. Wu YW, Colford JM. Chorioamnionitis as a risk factor for cerebral palsy: a meta-analysis. *JAMA* 2000; **284**: 1417–24.

54. Hopkins L, Smaill F. Antibiotic regimens for management of intraamniotic infection. *Cochrane Database Syst Rev* 2002; (3): CD003254.

55. ACOG Practice Bulletin. Clinical management guidelines for obstetricians–gynecologists. Number 55, September 2004. Management of postterm pregnancy. *Obstet Gynecol* 2004; **104**: 639–46.

56. ACOG Committee Opinion Number 346, October 2006: amnioinfusion does not prevent meconium aspiration syndrome. *Obstet Gynecol* 2006; **108**: 1053.

57. Rais-Bahrami K, Rivera O, Seale WR, *et al.* Effect of nitric oxide and high-frequency oscillatory ventilation in meconium aspiration syndrome. *Pediatr Crit Care Med* 2000; **1**: 166–9.

58. Dargaville PA, Copnell B. The epidemiology of meconium aspiration syndrome: incidence, risk factors, therapies, and outcome. *Pediatrics* 2006; **117**: 1712–21.

59. Fraser WD, Hofmeyr J, Lede R, *et al.* Amnioinfusion for the prevention of the meconium aspiration syndrome. *N Engl J Med* 2005; **353**: 909–17.

60. Chou MR, Kreiser D, Taslimi MM, *et al.* Vaginal versus ultrasound examination of fetal occiput position during the second stage of labor. *Am J Obstet Gynecol* 2004; **191**: 521–4.

61. Cruikshank DP, White CA. Obstetric malpresentations: twenty years' experience. *Am J Obstet Gynecol* 1973; **116**: 1097–104.

62. Hannah ME, Hannah WJ, Hewson SA, *et al.* Planned caesarean section versus planned vaginal birth for breech presentation at term: a randomised multicentre trial. Term Breech Trial Collaborative Group. *Lancet* 2000; **356**: 1375–83.

63. ACOG Committee Opinion: number 265, December 2001. Mode of term single breech delivery. *Obstet Gynecol* 2001; **98**: 1189–90.

64. ACOG Committee Opinion No. 340. Mode of term singleton breech delivery. *Obstet Gynecol* 2006; **108**: 235–7.

65. Whyte H, Hannah ME, Saigal S, *et al.* Outcomes of children at 2 years after planned cesarean birth versus planned vaginal birth for breech presentation at term: the International Randomized Term Breech Trial. *Am J Obstet Gynecol* 2004; **191**: 864–71.

66. ACOG practice patterns. External cephalic version. Number 4, July 1997. American College of Obstetricians and Gynecologists. *Int J Gynaecol Obstet* 1997; **59**: 73–80.

67. Hofmeyr GJ. Interventions to help external cephalic version for breech presentation at term. *Cochrane Database Syst Rev* 2004; (1): CD000184.

68. ACOG Practice Bulletin Number 49, December 2003. Dystocia and augmentation of labor. *Obstet Gynecol* 2003; **102**: 1445–54.

69. Kilpatrick SJ, Laros RK. Characteristics of normal labor. *Obstet Gynecol* 1989; **74**: 85–7.

70. Myles TD, Santolaya J. Maternal and neonatal outcomes in patients with a prolonged second stage of labor. *Obstet Gynecol* 2003; **102**: 52–8.

71. Cheng YW, Hopkins LM, Caughey AB. How long is too long: does a prolonged second stage of labor in nulliparous

women affect maternal and neonatal outcomes? *Am J Obstet Gynecol* 2004; **191**: 933–8.

72. Sung JF, Daniels KI, Brodzinsky L, *et al.* Cesarean delivery outcomes after a prolonged second stage of labor. *Am J Obstet Gynecol* 2007; **197**: 306.e1–5.

73. Holme A, Breen M, MacArthur C. Obstetric fistulae: a study of women managed at the Monze Mission Hospital, Zambia. *BJOG* 2007; **114**: 1010–17.

74. Menticoglou SM, Manning F, Harman C, *et al.* Perinatal outcome in relation to second-stage duration. *Am J Obstet Gynecol* 1995; **173**: 906–12.

75. Martin JA, Hamilton BE, Sutton PD, *et al.* Births: final data for 2002. *Natl Vital Stat Rep* 2003; **52**: 1–113.

76. ACOG Practice Bulletin. Clinical management guidelines for obstetrician–gynecologists, Number 70, December 2005. Intrapartum fetal heart rate monitoring. *Obstet Gynecol* 2005; **106**: 1453–60.

77. Vintzileos AM, Nochimson DJ, Guzman ER, *et al.* Intrapartum electronic fetal heart rate monitoring versus intermittent auscultation: a meta-analysis. *Obstet Gynecol* 1995; **85**: 149–55.

78. Nielsen PV, Stigsby B, Nickelsen C, *et al.* Intra- and inter-observer variability in the assessment of intrapartum cardiotocograms. *Acta Obstet Gynecol Scand* 1987; **66**: 421–4.

79. Blix E, Sviggum O, Koss KS, *et al.* Inter-observer variation in assessment of 845 labour admission tests: comparison between midwives and obstetricians in the clinical setting and two experts. *BJOG* 2003; **110**: 1–5.

80. Beaulieu MD, Fabia J, Leduc B, *et al.* The reproducibility of intrapartum cardiotocogram assessments. *Can Med Assoc J* 1982; **127**: 214–16.

81. Nelson KB, Dambrosia JM, Ting TY, *et al.* Uncertain value of electronic fetal monitoring in predicting cerebral palsy. *N Engl J Med* 1996; **334**: 613–18.

82. Thacker SB, Stroup D, Chang M. Continuous electronic heart rate monitoring for fetal assessment during labor. *Cochrane Database Syst Rev* 2001; (2): CD000063.

83. Clark SL, Hankins GD. Temporal and demographic trends in cerebral palsy: fact and fiction. *Am J Obstet Gynecol* 2003; **188**: 628–33.

Chapter

13

Fetal response to asphyxia

Laura Bennet and Alistair J. Gunn

Introduction

For most of the twentieth century the concept of perinatal brain damage centered around cerebral palsy and intrapartum asphyxia. It is only in the last 20 years that this view has been seriously challenged by clinical and epidemiological studies that have demonstrated that approximately 70–90% or more of cerebral palsy is unrelated to intrapartum events [1]. Many term infants who subsequently develop cerebral palsy are believed to have sustained asphyxial events in mid-gestation. In some cases, prenatal injury may lead to chronically abnormal heart-rate tracings and impaired ability to adapt to labor, which may be confounded with an acute event [2].

Furthermore, it has become clear that the various abnormal fetal heart-rate (FHR) patterns that have been proposed to be markers for potentially injurious asphyxia are consistently only very weakly predictive for cerebral palsy [3]. Although metabolic acidosis is more strongly associated with outcome, more than half of babies born with severe acidosis (base deficit > 16 mmol/L and pH < 7.0) do not develop encephalopathy, while conversely encephalopathy can still occur, although at low frequency, in association with relatively modest acidosis (BD 12–16 mmol/L) [4]. These data contrast with the presence of very abnormal fetal heart-rate tracings, severe metabolic acidosis [5], and acute cerebral lesions in the great majority of infants who *do* develop acute neonatal encephalopathy [6].

The key factor underlying all of these observations is the effectiveness of fetal adaptation to asphyxia. The fetus is, in fact, spectacularly good at defending itself against such insults, and injury occurs only in a very narrow window between intact survival and death. These adaptations work sufficiently well in the majority of cases that even the concept of "birth asphyxia" itself has been controversial. However, recent studies where cerebral function has been monitored from birth in infants with clinical evidence of compromise during labor have shown that many such children did have a precipitating episode in the immediate peripartum period, with evidence of acute evolving clinical encephalopathy [5], electroencephalographic (EEG) changes [7], cerebral lesions on magnetic resonance imaging (MRI) [6], mitochondrial oxidative activity,

and an increased rate of long-term cognitive or functional sequelae [8,9]. In those infants with evidence for acute perinatal asphyxial event(s) the link between asphyxia and long-term problems is the severity of early-onset encephalopathy. Newborns with mild encephalopathy are completely normal during follow-up, while at least 90% of those with severe (stage III) encephalopathy die or have severe handicap by 18 months of age. In contrast, only half of those with moderate (stage II) hypoxic–ischemic encephalopathy develop handicap; however, even those who do not develop neurological impairment are at risk of future academic failure [10].

Causes of pathological asphyxia

A number of events, some peculiar to labor, may result in asphyxia and fetal compromise, both antenatally and during labor. Broadly these may be grouped as chronic, acute catastrophic, and repeated hypoxia [5]. Chronic hypoxia may be caused by decreased fetal hemoglobin (e.g. fetomaternal or fetofetal hemorrhage), infection, and maternal causes such as systemic hypoxia and reduced uteroplacental blood flow due to hypotension. Immediate, catastrophic events include cord prolapse and to some extent cord entanglements, true knots in the cord, vasa previa, placental abruption, uterine rupture, and fetal entrapment, such as shoulder dystocia. The impact of asphyxia during placental abruption may be potentiated by fetal blood loss with fetal volume contraction. Finally, in labor, the fetus may be exposed to shorter but frequent episodes that may lead to a progressive decompensation over time [2].

Characteristics of perinatal asphyxial encephalopathy

The fetal response to asphyxia is not stereotypical. The fetal responses, and the ability of the fetus to avoid injury, depend upon the type of the insult (as above), the precise environmental conditions, and the maturity and condition of the fetus (Fig. 13.1). This review focuses on recent developments in our understanding of the factors that determine whether the brain is damaged after an asphyxial insult. We will briefly review the fundamental cellular mechanisms of cerebral damage and discuss in detail the systemic adaptations of the fetus to asphyxia in relation to the factors which can modulate the evolution of cerebral injury.

Fetal and Neonatal Brain Injury, 4th edition, ed. David K. Stevenson, William E. Benitz, Philip Sunshine, Susan R. Hintz, and Maurice L. Druzin. Published by Cambridge University Press. © Cambridge University Press 2009.

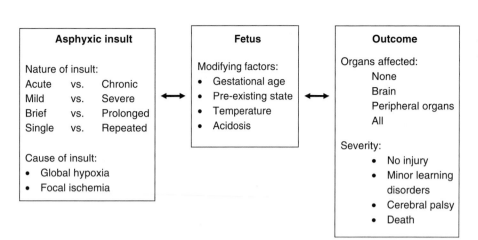

Fig. 13.1. Schema of the factors influencing the development of cerebral injury after perinatal asphyxia.

The pathogenesis of cell death
What initiates neuronal injury?

At the most fundamental level, injury requires a period of insufficient delivery of oxygen and substrates such as glucose (and other substrates in the fetus) such that neurons and glia cannot maintain homeostasis. Once the neurons' supply of high-energy metabolites such as ATP can no longer be maintained during hypoxia–ischemia, there is failure of the energy-dependent mechanisms of intracellular homeostasis, such as the Na^+,K^+-ATP-dependent pump. Neuronal depolarization occurs, leading to sodium and calcium entry into cells. This creates an osmotic and electrochemical gradient that in turn favors further cation and water entry, leading to cell swelling (cytotoxic edema). If sufficiently severe, this may lead to immediate lysis [11]. The swollen neurons may still recover, at least temporarily, if the hypoxic insult is reversed or the environment is manipulated. Evidence suggests that several additional factors act to increase cell injury during and following depolarization. These include the extracellular accumulation of excitatory amino acid neurotransmitters due to impairment of energy-dependent reuptake, which promote further receptor-mediated cell swelling and intracellular calcium entry, and the generation of oxygen free radicals and inflammatory cytokines [11,12]. Nevertheless, it is critical to appreciate that these factors appear to be injurious almost entirely in the presence of hypoxic cell depolarization. For example, glutamate is far more toxic during hypoxia (or mitochondrial dysfunction) than during normoxia [13]. Conversely, in vitro, hypoxia can still trigger cell death during glutamate receptor blockade, through apoptotic mechanisms [14].

If oxygen is reduced, but substrate delivery is effectively maintained (i.e., pure or nearly pure hypoxia), the cells will adapt in two ways to avoid or delay depolarization. Firstly, they can use anaerobic metabolism to support their production of high-energy metabolites for a time. The use of anaerobic metabolism is of course very inefficient since anaerobic glycolysis produces lactate and only two ATPs, whereas aerobic glycolysis produces 38 ATPs. Thus glucose reserves are rapidly consumed, and a metabolic acidosis develops, which,

as discussed further below, may have local and systemic consequences. In some circumstances the fetus may be able to benefit from increased circulating lactate. Many fetal tissues, such as the heart, get a high proportion of their substrate from sources other than glucose, particularly lactate [15], and the brain is able to oxidize lactate when its concentration is elevated [16]. Thus if hypoxia is mild or intermittent the circulating lactate may help support systemic metabolism during normoxic intervals. However, as lactate requires oxygen to be metabolized, clearly these alternative fuels cannot be used by the fetus during severe hypoxia/asphyxia.

Secondly, the brain can to some extent reduce non-obligatory energy consumption. This is clearly seen in neurons, where moderate hypoxia typically induces a switch to a high-voltage low-frequency EEG state requiring less oxygen consumption [17,18]. As an insult becomes more severe, neuronal activity ceases completely at a threshold above that which causes actual neuronal depolarization [19,20]. This regulated suppression of metabolic rate during hypoxia or ischemia, before energy stores are depleted, termed adaptive hypometabolism [21], is actively mediated through inhibitory neurotransmitters such as adenosine [20]. It is the duration of neuronal depolarization, rather than of suppression of the EEG per se, that ultimately determines the severity of injury [22]. Thus the brain remains protected as long as depolarization is avoided.

In contrast, under conditions where levels of both oxygen and substrate are reduced the options for the neuron are much more limited, since not only is there less oxygen, but there is also much less glucose available to support anaerobic metabolism. This may occur during pure ischemia (reduced tissue blood flow, such as occurs in stroke) but also, even more critically, during conditions of hypoxia–ischemia, i.e., a combination of reduced oxygen content with reduced tissue blood flow. In the fetus, hypoxia–ischemia commonly occurs due to hypoxic cardiac compromise and hypotension. Under these conditions depletion of cerebral high-energy metabolites will occur much more rapidly and profoundly, while at the same time there may actually be *less* acidosis, both because there is much less glucose available to be metabolized to lactate, and because the insult evolves more quickly.

These concepts help to explain the consistent observation, discussed later in this chapter, that most cerebral injury after acute perinatal insults occurs in association with hypotension and consequent tissue hypoperfusion or ischemia. In contrast, although asphyxial brain injury by definition requires exposure to an anaerobic environment, there is only a broad correlation between the severity of systemic acidosis and the severity of injury in any paradigm, at any age. Asphyxia is defined as the combination of impaired respiratory gas exchange (i.e., hypoxia and hypercapnia) accompanied by the development of metabolic acidosis. When we think about the impact on the brain of clinical asphyxia it will be critical to keep in mind that this definition tells us much about things that are relatively easily measured (fetal blood gases and systemic acidosis) and essentially nothing about the fetal blood pressure and perfusion of the brain, the key factors that contribute directly to brain injury.

Systemic and cardiovascular adaptation to asphyxia

The systemic adaptations of the fetus to whole-body asphyxia are critical to outcome. Although the focus of most of the classic studies in this area was to delineate the cardiovascular and cerebrovascular responses, more recently the relationship between particular patterns of asphyxia and neural outcome has been examined. The majority of experimental studies of the pathophysiology of fetal asphyxia have been performed in the chronically instrumented fetal sheep, in utero. The sheep is a highly precocial species, whose neural development approximates that of the term human around 0.8–0.85 of gestation [23,24]. Most studies have been performed at this age. The reader should note that the baseline heart rate of the fetal sheep is approximately 20 beats per minute higher than that of the human fetus.

Fetal adaptations and defense mechanisms

The fetus is highly adapted to intrauterine conditions, which include low partial pressures of oxygen and relatively limited supply of substrates compared with postnatal life. Although tissue myoglobin could in theory act as an oxygen store, in practice the fetus does not have appreciable tissue myoglobin levels except in the heart [25]. Myocardial myoglobin concentrations do increase in hypoxic fetuses, consistent with previous observations in postnatal animals. This appears to represent an intracellular compensatory mechanism for sustaining short-term mitochondrial oxygen delivery in a critical organ with high oxygen consumption [26].

Thus the fetus is largely dependent on a steady supply of oxygen, and consequently it has many adaptive features, some unique to the fetus, which help it to maximize oxygen availability to its tissues even during moderate hypoxia. Thanks to these adaptations, it normally exists with a surplus of oxygen relative to its needs. This surplus provides a significant margin of safety when oxygen delivery is impaired. These adaptive features include higher basal blood flow to organs; left shift of the oxygen dissociation curve, which increases the capacity of blood to carry oxygen and the amount of oxygen that can be extracted at typical fetal oxygen tensions; the capacity to significantly reduce energy-consuming processes; greater anaerobic capacity in many tissues; and the capacity to redistribute blood flow towards essential organs away from the periphery.

Additional structural features of the fetal circulation further support these adaptive features, including the systems of "shunts," such as the ductus arteriosus, and preferential blood flow streaming in the inferior vena cava to avoid intermixing of oxygenated blood from the placenta and deoxygenated blood in the fetal venous system. These features ensure maximal oxygen delivery to essential organs such as the brain and heart. The preferential streaming patterns may be augmented during hypoxia to help maintain oxygen delivery to these organs. Thus overall fetal oxygen consumption can be maintained at normal levels until uteroplacental blood flow falls below 50% [27]. Under these conditions, the fetus is able to maintain the removal of waste products of metabolism, mainly carbon dioxide and water, and thus avoids any oxygen debt and does not become acidotic [28].

Cerebral oxygen consumption is even more protected, and is little changed even if arterial oxygen content falls as low as 1.5 mmol/L (compared with about 4 mmol/L in the normal fetus), thanks to compensating increases in both cerebral blood flow (CBF) and oxygen extraction [29]. Nitric oxide (NO) has been shown to play a role in mediating the local increase in CBF [30,31].

Fetal responses to hypoxia

The response of the fetal sheep to moderate, stable hypoxia has been extensively evaluated [32,33]. Fetal isocapnic hypoxia is typically induced by reduction of maternal inspired oxygen fraction to 10–12%. This model permits the fetal responses to changes in oxygenation to be studied separately from the effects of hypercapnia and acidosis. In the late-gestation fetus the response to this degree of hypoxia is characterized by an initial transient moderate bradycardia followed by tachycardia and an increase in blood pressure (Fig. 13.2). There is a rapid redistribution of combined ventricular output (CVO), the sum of right and left ventricular outputs, in favor of the cerebral, myocardial, and adrenal vascular beds (central or vital organs, Fig. 13.2) at the expense of the gastrointestinal tract, renal, pulmonary, cutaneous, and skeletal beds (i.e., the periphery) [33]. The magnitude of the hemodynamic changes largely depends upon the magnitude of changes in arterial pH and blood gases [34].

The fetal cardiovascular response to hypoxia is initially mediated via reflex responses, which are rapid in onset, and via endocrine responses, which augment these reflexes but take much longer to become fully active. The afferent component of the reflex arc causing the initial bradycardia and increase in peripheral vasoconstriction during hypoxia is mediated by carotid chemoreceptors (chemoreflex). Hypoxia stimulates the carotid chemoreceptors, which are known to be

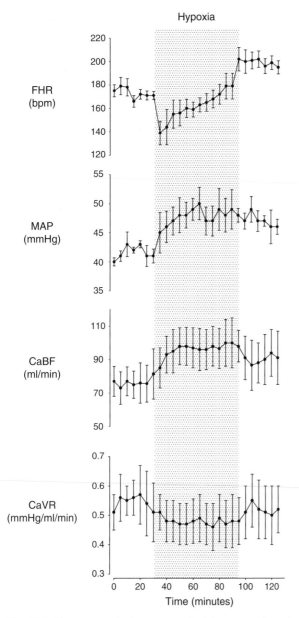

Fig. 13.2. The responses in the near-term fetal sheep to moderate isocapnic hypoxia for 60 minutes induced by altering the maternal inspired gas mixture, showing changes in fetal heart rate (FHR), mean arterial blood pressure (MAP), carotid blood flow (CaBF), and carotid vascular resistance (CaVR). Moderate hypoxia is associated with a sustained redistribution of blood flow away from peripheral organs to essential organs such as the brain. Data derived from Bennet *et al.* [74].

catecholamines, since it is reduced by sympathectomy [47] and abolished by α-adrenergic blockade [28,48–50]. The significant increase in peripheral vasoconstriction in turn mediates the rise in blood pressure observed during hypoxia. The rise in blood pressure during hypoxia is also augmented by circulating catecholamines released from the adrenal medulla, and in part other vasopressors such as arginine vasopressin [51] and angiotensin II [52]. There is also a large adrenocorticotropic and cortisol response to hypoxia [53,54]. Their role in the cardiovascular response to hypoxia is unclear, but cortisol has been shown to augment the actions of other vasopressors [55].

In addition to the cardiovascular responses, the fetus can also make changes to its behavior to help conserve energy. The fetus expends considerable energy making fetal breathing movements (FBMs), particularly in late gestation. In contrast to the neonate and adult, where hypoxia stimulates breathing, in the fetus hypoxia abolishes FBMs [56]. This inhibition is mediated through activation of neural networks that either arise from or pass through the upper pons [57,58] and thalamus [59]. Similarly, the fetus suspends other energy-consuming activities such as body and limb movements [56,60], as well as reducing cerebral requirements as discussed above [61].

Prolonged hypoxia

The effect of prolonged hypoxemia on cerebral metabolism in near-term fetal sheep has been studied during stepwise reductions of the maternal inspired oxygen concentration from 18% to 10–12% over four successive days [62]. Until the fetal arterial oxygen saturation was reduced to less than 30% of baseline, cerebral oxidative metabolism remained stable. At the lowest inspired oxygen concentration (with 3% CO_2) a progressive metabolic acidemia was induced. Initially, CBF increased, thus maintaining cerebral oxygen delivery as seen in acute hypoxia studies. Eventually, when the pH fell below 7.00 cerebral oxygen consumption fell to less than 50% of control values.

If mild to moderate hypoxia is continued the fetus may be able to fully adapt, as shown by normalization of FHR and blood pressure and the return of FBMs and body movements, but redistribution of blood flow is maintained [62,63]. This is consistent with the clinical situation of "brain sparing" in growth retardation. These fetuses can improve tissue oxygen delivery to near baseline levels by increasing hemoglobin synthesis, mediated by greater erythropoietin release [64].

Maturational changes in responses to hypoxia

Some aspects of the cardiovascular response to fetal hypoxia appear to be age-related. In the premature fetal sheep before 0.7 of gestation isocapnic hypoxia and hemorrhagic hypotension were not associated with hypertension, bradycardia, or peripheral vasoconstriction [65–68]. Even from late gestation to full term there is a further developmental increase in the magnitude and persistence of fetal bradycardia and in the magnitude of the femoral constrictor response to moderate hypoxia in fetal sheep [69]. Thus it has been suggested that

functional in utero [35–39]. During mild to moderate hypoxia the aortic chemoreceptors do not appear to play a role in these responses [40], although they may have a role during asphyxia [41]. The efferent limb of the fall in FHR is mediated by muscarinic (parasympathetic) pathways, as demonstrated by abolition of hypoxic bradycardia by vagotomy [42] or blockade with atropine [43,44]. The fall in FHR is then followed by a progressively developing tachycardia which is mediated by the increase in circulating catecholamines [45,46].

The reflex vasoconstriction is mediated in part by the sympathetic nervous system and partly by circulating peripheral vasomotor control starts to develop at 0.7 of gestation, coincident with maturation of neurohormonal regulators and chemoreceptor function [45,70]. However, when interpreting these results it is also important to consider that the preterm fetus has far greater anaerobic reserves and lower overall aerobic requirements than at term [66,71,72]. Thus relatively mild hypoxic insults may not be sufficient to elicit maximal responses by the preterm fetus. As discussed below (see *Maturational changes in fetal responses to asphyxia*), it is likely that the degree of hypoxia attained in these studies did not reduce tissue oxygen availability below the critical homeostatic threshold for this developmental stage.

The preterm fetus does respond to moderate hypoxia in a similar manner to that seen in term fetuses with regards to brain blood flow. Gleason and colleagues [66] have shown that hypoxia results in increased blood flow to cerebral hemispheres, cerebellum, and pons–medulla; furthermore, the increase in blood flow was sufficient to sustain cerebral oxygen consumption. However, in contrast to near-term fetuses, the increase in blood flow to the cerebral hemispheres was not sufficient to fully maintain oxygen delivery, and cerebral oxygen consumption was sustained in part by an increase in fractional extraction [66].

Fetal responses to asphyxia

Studies of asphyxia by definition involve both hypoxia and hypercapnia with metabolic acidosis. It is important to appreciate that these studies of asphyxia also involve a greater depth of hypoxia than is possible using maternal inhalational hypoxia. Further, asphyxia can be induced relatively abruptly, limiting the time available for adaptation. Brief, total clamping of the uterine artery or umbilical cord leads to a rapid reduction of fetal oxygenation within a few minutes [46,73,74]. In contrast, gradual partial occlusion induces a slow fetal metabolic deterioration without the initial fetal cardiovascular responses of bradycardia and hypertension; this is a function of the relative hypoxia attained [75]. During profound asphyxia, corresponding with a severe reduction of uterine blood flow to 25% or less and a fetal arterial oxygen content of less than 1 mmol/L, the fetal cardiovascular responses are substantially different to those during moderate hypoxia or asphyxia.

Two key phases of the cardiovascular responses of the fetus to such severe events can be distinguished: the initial, rapid chemoreflex-mediated adaptations [28,35,40,42], and a subsequent longer period of progressive hypoxic decompensation ultimately terminated by profound systemic hypotension (Fig. 13.3) with cerebral hypoperfusion (Fig. 13.4).

Initial, reflex responses to asphyxia

The initial responses include rapid, sustained bradycardia and generalized vasoconstriction involving essentially all organs [45]. In marked contrast to the increase in CBF during moderate hypoxia, during asphyxia CBF does not increase or may even fall despite a marked initial increase in fetal blood pressure, due to significant cerebral vasoconstriction

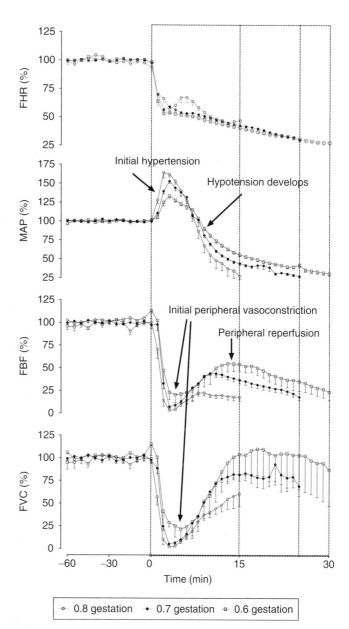

Fig. 13.3. The responses of fetal sheep to severe asphyxia induced by complete umbilical cord occlusion. Fetal heart rate (FHR, % baseline), mean arterial pressure (MAP, % baseline), femoral blood flow (FBF, % baseline), and femoral vascular conductance (FVC, % baseline) in 0.6 gestation (0.6 ga), 0.7 gestation (0.7 ga), and 0.85 gestation (0.85 ga) fetuses. Conductance is the reciprocal of resistance, i.e., a reduction in conductance indicates increased vascular resistance to flow. FHR and MAP data represent 5-minute averages before occlusion and 1-minute averages during occlusion, and are expressed as percentage of baseline. Umbilical cord occlusion begins at 0 min and ends for each group as indicated by the dotted rectangles. Data are mean ± SEM. Between-group comparisons by one-way ANOVA and LSD test, [a] $p < 0.05$, 0.6 ga vs. 0.7 ga; [b] $p < 0.05$, 0.6 ga vs. 0.85 ga; [c] $p < 0.05$, 0.7 ga vs. 0.85 ga; data derived from Wassink *et al.* [88].

(Fig. 13.4) [74,76,77]. The factors mediating this increase in cerebral vascular resistance are not clearly understood. However, while the failure of CBF to increase may seem counterintuitive, it should be remembered it occurs in conjunction with profound suppression of brain activity. This suppression is mediated by activation of the adenosine A1 receptor, and if it is blocked neural injury is exacerbated [20]. Further, blood

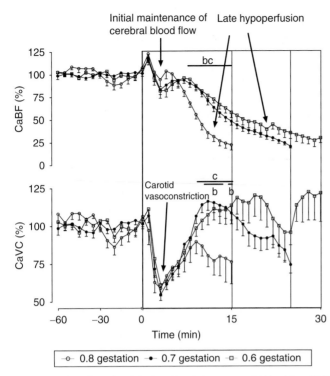

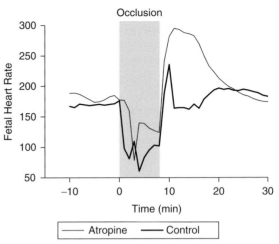

Fig. 13.4. The effect of umbilical cord occlusion on carotid blood flow (CaBF, % baseline, top panel) and carotid vascular conductance (CaVC, % baseline, bottom panel) in 0.6 gestation (0.6 ga), 0.7 gestation (0.7 ga), and 0.85 gestation (0.85 ga) fetuses. CaBF and CaVC data represent 5-minute averages before occlusion and 1-minute averages during occlusion, and are expressed as percentage of baseline. Umbilical cord occlusion for each group begins at 0 min and ends as indicated by the rectangles. Data are mean ± SEM. Between-group comparisons by one-way ANOVA and LSD test, [a] $p < 0.05$, 0.6 ga vs. 0.7 ga; [b] $p < 0.05$, 0.6 ga vs. 0.85 ga; [c] $p < 0.05$, 0.7 ga vs. 0.85 ga (unpublished data).

Fig. 13.5. An example showing the contribution of the parasympathetic system to bradycardia during 8 minutes of severe asphyxia in near-term sheep fetuses. Pretreatment with atropine delayed the fall in heart rate until the third minute after the start of umbilical occlusion, in contrast with the immediate bradycardia seen in the control fetus. This abrupt, delayed fall in FHR in the atropine-treated fetus was due to transient atrioventricular blockade. This was followed by partial recovery due to resolution of the AV block, but a progressive fall from the fourth minute onward. Similar results are seen with vagotomy. Thus, the typical variable deceleration which lasts for approximately 1 minute is entirely chemoreflexly mediated, whereas prolonged decelerations involve an increasing proportion of true hypoxic myocardial depression.

flow within the brain is preferentially redirected during asphyxia to protect structures important for survival such as the brainstem, at the expense of the cerebrum; speculatively, this redirection may help maintain autonomic function [70]. Furthermore, reduced oxygen content physically limits oxygen extraction from the blood. The combination of these two factors, restricted CBF and reduced oxygen extraction, in turn profoundly reduces cerebral oxygen consumption below even minimum cerebral requirements [45].

The initial bradycardia and intense peripheral vasoconstriction in the late-gestation fetus during asphyxia are mediated via afferent input from the carotid chemoreceptors leading to activation of the efferent parasympathetic and sympathetic systems, respectively. Selective chemodenervation attenuates the initial rate of fall in heart rate during asphyxia, but does not abolish the bradycardia and has little effect on blood pressure [41], providing further evidence for the operation of the vagal chemoreflexes during oxygen deprivation, but demonstrating that they are less important during profound asphyxia than moderate hypoxemia. In contrast, complete vagal blockade markedly delays the onset of bradycardia during umbilical cord occlusion [42], as shown in Figure 13.5. These data suggest that there are substantial additional afferent inputs which are not well understood at present.

Speculatively, one factor might be greater recruitment of aortic chemoreceptors during severe hypoxia [45].

Fetal decompensation

Ultimately, during sustained severe hypoxia, fetal bradycardia does develop despite full parasympathetic blockade or vagotomy, and the fall is maintained, in contrast with moderate hypoxia, where there is a progressive later rise in FHR during the insult. These experimental data are consistent with the clinical observation by Caldeyro-Barcia and colleagues that late decelerations during labor are not abolished by atropine [78]. This indicates that in contrast with the initial reflex-mediated bradycardia in the first few minutes of profound asphyxia, continuing bradycardia must be related to severe myocardial hypoxia with depletion of myocardial anaerobic stores such as glycogen [43].

Clinical implications

These data indicate that the chemoreflexes which mediate the early FHR deceleration are highly sensitive indicators of hypoxemia. However, except in the case of very prolonged periods of bradycardia, they are poor indicators of fetal well-being or tolerance to hypoxia. Decelerations due to true myocardial hypoxia do not occur unless hypoxia is continued for a pathologically long time or, we may speculate, unless the fetus is chronically hypoxic with low reserves of myocardial glycogen. The depth to which FHR falls is broadly related to the severity of the hypoxia [79]. Shallow decelerations indicate a modest reduction in uteroplacental flow, while a deep deceleration indicates near total or total abolition of uteroplacental flow [79]. Unfortunately, once deep decelerations are established, there is relatively little further change in the shape of the deceleration despite repeated decelerations and the consequent development of hypotension [80]. Detailed analysis suggests that developing fetal acidosis during continuing occlusion is associated with relatively subtle changes including an increase in FHR between occlusion and more rapid fall in FHR during each deceleration [81]. In contrast, major changes in the shape of the deceleration tend to be near-terminal events [80]. Thus all we can say from inspecting the typical variable deceleration is that the fetus has been exposed to a brief period of deeper hypoxia [2].

The decompensation phase

The initial phase, with peripheral vasoconstriction and hypertension, is only sustained for the first 5–6 minutes of occlusion and is followed, not by overt vasodilatation, but rather by a return of peripheral perfusion to control values [76,82–85]. This is unlikely to be due to local accumulation of metabolites, since a similar biphasic pattern occurs even during a more moderate insult such as partial umbilical cord occlusion [86]. Preliminary data from this paradigm in preterm fetal sheep suggest that loss of renal vasoconstriction is closely associated in time with attenuation of the renal sympathetic response to asphyxia [87], suggesting a primarily central mechanism.

Loss of initial vasoconstriction is associated with a further, progressive fall in heart rate, and a rapid fall in fetal blood pressure, leading to overt hypotension [88]. There is no evidence for continuing reflex mechanisms at this time [42]. Likely contributors to impaired cardiac function include hypoxia, acidosis, depletion of myocardial glycogen, and cardiomyocyte injury [89]. Once glycogen is depleted, there is rapid loss of high-energy metabolites such as ATP in mitochondria [71]. During a shorter episode of asphyxia, e.g., 5 minutes, the fetus may not become hypotensive. If the insult is repeated before myocardial glycogen can be replenished, successive periods of asphyxia are associated with increasing duration of hypotension [80].

Another possible factor leading to impaired contractility during asphyxia is myocardial injury, which has been found after severe birth asphyxia in limited case series [90,91]. Studies in adult animals have shown that there may be a significant delay in recovery of cardiac contractility after reperfusion from brief ischemia in the absence of necrosis. This delayed recovery, termed "myocardial stunning," may contribute to the progressive myocardial dysfunction and to delayed recovery of heart rate after exposure to a series of repeated umbilical cord occlusions in the fetal lamb [89].

Slow-onset asphyxia

During gradually induced asphyxia, even to arterial oxygen contents of less than 1 mmol/L, fetal adaptation may be closer to that seen with hypoxia associated with acidosis, with umbilical blood flow maintained, but blood flow to the fetal body reduced by 40% [34,92]. Progressive reduction of uterine perfusion over a 3–4 hour period in near-term fetal sheep led to a mean pH < 7.00, serum lactate levels > 14 mmol/L,

with a fetal mortality of 53%. Surviving animals remained normotensive and normoglycemic, and CBF was more than doubled. Interestingly, in surviving fetuses neuronal damage was limited to selective loss of the very large, metabolically active cerebellar Purkinje cells [75].

Uterine contractions and brief repeated asphyxia

Although the fetus can be exposed to a wide range of insults during labor, the key distinctive characteristic of labor is the development of brief, intermittent, repetitive episodes of asphyxia, which is almost entirely related to uterine contractions [2]. In turn, the effects of repeated hypoxia may be amplified by fetal vulnerability, for example due to intrauterine growth retardation and/or chronic hypoxia or by greater severity of contractions, as discussed next. Even a normal fetus, with normal placental function, may not be able to fully adapt to hyperstimulation causing brief but severe asphyxia repeated at an excessive frequency.

Uterine contractions have such a significant impact on fetal gas exchange during labor that it is worth examining their effect in detail. Fetal heart-rate decelerations are not seen in most antenatal recordings of the fetal heart rate. When they occur more than sporadically they indicate that further assessment of fetal condition is urgently required [2,93]. However, during labor decelerations are common, particularly in second stage, and in the great majority of cases are mild and require no special action or intervention. The vast majority of intrapartum decelerations occur as a direct consequence of uterine contractions and consequent reductions in uterine or fetal placental blood flow and fetal oxygenation. Doppler studies have shown that uterine contractions are associated with increased intrauterine pressure and a nearly linear fall in maternal uterine artery blood flow [94]. Indeed, even physiological prelabor contractions are associated with a marked increase in maternal uterine vascular resistance [95]. The impact of contractions on umbilical blood flow in humans is not fully described and is likely to be more complex than changes in uterine artery blood flow. However, experimentally, fetal hypoxia is associated with reduced umbilical venous blood flow [96–98]. Consistent with this, umbilical resistance increased significantly during contractions in human fetuses with a positive oxytocin challenge test, i.e., at-risk fetuses who developed FHR decelerations [99], suggesting that uterine contractions sufficient to cause an FHR deceleration are likely to be associated with reduced umbilical as well as uterine artery blood flow.

Even during normal labor there is intermittent reduction of placental gas exchange. This reduction is associated with a consistent fall in pH and oxygen tension, and a rise in carbon dioxide and base deficit in normal, uncomplicated labor [100–102]. Typically, the second stage of normal labor will be the time of greatest asphyxic stress for the fetus, accompanied by a more rapid decline in pH [100] and transcutaneous oxygen tension [101,103] and a rise in transcutaneous carbon dioxide tension [104]. Thus, in a technical sense, essentially all fetuses may be said to be exposed to "asphyxia" during labor. Fortunately it is usually mild and well tolerated by the fetus. Unfortunately, both the lay public and many clinicians associate the term "asphyxia" with the development of severe metabolic acidosis, postasphyxial encephalopathy, and other end-organ damage or death. In our haste to avoid using the term, the normal nature of labor and its effects on the fetus are often not fully appreciated.

Most fetuses enter labor with a large reserve of placental capacity that helps accommodate the repeated brief reductions in oxygen supply during contractions. Although contraction strength is important, once labor is established contraction frequency and duration are the key factors which determine the rate at which fetal asphyxia develops during labor. The proportion of time the uterus spends at resting tone compared with contracting tone will determine the extent to which fetal gas exchange can be restored between contractions [101]. Any intervention that increases the frequency and/or duration of uterine contractions clearly places the fetus at increased risk of compromise. For example, studies using near-infrared spectroscopy showed a progressive fall in cerebral oxygen saturation when contractions occurred more frequently than every 2.3 minutes [103]. The effects of repeated hypoxia may be amplified in vulnerable fetuses, for example in those with pre-existing placental insufficiency [105]. Conversely, even a normal fetus with normal placental function may be unable to fully adapt to tonic contractions or uterine hyperstimulation related to oxytocin infusion used for induction or augmentation, or prostaglandin preparations for induction of labor [106,107].

Experimental studies of brief repeated asphyxia

Brief repeated asphyxia has been produced in the fetal sheep by repeated complete occlusion of the umbilical cord at frequencies chosen to represent different stages of labor. This allows us to examine not only FHR and blood gas changes but also the accompanying blood pressure changes and the effects on cerebral perfusion, information which is not available clinically. Recent studies compared the effect of 1 minute of umbilical cord occlusion repeated every 5 minutes (1 : 5 group) with that of 1-minute occlusions repeated every 2.5 minutes (1 : 2.5 group). The former frequency of decelerations every 5 minutes is consistent with early labor, while the latter, with decelerations every 2.5 minutes, is consistent with late first-stage and second-stage labor. The fetal heart rate and blood pressure changes were monitored continuously, as shown in Figure 13.6, and occlusions were continued for 4 hours or until the development of fetal hypotension (a mean arterial blood pressure [MAP] < 20 mmHg) [108–112].

1 : 5 occlusion series

The onset of each occlusion (Fig. 13.6a) was accompanied by a variable FHR deceleration with rapid return to baseline levels between occlusions [81,105]. Fetal mean arterial pressure (MAP) rose at the onset of each occlusion and never fell below baseline levels during the occlusions. There was a sustained elevation in baseline MAP between occlusions. A small fall in

pH and rise in base deficit (BD) and lactate occurred in the first 30 minutes of occlusions (pH 7.34 ± 0.07, BD 1.3 ± 3.9 mmol/L, lactate 4.5 ± 1.3 mmol/L). Subsequently these values remained stable despite a further 3.5 hours of occlusions. This experiment demonstrated the remarkable capacity of the healthy fetus to fully adapt to a low frequency of repeated episodes of severe hypoxia.

1 : 2.5 occlusion series

Although this paradigm was also associated with variable decelerations, the outcome in this group was substantially different (Fig. 13.6b) [108]. The rapid occlusion frequency provided only a brief period of recovery between occlusions, which was insufficient to allow full recovery of fetal cellular metabolism and replenishment of glycogen stores [113]. Three distinctive phases of the fetal response to occlusions were observed in this 1 : 2.5 occlusion series, as follows.

First 30-minute period. During the first three occlusions there was a sustained rise in MAP during occlusions followed by recovery to baseline once the occlusion ended. After the third occlusion, all fetuses developed a biphasic blood pressure response to successive occlusions, with initial hypertension followed by a fall in MAP reaching a nadir a few seconds after release of the occluder. However, minimum MAP did not fall below baseline values. Over this initial 30 minutes pH fell from 7.40 ± 0.01 to 7.25 ± 0.02, BD rose from −2.6 ± 0.6 to 3.3 ± 1.1 mmol/L, and lactate rose from 0.9 ± 0.1 to 3.9 ± 0.6 mmol/L.

Middle 30-minute period. In the middle 30 minutes minimum FHR during occlusions fell and inter-occlusion baseline rose, compared to the first 30 minutes. Although the minimum MAP did fall over the course of this phase, it never fell below baseline levels. Despite a stable blood pressure response, without hypotension, the metabolic acidosis slowly worsened: pH fell to 7.09 ± 0.03, BD rose to 13.6 ± 1.2 mmol/L, and lactate rose to 9.9 ± 0.7 mmol/L.

Final 30-minute period. Finally, in the last 30 minutes minimum FHR during decelerations continued to fall compared to the mid 30 minutes, but there was no further rise in inter-occlusion (baseline) FHR. Minimum MAP fell below baseline levels and the degree of hypotension became greater with successive occlusions. All animals developed a severe metabolic acidosis, with pH 6.92 ± 0.03, BD 19.2 ± 1.5 mmol/L, and lactate 14.6 ± 0.8 mmol/L by the end of occlusions. Studies were stopped after a mean of 183 ± 43 minutes (range 140–235 minutes).

The key difference in outcome between these protocols was that frequent occlusions (1 minute every 2.5 minutes) were associated with focal neuronal damage in the parasagittal cortex, the thalamus, and the cerebellum, whereas no damage was seen after less frequent occlusions (1 minute every 5 minutes) [109]. These findings are highly consistent with clinical evidence that fetal intracerebral oxygenation is impaired

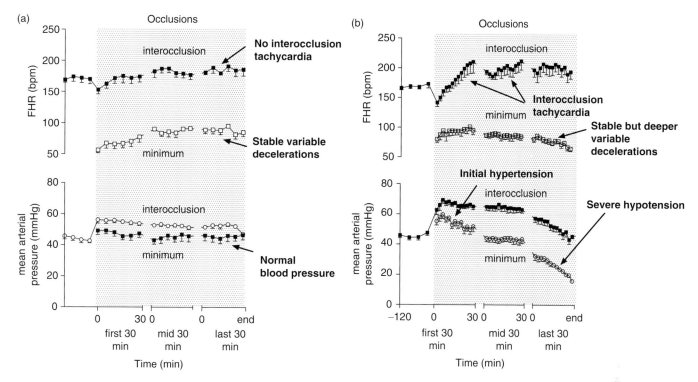

Fig. 13.6. Fetal heart rate (FHR) and mean arterial pressure (MAP) changes occurring in near-term fetal sheep exposed to (a) 1-minute umbilical cord occlusions repeated every 5 minutes for 4 hours (1:5 group) and (b) 1-minute occlusions repeated every 2.5 minutes (1:2.5 group) until fetal MAP fell < 20 mmHg. The minimum FHR and MAP during each occlusion, and the inter-occlusion FHR and MAP, are shown. As the individual experiments in the 1:2.5 group were of unequal duration, the data in both groups are presented for three time intervals: the first 30 minutes, the middle 30 minutes (defined as the median ± 15 min), and the final 30 minutes of occlusions. In the 1:5 group there was no significant change in inter-occlusion baseline FHR, and minimum MAP during occlusions never fell below pre-occlusion levels. A small fall in pH and rise in base deficit (BD) and lactate occurred in the first 30 minutes of occlusions (pH 7.34 ± 0.07, BD 1.3 ± 3.9 mmol/L, lactate 4.5 ± 1.3 mmol/L), but no subsequent change occurred despite a further 3.5 hours of occlusions. In the 1:2.5 group inter-occlusion FHR rose in the first and mid 30 minutes. Minimum MAP fell steadily in the first 30 minutes, stabilized in the mid 30 minutes and fell progressively in the last 30 minutes. All animals developed a severe metabolic acidosis, with pH 6.92 ± 0.03, BD 19.2 ± 1.46 mmol/L, and lactate 14.6 ± 0.8 mmol/L by the end of occlusions. Data derived from Westgate *et al.* [110,112,174].

during short contraction intervals (< 2.3 minutes) in labor [103]. Thus a prolonged series of brief variable decelerations can ultimately lead to severe, repeated hypotension and profound metabolic acidosis even in healthy singleton fetuses, if they are repeated sufficiently frequently. There are changes in the pattern of the FHR during the period of deterioration; however, they develop progressively and surprisingly slowly, even during frequent occlusions.

Maturational changes in fetal responses to asphyxia

The premature fetus at 90 days' gestation, prior to the onset of cortical myelination, can tolerate extended periods of up to 20 minutes of umbilical cord occlusion without neuronal loss [114,115]. The very prolonged cardiac survival during profound asphyxia (up to 30 minutes, Fig. 13.3) [116] corresponds with the maximal levels of cardiac glycogen that are seen near mid-gestation in the sheep and other species including humans [71]. Interestingly, while the premature fetal response to hypoxia appears to be different to that seen at term, the overall cardiovascular and cerebrovascular response during asphyxia was very similar to that seen in more mature

fetuses, with sustained bradycardia, accompanied by circulatory centralization, initial hypertension, then a progressive fall in pressure [82,84,88,116]. As also reported in the term fetus, there was no increase in blood flow to the brain during this initial phase, and again this was due to a significant increase in vascular resistance rather than to hypotension (Fig. 13.4). In contrast to the term fetus, at 0.6 and 0.7 gestation there is a delay in the suppression of neural activity [88,116]. Speculatively, the delay is indicative of the relative anaerobic tolerance of the preterm brain (discussed further in Chapter 4). As shown in Figures 13.3 and 13.4, as in the term fetus, once blood pressure begins to fall, blood flow to the brain falls in parallel, although the fall in blood pressure and blood flow is relatively slower in the less mature fetuses [88]. The fall in pressure is partly a function of the loss of redistribution of blood flow, as seen in Figure 13.3, with a rise in femoral blood flow (FBF). Similar responses are also seen in the kidney and gut [82,84]. Preliminary data from telemetry recordings of renal sympathetic nerve activity suggest that, in the kidney at least, the loss of vasoconstriction is closely associated in time with attenuation of the renal sympathetic response to asphyxia [87].

In the latter half of maximum survivable interval of asphyxia in the preterm fetus there is progressive failure of CVO, with a fall in both central and peripheral perfusion, both associated with falling blood pressure. This phase is much less likely to be seen for any significant duration in the term fetus, as glycogen stores in the term fetus are depleted more quickly [71]. Thus, at 0.6 gestation the majority of fetuses survived up to 30 minutes [116]. In contrast, term fetuses are unable to survive such prolonged periods of sustained hypotension, and typically will recover spontaneously from a maximum of 10–12 minutes of cord occlusion, whereas after a 15-minute period of complete umbilical artery occlusion the majority of fetuses either died or required active resuscitation with adrenaline after release of occlusion [73,74,88]. As a consequence of this extended survival during severe asphyxia the premature fetus is exposed to profound and prolonged hypotension and hypoperfusion. It may be speculated that during this final phase of asphyxia there is a catastrophic failure of redistribution of blood flow within the fetal brain which places previously protected areas of the brain such as the brainstem at risk of injury [117], consistent with clinical reports [118].

After the end of asphyxia a brief period of arterial hypertension and hyperperfusion occurs, followed by delayed hypoperfusion, despite normalization of blood pressure [84,116,119]. Although the significance of this consistent finding remains controversial, in the fetal sheep, for example, it was associated with suppression of cerebral metabolism, and increased cerebral oxygen tension, suggesting that postasphyxial hypoperfusion is actively mediated and reflects suppressed cerebral metabolism (see also Chapter 42) [120]. The brain is not the only organ to be affected. Recent experimental evidence shows that profound hypoperfusion also occurs in renal, gut, and femoral beds [84,119]. In the gut at least, the sympathetic nervous system plays a key role in mediating this vasoconstriction, and the data suggest that peripheral vasoconstriction may in part be acting to support the heart during recovery [119]. This may be advantageous in the fetus, where the gut and kidney are not vital to survival. However, postnatally, poor perfusion of the kidneys and gut, and associated functional impairment, are considered major problems in the first days of life in very preterm infants. These complications can be associated with a substantial mortality and further problems such as reduced kidney growth and chronic renal problems in later childhood [121].

Acute on chronic hypoxia/asphyxia

In addition to its potential impact on neurodevelopment (as outlined below), chronic hypoxia may also adversely affect the ability of the fetus to adapt to acute insults. Clinically, antenatal hypoxia [122–124], for example due to growth retardation and multiple pregnancy, is associated with an increased incidence of stillbirth, metabolic acidosis during labor, and subsequent abnormal neurodevelopment [124]. Although this clinical experience strongly suggests that such infants are likely to be compromised by otherwise well-tolerated labor, intriguingly, experimental studies seem to suggest improved or greater cardiovascular adaptation to moderate induced hypoxemia. When chronically hypoxic fetal sheep were exposed to a further episode of acute hypoxia, they exhibited more pronounced centralization of circulation [125], with enhanced femoral vasoconstriction [126]. This was associated with greater increases in plasma noradrenalin and vasopressin [126]. It is important to note, however, that these studies tested the response to mild to moderate hypoxia only, rather than to labor-like or profound hypoxic insults. Thus it may be speculated that these greater reflex responses reflect reduced fetal reserve that would be exposed during a more severe insult [125].

As discussed above (Fig. 13.6a), normoxic fetal sheep are easily able to adapt to 1-minute occlusions of the umbilical cord repeated every 5 minutes for 4 hours, with only minimal acidosis and without hypotension. In contrast, during the same insult chronically hypoxic fetuses from multiple pregnancies developed severe, progressive metabolic acidosis (pH 7.07 ± 0.14 vs. 7.34 ± 0.07 in previously normoxic fetuses) and hypotension (a nadir of 24 ± 2 mmHg vs. 45.5 ± 3 mmHg after 4 hours of occlusion) [105]. The fetuses with pre-existing hypoxia were smaller on average, and had lower blood glucose values and higher $PaCO_2$ values. These data support the clinical concept that fetuses with chronic placental insufficiency are vulnerable even to relatively infrequent periods of additional hypoxia in early labor.

Less obvious adverse intrauterine events may also modify fetal responses to hypoxia. There is considerable interest in the effects of stimuli such as maternal undernutrition and steroid exposure, particularly at critical times in pregnancy, not only on the fetal responses to challenges to its environment such as hypoxia, but also on risks for adverse health outcomes in adult life [127]. Intriguingly, mild maternal undernutrition that does not alter fetal growth may still affect development of fetal hypothalamic–pituitary–adrenal function, with reduced pituitary and adrenal responsiveness to moderate hypoxia [128]. Exposure to glucocorticoids may also detrimentally alter the responses to hypoxia [129,130] and ischemia [131].

Does gender modify fetal responses to asphyxia?

Numerous studies have confirmed that there is an increased risk of perinatal mortality and morbidity in boys compared to girls at all stages of gestation [132–134]. The mechanisms mediating the influence of gender on perinatal death and disability are poorly understood but are likely to be multifactorial, affecting the intrinsic responses of cells to hypoxia–ischemia and fetal physiological adaptation. Sexual dimorphism exists in the normal developing mammalian brain, and increasingly studies show that there are sex-related differences in the neuronal and glial responses to hypoxia–ischemia, to the induction of cell death pathways, and to neuroprotective treatments [135–138]. In the adult, estrogen is believed to play a key role in protecting females from injury, and there is increasing evidence that estradiol also plays a significant neuroprotective role in the developing brain [139]. There may be differential effects of other endogenous neuroprotective factors [140].

There are some data suggesting that male fetuses may be less able to physiologically adapt to hypoxia. Males fetuses have higher rates of abnormal FHR recordings, metabolic acidosis, and need for operative intervention or resuscitation in labor [133,141–144]. Male fetuses on average are bigger, grow faster, and have a higher metabolic rate than females [145,146], suggesting that when oxygen is limited they might deplete available resources more rapidly. Further, there is evidence that males have relatively delayed maturation of some aspects of autonomic nervous system function, such as adrenal medullary and lung β-receptor maturation in fetal rabbits [147]. Consistent with this, preterm boys are reported to have lower plasma catecholamine levels after exposure to asphyxia at birth than girls [148].

Recent data in healthy singleton preterm fetal sheep have shown that most fetuses, regardless of sex, can survive a prolonged, near-terminal episode of acute asphyxia of a defined duration (25 minutes) induced by umbilical cord occlusion [149]. Neither the average responses nor the incidence of failure to complete the full period of umbilical cord occlusion were significantly different between male and female fetuses. However, significantly more male fetuses developed profound hypotension (< 8 mmHg) before the end of the occlusion period and, intriguingly, male but not female fetuses showed a significant correlation between postmortem weight and severity of the fall in arterial blood pressure after 15 minutes of occlusion. This is consistent with the clinical observation that relatively small reductions in birthweight are associated with a significantly greater mortality in boys than in girls [132]. Interestingly, in the study of fetal sheep, male fetuses that did not tolerate prolonged umbilical cord occlusion had significantly lower $PaCO_2$ and lactate levels near the end of occlusion than males that did tolerate the full period of occlusion [149], consistent with a previous report from near-term fetuses [76]. Thus these fetuses may have had reduced glycogen stores, and thus reduced anaerobic metabolism, leading to reduced CO_2 and lactate production [149].

Further, male and female fetuses that failed to tolerate prolonged occlusion showed different patterns of early and late adaptation that suggested altered chemoreflex and cardiac responses between the genders [149]. The males demonstrated slower and reduced initial peripheral vasoconstriction compared with fetuses that tolerated the full insult, and then developed earlier and significantly greater hypotension, associated with greater falls in heart rate and carotid and femoral blood flow. In contrast, females that did not tolerate the full insult showed a markedly more rapid onset of initial femoral vasoconstriction, and their subsequent falls in blood pressure and heart rate were intermediate between the full-occlusion fetuses and short-occlusion males. Collectively these data suggest that for some fetuses, mainly male, previously restricted growth trajectory or nutrition may have altered both metabolic reserves and autonomic function. For example, moderate maternal undernutrition in pregnant rats that had only a transient effect on growth of the pups has been associated with increased sympathetic nervous system activity in female,

but not male, rats [150]. Further, there may be sexual dimorphism in the sensitivity of cardiac cells to ischemia, as suggested by the observations in adult animals that females may have greater resistance to hypoxic–ischemic injury of cardiomyocytes [151].

Pathophysiological determinants of asphyxial injury

Recent studies using well-defined experimental paradigms of asphyxia in the near-term fetal sheep have explored the relationship between the distribution of neuronal damage and the type of insult. These studies suggest that while local cerebral hypoperfusion due to hypotension is required to cause injury, a number of factors, including the pattern of repetition of insults as well as fetal factors such as maturity, pre-existing metabolic state, and cerebral temperature (Fig. 13.1), markedly alter the impact of the insult on the brain.

Hypotension and the "watershed" distribution of neuronal loss

The development of hypotension is highly associated with neural injury during acute asphyxia (Fig. 13.7). This is readily understood, since reduced perfusion will reduce supply of glucose for anaerobic metabolism, compounding the reduction in oxygen delivery and concentration. The real-life importance of hypotension is supported both by the correlation of injury with arterial blood pressure across multiple paradigms and by the common patterns of neural damage.

The close relationship between changes in carotid blood flow (CaBF) and blood pressure during asphyxia is shown in Figures 13.3, 13.4, and 13.6. In these fetuses, MAP initially rose with intense peripheral vasoconstriction. At this time CaBF was maintained. As cord occlusion was continued MAP eventually fell, probably as a function of impaired cardiac contractility and failure of peripheral redistribution. Once MAP fell below baseline, carotid blood flow fell in parallel, consistent with the known relatively narrow low range of autoregulation of cerebrovasculature in the fetus [46].

In the near-term fetus neural injury has been commonly reported in areas such as the parasagittal cortex, the dorsal horn of the hippocampus, and the cerebellar neocortex after a range of insults including pure ischemia, prolonged single complete umbilical cord occlusion, and prolonged partial

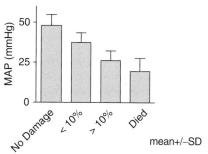

Fig. 13.7. The relationship between hypotension and neuronal damage. The severity of fetal systemic hypotension during asphyxia, induced by partial common uterine artery occlusion, is closely related to the degree of neuronal loss in the near-term fetal sheep. MAP, mean arterial pressure. Data derived from Gunn et al. [153].

153

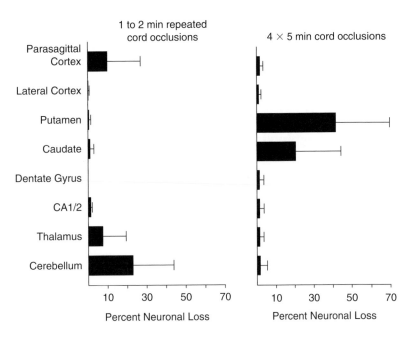

Fig. 13.8. The distribution of neuronal loss assessed after 3 days' recovery from two different patterns of prenatal asphyxia in near-term fetal sheep. The panel on the left shows the effects of brief (1 or 2 minute) cord occlusions repeated at frequencies consistent with established labor. Occlusions were terminated after a variable time, when the fetal blood pressure fell below 20 mmHg for two successive occlusions. This insult led to damage in the watershed regions of the parasagittal cortex and cerebellum [109]. The panel on the right shows the effect of 5-minute episodes of cord occlusion, repeated four times, at intervals of 30 minutes. This paradigm is associated with selective neuronal loss in the putamen and caudate nucleus, which are nuclei of the striatum [80]. CA 1/2 and the dentate gyrus are regions of the hippocampus. Mean ± SD.

asphyxia and repeated brief cord occlusion (e.g., as illustrated in the left panel of Figure 13.8) [73,75,109,152,153]. These areas are "watershed" zones within the borders between major cerebral arteries, where perfusion pressure is least, and in both adults and children lesions in these areas are typically seen after systemic hypotension [154].

There are some data suggesting that limited, or localized white- or gray-matter injury may occur even when significant hypotension is not seen [75,155], particularly when hypoxia is very prolonged [156]. Clearly there may have been some relative hypoperfusion in these studies. Nevertheless, there is a strong correlation between either the depth or duration of hypotension and the amount of neuronal loss within individual studies of acute asphyxia (e.g., Fig. 13.7) [80,109,153,155]. This is also seen between similar asphyxial paradigms causing severe fetal acidosis which have been manipulated to either cause fetal hypotension [153] or not [75]. In fetal lambs exposed to prolonged severe partial asphyxia, as judged by the degree of metabolic compromise, neuronal loss occurred only in those in which one or more episodes of acute hypotension occurred [153]. In contrast, in a similar study where an equally "severe" insult was induced gradually and titrated to maintain normal or elevated blood pressure throughout the insult no neuronal loss was seen except in the cerebellum [75].

The pattern of injury: repeated insults

One apparent exception to a general tendency to a "watershed" distribution after global asphyxial insults in the near-term fetus is the selective neuronal loss in striatal nuclei (putamen and caudate nucleus, Fig. 13.8, right panel) which develops when relatively prolonged periods of asphyxia or ischemia are repeated [109,157]. Whereas 30 minutes of continuous cerebral ischemia leads to predominantly parasagittal cortical neuronal loss, with only moderate striatal injury, when the

insult was divided into three episodes of ischemia, a greater proportion of striatal injury was seen relative to cortical neuronal loss (Fig. 13.9) [157]. Intriguingly, significant striatal involvement was also seen after prolonged partial asphyxia in which distinct episodes of bradycardia and hypotension occurred [153]. Given that both parasagittal-predominant and basal-ganglia-predominant injury are seen on early MRI scans in term infants with encephalopathy [158], this mode of injury is likely to be clinically important.

The striatum is not in a watershed zone but rather within the territory of the middle cerebral artery. Thus it is likely that the pathogenesis of striatal involvement in the near-term fetus is related to the precise timing of the relatively prolonged episodes of asphyxia and not to more severe local hypoperfusion. Speculatively, the apparent vulnerability of the medium-sized neurons of the striatum to this type of insult may be related to a greater release of glutamate into the striatal extracellular space after repeated insults compared with a single insult of the same cumulative duration. Consistent with this, immunohistochemical techniques have shown that inhibitory striatal neurons were primarily affected [157].

Pre-existing metabolic status and chronic hypoxia

While the original studies of factors influencing the degree and distribution of brain injury, primarily by Myers [117], focused on metabolic status, the issue remains controversial. It has been suggested, for example, that hyperglycemia is protective against hypoxia–ischemia in the infant rat [159,160], but not in the piglet [161]. The extreme differences between these neonatal species in the degree of neural maturation and activity of cerebral glucose transporters may underlie the different outcomes [160]. The most common metabolic disturbance to the fetus is intrauterine growth retardation (IUGR) associated with placental dysfunction. Although there is reasonable clinical information that IUGR is usually

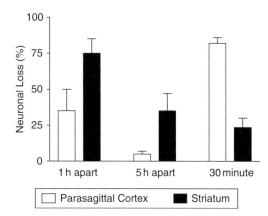

Fig. 13.9. The effects of different intervals between insults on the distribution of cerebral damage after ischemia in the near-term fetal sheep. Cerebral ischemia was induced by carotid occlusion for 10 minutes, repeated three times, at intervals of either 1 or 5 hours, compared with a single continuous episode of 30 minutes' occlusion. The divided insults were associated with a preponderance of striatal injury, whereas a single episode of 30 minutes of carotid occlusion was associated with severe cortical neuronal loss. Increasing the interval to 5 hours nearly completely abolished cortical injury, but was still associated with significant neuronal loss in the striatum. Data derived from Mallard et al. [175].

associated with a greater risk of brain injury, recent studies have suggested a greatly reduced rate of encephalopathy in this group over time [5]. This would suggest that the apparently increased sensitivity to injury is mostly due to reduced aerobic reserves, leading to early onset of systemic compromise during labor.

Neural maturation is markedly altered in IUGR, with some aspects delayed and others advanced [162,163]. This is likely to influence the response to asphyxia, but also to introduce a confounding independent effect on neural development. Severe growth retardation has been associated with altered neurotransmitter expression, reduced cerebral myelination, altered synaptogenesis, and smaller brain size [164]. The effect of the timing and severity of placental restriction has been examined in a range of studies in fetal sheep [156]. Chronic mild growth retardation due to periconceptual placental restriction was associated with delayed formation of neuronal connections in the hippocampus, cerebellum, and visual cortex, but did not alter neuronal migration or numbers. In contrast, in studies in the near-mid-gestation fetus, hypoxia induced by a variety of methods was associated with a reduction in numbers of Purkinje cells in the cerebellum and delayed development of neural processes. With more severe hypoxia the cortex and hippocampus were also affected and there was reduced subcortical myelination. The cerebellum develops later in gestation than the hippocampus, and thus appears to be more susceptible to the effects of hypoxia at this stage of development [156].

Temperature and hypoxia–ischemia

Hypothermia during experimental cerebral ischemia is consistently associated with potent, dose-related, long-lasting neuroprotection [165]. Conversely, hyperthermia of even 1–2 °C extends and markedly worsens damage, and promotes

pan-necrosis [166,167]. Although the majority of studies of hyperthermia have involved ischemia in adult rodents, similar results have been reported from studies of ischemia or hypoxia–ischemia in the newborn piglet and 7-day-old rat [168].

The impact of cerebral cooling or warming by only a few degrees is disproportionate to the known changes in brain metabolism (approximately a 5% change in oxidative metabolism per °C) [169], suggesting that changes in temperature modulate the secondary factors that mediate or increase ischemic injury [166,170]. Mechanisms that are likely to be involved in the worsening of ischemic injury by hyperthermia include greater release of oxygen free radicals and excitatory neurotransmitters such as glutamate, enhanced toxicity of glutamate on neurons, increased dysfunction of the blood–brain barrier, and accelerated cytoskeletal proteolysis [165]. The efficacy of postasphyxial hypothermia is discussed in Chapter 42.

Pyrexia in labor: chorioamnionitis and hyperthermia

These data logically lead to the concept that although mild pyrexia during labor might not necessarily be harmful in most cases, in those fetuses also exposed to an acute hypoxic–ischemic event it would be expected to accelerate and worsen the development of encephalopathy. Case–control and case-series studies strongly suggest that maternal pyrexia is indeed associated with an approximately fourfold increase in risk for unexplained cerebral palsy, or newborn encephalopathy [168].

Clearly, this association could potentially be mediated by maternal infection or by the fetal inflammatory reaction. However, maternal pyrexia was a major component of the operational definition of chorioamnionitis in all of these studies, and in several studies pyrexia was either considered sufficient for diagnosis even in isolation, or was the only criterion [168]. Consistent with the hypothesis that pyrexia can have a direct adverse effect, in a case–control study of 38 term infants with early-onset neonatal seizures, in whom sepsis or meningitis was excluded, and 152 controls, intrapartum fever was associated with a comparable 3.4-fold increase in the risk of unexplained neonatal seizures in a multifactorial analysis [171]. Finally, it is very interesting to note that although exposure to lipopolysaccharide (LPS) at the time of hypoxia–ischemia in adult rats worsened injury, this effect was not seen when LPS-induced hyperthermia was prevented [172]. Thus part of the adverse effects of chorioamnionitis may be mediated by hyperthermia.

Concluding thoughts

One of the most important issues in perinatology is to identify the fetus at risk of decompensation at an early enough stage that we may intervene and prevent actual injury or death. The ability to measure fetal pH or oxygenation at any single point in time generally provides little information about how well maintained fetal heart or brain function is at that point.

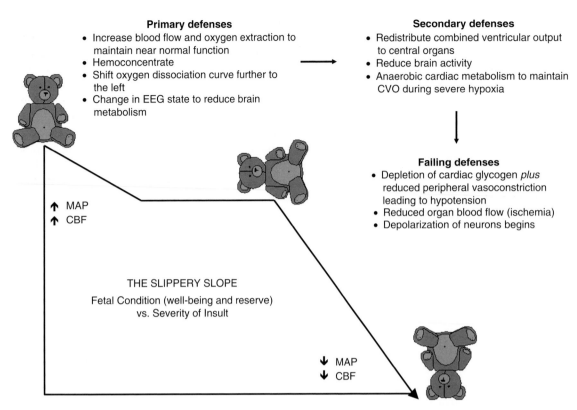

Primary defenses
- Increase blood flow and oxygen extraction to maintain near normal function
- Hemoconcentrate
- Shift oxygen dissociation curve further to the left
- Change in EEG state to reduce brain metabolism

Secondary defenses
- Redistribute combined ventricular output to central organs
- Reduce brain activity
- Anaerobic cardiac metabolism to maintain CVO during severe hypoxia

Failing defenses
- Depletion of cardiac glycogen *plus* reduced peripheral vasoconstriction leading to hypotension
- Reduced organ blood flow (ischemia)
- Depolarization of neurons begins

↑ MAP
↑ CBF

THE SLIPPERY SLOPE

Fetal Condition (well-being and reserve)
vs. Severity of Insult

↓ MAP
↓ CBF

Fig. 13.10. The slippery slope. A conceptual outline of fetal adaptations to episodes of asphyxia. The impact of asphyxia on the fetus depends greatly on the quality of fetal adaptation, which certainly depends partly on the severity of the insult, and how long it has continued for, but also where the fetus starts on the slope, i.e., its pre-existing reserves. With a sufficiently severe insult, e.g., very frequent, more prolonged contractions, even a very healthy fetus will ultimately become profoundly acidotic and develop intermittent hypotension, but only after a prolonged period where cerebral and cardiac perfusion are maintained. In contrast, a chronically hypoxic fetus, or one that has recent exposure to hypoxia that has depleted its cardiac glycogen, may develop hypotension nearly from very shortly after the start of the insult.

Impaired gas exchange and mild asphyxia are a normal part of labor, and the normal fetus has an enormous ability to respond to the consequent intervals of hypoxia/asphyxia while maintaining the function of essential organs such as the brain and the heart.

What sort of fetal problem are we trying to detect? If the fetus is being monitored in any way, there is no difficulty in detecting the prolonged bradycardia that accompanies an acute, catastrophic event of whatever cause, such as abruption or prolapse of the umbilical cord. Such events account for approximately 25% of cases of moderate to severe postasphyxial encephalopathy and are seldom predictable or even potentially preventable [5].

Thus the major clinical problem is to identify the fetuses whose adaptation to repeated asphyxia is beginning to fail. Conceptually, the fetus can be thought of as being on a "slippery slope" (Fig. 13.10). The fetal condition or reserve determines the fetus's position on the slope, while the effectiveness of the primary defenses and the severity of the insults determine how quickly the fetus moves down the slope (decompensation). Healthy fetuses are at the very top of the slope with considerable reserves for initial adaptation before significant hypoperfusion develops, while others start further down, closer to the final catastrophic failure of adaptation that leads to death or injury. When compensation begins to fail,

the pattern of the insult interacts with fetal maturity, aerobic reserve, and environmental temperature, both to determine how serious the decompensation is and to localize any injury. With sufficient spacing between short (1-minute) periods of profound asphyxia, a healthy fetus may be able to defend its central organs almost indefinitely. In contrast, and not surprisingly, a growth-retarded or previously hypoxic fetus may have very limited reserves and begin to decompensate very early, and yet show a similar pattern of variable decelerations to the healthy fetus.

How can we identify the fetus whose adaptations are failing? The options are limited because access to the fetus is limited. Traditionally, we try to assess fetal condition by assessing changes in fetal heart rate and occasionally fetal scalp pH measurements. Although fetal heart-rate changes have an excellent negative predictive value, the positive predictive value of heart-rate changes in isolation is very low. As we discuss above, the development of severe variable decelerations simply indicates transient exposure to hypoxia, regardless of whether the fetus is still in the initial stage of adaptation or is beginning to decompensate. Delayed recovery from the decelerations with continued occlusions occurs only in a minority of fetuses, at a time that is very close to terminal hypoxic cardiac arrest [2]. Nevertheless, more subtle features of decelerations may be useful [2].

Similarly, both the experimental studies reviewed above and clinical experience [173] show that there is, and can be, no close, intrinsic pathophysiological relationship between the severity of metabolic acidosis and fetal compromise. Peripheral acidosis is primarily a consequence of peripheral vasoconstriction, and reflects peripheral oxygen debt which occurs during redistribution of combined ventricular output. Thus severe acidosis may accompany both successful protection of the brain and catastrophic failure [109]. Conversely, brief but intense insults such as complete cord occlusion may cause brain injury in association with comparatively modest acidosis [20].

In contrast, there are very strong relationships, both within and between paradigms, between the development and severity of fetal blood pressure and impairment of cerebral perfusion, and the development of subsequent cerebral injury. The impact of hypotension is directly related both to its depth and to its cumulative duration, in relation to the brain's metabolic requirements given its developmental stage. Thus, ideally, we would like to measure fetal blood pressure, but this is not feasible at present. Newer methods for fetal surveillance include fetal pulse oximetry, near-infrared spectroscopy, more detailed analysis of the fetal electrocardiogram, and assessment of Doppler velocity waveforms. At present these techniques still provide only indirect measurements of the key variables, fetal blood pressure and perfusion, and it remains unclear whether they are superior to systematic monitoring of fetal heart rate [2]. As the critical events that lead to clinically significant perinatal hypoxic–ischemic encephalopathy are clarified by innovative experimental approaches, our ability to recognize significant prenatal events and to intervene appropriately will also improve.

Acknowledgments

The work reported in this review has been supported by the Health Research Council of New Zealand, the Lottery Health Board of New Zealand, the Auckland Medical Research Foundation, and the March of Dimes Birth Defects Trust.

References

1. MacLennan A. The International Cerebral Palsy Task Force. A template for defining a causal relation between acute intrapartum events and cerebral palsy: international consensus statement. *BMJ* 1999; **319**: 1054–9.

2. Westgate JA, Wibbens B, Bennet L, *et al.* The intrapartum deceleration in center stage: a physiological approach to interpretation of fetal heart rate changes in labor. *Am J Obstet Gynecol* 2007; **197**: e1–e11.236.

3. Nelson KB, Dambrosia JM, Ting TY, *et al.* Uncertain value of electronic fetal monitoring in predicting cerebral palsy. *N Engl J Med* 1996; **334**: 613–18.

4. Low JA, Lindsay BG, Derrick EJ. Threshold of metabolic acidosis associated with newborn complications. *Am J Obstet Gynecol* 1997; **177**: 1391–4.

5. Westgate JA, Gunn AJ, Gunn TR. Antecedents of neonatal encephalopathy with fetal acidaemia at term. *Br J Obstet Gynaecol* 1999; **106**: 774–82.

6. Cowan F, Rutherford M, Groenendaal F, *et al.* Origin and timing of brain lesions in term infants with neonatal encephalopathy. *Lancet* 2003; **361**: 736–42.

7. Hellstrom-Westas L, Rosen I, Svenningsen NW. Predictive value of early continuous amplitude integrated EEG recordings on outcome after severe birth asphyxia in full term infants. *Arch Dis Child Fetal Neonatal Ed* 1995; **72**: F34–8.

8. Roth SC, Baudin J, Cady E, *et al.* Relation of deranged neonatal cerebral oxidative metabolism with neurodevelopmental outcome and head circumference at 4 years. *Dev Med Child Neurol* 1997; **39**: 718–25.

9. Gluckman PD, Wyatt JS, Azzopardi D, *et al.* Selective head cooling with mild systemic hypothermia to improve neurodevelopmental outcome following neonatal encephalopathy. *Lancet* 2005; **365**: 663–70.

10. Robertson CM, Finer NN. Long-term follow-up of term neonates with perinatal asphyxia. *Clin Perinatol* 1993; **20**: 483–500.

11. Johnston MV. Excitotoxicity in perinatal brain injury. *Brain Pathol* 2005; **15**: 234–40.

12. Hagberg H, Mallard C. Effect of inflammation on central nervous system development and vulnerability. *Curr Opin Neurol* 2005; **18**: 117–23.

13. Deng W, Yue Q, Rosenberg PA, *et al.* Oligodendrocyte excitotoxicity determined by local glutamate accumulation and mitochondrial function. *J Neurochem* 2006; **98**: 213–22.

14. Niquet J, Seo DW, Allen SG, *et al.* Hypoxia in presence of blockers of excitotoxicity induces a caspase-dependent neuronal necrosis. *Neuroscience* 2006; **141**: 77–86.

15. Fisher DJ, Heymann MA, Rudolph AM. Fetal myocardial oxygen and carbohydrate consumption during acutely induced hypoxemia. *Am J Physiol* 1982; **242**: H657–61.

16. Turbow RM, Curran-Everett D, Hay WW, Jr., *et al.* Cerebral lactate metabolism in near-term fetal sheep. *Am J Physiol* 1995; **269**: R938–42.

17. Blood AB, Hunter CJ, Power GG. Adenosine mediates decreased cerebral metabolic rate and increased cerebral blood flow during acute moderate hypoxia in the near-term fetal sheep. *J Physiol* 2003; **553**: 935–45.

18. Harding R, Rawson JA, Griffiths PA, *et al.* The influence of acute hypoxia and sleep states on the electrical activity of the cerebellum in the sheep fetus. *Electroencephalogr Clin Neurophysiol* 1984; **57**: 166–73.

19. Astrup J, Symon L, Branston NM, *et al.* Cortical evoked potential and extracellular K+ and H+ at critical levels of brain ischemia. *Stroke* 1977; **8**: 51–7.

20. Hunter CJ, Bennet L, Power GG, *et al.* Key neuroprotective role for endogenous adenosine A1 receptor activation during asphyxia in the fetal sheep. *Stroke* 2003; **34**: 2240–5.

21. Mortola JP. Implications of hypoxic hypometabolism during mammalian ontogenesis. *Respir Physiol Neurobiol* 2004; **141**: 345–56.

22. Li J, Takeda Y, Hirakawa M. Threshold of ischemic depolarization for neuronal injury following four-vessel occlusion in the rat cortex. *J Neurosurg Anesthesiol* 2000; **12**: 247–54.

23. Barlow RM. The foetal sheep: morphogenesis of the nervous system and histochemical aspects of myelination. *J Comp Neurol* 1969; **135**: 249–62.

24. McIntosh GH, Baghurst KI, Potter BJ, *et al.* Foetal brain development in the sheep. *Neuropathol Appl Neurobiol* 1979; **5**: 103–14.

25. Longo LD, Koos BJ, Power GG. Fetal myoglobin: quantitative determination and importance for oxygenation. *Am J Physiol* 1973; **224**: 1032–6.

26. Guiang SF, Widness JA, Flanagan KB, *et al.* The relationship between fetal arterial oxygen saturation and heart and skeletal muscle myoglobin concentrations in the ovine fetus. *J Dev Physiol* 1993; **19**: 99–104.

27. Wilkening RB, Meschia G. Fetal oxygen uptake, oxygenation, and acid–base balance as a function of uterine blood flow. *Am J Physiol* 1983; **244**: H749–55.

28. Giussani DA, Spencer JA, Moore PJ, *et al.* Afferent and efferent components of the cardiovascular reflex responses to acute hypoxia in term fetal sheep. *J Physiol* 1993; **461**: 431–49.

29. Peeters LL, Sheldon RE, Jones MD, Jr., *et al.* Blood flow to fetal organs as a function of arterial oxygen content. *Am J Obstet Gynecol* 1979; **135**: 637–46.

30. Green LR, Bennet L, Hanson MA. The role of nitric oxide synthesis in cardiovascular responses to acute hypoxia in the late gestation sheep fetus. *J Physiol* 1996; **497**: 271–7.

31. Hunter CJ, Blood AB, White CR, *et al.* Role of nitric oxide in hypoxic cerebral vasodilatation in the ovine fetus. *J Physiol* 2003; **549**: 625–33.

32. Giussani DA, Spencer JAD, Hanson MA. Fetal and cardiovascular reflex responses to hypoxaemia. *Fetal Matern Med Rev* 1994; **6**: 17–37.

33. Jensen A, Garnier Y, Berger R. Dynamics of fetal circulatory responses to hypoxia and asphyxia. *Eur J Obstet Gynecol Reprod Biol* 1999; **84**: 155–72.

34. Cohn HE, Sacks EJ, Heymann MA, *et al.* Cardiovascular responses to hypoxemia and acidemia in fetal lambs. *Am J Obstet Gynecol* 1974; **120**: 817–24.

35. Itskovitz J, Rudolph AM. Denervation of arterial chemoreceptors and baroreceptors in fetal lambs in utero. *Am J Physiol* 1982; **242**: H916–20.

36. Giussani DA, Riquelme RA, Moraga FA, *et al.* Chemoreflex and endocrine components of cardiovascular responses to acute hypoxemia in the llama fetus. *Am J Physiol* 1996; **271**: R73–83.

37. Siassi B, Wu PY, Blanco C, *et al.* Baroreceptor and chemoreceptor responses to umbilical cord occlusion in fetal lambs. *Biol Neonate* 1979; **35**: 66–73.

38. Blanco CE, Dawes GS, Hanson MA, *et al.* The response to hypoxia of arterial chemoreceptors in fetal sheep and new-born lambs. *J Physiol* 1984; **351**: 25–37.

39. Boekkooi PF, Baan J, Teitel D, *et al.* Chemoreceptor responsiveness in fetal sheep. *Am J Physiol* 1992; **263**: H162–7.

40. Bartelds B, van Bel F, Teitel DF, *et al.* Carotid, not aortic, chemoreceptors mediate the fetal cardiovascular response to acute hypoxemia in lambs. *Pediatr Res* 1993; **34**: 51–5.

41. Jensen A, Hanson MA. Circulatory responses to acute asphyxia in intact and chemodenervated fetal sheep near term. *Reprod Fertil Dev* 1995; **7**: 1351–9.

42. Barcroft J. The development of vascular reflexes. In *Researches on Prenatal Life*. London: Blackwell, 1946: 123–44.

43. Caldeyro-Barcia R, Medez-Bauer C, Poseiro J, *et al.* Control of the human fetal heart rate during labour. In Cassels D, ed., *The Heart and Circulation in the Newborn and Infant*. New York, NY: Grune & Stratton, 1966: 7–36.

44. Parer JT. The effect of atropine on heart rate and oxygen consumption of the hypoxic fetus. *Am J Obstet Gynecol* 1984; **148**: 1118–22.

45. Hanson MA. Do we now understand the control of the fetal circulation? *Eur J Obstet Gynecol Reprod Biol* 1997; **75**: 55–61.

46. Parer JT. Effects of fetal asphyxia on brain cell structure and function: limits of tolerance. *Comp Biochem Physiol A Mol Integr Physiol* 1998; **119**: 711–16.

47. Iwamoto HS, Rudolph AM, Mirkin BL, *et al.* Circulatory and humoral responses of sympathectomized fetal sheep to hypoxemia. *Am J Physiol* 1983; **245**: H767–72.

48. Paulick RP, Meyers RL, Rudolph CD, *et al.* Hemodynamic responses to alpha-adrenergic blockade during hypoxemia in the fetal lamb. *J Dev Physiol* 1991; **16**: 63–9.

49. Lewis AB, Donovan M, Platzker AC. Cardiovascular responses to autonomic blockade in hypoxemic fetal lambs. *Biol Neonate* 1980; **37**: 233–42.

50. Reuss ML, Parer JT, Harris JL, *et al.* Hemodynamic effects of alpha-adrenergic blockade during hypoxia in fetal sheep. *Am J Obstet Gynecol* 1982; **142**: 410–15.

51. Giussani DA, Riquelme RA, Sanhueza EM, *et al.* Adrenergic and vasopressinergic contributions to the cardiovascular response to acute hypoxaemia in the llama fetus. *J Physiol* 1999; **515**: 233–41.

52. Green LR, McGarrigle HH, Bennet L, *et al.* Angiotensin II and cardiovascular chemoreflex responses to acute hypoxia in late gestation fetal sheep. *J Physiol* 1998; **507**: 857–67.

53. Green JL, Figueroa JP, Massman GA, *et al.* Corticotropin-releasing hormone type I receptor messenger ribonucleic acid and protein levels in the ovine fetal pituitary: ontogeny and effect of chronic cortisol administration. *Endocrinology* 2000; **141**: 2870–6.

54. Fraser M, Braems GA, Challis JR. Developmental regulation of corticotrophin receptor gene expression in the adrenal gland of the ovine fetus and newborn lamb: effects of hypoxia during late pregnancy. *J Endocrinol* 2001; **169**: 1–10.

55. Tangalakis K, Lumbers ER, Moritz KM, *et al.* Effect of cortisol on blood pressure and vascular reactivity in the ovine fetus. *Exp Physiol* 1992; **77**: 709–17.

56. Dawes GS. The central control of fetal breathing and skeletal muscle movements. *J Physiol* 1984; **346**: 1–18.

57. Gluckman PD, Johnston BM. Lesions in the upper lateral pons abolish the hypoxic depression of breathing in unanaesthetized fetal lambs in utero. *J Physiol* 1987; **382**: 373–83.

58. Dawes GS, Gardner WN, Johnston BM, *et al.* Breathing in fetal lambs: the effect of brain stem section. *J Physiol* 1983; **335**: 535–53.

59. Koos BJ, Chau A, Matsuura M, *et al.* Thalamic locus mediates hypoxic inhibition of breathing in fetal sheep. *J Neurophysiol* 1998; **79**: 2383–93.

60. Natale R, Clewlow F, Dawes GS. Measurement of fetal forelimb movements in the lamb in utero. *Am J Obstet Gynecol* 1981; **140**: 545–51.

61. Richardson BS. The effect of behavioral state on fetal metabolism and blood flow circulation. *Semin Perinatol* 1992; **16**: 227–33.

62. Richardson BS, Bocking AD. Metabolic and circulatory adaptations to chronic hypoxia in the fetus. *Comp Biochem*

Physiol A Mol Integr Physiol 1998; **119**: 717–23.

63. Danielson L, McMillen IC, Dyer JL, *et al.* Restriction of placental growth results in greater hypotensive response to alpha-adrenergic blockade in fetal sheep during late gestation. *J Physiol* 2005; **563**: 611–20.

64. Kitanaka T, Alonso JG, Gilbert RD, *et al.* Fetal responses to long-term hypoxemia in sheep. *Am J Physiol* 1989; **256**: R1348–54.

65. Boddy K, Dawes GS, Fisher R, *et al.* Foetal respiratory movements, electrocortical and cardiovascular responses to hypoxaemia and hypercapnia in sheep. *J Physiol* 1974; **243**: 599–618.

66. Gleason CA, Hamm C, Jones MD, Jr. Effect of acute hypoxemia on brain blood flow and oxygen metabolism in immature fetal sheep. *Am J Physiol* 1990; **258**: H1064–9.

67. Iwamoto HS, Kaufman T, Keil LC, *et al.* Responses to acute hypoxemia in fetal sheep at 0.6–0.7 gestation. *Am J Physiol* 1989; **256**: H613–20.

68. Matsuda Y, Patrick J, Carmichael L, *et al.* Effects of sustained hypoxemia on the sheep fetus at midgestation: endocrine, cardiovascular, and biophysical responses. *Am J Obstet Gynecol* 1992; **167**: 531–40.

69. Fletcher AJ, Gardner DS, Edwards M, *et al.* Development of the ovine fetal cardiovascular defense to hypoxemia towards term. *Am J Physiol Heart Circ Physiol* 2006; **291**: H3023–34.

70. Jensen A. The brain of the asphyxiated fetus: basic research. *Eur J Obstet Gynecol Reprod Biol* 1996; **65**: 19–24.

71. Shelley HJ. Glycogen reserves and their changes at birth and in anoxia. *Br Med Bull* 1961; **17**: 137–43.

72. Szymonowicz W, Walker AM, Cussen L, *et al.* Developmental changes in regional cerebral blood flow in fetal and newborn lambs. *Am J Physiol* 1988; **254**: H52–8.

73. Mallard EC, Gunn AJ, Williams CE, *et al.* Transient umbilical cord occlusion causes hippocampal damage in the fetal sheep. *Am J Obstet Gynecol* 1992; **167**: 1423–30.

74. Bennet L, Peebles DM, Edwards AD, *et al.* The cerebral hemodynamic response to asphyxia and hypoxia in the near-term fetal sheep as measured by near infrared spectroscopy. *Pediatr Res* 1998; **44**: 951–7.

75. de Haan HH, van Reempts JL, Vles JS, *et al.* Effects of asphyxia on the fetal

76. Jensen A, Hohmann M, Kunzel W. Dynamic changes in organ blood flow and oxygen consumption during acute asphyxia in fetal sheep. *J Dev Physiol* 1987; **9**: 543–59.

77. Ley D, Oskarsson G, Bellander M, *et al.* Different responses of myocardial and cerebral blood flow to cord occlusion in exteriorized fetal sheep. *Pediatr Res* 2004; **55**: 568–75.

78. Mendez-Bauer C, Poseiro JJ, Arellano-Hernandez G, *et al.* Effects of atropine of the heart rate of the human fetus during labor. *Am J Obstet Gynecol* 1963; **85**: 1033–53.

79. Itskovitz J, LaGamma EF, Rudolph AM. Heart rate and blood pressure responses to umbilical cord compression in fetal lambs with special reference to the mechanism of variable deceleration. *Am J Obstet Gynecol* 1983; **147**: 451–7.

80. de Haan HH, Gunn AJ, Williams CE, *et al.* Magnesium sulfate therapy during asphyxia in near-term fetal lambs does not compromise the fetus but does not reduce cerebral injury. *Am J Obstet Gynecol* 1997; **176**: 18–27.

81. Bennet L, Westgate JA, Lui YC, *et al.* Fetal acidosis and hypotension during repeated umbilical cord occlusions are associated with enhanced chemoreflex responses in near-term fetal sheep. *J Appl Physiol* 2005; **99**: 1477–82.

82. Bennet L, Quaedackers JS, Gunn AJ, *et al.* The effect of asphyxia on superior mesenteric artery blood flow in the premature sheep fetus. *J Pediatr Surg* 2000; **35**: 34–40.

83. Wibbens B, Westgate JA, Bennet L, *et al.* Profound hypotension and associated ECG changes during prolonged cord occlusion in the near term fetal sheep. *Am J Obstet Gynecol* 2005; **193**: 803–10.

84. Quaedackers JS, Roelfsema V, Hunter CJ, *et al.* Polyuria and impaired renal blood flow after asphyxia in preterm fetal sheep. *Am J Physiol Regul Integr Comp Physiol* 2004; **286**: R576–83.

85. Wibbens B, Bennet L, Westgate JA, *et al.* Pre-existing hypoxia is associated with a delayed but more sustained rise in T/QRS ratio during prolonged umbilical cord occlusion in near-term fetal sheep. *Am J Physiol Regul Integr Comp Physiol* 2007; **293**: R1287–93.

86. Giussani DA, Unno N, Jenkins SL, *et al.* Dynamics of cardiovascular responses to repeated partial umbilical

cord compression in late-gestation sheep fetus. *Am J Physiol* 1997; **273**: H2351–60.

87. Bennet L, Booth L, Malpas SC, *et al.* A role for renal sympathetic neural activity in regulating blood flow after hypoxia in preterm fetal sheep. Presented at the 2006 Pediatric Academic Societies' Annual Meeting. April 29–May 2, 2006.

88. Wassink G, Bennet L, Booth LC, *et al.* The ontogeny of hemodynamic responses to prolonged umbilical cord occlusion in fetal sheep. *J Appl Physiol* 2007; **103**: 1311–17.

89. Gunn AJ, Maxwell L, de Haan HH, *et al.* Delayed hypotension and subendocardial injury after repeated umbilical cord occlusion in near-term fetal lambs. *Am J Obstet Gynecol* 2000; **183**: 1564–72.

90. Costa S, Zecca E, De Rosa G, *et al.* Is serum troponin T a useful marker of myocardial damage in newborn infants with perinatal asphyxia? *Acta Paediatr* 2007; **96**: 181–4.

91. Primhak RA, Jedeikin R, Ellis G, *et al.* Myocardial ischaemia in asphyxia neonatorum: electrocardiographic, enzymatic and histological correlations. *Acta Paediatr Scand* 1985; **74**: 595–600.

92. Parer JT. The effect of acute maternal hypoxia on fetal oxygenation and the umbilical circulation in the sheep. *Eur J Obstet Gynecol Reprod Biol* 1980; **10**: 125–36.

93. Parer JT. *Handbook of Fetal Heart Rate Monitoring*, 2nd edn. Philadelphia, PA: Saunders, 1997.

94. Janbu T, Nesheim BI. Uterine artery blood velocities during contractions in pregnancy and labour related to intrauterine pressure. *Br J Obstet Gynaecol* 1987; **94**: 1150–5.

95. Oosterhof H, Dijkstra K, Aarnoudse JG. Uteroplacental Doppler velocimetry during Braxton Hicks' contractions. *Gynecol Obstet Invest* 1992; **34**: 155–8.

96. Tchirikov M, Eisermann K, Rybakowski C, *et al.* Doppler ultrasound evaluation of ductus venosus blood flow during acute hypoxemia in fetal lambs. *Ultrasound Obstet Gynecol* 1998; **11**: 426–31.

97. Morrow RJ, Bull SB, Adamson SL. Experimentally induced changes in heart rate alter umbilicoplacental hemodynamics in fetal sheep. *Ultrasound Med Biol* 1993; **19**: 309–18.

98. Arbeille P, Maulik D, Fignon A, *et al.* Assessment of the fetal PO2 changes by

cerebral and umbilical Doppler on lamb fetuses during acute hypoxia. *Ultrasound Med Biol* 1995; **21**: 861–70.

99. Li H, Gudmundsson S, Olofsson P. Acute increase of umbilical artery vascular flow resistance in compromised fetuses provoked by uterine contractions. *Early Hum Dev* 2003; **74**: 47–56.

100. Modanlou H, Yeh SY, Hon EH. Fetal and neonatal acid–base balance in normal and high-risk pregnancies: during labor and the first hour of life. *Obstet Gynecol* 1974; **43**: 347–53.

101. Huch A, Huch R, Schneider H, *et al.* Continuous transcutaneous monitoring of fetal oxygen tension during labour. *Br J Obstet Gynaecol* 1977; **84**: 1–39.

102. Wiberg N, Kallen K, Olofsson P. Physiological development of a mixed metabolic and respiratory umbilical cord blood acidemia with advancing gestational age. *Early Hum Dev* 2006; **82**: 583–9.

103. Peebles DM, Spencer JA, Edwards AD, *et al.* Relation between frequency of uterine contractions and human fetal cerebral oxygen saturation studied during labour by near infrared spectroscopy. *Br J Obstet Gynaecol* 1994; **101**: 44–8.

104. Katz M, Lunenfeld E, Meizner I, *et al.* The effect of the duration of the second stage of labour on the acid–base state of the fetus. *Br J Obstet Gynaecol* 1987; **94**: 425–30.

105. Westgate J, Wassink G, Bennet L, *et al.* Spontaneous hypoxia in multiple pregnancy is associated with early fetal decompensation and greater T wave elevation during brief repeated cord occlusion in near-term fetal sheep. *Am J Obstet Gynecol* 2005; **193**: 1526–33.

106. Brotanek V, Hendricks CH, Yoshida T. Changes in uterine blood flow during uterine contractions. *Am J Obstet Gynecol* 1969; **103**: 1108–16.

107. Winkler M, Rath W. A risk-benefit assessment of oxytocics in obstetric practice. *Drug Saf* 1999; **20**: 323–45.

108. de Haan HH, Gunn AJ, Gluckman PD. Fetal heart rate changes do not reflect cardiovascular deterioration during brief repeated umbilical cord occlusions in near-term fetal lambs. *Am J Obstet Gynecol* 1997; **176**: 8–17.

109. de Haan HH, Gunn AJ, Williams CE, *et al.* Brief repeated umbilical cord occlusions cause sustained cytotoxic cerebral edema and focal infarcts in near-term fetal lambs. *Pediatr Res* 1997; **41**: 96–104.

110. Westgate JA, Gunn AJ, Bennet L, *et al.* Do fetal electrocardiogram PR–RR changes reflect progressive asphyxia after repeated umbilical cord occlusion in fetal sheep? *Pediatr Res* 1998; **44**: 297–303.

111. Westgate JA, Bennet L, de Haan HH, *et al.* Fetal heart rate overshoot during repeated umbilical cord occlusion in sheep. *Obstet Gynecol* 2001; **97**: 454–9.

112. Westgate JA, Bennet L, Brabyn C, *et al.* ST waveform changes during repeated umbilical cord occlusions in near-term fetal sheep. *Am J Obstet Gynecol* 2001; **184**: 743–51.

113. Hokegard KH, Eriksson BO, Kjellmer I, *et al.* Myocardial metabolism in relation to electrocardiographic changes and cardiac function during graded hypoxia in the fetal lamb. *Acta Physiol Scand* 1981; **113**: 1–7.

114. Keunen H, Blanco CE, van Reempts JL, *et al.* Absence of neuronal damage after umbilical cord occlusion of 10, 15, and 20 minutes in midgestation fetal sheep. *Am J Obstet Gynecol* 1997; **176**: 515–20.

115. George S, Gunn AJ, Westgate JA, *et al.* Fetal heart rate variability and brainstem injury after asphyxia in preterm fetal sheep. *Am J Physiol Regul Integr Comp Physiol* 2004; **287**: R925–33.

116. Bennet L, Rossenrode S, Gunning MI, *et al.* The cardiovascular and cerebrovascular responses of the immature fetal sheep to acute umbilical cord occlusion. *J Physiol* 1999; **517**: 247–57.

117. Myers RE. Experimental models of perinatal brain damage: relevance to human pathology. In Gluck L, ed., *Intrauterine Asphyxia and the Developing Fetal Brain*. Chicago, IL: Year Book Medical, 1977: 37–97.

118. Barkovich AJ, Sargent SK. Profound asphyxia in the premature infant: imaging findings. *AJNR Am J Neuroradiol* 1995; **16**: 1837–46.

119. Quaedackers JS, Roelfsema V, Heineman E, *et al.* The role of the sympathetic nervous system in post-asphyxial intestinal hypoperfusion in the preterm sheep fetus. *J Physiol* 2004; **557**: 1033–44.

120. Jensen EC, Bennet L, Hunter CJ, *et al.* Post-hypoxic hypoperfusion is associated with suppression of cerebral metabolism and increased tissue oxygenation in near-term fetal sheep. *J Physiol* 2006; **572**: 131–9.

121. Bennet L, Booth L, Malpas SC, *et al.* Acute systemic complications in the preterm fetus after asphyxia: the role of cardiovascular and blood flow responses. *Clin Exp Pharmacol Physiol* 2006; **33**: 291–9.

122. Pardi G, Cetin I, Marconi AM, *et al.* Diagnostic value of blood sampling in fetuses with growth retardation. *N Engl J Med* 1993; **328**: 692–6.

123. Nicolaides KH, Economides DL, Soothill PW. Blood gases, pH, and lactate in appropriate- and small-for-gestational-age fetuses. *Am J Obstet Gynecol* 1989; **161**: 996–1001.

124. Soothill PW, Ajayi RA, Campbell S, *et al.* Fetal oxygenation at cordocentesis, maternal smoking and childhood neuro-development. *Eur J Obstet Gynecol Reprod Biol* 1995; **59**: 21–4.

125. Block BS, Llanos AJ, Creasy RK. Responses of the growth-retarded fetus to acute hypoxemia. *Am J Obstet Gynecol* 1984; **148**: 878–85.

126. Gardner DS, Fletcher AJ, Bloomfield MR, *et al.* Effects of prevailing hypoxaemia, acidaemia or hypoglycaemia upon the cardiovascular, endocrine and metabolic responses to acute hypoxaemia in the ovine fetus. *J Physiol* 2002; **540**: 351–66.

127. McMillen IC, Robinson JS. Developmental origins of the metabolic syndrome: prediction, plasticity, and programming. *Physiol Rev* 2005; **85**: 571–633.

128. Hawkins P, Steyn C, McGarrigle HH, *et al.* Effect of maternal nutrient restriction in early gestation on responses of the hypothalamic–pituitary–adrenal axis to acute isocapnic hypoxaemia in late gestation fetal sheep. *Exp Physiol* 2000; **85**: 85–96.

129. Jellyman JK, Gardner DS, Edwards CM, *et al.* Fetal cardiovascular, metabolic and endocrine responses to acute hypoxaemia during and following maternal treatment with dexamethasone in sheep. *J Physiol* 2005; **567**: 673–88.

130. Jellyman JK, Gardner DS, McGarrigle HH, *et al.* Pituitary–adrenal responses to acute hypoxemia during and after maternal dexamethasone treatment in sheep. *Pediatr Res* 2004; **56**: 864–72.

131. Elitt CM, Sadowska GB, Stopa EG, *et al.* Effects of antenatal steroids on ischemic brain injury in near-term ovine fetuses. *Early Hum Dev* 2003; **73**: 1–15.

132. Joseph KS, Wilkins R, Dodds L, *et al.* Customized birth weight for gestational

age standards: perinatal mortality patterns are consistent with separate standards for males and females but not for blacks and whites. *BMC Pregnancy Childbirth* 2005; **5**: 3.

133. Sheiner E, Levy A, Katz M, *et al.* Gender does matter in perinatal medicine. *Fetal Diagn Ther* 2004; **19**: 366–9.

134. Di Renzo GC, Rosati A, Sarti RD, *et al.* Does fetal sex affect pregnancy outcome? *Gend Med* 2007; **4**: 19–30.

135. Johnston MV, Hagberg H. Sex and the pathogenesis of cerebral palsy. *Dev Med Child Neurol* 2007; **49**: 74–8.

136. Renolleau S, Fau S, Charriaut-Marlangue C. Gender-related differences in apoptotic pathways after neonatal cerebral ischemia. *Neuroscientist* 2008; **14**: 46–52.

137. Hurn PD, Vannucci SJ, Hagberg H. Adult or perinatal brain injury: does sex matter? *Stroke* 2005; **36**: 193–5.

138. Nijboer CH, Groenendaal F, Kavelaars A, *et al.* Gender-specific neuroprotection by 2-iminobiotin after hypoxia–ischemia in the neonatal rat via a nitric oxide independent pathway. *J Cereb Blood Flow Metab* 2007; **27**: 282–92.

139. McCarthy MM. Estradiol and the developing brain. *Physiol Rev* 2008; **88**: 91–134.

140. Hussein MH, Daoud GA, Kakita H, *et al.* The sex differences of cerebrospinal fluid levels of interleukin 8 and antioxidants in asphyxiated newborns. *Shock* 2007; **28**: 154–9.

141. Dawes NW, Dawes GS, Moulden M, *et al.* Fetal heart rate patterns in term labor vary with sex, gestational age, epidural analgesia, and fetal weight. *Am J Obstet Gynecol* 1999; **180**: 181–7.

142. Ingemarsson I, Herbst A, Thorngren-Jerneck K. Long term outcome after umbilical artery acidaemia at term birth: influence of gender and duration of fetal heart rate abnormalities. *Br J Obstet Gynaecol* 1997; **104**: 1123–7.

143. Bekedam DJ, Engelsbel S, Mol BW, *et al.* Male predominance in fetal distress during labor. *Am J Obstet Gynecol* 2002; **187**: 1605–7.

144. Thorngren-Jerneck K, Herbst A. Low 5-minute Apgar score: a population-based register study of 1 million term births. *Obstet Gynecol* 2001; **98**: 65–70.

145. Clarke CA, Mittwoch U. Changes in the male to female ratio at different stages of life. *Br J Obstet Gynaecol* 1995; **102**: 677–9.

146. Mittwoch U. The elusive action of sex-determining genes: mitochondria to the rescue? *J Theor Biol* 2004; **228**: 359–65.

147. Padbury JF, Hobel CJ, Lam RW, *et al.* Sex differences in lung and adrenal neurosympathetic development in rabbits. *Am J Obstet Gynecol* 1981; **141**: 199–204.

148. Greenough A, Lagercrantz H, Pool J, *et al.* Plasma catecholamine levels in preterm infants: effect of birth asphyxia and Apgar score. *Acta Paediatr Scand* 1987; **76**: 54–9.

149. Bennet L, Booth LC, Ahmed-Nasef N, *et al.* Male disadvantage? Fetal sex and cardiovascular responses to asphyxia in preterm fetal sheep. *Am J Physiol Regul Integr Comp Physiol* 2007; **293**: R1280–6.

150. Jansson T, Lambert GW. Effect of intrauterine growth restriction on blood pressure, glucose tolerance and sympathetic nervous system activity in the rat at 3–4 months of age. *J Hypertens* 1999; **17**: 1239–48.

151. Ranki HJ, Budas GR, Crawford RM, *et al.* Gender-specific difference in cardiac ATP-sensitive K(+) channels. *J Am Coll Cardiol* 2001; **38**: 906–15.

152. Gunn AJ, Gunn TR, de Haan HH, *et al.* Dramatic neuronal rescue with prolonged selective head cooling after ischemia in fetal lambs. *J Clin Invest* 1997; **99**: 248–56.

153. Gunn AJ, Parer JT, Mallard EC, *et al.* Cerebral histologic and electrocorticographic changes after asphyxia in fetal sheep. *Pediatr Res* 1992; **31**: 486–91.

154. Torvik A. The pathogenesis of watershed infarcts in the brain. *Stroke* 1984; **15**: 221–3.

155. Ikeda T, Murata Y, Quilligan EJ, *et al.* Physiologic and histologic changes in near-term fetal lambs exposed to asphyxia by partial umbilical cord occlusion. *Am J Obstet Gynecol* 1998; **178**: 24–32.

156. Rees S, Mallard C, Breen S, *et al.* Fetal brain injury following prolonged hypoxemia and placental insufficiency: a review. *Comp Biochem Physiol A Mol Integr Physiol* 1998; **119**: 653–60.

157. Mallard EC, Williams CE, Johnston BM, *et al.* Repeated episodes of umbilical cord occlusion in fetal sheep lead to preferential damage to the striatum and sensitize the heart to further insults. *Pediatr Res* 1995; **37**: 707–13.

158. Miller SP, Ramaswamy V, Michelson D, *et al.* Patterns of brain injury in term neonatal encephalopathy. *J Pediatr* 2005; **146**: 453–60.

159. Simpson IA, Carruthers A, Vannucci SJ. Supply and demand in cerebral energy metabolism: the role of nutrient transporters. *J Cereb Blood Flow Metab* 2007; **27**: 1766–91.

160. Vannucci SJ, Maher F, Simpson IA. Glucose transporter proteins in brain: delivery of glucose to neurons and glia. *Glia* 1997; **21**: 2–21.

161. LeBlanc MH, Huang M, Vig V, *et al.* Glucose affects the severity of hypoxic–ischemic brain injury in newborn pigs. *Stroke* 1993; **24**: 1055–62.

162. Cook CJ, Gluckman PD, Williams C, *et al.* Precocial neural function in the growth-retarded fetal lamb. *Pediatr Res* 1988; **24**: 600–4.

163. Stanley OH, Fleming PJ, Morgan MH. Abnormal development of visual function following intrauterine growth retardation. *Early Hum Dev* 1989; **19**: 87–101.

164. Kramer MS, Olivier M, McLean FH, *et al.* Impact of intrauterine growth retardation and body proportionality on fetal and neonatal outcome. *Pediatrics* 1990; **86**: 707–13.

165. Gunn AJ. Cerebral hypothermia for prevention of brain injury following perinatal asphyxia. *Curr Opin Pediatr* 2000; **12**: 111–15.

166. Busto R, Dietrich WD, Globus MY, *et al.* Small differences in intraischemic brain temperature critically determine the extent of ischemic neuronal injury. *J Cereb Blood Flow Metab* 1987; **7**: 729–38.

167. Minamisawa H, Smith ML, Siesjo BK. The effect of mild hyperthermia and hypothermia on brain damage following 5, 10, and 15 minutes of forebrain ischemia. *Ann Neurol* 1990; **28**: 26–33.

168. Gunn AJ, Bennet L. Is temperature important in delivery room resuscitation? *Semin Neonatol* 2001; **6**: 241–9.

169. Laptook AR, Corbett RJ, Sterett R, *et al.* Quantitative relationship between brain temperature and energy utilization rate measured in vivo using 31P and 1H magnetic resonance spectroscopy. *Pediatr Res* 1995; **38**: 919–25.

170. Towfighi J, Housman C, Heitjan DF, *et al.* The effect of focal cerebral cooling

on perinatal hypoxic–ischemic brain damage. *Acta Neuropathol (Berl)* 1994; **87**: 598–604.

171. Lieberman E, Eichenwald E, Mathur G, *et al.* Intrapartum fever and unexplained seizures in term infants. *Pediatrics* 2000; **106**: 983–8.

172. Thornhill J, Asselin J. Increased neural damage to global hemispheric hypoxic ischemia (GHHI) in febrile but not nonfebrile lipopolysaccharide *Escherichia coli* injected rats. *Can J Physiol Pharmacol* 1998; **76**: 1008–16.

173. Low JA. Intrapartum fetal asphyxia: definition, diagnosis, and classification. *Am J Obstet Gynecol* 1997; **176**: 957–9.

174. Westgate JA, Bennet L, Gunn AJ. Fetal heart rate variability changes during brief repeated umbilical cord occlusion in near term fetal sheep. *Br J Obstet Gynaecol* 1999; **106**: 664–71.

175. Mallard EC, Williams CE, Gunn AJ, *et al.* Frequent episodes of brief ischemia sensitize the fetal sheep brain to neuronal loss and induce striatal injury. *Pediatr Res* 1993; **33**: 61–5.

Antepartum evaluation of fetal well-being

Deirdre J. Lyell and Maurice L. Druzin

Introduction

In the USA, nearly 50% of all perinatal death occurs prior to birth [1]. While fetal death from acute events such as cord accidents cannot be predicted, identifying, testing, and intervening for the fetus at risk for chronic in utero compromise may prevent neonatal and infant morbidity. This chapter discusses the antenatal assessment of fetal well-being.

An antepartum fetal test should reduce perinatal morbidity and mortality, and reassure parents. The test of choice depends on gestational age. When a fetus at risk for acidosis and asphyxia has reached viability, one of several tests may be employed for screening, including the non-stress test (NST), the contraction stress test (CST), fetal movement monitoring, the biophysical profile (BPP), and Doppler ultrasound. The sensitivity of these tests is generally high, while the specificity is highly variable. Diagnostic ultrasound and prenatal diagnostic procedures such as chorionic villus sampling (CVS) or amniocentesis are the most common tests performed during the early stages of pregnancy to identify chromosomal or major fetal anomalies.

The purpose of this chapter is to discuss common antepartum screening tests, including a description of each test, its indication, and its accuracy.

Perinatal mortality

Since 1965, the perinatal mortality rate (PMR) in the USA has fallen steadily, and the pattern of perinatal death has changed considerably. Improved techniques of antepartum fetal evaluation likely contribute to the decreasing PMR.

The PMR is defined in several ways. According to the National Center for Health Statistics (NCHS), the PMR is the number of late fetal deaths (28 weeks' gestation or more) plus early neonatal deaths per 1000 live births [2]. The World Health Organization (WHO) defines the PMR as the number of deaths of fetuses and live births weighing at least 500 g per 1000 live births. If the weight is unavailable, a fetus is counted if the gestational age is 22 weeks or greater, or if the crown-to-heel length is 25 cm or more in a newborn that dies before day seven of life, per 1000 live births. The American College of

Obstetricians and Gynecologists (ACOG) has recommended including in PMR statistics only fetuses and neonates weighing 500 g or more [3]. For international comparisons, ACOG recommends counting fetuses and neonates weighing 1000 g or more at delivery. Fetal death refers to the intrauterine death of a fetus prior to delivery, regardless of the duration of pregnancy, where the pregnancy was not electively terminated or induced [4]. Fetal death prior to 20 completed weeks of gestation is referred to as early fetal death, between 20 and 27 weeks is referred to as intermediate, and beyond 28 weeks is referred to as late. The fetal mortality rate (FMR) generally refers to fetal deaths of 20 weeks or beyond per 1000 live births [4].

Using the NCHS definition, the PMR has consistently declined in the USA in recent years. The PMR was 8.7 in 1991, 7.3 in 1997, and 6.7 in 2004 [4]. The fetal mortality rate (FMR) has fallen an average of 1.4% per year from 1990 to 2004. The greatest decline occurred in the FMR for gestations of 28 weeks or greater, and it has changed very little for gestations of 20–27 weeks. During the same period, the infant mortality rate has declined by an average of 2.8% per year, although not much change has been seen since 2000.

The PMR and FMR have declined among members of all races, though significant differences remain. The PMR for non-Hispanic blacks has been more than double that of non-Hispanic whites. In 1991 it was 15.7 versus 7.4, and in 2004 it was 12.2 versus 5.5. The increased PMR among blacks includes higher rates of both fetal and neonatal deaths. The reasons for the disparity in outcomes between these groups are not well understood, but differences in preterm delivery, income, access to care, stress and racism, cultural factors, and maternal preconceptional health have all been cited [4].

The infant mortality rate (infant death prior to 1 year of age/1000) was the lowest ever in 2004, at 6.78 infant deaths per 1000 live births [5]. Most of this decline was achieved by 2000, when the rate was 6.89 compared with 7.57 in 1995. Infant mortality during the past 20 years can be attributed most frequently to birth defects. In 1995, malformations were responsible for 22% of all infant deaths, one-third of which were caused by cardiac anomalies; chromosomal, respiratory, and nervous system defects were responsible for approximately 15% each [6]. In 2004, 20% of infant deaths were attributed to congenital malformations and chromosomal anomalies, followed by low birthweight (17%), sudden infant

Fetal and Neonatal Brain Injury, 4th edition, ed. David K. Stevenson, William E. Benitz, Philip Sunshine, Susan R. Hintz, and Maurice L. Druzin. Published by Cambridge University Press. © Cambridge University Press 2009.

death syndrome (SIDS, 8%), maternal complications of pregnancy (6%), and unintentional injuries (4%) [5].

The decline in the FMR may be attributed to improved methods of antepartum fetal surveillance, the prevention of Rh sensitization, improved ultrasound detection of intrauterine growth restriction (IUGR) and fetal anomalies, and improved care of maternal diabetes mellitus and pre-eclampsia. In Canada, Fretts and colleagues [7,8] analyzed the cause of fetal death among 94 346 total deliveries weighing at least 500 g at the Royal Victoria Hospital in Montreal from 1961 to 1993. Overall, the fetal death rate declined by 70%, from 11.5/1000 in the 1960s to 3.2/1000 in 1990–93. Significant declines were seen in fetal deaths due to antepartum asphyxia (13.1 to 1.2/1000), Rh disease (4.3 to 0.7/1000), lethal anomalies (10.8 to 5.4/1000), and intrauterine growth restriction (17.9 to 7.0/1000). Fetal death due to anomalies declined primarily because of improved ultrasonographic detection and early pregnancy termination.

The pattern of perinatal death in the USA has also changed during the past 30 years. According to data collected between 1959 and 1966 by the Collaborative Perinatal Project, 30% of perinatal deaths were attributed to complications of the cord and placenta [9]. Other major causes of perinatal death were unknown (21%), maternal and fetal infection (17%), prematurity (10%), congenital anomalies (8%), and erythroblastosis fetalis (4%). Lammer and colleagues [10] reviewed the causes of 574 fetal deaths in Massachusetts in 1982. Overall, 30% of fetal death was attributed to maternal disease such as hypertension and diabetes, 28% to hypoxia, 12% to congenital anomalies, and 4% to infection. Ten percent of fetal death occurred in multiple gestations, giving a fetal mortality rate of 50/1000, seven times the rate among singleton pregnancies. Fetal death was higher among women who were older than age 34, younger than age 20, unmarried, black, of parity of five or greater, and in those who received no prenatal care or care in the third trimester only. Data from Denmark also confirmed that the highest fetal death rate was found in teenagers and women over age 35 [11,12].

Most fetal deaths occur before 32 weeks' gestation. However, as pregnancy progresses, the risk of intrauterine fetal demise increases among high-risk patients. To plan a strategy for antepartum fetal testing, one must examine the risk of fetal death in a population of women still pregnant at that point in pregnancy [13,14]. When this approach is taken, one finds that fetuses at 40–41 weeks are at a threefold greater risk of intrauterine death than are fetuses at 28–31 weeks, and fetuses at 42 weeks or more are at a 12-fold greater risk [14].

Sensitivity, specificity, positive and negative predictive value

Any test of fetal well-being should ideally meet several criteria:
(1) The test reliably predicts the fetus at risk for hypoxia.
(2) The test reduces the risk of fetal death.
(3) A false-positive test does not materially increase the risk of poor outcome to the patient or the fetus.

(4) If an abnormality is detected, treatment options are available.
(5) The test provides information not already apparent from the patient's clinical status.
(6) The information is helpful to patient management.

Screening tests are applied broadly to healthy patients. The small screen-positive group subsequently undergoes more costly, potentially more invasive, confirmatory testing. In obstetrics, the positive predictive value (PPV) of most tests is limited by a low prevalence of conditions which lead to intrauterine fetal death, and by the variability of the normal fetal neurologic state.

When fetal tests are applied widely to populations with low disease prevalence, the tests' PPV is generally low. Because a missed diagnosis of fetal hypoxia may result in lifelong neurologic problems, most obstetricians accept tests of low PPV in clinical practice. While tests of high PPV are ideal, the low prevalence of the most worrisome obstetric conditions, coupled with the need to identify all fetuses at risk, has created acceptance of tests which have a high false-positive rate and a low positive predictive value. When interpreting the results of studies of antepartum testing, the obstetrician must consider the application of that test to his or her own population. If the population is at greater risk of poor fetal outcomes, the likelihood is greater that an abnormal test will be associated with an abnormal fetus. If the population is generally low-risk, an abnormal test will more likely be associated with a false-positive diagnosis.

Given the frequency of false-positive tests in obstetrics, to act upon a single test could result in iatrogenic prematurity. In this setting, multiple tests may be helpful. Multiple normal tests tend to exclude disease, while additional abnormal tests support the diagnosis of disease and may merit intervention.

The fetal neurologic state

During the third trimester, the normal fetal neurologic state varies markedly [15,16], and this limits the sensitivity of fetal testing. The fetus may spend up to 25% of its time in quiet sleep, a condition during which fetal testing may appear non-reassuring. During quiet, non-rapid eye movement (REM) sleep, the fetal heart rate slows and heart-rate variability is reduced. Breathing and startle movements may be infrequent. Electrocortical activity recordings reveal high-voltage, low-frequency waves. Near term, periods of quiet sleep may last 20 minutes, and those of active sleep approximately 40 minutes [16]. The mechanisms that control these periods of rest and activity in the fetus are not well established. Active sleep, in which the fetus spends approximately 60–70% of its time, is associated with REM. The fetus exhibits regular breathing movements, intermittent abrupt movements of its head, limbs, and trunk, increased variability of its heart rate, and frequent accelerations with movement, all of which are reassuring, as discussed below.

Biophysical techniques of fetal evaluation

During the 1970s and early 1980s biochemical tests such as human placental lactogen and estriol were considered the optimal methods of fetal evaluation. These tests have since fallen out of favor, replaced by more sensitive and less cumbersome biophysical surveillance techniques. The most commonly used tests are the CST, the NST, maternal perception of fetal movement, and the BPP.

Antenatal tests are limited in their scope. They can often identify chronic events such as progressive metabolic acidosis, though the point at which a fetus experiences long- or short-term negative sequelae from mild acidemia is unknown. Antenatal tests may not predict acute events such as umbilical cord accidents or placental abruption. The tests may be influenced by prematurity, maternal medication exposure, fetal sleep–wake cycle, and fetal anomalies.

Contraction stress test

The first widely adopted test of fetal well-being was the CST, also called the oxytocin challenge test. The CST mimics the first stage of labor with uterine contractions, and thus indirectly assesses fetal–placental reserve. Uterine contractions reduce blood to the intervillous space, causing transient fetal hypoxia. The fetus at risk for uteroplacental insufficiency will demonstrate an abnormal response to contractions, forming the basis for this test. If fetal and placental reserve is poor, the fetus will often develop evidence of hypoxia that is not physiologic and may manifest late decelerations. A well-oxygenated fetus with good reserve should tolerate contractions without evidence of pathological hypoxia. The CST is performed during the antepartum period.

The CST should take place in the labor and delivery suite, or in an adjacent area with easy access to labor and delivery. The patient is placed in the semi-Fowler's position at a 30–45° angle, with a slight left tilt in order to avoid supine hypotension. Baseline fetal heart rate and uterine tone are simultaneously recorded for at least 10 minutes. Following this, the fetal heart rate is observed during three contractions of at least 40 seconds' duration within 10 minutes. If there are no spontaneous uterine contractions, oxytocin is administered by an infusion pump at a rate of 0.5 mIU/min. The infusion rate is doubled every 20 minutes until adequate contractions have been achieved [17]. Nipple stimulation may be used to initiate or augment contractions, and may reduce testing time by half when used with oxytocin [18]. In one technique, the patient is instructed to rub one nipple through her clothing for 2 minutes, or until a contraction appears. If a contraction does not appear she should stop for 5 minutes and then repeat the process.

Although the CST has never been shown to cause premature labor [19], it is contraindicated when preterm labor is a significant risk, such as in the setting of premature rupture of the membranes, cervical insufficiency, or multiple gestation. The CST should also be avoided when labor is contraindicated, such as among patients with a prior classical cesarean delivery, placenta previa, or extensive uterine surgery.

How to interpret the test

The contraction stress test is interpreted as follows [20]:

Negative (normal): no late or significant variable
   decelerations

Positive: late decelerations following 50% or more
   contractions (regardless of contraction frequency)
Unsatisfactory: fewer than three contractions in 10
   minutes, or a tracing that cannot be interpreted
Equivocal suspicious: intermittent late decelerations or
   suspicious variable decelerations
Equivocal hyperstimulatory: fetal heart-rate decelerations
   in the presence of contractions lasting more than 90
   seconds or more frequent than every 2 minutes

A negative (normal) CST is associated with good fetal outcome, permitting the obstetrician to prolong a high-risk pregnancy safely. The incidence of perinatal death within 1 week of a negative test is less than 1/1000 [21,22]. A suspicious or equivocal CST should be repeated within 24 hours. A positive CST merits further evaluation and possibly delivery, as it may indicate uteroplacental insufficiency. Variable decelerations seen during the CST suggest cord compression, often associated with oligohydramnios. In such cases, ultrasonography should be performed to assess amniotic fluid volume. Low amniotic fluid may reflect chronic stress, as fetal blood is shunted preferentially to the brain and away from the kidneys. A positive CST has been associated with an increased incidence of intrauterine death, late decelerations in labor, low 5-minute Apgar, IUGR, and meconium-stained amniotic fluid [22].

The CST is limited by a high false-positive rate. Supine hypotension decreases uterine perfusion and may cause transient fetal heart-rate abnormalities, heart-rate tracings may be misinterpreted, oxytocin or nipple stimulation may cause uterine hyperstimulation, or the fetal condition may improve after the CST has been performed.

In addition to high-risk pregnancies, the CST has also been used to assess low-risk post-term pregnancies. There were no perinatal deaths among 679 prolonged pregnancies evaluated primarily with the CST [23]. When both the NST and the nipple-stimulation CST were used to determine the need for delivery, there were no antepartum deaths in a series of 819 patients tested at 40 weeks or more [24].

Druzin *et al.* found the CST to be most beneficial as a test to follow up a non-reactive NST [24]. In other situations, the CST did not significantly improve antepartum or intrapartum outcome. Merrill *et al.* evaluated all non-reactive NSTs with a CST and found that if the CST was negative and a biophysical profile (to be discussed later) was 6 or greater, the pregnancy could be prolonged for up to 13 days [25]. This approach should be used only when prematurity is an issue and when careful follow-up with daily assessment can be performed reliably.

The CST obtained between 28 and 33 weeks' gestation appears as accurate as a test performed at a greater gestational age.

The non-stress test

Fetal heart-rate monitoring, or cardiotocography, was developed during the 1960s as a means of evaluating the fetus in labor. The concept of fetal monitoring was eventually extrapolated to the developing fetus with the NST, CST, and BPP. The antenatal use of the NST in the assessment of fetal well-being has become an integral part of obstetric care [17].

The NST is based on the observation that fetal heart-rate accelerations reflect fetal well-being [26]. A "reactive" test is defined as the occurrence of two accelerations of 15 beats/minute above the fetal heart-rate baseline, lasting at least 15 seconds, during any 20-minute period. A "non-reactive" test is one that does not meet the aforementioned criteria. A reactive NST suggests the absence of fetal hypoxia or asphyxia. The incidence of stillbirth within 1 week of a normal test, corrected for lethal congenital anomalies and unpredictable causes of in utero demise such as cord accidents or placental abruption, is approximately 1.9/1000 [22].

The basis for the NST

The premise behind the NST is that the well-oxygenated non-acidotic, non-impaired fetus will temporarily accelerate its heart rate in response to movement. Regulation of the fetal heart rate and variability is complex and not entirely understood. The fetal heart rate is modulated by the vagal nerve and the sympathetic nervous system. As in the adult, the fetal heart has intrinsic pacemakers, including the sinoatrial (SA) and atrioventricular (AV) nodes. Both nodes are normally under continuous influence of the vagus nerve, which prevents the fetal heart from beating at its more rapid intrinsic rate. The interplay between the sympathetic and parasympathetic nervous systems results in beat-to-beat variability of the fetal heart rate, an important clinical predictor of fetal well-being.

In sheep, vagal influence increases fourfold during acute hypoxia [27], while the influence of the sympathetic nervous system increases to a lesser degree. In sum, vagal influence over the fetal heart dominates sympathetic influence during hypoxia. Baroreceptors located in the aortic arch and carotid sinus immediately signal the vagus or glossopharyngeal nerve, increasing vagal influence and slowing the heart rate. Fetal hypoxia results in a compensatory bradycardia with hypertension. The fetus also has functioning chemoreceptors in the medulla oblongata and carotid and aortic bodies. Interaction between the fetal chemoreceptors is poorly understood [27].

Uterine contractions reduce blood flow to the intervillous space, causing transient hypoxia. Using a sheep model, Parer demonstrated that the abrupt cessation of uterine blood flow for 20 seconds in normally oxygenated sheep resulted in a delayed deceleration in the fetal heart rate, known now as a late deceleration [27]. Pretreatment with atropine abolished any change in the fetal heart rate. The author concluded that chemoreceptors signal the vagus nerve to slow the heart during hypoxemic conditions, resulting in a deceleration of the heart rate following the contraction peak. Repetitive late decelerations suggest fetal hypoxemia.

When under hypoxic conditions, the fetus redistributes blood to its vital organs: the brain, heart, and adrenal glands. Blood is shunted away from the gut, spleen, and kidneys, leading to oligohydramnios. This, along with compensatory mechanisms such as decreased total oxygen consumption and anaerobic glycolysis, allows the fetus to survive for periods of up to 30 minutes in conditions of decreased oxygen.

Loss of reactivity is associated most commonly with a fetal sleep cycle, but may result from any cause of central nervous system depression, the most ominous being fetal acidosis.

When to perform the NST

The NST, or cardiotocography, can identify the suboptimally oxygenated fetus, and provides the opportunity for intervention before progressive metabolic acidosis results in morbidity or death. Patients with risk factors for uteroplacental insufficiency should undergo NST. In general, this includes maternal disease such as diabetes, hypertensive disorders, Rh sensitization, antiphospholipid syndrome, poorly controlled hyperthyroidism, hemoglobinopathies, chronic renal disease, systemic lupus erythematosus, and pulmonary disease, as well as fetal–placental conditions such as IUGR, decreased movement, oligo- or polyhydramnios, and finally other situations of increased risk such as multiple gestation, pregnancies past their due date, poor obstetric history, and bleeding.

Identifying the appropriate time to initiate fetal testing depends on several factors, including the prognosis for neonatal survival, the risk of intrauterine fetal death, the degree of maternal disease, and the potential for a false-positive test leading to iatrogenic prematurity. Most high-risk patients begin NSTs between 32 and 34 weeks, and are tested weekly.

The NST is generally not recommended prior to 26 weeks [20]. An NST should be performed only after viability, when intervention for a non-reassuring test is an option. The limit of viability is poorly defined. Recent survival rates of neonates born at 22 and 23 weeks have been reported at 21% and 30% respectively [28]. However, given the significant morbidity associated with birth at these gestational ages, testing and intervention prior to 24 weeks' gestation are controversial and should be evaluated on a case-by-case basis.

How to perform the test

The fetal heart rate is monitored using a Doppler ultrasound transducer attached with a belt to the maternal abdomen. At the same time, a tocodynameter is applied to the maternal abdomen to monitor for uterine contractions or fetal movement. Signals from the Doppler transducer and tocodynameter are then relayed to tracing paper. Ideally, the patient should not have smoked cigarettes recently, as this has been shown to interfere with the NST [29].

How to interpret the test

Using the most common definition, a normal or "reactive" test is when the fetal heart rate accelerates 15 beats/minute from the baseline, for 15 seconds, twice during a 20-minute period [30]. A non-reactive NST is one that lacks these accelerations during 40 minutes of testing.

A reactive NST is associated with fetal survival for at least 1 week in more than 99% of patients [31]. In the largest series of NSTs, the stillbirth rate among 5861 tests was 1.9/1000, when corrected for lethal anomalies and unpredictable causes of demise [32]. The negative predictive value of the NST is 99.8% [22]. The low false-negative rate depends on the appropriate follow-up of significant changes in maternal status or perception of fetal movement. The false-positive rate of the non-reactive NST is quite high. A non-reactive NST must be evaluated further, unless the fetus is extremely premature.

The fetal ability to generate a reactive heart-rate tracing depends on gestational age, as it likely reflects the maturation of the parasympathetic and sympathetic nervous systems. Druzin et al. demonstrated that, among women who delivered infants with normal Apgar scores, 73% had non-reactive NSTs between 20 and 24 weeks' gestation, 50% were non-reactive between 24 and 32 weeks, and 88% became reactive by 30 weeks. Between 32 and 36 weeks, 98% were reactive [33].

The high incidence of the false-positive non-reactive NST is primarily due to the normal quiet fetal sleep state. The near-term fetus has four neurologic states, described as 1F, 2F, 3F, and 4F. State 1F is a period of quiet sleep in which the fetus spends approximately 25% of its time. This state may last up to 70 minutes. During this time the fetal heart rate has few accelerations and reduced variability, and the fetus demonstrates only occasional gross body movements. The fetus spends 60–70% of its time in state 2F, or active sleep. During this time, heart-rate variability and accelerations are increased, as are body and eye movements. During state 3F, eye and body movements are common, but accelerations are diminished. State 4F is characterized by continuous movement, and constant fetal heart-rate accelerations and variability are seen. While a non-reactive NST may reflect sleep state 1F, it alternatively might indicate fetal compromise and must be evaluated further.

Fetal bradycardia during routine antepartum testing is potentially ominous, and merits further evaluation or delivery. Bradycardia, defined in some studies as a slowing of the fetal heart rate of 40–90 beats/minute lasting for at least 60 seconds, has been associated with stillbirth [34], significant cord compression, meconium passage, congenital abnormalities, and abnormal heart-rate patterns in labor [35]. In a study of 121 cases of antepartum fetal bradycardia managed by active intervention and delivery, there were no fetal deaths [35].

Efficacy

To date there are no prospective, double-blinded, randomized controlled trials of the use of the NST to reduce perinatal morbidity or mortality. The NST was widely adopted without demonstration of benefit among well-conducted trials. Observational studies have shown a correlation between abnormal NSTs and poor fetal outcome [36].

Four randomized controlled trials of the NST among intermediate- and high-risk patients failed to show reduction in perinatal morbidity or mortality due to asphyxia [37–40]. The study populations ranged from 300 to 550 patients, and lacked sufficient power to assess low-prevalence events such as perinatal mortality. A meta-analysis of these four trials also lacked the power to demonstrate a difference [41]. The meta-analysis demonstrated a trend toward increased perinatal morbidity among the tested group, although most of the deaths in the tested group were considered unavoidable, and reflect a weakness of the studies. NST did not lead to early delivery when compared to controls. The authors of the meta-analysis acknowledge that these trials are old, dating from the introduction and widespread use of NST, were not double-blinded, and vary in quality. Practice styles and interpretation of the tests may have since changed.

Given the current medical–legal climate, a randomized, double-blinded controlled trial is unlikely to be performed, as use of the NST has become the standard of care. Further, given the fact that adverse outcomes such as fetal death are uncommon even among high-risk populations, any investigation would require enormous patient enrollment [42].

Several retrospective studies have suggested that the NST decreases perinatal mortality in the tested, high-risk population. Schneider et al. reviewed their experience with antenatal testing from 1974 to 1983, before antenatal testing was widespread [43]. The authors utilized the contraction stress test for the first two years of the study period, and the NST for the remaining seven years. They found that perinatal mortality was 2.24% in the non-tested population and 0.12% in the high-risk tested population. Studies such as these fueled the widespread adaptation of the NST as a means of fetal assessment.

Vibroacoustic stimulation

To determine whether a non-reactive NST is due to the quiet fetal sleep state or to fetal compromise, vibroacoustic stimulation (VAS) is performed. VAS entails the application of a vibratory stimulus to the patient's abdomen above the fetal vertex for at least 3 seconds, creating a startle response in the non-compromised fetus. VAS results in fetal heart accelerations [44], reducing testing time and the incidence of non-reactive tests [45]. VAS increases the NST's positive predictive value without adversely affecting perinatal outcome [46–48].

VAS reduces the incidence of "false" non-reactive non-stress tests without changing the predictive reliability of the test [44]. Smith et al. found the incidence of fetal death within 7 days of a VAS-induced reactive NST was similar to that of a spontaneously reactive NST (1.9 vs. 1.6/1000 fetuses). There were no significant differences in Apgar scores, operative intervention, or meconium staining between groups.

The fetal response to VAS relies on an intact and mature auditory system. Anencephalic fetuses do not manifest heart-rate accelerations in response to VAS [49]. The blink–startle response to VAS does not occur prior to 24 weeks, and is seen consistently only after 28–31 weeks [50,51]. The incidence of reactivity after VAS increases significantly after 26 weeks [52].

The intensity and duration of the stimulus are important. A stimulus lasting for 3–5 seconds significantly increases fetal heart-rate accelerations, while no difference is seen with a 1-second VAS [53].

If VAS fails to achieve a reactive NST, a BPP should be performed, as described later in this chapter.

Though it is deemed safe, a case of supraventricular tachycardia was reported following VAS in a fetus with premature atrial contractions [54]. After 4 minutes the tachyarrhythmia reverted to baseline. The authors cautioned against the use of VAS among fetuses with arrhythmias.

In lieu of VAS, manual fetal manipulation, the manual stimulation test (MST), is used in some parts of the world to reduce the incidence of a non-reactive fetal tracing. Previous trials did not show a benefit to MST [55]. However, one recent study compared the MST to an NST alone and found that the time to reactivity was shorter and the incidence of reactivity was greater [56].

Maternal perception of fetal movement

Maternal perception of fetal movement, or fetal "kick counts," is an inexpensive, easily implemented, reliable test of fetal well-being, and may be ideal for routine antepartum fetal surveillance.

The normal fetus is active. Studies using real-time ultrasound show that, during the third trimester, the fetus generates gross body movements 10% of the time, making 30 such movements each hour [57]. Most women can perceive 70–80% of gross body movements. The fetus also makes fine body movements, more difficult to perceive, such as limb flexion and extension, sucking, and hand grasping. Fine body movements probably reflect more coordinated central nervous function. Decreased maternal perception of fetal movement often precedes fetal death, sometimes by several days [58]. Cessation of fetal movement has been correlated with a mean umbilical venous pH of 7.16 [59]. Several studies have shown that maternal awareness of changes in fetal activity can prevent unexplained fetal death.

There are several protocols for monitoring fetal movement. Using Cardiff Count-to-Ten, a woman starts counting fetal movements in the morning and records the time needed to reach ten movements. The optimal number of fetal movements has not been established. However, there were at least ten movements per 12-hour period in 97.5% of movement periods recorded by women who delivered healthy babies [58]. The ACOG recommends having the patient count movements while lying on her side. Her perception of ten movements within 2 hours is considered acceptable [20].

Fetal movement-counting protocols have been shown to decrease fetal demise. In a prospective, randomized trial, 1562 women counted movements three times a week, 2 hours after their largest meal, starting after 32 weeks' gestation. Fewer than three fetal movements each hour prompted further evaluation with NST and ultrasound. One stillbirth occurred in the monitored group, while ten occurred in a comparable control group of 1549 women ($p < 0.05$) [60]. In a cohort study, Moore and Piacquadio demonstrated a substantial reduction in fetal death using the Cardiff Count-to-Ten approach [61]. Women were asked to monitor fetal movements in the evening, typically a time of increased activity. On average, women observed ten movements by 21 minutes. Patients who failed to perceive ten movements within 2 hours were told to report immediately to the hospital for further evaluation. Compliance was greater than 90%. As a control, the

authors used a 7-month period preceding the study when no instructions were given regarding fetal movement counting. The fetal death rate during the study period was 2.1/1000, substantially lower than the 8.7/1000 among 2519 patients during the control period. Of the 290 patients who presented with decreased fetal movement in the Cardiff Count-to-Ten group, only one presented after fetal death had occurred. Antepartum testing to assess patients with decreased fetal activity increased 13% during the study period. During the control period, 247 women presented to the hospital with decreased fetal movement, 11 of whom had already suffered an intrauterine fetal death [61]. The study of intensive maternal surveillance was expanded to include almost 6000 patients. A fetal death rate of 3.6/1000 was achieved – less than half the rate observed during the control period [62].

The only other prospective, randomized trial in the literature suggests that there is no benefit to increased surveillance of fetal activity. Grant and coworkers randomized 68 000 European women to fetal movement counting using the Cardiff Count-to-Ten method, or to standard care [63]. Women counted movements for nearly 3 hours per day. Approximately 7% of patients experienced at least one episode of decreased movement. The antepartum death rate for normal, singleton fetuses was equal in both groups (2.9/1000 among the study group vs. 2.7/1000 among controls). This study contains serious flaws and should be interpreted with caution. Compliance for reporting decreased fetal movement among the study group was low – only 46%. Compliance was even lower among study patients who suffered a fetal death. Of the 17 study patients who later experienced an intrauterine fetal demise, none received emergency intervention when she presented to the hospital complaining of decreased fetal movement. Why? Grant *et al.* ascribed the lack of intervention to errors of clinical judgment and to falsely reassuring follow-up testing [63]. One might conclude that this large prospective study disproves the benefit of fetal kick counts. To the contrary, the study demonstrates the need for appropriate interventions, and follow-up of patients who complain of decreased fetal activity.

Maternal perception of fetal movement is influenced by several factors. An anterior placenta, polyhydramnios, and maternal obesity can decrease perception of fetal movement [64]. Movements lasting 20–60 seconds are more likely to be felt by the mother [65]. Fetal anomalies, sometimes associated with polyhydramnios, were linked in one study with decreased movement perception in 26% of cases, as compared with 4% of normal controls [66].

Fetal activity does not increase in response to food or glucose administration, despite popular belief [67,68]. To the contrary, hypoglycemia is associated with increased fetal movement [69]. Normal fetal activity ranges widely, and each mother and fetus serve as their own control. Fetal movements tend to peak between 9 p.m. and 1 a.m., when maternal glucose levels are falling [70].

Intensive maternal surveillance of fetal activity helps to identify fetuses at risk for death due to chronic insult. "Kick counts" are unlikely to prevent an acute event such as fetal death caused by cord prolapse. Charting fetal movement may increase anxiety for some, but generally reassures most women and may enhance maternal–fetal attachment [71,72]. When educated and encouraged, women are more likely to present early if they experience decreased fetal movement.

The biophysical profile

The discovery that decreased fetal activity is associated with hypoxia, combined with the 1970s development of B-mode ultrasound, which allowed for real-time observation of the fetus, led to the creation of the BPP. Hypoxic animals reduce activity in order to conserve oxygen. By decreasing movement and employing other protective mechanisms, the hypoxic fetus can reduce oxygen consumption by up to 19% minutes into a hypoxic event [73]. Observation of such reduction in movement can provide clues into the fetus's acid–base status.

The BPP is based upon a ten-point score. The fetus receives two points for the presence of each of the following:

(1) Reactive NST

(2) Fetal breathing movement

(3) Gross body movement

(4) Fetal tone

(5) Amniotic fluid volume

The lower the BPP, the greater the risk of fetal asphyxia.

A BPP is typically performed to evaluate a non-reactive or non-reassuring NST. It may be used for other indications, such as the evaluation of a fetus with an abnormal cardiac rhythm. Given the variation in the normal fetal neurologic state, an abnormal test should be evaluated by extending the testing time or repeating the test shortly thereafter in order to distinguish quiet sleep from asphyxia. VAS during the BPP can change the fetal behavioral state and improve the score without increasing the false-negative rate [74].

An abnormal BPP can predict an arterial cord pH of less than 7.20 with 90% sensitivity, 96% specificity, 82% positive predictive value, and 98% negative predictive value [75], and has been significantly associated with development of cerebral palsy [76]. The incidence of cerebral palsy was 0.7/1000 live births when the BPP was normal, 13.1/1000 live births when the score was 6, and 333/1000 live births when the score was zero in a study which controlled for birthweight and gestational age. The incidence of intrauterine fetal demise within 7 days of a normal BPP ranges from 0.411 to 1.01 per 1000 [77].

The BPP correlates well with acid–base status. Manning et al. performed BPPs immediately prior to cordocentesis and found that a non-reactive NST with an otherwise normal BPP correlated with a mean umbilical vein pH of 7.28 ($\pm$ 0.11) [59]. Fetuses with abnormal movement had an umbilical vein pH of 7.16 ($\pm$ 0.08). Vintzileos et al. evaluated 124 patients undergoing cesarean delivery prior to labor [75]. All patients underwent a BPP prior to surgery, followed by cord pH at delivery. Reasons for delivery included severe pre-eclampsia, growth restriction, placenta previa, breech presentation, fetal

macrosomia, and elective repeat cesarean section. The earliest biophysical signs of acidosis were a non-reactive NST and loss of fetal breathing movements. Among patients with a BPP of 8 or more, the mean arterial pH was 7.28; it was 6.99 among nine fetuses with BPPs of 4 or less. These data suggest that the NST is the most sensitive of the biophysical tests, followed by fetal breathing movements. Fetal movement is the least sensitive, ceasing at the lowest pH. Manning et al. postulate that the graded biophysical response to hypoxia is due to variation in sensitivity of the central nervous system regulatory centers [78]. When the other four components are normal, the NST may be eliminated from testing without fetal compromise [78].

Chronic hypoxemia may lead to an adaptive fetal response, lowering the pH threshold for the fetal biophysical response. This might explain why a chronically stressed fetus can die shortly after a reactive NST, and why oligohydramnios, which often reflects chronic hypoxia and reshunting of blood from the kidneys to the brain, is associated with increased morbidity and mortality regardless of other test results. The lowered threshold likely results from a shift in the hemoglobin dissociation curve, improved fetal extraction of maternal oxygen, and an increase in fetal hemoglobin. Manning postulates that resetting of the central nervous system threshold may occur in part because some biophysical activity is necessary, especially for limb and lung development [77].

Recent studies suggest that antenatal corticosteroids may adversely affect the BPP, decreasing the score. Antenatal steroids are administered between 24 and 34 weeks, when premature delivery is anticipated. Kelly et al. reported that BPP scores were decreased in one-third of fetuses who received steroids between 28 and 34 weeks [79]. The effect was seen within 48 hours of corticosteroid administration. Repeat BPPs performed within 24–48 hours were normal in cases where the BPP score had decreased by 4 points. Neonatal outcome was not affected. Similarly, Deren et al. reported transient suppression of heart-rate reactivity, breathing movements, and movement when corticosteroids were administered at less than 34 weeks' gestation, all of which returned to normal by 48–96 hours [80]. This effect must be considered at institutions where BPPs are used to evaluate the fetus.

A modified BPP, which uses only the NST and amniotic fluid index, may be used in lieu of the full BPP to identify the at-risk fetus [81]. The amniotic fluid index is an ultrasound measurement, calculated by adding the length of the largest vertical fluid pockets free of umbilical cord in the four quadrants of the gravid uterus. If either the NST is non-reactive or the amniotic fluid index is less than 5.0, further evaluation is mandated. Delivery is indicated if the fetus is full-term.

Doppler

Doppler ultrasound is used primarily to assess placental insufficiency and IUGR [82,83].

Blood flow through arteries supplying low-impedance vascular beds, such as the placenta, normally flow forward during systole and diastole. Diastolic forward flow in the umbilical artery is high during a normal pregnancy, and increases more than systolic flow. As gestation advances, placental resistance normally decreases, and the systolic to diastolic (S/D) ratio should decrease [84]. An increased S/D ratio suggests an increased placental resistance [85,86].

If the placenta is compromised, diastolic flow may be absent or reversed. This eventually leads to IUGR. Absent end-diastolic flow is associated with increased perinatal morbidity and mortality. Reversed end-diastolic flow is even more predictive of poor perinatal outcome. Farine et al. summarized data from 31 studies of 904 fetuses demonstrating absent or reversed end-diastolic velocities [87]. Perinatal mortality was 36%. Eighty percent of the fetuses weighed less than the 10th percentile for gestational age. Abnormal karyotypes were found in 6%, and malformations in 11%. Absent or reversed end-diastolic flow in the umbilical artery, while not an indication for immediate delivery, is considered an indication for intensive ongoing fetal surveillance. Delivery is usually based on results of fetal heart-rate monitoring or of the BPP, depending on maternal condition and gestational age.

Studies support the use of Doppler to assess high-risk pregnancies. A metaanalysis of six published randomized controlled clinical trials of 2102 fetuses followed with Doppler compared to 2133 controls demonstrated a reduction in perinatal mortality with Doppler [88]. An analysis of 12 published and unpublished randomized controlled clinical trials in 7474 high-risk patients revealed fewer antenatal admissions, inductions of labor, cesarean deliveries for fetal distress, and a lower perinatal mortality among high-risk pregnancies monitored with Doppler [89]. A report by Neilson and Alfirevic confirmed these findings [90]. Doppler ultrasound appears to reduce perinatal mortality without increasing maternal or neonatal morbidity among patients with high-risk pregnancies [91]. Among patients with IUGR, Doppler was a better predictor of fetal acid–base status than the NST and BPP

[92]. Studies of the use of Doppler ultrasound in low-risk pregnancies have not shown a benefit [93].

Researchers have investigated the utility of Doppler studies of several different arteries, including the middle cerebral and splenic arteries. The umbilical arteries are most commonly used because of their large size, lack of branches, and length, making them easy to study. Doppler studies are commonly conducted later in pregnancy. Prior to 15 weeks' gestation one cannot consistently identify diastolic flow in the umbilical artery [94].

Fetuses with congenital malformations and chromosomal abnormalities may demonstrate markedly abnormal Doppler studies.

Summary

Ideally, antepartum testing of fetal well-being should reduce perinatal morbidity and mortality. The predictive value of antepartum fetal tests is determined by the prevalence of an abnormal condition. When a test is applied widely to a low-prevalence population, the positive predictive value of the test is reduced. In obstetrics, the severe consequences of a missed diagnosis justify interventions based on a potentially false-positive fetal testing. The complete clinical situation should be considered when decisions are made to intervene in a pregnancy based on results of fetal evaluation techniques.

The incidence of stillbirth within 1 week of a negative CST is less than 1/1000, and for a reactive NST it is 1.9/1000.

The high false-positive rate of antepartum fetal tests is due in part to the fact that the near-term fetus spends approximately 25% of its time in a quiet sleep state. To design a strategy to reduce perinatal morbidity and mortality, maneuvers such as VAS, serial testing, and careful selection of patients tested should be employed, given the high false-positive rates and low prevalence of the most serious conditions.

References

1. Centers for Disease Control and Prevention, NCHS, National Vital Statistics System. *Vital Statistics of the United States. Vol. II, Mortality, Part A: Infant Mortality Rates, Fetal Mortality Rates, and Perinatal Mortality Rates, According to Race. United States, Selected Years 1950-1998*. Washington, DC: US Government Printing Office, 2000.

2. Fried A, Rochat R. Maternal mortality and perinatal mortality: definitions, data, and epidemiology. In Sachs B, ed., *Obstetric Epidemiology*. Littleton, MA: PSG, 1985: 35.

3. American College of Obstetricians and Gynecologists. *Perinatal and Infant Mortality Statistics. Committee Opinion 167*. Washington, DC: ACOG, 1995.

4. MacDorman MF, Munson ML, Kirmeyer S. Fetal and perinatal mortality, United States, 2004. *Natl Vital Stat Rep* October 11, 2007; **56** (3).

5. Matthews TJ, MacDorman MF. Infant mortality statistics from the 2004 period: linked birth/infant death data set. *Natl Vital Stat Rep* June 13, 2007; **55** (14).

6. Centers for Disease Control and Prevention. Trends in infant mortality attributable to birth defects: United States, 1980–1995. *MMWR Morb Mortal Wkly Rep* 1998; **47**: 773–8.

7. Fretts RC, Boyd ME, Usher RH, *et al.* The changing pattern of fetal death, 1961–1988. *Obstet Gynecol* 1992; **79**: 35–9.

8. Fretts RC, Schmittdiel J, McLean FH, *et al.* Increased maternal age and the risk

of fetal death. *N Engl J Med* 1995; **333**: 953–7.

9. Naeye RL. Causes of perinatal mortality in the United States Collaborative Perinatal Project. *JAMA* 1977; **238**: 228–9.

10. Lammer EJ, Brown LE, Anderka MR, *et al.* Classification and analysis of fetal deaths in Massachussetts. *JAMA* 1989; **261**: 1757–62.

11. Nybo Andersen AM, Wohlfahrt J, Christens P, *et al.* Maternal age and fetal loss: population based register linkage study. *BMJ* 2000; **320**: 1708–12.

12. Stein Z, Susser M. The risks of having children later in life. *BMJ* 2000; **320**: 1681–2.

13. Grant A, Elbourne D. Fetal movement counting to assess fetal well-being. In

Chalmers I, Enkin M, Keirse MJNC, eds., *Effective Care in Pregnancy and Childbirth*. Oxford: Oxford University Press, 1989: 440.

14. Cotzias CS, Paterson-Brown S, Fisk NM. Prospective risk of unexplained stillbirth in singleton pregnancies at term: population based analysis. *BMJ* 1999; **319**: 282–8.

15. Manning FA. Assessment of fetal condition and risk: analysis of single and combined biophysical variable monitoring. *Semin Perinatol* 1985; **9**: 168–83.

16. Van Woerden EE, VanGeijn HP. Heart-rate patterns and fetal movements. In Nijhuis J, ed., *Fetal Behaviour*. New York, NY: Oxford University Press, 1992: 41.

17. Antepartum fetal surveillance. ACOG Technical Bulletin Number 188: January 1994. *Int J Gynaecol Obstet* 1994; **44**: 289–94.

18. Huddleston JF, Sutliff G, Robinson D. Contraction stress test by intermittent nipple stimulation. *Obstet Gynecol* 1984; **63**: 669–73.

19. Braly P, Freeman R, Garite T, *et al.* Incidence of premature delivery following the oxytocin challenge test. *Am J Obstet Gynecol* 1981; **141**: 5–8.

20. ACOG practice bulletin. Antepartum fetal surveillance. Number 9, October 1999. Clinical management guidelines for obstetrician–gynecologists. *Int J Gynaecol Obstet* 2000; **68**: 175–85.

21. Nageotte MP, Towers CV, Asrat T, *et al.* The value of a negative antepartum test: contraction stress test and modified biophysical profile. *Obstet Gynecol* 1994; **84**: 231–4.

22. Freeman R, Anderson G, Dorchester W. A prospective multi-institutional study of antepartum fetal heart rate monitoring. I. Risk of perinatal mortality and morbidity according to antepartum fetal heart rate test results. *Am J Obstet Gynecol* 1982; **143**: 771–7.

23. Freeman R, Garite T, Mondanlou H, *et al.* Postdate pregnancy: utilization of contraction stress testing for primary fetal surveillance. *Am J Obstet Gynecol* 1981; **140**: 128–35.

24. Druzin ML, Karver ML, Wagner W, *et al.* Prospective evaluation of the contraction stress test and non stress tests in the management of post-term pregnancy. *Surg Gynecol Obstet* 1992; **174**: 507–12.

25. Merrill PM, Porto M, Lovett SM, *et al.* Evaluation of the non-reactive positive contraction stress test prior to 32 weeks: the role of the biophysical profile. *Am J Perinatol* 1995; **12**: 229–37.

26. Hammacher K. The clinical significance of cardiotocography. In Huntingford P, Huter K, Saling E, eds., *Perinatal Medicine. 1st European Congress, Berlin.* San Diego, CA: Academic Press, 1969: 80.

27. Parer JT. Fetal heart rate. In Creasy RK, Resnick R, eds., *Maternal–Fetal Medicine: Principles and Practice*, 3rd edn. Philadelphia, PA: Saunders, 1994.

28. Lemons JA, Bauer CR, Oh W. Very low birth weight outcomes of the National Institute of Child Health and Human Development Neonatal Research Network, January 1995 through December 1996. *Pediatrics* 2001; **107**: 1.

29. Graca LM, Cardoso CG, Clode N, *et al.* Acute effects of maternal cigarette smoking on fetal heart rate and fetal body movements felt by the mother. *J Perinat Med* 1991; **19**: 385–90.

30. Lavery J. Nonstress fetal heart rate testing. *Clin Obstet Gynecol* 1982; **25**: 689–705.

31. Schifrin B, Foye G, Amato J, *et al.* Routine fetal heart rate monitoring in the antepartum period. *Obstet Gynecol* 1979; **54**: 21–5.

32. Miller DA, Rabello YA, Paul RH. The modified biophysical profile: antepartum testing in the 1990s. *Am J Obstet Gynecol* 1996; **174**: 812–7.

33. Druzin ML, Fox A, Kogut E, *et al.* The relationship of the nonstress test to gestational age. *Am J Obstet Gynecol* 1985; **153**: 386–9.

34. Dashow EE, Read JA. Significant fetal bradycardia during antepartum heart rate testing. *Am J Obstet Gynecol* 1984; **148**: 187–90.

35. Druzin ML. Fetal bradycardia during antepartum testing. *J Reprod Med* 1989; **34**: 1.

36. Phelan JP. The nonstress test: a review of 3000 tests. *Am J Obstet Gynecol* 1981; **139**: 7–10.

37. Brown VA, Sawers RS, Parsons RJ, *et al.* The value of antenatal cardiotocography in the management of high risk pregnancy: a randomised controlled trial. *Br J Obstet Gynaecol* 1982; **89**: 716–22.

38. Flynn A, Kelly J, Mansfield H, *et al.* A randomized controlled trial of non-stress antepartum cardiotocography. *Br J Obstet Gynaecol* 1982; **89**: 427–33.

39. Kidd L, Patel N, Smith R. Non-stress antenatal cardiotocography: a prospective randomized clinical trial. *Br J Obstet Gynaecol* 1985; **92**: 1156–9.

40. Lumley J, Lester A, Anderson I, *et al.* A randomised trial of weekly cardiotocography in high risk obstetric patients. *Br J Obstet Gynaecol* 1993; **90**: 1018–26.

41. Pattison N, McCowan L. Cardiotocography for antepartum fetal assessment. *Cochrane Database Syst Rev* 2000; (2): CD001068.

42. Thornton JG, Lilford RJ. Do we need randomised trials of antenatal tests of fetal wellbeing? *Br J Obstet Gynaecol* 1993; **100**: 197–200.

43. Schneider EP, Hutson JM, Petrie RH. An assessment of the first decade's experience with antepartum fetal heart rate testing. *Am J Perinatol* 1988; **5**: 134.

44. Smith CV, Phelan JP, Nguyen HN, *et al.* Continuing experience with the fetal acoustic stimulation test. *J Reprod Med* 1988; **33**: 365–8.

45. Sarno AP, Bruner JP. Fetal acoustic stimulation as a possible adjunct to diagnostic ultrasound: a preliminary report. *Obstet Gynecol* 1990; **76**: 668–90.

46. Tan KH, Smyth R. Fetal vibroacoustic stimulation for the facilitation of tests of fetal wellbeing. *Cochrane Database Syst Rev* 2001; (1): CD002963.

47. Serafini P, Lindsay MBJ, Nagey DA, *et al.* Antepartum fetal heart rate response to sound stimulation, the acoustic stimulation test. *Am J Obstet Gynecol* 1984; **148**: 41–5.

48. Divon MY, Platt LD, Cantrell CJ. Evoked fetal startle response: a possible intrauterine neurological examination. *Am J Obstet Gynecol* 1985; **153**: 454–6.

49. Ohel G, Simon A, Linder N, *et al.* Anencephaly and the nature of fetal response to vibroacoustic stimulation. *Am J Perinatol* 1986; **3**: 345–6.

50. Birnholz JC, Benacerraf BR. The development of fetal hearing. *Science* 1983; **148**: 41–5.

51. Crade M, Lovett S. Fetal response to sound stimulation: preliminary report exploring use of sound stimulation in routine obstetrical ultrasound examination. *J Ultrasound Med* 1988; **7**: 499–503.

52. Druzin ML, Edersheim TG, Hutson JM. The effect of vibroacoustic stimulation

on the nonstress test at gestational ages of thirty-two weeks or less. *Am J Obstet Gynecol* 1989; **161**: 1476–8.

53. Pietrantoni M, Angel JL, Parsons MT, *et al.* Human fetal response to vibroacoustic stimulation as a function of stimulus duration. *Obstet Gynecol* 1991; **78**: 807–11.

54. Patrick J, Campbell K, Carmichael L, *et al.* Patterns of gross fetal body movements over 24-hour observation intervals during the last 10 weeks of pregnancy. *Am J Obstet Gynecol* 1982; **142**: 363–71.

55. Pearson JF, Weaver JB. Fetal activity and fetal wellbeing: an evaluation. *Br Med J* 1976; **1**: 1305–7.

56. Laventhal NT, Dildy GA, Belfort MA. Fetal tachyarrhythmia associated with vibroacoustic stimulation. *Obstet Gynecol* 2003; **101**: 1116–18.

57. Tan KH, Sabaphy A. Fetal manipulation for facilitating tests of fetal wellbeing. *Cochrane Database Syst Rev* 2001; (4): CD003396.

58. Piyamongkol W, Trungtawatchai S, Chanprapaph P, *et al.* Comparison of the manual stimulation test and the nonstress test: a randomized controlled trial. *J Med Assoc Thai* 2006; **89**: 1999–2002.

59. Manning FA, Snijders R, Harman CR, *et al.* Fetal biophysical profile score. VI. Correlation with antepartum umbilical venous pH. *Am J Obstet Gynecol* 1993; **169**: 755–63.

60. Neldam S. Fetal movements as an indicator of fetal well being. *Dan Med Bull* 1983; **30**: 274–8.

61. Moore TR, Piacquadio K. A prospective evaluation of fetal movement screening to reduce the incidence of antepartum fetal death. *Am J Obstet Gynecol* 1989; **160**: 1075–80.

62. Elbourne D, Grant A. Study results vary in count-to-10 method of fetal movement screening. *Am J Obstet Gynecol* 1990; **163**: 264–5.

63. Grant A, Valentin L, Elbourne D. Routine formal fetal movement counting and risk of antepartum late death in normally formed singletons. *Lancet* 1989; **2**: 345–9.

64. Sorokin Y, Kierker L. Fetal movement. *Clin Obstet Gynecol* 1982; **25**: 719–34.

65. Johnson TR, Jordan ET, Paine LL. Doppler recordings of fetal movement: II. Comparison with maternal perception. *Obstet Gynecol* 1990; **76**: 42–3.

66. Rayburn W, Barr M. Activity patterns in malformed fetuses. *Am J Obstet Gynecol* 1982; **142**: 1045–8.

67. Phelan JP, Kester R, Labudovich ML. Nonstress test and maternal glucose determinations. *Obstet Gynecol* 1982; **60**: 437–9.

68. Druzin ML, Foodim J. Effect of maternal glucose ingestion compared with maternal water ingestion on the nonstress test. *Obstet Gynecol* 1982; **67**: 425–6.

69. Holden K, Jovanovic L, Druzin M, *et al.* Increased fetal activity with low maternal blood glucose levels in pregnancies complicated by diabetes. *Am J Perinatol* 1984; **1**: 161–4.

70. Schwartz RM, Luby AM, Scanlon JW, *et al.* Effect of surfactant on morbidity, mortality and resource use in newborn infants weighing 500–1500 grams. *N Engl J Med* 1994; **330**: 1476–80.

71. Draper J, Field S, Thomas H. Women's views on keeping fetal movement charts. *Br J Obstet Gynaecol* 1986; **93**: 334–8.

72. Mikhail MS, Freda MC, Merkatz RB, *et al.* The effect of fetal movement counting on maternal attachment to fetus. *Am J Obstet Gynecol* 1991; **165**: 988–91.

73. Rurak DW, Gruber NC. Effect of neuromuscular blockade on oxygen consumption and blood gases. *Am J Obstet Gynecol* 1983; **145**: 258–62.

74. Inglis SR, Druzin ML, Wagner WE, *et al.* The use of vibroacoustic stimulation during the abnormal or equivocal biophysical profile. *Obstet Gynecol* 1993; **82**: 371–4.

75. Vintzileos AM, Gaffrey SE, Salinger IM, *et al.* The relationship between fetal biophysical profile score and cord pH in patients undergoing cesarean section before the onset of labour. *Obstet Gynecol* 1987; **70**: 196–201.

76. Manning F. Fetal assessment by evaluation of biophysical variables: fetal biophysical profile score. In Creasy R, Resnik R, eds., *Maternal–Fetal Medicine*, 3rd edn. Philadelphia, PA: Saunders, 1999.

77. Manning FA. Fetal biophysical profile. *Obstet Gynecol Clin North Am* 1999; **26**: 557–77.

78. Manning FA, Morrison I, Lange IR, *et al.* Fetal biophysical profile scoring: selective use of the nonstress test. *Am J Obstet Gynecol* 1987; **156**: 709–12.

79. Kelly MK, Schneider EP, Petrikovsky BM, *et al.* Effect of antenatal steroid administration on the fetal biophysical profile. *J Clin Ultrasound* 2000; **28**: 224–226.

80. Deren O, Karaer C, Onderoglu L, *et al.* The effect of steroids on the biophysical profile and Doppler indices of umbilical and middle cerebral arteries in healthy preterm fetuses. *Eur J Obstet Gynecol Reprod Biol* 2001; **99**: 72–6.

81. Nageotte MP, Towers CV, Asrat T, *et al.* Perinatal outcome with the modified biophysical profile. *Am J Obstet Gynecol* 1994; **170**: 1672–6.

82. McCowan LME, Harding JE, Stewart AW, *et al.* Umbilical artery Doppler studies in small for gestational age babies reflect disease severity. *BJOG* 2000; **107**: 916–25.

83. Pollack RN, Divon MY. Intrauterine growth retardation: diagnosis. In Copel JA, Reed KL, eds., *Doppler Ultrasound in Obstetrics and Gynecology*. New York, NY: Raven Press, 1995: 171.

84. Itskovitz J. Maternal–fetal hemodynamics. In Maulik D, McNellis D, eds., *Reproductive and Perinatal Medicine (VIII). Doppler Ultrasound Measurement of Maternal–Fetal Hemodynamics*. Ithaca, NY: Perinatology Press, 1987: 13.

85. Morrow R, Ritchie K. Doppler ultrasound fetal velocimetry and its role in obstetrics. *Clin Perinatol* 1989; **16**: 771.

86. Copel JA, Schlafer D, Wentworth R, *et al.* Does the umbilical artery systolic/diastolic ratio reflect flow or acidosis? *Am J Obstet Gynecol* 1990; **163**: 751.

87. Farine D, Kelly EN, Ryan G, *et al.* Absent and reversed umbilical artery end-diastolic velocity. In Copel JA, Reed KL, eds., *Doppler Ultrasound in Obstetrics and Gynecology*. New York, NY: Raven Press, 1995: 187.

88. Giles WB, Bisets A. Clinical use of Doppler in pregnancy: information from six randomized trials. *Fetal Diagn Ther* 1993; **8**: 247–55.

89. Alfirevic Z, Neilson JP. Doppler ultrasonography in high-risk pregnancies: systematic review with meta-analysis. *Am J Obstet Gynecol* 1995; **172**: 1379.

90. Neilson JP, Alfirevic Z. Doppler ultrasound for fetal assessment in high risk pregnancies. *Cochrane Database Syst Rev* 2000; (2): CD000073.

91. Divon MY, Ferber A. Evidence-based antepartum fetal testing. *Prenat Neonatal Med* 2000; **5**: 3–8.

92. Turan S, Turan OM, Berg C, *et al.* Computerized fetal heart rate analysis, Doppler ultrasound and biophysical profile score in the prediction of acid–base status of growth-restricted fetuses. *Ultrasound Obstet Gynecol* 2007; **30**: 750–6.

93. Goffinet F, Paris-Llado J, Nisand I, *et al.* Umbilical after Doppler velocimetry in unselected and low risk pregnancies: a review of randomized controlled trials. *Br J Obstet Gynaecol* 1997; **104**: 425.

94. Rizzo G, Arduini D, Romanini C. First trimester fetal and uterine Doppler. In Copel JA, Reed KL, eds., *Doppler Ultrasound in Obstetrics and Gynecology*. New York, NY Raven Press, 1995: 105.

Intrapartum evaluation of the fetus

Israel Hendler and Daniel S. Seidman

Introduction

The preliminary estimate of total births in the USA for 2005 was 4 138 349 [1]. Intrapartum fetal heart-rate (FHR) monitoring was used in more than 85% of the deliveries. Fetal heart-rate monitoring was introduced into clinical practice in the 1970s. At that time, obstetric providers and researchers in fetal physiology believed electronic fetal monitoring (EFM) would identify changes in the FHR and/or rhythm that reflect fetal acidosis [2]. It was presumed that detection would be early enough to allow clinical intervention that would prevent perinatal asphyxia. Despite 30 years of widespread use and multiple randomized clinical trials, FHR monitoring has not yet been shown to decrease perinatal mortality other than by decreasing intrapartum fetal deaths [3]. Moreover, some experts believe that the use of EFM leads to over-detection of non-reassuring FHR patterns, thereby directly contributing to the escalating rate of cesarean-section deliveries in the USA [4], which by 2005 increased to 30.3% [1]. We will review the physiology underlying FHR patterns, and the possible reasons why randomized trials of EFM have so far failed to demonstrate efficacy. The current knowledge that guides interpretation of EFM in the intrapartum period will be discussed, with special emphasis on newer methods for intrapartum fetal surveillance.

The history of EFM

The common practice of monitoring FHR during labor was stimulated in 1862 by William Little, a London orthopedic surgeon who took care of spastic infants [5]. He expressed the view that "the process of birth was responsible for the pathology of cerebral palsy." In 1950, Edward Hon, a physician and engineer, invented the "internal" monitor and electrode to collect electrocardiographic information [6].

Soon thereafter, FHR monitoring was rapidly incorporated into routine use. Unfortunately, clinical practice proceeded before controlled trials could establish a true cause-and-effect relationship between specific FHR patterns and fetal acidemia.

In 1969 it was claimed that 90% of all fetal distress was caused by umbilical cord compression, and that electronically monitoring the entire birth process from labor to delivery could save as many as 20 000 babies a year and reduce the number of injured babies by 50% [7]. A cost analysis published in 1975 concluded that EFM could enhance the quality of maternal–fetal health care, although it was clearly cited that "to date, there has been no definitive well-controlled study which has scientifically proven the value of this technique" [8]. A number of studies published in the 1970s pointed to the decline in perinatal morbidity and mortality that had occurred since the introduction of EFM, and attributed this decline to EFM. During a 10-year period from 1970 to 1979, the obstetric service at the University of Southern California found that after EFM was introduced in 1969 their perinatal mortality rate decreased. The cesarean delivery rate increased as well during this period, but the authors did not ascribe this increase to EFM [9].

In 1976, a prospective randomized study in Denver of 483 high-risk patients in labor, monitored either electronically or with intermittent auscultation, found that the cesarean rate was significantly increased in the EFM group (16.5% vs. 6.8%), but there was no difference in neonatal morbidity and mortality [10]. However, in 1979 a meta-analysis of 10 non-randomized studies concluded that "there is now compelling evidence that the intrapartum stillbirth rate will decrease by 1–2 in 1000, and neonatal deaths will be halved if monitoring is widely used" [11]. The largest randomized study to date was performed in Dublin between 1981 and 1983, with 12 964 women randomized to either EFM or auscultation [12]. The cesarean delivery rate was 2.4% in the EFM group and 2.2% in the auscultation group. There were 14 stillbirths and neonatal deaths in each group. There were no apparent differences in the rates of low Apgar scores, need for resuscitation, or transfer to the special-care nursery. Cases of neonatal seizures and persistent abnormal neurological signs followed by survival were twice as frequent in the intermittent-auscultation group. However, when the nine children from the EFM group and the 21 children from the intermittent auscultation group who survived after neonatal seizures were followed up at 4 years of age, there were three children with cerebral palsy (CP) in each group [13].

In 1995, Thacker et al. reviewed the results of 12 randomized trials between 1966 and 1994 with 58 855 patients and

Fetal and Neonatal Brain Injury, 4th edition, ed. David K. Stevenson, William E. Benitz, Philip Sunshine, Susan R. Hintz, and Maurice L. Druzin. Published by Cambridge University Press. © Cambridge University Press 2009.

found that newborns who were monitored electronically had a relative risk of 0.5 for seizures compared to a randomized group of patients managed by auscultation during labor (1.1% vs. 0.8% of the newborns, respectively) [14]. With the exception of the reduction in the rate of neonatal seizures, the use of EFM had no measurable impact on morbidity and mortality. The long-term impact of the reduction in seizures was not demonstrated. In fact, the majority of newborns in some of these trials who developed CP were not in the group of those fetuses who had FHR tracings that were considered ominous. The value of EFM in this meta-analysis was uncertain. These authors pointed out that EFM was introduced into widespread clinical practice before evidence from randomized controlled trials demonstrated either efficacy or safety, and that widespread diffusion of this technology before efficacy was determined may have led to misuse, misunderstanding, and misinformation regarding malpractice litigation.

FHR monitoring may have high sensitivity for the detection of fetal acidosis, but several of the FHR patterns presumed "abnormal" do not reflect fetal acidosis, and the specificity of this tool for the detection of hypoxic–ischemic injury is very low. Moreover, only about 10% of the children with CP had an asphyxial event during labor.

In a 2001 meta-analysis by the Cochrane Collaboration of 13 published randomized controls trials addressing the efficacy and safety of EFM, four trials were excluded for not fulfilling selection criteria, and only one showed a significant decrease in perinatal mortality with EFM compared with intermittent auscultation [15]. This meta-analysis deduced that the routine use of continuous EFM reduced the incidence of neonatal seizures (relative risk [RR] 0.51, 95% CI 0.32–0.82), but had no impact on the incidence of CP (RR 1.66, 95% CI 0.92–3.00) or perinatal death (RR 0.89, 95% CI 0.60–1.33). In view of the increase in cesarean (RR 1.41, 95% CI 1.23–1.61) and operative vaginal delivery (RR 1.20, 95% CI 1.11–1.30), and the lack of long-term pediatric benefit, EFM was not superior to auscultation.

In a separate study, 78 term singleton children with the diagnosis of moderate–severe CP at the age of 3 years were compared to 300 randomly selected term controls [16]. Although late decelerations (odds ratio [OR] 3.9, 95% CI 1.7–9.3) and decreased beat-to-beat variability (OR 2.7, 95% CI 1.1–5.8) were associated with an increased risk of CP, 57 of 78 (73%) children with CP did not have either of these abnormalities. The 21 children with CP with those severe changes on EFM represented only 0.2% of singleton infants at term who had these EFM findings, for a false-positive rate of 99.8%.

Recently, Larma et al. investigated the ability of EFM to detect metabolic acidosis, which may be associated with hypoxic–ischemic encephalopathy (HIE) [17]. For the identification of HIE, the sensitivity, specificity, and positive and negative predictive values for bradycardia, decreased variability, non-reactivity, and for all three abnormalities combined are shown in Table 15.1. The authors concluded that fetal metabolic acidosis and HIE are associated with significant

Table 15.1. Sensitivity, specificity, positive predictive value (PPV), and negative predictive value (NPV) for bradycardia, decreased variability, non-reactivity, and for all three abnormalities combined for the identification of hypoxic–ischemic encephalopathy (HIE)

	Bradycardia	Decreased variability	Non-reactivity	Combined
Sensitivity	15.4%	53.8%	92.3%	7.7%
Specificity	98.9%	79.8%	61.7%	98.9%
PPV	66.7%	26.9%	2.7%	50.0%
NPV	89.4%	92.6%	82.9%	88.6%

Source: Modified from Larma et al. [17].

increases in EFM abnormalities, but their predictive ability to identify these conditions is low.

Despite the apparent lack of efficacy, the use of EFM during labor has continued to grow in hospital settings, and interpretation is being refined as knowledge of fetal physiology grows.

Physiology of the fetal heart rate
Fetal oxygenation

The transfer of oxygen and carbon dioxide (CO_2) between the fetal and maternal circulations depends upon the structure and adequate function of the uterine vasculature, intervillous space, fetal placenta, and umbilical cord. The fetal umbilical vein blood, which carries oxygenated blood from the placenta to the fetus, has about the same partial pressure of oxygen (PO_2) as that in maternal uterine vein blood – approximately 35 mmHg. Although the system of gas exchange across the placenta is efficient, the PO_2 in fetal oxygenated blood is low relative to arterial values in adults [18].

There are several physiologic mechanisms that enable the fetus to maintain normal metabolism in an environment with low PO_2 [18–21]:

(1) High blood flow due to high heart rate. For instance, fetal myocardial oxygen needs are met through a 60% greater resting myocardial blood flow than that of the adult.

(2) Fetal hemoglobin (HbF) can bind oxygen even at a low PO_2, and therefore more oxygen can be transported at a low PO_2.

(3) Fetal blood has more Hb than adult blood. The extra "carrying capacity" allows the fetus to extract maximal amounts of oxygen.

(4) The pattern of blood flow in the fetus allows overperfusion of some organs with higher oxygen requirements, e.g., cerebral blood flow.

The most common etiologies of interruption of oxygen delivery to the fetus during labor are acute decreases in uterine blood flow secondary to uterine contractions, or decreases in umbilical blood flow secondary to cord occlusion. The fetus is able to maintain normal aerobic metabolism during transient decreases in blood flow to the uterus. Certain FHR patterns, namely variable decelerations, have been ascribed to transient umbilical cord compression in the fetus during labor, and manipulation of maternal position either to the lateral or Trendelenburg position can sometimes abolish these patterns. Under normal conditions, the fetus compensates for short-term transient decreases in PO_2 without altering normal metabolic function [20].

Role of the autonomic nervous system

The parasympathetic and sympathetic nervous systems comprise the autonomic nervous system, which regulates the FHR. FHR changes result from moment-to-moment autonomic modulation from medullary cardiorespiratory centers in response to inputs from:

Chemoreceptors

Baroreceptors

Central nervous system activities, such as arousal and sleep

Hormonal regulation

Blood volume control

Parasympathetic nervous system

The parasympathetic innervation of the heart is primarily mediated by the vagus nerve, which originates in the medulla oblongata. Fibers from this nerve supply the sinoatrial (SA) and atrioventricular (AV) nodes. The two parasympathetic influences on the heart are:

(1) A *chronotropic* effect that slows FHR. Stimulation of the vagus nerve results in a relative slowing of SA node firing and a decrease in FHR. Medications (e.g., atropine) that block the release of acetylcholine from the vagus nerve lead to a relative increase in SA node firing and acceleration of the FHR (by approximately 20 beats per minute [bpm]) at term.

(2) An *oscillatory* effect that alters R-wave intervals, resulting in FHR variability.

Sympathetic nervous system

Sympathetic nerves are distributed throughout the myocardium of the term fetus. Stimulation of the sympathetic nerves to the heart releases norepinephrine, resulting in an increase in heart rate and in cardiac contractility, a combination that results in an increase in cardiac output. Blockade of sympathetic activity decreases baseline FHR and blunts accelerations.

Effect of gestational age on FHR

The parasympathetic nervous system exerts a progressively greater influence on FHR as gestational age advances (i.e., advancing gestational age is associated with slowing of the baseline heart rate). As an example, at 20 weeks of gestation the average FHR is 155 bpm, while at 30 weeks it is 144 bpm.

Maturation of the autonomic nervous system is accompanied by increasing heart-rate variability with a pronounced increase of parasympathetic activity. FHR variability is rarely present before 24 weeks of gestation, while the absence of variability is abnormal after 28 weeks of gestation since the parasympathetic nervous system is developed by the third trimester. Regardless of gestational age, loss of variability is an abnormal finding once a fetus has demonstrated that its heart rate responds to the oscillatory input from the parasympathetic nervous system.

Advancing gestational age is also associated with increased frequency and amplitude of FHR accelerations, which are modulated by the sympathetic nervous system [22,23]. Fifty percent of normal fetuses demonstrate accelerations with fetal movements at 24 weeks; this proportion rises to over 95% at 30 weeks of gestation [24]. Before 30 weeks, however, accelerations are typically only 10 bpm for 10 seconds rather than the 15 bpm sustained for 15 seconds noted after 30 weeks.

Chemoreceptors, baroreceptors, and cardiac output

Chemoreceptors are found in the carotid and aortic bodies of the aorta and the carotid sinus. In the adult, when the central chemoreceptors perceive a decrease in circulating oxygen, a reflex tachycardia is initiated, presumably to circulate more blood. The fetus, in contrast, responds to hypoxia with a decrease in heart rate. The cardiovascular responses to hypoxia in the fetus are instituted rapidly and are mediated by both neural and hormonal mechanisms. Baroreceptors in the aortic arch and carotid sinus are small stretch receptors sensitive to changes in blood pressure. When blood pressure rises, impulses from the baroreceptors are sent to the brainstem via afferent fibers in the vagus nerve and impulses returned via vagal efferent fibers, rapidly resulting in a slowing of the FHR.

Cardiac output depends on heart rate, preload, afterload, and intrinsic contractility [25,26]. Each of these four determinants interacts dynamically to modulate the fetal cardiac output during physiologic conditions. The Frank–Starling mechanism is probably not well developed in the fetal heart. Because the fetal cardiac muscle is less developed than that of the adult, increases or decreases in preload do not initiate compensatory changes in stroke volume [27]. In addition, the fetal heart function appears to be highly sensitive to changes in the afterload, represented by the fetal arterial blood pressure. Increases in afterload elicit a dramatic reduction in the stroke volume or cardiac output. In clinical practice, it is reasonable to assume that, at small variations of heart rate, there are relatively small effects on the cardiac output in the fetus. However, at extremes (for example, a tachycardia above 240 bpm or a bradycardia below 60 bpm), cardiac output and umbilical blood flow are substantially decreased.

Other factors, which either directly or indirectly alter FHR and the fetal circulation, include central nervous system activity (sleep–wake cycles change the FHR variability), hormones, and blood volume shifts. The primary hormones involved in regulation of FHR, cardiac contractility, and distribution of blood flow in the fetus include epinephrine, norepinephrine, the renin–angiotensin system, arginine vasopressin, prostaglandins, melanocyte-stimulating hormone, atrial natriuretic hormone, neuropeptide Y, and thyrotropin-releasing hormone. In addition, nitric oxide (NO) and adenosine can affect the fetal circulation.

Table 15.2. Definitions of fetal heart-rate patterns

Pattern	Definition

Baseline	• The mean FHR rounded to increments of 5 bpm during a 10-min segment, excluding:
	  Periodic or episode changes
	  Periods of marked FHR variability
	  Segments of baseline that differ by more than 25 bpm
	• The baseline must be for a minimum of 2 min in any 10-min segment

Baseline variability	• Fluctuations in the FHR of 2 cycles per min or greater
	• Variability is visually quantitated as the amplitude of peak-to-trough in bpm
	  Absent – amplitude range undetectable
	  Minimal – amplitude range detectable but 5 bpm or fewer
	  Moderate (normal) – amplitude range 6–25 bpm
	  Marked – amplitude range > 25 bpm

Acceleration	• A visually apparent increase (onset to peak in < 30 sec) in the FHR from the most recent calculated baseline • The duration of an acceleration is defined as the time from the initial change in FHR from the baseline to the return of the FHR to the baseline • At 32 wks of gestation and beyond, an acceleration has an acme of 15 bpm or more above baseline, with a duration of 15 sec or more, but < 2 min • Before 32 wks of gestation, an acceleration has an acme of 10 bpm or more above baseline, with a duration of 10 sec or more, but < 2 min • Prolonged acceleration lasts 2 min or more but < 10 min • If an acceleration lasts 10 min or longer, it is baseline change
Bradycardia	• Baseline FHR < 110 bpm
Early deceleration	• In association with a uterine contraction, a visually apparent, gradual (onset to nadir 30 sec or more) decrease in FHR with return to baseline
Tachycardia	• Baseline FHR > 160 bpm
Variable deceleration	• An abrupt (onset to nadir 30 sec or more), visually apparent decrease in the FHR below the baseline • The decrease in FHR is 15 bpm or more, with a duration of 15 sec or more, but < 2 min
Prolonged deceleration	• Visually apparent decrease in the FHR below the baseline • Deceleration is 15 bpm or more, lasting 2 min or more but less than 10 min from onset to return to baseline

Notes:
FHR, fetal heart rate; bpm, beats per minute. Reprinted from the ACOG Practice Bulletin No. 70. American College of Obstetricians and Gynecologists. *Obstet Gynecol* 2005; **106**: 1453–61.

Characteristics of the normal fetal heart rate

The baseline features of the FHR, that is, those predominant characteristics which can be recognized between uterine contractions, are listed in Table 15.2 [28,29].

Baseline rate

The baseline FHR is the approximate mean FHR rounded to 5 bpm during a 10-minute segment, excluding:

Periodic or episodic changes

Periods of marked FHR variability

Segments of the baseline that differ by 25 bpm

In any 10-minute window, the minimum baseline duration must be at least 2 minutes, otherwise the baseline for that period is indeterminate or *saltatoric*, in which case one may need to refer to the previous 10-minute segment(s). The normal baseline FHR is considered to be between 110 and 160 bpm. Values below 110 bpm are termed *bradycardia* and those above 160 bpm are termed *tachycardia*.

Variability

Variability refers to the irregularity in the line seen when examining an FHR monitor tracing. The FHR variability represents a slight difference in time interval between each beat as counted and recorded by the monitor. If all intervals between heart beats were identical, the line would be regular or smooth. Baseline variability is defined as fluctuations in the baseline FHR of 2 cycles per minute or greater. Variability is a critical determinant of adequate perfusion and/or function in the central nervous system [2].

Accelerations

An acceleration is a visually apparent abrupt increase in FHR above the baseline, defined as onset of acceleration to peak in 30 seconds. The increase is calculated from the most recently determined portion of the baseline. The acme is 15 bpm above the baseline, and the acceleration lasts between 15 seconds and 2 minutes from the onset to return to baseline (Fig. 15.1).

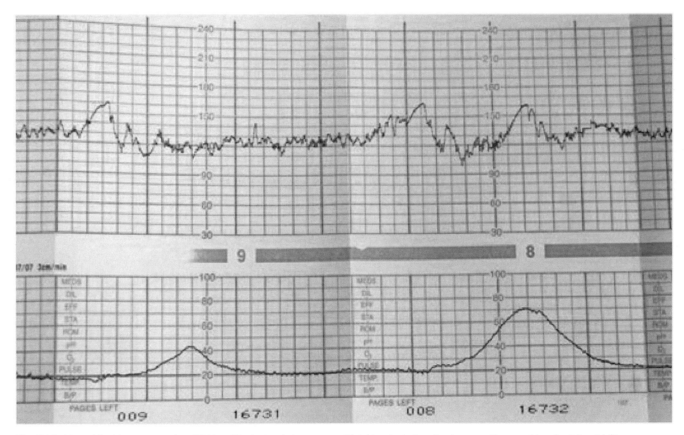

Fig. 15.1. Normal fetal heart-rate tracing. Within a 20-minute window a normal fetal heart-rate baseline is seen with normal (moderate) variability and two accelerations. *See color plate section.*

Before 32 weeks of gestation, accelerations are defined as having an acme 10 bpm above the baseline and duration of at least 10 seconds [29]. A prolonged acceleration is more than 2 and less than 10 minutes in duration. There is a close association between the presence of accelerations and normal FHR variability, and both accelerations and normal variability have the same positive prognostic significance of normal fetal oxygenation. A recent study of 97 fetuses with birthweights < 1200 g demonstrated that the absence of two FHR accelerations of 10 bpm for 10 seconds twice in a 20-minute window, 1 hour before delivery, was associated with intraventricular hemorrhage (IVH) and/or periventricular leukomalacia (PVL) ($p < 0.01$). Both are associated with a significant risk for mental and psychomotor delays by Bayley testing ($p < 0.001$) [30].

Fetal response to hypoxia/asphyxia

Fetal response to hypoxia is complicated, since there are a number of physiologic control mechanisms that are activated in response to acute hypoxia. These include both baroreceptors and chemoreceptors, as well as sympathetic and parasympathetic influences [31]. Fetal bradycardia occurs promptly in response to fetal hypoxia secondary to maternal hypoxia, reduced uterine blood flow, or umbilical cord occlusions. This bradycardia is variably associated with hypertension and therefore can occur as a result of activation of either

chemoreceptors or baroreceptors. When fetal hypoxemia is maintained in pregnant sheep, there is a gradual return of the FHR to normal followed by a tachycardia that is associated with elevations in fetal catecholamine levels. FHR returns to normal levels after 12–16 hours of hypoxia in the absence of progressive acidemia secondary to reduced uterine blood flow. A similar adaptation takes place with FHR variability.

Augmented β-adrenergic activity may be important in maintaining cardiac output and umbilical blood flow during hypoxia, by increasing the inotropic effect on the heart. α-Adrenergic activity is important in determining regional distribution of blood flow in the hypoxic fetus by selective vasoconstriction.

The initial response to hypoxia includes a decrease in fetal oxygen consumption to values as low as 60% of control. This decrease is rapidly instituted, stable for periods up to 45 minutes, proportional to the degree of hypoxia, and rapidly reversible on cessation of maternal hypoxia. It is accompanied by a fetal bradycardia of about 30 bpm below control and an increase in fetal arterial blood pressure. If hypoxia persists, metabolic acidosis develops. This is due to lactic acid accumulation as a result of anaerobic metabolism primarily in those partially vasoconstricted beds where oxygenation is inadequate for normal basic needs [23].

The fetus responds to hypoxia with a redistribution of blood flow favoring certain vital organs – namely, heart, brain,

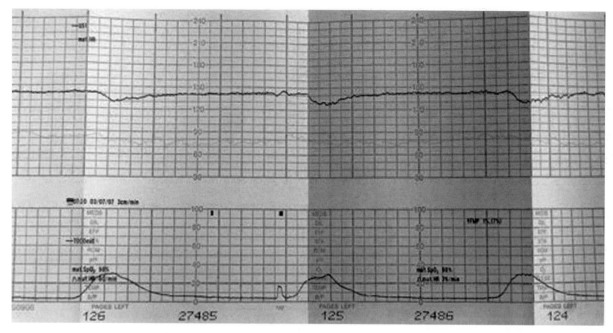

Fig. 15.2. Late decelerations with decreased variability and normal baseline.

and adrenal glands – and a decrease in blood flow to the gut, spleen, kidneys, and carcass [24]. In addition, there is bradycardia, decreased total oxygen consumption, and anaerobic glycolysis. These compensatory mechanisms enable a fetus to survive moderately long periods (e.g., 30–60 minutes) of limited oxygen supply, without damage to vital organs. The response of blood flow to oxygen availability achieves a constancy of oxygen delivery in the fetal cerebral circulation and in the fetal myocardium.

During more severe asphyxia or sustained hypoxemia, the responses described above are no longer maintained, and decreases in cardiac output, arterial blood pressure, and blood flow to the brain and heart have been described [31].

Variant fetal heart-rate patterns
Periodic patterns: late, early, and variable decelerations

Periodic patterns are the alterations in FHR that are associated with uterine contractions. The three characteristic periodic patterns seen are late decelerations, early decelerations, and variable decelerations. Prolonged decelerations are a subcategory of variable or late decelerations. Episodic decelerations are similar to periodic patterns, but do not have the same constant association with contractions [29].

Late deceleration of the FHR is a visually apparent gradual decrease (defined as onset of deceleration to nadir in more than 30 seconds) and return to baseline FHR associated with a uterine contraction. It is delayed in timing, with the nadir of the deceleration late in relation to the peak of the contraction. In most cases the onset, nadir, and recovery are all late in

relation to the beginning, peak, and ending of the contraction, respectively (Fig. 15.2) [29].

Originally, all late decelerations were thought to represent the fetal response to decreased oxygenation in the presence of significant uteroplacental insufficiency. More recent research has identified two different mechanisms. Late decelerations that have retained variability are neurogenic in origin. When a well-oxygenated fetus has an acute reduction in oxygenation during a contraction, chemoreceptors detect the hypoxemia and initiate the vagal bradycardiac response. It takes a short time for hypoxemia to develop in this setting, thus the chemoreceptor reflex occurs as the hypoxemia is detected. The FHR baseline has a slower decline and the nadir of the deceleration is "late" relative to the peak of the contraction. Because the fetus is centrally well oxygenated and not acidemic, variability is retained [32]. Late decelerations with decreased or absent variability are possibly asphyxial. Late decelerations with absent variability occur when there is insufficient oxygen for myocardial metabolism and/or normal cerebral function. These are likely to occur in the fetus with chronic and prolonged placental insufficiency [31].

Early deceleration of the FHR is similar to late deceleration in shape and duration. However, the nadir of the deceleration is coincident to the peak of the contraction. In most cases the onset, nadir, and recovery are all coincident to the beginning, peak, and ending of the contraction respectively. Early decelerations are caused by fetal head compression during uterine contraction, resulting in vagal stimulation and slowing of the heart rate. They are not associated with significant fetal acidemia [31].

Variable decelerations are visually apparent abrupt decreases in FHR from the baseline, defined as onset of deceleration to beginning of nadir less than 30 seconds [33].

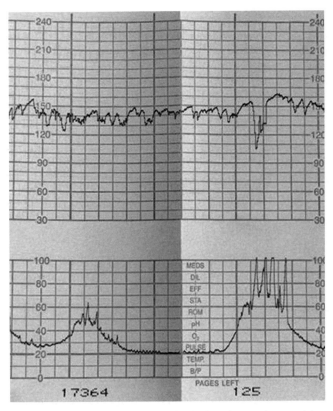

Fig. 15.3. Mild variable deceleration. The depth is above 80 bpm, and the duration is less than 30 seconds.

The decrease in FHR below the baseline is at least 15 bpm, lasting (from baseline to baseline) between 15 seconds and 2 minutes. When variable decelerations are associated with uterine contractions their onset, depth, and duration commonly vary with successive uterine contractions (Fig. 15.3).

Variable decelerations are secondary to umbilical cord compression that causes baroreceptor stimulation. Umbilical cord compression causes an increase in blood pressure secondary to umbilical artery occlusion. The sudden increase in blood pressure stimulates baroreceptors in the aortic arch. The baroreceptor reflex through the vagus to the medulla oblongata and back to the pacemaker of the heart is extremely fast and the bradycardial response is quick, thus the abrupt descent of the FHR. If variable decelerations are persistent and/or severe, one may see the development of tachycardia, late return to baseline with progressive decelerations, and/or decreased variability. The evolution of moderate variables to variables with or absent variability reflects developing fetal acidemia. Variable decelerations may be classified according to their depth and duration as mild, when the depth is above 80 bpm and the duration is less than 30 seconds; moderate, when the depth is between 70 and 80 bpm and the duration is between 30 and 60 seconds (Fig. 15.3); and severe, when the depth is below 70 bpm and the duration is longer than 60 seconds (Fig. 15.4). Variable decelerations are generally associated with a favorable outcome [34].

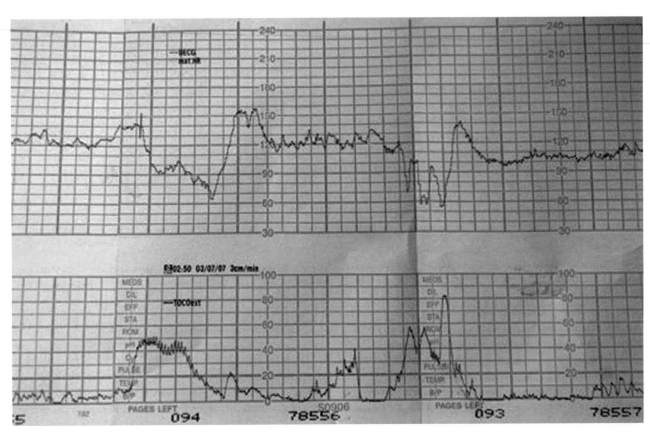

Fig. 15.4. Severe variable decelerations. The depth is below 70 bpm and the duration is longer than 60 seconds.

Episodic decelerations: prolonged deceleration

A prolonged deceleration is a subcategory of the variable deceleration. The decrease in FHR below the baseline is at least 15 bpm, lasting more than 2 minutes, but less than 10 minutes [29]. The definition refers to a change in baseline rate (e.g., bradycardia) if the prolonged deceleration is longer than 10 minutes in duration. Prolonged decelerations can lead to hypoxia. These patterns may reflect a stepwise decrease in fetal oxygenation secondary to an acute asphyxial insult [31]. The stimulus may be anything that causes a sudden drop in blood flow to the intervillous space (e.g., maternal hypotension or tetanic contractions).

Changes in baseline rate: tachycardia and bradycardia

Non-asphyxial causes of fetal tachycardia include the administration of some drugs such as β-sympathomimetics or atropine. Non-asphyxial causes that may develop into asphyxia include maternal fever, fetal infection, and fetal cardiac tachyarrhythmia. Tachycardia signifying fetal acidemia is most frequently seen with absent variability, recurrent late decelerations, recurrent variable decelerations or a combination of the above patterns [35]. Mild tachycardia with normal variability and no periodic changes is not associated with fetal acidemia [36–39]. Tachycardia can also be seen transiently when the fetus recovers from an acute hypoxic stress. This tachycardia is considered a physiologic response secondary to adrenal stimulation with release of catecholamines.

By definition, bradycardia refers to a baseline rate of less than 110 bpm [31]. Uncomplicated bradycardias of more than 80 bpm with retained variability are not associated with fetal acidemia [35–37,40]. Non-asphyxial causes of bradycardia include complete heart block and treatment with significant doses of β-adrenergic blockers. Occasionally a fetus will have a baseline below 110 bpm without pathologic implications.

Like the patterns described above, bradycardial episodes in the fetus may cause hypoxia or they may be the cause of hypoxia. Bradycardias that occur during the final moments of the second stage (end-stage bradycardias) are an example of an FHR pattern that can lead to hypoxia if sufficiently prolonged and severe. These bradycardias can be secondary to head compression and vagal stimulation or secondary to acute umbilical cord occlusion. The fetus can tolerate end-stage bradycardias as long as the baseline remains above 80 bpm and the variability is retained [41,42].

If a bradycardia becomes severe, oxygen and CO_2 transfer will become impaired, a metabolic acidosis will develop, and variability will diminish. Bradycardias that result from severe hypoxia do not return to baseline and have decreased or absent variability [37,43]. The progressive flat-line bradycardia can be seen following a period of severe late or variable decelerations. This evolution from severe periodic changes to the progressive bradycardia with minimal or absent variability is associated with metabolic acidemia and eventually fetal hypotension. It may be seen in uterine rupture, extensive placental abruption, or just prior to fetal death.

Sinusoidal patterns

The sinusoidal pattern was first described in a group of severely affected Rh-isoimmunized fetuses [44], but has subsequently been noted in association with fetuses who are anemic for other reasons, such as fetal–maternal bleeding, and in severely asphyxiated infants. This pattern appears as a regular, smooth sine-wave-like baseline, with a frequency of approximately 3–6 per minute and an amplitude range of up to 30 bpm (Fig. 15.5). The regularity of the waves distinguishes it from long-term variability complexes, which are more crudely shaped and irregular. In addition, sinusoidal patterns exhibit an absence of beat-to-beat or short-term variability. The essential characteristic of a true sinusoidal pattern is extreme regularity and smoothness [34].

Sinusoidal patterns have also been described in cases of normal infants born without depression or acid–base abnormalities, although in these cases there is dispute about whether the patterns are truly sinusoidal or whether, because of the moderately irregular pattern, they are variants of long-term variability. Such patterns, called *pseudosinusoidal*, are sometimes seen after administration of narcotics to the mother.

The presence of a sinusoidal pattern in an Rh-sensitized patient suggests fetal anemia, generally with a hematocrit below 25%. In cases of fetal–maternal bleeding, the appearance of a striking sinusoidal pattern has given rise to the belief that the pattern is caused by acute anemia, rather than a slow development of anemia, as seen usually with erythroblastosis fetalis [34]. However, there may be a less striking blunted variant in Rh-affected babies. As yet there is little evidence for this, although the association of the acute anemia in fetal arginine vasopression levels is consistent with the theory. If the pattern is irregularly sinusoidal or pseudosinusoidal, intermittently present, and not associated with intervening periodic decelerations, it is unlikely to indicate fetal compromise [34].

Absent or minimal variability

Minimal variability can be secondary to fetal sleep, medication, or early hypoxia. Minimal variability without decelerations is almost always non-asphyxial [45]. Absent variability can be asphyxial or non-asphyxial as well. Examples of non-asphyxial causes include central nervous system depressants, anencephaly, defective cardiac conduction system, and congenital or acquired neurologic abnormalities. Conversely, absent variability is seen when the fetus has cerebral asphyxia with accompanying loss of either fine-tuning within the cardioregulatory center in the brain and/or direct myocardial depression. Loss of variability, especially in the presence of other periodic patterns during labor, is the most sensitive indicator of metabolic acidemia in a fetus (Fig. 15.6) [32,36,40,46,47].

In summary, when assessing periodic or episodic FHR patterns, variability is the key reflection of intact cerebral

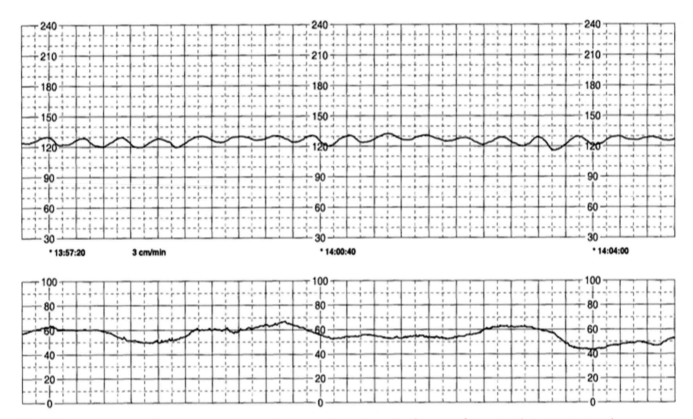

Fig. 15.5. Sinusoidal patterns. This pattern is a regular, smooth sine-wave-like baseline, with a frequency of approximately 3–6 per minute and an amplitude range of up to 30 bpm.

oxygenation. Periodic FHR patterns have specific physiologic mechanisms but, because such variant patterns are common during labor, the degree of hypoxia or asphyxia experienced by an individual fetus is not well predicted by them.

Inter- and intra-observer variability

There is a wide variation in the way obstetricians interpret and respond to EFM tracings. When four obstetricians, for example, examined 50 cardiotocograms, the inter-observer variability was wide (they agreed in only 22% of the cases) [48], as was the intra-observer variability. When the same individuals re-analyzed these tracings 2 months later, the clinicians interpreted 21% of the tracings differently than they did during the first evaluation [49]. However, when the tracing is reassuring, there is less inter- and intra-observer variability [50]. On the other hand, knowledge of the neonatal outcome and retrospective review of fetal tracing significantly influences the analysis of the FHR tracing [51].

Role of EFM in predicting perinatal asphyxia

The link between the FHR pattern and the actual acid–base status of the fetus is not well defined. Thirty-nine percent of the intrapartum FHR tracings obtained during labor display periodic FHR patterns, yet only 2% of all newborns have evidence of metabolic acidemia (pH 7.1 with a base excess of 12 mmol/L) [35,52].

The original outcome measures used in early studies of FHR monitoring were intrapartum stillbirth and CP. FHR

monitoring has been associated with a virtual disappearance of intrapartum stillbirths. Prior to the introduction of FHR monitoring, approximately one-third of all stillbirths, or 3/1000 births, occurred in the intrapartum period [53]. Currently, the overall incidence of intrapartum stillbirth is at most 0.5/1000 births. The hope that EFM during labor would abolish CP through the diagnosis of "fetal distress" and early intervention has proven to be an unrealistic goal because the majority of children with CP develop the disorder prior to labor. In fact, the incidence of CP due to intrapartum asphyxia is of the order of 0.025%, i.e., more than 1000-fold less than the incidence of variant FHR patterns during labor [13,54–56].

However, normal baseline rate, moderate variability, accelerations, and absence of periodic patterns are highly predictive of the absence of fetal acidemia. Absent variability with severe bradycardia, late decelerations (mild or severe), and/or severe variable decelerations are predictive of newborn acidemia. Decreased or minimal variability with pathological patterns may also be predictive of newborn acidemia.

In summary, CP and neonatal seizures are extremely rare events, and variant heart-rate patterns are common. Although there are no specific FHR patterns or group of patterns that reliably predict brain damage, there is a growing literature that suggests a correlation between absent variability with severe periodic decelerations or bradycardia and progressive metabolic acidemia in the fetus. The degree of acidemia that reliably predicts newborn complications is as yet to be defined.

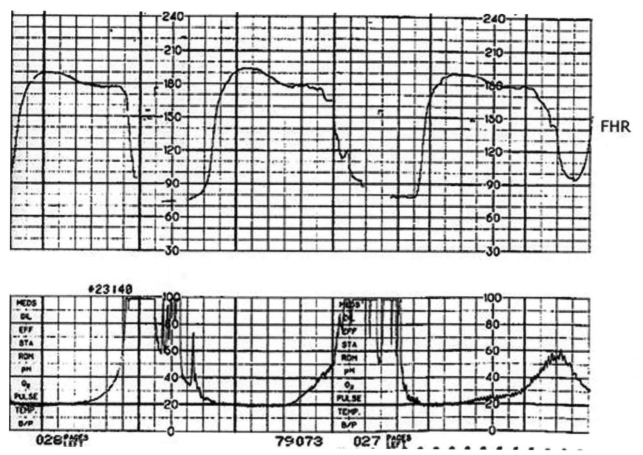

Fig. 15.6. No variability and decelerations. Loss of variability, especially in the presence of other periodic patterns during labor, is the most sensitive indicator of metabolic acidemia in a fetus.

The current recommendations for the use of FHR monitoring during labor by the American College of Obstetricians and Gynecologists (ACOG) are [31]:

(1) The false-positive rate of EFM for predicting adverse outcomes is high.

(2) The use of EFM is associated with an increase in the rate of operative interventions (vacuum, forceps, and cesarean delivery).

(3) The use of EFM does not result in a reduction of CP rates.

(4) The labor of parturients with high-risk conditions should be monitored continuously.

Management of non-reassuring fetal heart rate

In the case of an EFM tracing with decreased or absent variability without spontaneous accelerations, an effort should be made to elicit one. A meta-analysis of 11 studies of intrapartum fetal stimulation noted that four techniques are available to stimulate the fetus: (1) fetal scalp sampling, (2) Allis clamp scalp stimulation, (3) vibroacoustic stimulation, and (4) digital scalp stimulation [57].

Vibroacoustic stimulation and scalp stimulation are the preferred methods to be used since they are less invasive than the other two methods. When there is an acceleration following stimulation, acidosis is unlikely and labor can continue. When a non-reassuring FHR tracing persists and neither spontaneous nor stimulated accelerations are present, a scalp blood sample for the determination of pH or lactate can be considered. Fetal blood sampling from the fetal scalp after adequate dilation of the cervix was developed at about the same time as continuous electronic FHR monitoring, and, in fact, for a time was a competitor to FHR monitoring for primary screening of fetal condition during labor. Later, a combination of the two techniques, with FHR monitoring as the screening tool and fetal blood sampling as a follow-up in cases of uncertainty, was recommended by a number of investigators. Such an approach was utilized with great enthusiasm by tertiary institutions. However, the sensitivity and positive predictive value of a low scalp pH (defined in the study as less than 7.21, because it was the 75th percentile) to predict umbilical arterial pH less than 7 were 36% and 9%, respectively. More importantly, the sensitivity and positive predictive value of a low scalp pH to identify a newborn with HIE were 50% and 3%, respectively [58]. These results made the technique impractical, and it never penetrated to any great extent to community hospitals, where the vast majority of the USA's 4 million births per year are carried out.

Fetal pulse oximetry

In May 2000, the Food and Drug Administration (FDA) granted conditional approval of the OxiFirst Fetal Oxygen Saturation Monitoring System™ for use as an adjunct to EFM [59]. This new technology was designed to improve knowledge of the fetal condition by continuously measuring fetal oxygen saturation in the presence of a non-reassuring FHR pattern. With this technology, a specialized sensor that is positioned against the fetal face is inserted through the dilated cervix after the membranes have ruptured. Once in contact with the fetal skin, the device permits continuous measurement of fetal oxygen saturation during labor [60]. Conditional approval of the device was based primarily on the results of a trial in which 1010 women with labors complicated by non-reassuring FHR patterns were randomly assigned to either EFM alone or EFM plus continuous fetal pulse oximetry [61]. There was a reduction in the rate of cesarean delivery for the indication of a non-reassuring FHR from 10.2% to 4.5% ($p = 0.007$) when fetal oximetry was used. However, the rate of cesarean delivery for the indication of dystocia in the oximetry group more than doubled, and thus there was no overall difference in the rate of cesarean delivery between the two groups. The discrepancy in the effect of the oximeter between the two indications for cesarean delivery was unanticipated and not easily explained. In 2003, the Maternal–Fetal Medicine Network of the NICHD published a randomized controlled multicenter study of more than 5000 women delivering at 14 university hospitals throughout the USA [62]. Knowledge of intrapartum fetal oxygen saturation had no significant effect on the rates of cesarean delivery overall, or specifically for the indications of a non-reassuring FHR or dystocia, nor did it significantly affect infant outcomes. Findings for the subgroup of women with FHR abnormalities before randomization were similar to those for the overall cohort [62]. Currently ACOG does not support the routine use of fetal pulse oximetry in clinical practice [31].

ST-waveform analysis (STAN)

ST-waveform changes in the fetal electrocardiogram (FECG) can provide continuous information during labor about myocardial function, and in particular regarding fetal hypoxia [63]. When the fetal heart utilizes myocardial glycogen by anaerobic metabolism, there is an increase in the T-wave amplitude. An elevation of the ST segment and T wave, quantified by the ratio between T-wave and QRS amplitudes (T/QRS), identifies fetal heart muscle responding to hypoxia by a surge of stress hormones (catecholamines) that leads to utilization of glycogen stored in the heart as an extra source of energy. However, when the heart is not fully capable of responding to stress, ST-segment depression and negative T waves can be observed. The ST waveform of the FECG provides continuous information on the ability of the fetal heart muscle to respond to the stress of labor. The STAN S21™ and S31 (Neoventa Medical, Mölndal, Sweden) saw the full use of digital signal processing with automatic detection of ST changes. It combines visual assessment of FHR tracings with automated analysis of the FECG. STAN uses computerized FECG analysis to detect ST-interval changes that may predict myocardial hypoxia.

In 2001, the first Swedish randomized controlled trial regarding the use of STAN S21 was published [64]. The size of the trial allowed an assessment of outcome related to mode of surveillance among the 351 babies that were admitted to the special-care baby unit. The use of STAN during labor in accordance with fetal heart monitoring reduced neonatal mortality/morbidity as a consequence of adverse events in labor from 1.0% to 0.017% (OR 0.17, 95% CI 0.03–0.78, $p < 0.01$). Moreover, there was a significant reduction of moderate or severe neonatal encephalopathy in term newborns with the use of STAN clinical guidelines from 3.3/1000 to 0.4/1000 (OR 0.12, 95% CI 0.01–0.94, $p < 0.02$). Data from two large randomized controlled trials[65–67], including 6826 cases, have shown that with the support of ST-waveform analysis the number of babies born with cord-artery metabolic acidosis could be reduced from 1.46% to 0.65% (OR 0.44, $p < 0.003$). At the same time, operative delivery for fetal distress rates was reduced from 9.2 to 6.8% (OR 0.72, $p < 0.001$) and the rate of moderate or severe encephalopathy was reduced from 3.3/1000 to 0.5/1000. Thus the use of STAN was shown to reduce the rate of cesarean deliveries for non-reassuring FHR concomitantly with the rate of neonatal encephalopathy.

Currently, more than 200 European hospitals are using the STAN methodology as an adjunct to FHR analysis. It was recently shown that the use of STAN for decision support by trained US clinicians was similar to the level of STAN expert clinicians, suggesting that this system was transportable to the different labor environments found in American hospitals [68].

Current recommendations

Recently, a two-day workshop was convened to update the definition, interpretation, and research guidelines of EFM. Subsequently, a three-tier fetal heart rate interpretation system was published [69]. Category I was strongly predictive of normal fetal acid–base status, and category III reflected abnormalities that required prompt evaluation and therapy. Category II reflected intermediate findings that were not predictive of abnormal fetal acid–base status, but required continued surveillance re-evaluation.

Except for the most extreme situations associated with markedly abnormal fetal heart-rate patterns, there are few, if any, specific FHR patterns that can reliably predict intrapartum asphyxia in the fetus who is acidemic or who is becoming acidemic. The ultimate goal of monitoring would be the detection of problems before the fetus is irreversibly damaged. The future use of STAN combined with FHR monitoring may help us achieve at last the goal of decreasing the rate of neonatal encephalopathy while decreasing the rate of cesarean delivery for presumed fetal distress.

N.B. Sections of this chapter have been adapted from the chapter by Pare and King which was published in 2003, in the third edition of this text.

References

1. Martin JA, Hamilton BE, Sutton PD, *et al.* Births: final data for 2005. *Natl Vital Stat Rep* 2007; **56**: 1–103.

2. Benson RC, Shubeck F, Deutschberger J, *et al.* Fetal heart rate as a predictor of fetal distress: a report from the collaborative project. *Obstet Gynecol* 1968; **32**: 259–66.

3. Banta DH, Thacker SB. Historical controversy in health technology assessment: the case of electronic fetal monitoring. *Obstet Gynecol Surv* 2001; **56**: 707–19.

4. Wenske P. Doctor told to pay $2 million. *Daily Oklahoman* 1981 June 17.

5. Little WJ. On the influence of abnormal parturition, difficult labors, premature birth, and asphyxia neonatorum, on the mental and physical condition of the child, especially in relation to deformities. *Trans Obstet Soc Lond* 1862; **3**: 293–344.

6. Hon EH. The electronic evaluation of the fetal heart rate: preliminary report. *Am J Obstet Gynecol* 1958; **75**: 1215–30.

7. Interview with Dr. Edward Hon. Watching the unborn inside the womb: high-risk mothers and the graph that raises their babies' chances. *Life Magazine* 1969 July 25: 63–5.

8. Quilligan EJ, Paul RH. Fetal monitoring: is it worth it? *Obstet Gynecol* 1975; **45**: 96–100.

9. Yeh SY, Diaz F, Paul RH. Ten-year experience of intrapartum fetal monitoring in Los Angeles County/ University of Southern California Medical Center. *Am J Obstet Gynecol* 1982; **143**: 496–500.

10. Haverkamp AD, Thompson HE, McFee JG, *et al.* The evaluation of continuous fetal heart rate monitoring in high-risk pregnancy. *Am J Obstet Gynecol* 1976; **125**: 310–20.

11. Parer JT. Fetal heart-rate monitoring. *Lancet* 1979; **2**: 632–3.

12. MacDonald D, Grant A, Sheridan-Pereira M, *et al.* The Dublin randomized controlled trial of intrapartum fetal heart rate monitoring. *Am J Obstet Gynecol* 1985; **152**: 524–39.

13. Grant A, O'Brien N, Joy MT, *et al.* Cerebral palsy among children born during the Dublin randomised trial of intrapartum monitoring. *Lancet* 1989; **2**: 1233–6.

14. Thacker SB, Stroup DF, Peterson HB. Efficacy and safety of intrapartum electronic fetal monitoring: an update. *Obstet Gynecol* 1995; **86**: 613–20.

15. Thacker SB, Stroup D, Chang M. Continuous electronic heart rate monitoring for fetal assessment during labor. *Cochrane Database Syst Rev* 2001; (2) CD000063.

16. Nelson KB, Dambrosia JM, Ting TY, *et al.* Uncertain value of electronic fetal monitoring in predicting cerebral palsy. *N Engl J Med* 1996; **334**: 613–18.

17. Larma JD, Silva AM, Holcroft CJ, *et al.* Intrapartum electronic fetal heart rate monitoring and the identification of metabolic acidosis and hypoxic-ischemic encephalopathy. *Am J Obstet Gynecol* 2007; **197**: 301. e1–8.

18. Martin CB, Gingerich B. Uteroplacental physiology. *JOGN Nurs* 1976; **5**: 16–25s.

19. Jepson JH. Factors influencing oxygenation in mother and fetus. *Obstet Gynecol* 1974; **44**: 906–14.

20. Parer JT. *Handbook of Fetal Heart Rate Monitoring*, 2nd edn. Philadelphia, PA: Saunders, 1997.

21. Richardson BS. Fetal adaptive responses to asphyxia. *Clin Perinatol* 1989; **16**: 595–611.

22. Park MI, Hwang JH, Cha KJ, *et al.* Computerized analysis of fetal heart rate parameters by gestational age. *Int J Gynaecol Obstet* 2001; **74**: 157–64.

23. Sadovsky G, Nicolaides KH. Reference ranges for fetal heart rate patterns in normoxaemic nonanaemic fetuses. *Fetal Ther* 1989; **4**: 61–8.

24. Pillai M, James D. The development of fetal heart rate patterns during normal pregnancy. *Obstet Gynecol* 1990; **76**: 812–16.

25. Anderson PA, Glick KL, Killam AP, *et al.* The effect of heart rate on in utero left ventricular output in the fetal sheep. *J Physiol* 1986; **372**: 557–73.

26. Anderson PA, Killam AP, Mainwaring RD, *et al.* In utero right ventricular output in the fetal lamb: the effect of heart rate. *J Physiol* 1987; **387**: 297–316.

27. Rudolph AM, Heymann MA. Control of the foetal circulation. In Comline KS, Cross KW, Dawes GS, *et al.*, eds., *Fetal and Neonatal Physiology: Proceedings of the Barcroft Centenary Symposium.* Cambridge: Cambridge University Press, 1973: 89–111.

28. Hon EH, Quilligan EJ. The classification of fetal heart rate. II. A revised working classification. *Conn Med* 1967; **31**: 779–84.

29. National Institute of Child Health and Human Development Research Planning Workshop. Electronic fetal heart rate monitoring: research guidelines for interpretation. *Am J Obstet Gynecol* 1997; **17**: 1385–90.

30. Vlastos EJ, Tomlinson TM, Bildirici I, *et al.* Fetal heart rate accelerations and the risk of cerebral lesions and poor neurodevelopmental outcome in very low birthweight neonates. *Am J Perinatol* 2007; **24**: 83–8.

31. American College of Obstetricians and Gynecologists. Intrapartum fetal heart rate monitoring. ACOG Practice Bulletin No. 70. *Obstet Gynecol* 2005; **106**: 1453–61.

32. Paul RH, Suidan AK, Yeh S, *et al.* Clinical fetal monitoring. VII. The evaluation and significance of intrapartum baseline FHR variability. *Am J Obstet Gynecol* 1975; **123**: 206–10.

33. Ball RH, Parer JT. The physiologic mechanisms of variable decelerations. *Am J Obstet Gynecol* 1992; **166**: 1683–9.

34. Parer JTP, King T. Whither fetal heart rate monitoring? *Obstet Gynecol Fertil* 1999; **22**: 149–92.

35. Krebs HB, Petres RE, Dunn LJ, *et al.* Intrapartum fetal heart rate monitoring. I. Classification and prognosis of fetal heart rate patterns. *Am J Obstet Gynecol* 1979; **133**: 762–72.

36. Beard RW, Filshie GM, Knight CA, *et al.* The significance of the changes in the continuous fetal heart rate in the first stage of labour. *J Obstet Gynaecol Br Commonw* 1971; **78**: 865–81.

37. Berkus MD, Langer O, Samueloff A, *et al.* Electronic fetal monitoring: what's reassuring? *Acta Obstet Gynecol Scand* 1999; **78**: 15–21.

38. Low JA, Victory R, Derrick EJ. Predictive value of electronic fetal monitoring for intrapartum fetal asphyxia with metabolic acidosis. *Obstet Gynecol* 1999; **93**: 285–91.

39. Tejani N, Mann LI, Bhakthavathsalan A, *et al.* Correlation of fetal heart rate–uterine contraction patterns with fetal scalp blood pH. *Obstet Gynecol* 1975; **46**: 392–6.

40. Low JA, Cox MJ, Karchmar EJ, *et al.* The prediction of intrapartum fetal metabolic acidosis by fetal heart rate

monitoring. *Am J Obstet Gynecol* 1981; **139**: 299–305.

41. Gilstrap LC, Hauth JC, Hankins GD, *et al.* Second-stage fetal heart rate abnormalities and type of neonatal acidemia. *Obstet Gynecol* 1987; **70**: 191–5.

42. Gull I, Jaffa AJ, Oren M, *et al.* Acid accumulation during end-stage bradycardia in term fetuses: how long is too long? *Br J Obstet Gynaecol* 1996; **103**: 1096–101.

43. Dellinger EH, Boehm FH, Crane MM. Electronic fetal heart rate monitoring: early neonatal outcomes associated with normal rate, fetal stress, and fetal distress. *Am J Obstet Gynecol* 2000; **182**: 214–20.

44. Rochard F, Schifrin BS, Goupil F, *et al.* Nonstressed fetal heart rate monitoring in the antepartum period. *Am J Obstet Gynecol* 1976; **126**: 699–706.

45. Parer JT, Livingston EG. What is fetal distress? *Am J Obstet Gynecol* 1990; **162**: 1421–7.

46. Clark SL, Gimovsky ML, Miller FC. The scalp stimulation test: a clinical alternative to fetal scalp blood sampling. *Am J Obstet Gynecol* 1984; **148**: 274–7.

47. Wood C, Ferguson R, Leeton J, *et al.* Fetal heart rate and acid–base status in the assessment of fetal hypoxia. *Am J Obstet Gynecol* 1967; **98**: 62–70.

48. Helfand M, Marton K, Ueland K. Factors involved in the interpretation of fetal monitor tracings. *Am J Obstet Gynecol* 1985; **151**: 737–44.

49. Nielsen PV, Stigsby B, Nickelsen C, *et al.* Intra- and inter-observer variability in the assessment of intrapartum cardiotocograms. *Acta Obstet Gynecol Scand* 1987; **66**: 421–4.

50. Blix E, Sviggum O, Koss KS, *et al.* Inter-observer variation in assessment of 845 labour admission tests: comparison between midwives and obstetricians in the clinical setting and two experts. *BJOG* 2003; **110**: 1–5.

51. Zain HA, Wright JW, Parrish GE, *et al.* Interpreting the fetal heart rate tracing: effect of knowledge of neonatal outcome. *J Reprod Med* 1998; **43**: 367–70.

52. Helwig JT, Parer JT, Kilpatrick SJ, *et al.* Umbilical cord blood acid–base state: what is normal? *Am J Obstet Gynecol* 1996; **174**: 1807–14.

53. Lilien AA. Term intrapartum fetal death. *Am J Obstet Gynecol* 1970; **107**: 595–603.

54. Nelson KB. What proportion of cerebral palsy is related to birth asphyxia? *J Pediatr* 1988; **112**: 572–4.

55. Paneth N, Kiely J. The frequency of cerebral palsy: a review of population studies in industrial nations since 1950. In Stanley FJ, Alberman E, eds., *The Epidemiology of the Cerebral Palsies*. Philadelphia, PA: Lippincott, 1984: 46–56.

56. Shy KK, Luthy DA, Bennett FC, *et al.* Effects of electronic fetal-heart-rate monitoring, as compared with periodic auscultation, on the neurologic development of premature infants. *N Engl J Med* 1990; **322**: 588–93.

57. Skupski DW, Rosenberg CR, Eglinton GS. Intrapartum fetal stimulation tests: a meta-analysis. *Obstet Gynecol* 2002; **99**: 129–34.

58. Goodwin TM, Milner-Masterson L, Paul RH. Elimination of fetal scalp blood sampling on a large clinical service. *Obstet Gynecol* 1994; **83**: 971–4.

59. Yam J, Chua S, Arulkumaran S. *Summary minutes: Meeting of the Obstetrics and Gynecology Devices Advisory Panel, open session*, June 9, 2003. www.fda.gov/ohrms/dockets/ac/03/minutes/3963m1_summary%20minutes.pdf.

60. Yam J, Chua S, Arulkumaran S. Intrapartum fetal pulse oximetry. Part I: Principles and technical issues. *Obstet Gynecol Surv* 2000; **55**: 163–72.

61. Garite TJ, Dildy GA, McNamara H, *et al.* A multicenter controlled trial of fetal pulse oximetry in the intrapartum management of nonreassuring fetal heart rate patterns. *Am J Obstet Gynecol* 2000; **183**: 1049–58.

62. Bloom SL, Spong CY, Thom E, *et al.* Fetal pulse oximetry and cesarean delivery. *N Engl J Med* 2006; **355**: 2195–202.

63. Rosen KG, Amer-Wahlin I, Luzietti R, *et al.* Fetal ECG waveform analysis. *Best Pract Res Clin Obstet Gynaecol* 2004; **18**: 485–514.

64. Amer-Wahlin I, Bordahl P, Eikeland T, *et al.* ST analysis of the fetal electrocardiogram during labor: Nordic observational multicenter study. *J Matern Fetal Neonatal Med* 2002; **12**: 260–6.

65. Amer-Wahlin I, Hellsten C, Noren H, *et al.* Cardiotocography only versus cardiotocography plus ST analysis of fetal electrocardiogram for intrapartum fetal monitoring: a Swedish randomised controlled trial. *Lancet* 2001; **358**: 534–8.

66. Neilson JP. Fetal electrocardiogram (ECG) for fetal monitoring during labour. *Cochrane Database Syst Rev* 2003; (2): CD000116.

67. Westgate J, Harris M, Curnow JS, *et al.* Plymouth randomized trial of cardiotocogram only versus ST waveform plus cardiotocogram for intrapartum monitoring in 2400 cases. *Am J Obstet Gynecol* 1993; **169**: 1151–60.

68. Devoe LD, Ross M, Wilde C, *et al.* United States multicenter clinical usage study of the STAN 21 electronic fetal monitoring system. *Am J Obstet Gynecol* 2006; **195**: 729–34.

69. Macones G, Hankins G, Spong C, *et al.* The 2008 National Institute of Child Health and Human Development workshop report on electronic fetal monitoring: update on definitions, interpretations, and research guidelines. *Obstet Gynecol* 2008; **112**: 661–6.

Clinical manifestations of hypoxic–ischemic encephalopathy

Jin S. Hahn

Introduction

Hypoxic–ischemic encephalopathy (HIE) is a well-recognized clinical syndrome and the most common cause of acute neurological impairment and seizures in the neonatal period [1–5]. Neonatal encephalopathy is a term used to describe newborns with acute neurological syndromes and encephalopathy that may be caused by diverse processes including hypoxia–ischemia, infections, inflammation, trauma, and metabolic disorders. Neonatal encephalopathy due to perinatal asphyxia can lead to neurological sequelae and cerebral palsy, but recent literature has shown that only a small percentage of children with cerebral palsy had intrapartum asphyxia as a possible etiology [6–8]. More emphasis has been placed on antenatal events as having a greater association with cerebral palsy [9]. Although newborns with neonatal encephalopathy may have antenatal risk factors associated with other findings, such as delayed onset of respiration, arterial cord blood pH less than 7.1, and multiorgan failure, the MRI most often shows signs of acute perinatal insult [10]. Therefore, hypoxic–ischemic injury during the perinatal period can lead to a neurological syndrome in the newborn period, i.e., HIE, and subsequent neurological sequelae in the survivors [11]. Recognizing and understanding hypoxic–ischemic encephalopathy are therefore important.

Clinical features and management

The clinical features in the infant with HIE are presented here by first describing a general approach to the evaluation. Then the specific clinical features, diagnostic studies, prognosis, and management of these infants are described.

General evaluation

The initial assessment of the infant with suspected HIE relies on obtaining a thorough history and carrying out a careful physical examination. The history should be directed toward determining whether there were any specific antenatal factors that might account for the disorder. Review of the maternal history, fetal monitoring studies, fetal ultrasonographic findings, and fetal acid–base measurements are essential. Information

regarding examination of the placenta should also be obtained. Special attention should be paid to any possible history of maternal infection and chorioamnionitis.

A general physical examination is required to establish the infant's gestational age, cardiopulmonary status, presence of congenital anomalies, and growth parameters. A carefully performed neurologic examination is essential to obtain information about the infant's current status. This information is used to determine additional evaluations that are critical in establishing a prognosis. Many studies have shown that the neonatal neurologic examination is a valuable predictor of outcome [2,12]. A detailed neurologic examination provides the most information in regard to the localization and severity of the encephalopathy, but a clinical grading of encephalopathy, used in several studies of asphyxiated newborns, should be performed initially [12].

Neurologic assessment in hypoxic–ischemic encephalopathy

If the degree of hypoxic–ischemic insult at or shortly before delivery is of sufficient magnitude to cause long-term neurological sequelae, newborns will manifest signs of neurological dysfunction shortly after birth, often within hours. Conversely, the absence of significant neonatal encephalopathy during the newborn period implies the absence of significant hypoxic–ischemic insult during the intrapartum period.

Neurological dysfunctions due to hypoxic–ischemic insult include altered level of consciousness and reactivity, altered tone, and seizures. There is a correlation between the severity and duration of the hypoxic–ischemic insult and the severity of the encephalopathy. Careful documentation of the neurologic examination and grading of the encephalopathy will help determine the severity of the hypoxic–ischemic insult and ultimate outcome.

Several grading systems have been developed to assess the severity of HIE. One of the more widely used scales is the staging system developed by Sarnat and Sarnat, in which the clinical stages of HIE are divided into three levels [13]. An updated version has been used by the NICHD Neonatal Research Network to identify newborn infants who may be eligible for neuroprotective treatments [14]. The major clinical features that are used in the assessment are the infant's level of consciousness, cranial nerve findings, muscle tone, deep tendon reflexes, neonatal reflexes, spontaneous motor activity,

Fetal and Neonatal Brain Injury, 4th edition, ed. David K. Stevenson, William E. Benitz, Philip Sunshine, Susan R. Hintz, and Maurice L. Druzin. Published by Cambridge University Press. © Cambridge University Press 2009.

Table 16.1. Clinical staging and outcome of hypoxic–ischemic encephalopathy

Severity of encephalopathy	Mild	Moderate	Severe
Level of consciousness	Alert or hyperalert	Lethargy	Stupor or coma
Tone	Normal or hypertonia	Hypotonia (focal or general)	Flaccidity
Tendon reflexes	Increased	Increased	Depressed or absent
Primitive reflexes			
Suck	Weak	Weak to absent	Absent
Moro	Exaggerated	Incomplete	Absent
Autonomic function			
Pupils	Dilated	Constricted	Deviated, dilated or nonreactive to light
Heart Rate	Tachycardia	Bradycardia	Variable
Respiration	Normal	Periodic breathing	Apnea
Others	Irritability, jitteriness	Brainstem dysfunction	± Elevated intracranial pressure
Seizures	Absent	±	Frequent, often refractory to anticonvulsants
EEG background	Normal	Low voltage, periodic or paroxysmal	Periodic or isoelectric
Outcome	Normal	20–40% abnormal	Death or 100% abnormal

Notes:
Based on Sarnat & Sarnat [13], Roland & Hill [4], and Shankaran et al. [14].

and autonomic function (Table 16.1). The degree of encephalopathy is then graded as mild, moderate, or severe.

Infants with a *mild* degree of encephalopathy (stage 1) often have variable levels of consciousness with periods of irritability and "hyperalertness." They often feed poorly, have disturbed sleep–wake cycles with a preponderance of active sleep, and are described as "jittery." Jitteriness is best described as a spontaneous or stimulus-induced myoclonus (non-epileptic). Findings on the cranial nerve examination are normal. Muscle tone is normal or increased and the deep tendon reflexes are hyperactive. The Moro reflex is often exaggerated, but other neonatal reflexes are normal. Pupillary dilation and tachycardia are frequently observed. Mild encephalopathy usually lasts for less than 24 hours and is generally associated with a favorable prognosis [13,15].

Newborn term infants with *moderate* encephalopathy (stage 2) manifest lethargy, hypotonia, hyporeflexia, and seizures [16,17]. Although lethargic, they can be aroused with auditory and tactile stimuli. Feeding is extremely poor. Muscle tone is decreased, with a prominent head lag, a positive scarf sign, and a poor response to the Landau maneuver. Exaggerated deep tendon reflexes with clonus are elicited. Jaw clonus may be observed. Cranial nerve examination reveals a weak suck and decreased gag reflex. Spontaneous motor activity is decreased, and the observed movements may include spontaneous myoclonus or show signs of extrapyramidal dysfunction. Pupils are often constricted, and periodic breathing associated with bradycardia may be present. Seizures may occur and must be differentiated from other abnormal movements and behavior. The duration of moderate encephalopathy is usually 2–14 days. Recovery is heralded by disappearance of myoclonus, increased alertness, and improved suck. Neurologic sequelae occur in approximately 20–40% of infants with moderate encephalopathy, especially if the abnormal neurologic signs persist for over 1 week [16,18].

Infants who are profoundly affected display *severe* encephalopathy (stage 3), characterized by stupor or coma, flaccidity, and unresponsiveness to noxious stimuli [13]. They also have episodic decerebrate (extensor) posturing and poor brainstem function. Deep tendon and neonatal reflexes are absent. The pupils are poorly reactive or fixed, and the oculocephalic reflex and sucking reflex are absent. Seizures are very common. The infant often has bradycardia, systemic hypotension, irregular respirations, periodic breathing, and apnea. The duration of this stage ranges from hours to weeks. Mortality rate is high, and nearly all of the survivors will develop neurologic sequelae [14]. If the infant recovers, a period of extensor hypertonia and brainstem dysfunction (abnormal swallowing, sucking movements) may occur.

Newborns with perinatal asphyxia may transition from one stage to another. Most infants who initially manifest mild encephalopathy also develop moderate encephalopathy before recovering [13]. More severely asphyxiated infants begin in the moderate encephalopathic state shortly after delivery. Often the clinical manifestations of severe encephalopathy may not be apparent until day 2 or 3 after birth, when cerebral edema is at its maximum. Clinically, when severe cerebral edema is present, the anterior fontanel is often bulging or tense and the cranial sutures are splayed.

During the first week, infants with moderate or severe encephalopathy may show signs of neurological improvement. However, abnormalities in tone, bulbar function, hyperactive reflexes, and seizures may persist for days or weeks. If infants remain in moderate or severe encephalopathic states for more than 7 days, there is a high incidence of long-term neurological sequelae [13].

Laboratory evaluations

Laboratory investigations of the asphyxiated infant should include measurements of cord blood gases, arterial blood gas and pH levels, serum electrolyte levels (including calcium and magnesium), and serum glucose, blood urea nitrogen, creatinine levels, and hepatic enzyme levels. Measurements of several other metabolic indicators of the degree of insult can be carried out, including cerebrospinal fluid (CSF) lactate and serum catecholamine levels [19,20]. The abnormalities found in the majority of these parameters reflect the severity of the systemic asphyxial insult rather than the severity of the insult to the brain. A lumbar puncture with measurement of CSF opening pressure, cell count, and protein and glucose level should be performed. Other biochemical indicators of neuronal injury in the CSF include elevated creatine kinase brain isoenzyme (CK-BB) and neuron-specific enolase. However, these tests have not been widely used in the clinical setting.

Electroencephalography

The electroencephalogram (EEG) is a valuable measure of cerebral function that can be performed at the bedside. It complements the clinical examination in establishing the severity of the encephalopathy and in determining the prognosis [21]. The diagnosis of seizures in this age group is dependent on the EEG, since a significant number of abnormal behavior patterns thought to represent seizures actually represent non-epileptic phenomena [3,22]. Furthermore, the clinical seizure type in these infants may often be subtle and fragmentary or masked by anticonvulsant therapy, making the EEG essential for the diagnosis of seizures. The EEG is also helpful in assessing the degree of cerebral dysfunction and providing information about neurological prognosis. Severely depressed backgrounds, such as suppression-burst pattern or isoelectric pattern, indicate severe cerebral dysfunction and usually portend a poor prognosis. The presence of status epilepticus on the EEG also carries an unfavorable prognosis. EEG patterns with less severe background disturbance that revert to normal after the first week usually indicate a more favorable prognosis. The application of EEG in the evaluation of the encephalopathic newborn is described in detail in Chapter 17.

Other neurophysiologic measures of nervous system function, such as somatosensory, brainstem, and visual evoked responses, have been applied in the past to evaluating the asphyxiated newborn, but are not routinely used as part of the acute evaluation [23–26]. Continuous amplitude-integrated EEG has been used to monitor neonates with HIE. This method, which simplifies bedside interpretation of the EEG background, can be useful for identifying infants with more severe encephalopathy and worse outcomes [27].

Neuroimaging studies

Neuroimaging studies are an essential component of the assessment of the newborn with HIE. It is helpful for determining the nature, severity, and extent of the hypoxic–ischemic brain injury.

Cranial ultrasonography has proven to be a valuable technique in the diagnosis of intraventricular hemorrhage (IVH) and periventricular leukomalacia (PVL). This study can be readily carried out at the bedside in newborns. However, since IVH and PVL tend to affect premature infants primarily, it may not be as useful in term infants with hypoxic–ischemic insults.

Computed tomography (CT) is widely used to assess the nature and extent of cerebral injury, especially in term infants. It is more useful in assessing cortical and hemorrhagic injury. It can be obtained rapidly, often without need for sedation. CT scans in asphyxiated newborns may show focal or multifocal areas of decreased attenuation in the cerebral gray or white matter. These abnormal areas likely represent areas of ischemia or cerebral edema. Diffuse cerebral edema can manifest as loss of gray–white matter differentiation, effacement of sulcal spaces, and slit-like ventricles. CT is also useful for detecting acute intracranial hemorrhage.

Magnetic resonance imaging (MRI) has become the method of choice to assess the newborn brain. MRI has been used to document in the neonate various clinicopathologic syndromes of hypoxic–ischemic brain injury, including basal ganglia injury, parasagittal cerebral injury, PVL, focal ischemic lesions, and selective neuronal necrosis [28–30]. Diffusion-weighted MRI and magnetic resonance spectroscopy have also been used to assess the extent of cerebral injury and to provide prognostic information [31,32]. The disadvantages of MRI include the prolonged scanning time and impaired ability to monitor the mechanically ventilated sick newborns. The use of newer MRI-compatible incubators and monitors may facilitate obtaining MRI studies. Further details on neuroimaging studies in the newborn are available in Chapter 18.

Patterns of injury and clinical syndromes

The cerebral injury from perinatal asphyxia results in specific patterns of regional injury, the topography of which is maturation-dependent. This regional vulnerability is caused in part by dysregulation of cellular processes that are critical for normal brain development. For example, the increased density of glutamate receptors normally present in the rapidly developing brain regions (e.g., the basal ganglia) renders these areas exquisitely sensitive to hypoxic–ischemic insults. The specific type of lesion also varies with the characteristics of the primary insult and the subsequent management. Recent neuroimaging studies with MRI have correlated the specific patterns of neuroradiologic alterations with the specific clinicopathologic syndromes. Recognition of these disorders provides an understanding of the mechanisms leading to their development and allows prediction of possible neurologic disabilities. The neuropathologic changes can be divided into lesions that are the result of primary damage to specific types of cells and structures and those due to hemorrhage.

The pathologic changes observed in the term infant are different from those seen in the premature infant (Table 16.2).

Table 16.2. Patterns of injury in neonatal hypoxic–ischemic encephalopathy

Full-term newborn	Preterm newborn
Parasagittal border-zone "watershed" lesions	Intraventricular or periventricular hemorrhage
Necrosis of deep gray nuclei	Periventricular leukomalacia
Basal ganglia	
Thalamus	
Diencephalon	
Perirolandic gyri and posterior limb of internal capsule	
Brainstem necrosis	
Selective nuclei	
Diffuse cerebral edema	
Focal brain injury	
Arterial occlusion	
Venous occlusion	

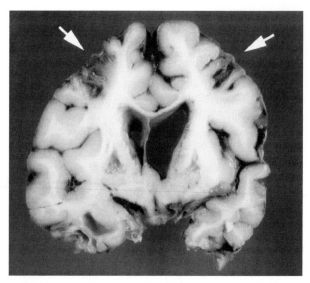

Fig. 16.1. Coronal section of a 13-year-old boy who had spastic quadriplegia and mental retardation as a result of perinatal brain injury shows bilateral parasagittal (border-zone) atrophy and necrosis (arrows). The cortex in these regions shows thinning (ulegyria) and laminar necrosis that are consistent with remote anoxic/ischemic injury.

The term infant most commonly is observed to have neuropathologic changes involving primarily the gray matter and specific neuroanatomic structures in both the cortical and subcortical regions. IVH occurs in the term infant, but the pathogenic mechanisms are different from those in the preterm infant. On the contrary, periventricular or intraventricular hemorrhage is the most common neuropathologic finding in the premature infant. Pathologic changes in the white matter are the next most common disorder, followed by lesions involving selected neuronal populations.

The patterns of brain injury observed in the term newborn can be categorized into lesions involving four major areas of the central nervous system: the cortex, deep gray matter nuclei, brainstem, and cerebellum. There is often an overlap of these pathologic processes, but primary involvement of one of these regions results in specific clinical characteristics both acutely and over the long term. The clinicopathologic correlates of the major types of hypoxic–ischemic brain injury are presented here.

Parasagittal border-zone injury

This form of cortical injury resulting from a general decrease in the cerebral blood flow (ischemia) is referred to as the *watershed* infarction, since the disorder involves the border zones of the three major arterial supply zones. The injury is bilateral, and usually symmetrical. *Ulegyria*, a term describing cortical gyri that are atrophic, particularly at the depth of sulci, is the chronic lesion resulting from this particular brain injury (Fig. 16.1). In one autopsy series of neurologically handicapped children 30 of 153 subjects had this lesion in the parasagittal watershed region [33]. This type of injury most often affects the term infant and appears to be due to mild-to-moderate hypotension in the peripartum period [30]. The hypotension leads to subacute, *partial hypoxic–ischemic* injury that primarily involves the vascular border zones. More prolonged partial hypoxic–ischemic injury may lead to a more

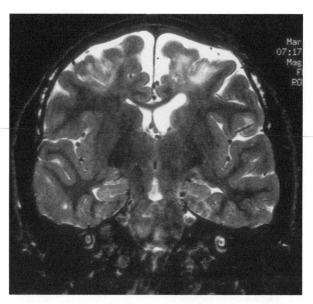

Fig. 16.2. Coronal T2-weighted MRI (TE 93/Ef, TR6000) of a 12-year-old girl who had a history of neonatal hypoxic–ischemic encephalopathy and seizures shows bilateral parasagittal signal hyperintensities consistent with border-zone ischemia.

diffuse neuronal necrosis, with relative sparing of the deep gray matter.

Cortical infarcts in the watershed regions are difficult to diagnose in the neonatal period. This is most likely because CT and ultrasound techniques do not visualize this region well. Radioisotope studies and positron emission tomography have identified infants with decreased cerebral blood flow in the parasagittal cortex [34,35]. MRI is useful in identifying these infants earlier in the course, especially when coronal images are obtained (Fig. 16.2).

Newborns with parasagittal injury often have a moderate encephalopathy in the neonatal period and may show evidence of weakness of the shoulder girdles and the proximal extremities. Seizures can be observed, especially in more severely affected infants. The neurologic sequelae often include a spastic quadriparesis with varying degrees of intellectual impairment. The topographic localization (i.e., preferential injury to the parietal, posterior temporal, and occipital cortices) may account for the frequent occurrence of language and visuospatial disabilities.

Selective injury

Deep gray nuclei

Lesions in the deep gray nuclei (thalamus and basal ganglia) have been described for more than a century in children with presumed birth injury who exhibited choreoathetosis and dystonia [36]. Infants with this pathologic lesion have been identified in the neonatal period by neuroimaging studies (Fig. 16.3) [37].

Acute near-total asphyxia can lead to specific symmetric lesions in the putamen and the thalamus with sparing of the globus pallidus [38]. The posterior putamen and lateral thalami are more affected. The mechanism for this pattern appears to be due to impairment of energy substrates that selectively

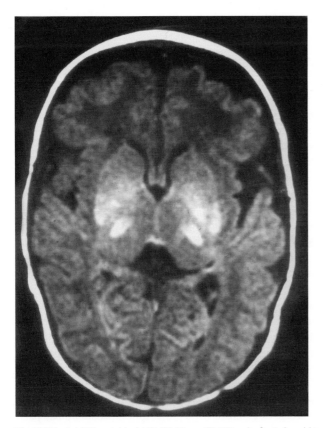

Fig. 16.3. Axial T1-weighted MRI (TE 16 ms, TR 600 ms) of a 7-day-old term infant who had an unexplained cardiorespiratory arrest at 12 hours of age shows bilateral, symmetric areas of high signal intensity in the basal ganglia and thalami. These areas were low in signal intensity on T2-weighted images. At 1 year of age this child manifested hypotonia, ataxia, and bulbar dysfunction.

damage areas with higher metabolic requirements [30]. This type of injury may occur in the setting of severe umbilical cord prolapse, uterine rupture, or severe placental abruption. Affected newborns often manifest evidence of brainstem dysfunction, such as facial diplegia and abnormal eye movements due to concomitant brainstem injury (see below). Children with this type of injury later often develop extrapyramidal cerebral palsy manifested by dystonia, rigidity, axial hypotonia, dysphagia, and abnormal vocalization.

Early in the course there is often hemorrhage and infarction in these structures on neuropathology. Eventually cystic changes develop, particularly in the neostriatum. The neurons and penetrating vessels become calcified. The basal ganglia and thalamus develop a chronic pathologic lesion termed *status marmoratus*. This lesion, characterized by neuronal loss, gliosis, and hypermyelination, was observed in 173 of 198 cases of presumed perinatal birth injury in one report [39]. The lesions are probably the result of both impairment of blood flow through the deep penetrating arteries and the high level of metabolic activity of this structure. These children usually have a poor long-term outcome. Infants with status marmoratus of the basal ganglia develop choreoathetosis, dystonia, tremor, and intellectual deficits. The movement disorder has a delayed onset and may deteriorate over a period of 1–2 years.

In infants that manifest injury to the basal ganglia and thalamus, there is often concomitant injury to the corticospinal tract and hippocampi. Abnormal MR signals are often seen in the posterior limbs of the internal capsules bilaterally. The perirolandic cortex is also often affected, resulting in abnormal MR signal and loss of gray–white differentiation in the perirolandic gyri.

Brainstem

Pathologic changes of the brainstem are rarely isolated, and other structures, especially the thalamus, are also involved. Brainstem injury usually occurs in the setting of acute hypotension [40]. Selective necrosis of specific brainstem nuclei has been observed, and the nuclei adjacent to the floor of the fourth ventricle are more often affected. These nuclei include the inferior colliculi, fifth and seventh cranial nerve nuclei, and nucleus ambiguus (ninth and tenth cranial nerves). An MRI pattern involving the dorsomesencephalic structure has been recognized but appears to occur relatively infrequently [30].

Cerebellum

The cerebellum is especially vulnerable to hypoxic–ischemic insult, and the Purkinje cells are the most vulnerable type of cell. The cerebellum is often affected by bilateral lesions at the boundaries of the superior and inferior cerebellar arterial zones or by lesions of the foliar cortex. White-matter edema and small hemorrhages accompany the neuronal loss. Chronic lesions are referred to as cerebellar sclerosis. In this condition there is a loss of Purkinje cells and an increase in Bergmann's astrocytes. The folia are narrowed and there is an increased space between them.

Cerebellar involvement is often observed concurrently with deep gray nuclei and brainstem lesions. Impairment of the posterior circulation due to hyperextension of the neck at the time of delivery has been suggested as being a factor in the pathogenesis of this lesion [41]. Hypotonia and ataxia are observed as sequelae of cerebellar involvement. Intellectual impairment is common and may be severe.

Infants with disease involving the deep gray matter nuclei, brainstem, and cerebellum usually have moderate to severe encephalopathy in the neonatal period. A history of an acute process that causes near-total asphyxia, such as severe umbilical cord prolapse, uterine rupture, or significant placental abruption, is often found. Acutely, bifacial weakness, gaze abnormalities, and tongue fasciculations have been described in an infant with brainstem involvement due to "acute" near-total asphyxia [42–44]. Infants with more extensive brainstem involvement may require prolonged ventilatory support. Infants with brainstem involvement have bulbar dysfunction associated with poor feeding, failure to thrive, and recurrent aspiration. Interestingly, in this pattern of injury there may be complete or relative sparing of the cortex and white matter. Also, since the hypoxic–ischemic insult occurs acutely, there is little time for shunting of blood away from extracerebral organs. Hence there is less evidence of multiorgan dysfunction.

Although there seems to be different topographic distribution of injury caused by hypotension (parasagittal border-zone injury) and acute near-total asphyxia (deep gray nuclei and brainstem), there is often an overlap between the two pathophysiologic syndromes. Furthermore, when the nature of the hypoxic–ischemic injury is severe and prolonged, diffuse injury to the brain occurs. This manifests in the first few days as diffuse cytotoxic edema on MRI in addition to the thalamic and basal ganglia injury [30]. Neurologic examination reveals encephalopathy, brainstem dysfunction, flaccid quadriparesis, and respiration abnormalities. The majority of infants require mechanical ventilation. As the encephalopathy evolves, the infants are described as having clinical seizures, the brainstem signs persist, and temperature instability may be observed. The injured areas will evolve into multicystic encephalomalacia.

Focal brain injury

Cortical injury may result from occlusion of an artery (i.e., ischemic stroke) resulting in necrosis of all cellular elements in the distribution of a single vessel. Arterial occlusions occur most often in the term infant and have been observed in 5–9% of autopsy series [45,46]. The middle cerebral artery is most frequently involved. Most are thought to be due to embolic or thrombotic processes. Although the actual etiology is infrequently found, coagulopathy, congenital heart disease, and trauma are common associated disorders. As the infarction evolves, there is dissolution of brain parenchyma and formation of a cavity (porencephalic cyst). If multiple vessels are involved, multicystic encephalomalacia or hydranencephaly may result.

Infants with neonatal strokes often present with early-onset seizures with absence or only a mild degree of encephalopathy [47,48]. Neonatal strokes are the second most common cause of seizures in the newborn period after global hypoxic–ischemic insult, and often occur in the absence of intrapartum difficulties [10]. Focal clonic seizures are often exhibited, and these seizures can be readily diagnosed by clinical criteria [3]. Focal findings may be noted on neurologic examination, but are often subtle. The EEG usually demonstrates lateralized abnormalities and allows assessment of the severity of the encephalopathy in other cortical regions. CT and MRI show a wedge-shaped area of abnormal signal that is in the distribution of a single artery. Diffusion-weighted MRI provides a sensitive way of detecting infarcts early in the course.

Infants may develop spastic hemiparesis as a long-term sequela. Because of the frequent involvement of the middle cerebral artery distribution, the upper extremities are more impaired. The extent and location of the pathologic lesion are important factors in determining whether intellectual impairment and epilepsy will also develop [49].

Focal cerebral injury may also occur with venous occlusions. Venous occlusions often involve the sinuses or major veins, leading to superficial cortical infarcts, which are frequently hemorrhagic. MRI has been particularly useful for diagnosing venous sinus thrombosis and focal injury due to venous occlusions [50]. Venous sinus thrombosis may also cause secondary intraventricular (choroid plexus) hemorrhages in the term newborn. A more severe encephalopathy is noted with venous occlusion because of frequently associated hemorrhage. Seizures are also common [50,51].

White-matter injury

Preterm infants have a predilection for white-matter injury as a result of hypoxic–ischemic insult. *Periventricular leukomalacia* (PVL) is the term frequently used to describe this disorder, which is characterized by necrosis of the white matter and may include hemorrhage [52]. The lesion is readily identified by ultrasonography, and prospective studies have determined that the incidence is 4–26% in low-birthweight infants [53–55]. Grossly, the acute lesions are characterized by white or white-yellow spots in the periventricular white matter, which occasionally show hemorrhagic infiltration. Microscopically, focal coagulative necrosis is observed. Petechial hemorrhages may also be seen within these lesions. These areas often develop into cystic lesions and later contract into gliotic scars (Fig. 16.4). The lesions are observed most frequently in the corona radiata, occipital and temporal horns of the lateral ventricles, and just anterior to the anterior horn of the lateral ventricles. In the term infant the lesions are usually hemorrhagic and are associated with a coagulopathy or congenital heart disease.

The clinical characteristics of infants with PVL include decreased tone in the lower extremities associated with increased neck extensor tone [56]. Apnea, pseudobulbar palsy with poor feeding, and irritability have been described. Clinical seizures without electroencephalographic confirmation have been reported in 10–30% of the infants. The diagnosis of PVL can be made by ultrasonography, but MRI in later

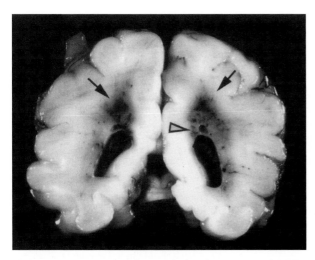

Fig. 16.4. Coronal section of a 1-week-old infant (gestational age 34 weeks) shows periventricular leukomalacia with bilateral areas of congestion and hemorrhage (arrows) in the white matter and a periventricular cyst (arrowhead). The pregnancy was complicated by non-immune hydrops, and an ultrasound study on the first day after birth revealed extensive bilateral periventricular cysts.

infancy better defines the extent of the disease and the associated abnormalities of myelination [57]. Spastic diplegia with varying degrees of intellectual impairment, especially visual–motor dysfunction, is the usual sequela.

Periventricular/intraventricular hemorrhages

Periventricular or intraventricular hemorrhage is the most common neuropathologic change observed in the premature infant. It is observed in 31–43% of low-birthweight infants in prospective neuroimaging studies [58,59]. The hemorrhage arises from the germinal matrix at the ventromedial angle of the lateral ventricle. Cerebral hypoxic ischemia leads to impaired autoregulation of cerebral blood flow and injury to the germinal matrix and capillary endothelium, which have a

high level of oxidative metabolism. Changes in the systemic blood pressure, platelet and coagulation disturbances, and increased cerebral venous pressure also contribute to the pathogenesis of this lesion.

The pathologic findings include subarachnoid hemorrhage with blood in the basal and pontine cisterns and cisterna magna. The hemorrhage may range from a small area of bleeding in the subependymal matrix zone to massive distension of the ventricular system associated with extension of blood into the centrum semiovale. Hydrocephalus may be a complication in infants with this disorder. The hydrocephalus is often secondary to an obstruction at the aqueduct or the foramina exiting from the fourth ventricle, or it may be due to impairment of reabsorption of cerebrospinal fluid over the convexities.

IVH in the term infant often arises from the choroid plexus, and trauma, venous thrombosis, and hypoxia are thought to be important pathogenic factors [60,61]. In 25% of term infants with this disorder there is no identifiable cause for the hemorrhage [61].

Periventricular or intraventricular hemorrhages are often clinically silent in the preterm neonate. Severe hemorrhage may present with an acute syndrome, characterized by rapid deterioration of the level of consciousness, brainstem dysfunction, decerebrate posturing, and tonic seizures. A subacute presentation is more common, with intermittent neurologic symptoms superimposed on slowly progressive encephalopathy. The newborn may have episodes of abnormal eye movements, hypotonia, and decreased spontaneous motor activity. A fall in the hematocrit level is often an important sign. Ultrasonography is usually diagnostic and can be done serially at the bedside.

The prognosis is extremely variable, and many infants have no sequelae. The prognosis is most closely correlated with the degree of parenchymal involvement rather than the extent of the hemorrhage.

References

1. Finer NN, Robertson CM, Peters KL, *et al.* Factors affecting outcome in hypoxic–ischemic encephalopathy in term infants. *Am J Dis Child* 1983; **137**: 21–5.

2. Finer NN, Robertson CM, Richards RT, *et al.* Hypoxic–ischemic encephalopathy in term neonates: perinatal factors and outcome. *J Pediatr* 1981; **98**: 112–17.

3. Mizrahi EM, Kellaway P. Characterization and classification of neonatal seizures. *Neurology* 1987; **37**: 1837–44.

4. Roland EH, Hill A. Clinical aspects of perinatal hypoxic–ischemic brain injury. *Semin Pediatr Neurol* 1995; **2**: 57–71.

5. Vannucci R. Hypoxic–ischemic encephalopathy. *Am J Perinatol* 2000; **17**: 113–20.

6. Blair E, Stanley FJ. Intrapartum asphyxia: a rare cause of cerebral palsy. *J Pediatr* 1988; **112**: 515–19.

7. Nelson KB, Ellenberg JH. Antecedents of cerebral palsy: multivariate analysis of risk. *N Engl J Med* 1986; **315**: 81–6.

8. Nelson KB. What proportion of cerebral palsy is related to birth asphyxia? *J Pediatr* 1988; **112**: 572–4.

9. Naeye RL, Peters EC. Antenatal hypoxia and low IQ values. *Am J Dis Child* 1987; **141**: 50–4.

10. Cowan F, Rutherford M, Groenendaal F, *et al.* Origin and timing of brain lesions in term infants with neonatal encephalopathy. *Lancet* 2003; **361**: 736–42.

11. Allan WC, Riviello JJ. Perinatal cerebrovascular disease in the neonate. *Pediatr Clin North Am* 1992; **39**: 621–50.

12. Levene MI, Grindulis H, Sands C, *et al.* Comparison of two methods of predicting outcome in perinatal asphyxia. *Lancet* 1986; **1**: 67–9.

13. Sarnat HB, Sarnat MS. Neonatal encephalopathy following fetal distress: a clinical and electroencephalographic study. *Arch Neurol* 1976; **33**: 696–705.

14. Shankaran S, Laptook AR, Ehrenkranz RA, *et al.* Whole-body hypothermia for neonates with hypoxic–ischemic encephalopathy. *N Engl J Med* 2005; **353**: 1574–84.

15. Hill A, Volpe JJ. Perinatal asphyxia: clinical aspects. *Clin Perinatol* 1989; **16**: 435–57.

16. Robertson C, Finer N. Term infants with hypoxic–ischemic encephalopathy: outcome at 3.5 years. *Dev Med Child Neurol* 1985; **27**: 473–84.

17. Ishikawa T, Ogawa Y, Kanayama M, *et al.* Long-term prognosis of asphyxiated full-term neonates with CNS complications. *Brain Dev* 1987; **9**: 48–53.

18. Hill A. Current concepts of hypoxic–ischemic cerebral injury in the term newborn. *Pediatr Neurol* 1991; **7**: 317–25.

19. Fernandez F, Verdu A, Quero J, *et al.* Cerebrospinal fluid lactate levels in term infants with perinatal hypoxia. *Pediatr Neurol* 1986; **2**: 39–42.

20. Nylund L, Dahlin I, Lagercrantz H. Fetal catecholamines and the Apgar score. *J Perinat Med* 1987; **15**: 340–4.

21. Takeuchi T, Watanabe K. The EEG evolution and neurological prognosis of neonates with perinatal hypoxia. *Brain Dev* 1989; **11**: 115–20.

22. Scher MS, Painter MJ, Bergman I, *et al.* EEG diagnosis of neonatal seizures: clinical correlations and outcome. *Pediatr Neurol* 1989; **5**: 17–24.

23. Majnemer A, Rosenblatt B, Riley P, *et al.* Somatosensory evoked response abnormalities in high-risk newborns. *Pediatr Neurol* 1987; **3**: 350–5.

24. Majnemer A, Rosenblatt B, Riley PS. Prognostic significance of multimodality evoked response testing in high-risk newborns. *Pediatr Neurol* 1990; **6**: 367–74.

25. Stockard JE, Stockard JJ, Kleinberg F, *et al.* Prognostic value of brainstem auditory evoked responses in neonates. *Arch Neurol* 1983; **40**: 360–5.

26. Whyte HE, Taylor MJ, Menzies R, *et al.* Prognostic utility of visual evoked potentials in term asphyxiated neonates. *Pediatr Neurol* 1986; **2**: 220–3.

27. Toet MC, Hellström-Westas L, Groenendaal F, *et al.* Amplitude integrated EEG 3 and 6 hours after birth in full term neonates with hypoxic-ischemic encephalopathy. *Arch Dis Child Fetal Neonatal Ed* 1999; **81**: F19–23.

28. Kuenzle C, Baenziger O, Martin E, *et al.* Prognostic value of early MR imaging in term infants with severe perinatal asphyxia. *Neuropediatrics* 1994; **25**: 191–200.

29. Baenziger O, Martin E, Steinlin M, *et al.* Early pattern recognition in severe perinatal asphyxia: a prospective MRI study. *Neuroradiology* 1993; **35**: 437–42.

30. Triulzi F, Parazzini C, Righini A. Patterns of damage in the mature neonatal brain. *Pediatr Radiol* 2006; **36**: 608–20.

31. Hüppi PS, Murphy B, Maier SE, *et al.* Microstructural brain development after perinatal cerebral white matter injury assessed by diffusion tensor magnetic resonance imaging. *Pediatrics* 2001; **107**: 455–60.

32. Robertson RL, Ben-Sira L, Barnes PD, *et al.* MR line-scan diffusion-weighted imaging of term neonates with perinatal brain ischemia. *Am J Neuroradiol* 1999; **20**: 658–70.

33. Myer JE. Uber die Lokalisation frühkindlicher Hirnshäden in arteriellen Grenzgebieten. *Arch Psychiatr Zeitschr Neurol* 1953; **190**: 328–41.

34. Volpe JJ, Herscovitch P, Perlman JM, *et al.* Positron emission tomography in the asphyxiated term newborn: parasagittal impairment of cerebral blood flow. *Ann Neurol* 1985; **17**: 287–96.

35. Volpe JJ, Pasternak JF. Parasagittal cerebral injury in neonatal hypoxic–ischemic encephalopathy: clinical and neuroradiological features. *J Pediatr* 1979; **91**: 472–6.

36. Friede RL. *Developmental Neuropathology*, 2nd edn. New York, NY: Springer-Verlag, 1989.

37. Voit T, Lemburg P, Neuen E, *et al.* Damage of thalamus and basal ganglia in asphyxiated full-term neonates. *Neuropediatrics* 1987; **18**: 176–81.

38. Johnston MV, Hoon AH. Possible mechanisms in infants for selective basal ganglia damage from asphyxia, kernicterus, or mitochondrial encephalopathies. *J Child Neurol* 2000; **15**: 588–91.

39. Malamud N, Hirano A. *Atlas of Neuropathology*, 2nd edn. Berkeley, CA: University of California Press, 1974.

40. Gilles FH. Hypotensive brain stem necrosis: selective symmetrical necrosis of tegmental neuronal aggregates following cardiac arrest. *Arch Pathol* 1969; **88**: 32–41.

41. Rorke LB. *Pathology of Perinatal Brain Injury*. New York, NY: Raven Press, 1982.

42. Roland EH, Hill A, Norman MG, *et al.* Selective brainstem injury in an asphyxiated newborn. *Ann Neurol* 1988; **23**: 89–92.

43. Pasternak JF, Gorey MT. The syndrome of acute near-total intrauterine asphyxia in the term infant. *Pediatr Neurol* 1998; **18**: 391–8.

44. Natsume J, Watanabe K, Kuno K, *et al.* Clinical, neurophysiologic, and neuropathological features of an infant with brain damage of total asphyxia type (Myers). *Pediatr Neurol* 1995; **13**: 61–4.

45. Barmada MA, Moossy J, Shuman RM. Cerebral infarcts with arterial occlusion in neonates. *Ann Neurol* 1979; **6**: 495–502.

46. Banker BQ. Cerebral vascular disease in infancy and childhood. I. Occlusive vascular disease. *J Neuropathol Exp Neurol* 1961; **20**: 127–40.

47. Clancy R, Malin S, Laraque D, *et al.* Focal motor seizures heralding stroke in full-term neonates. *Am J Dis Child* 1985; **139**: 601–6.

48. Koelfen W, Freund M, Varnholt V. Neonatal stroke involving the middle cerebral artery in term infants: clinical presentation, EEG and imaging studies, and outcome. *Dev Med Child Neurol* 1995; **37**: 204–12.

49. Levine SC, Huttenlocher P, Banich MT, *et al.* Factors affecting cognitive function of hemiplegic children. *Dev Med Child Neurol* 1987; **29**: 27–35.

50. Rivkin MJ, Anderson ML, Kaye EM. Neonatal idiopathic cerebral venous thrombosis: an unrecognized cause of transient seizures or lethargy. *Ann Neurol* 1992; **32**: 51–6.

51. Wong VK, LeMesurier J, Franceschini R, *et al.* Cerebral venous thrombosis as a cause of neonatal seizures. *Pediatr Neurol* 1987; **3**: 235–7.

52. Banker BQ, Larroche JC. Periventricular leukomalacia of infancy. *Arch Neurol* 1962; **7**: 386–410.

53. Guzzetta F, Shackleford GD, Volpe S, *et al.* Periventricular intraparenchymal echodensities in the premature newborn: critical determination of neurologic outcome. *Pediatrics* 1986; **78**: 995–1006.

54. Fawer CL, Calame A, Perentes E, *et al.* Periventricular leukomalacia: a correlation study between real-time ultrasound and autopsy findings. *Neuroradiology* 1985; **27**: 292–300.

55. Trounce JQ, Rutter N, Levene MI. Periventricular leucomalacia and intraventricular haemorrhage in the preterm neonate. *Arch Dis Child* 1986; **16**: 1196–202.

56. Trounce JQ, Shaw DE, Leverne MI, *et al.* Clinical risk factors and periventricular

leucomalacia. *Arch Dis Child* 1988; **63**: 17–22.

57. De Vries LS, Connell JA, Dubowitz LMS, *et al.* Neurological, electrophysiological and MRI abnormalities in infants with extensive cystic leukomalacia. *Neuropediatrics* 1987; **18**: 61–6.

58. Dolfin T, Skidmore MB, Fong KW, *et al.* Incidence, severity, and timing of subependymal and intraventricula hemorrhages in preterm infants born in a perinatal unit as detected by serial real-time ultrasound. *Pediatrics* 1983; **71**: 541–6.

59. Enzmann D, Murphy-Irwin K, Stevenson D, *et al.* The natural history of subependymal germinal matrix hemorrhage. *Am J Perinatol* 1985; **2**: 123–33.

60. Scher MS, Wright FS, Lockman LA, *et al.* Intraventricular haemorrhage in the full-term neonate. *Arch Neurol* 1982; **39**: 769–72.

61. Volpe JJ. Intracranial hemorrhage: subdural, primary subarachnoid, intracerebellar, intraventricular (term infant), and miscellaneous. In *Neurology of the Newborn*, 4th edn. Philadelphia, PA: Saunders. 2001: 397–427.

The use of EEG in assessing acute and chronic brain damage in the newborn

Donald M. Olson and Alexis S. Davis

Introduction

The goal of this chapter is to help the reader understand the fundamentals of neonatal electroencephalography (EEG), including the source of EEG signals and the technical aspects of a well-performed EEG. Particular attention will be paid to (1) maturational features which correlate with the infant's conceptional age, (2) abnormal findings indicative of encephalopathies of various causes, and (3) the value of the EEG in determining the prognosis for normal and abnormal neurological outcome. The role of EEG in neonatal seizures is covered more thoroughly in Chapter 43.

Value of the EEG

The EEG is a valuable tool for assessing neonatal brain function. It has unique properties compared to many other diagnostic tests of brain function. It can resolve temporal aspects of brain function more effectively than computed tomography (CT), magnetic resonance imaging (MRI), or even the bedside neurological examination. There is no other test that can so precisely discriminate between epileptic seizures and non-epileptic events in the neonate. It provides information about the severity of brain dysfunction (encephalopathy). Serial EEGs provide information about the course and effectiveness of treatment. Sometimes the EEG helps distinguish between various etiologies of encephalopathy.

Indication for EEG

An EEG in the neonate should be considered when questions arise regarding the cause of a child's abnormal neurological responses. There are many scenarios in which the EEG provides much-needed information that is otherwise difficult or impossible to obtain. For example, it is difficult to perform an adequate bedside neurological assessment of a neonate paralyzed due to neuromuscular blocking agents or an infant who is deeply sedated. The degree of neurological dysfunction may be assessed by means of the EEG. Some very ill infants would benefit from neuroimaging studies, but such studies can be challenging because of instability of the infant or the difficulty of moving an intubated and ventilated baby between the

Fetal and Neonatal Brain Injury, 4th edition, ed. David K. Stevenson, William E. Benitz, Philip Sunshine, Susan R. Hintz, and Maurice L. Druzin. Published by Cambridge University Press. © Cambridge University Press 2009.

neonatal intensive care unit (NICU) and the radiology suite. Since the EEG is performed at the bedside, it can be helpful in these situations.

Another setting where the EEG is particularly valuable is when there is a question about seizures. In the case of the paralyzed or sedated infant, sudden and transient changes in vital signs may raise the suspicion of seizures though no obvious seizure-like movements are observed. The EEG is the only means of determining if frequent subtle (or "subclinical") seizures are present [1]. Even in non-paralyzed newborns, it is often difficult to distinguish neonatal seizures from other non-epileptic clinical behavior. Therefore, the EEG is helpful in most neonates who are having abnormal paroxysmal behaviors.

Timing of the EEG

An EEG should be obtained early in the course of an infant at risk for encephalopathy or seizures. It provides a starting point for later reference. If obtained when the baby is initially recognized as being neurologically "at risk," the EEG provides some prognostic information and can suggest the timing of the brain insult [2–5]. However, an EEG obtained within hours of an acute insult such as hypoxia or hypotension may only be transiently abnormal. Hence, serial EEGs are often of benefit.

Serial EEGs are valuable when prior EEGs show evidence of a severe encephalopathy, since persistence or improvement in the EEG findings has prognostic value and may provide evidence of the success (or failure) of various treatments [6]. Serial EEGs are also useful when previous recordings have identified frequent seizures and the treating physician needs to know whether the treatment has been adequate.

Technical considerations
General description

The EEG measures the "potential difference" (voltage) between areas on the baby's scalp. The electrical activity measured consists of the summed membrane potentials caused by many synapses on cortical neurons, not the individual neuronal action potentials [7]. The activity recorded originates mainly from the cerebral cortex, particularly that close to the skull. However, some deeper centers act as pacemakers and cause changes in the EEG in various states of sleep and arousal. Scalp EEG abnormalities are sometimes strongly correlated with underlying pathology in deeper structures [8–12]. Other clinical neurophysiology tests directly measure neuronal activity from deeper structures such as the brainstem during brainstem auditory evoked responses or potentials (BAERs) or the spinal cord and brainstem during somatosensory evoked potentials (SEPs) [13,14].

Electrodes and application

Recording electrodes are usually applied with an electrolyte paste that holds the metal disk-shaped electrodes in place. The paste also has favorable electrical conduction properties. In order to keep the impedance low, the area to which the electrode will be attached needs to be cleaned. Sometimes, especially in very premature babies, particular care must be paid to the infant's thin, easily abraded skin during preparation for electrode application. A special glue, collodion, is occasionally used to secure the electrodes, particularly during more prolonged recordings, but in neonates gluing is seldom necessary.

The standard method of electrode placement is referred to as the *international 10–20 system* [15,16]. This allows reliable electrode placements relative to the underlying brain structures, as well as consistent placements for serial EEG studies in a given infant. Standard electrode locations are designated by a combination of letters and numbers. *F, Fp, T, C, P,* and *O* correspond to frontal, frontopolar, temporal, central, parietal, and occipital locations, respectively. Odd numbers indicate the left side of the head, and even numbers the right. The letter *z* indicates the midline of the head. In neonates the number of electrodes is reduced because of the small head size and the relatively wide electrical fields of the activity measured in babies (Fig. 17.1). For neonatal recordings the frontopolar electrodes are placed slightly posterior to their relative positions on the adult scalp and are sometimes designated *Fp3* and *Fp4* [17,18]. Placement often has to be modified slightly because of scalp intravenous lines, surgical dressings, or movement restricted by such procedures as carotid catheterization for extracorporeal membrane oxygenation (ECMO).

Neonatal EEG should almost always be accompanied by simultaneous polygraphic recording of physiologic variables, including eye movement, electromyogram (EMG: usually from the submental muscle on the chin, just below the lower lip), electrocardiogram (ECG), and respiration [18]. These tracings permit the interpreter to determine the baby's sleep state and, in the case of the respiration recording, correlate apnea with the presence or absence of seizures [19–22].

Recordings in neonates can be performed using a single montage (arrangement of the EEG channels on the display), since there is a reduced number of electrodes compared with adult EEG recordings [18,23]. With modern digital EEG instruments, the EEG can be displayed in various other montages if the need arises. Other technical differences address the fact that the predominant frequencies of the EEG activity in neonates are much slower than in older children and adults. Neonatal EEG recordings are often displayed using a compressed display with 20 seconds of EEG per page (slower paper speed). A display of at least 16 channels is recommended. Because slow frequencies constitute the majority of neonatal EEG activity, slow-frequency filters should be minimal.

Sedation

Sedation is seldom needed as a routine part of the neonatal EEG. While it is desirable to record awake, quiet, and active sleep states, careful preparation and communication with the NICU nursing team ahead of time, and a patient approach by the technologist, will usually suffice. If the neonate is taking oral feedings, timing the EEG shortly after a feeding can eliminate the need for sedation in the majority of cases. If sedation is required, chloral hydrate is most commonly used for EEG since it is relatively short-acting and has little effect on the EEG [23]. However, some concerns about excessive sedation and possible toxicity of chloral hydrate metabolites have been raised [24,25].

Duration to obtain sleep states

Most neonatal EEGs will last between 45 and 60 minutes. To be considered adequate an EEG will ideally include all the

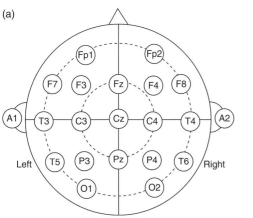
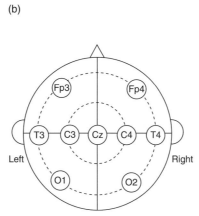

(a)

(b)

Fig. 17.1. Electrode nomenclature using the international 10–20 system. (a) Most commonly used electrodes for recordings outside the neonatal period. (b) More limited set of electrodes used for neonates. Note the slightly more lateral placement of the frontopolar electrodes.

stages of sleep that are likely to occur in a neonate of a given conceptional age. In the term infant these will include active sleep, transitional sleep, and quiet sleep, as well as wakefulness. By 32–34 weeks' conceptional age most normal infants have easily identifiable sleep states. The earliest stage of sleep, active sleep after wakefulness, may last up to 40 minutes; hence the duration of the recording may need to be as long as 60 minutes to try and record all sleep stages. Since this is longer than most recording done on adults and older children in the EEG laboratory, the EEG technologist and the NICU staff will have to plan accordingly.

Technologist

Working in a challenging environment

The NICU is a far-from-ideal recording location. There are many pieces of electrical equipment that can cause electrical artifacts to appear on the EEG. Mechanical devices such as ventilator tubing may vibrate and cause a rhythmic movement artifact that can be mistaken for seizures. Because of noise, bright lights, and the constant bustle of the NICU, getting a baby to sleep and keeping him or her asleep can be challenging. It is worthwhile for the technologist to contact the baby's nurse ahead of time and coordinate the EEG for just after a feeding or routine sedation – a time the infant is more likely to fall asleep.

Dealing with artifacts

Artifacts are a normal part of any EEG recording. A baby's movements are a common source of artifact and constitute an important and necessary component of the recording in the neonate. Artifacts are commonly caused by movement near the child (e.g., a nurse working with the baby; fluid bubbling in ventilator tubing), and nearby electrical equipment (60 Hz electrical noise). Many artifacts seen on EEG are rhythmic in appearance and may be mistaken for seizures. An experienced technologist will carefully evaluate the tracing during the recording, and document movements that cause artifacts. He or she will work with the nursing staff in the NICU to decrease artifacts, e.g., by repositioning the baby, moving nearby power cords, or turning off a high-frequency ventilator for a few seconds if medically safe.

Age of infant

Knowing the age of the infant is very important when interpreting the neonatal EEG. Because the EEG changes so dramatically between 24 weeks' gestational age and term, and because "dysmature" EEG findings are a frequently reported abnormality, correct assessment of the age of the neonate is critical. The *conceptional age* is the most important value to calculate: the baby's gestational age plus chronological (legal) age (in weeks) is noted at the beginning of the EEG. This permits the interpreting physician to look for characteristic patterns normally seen at a given conceptional age [26,27].

Documenting behavior during recording

The neonatologist may be asking, "Are tongue thrusting or apneic spells seizures?" Correlating rhythmic or unusual body movements with paroxysmal EEG findings is frequently the most important aspect of EEG interpretation. Careful documentation of the baby's behavior and the staffs' movement near the bed is important when interpreting neonatal (and indeed all) EEGs. The corollary is the importance of documenting any movement (or lack of movement) while rhythmic, seizure-like patterns are present on the EEG. For example, a small amount of water condensed in ventilator tubing can induce a prominent rhythmic pattern (artifact) on the EEG that might be confused with a seizure. Using an EEG recording system that includes simultaneous video recording can be very helpful [28].

Interpretation by electroencephalographer

The accuracy of EEG interpretation is very dependent upon the skill and experience of the physicians reading the recording. They should be familiar with the normal maturational changes expected at various conceptional ages. Recognizing common artifacts will prevent interpreting these as abnormalities. Without experience in recognizing normal versus abnormal findings such as frequency of sharp waves or degree of "discontinuity" of the background, interpretation can be arduous despite the availability of good atlases of neonatal EEG. Electrographic seizures may be quite subtle on the EEG itself, and the interpreting physician should be experienced enough to differentiate normal rhythmic activity from brief, abnormal rhythmic activity and more sustained rhythmic evolving seizure activity [29].

Maturational features

Introduction

Time of rapid anatomical maturation of the brain

Brain maturation occurs rapidly during the last trimester of fetal life and in the early weeks of postnatal life. The cortical surface is almost smooth with a simple sulcal pattern at 26–28 weeks' conceptional age. By contrast, the full-term newborn has a complex pattern of cortical gyri and sulci [30]. There are also rapid and dramatic changes in myelin formation [31]. The EEG features of normal newborns correlate well with the anatomic, MRI, and ultrasound-defined maturation of the brain [32].

EEG changes correspond to brain maturation

It is not surprising, then, that the EEG undergoes similarly rapid and dramatic changes during the first weeks of life. Certain EEG patterns appear and others disappear during the last trimester and the first months of life. The most marked changes occur between 24 weeks' gestational age and 1 month after term [33–35]. These maturational changes are similar whether the infant is in utero or born prematurely [26]. In other words, the EEG of a 12-week-old infant born at 28 weeks' gestational age and that of a 2-day-old infant of

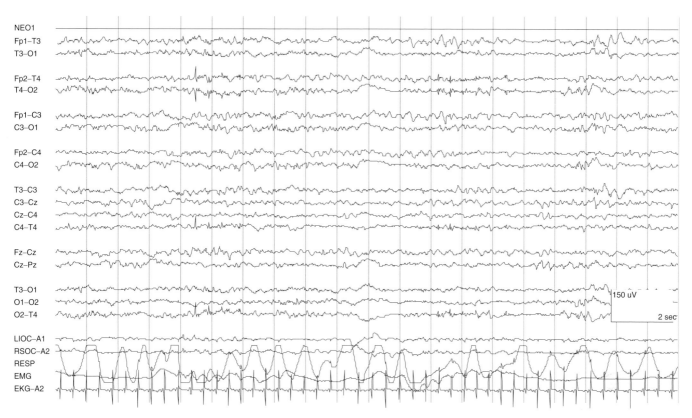

Fig. 17.2. Active sleep recorded in an infant of 39 weeks' conceptional age. Note irregular respirations, eye movement, and continuous, low-voltage EEG.

40 weeks' gestational age will be very similar. For this reason, it is important that the EEG technologist and interpreting physician have as accurate an idea as possible about the infant's gestational and chronological age. Specific EEG patterns are prominent features of normal neonates at particular ages. These include such features as "delta brushes," "frontal sharp transients," and "temporal theta bursts." These patterns appear and disappear at various conceptional ages in a predictable fashion. Similarly, the overall background pattern of the EEG changes with conceptional age. In particular, the degree of "discontinuity" evolves in a predictable way [34,36]. Deviations in the evolution of these specific EEG patterns and the overall background pattern represent evidence of an encephalopathy [37–40].

Ontogeny of sleep stage

Sleep states are important to identify in the newborn. Certain EEG patterns correlate with a given sleep state, and a "discordance" between the EEG pattern and the sleep state is evidence of an encephalopathy. The two main sleep states in the neonate are active sleep and quiet sleep. Active sleep is the equivalent of REM sleep in older children and adults. Quiet sleep is the equivalent of non-REM sleep. It is important to understand that sleep states are identified by the physiologic changes observable in the infant, and not by the EEG pattern.

Active sleep can first be identified between 27 and 31 weeks' conceptional age [33,34]. It is characterized by rapid eye movements, irregular respirations, loss of muscle tone,

and frequent small body and limb movements. The EEG background is continuous during active sleep (Fig. 17.2).

Quiet sleep appears between 31 and 34 weeks' conceptional age. It is characterized by regular respiration, little motor activity, absence of eye movements, and subtle tonic muscle activity. The EEG background during quiet sleep is discontinuous, but becomes more continuous as the conceptional age increases (Fig. 17.3).

Discontinuity of the background

The degree of discontinuity is one of the main features that distinguishes among normal infants of varying conceptional ages [32,38,41,42]. Premature infants between 24 and 28 weeks' conceptional age normally have very discontinuous tracings [34]. The "interburst intervals," the low-amplitude portions of the tracing between bursts of brain activity, are virtually flat at 26 weeks' conceptional age. On the other hand, the discontinuity normally present in quiet sleep of an infant of 42 weeks' conceptional age will be subtle, with the interburst intervals only slightly suppressed compared to the higher-amplitude epochs. Discontinuity is limited to quiet sleep by 36 weeks' conceptional age. Excessive discontinuity is a "dysmature feature" that indicates a degree of encephalopathy. It is not a very specific finding with regard to etiology or prognosis, however. It is important to realize that various neuroactive medications, such as barbiturates, may increase the interburst intervals and produce an excessively discontinuous pattern. If the infant is

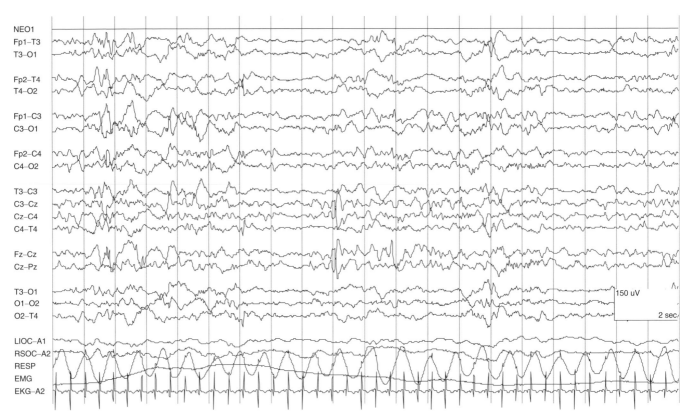

Fig. 17.3. Quiet sleep recorded in the same infant as in Figure 17.2. Note regular respirations, absence of eye movements and higher-amplitude, somewhat discontinuous EEG.

on such medications, the EEG must be interpreted with these caveats.

Another important feature of the discontinuity is the synchrony of the bursts. Even at a very early conceptional age, the bursts will almost entirely be synchronous between the two hemispheres [34]. Poor interhemispheric synchrony indicates an encephalopathy, but is not specific for etiology [5,42].

Specific patterns

Delta brushes

The delta brush is a pattern consisting of a short run of high-frequency EEG activity superimposed on a slower (delta frequency) wave (Fig. 17.4). This distinct pattern is most common at about 32–34 weeks and is rarely present after 40–44 weeks. They occur predominantly in active or quiet sleep depending on the infant's conceptional age. The frequency with which delta brushes occur during active and quiet sleep at various conceptional ages has been carefully quantified [35,43]. An excessive number of delta brushes in a particular sleep state at a particular conceptional age is a non-specific encephalopathic feature.

Frontal sharp transients and sporadic sharp waves

Sharp waves in the neonate do not have the same significance as they do in adults. In adults, sharp waves usually connote an increased risk of seizures. This is not the case with neonates. They normally have occasional sharp waves present during the

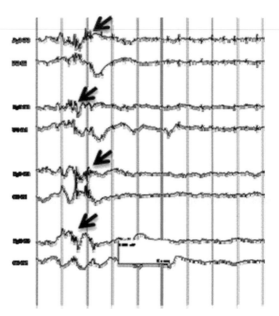

Fig. 17.4. Delta brushes (arrows) in EEG of an infant of 34 weeks' conceptional age.

EEG. As with other patterns already discussed, the frequency of their occurrence varies with sleep state and conceptional age. When they are persistently focal, they suggest a focal brain abnormality. Repetitive bursts of sharp waves, especially when there is a stereotyped evolution of the frequency and

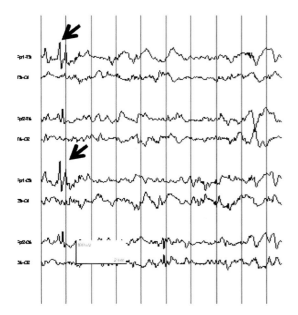

Fig. 17.5. Frontal sharp transients in EEG of an infant of 39 weeks' conceptional age.

amplitude, have been characterized as "brief ictal rhythmic discharges," and indicate a higher risk of seizures [44,45].

Another prominent sharp wave that is usually distinguished from the sporadic sharp waves described above is frontal sharp transients. These are high-amplitude monophasic or biphasic sharp waves which are, of course, maximum over the frontal regions (Fig. 17.5). They are a prominent feature of active sleep and transitional sleep states in more mature neonates [35,46].

Theta bursts
The temporal theta burst, or temporal "saw tooth" pattern, is a normal feature of the EEG of younger conceptional-age infants. This sometimes dramatic pattern of rhythmic, sharply contoured theta waves is maximum between 27 and 32 weeks' conceptional age [35]. Other theta patterns described in EEGs of normal premature infants are maximum over the occipital and frontal regions [47,48]. The absence of these normally seen rhythms in the very premature infant suggests an encephalopathic process [49].

Midline rhythms
Various types of rhythmic or sharp EEG patterns occurring at the midline of the scalp can have a striking appearance but are still quite normal. Among these are single sharp waves, trains of 4–8 Hz sharp patterns, and runs of alpha-frequency waves lasting up to 3 seconds. They occur across a wide range of conceptional ages from 27 to 46 weeks. Though easily mistaken for abnormal rhythmic sharp EEG patterns, they are an occasionally seen feature of normal neonates and have been characterized as "Fz theta/alpha bursts" [49,50].

EEG in diffuse encephalopathy
EEG is often used to determine the severity and progression of encephalopathies in neonates. Most of the time, the EEG findings are not specific for a particular cause such as hypoxia or infection. Certain patterns, such as a dysmature background or burst–suppression, can occur in a variety of disorders. However, the degree of abnormality and the persistence or resolution of the abnormal finding are helpful in determining the timing of an insult, the cause, and the prognosis [51].

Grading encephalopathy using the EEG
The encephalopathy is most often referred to as "mild," "moderate," or "severe." The criteria for distinguishing between these categories may vary somewhat from one EEG laboratory to another, but it will generally be agreed that a severely abnormal EEG in a neonate comprises one of two patterns: burst–suppression or low-voltage undifferentiated (flat) pattern with no apparent EEG activity over 20 mV (Figs. 17.6, 17.7). These patterns are usually invariant, i.e., there is no spontaneous variability and no reactivity to vigorous stimulation [38,52].

It is important to distinguish a burst–suppression pattern from normal discontinuity present in neonates at lower conceptional ages. For instance, the interburst intervals of a 26-week conceptional-age infant may appear very flat and suggest burst–suppression. However, there will generally be clear variability and reactivity if appropriate stimuli are administered during the recording. The bursts themselves will not look as abnormal in the normal premature infant as in a burst–suppression recording, since the latter will usually be very high in amplitude and contain bursts of abnormal repetitive sharp waves and will lack normal patterns.

An EEG may be considered severely abnormal because of other findings that have been shown to have prognostic significance: positive rolandic sharp waves, electrographic seizures, marked interhemispheric voltage asymmetry, or excessively slow background with absence of the patterns expected at the particular conceptional age [51]. The prognostic significance of these various EEG patterns as they relate to outcomes is provided in Table 17.1.

Specificity of the "encephalopathic" EEG
The cause of the encephalopathy will most often be apparent from the baby's history. The EEG itself seldom gives specific information about the underlying cause. A severely abnormal EEG may be seen in hypoxia, various metabolic abnormalities, infections, and brain malformations.

Prognostic value of the encephalopathic EEG
A single severely abnormal EEG is usually predictive of an abnormal neurological outcome [53,54]. However, under certain circumstances, the prognostic value of a severely abnormal EEG is limited. For example, if an infant has received a large amount of neuroactive medication, the EEG may be flat or have a burst–suppression pattern. Immediately after an acute hypoxic event, hypotension, or other acute

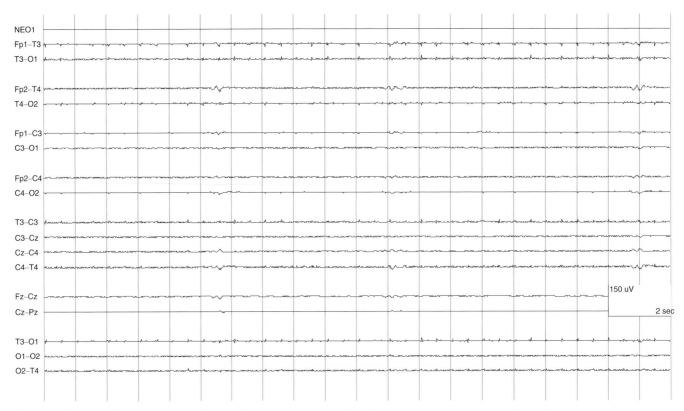

Fig. 17.6. Very low-voltage, non-reactive EEG pattern from a 3-day-old term infant with severe hypoxic–ischemic encephalopathy.

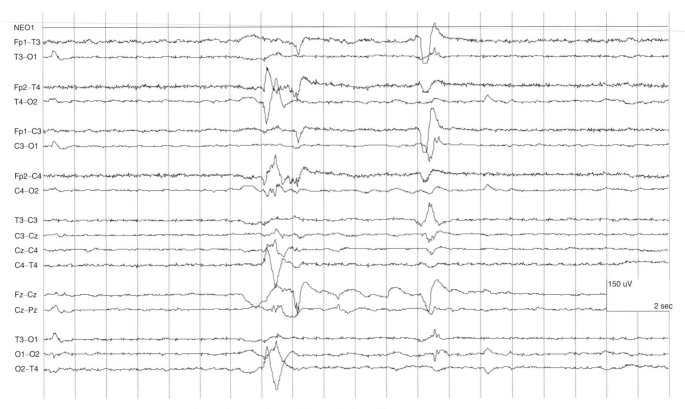

Fig. 17.7. Burst–suppression EEG pattern. Same infant as in Figure 17.6, now 11 days old.

Table 17.1. Various encephalopathic EEG patterns and their prognostic significance

EEG background patterns	Percent with favorable outcome
Isoelectric	0–5
Burst–suppression	0–15
Low-voltage undifferentiated	15–30
Excessively discontinuous	40–50
Diffuse slow activity	15–20

metabolic derangement (hypoglycemia, hypothermia), the EEG may appear severely abnormal although the cause is reversible and did not persist long enough to produce a significant degree of permanent brain injury. It is important to know the clinical circumstances during and just prior to obtaining the EEG.

Serial EEGs are helpful for determining the neurological prognosis. Clancy and Chung found that serial recordings provided more useful prognostic information than did any single recording [55]. Aso and colleagues studied 32 infants who underwent autopsy and were found to have periventricular–intraventricular hemorrhage [56]. Twenty-seven had parenchymal pathology including periventricular leukomalacia, ischemic neuronal sclerosis, pontosubicular necrosis, cerebral infarction, or cerebral hemorrhage. The severity of the pathological changes was highly correlated with the grading of the severity of the EEG background abnormalities. In a study of 119 near-term infants with severe respiratory failure, a burst–suppression pattern or electrographic seizures on two or more recordings was predictive of a poor prognosis (death, severely abnormal developmental score, or cerebral palsy), but a single such recording in this series was not predictive [57].

Timing of a brain insult may be suggested by an abnormally dysmature EEG. Tharp described a case of an infant whose abnormal EEG at several hours of age showed many dysmature features. The delivery was complicated by an abnormal fetal heart rate suggesting fetal distress, and the question was whether the intrapartum distress was the cause of the infant's severe encephalopathy. The infant died and the autopsy revealed changes that had occurred 7–10 days prior to death [26].

Timing of an insult may also be suggested by the changes (or lack of changes) that occur over time. It takes several days for positive rolandic sharp waves (PRSW) to appear in cases of periventricular leukomalacia [58,59]. If such findings are present in the first days of life and persist with little change, it suggests that the insult occurred prior to delivery. If the changes are more dynamic, i.e., appear then disappear on serial EEGs over several weeks, the likelihood is that the encephalopathy was more acute.

ECMO is a situation where EEG can be useful for helping follow the child's encephalopathic condition. Infants undergoing ECMO are often quite encephalopathic from their original insult or are pharmacologically paralyzed, so clinical assessment can be difficult. In children undergoing ECMO, two or more severely abnormal EEG patterns (burst–suppression or electrographic seizure tracings) are strongly predictive of an abnormal neurological outcome [57]. The majority of the infants in this study by Graziani *et al.* had moderate to severe EEG abnormalities before ECMO. The authors concluded that fetal and neonatal complications that were associated with the severe cardiorespiratory failure were responsible in large part for the neurologic sequelae in ECMO survivors.

Another question specific to ECMO is whether cannulation of the right common carotid artery damages the right cerebral hemisphere. Studies looking at EEGs performed during ECMO have not shown a predilection for lateralized abnormalities over the right side, and therefore conclude that carotid artery cannulation is relatively safe [60,61].

The amplitude-integrated EEG (aEEG) is often used for monitoring brain activity in the ICU setting. It comprises a simplified display of EEG displayed graphically and provides an impression of cerebral activity over a longer time span than routine EEG displays. The EEG signal is acquired from just 1–2 scalp locations, usually the central-parietal regions. The EEG signal is displayed in a time-compressed fashion on a semi-logarithmic scale (Fig. 17.8). Most devices simultaneously display the raw EEG tracing, and two-channel devices permit interhemispheric comparisons.

The display shows the degree of continuity of the cerebral activity. In general, there is good correlation between aEEG and EEG for the assessment of background activity [62]. Because of the time-compressed nature of the data output, sleep–wake cycles can be documented, and these may be important predictors in the recovery of the hypoxic–ischemic infant or the maturation of the preterm CNS [63,64]. In general, lower voltages and increased bandwidth indicate depressed brain activity, but may also be consistent with an immature pattern. As with the standard EEG, clinical interventions that may affect aEEG voltages include surfactant administration, tracheal suctioning, sedative and paralytic medication, hypotension, acidosis, hypoglycemia, and pneumothorax [65].

Use of aEEG in the neonatal population began in the 1980s, with initial studies focusing on monitoring of asphyxiated newborns [66]. Continuous aEEG has been used to monitor seizures and to document the efficacy of pharmacologic interventions. While this can be a valuable adjunct to routine EEG monitoring, there are limitations, such as a likelihood that aEEG will miss short-duration, low-amplitude seizures, and those localized outside the area monitored by the aEEG [67]. Seizures on aEEG may appear as a distinctive deviation from the baseline activity, but this needs to be correlated initially with confirmed seizure activity on the source EEG tracing in order to avoid misinterpreting such things as rhythmic artifact as seizures.

There is increasing use of aEEG to investigate the maturation of the preterm CNS. Correlations between aEEG findings and preterm brain injury such as intraventricular hemorrhage and posthemorrhagic hydrocephalus have also been reported [68,69].

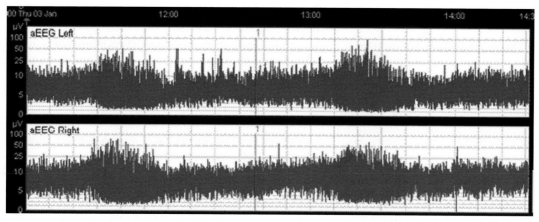

Fig. 17.8. Amplitude-integrated EEG in a healthy term infant. Example shows 3.5-hour recording. Broad portions of band correlate with quiet sleep; narrow portions correlate with active sleep. *See color plate section.*

Amplitude-integrated EEG recording has predictive value in the management of term newborns with hypoxic–ischemic encephalopathy (HIE). Recovery of background voltage patterns and the onset of sleep–wake cycles on aEEG have been shown to be predictive of neurodevelopmental outcome at 18–22 months of age. The earlier the recovery of sleep–wake cycles occurs, the better the outcome [63,70]. Neurologic examination coupled with aEEG demonstrated an enhanced capability to predict persistent encephalopathy in this patient population [71]. A study of brain cooling for the treatment of HIE enrolled infants with moderate to severe neonatal encephalopathy and abnormal aEEG. Head cooling was of no benefit in infants with the most severely abnormal aEEG [72]. These studies indicate that aEEG can help in the selection of patients most likely to benefit from hypothermia. A meta-analysis demonstrated the ability of aEEG to predict poor outcome with 91% sensitivity in infants with HIE [73].

Correlation with specific disorders
Brain malformations
Lissencephaly
Lissencephaly, a disturbance of neuronal migration associated with agyria or pachygyria, is associated with an abnormal EEG pattern in the neonatal period. Abnormal high-amplitude rhythmic fast frequencies have been described. There may be poor reactivity to stimulation and absent sleep–wake changes [74,75].

Aicardi syndrome
Aicardi syndrome comprises agenesis of the corpus callosum, characteristic ocular lesions, and infantile spasms. EEG findings in the neonatal period include abnormal, poorly synchronized bursts, usually in the setting of burst–suppression [76,77].

Holoprosencephaly
Holoprosencephaly, a malformation of the brain characterized by some degree of failure of separation of the forebrain, may show suggestive EEG changes in the neonatal period as well. The EEG in the region of the dorsal cyst is low-voltage or isoelectric. The EEG in regions overlying the cortical tissue shows prolonged runs of rhythmic alpha and theta patterns, as well as fast beta (ictal) discharges. Multifocal spikes and polyspikes can also be seen, especially when cortical malformations accompany holoprosencephaly [77].

Metabolic encephalopathies
Maple syrup urine disease
A unique, mu-like rhythm has been described in association with maple syrup urine disease. This pattern, characterized by rhythmic 5–7 Hz activity, can be distinguished from similar patterns occurring in normal infants and those with other encephalopathies, so it may be relatively specific for maple syrup urine disease [78].

Pyridoxine dependency
The EEG may be particularly suggestive of pyridoxine dependency in the setting of medically refractory neonatal seizures. In one study, burst–suppression and a pattern of high-amplitude bilateral slow waves were very suggestive of pyridoxine dependence [79,80]. Furthermore, the response to treatment (with pyridoxine) provides additional evidence for this disorder.

Non-ketotic hyperglycinemia
The EEG may be suggestive of non-ketotic hyperglycinemia. A burst–suppression pattern is common, and may evolve over time to hypsarrhythmia. A burst–suppression pattern with superimposed midline seizures and cortical myoclonus has been described in one study [81–83].

Hyperammonemia
A burst–suppression pattern, excessive discontinuity (short of true burst–suppression), or a pattern of multifocal sharp waves may be present in the setting of citrullinemia or ornithine transcarbamylase deficiency. The improvement (or worsening) of the EEG during therapeutic interventions can provide evidence of the treatment efficacy [55,84].

Intraventricular hemorrhage
The EEG has a limited role in the diagnosis of intraventricular hemorrhage, but has proven helpful in assessing the prognosis

for neurological outcome [85]. The EEG can provide prognostic information beyond that apparent from brain-imaging studies [86]. In a series of 88 EEGs from 35 infants with autopsy-proven intraventricular hemorrhage, the EEG correlated better with the overall brain abnormalities than with the grade of intraventricular hemorrhage [56]. In another study, the continuity of background activity was not affected by intraventricular hemorrhage, but there was depression of the EEG background activity during the onset or extension of periventricular–intraventricular hemorrhage [87].

Periventricular leukomalacia

PRSW are an EEG pattern associated with deep white-matter injury. A number of studies have shown the predictive value of PRSW [88]. PRSW have been associated with periventricular leukomalacia. In a study of 301 premature infants, the absence of PRSW was correlated with a favorable motor development in 98.2% [10]. When very frequent (2/minute), they were strongly predictive of severe spastic diplegia. They were not specifically associated with social and language developmental abnormalities. PRSW also precede the appearance of the typical changes of cystic periventricular leukomalacia as detected by ultrasound, though ultrasound-detected echodensities may appear earlier [89].

Stroke

Focal or hemispheric voltage attenuation may occur when infants have had large-vessel infarction [90–92]. In some cases EEG changes will precede those on ultrasound or CT.

Infectious disease

Encephalitis

Herpes simplex meningoencephalitis is a potentially devastating infectious disease in infants. EEG changes are often non-specific, but a pattern of temporal or multifocal periodic sharp waves has been described in infants (though this periodic pattern is more common in older children and adults) [93,94]. EEG changes are likely to precede changes on neuroimaging studies, and the imaging changes most characteristic of neonatal herpes may only be apparent late [95,96].

The EEG in other forms of encephalitis often shows abnormalities, but most reports are case reports, and findings are usually non-specific [97,98]. Presumably the background EEG changes again support a neurological prognostication [52].

Meningitis

Meningitis can cause devastating brain injury in the neonate. The EEG has been a useful tool for helping predict long-term neurological outcome in neonates with meningitis [99,100]. In a study of 29 infants with culture-proven meningitis, the degree of background abnormality correlated with outcome. Infants with normal or mildly abnormal background EEGs were normal at follow-up, whereas those with markedly abnormal EEGs died or had severe neurological sequelae. EEG patterns were non-specific, although some well-recognized patterns such as PRSW suggested a more specific pathology [90].

Maternal drug use

Scher and colleagues have reported the effects of cocaine and other illicit drugs on the EEG of neonates [101]. Cocaine produced abnormalities in the spectral correlations between homologous brain regions at birth, while alcohol, marijuana, and tobacco use were found to affect state regulation and cortical activities.

Conclusion

When obtained in a timely manner, and when appropriate questions are being asked, the EEG will provide useful information about acute and chronic brain processes in the neonate. This chapter has stressed the importance of looking at the EEG in the context of the clinical setting and in conjunction with other diagnostic studies. Not enough emphasis can be placed on the importance of clear communication between the clinicians caring for the infant, the EEG technologist, and the electroencephalographer.

References

1. Mizrahi EM. Pediatric electroencephalographic video monitoring. *J Clin Neurophysiol* 1999; **16**: 100–10.

2. Hayakawa F, Okumura A, Kato T, *et al.* Determination of timing of brain injury in preterm infants with periventricular leukomalacia with serial neonatal electroencephalography. *Pediatrics* 1999; **104**: 1077–81.

3. Itakura A, Kurauchi O, Hayakawa F, *et al.* Timing of periventricular leukomalacia using neonatal electroencephalography. *Int J Gynaecol Obstet* 1996; **55**: 111–15.

4. Marret S, Jeannot E, Parain D, *et al.* [Positive rolandic sharp waves, periventricular ischemia and neurologic outcome. Prospective study in 66 premature infants]. *Arch Fr Pediatr* 1989; **46**: 249–53.

5. Watanabe K, Hayakawa F, Okumura A. Neonatal EEG: a powerful tool in the assessment of brain damage in preterm infants. *Brain Dev* 1999; **21**: 361–72.

6. Bellieni CV, Ferrari F, De Felice C, *et al.* EEG in assessing hydroxycobalamin therapy in neonatal methylmalonic aciduria with homocystinuria. *Biol Neonate* 2000; **78**: 327–30.

7. Brazier MAB. *Electrical Activity of the Nervous System*, 4th edn. Baltimore, MD: Williams and Wilkins, 1977.

8. Marret S, Parain D, Menard JF, *et al.* Prognostic value of neonatal electroencephalography in premature newborns less than 33 weeks of gestational age. *Electroencephalogr Clin Neurophysiol* 1997; **102**: 178–85.

9. Chung HJ, Clancy RR. Significance of positive temporal sharp waves in the neonatal electroencephalogram. *Electroencephalogr Clin Neurophysiol* 1991; **79**: 256–63.

10. Marret S, Parain D, Jeannot E, *et al.* Positive rolandic sharp waves in the EEG of the premature newborn: a five year prospective study. *Arch Dis Child* 1992; **67**: 948–51.

11. Novotny EJ, Tharp BR, Coen RW, *et al.* Positive rolandic sharp waves in the EEG of the premature infant. *Neurology* 1987; **37**: 1481–6.

12. Cukier F, Andre M, Monod N, et al. [Contribution of EEG to the diagnosis of intraventricular hemorrhages in the premature infant]. Rev Electroencephalogr Neurophysiol Clin 1972; 2: 318–22.

13. Levy SR. Brainstem auditory potentials in pediatrics. In Chiappa KH, ed., Evoked Potentials in Clinical Medicine, 3rd edn. Philadelphia, PA: Lippincott-Raven, 1997: 269–78.

14. Levy SR. Somatosensory evoked potentials in pediatrics. In Chiappa KH, ed., Evoked Potentials in Clinical Medicine, 3rd edn. Philadelphia, PA: Lippincott-Raven, 1997: 453–70.

15. Jasper HH. The ten twenty electrode system of the international federation. Electroencephalogr Clin Neurophysiol 1958; 10: 371–5.

16. Nuwer MR. Recording electrode site nomenclature. J Clin Neurophysiol 1987; 4: 121–33.

17. Hrachovy RA, Mizrahi EM, Kellaway P. Electroencephalography of the newborn. In Daly DD, Pedley TA, eds., Current Practice of Clinical Electroencephalography, 2nd edn. New York, NY: Raven Press, 1990: 201–42.

18. Guideline two: minimum technical standards for pediatric electroencephalography. Am J Electroneurodiagnostic Technol 2006; 46: 205–10.

19. Ramelli GP, Donati F, Bianchetti M, et al. Apnoeic attacks as an isolated manifestation of epileptic seizures in infants. Eur J Paediatr Neurol 1998; 2: 187–91.

20. Watanabe K, Hara K, Miyazaki S, et al. Apneic seizures in the newborn. Am J Dis Child 1982; 136: 980–4.

21. Hosain S, La Vega-Talbott M, Solomon G, et al. Apneic seizures in infants: role of continuous EEG monitoring. Clin Electroencephalogr 2003; 34: 197–200.

22. Tramonte JJ, Goodkin HP. Temporal lobe hemorrhage in the full-term neonate presenting as apneic seizures. J Perinatol 2004; 24: 726–9.

23. Hahn JS, Tharp, B. Neonatal and pediatric electroencephalography. In Aminoff M, ed., Electrodiagnosis in Clinical Neurology, 3rd edn. Edinburgh: Churchill Livingstone, 1999: 81–127.

24. Sing K, Erickson T, Amitai Y, et al. Chloral hydrate toxicity from oral and intravenous administration. J Toxicol Clin Toxicol 1996; 34: 101–6.

25. Pershad J, Palmisano P, Nichols M. Chloral hydrate: the good and the bad. Pediatr Emerg Care 1999; 15: 432–5.

26. Tharp BR. Electrophysiological brain maturation in premature infants: an historical perspective. J Clin Neurophysiol 1990; 7: 302–14.

27. Scher MS, Waisanen H, Loparo K, et al. Prediction of neonatal state and maturational change using dimensional analysis. J Clin Neurophysiol 2005; 22: 159–65.

28. Watemberg N, Tziperman B, Dabby R, et al. Adding video recording increases the diagnostic yield of routine electroencephalograms in children with frequent paroxysmal events. Epilepsia 2005; 46: 716–19.

29. Wical BS. Neonatal seizures and electrographic analysis: evaluation and outcomes. Pediatr Neurol 1994; 10: 271–5.

30. Dooling EC, Chi J, Gilles FH. Telencephalic development. In Gilles FH, Leviton A, Dooling EC, eds., The Developing Human Brain: Growth and Epidemiologic Neuropathology. Boston, MA: Wright-PSG, 1983: 117–82.

31. McArdle CB, Richardson CJ, Nicholas DA, et al. Developmental features of the neonatal brain: MR imaging. Part I. Gray–white matter differentiation and myelination. Radiology 1987; 162: 223–9.

32. Scher MS, Martin JG, Steppe DA, et al. Comparative estimates of neonatal gestational maturity by electrographic and fetal ultrasonographic criteria. Pediatr Neurol 1994; 11: 214–18.

33. Monod N, Tharp B. [The normal EEG of the neonate (author's transl)]. Rev Electroencephalogr Neurophysiol Clin 1977; 7: 302–15.

34. Selton D, Andre M, Hascoet JM. Normal EEG in very premature infants: reference criteria. Clin Neurophysiol 2000; 111: 2116–24.

35. Torres F, Anderson C. The normal EEG of the human newborn. J Clin Neurophysiol 1985; 2: 89–103.

36. Van Sweden B, Koenderink M, Windau G, et al. Long-term EEG monitoring in the early premature: developmental and chronobiological aspects. Electroencephalogr Clin Neurophysiol 1991; 79: 94–100.

37. Biagioni E, Bartalena L, Biver P, et al. Electroencephalographic dysmaturity in preterm infants: a prognostic tool in the early postnatal period. Neuropediatrics 1996; 27: 311–16.

38. Biagioni E, Bartalena L, Boldrini A, et al. Constantly discontinuous EEG patterns in full-term neonates with hypoxic–

ischaemic encephalopathy. Clinical Neurophysiology 1999; 110: 1510–15.

39. Hahn JS, Tharp BR. Winner of the Brazier Award: the dysmature EEG pattern in infants with bronchopulmonary dysplasia and its prognostic implications. Electroencephalogr Clin Neurophysiol 1990; 76: 106–13.

40. Hayakawa F, Okumura A, Kato T, et al. Disorganized patterns: chronic-stage EEG abnormality of the late neonatal period following severely depressed EEG activities in early preterm infants. Neuropediatrics 1997; 28: 272–5.

41. Scher MS, Steppe DA, Banks DL, et al. Maturational trends of EEG-sleep measures in the healthy preterm neonate. Pediatr Neurol 1995; 12: 314–22.

42. Wertheim D, Mercuri E, Faundez JC, et al. Prognostic value of continuous electroencephalographic recording in full term infants with hypoxic ischaemic encephalopathy. Arch Dis Child 1994; 71: F97–102.

43. Lombroso CT. Quantified electrographic scales on 10 pre-term healthy newborns followed up to 40–43 weeks of conceptional age by serial polygraphic recordings. Electroencephalogr Clin Neurophysiol 1979; 46: 460–74.

44. Oliveira AJ, Nunes ML, Haertel LM, et al. Duration of rhythmic EEG patterns in neonates: new evidence for clinical and prognostic significance of brief rhythmic discharges. Clin Neurophysiol 2000; 111: 1646–53.

45. Shewmon DA. What is a neonatal seizure? Problems in definition and quantification for investigative and clinical purposes. J Clin Neurophysiol 1990; 7: 315–68.

46. Nunes ML, Da Costa JC, Moura-Ribeiro MV. Polysomnographic quantification of bioelectrical maturation in preterm and ful{} term newborns at matched conceptional ages. Electroencephalogr Clin Neurophysiol 1997; 102: 186–91.

47. Hughes JR, Miller JK, Fino JJ, et al. The sharp theta rhythm on the occipital areas of prematures (STOP): a newly described waveform. Clin Electroencephalogr 1990; 21: 77–87.

48. Kuremoto K, Hayakawa F, Watanabe K. [Rhythmic alpha/theta bursts in the electroencephalogram of early premature infants. 1. The features in normal early premature infants]. No To Hattatsu 1997; 29: 239–43.

49. Kuremoto K, Hayakawa F, Watanabe K. [Rhythmic alpha/theta bursts in the

electroencephalogram of early premature infants. 2. Correlation with background EEG activity]. *No To Hattatsu* 1997; **29**: 244–8.

50. Zaret BS, Guterman B, Weig S. Circumscribed midline EEG activity in neurologically normal neonates. *Clin Electroencephalogr* 1991; **22**: 13–22.

51. Tharp BR, Cukier F, Monod N. The prognostic value of the electroencephalogram in premature infants. *Electroencephalogr Clin Neurophysiol* 1981; **51**: 219–36.

52. Holmes GL, Lombroso CT. Prognostic value of background patterns in the neonatal EEG. *J Clin Neurophysiol* 1993; **10**: 323–52.

53. Pressler RM, Boylan GB, Morton M, *et al*. Early serial EEG in hypoxic ischaemic encephalopathy. *Clin Neurophysiol* 2001; **112**: 31–7.

54. Zeinstra E, Fock JM, Begeer JH, *et al*. The prognostic value of serial EEG recordings following acute neonatal asphyxia in full-term infants. *Eur J Paediatr Neurol* 2001; **5**: 155–60.

55. Clancy RR, Chung HJ. EEG changes during recovery from acute severe neonatal citrullinemia. *Electroencephalogr Clin Neurophysiol* 1991; **78**: 222–7.

56. Aso K, Abdab-Barmada M, Scher MS. EEG and the neuropathology in premature neonates with intraventricular hemorrhage. *J Clin Neurophysiol* 1993; **10**: 304–13.

57. Graziani LJ, Streletz LJ, Baumgart S, *et al*. Predictive value of neonatal electroencephalograms before and during extracorporeal membrane oxygenation. *J Pediatr* 1994; **125**: 969–75.

58. Okumura A, Hayakawa F, Kato T, *et al*. Positive rolandic sharp waves in preterm infants with periventricular leukomalacia: their relation to background electroencephalographic abnormalities. *Neuropediatrics* 1999; **30**: 278–82.

59. Tich SN, d'Allest AM, Villepin AT, *et al*. Pathological features of neonatal EEG in preterm babies born before 30 weeks of gestational age. *Neurophysiol Clin* 2007; **37**: 325–70.

60. Kumar P, Gupta R, Shankaran S, *et al*. EEG abnormalities in survivors of neonatal ECMO: its role as a predictor of neurodevelopmental outcome. *Am J Perinatol* 1999; **16**: 245–50.

61. Trittenwein G, Plenk S, Mach E, *et al*. Quantitative electroencephalography values of neonates during and after venoarterial extracorporeal membrane

oxygenation and permanent ligation of right common carotid artery. *Artif Organs* 2006; **30**: 447–51.

62. Toet M, van der Meij W, de Vries L, *et al*. Comparison between simultaneously recorded amplitude integrated electroencephalogram (cerebral function monitor) and standard electroencephalogram in neonates. *Pediatrics* 2002; **109**: 772–9.

63. Osredkar D, Toet M, van Rooij L, *et al*. Sleep–wake cycling on amplitude-integrated electroencephalography in term newborns with hypoxic–ischemic encephalopathy. *Pediatrics* 2005; **115**: 327–32.

64. Kuhle S, Klebermass K, Olischar M, *et al*. Sleep–wake cycles in preterm infants below 30 weeks of gestational age: preliminary results of a prospective amplitude-integrated EEG study. *Wiener Klin Wochenschr* 2001; **113**: 219–23.

65. Hellstrom-Westas L, de Vries L, Rosen I. *An Atlas of Amplitude-Integrated EEGs in the Newborn*. New York, NY: Parthenon, 2003.

66. Bjerre I, Hellstrom-Westas L, Rosen I, *et al*. Monitoring of cerebral function after severe asphyxia in infancy. *Arch Dis Child* 1983; **58**: 997–1002.

67. Clancy R. Prolonged electroencephalogram monitoring for seizures and their treatment. *Clin Perinatol* 2006; **33**: 649–65.

68. Olischar M, Klebermass K, Kuhle S, *et al*. Progressive posthemorrhagic hydrocephalus leads to changes of amplitude-integrated EEG activity in preterm infants. *Childs Nerv Syst* 2004; **20**: 41–5.

69. Hellstrom-Westas L, Klette H, Thorngren-Jerneck K, *et al*. Early prediction of outcome with aEEG in preterm infants with large intraventricular hemorrhages. *Neuropediatrics* 2001; **32**: 319–24.

70. de Vries LS, Toet MC. Amplitude integrated electroencephalography in the full-term newborn. *Clin Perinatol* 2006; **33**: 619–32, vi.

71. Shalak L, Laptook A, Velaphi S, *et al*. Amplitude-integrated electroencephalography coupled with an early neurologic examination enhances prediction of term infants at risk for persistent encephalopathy. *Pediatrics* 2003; **111**: 351–7.

72. Gluckman P, Wyatt J, Azzopardi D, *et al*. Selective head cooling with mild systemic hypothermia after neonatal

encephalopathy: multicentre randomised trial. *Lancet* 2005; **365**: 663–70.

73. Spitzmiller R, Phillips T, Meinzen-Derr J, *et al*. Amplitude-Integrated EEG is useful in predicting neurodevelopmental outcome in full-term infants with hypoxic–ischemic encephalopathy: a meta-analysis. *J Child Neurol* 2007; **22**: 1069–78.

74. Bode H, Bubl R. [EEG changes in type I and type II lissencephaly]. *Klin Padiatr* 1994; **206**: 12–17.

75. Worle H, Keimer R, Kohler B. [Miller-Dieker syndrome (type I lissencephaly) with specific EEG changes]. *Monatsschr Kinderheilkd* 1990; **138**: 615–18.

76. Ohtsuka Y, Oka E, Terasaki T, *et al*. Aicardi syndrome: a longitudinal clinical and electroencephalographic study. *Epilepsia* 1993; **34**: 627–34.

77. Shah KN, Rajadhyaksha S, Shah VS, *et al*. EEG recognition of holoprosencephaly and Aicardi syndrome. *Indian J Pediatr* 1992; **59**: 103–8.

78. Tharp BR. Unique EEG pattern (comb-like rhythm) in neonatal maple syrup urine disease. *Pediatr Neurol* 1992; **8**: 65–8.

79. Nabbout R, Soufflet C, Plouin P, *et al*. Pyridoxine dependent epilepsy: a suggestive electroclinical pattern. *Arch Dis Child Fetal Neonatal Ed* 1999; **81**: F125–9.

80. Baxter P. Pyridoxine dependent epilepsy: a suggestive electroclinical pattern. *Arch Dis Child Fetal Neonatal Ed* 2000; **83**: F163.

81. Markand ON, Garg BP, Brandt IK. Nonketotic hyperglycinemia: electroencephalographic and evoked potential abnormalities. *Neurology* 1982; **32**: 151–6.

82. Scher MS, Bergman I, Ahdab-Barmada M, *et al*. Neurophysiological and anatomical correlations in neonatal nonketotic hyperglycinemia. *Neuropediatrics* 1986; **17**: 137–43.

83. Seppalainen AM, Simila S. Electroencephalographic findings in three patients with nonketotic hyperglycinemia. *Epilepsia* 1971; **12**: 101–7.

84. Brunquell P, Tezcan K, DiMario FJ. Electroencephalographic findings in ornithine transcarbamylase deficiency. *J Child Neurol* 1999; **14**: 533–6.

85. Clancy RR, Tharp BR, Enzman D. EEG in premature infants with intraventricular hemorrhage. *Neurology* 1984; **34**: 583–90.

86. Watanabe K, Hakamada S, Kuroyanagi M, *et al*. Electroencephalographic study of

intraventricular hemorrhage in the preterm newborn. *Neuropediatrics* 1983; **14**: 225–30.

87. van de Bor M, van Dijk JG, van Bel F, *et al.* Electrical brain activity in preterm infants at risk for intracranial hemorrhage. *Acta Paediatr* 1994; **83**: 588–95.

88. Hughes JR, Guerra R. The use of the EEG to predict outcome in premature infants with positive sharp waves. *Clin Electroencephalogr* 1994; **25**: 127–35.

89. Baud O, d'Allest AM, Lacaze-Masmonteil T, *et al.* The early diagnosis of periventricular leukomalacia in premature infants with positive rolandic sharp waves on serial electroencephalography. *J Pediatr* 1998; **132**: 813–17.

90. Chequer RS, Tharp BR, Dreimane D, *et al.* Prognostic value of EEG in neonatal meningitis: retrospective study of 29 infants. *Pediatr Neurol* 1992; **8**: 417–22.

91. Koelfen W, Freund M, Varnholt V. Neonatal stroke involving the middle cerebral artery in term infants: clinical presentation, EEG and imaging studies, and outcome. *Dev Med Child Neurol* 1995; **37**: 204–12.

92. Sreenan C, Bhargava R, Robertson CM. Cerebral infarction in the term newborn: clinical presentation and long-term outcome. *J Pediatr* 2000; **137**: 351–5.

93. Lai CW, Gragasin ME. Electroencephalography in herpes simplex encephalitis. *J Clin Neurophysiol* 1988; **5**: 87–103.

94. Sainio K, Granstrom ML, Pettay O, *et al.* EEG in neonatal herpes simplex encephalitis. *Electroencephalogr Clin Neurophysiol* 1983; **56**: 556–61.

95. Mikati MA, Feraru E, Krishnamoorthy K, *et al.* Neonatal herpes simplex meningoencephalitis: EEG investigations and clinical correlates. *Neurology* 1990; **40**: 1433–7.

96. Shian WJ, Chi CS. Magnetic resonance imaging of herpes simplex encephalitis. *Zhonghua Min Guo Xiao Er Ke Yi Xue Hui Za Zhi* 1996; **37**: 22–6.

97. Haddad J, Messer J, Gut JP, *et al.* Neonatal echovirus encephalitis with white matter necrosis. *Neuropediatrics* 1990; **21**: 215–17.

98. Kohyama J, Suzuki N, Kajiwara M, *et al.* A case of chronic epileptic encephalopathy of neonatal onset: a probable concern of human cytomegalovirus. *Brain Dev* 1993; **15**: 448–52.

99. Berg U, Bohlin AB, Malmborg AS. Neonatal meningitis caused by *Haemophilus influenzae* type c. *Scand J Infect Dis* 1981; **13**: 155–7.

100. Watanabe K, Hara K, Hakamada S, *et al.* The prognostic value of EEG in neonatal meningitis. *Clin Electroencephalogr* 1983; **14**: 67–77.

101. Scher MS, Richardson GA, Day NL. Effects of prenatal cocaine/crack and other drug exposure on electroencephalographic sleep studies at birth and one year. *Pediatrics* 2000; **105**: 39–48.

Neuroimaging in the evaluation of pattern and timing of fetal and neonatal brain abnormalities

Patrick D. Barnes

Introduction

In this updated review, current and advanced neuroimaging technologies are discussed, along with the basic principles of imaging diagnosis and guidelines for utilization in fetal, perinatal, and neonatal brain abnormalities [1,2]. This includes pattern of injury and timing issues, with special emphasis on neurovascular disease and the differential diagnosis. In the causative differentiation of static encephalopathies (e.g., cerebral palsy, CP) from progressive encephalopathies, specific categories and timing are addressed. These include developmental abnormalities, trauma, neurovascular disease, infections and inflammatory processes, and metabolic disorders. Although a rare but important cause of progressive perinatal encephalopathy, neoplastic processes are not considered in detail here. Molecular and genetic technologies continue to advance toward eventual clinical application.

Neuroimaging technologies and general utilization

Imaging modalities may be classified as structural or functional [1–12]. **Structural imaging** modalities provide spatial resolution based primarily on anatomic or morphologic data. **Functional imaging** modalities provide spatial resolution based upon physiologic, chemical, or metabolic data. Some modalities may actually be considered to provide both structural and functional information.

Ultrasonography (US) is primarily a structural imaging modality with some functional capabilities (e.g., Doppler: Fig. 18.1a,b) [1–8,13–26]. It is readily accessible, portable, fast, real-time and multiplanar. It is less expensive than other cross-sectional modalities and relatively non-invasive (non-ionizing radiation). It requires no contrast agent and infrequently needs patient sedation. The resolving power of US is based on variations in acoustic reflectance of tissues. Its diagnostic effectiveness, however, continues to be dependent upon the skill and experience of the operator and interpreter, and there are issues regarding inter-observer reliability and accuracy

[1–8,13–26]. Also, US requires a window or path unimpeded by bone or air for cranial and spinal imaging. The most common uses of US are (1) fetal and neonatal screening, (2) screening of the infant who cannot be examined in the radiology department (e.g., premature neonate with intracranial hemorrhage, ECMO, intraoperative), (3) when important adjunctive information is quickly needed (e.g., cystic versus solid, vascularity, vascular flow [Doppler: Fig. 18.1a,b], or increased intracranial pressure), and (4) for real-time guidance and monitoring of invasive diagnostic or therapeutic surgical and interventional procedures [1–8,13].

In recent years, advanced US techniques have been introduced into clinical practice [1–8,13]. The development of high-resolution transducers, improvements in color Doppler signal processing, and new scanning techniques have significantly improved our ability to visualize structural, vascular, and cerebrospinal fluid abnormalities in the neonatal brain. Examples are the mastoid view to better visualize the posterior fossa, power Doppler and transcranial Doppler (TCD) to evaluate intracranial hemodynamics (e.g., resistive indices, RI: Fig. 18.1a,b), and the graded fontanel compression Doppler technique to evaluate hydrocephalus. Another advance in US technology that has yet to be translated is the development of vascular US contrast agents to amplify reflected sound waves. Potential applications include the detection of slow flow and the assessment of organ perfusion. Computerized analysis of textural features is another development that has promised increased sensitivity and specificity, but has not been translated to clinical practice [13].

Computed tomography (CT) is also primarily a structural imaging modality that has some functional capabilities (e.g., CT angiography) [1–8]. Although using ionizing radiation, current-generation multidetector CT (MDCT) effectively collimates and restricts the x-ray exposure to the immediate volume of interest, particularly when using the ALARA standard for pediatric patients, which adjusts radiation dose relative to age, size, and anatomic region [27]. Direct imaging is usually restricted to the axial plane (Fig. 18.1c–e). Reformatting from axial sections to other planes (e.g., coronal or sagittal) is now the MDCT standard. Projection scout images may provide information similar to plain films but with less spatial resolution. CT of the pediatric CNS is usually done using either the conventional or the helical/spiral technique. CT

Fetal and Neonatal Brain Injury, 4th edition, ed. David K. Stevenson, William E. Benitz, Philip Sunshine, Susan R. Hintz, and Maurice L. Druzin. Published by Cambridge University Press. © Cambridge University Press 2009.

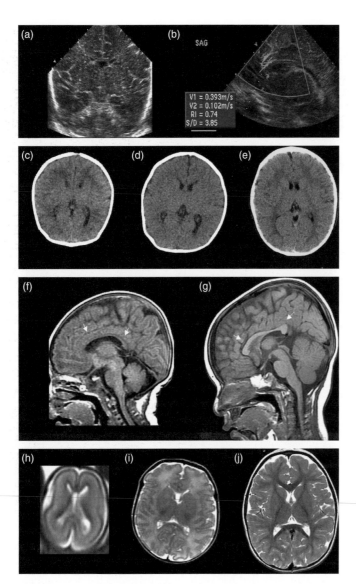

Fig. 18.1. Normal infant and child brain. Ultrasound (US) images of term neonate: (a) coronal US; (b) sagittal US + Doppler with resistive indices (RI). Computed tomography (CT) images of (c) term neonate, (d) 2-month-old infant, and (e) 2-year-old child show progress of maturation, including myelination. Sagittal T1 magnetic resonance images (MRIs) of (f) term neonate and (g) 1-year-old infant show progress in brain growth, myelination of the corpus callosum (arrows), and pituitary maturation. T2 MRIs of (h) 20-week fetus, (i) term neonate, and (j) 2-year-old child show progress in maturation, i.e., decreasing water content, increasing myelination and cortication. *See color plate section.*

requires sedation in infants and young children more often than does US but less often than MRI. The more rapid MDCT technology, however, has allowed a significant reduction in the need for sedation or anesthesia. The neonate or very young infant, for example, may be examined bundled while asleep after a feeding or during a nap. CT occasionally needs intravenous iodinated contrast enhancement, but cerebrospinal (CSF) contrast opacification is rarely needed. High-resolution bone and soft-tissue algorithms are important for demonstrating fine anatomy (e.g., skull base). Advances in computer display technology include image fusion, two-dimensional

reformatting, three-dimensional volumetric and reconstruction methods, segmentation, and surface rendering techniques. These high-resolution display techniques are used for CT angiography and venography, craniofacial and spinal imaging for surgical planning, and stereotactic image guidance of radiotherapy, interventional, and neurosurgical procedures.

The role of CT has been further redefined in the context of accessible and reliable US and MRI [1–12,15,28,29]. US is the procedure of choice for primary imaging or screening of the brain and spinal neuraxis in the neonate and young infant. When US does not satisfy the clinical inquiry, or an acoustic window is not available, then CT becomes the primary modality for brain imaging in children, especially in acute or emergent presentations. This is especially important for acute neurologic presentations. In these situations, CT is primarily used to screen for acute or subacute hemorrhage, focal or diffuse edema, herniation, fractures, hydrocephalus, tumor mass, or abnormal collection (blood, pus, air, CSF, etc.). Other primary indications for CT include the evaluation of bony or air-space abnormalities of the skull base, cranial vault, orbit, paranasal sinuses, facial bones, and temporal bone. Additionally, CT is the definitive procedure for detection and confirmation of calcification. It is also important in the bony evaluation of a localized spinal column abnormality (e.g., trauma). Contraindications to CT in childhood are unusual, particularly with the proper application of radiation protection (ALARA standard), the appropriate use of non-ionic contrast agents, the proper administration of sedation or anesthesia, and the use of vital monitoring.

When CT is used, intravenous enhancement for blood pool effect (e.g., CT angiography) or blood–brain barrier disruption is additionally recommended for the evaluation of suspected or known vascular malformation, neoplasm, abscess, or empyema [1–4,28,29]. Enhanced CT may help evaluate a mass or hemorrhage of unknown etiology and identify the membrane of a chronic subdural collection. By identifying the cortical veins, enhanced CT may distinguish prominent low-density subarachnoid collections (benign extracerebral collections or benign external hydrocephalus of infancy) from low-density subdural collections (e.g., chronic subdural hematomas or hygromas). It also may help differentiate infarction from neoplasm or abscess, serve as an indicator of disease activity, for example in degenerative or inflammatory disease and vasculitis, or provide a high-yield guide for stereotactic or open biopsy. Ventricular or subarachnoid CSF-contrast opacification may further assist in evaluating or confirming CSF compartment lesions or communication (e.g., arachnoid cyst or ventricular encystment). As a rule, MRI is the preferred alternative to contrast-enhanced CT in the circumstances just enumerated.

Nuclear Medicine (NM) is primarily a functional imaging technology [1–8]. NM involves imaging of the biological distributions of administered radioactive pharmaceuticals. Whereas positron emission tomography (PET) has the unique ability to provide specific metabolic tracers (e.g., oxygen utilization and glucose metabolism) the wider availability, relative simplicity, and rapid technical advancement of single photon emission computed tomography (SPECT) allows more practical functional assessment of the pediatric CNS. Clinical and investigative applications have included the assessment of brain development and maturation, focus localization in refractory childhood epilepsy (e.g., ictal perfusion SPECT, interictal PET), assessment of tumor progression versus treatment effects in childhood CNS neoplasia (perfusion and thallium SPECT, [18]FDG-PET), the evaluation of occlusive cerebrovascular disease for surgical revascularization (e.g., perfusion SPECT), the diagnosis of brain death (perfusion SPECT), the use of brain activation techniques (e.g., perfusion SPECT, PET) in the elucidation of childhood cognitive disorders, the assessment of CSF kinetics (e.g., in hydrocephalus, CSF leaks), and spinal-column screening (skeletal SPECT) [1–8].

Magnetic resonance imaging (MR, MRI) is both a structural and functional imaging modality [1–12]. MRI uses magnetic fields and radio waves. It is one of the less invasive or relatively non-invasive imaging technologies (Fig. 18.1f–j). Furthermore, the MRI signal is exponentially derived from multiple parameters (e.g., T1, T2, proton density, T2*, proton flow, proton relaxation enhancement, chemical shift, magnetization transfer, and molecular diffusion). MRI also employs many more basic imaging techniques than other modalities (e.g., spin echo, inversion recovery, gradient echo, and chemical shift imaging methods). Advancing MRI capabilities have further improved its sensitivity, specificity, and efficiency [1–12,30]. These include the fluid attenuation inversion recovery technique (FLAIR), fat-suppression short TI inversion recovery imaging (STIR), and magnetization transfer imaging (MTI) for increased structural resolution. Fast and ultrafast MRI techniques (fast spin echo, fast gradient echo, echo planar imaging, parallel imaging) have also been developed to reduce imaging

times, improve structural resolution, and provide functional resolution (e.g., fetal imaging). Important applications include MR vascular imaging (MR angiography and venography, MRA) and perfusion MRI (PMRI), diffusion-weighted imaging (DWI), CSF flow and brain/cord motion imaging, brain activation techniques, and MR spectroscopy (MRS). Fast and ultrafast imaging techniques are also being used for fetal/obstetrical imaging [31–36], morphometrics, treatment planning, and "real-time" MRI-guided surgical and interventional procedures.

The role of MRI in imaging of the developing CNS is defined by its superior sensitivity and specificity in a number of areas as compared to US and CT [1–12,15,19–24,26,28–36]. MRI has also obviated or redefined the roles of invasive procedures (e.g., myelography, ventriculography, cisternography, angiography). MRI provides multiplanar imaging with equivalent resolution in all planes without repositioning the patient. Bone does not interfere with soft-tissue resolution, although metallic objects often produce signal void or field distortion artifacts. Some ferromagnetic or electronic devices (e.g., ferrous aneurysm clips and pacemakers) pose a hazard, and MRI is usually contraindicated in these cases. MRI usually requires longer exam times than does US and CT, and patient sedation or anesthesia is often required in infants and younger children, since image quality is easily compromised by motion. However, MRI may be successfully done in a large percentage of stable neonates and young infants using the "bundle and feed" technique. MRI may not be as readily accessible to the critically ill pediatric patient as is US or CT, and it may not be feasible in emergencies or for intensive care cases unless magnet-compatible vital monitoring and support is available. This is particularly important for the unstable neonate (e.g., using an MRI-compatible incubator) [12] (Fig. 18.2a).

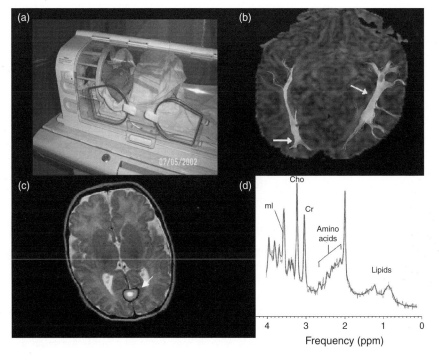

Fig. 18.2. Advanced MRI techniques: (a) MR-compatible incubator; (b) DTI white-matter tractography (arrows); (c) fMRI (primary visual cortex activation: arrow); (d) MR spectroscopy (see text). *See color plate section*. Courtesy of Ashok Panigrahy, MD, Children's Hospital Los Angeles [12].

MRI demonstrates superior sensitivity and specificity in a number of circumstances, particularly with the addition of new structural and functional techniques such as FLAIR, STIR, MTI, DWI, PMRI, and MRS [1–12,15,19–24,26,28–36]. The **FLAIR** sequence attenuates the signal from flowing water (i.e., CSF) and increases the conspicuity of non-fluid-water-containing lesions lying in close approximation to the CSF-filled subarachnoid and ventricular spaces. The **STIR** technique suppresses fat signal to provide improved conspicuity of water-containing lesions in regions where fat dominates (e.g., orbit, head and neck, spine). The **MTI** method suppresses background tissues and increases conspicuity for vascular flow enhancement (e.g., MRA) and gadolinium enhancement.

MRI is the imaging modality of choice in a number of clinical situations [1–12,15,19–24,26,28–36]. These include developmental delay (e.g., static encephalopathy vs. neurodegenerative disease); unexplained seizures (especially focal), unexplained neuroendocrine disorder, or unexplained hydrocephalus; the pretreatment evaluation of neoplastic processes and the follow-up of tumor response and treatment effects; suspected infectious, postinfectious, and other inflammatory or non-inflammatory encephalitides (e.g., encephalitis, postinfectious demyelination, vasculitis); migrational and other submacroscopic dysgeneses (e.g., cortical dysplasia); neurocutaneous syndromes (e.g., neurofibromatosis 1, tuberous sclerosis); intractable or refractory epilepsy; vascular diseases, hemorrhage, and the sequelae of trauma.

MRI frequently offers greater diagnostic specificity than does CT or US for delineating vascular and hemorrhagic processes. This includes the clear depiction of vascular structures and abnormalities based on proton flow parameters and software enhancements not requiring the injection of contrast agents (e.g., MRA). **MR angiography (MRA)** techniques may additionally be used to differentiate arterial from venous occlusive disease [1–12,15,19–24,26,28–36]. Using gradient recalled echo (GRE) magnetic susceptibility techniques, MRI also provides more specific identification and staging of hemorrhage and clot formation according to the evolution of hemoglobin breakdown. MRI is often reserved for more definitive evaluation of hemorrhage and as an indicator or guide for angiography in a number of special situations. MRI may be used to evaluate an atypical or unexplained intracranial hemorrhage by distinguishing hemorrhagic infarction from hematoma and by distinguishing among the types of vascular malformations (e.g., cavernous vs. arteriovenous malformations). MRA may obviate the need in some cases of vascular malformation for conventional angiography in the follow-up of surgery, interventional treatment, or radiosurgery.

In the evaluation of intracranial vascular anomalies (e.g., vascular malformation, aneurysm), MRI may identify otherwise unsuspected prior hemorrhage (i.e., hemosiderin) [1–12,15,19–24,26,28–36]. When CT demonstrates a non-specific focal high density (calcification vs. hemorrhage), MRI may provide further specificity, for example, by distinguishing an occult vascular malformation (e.g., cavernous malformation) from a neoplasm (e.g., glioma). It may further assist US or CT in differentiating benign infantile collections (i.e., external hydrocephalus) from subdural hematomas [28,29]. MRI often also provides definitive evaluation of muscular and cutaneous vascular anomalies (i.e., hemangiomas, vascular malformations) that arise in parameningeal locations (e.g., head and neck, paraspinal) and extend to involve the CNS directly or are associated with other CNS vascular or non-vascular abnormalities.

MR spectroscopy (MRS) offers a non-invasive in vivo approach to biochemical analysis [1–12,37–40] (Fig. 18.2d). Furthermore, MRS provides additional quantitative information regarding cellular metabolites, since signal intensity is linearly related to steady-state metabolite concentration. MRS can detect cellular biochemical changes prior to the detection of morphological changes by MRI or other imaging modalities. MRS may therefore provide further insight into both follow-up assessment and prognosis. With recent advances in instrumentation and methodology, and utilizing the high inherent sensitivity of hydrogen 1, single-voxel and multivoxel proton MRS is now carried out with relatively short acquisitions to detect low-concentration metabolites in healthy and diseased tissues. Phosphorus-31 spectroscopy has also been developed for pediatric use. Currently, MRS has been primarily used in the assessment of brain development and maturation (Fig. 18.3), perinatal brain injury, childhood CNS neoplasia versus treatment effects, and metabolic and neurodegenerative disorders [39–40].

Perfusion MRI (PMRI) has been developed to evaluate cerebral perfusion dynamics through the application of a dynamic contrast-enhanced T2*-weighted MR imaging technique [1–4,8,12,31,41]. This technique has been used to qualitate and quantitate normal and abnormal cerebrovascular dynamics of the developing brain by analyzing hemodynamic parameters including relative cerebral blood volume, relative cerebral blood flow, and mean transit time, all as complementary to conventional MR imaging. Non-contrast-enhanced methods of PMRI have also been developed (e.g., flow-activated inversion recovery, FAIR; arterial spin labeling, ASL; blood oxygen level determination, BOLD) [41]. Current and advanced applications of these perfusion techniques include the evaluation of ischemic cerebrovascular disease (e.g., hypoxia–ischemia, moyamoya, sickle cell disease), the differentiation of tumor progression from treatment effects, and brain activation imaging [1–4,8,12,31,41]. One of the most active areas of research is the localization of brain activity, an area previously dominated by NM including SPECT and PET.

Functional MRI (fMRI) is the terminology often applied to brain activation imaging in which local or regional changes in cerebral blood flow are displayed that accompany stimulation or activation of sensory (e.g., visual, auditory, somatosensory), motor, or cognitive centers [1–4,12]. fMRI is providing important information regarding the spatial distribution of sensory, motor, and cognitive function and functional impairment (Fig. 18.2c). Also, it may serve as a guide for safer and

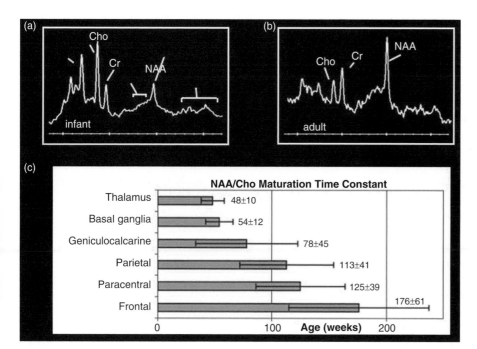

Fig. 18.3. H-1 MR spectroscopy of the developing brain with (a) infant spectra, (b) adult spectra, and (c) maturation time constants for brain regions. Dermon J, Barnes PD, Spielman D. Spatiotemporal mapping of cerebral maturation in childhood using 2D MR spectroscopic imaging. American Society of Neuroradiology, 2002.

more effective interventions including microneurosurgery or conformal radiotherapy, for example in the ablation of tumors, vascular malformations, and seizure foci. More recently, fMRI is being used to evaluate brain development and maturation in the neonate and young infant, including the effects of injury and post-injury repair and recovery [12].

Using echo planar or line-scan spin echo techniques, **diffusion-weighted imaging (DWI)** provides information based upon differences in the rate of diffusion of water molecules, and it is especially sensitive to cellular changes [1–12,30,40,42–53]. The rate of diffusion, or apparent diffusion coefficient (ADC), is higher for free or pure water than for macromolecular bound water. The ADC varies according to the microstructural or physiologic state of a tissue. Fractional anisotropy (FA) is a vector measurement of the directionality of diffusion using **diffusion tensor imaging** (**DTI**) methods and also varies with the microstructural environment, both developmentally and pathologically [53] (Fig. 18.2b). This method is especially helpful in assessing axonal development and injury, including myelination and synaptogenesis (connectivity). Current clinical applications of DWI and DTI include the assessment of brain maturation, the evaluation of acute injury, and the analysis of the sequelae of injury (Fig. 18.4). A particularly important application of DWI is in the early detection of diffuse and focal ischemic injury. The ADC of water is reduced within minutes of an ischemic insult and progressively so within the first hour. High-intensity abnormalities are demonstrated on DWI, along with low-intensity abnormalities on calculated ADC images, at a time when conventional MRI is negative, and this likely reflects cellular injury (e.g., necrosis) with primary or secondary energy failure. Further investigations are under way regarding the roles

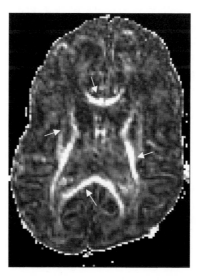

Fig. 18.4. DTI with FA map in preterm neonate as a quantitative display of white-matter development (arrows) of the internal capsule and corpus callosum [12].

of DWI, PMRI, and MRS in the early diagnosis and treatment of potentially reversible ischemic injury.

Motion-sensitive MRI techniques are not only used to evaluate vascular flow (e.g., MRA) and perfusion, but may also be used to demonstrate the effect of pulsatile cardiovascular flow on other fluid tissues (e.g., CSF) and on non-fluid tissues such as the brain and spinal cord. Using cardiac or pulse gating, these MRI techniques may be used to evaluate, preoperatively and postoperatively, abnormalities of CSF dynamics (e.g., hydrocephalus, hydrosyringomyelia), as well as abnormalities of brain motion (e.g., Chiari malformation), and spinal cord motion (e.g., tethered cord syndrome) [1–4]. A number of non-gated MRI techniques (e.g., propeller imaging) are also being used to reduce motion artifact and improve image quality.

Guidelines and principles of imaging diagnosis

Developmental abnormalities

Congenital abnormalities of the CNS may be developmental or acquired in origin, and may result from defective formation, postformational destruction, or disordered maturation [1,2,4,5,54]. These are probably best classified according to gestational timing (Table 18.1), and include disorders of dorsal and ventral neural tube formation; disorders of neuronal, glial, and mesenchymal formation; neuroclastic processes (encephaloclastic, myeloclastic); and disorders of maturation (myelination and cortical maturation). These are classified in six groups (I–VI) in Table 18.1. Developmental anomalies often detected by US (prenatal or postnatal) or CT are the *gross* formational macrostructural defects of categories I–IV and the *gross* neuroclastic macrostructural lesions of category V [1,2,4,5,54]. However, MRI always provides more complete delineation of these defects. This is especially true for those abnormalities involving the ventricular system or containing CSF. These include cephaloceles (Fig. 18.5), hydrocephalus, hydranencephaly, holoprosencephaly, absent septum pellucidum, hypogenesis of the corpus callosum (Figs. 18.5–18.7), porencephaly, open schizencephaly, the Dandy–Walker–Blake spectrum (Fig. 18.7), and arachnoid cysts. US may not clearly distinguish hydranencephaly (absent cerebral mantle) from severe hydrocephalus (attenuated cerebral mantle). This is usually clarified by CT or MRI (Fig. 18.8). Other gross macrostructural anomalies often detected by US or CT include Chiari II malformation, lissencephaly, and vascular malformations such as the Galenic malformation. Any "cystic" lesion detected by US should be examined with Doppler to determine if it is vascular in nature. Neuroclastic processes are destructive lesions of the already formed CNS and may result from a variety of prenatal or perinatal insults including hypoxia–ischemia and infection (Table 18.1). MRI may often demonstrate subtle macrostructural abnormalities not revealed by US or CT (e.g., periventricular leukomalacia) [1–12,15,17,19–24,26,33].

MRI is important when the US or CT fails to satisfy the clinical investigation. MRI often provides a more complete delineation of complex macrostructural CNS anomalies for diagnosis, treatment, prognosis, and genetic counseling [1,2,4,5,33,54]. In fact, ultrafast MRI techniques are being increasingly used prenatally to evaluate for fetal CNS abnormalities in at-risk pregnancies or as detected by obstetrical US [31–36] (Figs. 18.5–18.7). Furthermore, MRI is often indicated if more specific treatment is planned beyond simple shunting of hydrocephalus. Intraoperative guidance may be provided by real-time and Doppler US. Patients with craniosynostosis are best evaluated with 3DCT. Those with multiple suture involvement, especially when it is associated with craniofacial syndromes, may require more extensive evaluation beyond 3DCT, including CT venography, MRI, and MR venography (jugular venous steno-occlusive disease with collateralization).

MRI is often required to structurally delineate the more subtle macrostructural anomalies arising as disorders of

Table 18.1. Classification of CNS malformations by gestational timing

I. Disorders of dorsal neural tube development (3–4 weeks)

Anencephaly

Cephaloceles

Dermal sinus

Chiari malformations

Spinal dysraphism

Hydrosyringomyelia

II. Disorders of ventral neural tube development (5–10 weeks)

Holoprosencephalies

Agenesis septum pellucidum

Optic and olfactory hypoplasia/aplasia

Pituitary – hypothalamic hypoplasia/aplasia

Cerebellar hypoplasia/aplasia

Dandy Walker spectrum

Craniosynostosis

III. Disorders of migration and cortical organization (2–5 months)

Schizencephaly

Neuronal heterotopia

Agyria/pachygyria

Lissencephaly

Polymicrogyria

Agenesis corpus callosum

IV. Disorders of neuronal, glial, and mesenchymal proliferation, differentiation, and histiogenesis (2–6 months)

Micrencephaly

Megalencephaly

Hemimegalencephaly

Aqueductal anomalies

Colpocephaly

Cortical dysplasias

Neurocutaneous syndromes

Vascular anomalies

Malformative tumors

Arachnoid cysts

V. Encephaloclastic processes (> 5–6 months)

Hydranencephaly

Porencephaly

Multicystic encephalopathy

Encephalomalacia

Leukomalacia

Hemiatrophy

Hydrocephalus

Hemorrhage

Infarction

VI. Disorders of maturation (7 months – 2 years)

Hypomyelination

Delayed myelination

Dysmyelination

Demyelination

Cortical dysmaturity

Note:
See references [2,4,54].

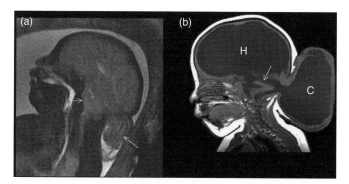

Fig. 18.5. (a) Fetal sagittal T2 MRI, showing cervico-occipital cephalocele (posterior arrow), Chiari III malformation (anterior arrow), agenesis of the corpus callosum, and microcephaly. (b) Neonatal sagittal T1 MRI, showing occipital meningoencephalocele (C) with kinked brainstem (arrow) and hydrocephalus (H).

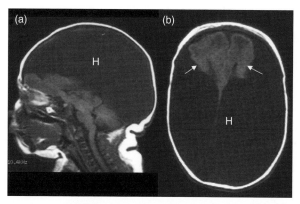

Fig. 18.8. Hydranencephaly on (a) sagittal and (b) axial T1 MRI. Only a small portion of cortex is present frontally (arrows).

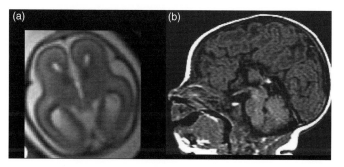

Fig. 18.6. Agenesis corpus callosum on (a) fetal axial T2 and (b) neonatal sagittal T1 MRI (see Fig. 18.1. f,g) [50].

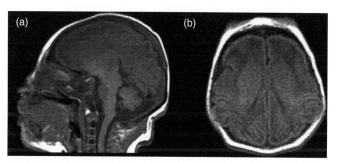

Fig. 18.9. Microlissencephaly: neonatal (a) sagittal and (b) axial T1 MRI, showing microcephaly with agyric cortex.

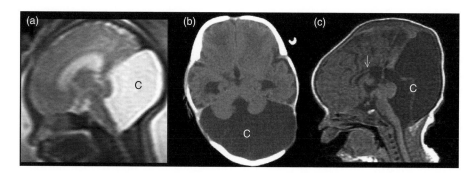

Fig. 18.7. Dandy–Walker cyst (C): (a) fetal sagittal T2 MRI; (b) neonatal axial CT; (c) sagittal T1 MRI with hypogenesis of the corpus callosum (arrow).

migration and cortical organization (category III: Fig. 18.9) or as disorders of proliferation, differentiation, and histiogenesis (category IV: Fig. 18.10) [1,2,4,5,33,54]. The perfusional and metabolic characteristics of these anomalies (e.g., focal cortical dysgenesis, hemimegalencephaly) may be investigated with SPECT and PET, respectively, in children with medically refractory partial epilepsy who are candidates for surgical ablation. For added precision, the SPECT or PET data may be fused with the MRI data to provide a higher-resolution spatial display of the functional information. MRS, DWI, DTI, and PMRI with fMRI are also contributing to the evaluation and treatment of these patients [4,12,30]. MRI is now the preferred modality for the screening and definitive evaluation

of the dysgenetic, neoplastic, and vascular manifestations of the neurocutaneous syndromes (Fig. 18.11). After initial screening with US or CT, MRI is also considered the primary technology for treatment planning and follow-up of vascular malformations and developmental tumors [1,2,4,30]. Although arachnoid cysts are often readily delineated by US or CT, MRI is usually necessary for confirmation (i.e., to exclude solid tumor) and for surgical planning. FLAIR or DWI may readily distinguish an arachnoid cyst from other lesions (e.g., dermoid–epidermoid, fibrillary astrocytoma). Maturation (i.e., myelination and cortical maturation) and disorders of maturation (category VI) may be precisely assessed only by MRI [1,2,4,5,30,33,54] (Fig. 18.1f–j). The MRI findings,

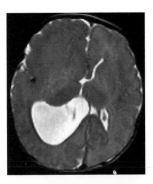

Fig. 18.10. Hemimegalencephaly: neonatal axial T2 MRI shows larger right hemisphere with unilateral ventriculomegaly and abnormal cortication.

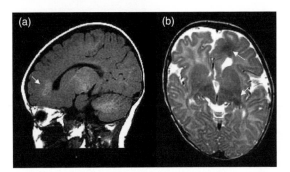

Fig. 18.11. Tuberous sclerosis with periventricular and subcortical tubers (arrows) on (a) neonatal sagittal T1 and (b) axial T2 MRI.

Table 18.2. Imaging patterns of hypoxic–ischemic encephalopathy (HIE)

Hemorrhage
Germinal matrix – intraventricular hemorrhage
Choroid plexus – intraventricular hemorrhage
Subarachnoid hemorrhage
Hemorrhagic infarctions
Partial prolonged HIE
Preterm: White-matter injury of prematurity (e.g., periventricular leukomalacia)
Term/full-term/post-term: Cortical/subcortical injury (borderzone, watershed, parasagittal)
Intermediate: combined or transitional pattern
Ulegyria
Cystic encephalomalacia
Profound HIE
Thalamic and basal ganglia injury
Brainstem injury
Cerebellar vermian injury
Hippocampal injury
Cerebral white-matter injury
Paracentral injury
Global injury (prolonged profound)
Combined profound and partial prolonged (or prolonged profound) HIE
Total asphyxia pattern (including cystic encephalomalacia)

Notes:
Depends on gestational age, chronological age, duration and severity of the insult.
See references [2–8].

however, are often non-specific regarding causation, particularly in the first year of life, because of the watery character of the immature brain. DTI and MRS may add specificity to the diagnostic evaluation of these infants [1–12,37–40] (Figs. 18.2–18.4).

Neurovascular disease

Neurovascular disease characteristically presents as an acute neurologic event (e.g., neonatal encephalopathy). However, a recently discovered but fixed deficit (e.g., hemiplegia, spastic diplegia, hypotonia) may be the first indication of a remote prenatal or perinatal neurovascular injury. Imaging assists in the clinical evaluation and differentiation of hypoxia–ischemia, hemorrhage, and occlusive vascular disease [1–12,30].

Hypoxia–ischemia

In general, the pattern of injury associated with hypoxic–ischemic encephalopathy (HIE), or other insults (e.g., reperfusion), varies with the severity and duration of the insult as well as with the gestational (or corrected) age (GA) of the fetus, neonate, or infant at the time of the insult or insults [1–12] (Table 18.2). Different brain structures are more vulnerable than others to the different types of HIE insults (e.g., partial prolonged, profound, combined) at different stages of brain development (e.g., formational vs. postformational GA, preterm vs. term vs. full-term or post-term GA). Brain tissues in the arterial border zones or watersheds (intervascular boundary zones), brain tissues with high metabolic demands, mature or actively maturing tissues, and tissues with higher concentrations of neuroexcitatory amino acids are particularly vulnerable to HIE and to other insults (e.g., hypoglycemia,

trauma, infection, seizures) [1–12,55–61]. Prenatal or perinatal partial prolonged HIE (e.g., one or more insults of hypoxia/hypoperfusion) may be associated with periventricular borderzone/watershed injury to the preterm fetus or neonate (e.g., 27–35 weeks GA) [1–12,55,57,62–75]. Subtypes of white-matter injury of prematurity (i.e., "encephalopathy of prematurity") include the classic focal/multifocal "cystic" type of periventricular leukomalacia (PVL), the focal/multifocal "noncystic" (gliotic) form of PVL, and the diffuse white-matter gliosis injury pattern (Figs. 18.12–18.15). The pathogenesis may include not only hypoxia–ischemia but other factors such as infectious or inflammatory processes (e.g., maternal infection, chorioamnionitis, funisitis, fetal inflammatory response, cytokine-mediated injury) whether occurring in the preterm, or term, fetus or neonate [7,66,70]. Prenatal or perinatal partial prolonged HIE during term gestation (e.g., 37–42 weeks GA) may produce a cortical and subcortical border-zone/watershed cerebral injury (Figs. 18.16, 18.17). A transitional partial prolonged HIE pattern (cortical/subcortical/periventricular) may be seen in the late preterm to early mid-term GA (e.g., 36–38 weeks) or with more severe injuries. Fetal or neonatal brain injury may also occur with more profound HIE insults (e.g., anoxia or circulatory arrest) and involve the thalami, basal ganglia (especially putamina), brainstem (especially midbrain), cerebellar vermis,

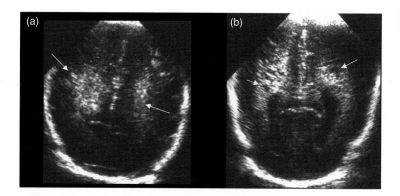

Fig. 18.12. Cystic PVL: (a) US, acute edema phase (confluent increased echoes – arrows); (b) US, subacute cystic phase (hypoechoic foci with surrounding increased echoes – arrows).

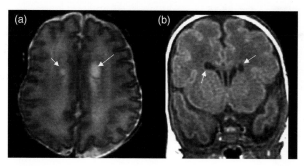

Fig. 18.13. Cystic PVL: (a) axial T2 and (b) coronal FLAIR MRI, chronic cystic phase (arrows).

hippocampi, paraventricular white matter, and perirolandic cortex [1–12,55,57,76–80] (Figs. 18.18, 18.19). This type of injury may also vary with GA (thalamic greater than putaminal involvement in the preterm GA; putaminal, hippocampal, and paracentral injury more common in the term GA). Combined partial prolonged plus profound HIE patterns (e.g., total asphyxia) may also occur [1–12,76–80] (Fig. 18.20).

US, CT, or MRI (e.g., DWI) may demonstrate evolving edema, necrosis, or hemorrhage in the hyperacute, acute, and subacute phases [1–12] (Figs. 18.12–18.20). The edema of non-hemorrhagic HIE (e.g., partial prolonged type) usually evolves over 1–7 days and often peaks between 36 and 72 hours (2–4 days by US, CT) following the insult(s) and depending upon reperfusion (and other "insults"). US may show hyperechogenicity, and CT may show hypodensities with decreased gray–white matter differentiation. Complete loss of gray–white differentiation may correlate with peak edema [60,61]. In the early phases of the injury, the neuroimaging findings may be non-specific as to causation. The differential diagnosis

includes HIE, multifocal occlusive vascular infarction, infection, metabolic derangement (e.g., hypoglycemia, hyperbilirubinemia, fluid-electrolyte imbalance), metabolic or connective tissue disorder, and venous thrombosis (e.g., coagulopathy) [1–12]. Associated hemorrhage may be subarachnoid, germinal matrix and intraventricular hemorrhage (e.g., preterm fetus or neonate), choroid plexus/intraventricular hemorrhage (e.g., term fetus or neonate), and cerebral or cerebellar hemorrhage (e.g., hemorrhagic infarction). Their imaging characteristics are described in the next section.

According to the evidence-based medical literature, the sensitivity and specificity of MRI depends on the techniques used and the timing of the imaging [2,4,6,40,45,78]. Conventional MRI may show characteristic T1 hypointensities/ T2 hyperintensities (12–48 hours), followed by T1 hyperintensities (as early as 2–4 days), and then T2 hypointensities (as early as 6–7 days). These T1 and T2 changes may last for a number of weeks to a month. DWI may be abnormal before conventional MRI and show restricted diffusion with decreased ADC as increased intensity on DWI and decreased intensity on ADC maps [2,8,40,45]. Diffusion abnormalities may tend to evolve for up to 2–3 weeks. Knowledge of these evolving intensity features is particularly important in order to avoid misinterpretation regarding pattern of injury and timing [40]. Doppler with resistive indices (e.g., RI < 60) or MRS (e.g., elevated lactate, elevated glutamate, elevated lipids, decreased N-acetyl-aspartate [NAA]) may provide additional early indicators of timing and outcome [2,6,8,14,37,40,81]. The more subtle ischemic PVL lesions (e.g., cystic phase) may be better delineated by US (2–6 weeks after insult(s)) than by CT or MRI, in which the density and intensity character of immature

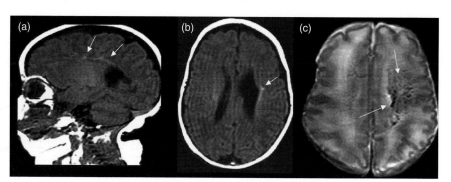

Fig. 18.14. Non-cystic PVL with foci of gliosis (arrows) as high intensities on (a) sagittal and (b) axial T1 MRI, plus mineralization or hemorrhages (arrows) as low intensities on (c) axial GRE MRI.

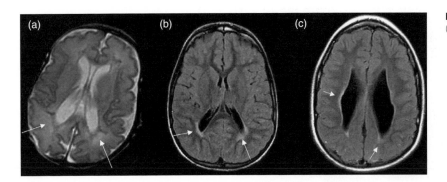

Fig. 18.15. Diffuse PVL (high intensities – arrows) on (a) near-term axial T2 and (b,c) older infant axial FLAIR MRI.

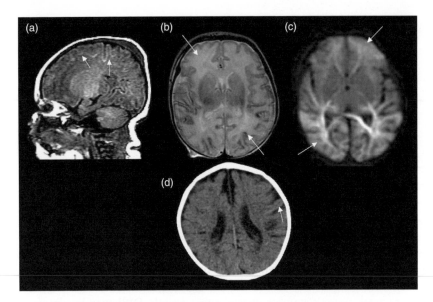

Fig. 18.16. Partial prolonged HIE: acute phase with watershed injury (arrows) on (a) sagittal T1, (b) axial T2, and (c) axial DWI; (d) chronic phase with cortical atrophy and ulegyria (arrow) on axial CT.

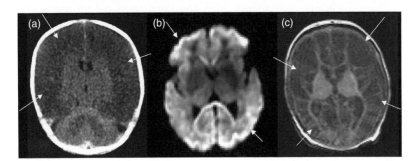

Fig. 18.17. Very severe partial prolonged HIE: acute–subacute phase with (a) low-density cerebral peak edema (arrows) on axial CT and (b) high-intensity cerebral restricted diffusion (arrows) on axial DWI; (c) chronic phase with cystic encephalomalacia (arrows) on axial T1.

white matter often obscures the injury. However, CT and MRI often show gray-matter injury better than US, and MRI demonstrates non-cystic white-matter injury better than US or CT [4,8,19–24,26]. Further developments of PMRI, DWI, and MRS have further improved the diagnostic sensitivity and specificity of MRI [4,8,12,30,40]. In fact, DWI has demonstrated restricted diffusion in the acute phase of PVL when US, CT, and conventional MRI are negative or non-specific. Such advances may facilitate the early institution of neuroprotective measures to treat potentially reversible primary injury (necrosis, apoptosis) and secondary injury (reperfusion, transneural degeneration) in HIE [82]. These advanced MRI techniques may also assist in distinguishing HIE from other causes of

encephalopathy, including common metabolic derangements (e.g., hypoglycemia, hyperbilirubinemia), rarer inborn errors of metabolism, and non-metabolic conditions (e.g., infection).

The long-term result of HIE is a static encephalopathy (i.e., CP) and imaging may demonstrate injury in the chronic phases (> 14–21 days after the insult(s)) including porencephaly, hydranencephaly, atrophy, chronic periventricular leukomalacia, cystic encephalomalacia, gliosis, or mineralization in a characteristic distribution as described above [1–12] (Figs. 18.12–18.20). The chronic changes are best demonstrated by MRI. In general, for pattern of injury and timing purposes, two pieces of imaging evidence are optimally desired: (1) late imaging, and preferably MRI, beyond 2–3 years of age

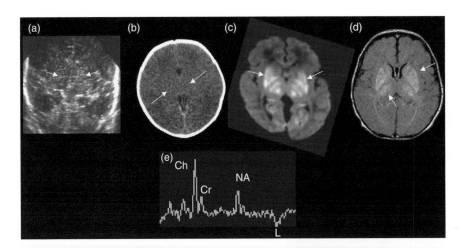

Fig. 18.18. Profound HIE: acute phase with (a) bilateral basal ganglia and thalamic hyperechogenicity (arrows) on US; (b) hypodensities (arrows) on CT; high intensities (arrows) on (c) axial DWI and (d) T1/FLAIR MRI; and (e) inverted lactate doublet (L) on MRS.

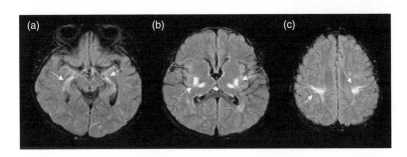

Fig. 18.19. Profound HIE: chronic phase with (a–c) bilateral hippocampal, putaminal, thalamic, and paracentral high intensities (arrows) on axial FLAIR MRI.

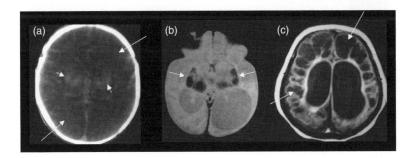

Fig. 18.20. Term combined HIE: subacute phase with (a) basal ganglia and thalamic high densities (short arrows) plus cerebral low densities (long arrows) on CT; chronic phase with (b) basal ganglia and thalamic hypointense mineralization (arrows) on axial GRE plus (c) hypointense cystic encephalomalacia (arrows) on axial T1 MRI.

when the brain is greater than 90% mature (no more water of immaturity), in order to get a final, permanent injury pattern for causative etiology and GA timing; and (2) early postnatal (and/or prenatal) imaging, and preferably MRI, in order to evaluate evolution in the acute, subacute, and chronic phases, so that timing as to "day range" relative to the perinatal and peripartum periods may be assessed [1–12,40].

Intracranial hemorrhage

Intracranial hemorrhage may result from parturitional trauma, HIE, a coagulopathy (e.g., thrombocytopenia, disseminated intravascular coagulopathy [DIC], extracorporal membrane oxygenation [ECMO]), vasoocclusive disease (e.g., thrombophilia with venous thrombosis), or it may be idiopathic [1–12,28,29,83]. Hemorrhage may occasionally be associated with infection (e.g., herpes simplex virus 2). Vascular malformations producing intracranial hemorrhage are rare in the neonate and young infant and usually not encountered until later childhood (i.e., arteriovenous malformations [AVM],

cavernous malformations, developmental venous anomalies, and telangiectasias) [1–12,28,29]. Aneurysms are exceedingly rare in children but may be developmental, associated with a syndrome (e.g., Turner syndrome), or related to trauma (e.g., dissection) or infection (i.e., mycotic aneurysm). The vein of Galen malformations are subclassified as choroidal, mural, and AVM types. They rarely hemorrhage, and more commonly present in infancy with congestive heart failure, cerebral ischemia, or hydrocephalus.

US or CT remains the primary imaging choice in acute situations [1–12,29]. As mentioned above, there may be subarachnoid hemorrhage, germinal matrix and intraventricular hemorrhage (e.g., premature fetus or neonate), choroid plexus/intraventricular hemorrhage (e.g., term fetus or neonate), and cerebral or cerebellar hemorrhage (e.g., hemorrhagic infarction). The hemorrhage usually appears hyperechoic on US and high-density on CT in the acute to subacute phases (range 3 hours – 7 days) unless there is associated coagulopathy. With evolution and resolution, the hemorrhage

Table 18.3. MRI of intracranial hemorrhage and thrombosis

Stage	Biochemical form	Site	T1 MRI	T2 MRI
Hyperacute (+ edema) [< 12 hours]	Fe II oxy Hb	Intact RBCs	Isointense–Low i	High i
Acute (+ edema) [1–3 days]	Fe II deoxy Hb	Intact RBCs	Isointense–Low i	Low i
Early subacute (+ edema) [3–7 days]	Fe III met Hb	Intact RBCs	High i	Low i
Late subacute (− edema) [1–2 weeks]	Fe III met Hb	Lysed RBCs (extracellular)	High i	High i
Early chronic (− edema) [> 2 weeks]	Fe III transferrin	Extracellular	High i	High i
Chronic (cavity)	Fe III ferritin and hemosiderin	Phagocytosis	Isointense–Low i	Low i

Notes:
RBCs, red blood cells; +, present; −, absent; Hb, hemoglobin; Fe II, ferrous; Fe III, ferric.
See references [2,4,29,84,98].

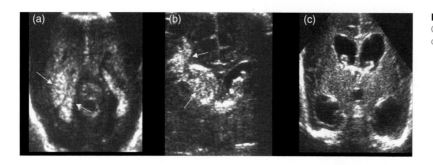

Fig. 18.21. (a) Hyperechoic grade III and (b) grade IV GMH–IVH (arrows), and (c) posthemorrhagic hydrocephalus on coronal US.

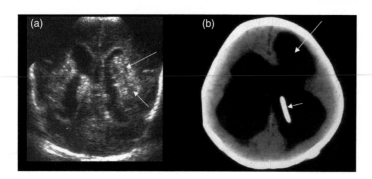

Fig. 18.22. (a) Hyperechoic grade IV IVH with periventricular hemorrhagic infarction (arrows) on coronal US; (b) posthemorrhagic hydrocephalus with porencephaly (long arrow) on axial CT with shunt catheter (short arrow).

becomes isoechoic to hypoechoic and isodense to hypodense (> 7–10 days).

MRI may offer more specific characterization of the hemorrhagic component with regard to timing (Table 18.3). Acute intracranial hemorrhage, particularly subarachnoid, may be specifically diagnosed by CT or lumbar puncture for CSF analysis. Although FLAIR may identify subarachnoid hemorrhage as hyperintensity and GRE may identify acute hemorrhage in any location as hypointensity, MRI often provides better specificity beyond the acute phases [2,4,29,84] (Table 18.3). Hemorrhagic manifestations and sequelae of HIE in the premature infant readily detected by US include germinal matrix hemorrhage (GMH grades I–IV), intraventricular hemorrhage (IVH), periventricular hemorrhagic infarction (a.k.a. grade IV), and posthemorrhagic hydrocephalus [1–13,25] (Figs. 18.21, 18.22). Choroid plexus hemorrhage and hemorrhagic infarction in the term infant are also easily demonstrated. Portable US may effectively delineate the potential hemorrhagic or ischemic sequelae of ECMO.

Although CT has been more reliable, high-resolution US using transfontanel and transcranial approaches, including the mastoid view, may detect extracerebral hemorrhage (subdural and subarachnoid) and posterior fossa collections (cerebellar or subdural) [1–13,25]. Color Doppler US, MRA, and CTA are all able to identify and distinguish the types of Galenic malformations, and provide follow-up (Fig. 18.23). Angiography is more specifically directed to the definitive interventional or surgical management of these and other vascular anomalies. Real-time Doppler US provides intraprocedural guidance and monitoring. The long-term sequelae of intracranial hemorrhage are often better demonstrated by MRI than by CT (e.g., hydrocephalus, atrophy, encephalomalacia, porencephaly, calcification, hemosiderin).

Occlusive neurovascular disease and sequelae
Occlusive neurovascular disease in the fetus, newborn, and infant may be arterial or venous in origin, and typically results in focal or multifocal lesions within the distribution of the

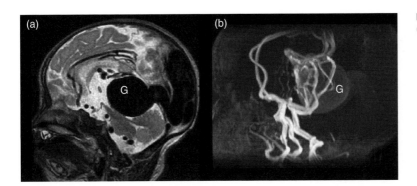

Fig. 18.23. Vein of Galen (G) vascular malformation (choroidal type) on (a) sagittal T2 and (b) lateral MRA.

Table 18.4. Occlusive neurovascular disease in the fetus, neonate, and infant

Idiopathic
Cardiac disease
Congenital
Acquired
Vascular maldevelopment
Atresia
Hypoplasia
Traumatic
Dissection
Vascular distortion
Air or fat emboli
Vasculopathy
Moyomoya
Fibromuscular dysplasia
Marfan syndrome
Takayasu arteritis
Kawasaki disease
Vasculitis
Polyarteritis nodosa
Lupus
Vasospasm
Migraine
Ergot poisoning
Subarachnoid hemorrhage
Drugs
Cocaine
Amphetamines
l-asparaginase
Oral contraceptives
Hypercoagulopathy (thrombophilias)
Protein S deficiency
Protein C deficiency
Antithrombin III deficiency
Factor V (Leiden) & prothrombin mutations
Antiphospholipid antibody (lupus, anticardiolipin)
Heparin cofactor II deficiency
Dehydration/hypernatremia
HIE/DIC
Sepsis/DIC
Polycythemia/hyperviscosity
Nephrotic syndrome
Oncologic disease
Hemolytic uremic syndrome
Hemoglobinopathies
Sickle cell disease
Infection
Meningoencephalitis
Sepsis
Metabolic disease
Homocystinuria
Dyslipoproteinemia
Fabry disease
Mitochondrial cytopathies
Familial lipid disorders
Other
Emboli from involuting fetal vasculature
Placental vascular anastomoses (twin gestation)
Co-twin fetal death
Fetofetal transfusion
ECMO
Catheterized vessel

Note:
See references [2–5,90].

occluded vessel or vessels [1–12] (Table 18.4). Arterial occlusive disease may be partial or complete, and may be due to embolization, thrombosis, or stenosis. The result may be ischemic infarction or hemorrhagic infarction followed by atrophy. Arterial occlusive disease may occur as a prenatal or perinatal event (emboli of placental origin, fetal heart, or involuting fetal vessels), as a complication of infection (e.g., meningitis), with congenital heart disease, or from a hypercoagulopathy (thrombophilias, prothrombotic disorders) [85–93]. The thrombophilias may be genetic or acquired,

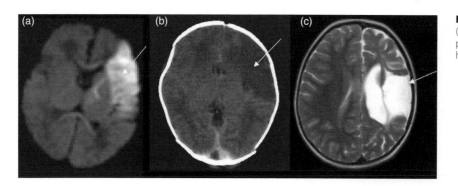

Fig. 18.24. Middle cerebal arterial infarction (arrows): (a) acute phase with edema on axial DWI; (b) subacute phase on CT; (c) chronic phase on axial T2 with hemiatrophy.

and include protein C and S deficiencies, activated protein C resistance, antiphospholipid antibody (lupus, anticardiolipin), antithrombin III deficiency, factor V Leiden, prothrombin gene mutation, methylene tetrahydrofolate reductase (MTHFR), homocysteine, factors VIII/IX/XI, anemia, polycythemia, and others. These are risk factors that are often provoked by "triggers" that may include acute systemic disease (e.g., dehydration, infection, trauma, hypoxia–ischemia) and chronic systemic disease (e.g., hematologic disorders, connective tissue disorders, lupus) [90]. Other causes include trauma (e.g., dissection), arteriopathies (e.g., moyamoya), and metabolic disorders (e.g., mitochondrial cytopathies). Conditions commonly associated with cortical or dural venous sinus occlusive disease include infection, dehydration, perinatal encephalopathy, cyanotic congenital heart disease, polycythemia, other hypercoagulable states, DIC, and trauma [1–12,85–94]. Color Doppler US may be used as a non-invasive tool for initial identification and monitoring of these infants. MRI is more sensitive and specific than US or CT for ischemic infarction, hemorrhagic infarction, and venous thrombosis [2–5,7,12,30,88,90] (Figs. 18.24, 18.25). MRA or CTA may also contribute to the diagnosis of arterial or venous occlusion and clarify (or obviate) the need for cerebral angiography, particularly when anticoagulation or thrombolysis is being considered. As mentioned earlier, PMRI, DWI, and MRS are contributing to the early diagnosis and timely treatment of ischemic insults. The long-term sequelae of infarction include atrophy, encephalomalacia, gliosis, mineralization, and porencephaly. These may be better shown by MRI than by CT.

Acute myelopathy due to HIE, vascular occlusion, hemorrhage, or vascular malformation is extremely rare in the perinatal period. Spinal MRI is the definitive procedure to evaluate spinal cord infarction or hemorrhage (see section on trauma, below). Spinal angiography is necessary to evaluate for vascular malformation in anticipation of interventional or surgical therapy [2,4].

Trauma

With improvements in resolution and the use of additional views (e.g., mastoid view), US may be used as the primary modality for evaluating the newborn with parturitional trauma. CT, however, is usually relied upon for delineating skull and scalp injury (e.g., subgaleal hematoma: Fig. 18.26), extracerebral hemorrhage (e.g., subarachnoid or subdural),

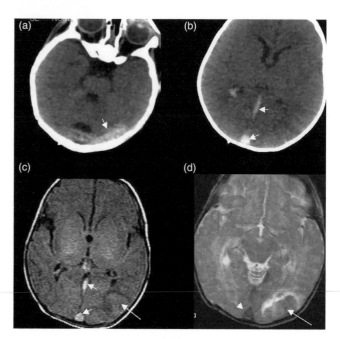

Fig. 18.25. Venous thromboses (short arrows) with hemorrhages and infarctions (long arrows) on (a,b) axial CT, (c) axial T1, (d) axial GRE in infant with hypercoagulable state.

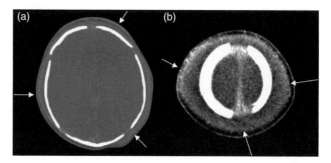

Fig. 18.26. Large bilateral subgaleal hematomas (arrows) on CT with (a) bone and (b) soft tissue algorithms.

posterior fossa hemorrhage, and direct (e.g., contusion, shear) versus indirect (e.g., HIE) brain injury [1–12,29,94–100]. CT is sufficiently sensitive and specific for acute hemorrhage and the complications or sequelae of fractures (e.g., depression, growing fracture, leptomeningeal cyst) (Fig. 18.27). Occasionally, skull films will demonstrate a skull fracture not shown by CT. It may occasionally be difficult to distinguish fracture

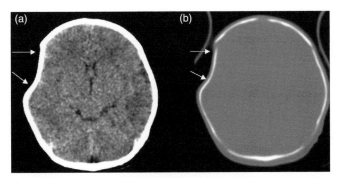

Fig. 18.27. Right frontal cranial depression (arrows) on CT with (a) soft tissue and (b) bone algorithms.

from sutures, synchondroses, and their variants or anomalies (e.g., fissures, accessory sutures, intrasutural bones). MDCT with 3D surface reconstructions may possibly be needed. MRI is probably necessary when neurologic deficits are present and the CT is negative or non-specific. In this situation MRI may reveal lesions such as brainstem infarction, traumatic axonal (shear) injury, and cortical contusion, or sequelae such as gliosis, microcystic encephalomalacia, and hemosiderin deposition. MRI is often more specific than CT for hemorrhage beyond the hyperacute/acute stage (Table 18.3). Color Doppler US, contrast-enhanced CT, or MRI may distinguish external hydrocephalus (dilated subarachnoid spaces) from chronic subdural hematomas (e.g., child abuse and its mimics) when non-enhanced CT demonstrates non-specific extracerebral collections [29]. Furthermore, hemosiderin as demonstrated by MRI is confirmation of a previous hemorrhage. In children with atypical intracranial hemorrhage on CT (e.g., hemorrhage out of proportion to the history of trauma, hemorrhage of varying age), MRI may show an existing vascular malformation, a hemorrhagic neoplasm, or other findings indicating the need for distinguishing child abuse from its mimics [29].

Initial evaluation of spine trauma (e.g., fracture/dislocation) may include plain films or US, but MDCT (including 2D reformatting and 3D surface reconstructions) is preferred. Abnormality on preliminary imaging, changing clinical signs, or unexplained brain injury may provide the indication for spinal MRI [2,4,29], including a STIR sequence. An existing spinal anomaly or mass should be ruled out. MRI is the procedure of choice to fully evaluate acute spinal injury (e.g., intraspinal hemorrhage, cord contusion, cord edema, transection, brachial plexus injury, ligamentous injury), and the sequelae of spinal injury (e.g., hydrosyringomyelia, cystic myelopathy, myelomalacia).

Infections and inflammatory processes

US or CT is often initially used to delineate CNS infection and its sequelae or complications. However, MRI is clearly superior for early detection, including the use of diffusion imaging, and for demonstrating the precise nature and extent of involvement using T2, FLAIR, GRE, and gadolinium-enhanced sequences (e.g., CMV) [1–12,101–103]. This includes meningoencephalitis

due to TORCH infections (i.e., toxoplasmosis, other [e.g., syphilis], rubella, cytomegalovirus [CMV], herpes simplex virus [HSV2], human immunodeficiency virus [HIV]), and neonatal meningitis (e.g., Group B *Streptococcus*, *Listeria*, Gram-negative) (Figs. 18.28–18.33). Less common but increasingly prevalent causes of subacute and chronic CNS inflammation are the granulomatous meningoencephalitic infections (e.g., tuberculosis, spirochete, fungal, parasitic), particularly in immunocompromised hosts. The imaging pattern is often asymmetric and progressive. Such findings may include subarachnoid exudate, ventriculitis, edema, cerebritis, infarction, hydrocephalus, effusion, empyema, abscess, and in the chronic phase cystic encephalomalacia, atrophy, gliosis, and calcification.

Recurrent infectious or non-infectious CNS infection (e.g., meningitis) may require investigation for a "parameningeal focus" (e.g., sinus or mastoid infection, dermal sinus, primitive neurenteric connection, CSF leak after trauma, dermoid–epidermoid) [1–12]. Brain abscess or empyema may be associated with Gram-negative meningitis (e.g., *Citrobacter*) in the neonate. Suppurative collections related to sinus infection, trauma, surgery, sepsis, the immunocompromised state, or uncorrected cyanotic congenital heart disease primarily occur in older children. MRI is the imaging modality of choice for definitive evaluation and follow-up. Multiplanar T2, FLAIR, GRE, and DWI sequences are often necessary, along with gadolinium-enhanced T1 images, in order to delineate collections requiring drainage. Contrast-enhanced stereotactic MRI or CT and intraoperative US may provide additional guidance for surgery.

Plain films or SPECT have been used in the past for screening of suspected spinal-column infection (discitis, osteomyelitis) [2,5]. MRI, however, is now preferred for definitive diagnosis, treatment planning, and follow-up. CT may further assist in the delineation of bony involvement. MRI is also the procedure of choice for evaluating spinal neuraxis infection. STIR sequences and fat-suppressed gadolinium-enhanced techniques are particularly important for demonstrating suppurative collections (e.g., epidural abscess).

Metabolic, toxic, and neurodegenerative disorders

In the evaluation of neonatal encephalopathy and developmental delay (e.g., static encephalopathy vs. progressive encephalopathy), MRI is the only modality that can provide an accurate assessment of brain maturation based on myelination and cortical development [2–5,7,8,12,30,38,39,104–107] (Figs. 18.1–18.4). The clinical hallmark of a metabolic, toxic, or neurodegenerative disorder is "progressive" neurologic impairment in the absence of another readily identifiable process. These are to be distinguished from the "non-progressive" encephalopathies, for example, due to maldevelopment, hypoxia–ischemia, or infection. These disorders may be exogenous and internal (e.g., hypoglycemia, hyperbilirubinemia) or external (e.g., fetal alcohol syndrome). The endogenous disorders (e.g., inborn errors of metabolism) are not as

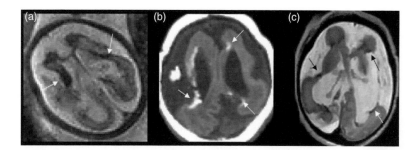

Fig. 18.28. Congential CMV on (a) fetal T2 and (b) neonatal T1 + (c) GRE MRI including dysplastic (microcephaly, undergyration) and encephaloclastic (cavitations) components plus T1 hyperintense/T2 hypointense mineralization (arrows).

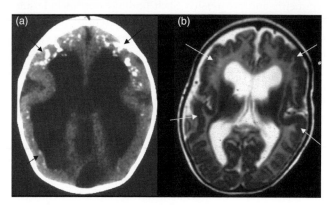

Fig. 18.29. Congenital CMV: (a) calcification (arrows) on CT; (b) diffuse polymicrogyria (arrows) on axial T2 MRI.

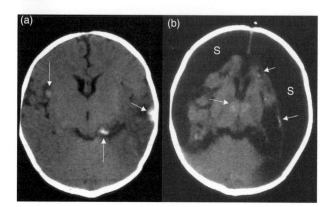

Fig. 18.32. HSV2 encephalitis on CT: (a) subacute phase, including hemorrhages (arrows); (b) chronic phase, with encephalomalacia, subdural collections (s), and calcifications (arrows).

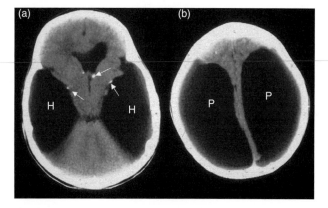

Fig. 18.30. Congenital toxoplasmosis: (a,b) CT with hydrocephalus (H), porencephaly (P), and calcifications (arrows).

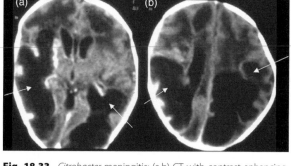

Fig. 18.33. *Citrobacter* meningitis: (a,b) CT with contrast-enhancing abscesses (arrows), ventriculitis, and hydrocephalus.

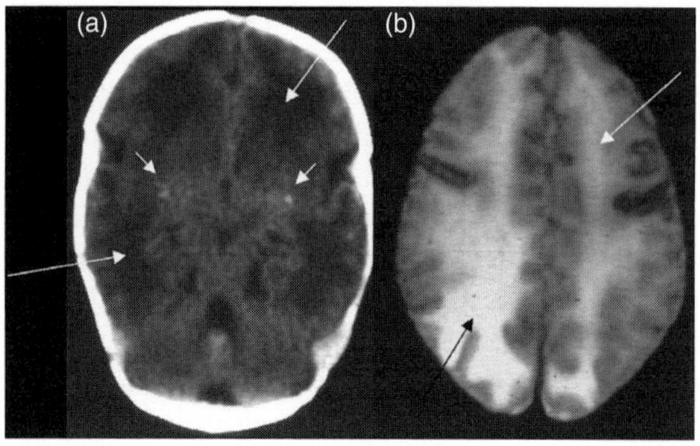

Fig. 18.31. Congenital rubella on (a) CT and (b) T2 MRI, including calcifications (short arrows) and leukoencephalitis (long arrows) with white-matter low densities and T2 high intensities.

rare as previously considered, and some are specifically treatable. Many are genetic and heredofamilial disorders such that genetic counseling and prenatal screening are important. Metabolic disorders may be classified in a number of ways including anatomic predilection (e.g., gray matter, white matter, both) and metabolic defect. Diagnosis is primarily a clinical one and may involve metabolic testing, genetic evaluation, or biopsy of CNS or extra-CNS tissues. MRI is superior to US and CT in evaluating disease extent and anatomic distribution. Occasionally MRI may demonstrate characteristic imaging findings (e.g., kernicterus, Zellweger disease). MRS contributes to the specific metabolic characterization of these disorders [39]. Stereotactic CT or MRI may serve as a guide for biopsy.

The classification of metabolic diseases may be biochemical, molecular, genetic, pathological, or clinical [2–5,7,8,12, 30,38,39,104–113] (Table 18.5). These disorders are often

Table 18.5. Metabolic, toxic, and neurodegenerative disorders

Lysosomal disorders

  Lipidoses

    Fabry, Gaucher's and Niemann–Pick disease

    GM$_1$ gangliosidosis

    GM$_2$ gangliosidosis (Tay–Sachs and Sandhoff diseases)

    Neuronal ceroid lipofuscinosis

  Mucopolysaccharidoses (MPS)

    Hurler, Scheie, Hurler–Scheie

    Hunter

    Sanfilippo A–D

    Morquio A & B

    Matoreaux-Lamy

    Sly

  Mucolipidoses

    Mannosidosis, Fucosidosis, Sialidosis

  Lysosomal leukodystrophies

    Metachromatic leukodystrophy

    Globoid cell leukodystrophy (Krabbe)

Peroxisomal disorders

  Adrenoleukodystrophy complex

  Neonatal leukodystrophy

  Zellweger syndrome

  Infantile Refsum's syndrome

  Rhizomelic chondrodysplasia punctata

  Hyperpipecolic acidemia

  Cerebrotendinous xanthomatosis

Other leukodystrophies

  Pelizaeus–Merzbacher disease

  Canavan's disease

  Alexander's disease

  Cockayne's syndrome

  Leukodystrophy with calcifications

Mitochondrial (respiratory oxidative) disorders

  Leigh's disease

  Kearns–Sayre syndrome

  MELAS syndrome

  MERRF syndrome

  Alper's syndrome (poliodystrophy)

  Menkes' disease (trichopoliodystrophy)

  Marinesco-Sjogren syndrome

  Infantile bilateral striatal necrosis

  Lebers hereditary optic atrophy

  L-Carnitine deficiency

Amino acid disorders

  Phenylketonuria

  Homocystinuria

  Non-ketotic hyperglycinemia

  Maple syrup urine disease

  Glutaric aciduria, type I

  Glutaric aciduria, type II

  Methylmalonic and propionic acidurias

  Urea cycle defects (e.g., OTC deficiency)

  Oculocerebrorenal syndrome

  Pyridoxine dependency

Carbohydrate and other storage disorders

  Galactosemia

  Glycogen storage diseases (i.e. Pompe)

  Carbohydrate-deficient glycoprotein syndrome

  Niemann-Pick

  Gaucher

  Farber

  Infantile sialidosis

Liver metabolic disorders

  Wilson's disease (hepatolenticular degeneration)

  PKAN

  Hyperbilirubinemia (see toxic encephalopathies)

  Hepatocerebral syndromes (see toxic encephalopathies)

Diseases of the cerebellum, brainstem, and spinal cord

  Friedreich's ataxia

  Olivopontocerebellar atrophies

  Ataxia–telangiectasia

  Carbohydrate-deficient glycoprotein syndrome

  Infantile neuraxonal dystrophy

Other metabolic and neurodegenerative diseases

  Juvenile multiple sclerosis

  Molybdenum cofactor deficiency

  3-Hydroxy-3-methylglutaryl-coenzyme A lyase deficiency

  Idiopathic leukoencephalopathy

Diseases of the basal ganglia

  Sulfite oxidase deficiency

  Parathyroid disease

  Tuberous sclerosis

  Down's syndrome

  Progressive encephalopathy with basal ganglia calcifications and CSF lymphocytosis

Inflammatory, toxic, and anoxic conditions

  Radiation therapy

  Renal tubular acidosis and osteoporosis

  Huntington's disease

  Fahr's disease

  PKAN

  Cockayne

  Wilson

Toxic encephalopathies

  Exogenous internal toxicities

    Hyperbilirubinemia

    Hepatocerebral syndromes

    Hypoglycemia

    Hypothermia and hyperthermia

    Paraneoplastic toxins

    Hemolytic uremic syndrome

    Uremia

    Ion imbalance disorders

    Endocrinopathies

    Porphyria

  Exogenous external toxicities

    Vitamin deficiencies/depletions

      Vitamin B$_1$

      Folate

      Vitamin B$_{12}$

      Biotin

      Vitamin K

      Vitamin C

      Vitamin D

    Toxins

      Mercury poisoning

      Methanol

      Toluene

      Carbon monoxide

      Cyanides and sulfides

      Lead

      Alcohol

      Cocaine and heroin

    Anticonvulsants

    Drug-induced

      Methotrexate

      Cyclosporine

      Tacrolimus

      Carmustine, cytosine arabiniside

Note:
See references [2,4,5,106,107].

categorized according to the metabolic defect. Such a classification includes the lysosomal disorders (e.g., Krabbe), peroxisomal defects (e.g., Zellweger), the mitochondrial disorders (e.g., Leigh, Menkes), organic and aminoacidopathies (e.g., non-ketotic hyperglycinemia), disorders of carbohydrate metabolism (e.g., glycogen storage disease), liver metabolic disorders, and miscellaneous. Certain clinical features that assist in directing the initial evaluation of these patients may also provide a basis for classification (e.g., macrocephaly in maple syrup urine disease). The ideal radiological classification would categorize the diseases by the anatomic distribution of the pathological process using CT and MRI. Unfortunately, most of these conditions affect multiple sites, and considerable overlap in appearance is found. However, a practical imaging classification may be based on the predominant areas of involvement including the white matter (subcortical, periventricular), gray matter (cortical, deep), basal ganglia, brainstem, cerebellum, spinal cord, and peripheral nervous system [2,5,12,7,8,12,39, 104–107].

Disorders primarily affecting cortical gray matter

Endogenous metabolic disorders which primarily, or predominantly, affect the cortical gray matter include the storage diseases that result from lysosomal enzyme defects [2,5,39,107]. However, these findings are often non-specific, and the differential diagnosis may include diffuse cortical atrophy due to any number of causes. Other considerations include the end stage of a static encephalopathy (e.g., post-HIE or post-infection), or "atrophy" related to chronic systemic disease, malnutrition, or certain types of therapy (e.g., steroids).

Disorders primarily affecting deep gray matter

Metabolic disorders may primarily involve the deep gray matter (including mineralization) [2,5,39,107,110–113]. Those disorders primarily involving the corpus striatum (i.e., caudate and putamen) include the mitochondrial disorders, organic and aminoacidopathies, juvenile Huntington's disease, Wilson disease, and Cockayne's syndrome. Those disorders primarily involving the globus pallidus include the aminoacidopathies, hyperbilirubinemia, pentothenate kinase associated neuro-degeneration (PKAN, formerly Hallervorden–Spatz disease), and toxic exposure (e.g., carbon dioxide) (Figs. 18.34, 18.35). It is unusual to see isolated involvement of the thalami in any of the metabolic disorders. However, thalamic involvement may be an early or dominant feature of Krabbe disease or

GM2 gangliosidosis. It may also be seen in the infantile form of Leigh disease along with extensive brainstem, basal ganglia, and cerebral white-matter involvement. In general, the differential diagnosis, depending on the clinical picture and timing of the imaging, may also include profound HIE, hypoglycemia, toxic exposure (e.g., methane, cyanide), osmolar myelinolysis, striatal necrosis, and meningoencephalitis.

Disorders primarily affecting white matter

Those disorders which primarily, or predominantly, affect the white matter are known as the leukoencephalopathies [2,5,39,107–109]. Traditionally, leukoencephalopathies have been divided into dysmyelinating and myelinoclastic disorders. In dysmyelinating disorders an intrinsic (inherited) enzyme deficiency results in the disturbed formation, destruction, or turnover of the essential components of myelin. They are also referred to as the leukodystrophies. The pattern of damage is symmetrical in both hemispheres, has diffuse margins, often spares the arcuate fibers, and consistently involves the cerebellar white matter. The leukodystrophies are primarily associated with the lysosomal and peroxisomal disorders (e.g., metachromatic leukodystrophy, Krabbe leukodystrophy, and the adrenoleukodystrophy complex [ALD]), and with diseases of white matter (e.g., Pelizaeus–Merzbacher, Canavan, Alexander, and Cockayne). Included in the differential diagnosis is infantile-onset leukoencephalopathy with swelling (macrocephaly) and mild clinical course. Early central white-matter involvement may suggest Krabbe (also, abnormal thalami), ALD, phenylketonuria, maple syrup urine disease (MSUD: Fig. 18.34), or Lowe syndrome. The lack of myelination

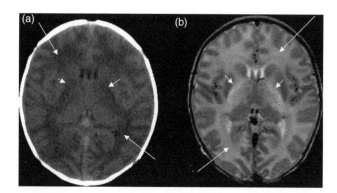

Fig. 18.34. Maple syrup urine disease in neonate with globus pallidus (short arrows) and white matter (long arrows) edema on (a) axial CT and (b) axial T2 MRI.

Fig. 18.35. Bilirubin encephalopathy and kernicterus on MRI with (a,b) globus pallidus and subthalamic T1 hyperintensity (arrows) in subacute phase, and (c) T2 hyperintensity (arrows) plus atrophy in chronic phase.

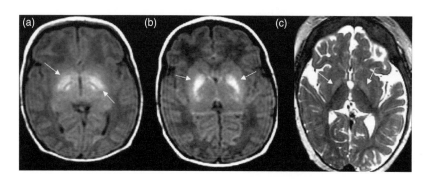

(hypomyelination) may suggest Pelizaeus–Merzbacher disease or Menkes' disease. In myelinoclastic disorders, the myelin sheath is intrinsically normal until it yields to exogenous or endogenous myelinotoxic factors. The pattern of damage is asymmetric, is sharply demarcated, irregularly involves the subcortical arcuate fibers, and may spare the cerebellum. Examples are the infectious and postinfectious demyelinating diseases (e.g., TORCH, HIV, SSPE, ADEM) and the vasculitides (e.g., lupus). Non-specific white-matter abnormalities may be seen with a variety of metabolic, neurodegenerative, infectious, postinfectious, toxic, and vascular processes. In this situation, the clinical findings must be relied upon. An important example is posterior reversible leukoencephalopathy (e.g., hypertension, transplant, cyclosporine, renal disease). Also, it is important to remember that the most common causes of cerebral white-matter abnormalities (particularly periventricular) and prominent Virchow–Robin spaces in children with developmental delay are the static leukoencephalopathies (e.g., maldevelopmental, undermyelination, postinflammatory, postischemic, idiopathic).

Disorders affecting both white matter and cortical gray matter

A number of metabolic disorders involve both gray and white matter [2,5,39,107–109]. Those disorders associated with cortical atrophy along with white-matter involvement include lysosomal disorders such as the lipidoses and mucopolysaccharidoses (also, associated skeletal dysplasia), and mitochondrial disorders such as Alper disease and Menkes' disease. If there is a diffuse cortical dysgenesis (e.g., lissencephaly, polymicrogyria) associated with white-matter abnormalities, then peroxisomal disorders such as Zellweger syndrome should be considered along with congenital infections (e.g., cytomegaloviral), and the congenital muscular dystrophies (e.g., Fukuyama, Walker–Warburg, Santavuori) (Fig. 18.36).

In hypoglycemia, there is predominant involvement of the parieto-occipital gray and white matter, and especially the primary visual cortex (Fig. 18.37). This pattern is to be distinguished from a predominant posterior border-zone HIE and from dural venous sinus thrombosis primarily in the distribution of the straight sinus, posterior superior sagittal sinus, and/or the inferior sagittal sinus.

Disorders affecting both white matter and deep gray matter

Disorders associated with deep gray-matter involvement, in addition to white-matter abnormalities, include those with primarily corpus striatum involvement (Leigh [Fig. 18.38], MELAS, Wilson's, Cockayne), those with predominant thalamic abnormalities (Krabbe, GM2 gangliosidoses), and those with primarily globus pallidus involvement (Canavan, MSUD, methylmalonic/propionic acidopathy, Kearns–Sayre) [2,5,39,107–113]. Sulfite oxidase deficiency also involves the basal ganglia and white matter and can mimic HIE [114] (Fig. 18.39). Included in

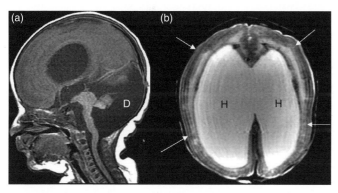

Fig. 18.36. Walker–Warburg with Dandy–Walker malformation (D) on (a) sagittal T1 plus (b) cobblestone lissencephaly (arrows) with extensive white-matter dysplasia and hydrocephalus (H) on axial T2 MRI.

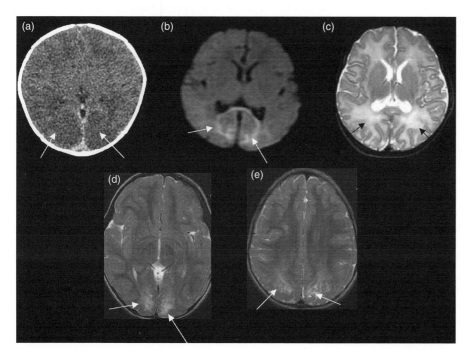

Fig. 18.37. Hypoglycemia with parieto-occipital involvement (arrows) in the subacute phase with edema as (a) low density on CT, and as high intensity on (b) DWI and (c) T2 MRI; also (d,e) the chronic phase with atrophy and gliosis on T2 MRI.

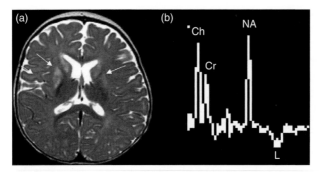

Fig. 18.38. Leigh syndrome with basal-ganglia lesions (arrows) and white-matter involvement: (a) axial T2 MRI; (b) lactate doublet (L) on MRS.

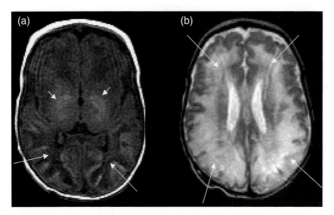

Fig. 18.39. Sulfite oxidase deficiency with thalamic (short arrows) and diffuse white-matter involvement (long arrows) on (a) axial T1 and (b) T2 MRI.

the differential diagnoses, depending on the clinical context, are profound HIE, osmolar myelinolysis, bilirubin encephalopathy (kernicterus), toxic exposure, and infectious or postinfectious processes (e.g., TORCH, HIV, ADEM).

MR spectroscopy (MRS) in metabolic disorders

Proton (hydrogen-1) MRS using both short and long TE acquisitions (e.g., TEs 35, 144) is being increasingly used clinically to evaluate brain development and maturation, as well as patients with metabolic and other disorders [12,38,39]. The normal MR brain spectra show an evolution from the immature infantile pattern (e.g., decreased N-acetyl-aspartate [NAA] relative to choline [Ch]) to the mature, adult pattern (e.g., increased NAA to Ch) (Fig. 18.3). Although many of the metabolic and neurodegenerative disorders have specific biochemical markers, most of the disorders have no differentiating features. Non-specific MRS abnormalities are those that reflect brain destruction and reactive changes including delayed maturation, neuronal loss, axonal degeneration, demyelination, and gliosis. Alterations in metabolites are often displayed as a ratio relative to the reference metabolite, creatine (Cr), an energy marker. In disorders in which there is predominant neuronal degeneration (i.e., loss of cell bodies, axons) and atrophy, or oligodendroglial loss, the major MRS finding is a decrease in N-acetyl-aspartate (NAA), a neuronal (neurons including axons) and immature oligodendroglial

marker. In disorders in which there is predominant loss of myelin sheaths with secondary axonal degeneration and gliosis (e.g., demyelination), the characteristic spectral abnormalities are characterized by elevated lipids, a marker for myelin destruction; elevated choline (Ch), a marker of membrane turnover (e.g., myelin, glial); variable increases in lactate (L), a marker of anaerobic glycolysis; elevated glutamate/glutamine (Glx), neuroexcitatory amino acid markers; and elevated myoinositols (mI), also an osmolyte and glial marker. Associated neuronal (e.g., axonal) or oligodendroglial damage is indicated by a decrease in NAA.

More specific MRS abnormalities may be seen in a number of disorders [39]. Abnormal MRS spectra have been reported with some of the lysosomal defects such as Niemann–Pick disease (abnormal lipid peak at 1.2 ppm), the mucopolysaccharidoses (decreased NAA late), and metachromatic leukodystrophy (decreased NAA, Ch, and Cr; increased mI and L). MRS abnormalities have been observed with a number of the peroxisomal disorders including adrenoleukodystrophy (decreased NAA with increased Ch, Glx, mI, lipids, and L) and Zellweger syndrome (decreased NAA with increased lipids and Glx). Other leukodystrophies associated with observed MRS findings are Canavan disease (increased NAA with decreased Ch and Cr plus increased mI and L), Alexander disease (decreased NAA with increased L), and Pelizaeus–Merzbacher disease (normal early; decreased NAA and increased Ch late). Primary and secondary disorders of energy metabolism have been associated with MRS findings of decreased NAA and increased L, including mitochondrial disorders such as Leigh disease and MELAS (Fig. 18.38). Similar findings, however, are present with acute/subacute hypoxia–ischemia (plus elevated Glx, decreased Cr, and increased lipids) (Fig. 18.18). Aminoacidopathies with reportedly abnormal spectra include phenylketonuria (increased phenylalanine peak at 7.37 ppm), maple syrup urine disease (abnormal peak at 0.9 ppm), and non-ketotic hyperglycinemia (elevated glycine peak at 3.55 ppm). Other metabolic disorders associated with abnormal MRS findings include the creatine deficiencies (decreased, absent Cr), hepatic encephalopathy (increased Glx with decreased inositols and Ch), and hyperosmolar states (increased inositols, Cr, and Ch). Neoplastic processes characteristically show elevated Ch/Cr, decreased NAA/Cr, and decreased NAA/Cr ratios. Inflammatory processes may be differentiated from neoplastic and other processes by the suppressed mI peak [12].

Summary

US and CT may provide important screening information, particularly with regard to hemorrhage, trauma, hydrocephalus, infection, and gross macrostructural anomalies. However, current and advanced MRI techniques provide more definitive macrostructural, microstructural, and functional imaging information in both the early and late assessment of fetal and neonatal CNS injuries.

References

1. Blankenburg FG, Barnes PD. Structural and functional imaging of hypoxic-ischemic injury (HII) in the fetal and neonatal brain. In Stevenson D, Benitz W, Sunshine P, eds., *Fetal and Neonatal Brain Injury*, 3rd edn. Cambridge: Cambridge University Press, 2003: 446–89.

2. Barnes P. State of the art: neuroimaging and the timing of fetal and neonatal brain injury. *J Perinatol* 2001; **21**: 44–60.

3. Winkler P, Zimmerman RA. *Perinatal Brain Injury. Neuroimaging: Clinical and Physical Principles*. New York, NY: Springer, 2000: 531–83.

4. Barkovich A. *Pediatric Neuroimaging*, 4th edn. Philadelphia, PA: Lippincott-Raven, 2005: 190–290.

5. Volpe JJ. *Neurology of the Newborn*, 4th edn. Philadelphia, PA: Saunders, 2001.

6. Ment L, Bada H, Barnes P, *et al.* Practice parameter: neuroimaging of the neonate. *Neurology* 2002; **58**: 1726–38.

7. Ferriero D. Neonatal brain injury. *N Engl J Med* 2004; **351**: 1985–95.

8. Barkovich A. MR imaging of the neonatal brain. *Neuroimaging Clin N Am* 2006; **16**: 117–36.

9. Rutherford M, Srinivasan L, Dyet L, *et al.* MRI in perinatal brain injury. *Pediatr Radiol* 2006; **36**: 582–92.

10. Zimmerman R, Bilaniuk L. Neuroimaging evaluation of cerebral palsy. *Clin Perinatol* 2006; **33**: 517–44.

11. Triulzi F, Parazzini C, Righini A. Patterns of damage in the mature neonatal brain. *Pediatr Radiol* 2006; **36**: 608–20.

12. Panigrahy A, Blumel S. Advances in MR neuroimaging techniques in the evaluation of neonatal encephalopathy. *Top Magn Reson Imaging* 2007; **18**: 3–30.

13. Barnes PD, Taylor GA. Imaging of the neonatal central nervous system. *Neurosurgery Clin North Am* 1998; **1**: 17–48.

14. Allison JW, Seibert JJ. Transcranial Doppler in the newborn with asphyxia. *Neuroimaging Clin N Am* 1999; **9**: 11–16.

15. Blankenberg FG, Loh N, Bracci P, *et al.* Sonography, CT, and MR imaging: a prospective comparison of neonates with suspected intracranial ischemia and hemorrhage. *AJNR Am J Neuroradiol* 2000; **21**: 213–18.

16. Debillon T, N'Guyen, Muet A, *et al.* Limitations of ultrasonography for diagnosing white matter damage in preterm infants. *Arch Dis Child Fetal Neonatal Ed* 2003; **88**: F275–9.

17. Laptook A, O'Shea M, Shankaran S, *et al.* Adverse neurodevelopmental outcomes among extremely low birth weight infants with normal head ultrasound. *Pediatrics* 2005; **115**: 673–80.

18. Pinto-Martin JA, Riolo S, Cnaan A, *et al.* Cranial ultrasound prediction of disabling and nondisabling cerebral palsy at age two in a low birthweight population. *Pediatrics* 1995; **95**: 249–54.

19. Maalouf EF, Duggan PJ, Counsell SJ, *et al.* Comparison of findings on cranial ultrasound and magnetic resonance imaging in preterm neonates. *Pediatrics* 2001; **107**: 719–27.

20. Sie LT, van der Knapp MD, van Wezel-Meijler G, *et al.* Early MR features of hypoxic-ischemic brain injury in neonates with periventricular densities on sonograms. *AJNR Am J Neuroradiol* 2000; **21**: 852–61.

21. Childs AM, Cornette L, Romenghi LA, *et al.* Magnetic resonance and cranial ultrasound characteristics of periventricular white matter abnormalities in newborn infants. *Clin Radiol* 2001; **56**: 647–55.

22. Roelants-van Rijn AM, Groenendaal F, Beek FJ, *et al.* Parenchymal brain injury in the preterm infant: comparison of cranial ultrasound, MRI and neurodevelopmental outcome. *Neuropediatrics* 2001; **32**: 80–9.

23. Inder TE, Anderson NJ, Spencer C, *et al.* White matter injury in the premature infant: a comparison between serial cranial sonographic and MR findings at term. *AJNR Am J Neuroradiol* 2003; **24**: 805–9.

24. Miller SP, Cozzio C, Goldstein RB, *et al.* Comparing the diagnosis of white matter injury in premature newborns with serial MR imaging and transfontanel ultrasonography findings. *AJNR Am J Neuroradiol* 2003; **24**: 1661–9.

25. Hintz SR, Slovis T, Bulas D, *et al.* Interobserver reliability and accuracy of cranial ultrasound scanning interpretation in premature infants. *J Pediatr* 2007; **150**: 592–6.

26. Mirmiran M, Barnes P, Keller K, *et al.* Neonatal brain MRI before discharge is better than serial cranial ultrasound in predicting cerebral palsy in very low birth weight preterm infants. *Pediatrics* 2004; **114**: 992–8.

27. Slovis T. Children, computed tomography radiation dose, and the As Low As Reasonably Achievable (ALARA) concept. *Pediatrics* 2003; **112**: 971–2.

28. Vertinzksy A, Barnes P. Macrocephaly, increased intracranial pressure, and hydrocephalus in the infant and young child. *Top Magn Reson Imaging* 2007; **18**: 31–52.

29. Barnes P, Krasnokutsky M. Imaging of the CNS in suspected or alleged nonaccidental injury, including the mimics. *Top Magn Reson Imaging* 2007; **18**: 53–74.

30. Mukherjee P. Advanced pediatric imaging. *Neuroimaging Clin N Am* 2006; **16**(1).

31. Levine D, Barnes PD, Robertson RR, *et al.* Fast MR imaging of fetal central nervous system abnormalities. *Radiology* 2003; **229**: 51–61.

32. Garel C, Delezide A, Elmaleh-Berges M, *et al.* Contribution of fetal MRI in the evaluation of cerebral ischemic lesions. *AJNR Am J Neuroradiol* 2004; **25**: 1563–1568.

33. Levine D, Barnes P. MR imaging of fetal CNS abnormalities. In Levine D, ed., *Atlas of Fetal MRI*. Boca Raton, FL: Taylor & Francis Group, 2005: 25–72.

34. Griffiths P, Widjaja E, Paley M, *et al.* Imaging of the fetal spine in utero: diagnostic accuracy and impact on management. *Pediatr Radiol* 2006; **36**: 927–33.

35. Garel C. New advances in fetal MR neuroimaging. *Pediatr Radiol* 2006; **36**: 621–5.

36. Glenn O, Barkovich J. Magnetic resonance imaging of the fetal brain and spine. Part 1. *AJNR Am J Neuroradiol* 2006; **27**: 1604–11; Part 2. *AJNR Am J Neuroradiol* 2006; **27**: 1807–14.

37. Barkovich AJ, Baranski K, Vigneron D, *et al.* Proton MR spectroscopy in the evaluation of asphyxiated term neonates. *AJNR Am J Neuroradiol* 1999; **20**: 1399–405.

38. Vigneron DB. Magnetic resonance spectroscopic imaging of human brain development. *Neuroimag Clin N Am* 2006; **16**; 75–86.

39. Cecil K. MR spectroscopy of metabolic disorders. *Neuroimaging Clin N Am* 2006; **16**: 87–116.

40. Barkovich A, Miller S, Bartha A. MR imaging, MR spectroscopy, and diffusion tensor imaging of sequential studies in neonates with encephalopathy. *AJNR Am J Neuroradiol* 2006; **27**: 533–47.

41. Wang J, Licht D. Pediatric perfusion MRI using arterial spin labeling. *Neuroimaging Clin N Am* 2006; **16**: 149–68.

42. Huppi PS, Maier SE, Peled S, *et al.* Microstructural development of human newborn cerebral white matter assessed in vivo by diffusion tensor magnetic resonance imaging. *Pediatr Res* 1998; **44**: 584–90.

43. Neil JJ, Shiran SI, McKinstry RC. Normal brain in human newborns: apparent diffusion coefficient and diffusion anisotropy measured by using diffusion tensor MR imaging. *Radiology* 1998; **209**: 57–66.

44. Johnson AJ, Lee BCP, Lin W. Echoplanar diffusion-weighted imaging in neonates and infants with suspected hypoxic–ischemic injury. *AJNR Am J Neuroradiol* 1999; **172**: 219–26.

45. Robertson RL, Ben-Sira L, Barnes PD, *et al.* MR line scan diffusion imaging of term neonates with perinatal brain ischemia. *AJNR Am J Neuroradiol* 1999; **20**: 1658–70.

46. Phillips MD, Zimmerman RA. Diffusion imaging in pediatric hypoxic-ischemic injury. *Neuroimaging Clin N Am* 1999; **9**: 41–52.

47. Inder T, Huppi PS, Zientara GP, *et al.* Early detection of periventricular leukomalacia by diffusion-weighted magnetic resonance imaging techniques. *J Pediatr* 1999; **134**: 631–4.

48. Inder TE, Huppi PS, Warfield S, *et al.* Periventricular white matter injury in the premature infant followed by reduced cerebral cortical gray matter volume at term. *Ann Neurol* 1999; **46**: 755–60.

49. Huppi PS, Murphy B, Maier SE, *et al.* Microstructural brain development after perinatal cerebral white matter injury assessed by diffusion tensor MR imaging. *Pediatrics* 2001; **107**: 455–60.

50. Arzoumanian Y, Mirmiran M, Barnes P, *et al.* Diffusion tensor brain imaging findings at term-equivalent age may predict neurologic abnormalities in low birth weight preterm infants. *AJNR Am J Neuroradiol* 2003; **24**: 1646–53.

51. Counsell S, Allsop J, Harrison M, *et al.* Diffusion-weighted imaging of the brain in preterm infants with focal and diffuse white matter abnormality. *Pediatrics* 2003; **112**: 1–7.

52. Sagar P, Grant PE. Diffusion-weighted imaging: pediatric clinical applications. *Neuroimaging Clin N Am* 2006; **16**: 45–74.

53. Mukherjee P, McKinstry R. Diffusion tensor imaging and tractography of human brain development. *Neuroimaging Clin N Am* 2006; **16**: 19–44.

54. van der Knaap M, Valk J. Classification of congenital abnormalities of the CNS. *AJNR Am J Neuroradiol* 1988; **9**: 315–26.

55. Barkovich AJ, Truwit CL. Brain damage from perinatal asphyxia: correlation of MR findings with gestational age. *AJNR Am J Neuroradiol* 1990; **11**: 1087–96.

56. Aida N, Nishimura G, Hachiya Y, *et al.* MR imaging of perinatal brain damage: comparison of clinical outcome with initial follow-up MR findings. *AJNR Am J Neuroradiol* 1992; **19**: 1909–22.

57. Barkovich A, Hallam D. Neuroimaging in perinatal hypoxic–ischemic injury. *Ment Retard Dev Disabil Res Rev* 1997; **3**: 28–41.

58. Cowan F, Rutherford M, Groenendaal F, *et al.* Origin and timing of brain lesions in term infants with neonatal encephalopathy. *Lancet* 2003; **361**: 736–42.

59. Miller S, Ramaswamy V, Michelson D, *et al.* Patterns of brain injury in term neonatal encephalopathy. *J Pediatr* 2005; **146**: 453–60.

60. Lupton BA, Hill A, Roland EH, *et al.* Brain swelling in the asphyxiated term newborn: pathogenesis and outcome. *Pediatrics* 1988; **82**: 139–46.

61. Vannucci RC, Christensen MA, Jager JY. Nature, time-course, and extent of cerebral edema in perinatal hypoxic–ischemic brain damage. *Pediatr Neurol* 1993; **9**: 29–34.

62. Pinto-Martin JA, Riolo S, Cnaan A, *et al.* Cranial ultrasound prediction of disabling and nondisabling cerebral palsy at age two in a low birthweight population. *Pediatrics* 1995; **95**: 249–54.

63. Goetz MC, Gretebeck RJ, Oh KS, *et al.* Incidence, timing and follow-up of periventricular leukomalacia. *Am J Perinatol* 1995; **12**: 325–7.

64. Valkama AM, Pääkkö ELE, Vainionpää LK, *et al.* Magnetic resonance imaging at term and neuromotor outcome in preterm infants. *Acta Paediatr* 2000; **89**: 348–55.

65. Perlman JM, Rollins N. Surveillance protocol for the detection of intracranial abnormalities in premature neonates. *Arch Pediatr Adolesc Med* 2000; **154**: 822–6.

66. Volpe JJ. Neurobiology of periventricular leukomalacia in the premature infant. *Pediatr Res* 2001; **50**: 553–62.

67. Panigrahy A, Barnes PD, Robertson RL, *et al.* Volumetric brain differences in children with periventricular T2-signal hyperintensities: a grouping by gestational age at birth. *AJR Am J Roentgenol* 2001; **177**: 695–702.

68. Miller SP, Hoque NN, Piecuch RE, *et al.* The spectrum of cerebellar hemorrhage in premature newborns. *Pediatr Res* 2003; **53**: 537A (abst #3040).

69. Austin NC, Woodward L, Spencer C, *et al.* Neurodevelopmental outcome at one year in a regional cohort of very low birth weight infants: correlation with MRI at term. *Pediatr Res* 2003; **53**: 398A (abst #2253).

70. Volpe JJ. Cerebral white matter injury of the premature infant: more common than you think. *Pediatrics* 2003; **112**: 176–80.

71. Inder TE, Wells SJ, Mogridge NB, *et al.* Defining the nature of the cerebral abnormalities in the premature infant: a qualitative magnetic resonance imaging study. *J Pediatr* 2003; **143**: 171–9.

72. Panigrahy A, Barnes PD, Robertson RL, *et al.* Quantitative analysis of the corpus callosum in children with cerebral palsy and developmental delay: correlation with cerebral white matter volume. *Pediatr Radiol* 2005; **35**: 1199–207.

73. Bodensteiner J, Johnsen S. MRI findings in children surviving extremely premature delivery and extremely low birthweight with cerebral palsy. *J Child Neurol* 2006; **21**: 743–7.

74. Dyet L, Kennea N, Counsell S, *et al.* Natural history of brain lesions in extremely preterm infants studied with serial MRI from birth and neurodevelopmental assessment *Pediatrics* 2006; **118**: 536–48.

75. Khwaja O, Volpe J. Pathogenesis of cerebral white matter injury of prematurity. *Arch Dis Child Fetal Neonatal Ed* 2008; **93**: F153–61.

76. Barkovich AJ. MR and CT evaluation of profound neonatal and infantile asphyxia. *AJNR Am J Neuroradiol* 1992; **13**: 959–72.

77. Barkovich AJ, Sargent SK. Profound asphyxia in the premature infant: imaging findings. *AJNR Am J Neuroradiol* 1995; **16**: 1837–46.

78. Barkovich AJ, Westmark K, Partridge C, *et al.* Perinatal asphyxia: MR findings in

the first 10 days. *AJNR Am J Neuroradiol* 1995; **16**: 427–39.

79. Roland EH, Poskitt K, *et al.* Perinatal hypoxic–ischemic thalamic injury: clinical features and neuroimaging. *Ann Neurol* 1998; **44**: 161–6.

80. Sargent M, Poskitt K, Roland E, *et al.* Cerebellar vermian atrophy after neonatal hypoxic–ischemic encephalopathy. *AJNR Am J Neuroradiol* 2004; **25**: 1008–15.

81. Boichot C, Walker P, Durand C, *et al.* Term neonate prognosis after perinatal asphyxia: contributions of MR imaging, MR spectroscopy, relaxation times, and ADCs. *Radiology* 2006; **239**: 839–48.

82. Shankaran S, Laptook A, Ehrenkranz R, *et al.* Whole-body hypothermia for neonates with hypoxic–ischemic encephalopathy. *N Engl J Med* 2005; **353**: 1574–84.

83. Bulas D, Glass P. Neonatal ECMO: neuroimaging and neurodevelopmental outcome. *Semin Perinatol* 2005; **29**: 58–65.

84. Zuerrer M, Martin E, Boltshauser E. MRI of intracranial hemorrhage in neonates and infants at 2.35 tesla. *Neuroradiology* 1991; **33**: 223–9.

85. DeVeber G, Andrew M, Adams C, *et al.* Cerebral sinovenous thrombosis in children. *N Engl J Med* 2001; **345**: 417–23.

86. Carvalho K, Bodensteiner J, Connolly P, *et al.* Cerebral venous thrombosis in children. *J Child Neurol* 2001; **16**: 574–85.

87. Lynch J, Hirtz D, deVeber G, *et al.* Report of the National Institute of Neurologic Disorders and Stroke Workshop on Perinatal and Childhood Stroke. *Pediatrics* 2002; **109**: 116–23.

88. DeVeber G. Arterial ischemic strokes in infants and children: an overview of current approaches. *Semin Thrombosis Hemostasis* 2003; **29**: 567–73.

89. Sebire G, Tabarki B, Saunders DE, *et al.* Cerebral venous thrombosis in children: risk factors, presentation, diagnosis, and outcome. *Brain* 2005; **128**: 477–89.

90. Kirton A, deVeber G. Cerebral palsy secondary to perinatal ischemic stroke. *Clin Perinatol* 2006; **33**: 367–86.

91. Fitzgerald K, Williams LS, Garg BP, *et al.* Cerebral sinovenous thrombosis in the neonate. *Arch Neurol* 2006; **63**: 405–9.

92. Barnes C, deVeber G. Prothrombotic abnormalities in childhood ischaemic stroke. *Thromb Res* 2006; **118**: 67–74.

93. Ehtisham A, Stern B. Cerebral venous thrombosis: a review. *Neurologist* 2006; **12**: 32–8.

94. Huang A, Robertson R. Spontaneous superficial parenchymal and leptomeningeal hemorrhage in term neonates. *AJNR Am J Neuroradiol* 2004; **25**: 469–75.

95. Govaert P, Vanhaesebrouck P, de Praeter C. Traumatic neonatal intracranial bleeding and stroke. *Arch Dis Child* 1992; **67**: 840–5.

96. Castillo M, Fordham LA. MR of neurologically symptomatic newborns after vacuum extraction delivery. *AJNR Am J Neuroradiol* 1995; **16**: 816–18.

97. Odita JC, Hebi S. CT and MRI characteristics of intracranial hemorrhage complicating breech and vacuum delivery. *Pediatr Radiol* 1996; **26**: 782–5.

98. Kleinman PK, Barnes PD. Head trauma. In Kleinman PK, ed., *Imaging of Child Abuse*, 2nd edn. St Louis, MO: Mosby-Year Book, 1998.

99. Alexander J, Leveno K, Hauth J, *et al.* Fetal injury associated with cesarean delivery. *Obstet Gynecol* 2006; **108**: 885–90.

100. Doumouchtsis S, Arulkumaran S. Head trauma after instrumental births. *Clin Perinatol* 2008; **35**: 69–83.

101. Teixeira J, Zimmerman R, Haselgrove J, *et al.* Diffusion imaging in pediatric central nervous system infections. *Neuroradiology* 2001; **43**: 1031–9.

102. Jan W, Zimmerman R, Bilaniuk L, *et al.* Diffusion-weighted imaging in acute bacterial meningitis in infancy. *Neuroradiology* 2003; **45**: 634–9.

103. DeVries L, Verboon-Maciolek M, Cowan F, *et al.* The role of cranial US and MRI in the diagnosis of infections of the central nervous system. *Early Hum Dev* 2006; **82**: 819–25.

104. Hoon AH. Neuroimaging in cerebral palsy: patterns of brain dysgenesis and injury. *J Child Neurol* 2005; **12**: 936–9.

105. Rodriguez D, Young Poussaint T. Neuroimaging of the child with developmental delay. *Top Magn Reson Imaging* 2007; **18**: 75–92.

106. Valk J, van der Knapp MS. Toxic encephalopathy. *AJNR Am J Neuroradiol* 1992; **13**: 747–60.

107. van der Knaap MS, Valk J. *Magnetic Resonance of Myelination & Myelin Disorders*, 3rd edn. New York, NY: Springer, 2005.

108. Barker P, Horska A. Neuroimaging in leukodystrophies. *J Child Neurol* 2004; **19**: 559–70.

109. Vanderver A. Tools for diagnosis of leukodystrophies and other disorders presenting with white matter disease. *Curr Neurol Neurosci Rep* 2005; **5**: 110–18.

110. Murakami Y, Yamashita Y, Matsuishi T, *et al.* Cranial MRI of neurologically impaired children suffering from neonatal hypoglycemia. *Pediatr Radiol* 1999; **29**: 23–7.

111. Alkalay A, Flores-Sarnat L, Sarnat H, *et al.* Brain imaging findings in neonatal hypoglycemia. *Clin Pediatr* 2005; **44**: 783–90.

112. Barkovich A, Ali F, Rowley H, *et al.* Imaging patterns of neonatal hypoglycemia. *AJNR Am J Neuroradiol* 1998; **19**: 523–8.

113. Govaert P, Lequin M, Swarte R, *et al.* Changes in globus pallidus with (pre) term kernicterus. *Pediatrics* 2003; **112**: 1256–63.

114. Dublin A, Hald J, Wootton-Gorges S. Isolated sulfite oxidase deficiency: MR imaging features. *AJNR Am J Neuroradiol* 2002; **23**: 484–5.

Ken Brady and Chandra Ramamoorthy

Introduction

Jobsis first described the measurement of cerebral oxyhemoglobin saturation using near-infrared spectroscopy (NIRS) in 1977 [1]. This work was immediately recognized for its profound clinical implications, especially in the neonatal arena, and the search for the ideal neurologic neonatal monitor began. In 1985, when the NIROS-SCOPE was used on three infants in the neonatal intensive care unit (NICU) at Duke University, Brazy *et al.* made the following claim:

> For effective measurement of cerebral oxygen sufficiency in a sick newborn, an instrument should be non-invasive, be adaptable at the bedside, not interfere with patient care, and give continuous rapid information. The signals should directly assess brain oxygen delivery and utilization and be sensitive to small changes. The NIROS-SCOPE appears to fulfill these basic requirements [2].

Available for many years, NIRS-based monitors of cerebral oxygenation have held the promise to fill the gap in neonatal neuromonitoring, but at this writing they are neither standard of care nor ubiquitous. Signs point to increased marketing of NIRS-based cerebral oximetry monitors to healthcare facilities in the United States, particularly to NICUs. In an effort to prepare clinicians for this impending deployment, we summarize in this chapter three decades of work done with NIRS to develop the cerebral oximeters available today.

Some view NIRS-based cerebral oximetry as purely an investigational tool. However, it is noteworthy that (1) the cerebral oximeter is frequently employed in the congenital cardiac surgical arena at major medical centers, and (2) competing companies have marketed cerebral oximeters that have been approved by the United States Food and Drug Administration (FDA). Moreover, based on the results of a show-of-hands survey following a lecture regarding cerebral oximetry that was presented during a meeting of congenital cardiac surgeons in 2007 (Congenital Heart Surgeons' Society Annual Meeting, October 28–29, 2007, Chicago, Illinois), practitioners in attendance unanimously reported the use of cerebral oximetry at their facilities. This informal survey occurred after the speaker had summarized the clinical data evaluating

cerebral oximetry and concluded that the data are insufficient to establish use of this device as the standard of care. At first blush, then, the consensus acceptance may seem counterintuitive. However, experience shows this to be a common fate of medical monitoring devices: without evidentiary data to support their outcome benefit, the medical community begins to use them nonetheless. Randomized trials of monitoring devices that are already in widespread use are practically and ethically difficult to perform, so without proven – or disproven – benefit, their use becomes the de facto standard of care. Unless a randomized controlled clinical trial is performed in the very near future with cerebral oximetry, we believe that this same outcome can be expected for NIRS-based cerebral oximetry in the NICU.

Theory

Light in the near-infrared spectrum has three physical properties that make it useful for diagnostic assessments: it penetrates tissue, it is non-ionizing, and it is absorbed differentially by relevant chromophores, depending on their oxygen-binding state. The excellent penetrance of light in the wavelength range of 650–950 nm is the result of minimal absorbance by the tissue, with the exception of a few species of chromophores. Within this spectroscopic window, tissue penetrance and chromophore absorption are both sufficient to assess tissue at the depth of the cerebral cortex. Unlike other forms of radiation with this degree of penetrance, near-infrared light is non-ionizing; therefore, it forms the substrate of a safe monitoring modality.

Two chromophores that absorb near-infrared light are hemoglobin and cytochrome. Hemoglobin has been the primary subject of NIRS-based monitoring attempts, because of its obvious central role in oxygen delivery to the brain. Cytochrome aa3 is the terminal enzyme in the mitochondrial electron transport system, and the oxidation–reduction state of cytochrome aa3 may reflect oxygen availability at the cellular level. Therefore, interest in measuring this parameter with NIRS persists. Although not marketed in the United States, the NIRO 500 cerebral oximeter (HamamatsuPhotonics; Hamamatsu City, Japan) is commercially available and does report the redox state of cytochrome aa3.

When near-infrared light is emitted across a tissue (e.g., brain) and detected at its exit of the tissue, absorption of the light can be used to calculate chromophore concentration

Fetal and Neonatal Brain Injury, 4th edition, ed. David K. Stevenson, William E. Benitz, Philip Sunshine, Susan R. Hintz, and Maurice L. Druzin. Published by Cambridge University Press. © Cambridge University Press 2009.

using variants of the Beer–Lambert equation, conceptually simplified:

$$A = -\log\left(I/I_0\right) = \varepsilon_\lambda L C$$

where A is absorbance, I_0 is the intensity of light before passing through the tissue, and I is the intensity of light after passing through the tissue. Absorbance of the near-infrared light by a particular chromophore is a function of the path length (L), the concentration of the chromophore in that path (C), and the molar absorptivity of the chromophore at the specific wavelength used (ε_λ).

Near-infrared absorption can be used to calculate oxygenated and deoxygenated hemoglobin concentration because the known molar absorptivities of the hemoglobin species for each wavelength differ according to the oxygenation state. Permutations of the equation exist to account for scattering of light outside of the interoptode vector and light absorption by other chromophores or non-chromophores. However, the basic principle remains: light of a known intensity is directed across a known path that contains a chromophore with known absorptive properties. The recovered light intensity is used to calculate absorbance, and absorbance is converted to concentration. Using multiple wavelengths of light allows for the separate measurement of oxygenated hemoglobin and total hemoglobin. Thus, the percentage of oxygenated hemoglobin is determined. These somewhat simplified relationships are applied to both arterial pulse oximeters and cerebral oximeters.

Intracranial and extracranial hemoglobin measurements are distinguished by the use of more than one sensing optode and the creation of varying path lengths. Shallow arcs of light travel across skin and skull but do not penetrate the cerebrum. Deep arcs of light cross skin, skull, dura, and cortex. Subtracting the absorbance measured in the narrow arc from that measured in the deep arc leaves absorbance that is due to intracerebral chromophores, and this processing renders the cerebral specificity of cerebral oximetry. Herein lies one of the distinguishing features of cerebral oximeters when compared to pulse oximeters. Cerebral oximeters use spatial resolution techniques to differentiate cortical from extracranial blood, where pulse oximeters differentiate pulsatile (arterial) from non-pulsatile (venous/capillary) blood. Although arterial oxygen saturation is useful for quantifying pulmonary function, it is not useful for determining the adequacy of substrate delivery to the brain. Cerebral venous oxygen saturation is the more illuminating measurement to describe the ratio of cerebral oxygen delivery to the cerebral metabolic rate of oxygen consumption ($CMRO_2$).

Regional cerebral oximetry is a reflection of all of the hemoglobin in the cerebral path length, which is estimated to include 70% venous, 5% capillary, and 25% arterial blood. Given these relative arterial and venous contributions, transcranial cerebral oximetry readings are consistently higher than, but closely correlated to, jugular venous oximetry readings [3,4]. In theory at least, a cerebral oximeter should be as useful as a jugular vein oximeter without the invasiveness. Low venous oxygen saturation in the brain is a sign of inadequate oxygen delivery for the $CMRO_2$ and signals ischemic conditions for the brain. Validation of NIRS-based monitors has focused on the potential of this modality to alert providers to the presence of an ischemic milieu.

Cerebral oximeters currently in clinical use

The ability of NIRS to accurately quantify the concentrations of oxygenated, deoxygenated, and total hemoglobin in the cortex has been a subject of considerable debate [5,6]. Two factors have consistently confounded the accuracy of cortical NIRS: first, variable scattering of the near-infrared light causes variations in the path length between the emitter and detector [7,8]; second, variability in tissue composition causes variable non-hemoglobin absorbance of the infrared light.

The three main monitors that are commercially available are the NIRO 500, the INVOS cerebral oximeter, and more recently the Foresight monitor. Each of them uses a differential path length factor that is a laboratory-derived estimation of the actual path length of near-infrared light as it is reflected between optodes. To resolve variations in path length due to light scattering, some experimental cerebral oximeters employ phase-shift analysis (in so-called frequency-domain NIRS or time-resolved NIRS) to calculate the actual path length [9,10]. Monitors also differ in the number of wavelengths used and therefore the number of chromophores quantified in the light path.

The INVOS cerebral oximeter (Somanetics; Troy, MI, USA) is the cerebral oximeter most commonly used in the United States, and it employs two wavelengths of light, 730 and 810 nm, to report the ratio of oxyhemoglobin to total hemoglobin (rSO_2i) in the light path. The equation used to determine rSO_2i requires an assumption that the noise from light-path variation and the noise from background absorption equally affect the calculation of oxyhemoglobin and deoxyhemoglobin concentrations. Therefore, it is believed that the effects are canceled in the ratio. Because of its inability to demonstrate an absolute calibration, the INVOS monitor is approved by the FDA as a trend-only monitoring device.

The NIRO 500 uses four wavelengths of light: 775, 810, 850, and 910 nm. Additional wavelengths allow for determination of cytochrome aa3 concentrations in addition to the hemoglobin species concentrations, and the NIRO series monitors report a tissue oxygen index, which is also the percentage of calculated oxygenated hemoglobin relative to total hemoglobin. Hamamatsu has not marketed a NIRS-based monitor with FDA approval in the United States, but its monitors are used elsewhere.

A more recent FDA approval for the Foresight monitor (Casmed; Branford, CT, USA) allows a claim for absolute cerebral oximetry measurements. Four light wavelengths are used in the instrument: 690, 778, 800, and 850 nm. The purpose of the additional wavelengths is to better discriminate non-hemoglobin sources of infrared absorption, which in theory leads to a more accurate calculation of oxygenated and total hemoglobin concentrations [11]. The Foresight monitor also reports the percentage of oxygenated hemoglobin relative to total hemoglobin as a cerebral tissue oxygen saturation ($S_{CT}O_2$).

In addition to differences in the light spectra used, the monitors listed above have differences in optode spacing and path-length calibrations. Because of these differences, studies of NIRS-based monitoring with one device do not provide data that are not necessarily applicable to the other devices. All of these monitors report a ratio of oxygenated to total hemoglobin in their output, so the effects of path length variability and background absorption are at least partially mitigated. When the absolute tissue concentrations of hemoglobins are used in attempts to quantify cerebral blood volume or cerebral blood flow, the inherent ambiguities in the measurements become more significant.

Validation of cerebral oximetry

The validation of cerebral oximetry will be discussed in two domains to explore the accuracy and potential impact of NIRS-based cerebral monitoring. Data that show the accuracy of NIRS when compared against gold-standard cerebral physiologic monitoring will be considered first, followed by a summary of data from clinical applications of cerebral oximetry.

Comparing cerebral oximetry to a gold standard

Oximetry reported by NIRS-based monitors has been validated by comparing non-invasive cerebral oximetry to the saturation of oxygen in the jugular vein ($SjvO_2$). The use of jugular vein oximetry as a gold standard for validation of the cerebral oximetry highlights one of the limitations in the validation process. Because no physiologic monitor other than the cerebral oximeter measures tissue oxygen saturation, the best standard for comparison is the jugular bulb oximeter – a monitor that has only a small clinical relevance in pediatrics. When considering the ratio of arterial to venous blood in brain tissue, it is understandable that cerebral oximetry monitors track – but normally read higher than – the jugular oxyhemoglobin saturation readings. Results have been inconsistent between studies, which have included small numbers of patients and/or animals.

In piglet studies of cerebral oximetry during deep hypothermic circulatory arrest, a strong correlation between cerebral oximetry and $SjvO_2$ was reported [12]. Reductions of cerebral oximetry have also been correlated to reductions in phosphate energy stores (adenosine triphosphate and phosphocreatine) quantified by mass spectroscopy in animals, suggesting a detrimental metabolic consequence to the low oximetry measurement [13].

When cerebral oximetry was compared with $SjvO_2$ in 40 children with congenital heart lesions only a modest association ($r = 0.69$) was found as well as a bias for high oximetry readings at lower $SjvO_2$ states and low oximetry readings at higher $SjvO_2$ states [7]. A similar study of 30 children undergoing cardiac catheterization reported a higher correlation ($r = 0.93$) over a range of $SjvO_2$ values from 31% to 83% [14]. In a study of 17 neonates on venovenous extracorporeal membrane oxygenation, NIRS-derived cerebral oximetry compared favorably against $SjvO_2$ [15].

Validating NIRS as a modality is complicated by the diversity of monitoring devices used. It is not clear that validating one monitor validates the others, as they use different optode configurations, wavelength spectra, and modifications of the Beer–Lambert equation to derive cerebral oximetry values. As noted above, evidence supports the conclusion that cerebral oximetry correlates with cerebral tissue oxygen saturation, but the first FDA approval was granted for monitoring trends only, as calibration of the absolute value of oximetry was not proven to be reliable. NIRS-based oximeters understandably have enjoyed the widest clinical application in the pediatric cardiac operating rooms, where a baseline can be established for each patient against which the changes in cerebral oximetry are compared during and after cardiopulmonary bypass. In the intensive care unit, establishing a baseline for an unstable patient can be more difficult. The absence of an absolute normal value for cerebral oximetry has been an obstacle to the implementation of NIRS-based neuromonitoring in the NICU. The recent FDA approval of the foresight device with an absolute rather than a trend monitor may have overcome this obstacle, but this device is relatively new and studies using the device in premature neonates are not yet published. Hence, despite a decade-long use of NIRS in the pediatric world, the relevance of cerebral oximetry still remains a question.

The ischemic threshold

To be useful as a monitor of cerebral ischemia, cerebral oximetry should alert the provider to injuriously low tissue oxygen levels. Defining the ischemic threshold in the absolute sense with the monitors in clinical use has been challenging.

A more rigorous definition of the ischemic threshold for cerebral oximetry was attained using frequency-domain NIRS in neonatal piglets. EEG abnormalities as well as perturbations of brain tissue ATP and lactate concentrations were used as a standard to quantify ischemic conditions. The baseline cerebral oximetry in the piglets was 68%. Cerebral oximetry correlated well with both sagittal sinus oximetry ($r = 0.98$) and cerebral blood flow measured by laser–Doppler ($r = 0.89$). Lactate levels increased at cerebral oximetry readings of $\leq 44\%$. Minor and major EEG abnormalities were seen at cerebral oximetry thresholds of 42% and 37% respectively, and ATP reductions occurred at cerebral oximetry readings $< 33\%$ [16]. Clinical studies commonly use a cerebral oximetry measurement of $\leq 45\%$, or a 20% reduction from baseline, as the ischemic threshold.

Relevance of cerebral oximetry to clinical outcome

NIRS-based cerebral oximetry has already found acceptance in the congenital cardiac surgery specialty, notwithstanding the limited data to suggest that it has a measureable impact on outcome. Therefore, data that support the use of cerebral oximetry are largely limited to children undergoing heart surgery, and are observational in design.

In a study of 26 infants undergoing cardiopulmonary bypass (CPB) and deep hypothermic circulatory arrest, neurologic complications were reported in three patients who had lower intraoperative cerebral oximetry than their counterparts who did not have neurologic complications [17].

In a non-randomized prospective study, 250 children had multimodal neuromonitoring, including EEG, transcranial middle cerebral artery ultrasonography (TCD), and cerebral oximetry during cardiac surgery. The authors reported that cerebral desaturations from baseline (20% reduction) were the most common (58%) recorded monitoring event, followed by TCD changes. Interventions by the cardiac team consisting of anesthesiologists, surgeons, and perfusionists were recorded along with monitoring events. Postoperative gross neurologic sequelae were noted in 26% of patients with monitoring events that were not treated, but were only seen in 6% of cases when monitoring changes prompted therapy. Disturbingly, 7% of patients without any monitoring events also had adverse neurologic sequelae [18].

More recently, cerebral oximetry readings of < 45% for a cumulative time exceeding 180 minutes were shown to be associated with new ischemic lesions in 22 patients with hypoplastic left heart syndrome who had the Norwood procedure. Magnetic resonance imaging was performed before and 9 days after surgery in this cohort, and 73% of patients had new lesions, or worsening of lesions, detected preoperatively [19]. No long-term outcome studies exist to show the clinical significance of these MRI changes. Similarly, McQuillen et al. reported new white-matter injury (WMI) that correlated with prolonged periods of cerebral desaturation in neonates undergoing open heart surgery [20].

Initial studies of CPB and deep hypothermic circulatory arrest with near-infrared monitoring were observational [21,22]. These studies are important because their results were consistent with our understanding of bypass and circulatory arrest, a consistency that was considered validation of the monitoring modality. The studies also contributed to an understanding of the physiology of injury in this setting. Cerebral oxygenation was monitored using NIRS during CPB in 15 pediatric patients who ranged in age from 1 day to 6 years. Oxyhemoglobin, hemoglobin, and oxidized cytochrome aa3 were compared between nine patients who had undergone repairs during deep hypothermic CPB without circulatory arrest, and six patients who had CPB with deep hypothermic circulatory arrest. The authors found that, in the continuous-bypass group, oxyhemoglobin decreased during CPB and cooling but returned to control levels during rewarming. However, in the group with deep hypothermic circulatory arrest, both oxidized cytochrome aa3 and oxyhemoglobin decreased dramatically during circulatory arrest; oxidized cytochrome aa3 did not return to baseline levels and deoxyhemoglobin was elevated, even upon rewarming and initiation of CPB. These findings indicate that brain cellular metabolism may undergo sustained impairment after deep

hypothermic cardiac arrest, and that it may persist even after adequate flow and oxygenation have been established [21,22].

Neonates with patent ductus arteriosus (PDA) were monitored during pharmacologic ductus closure with indomethacin. Regional cerebral oxygen tissue saturation and arterial blood pressure levels were both significantly lower than those of matched controls who did not have a PDA (33 ± 5 mmHg vs. 38 ± 6 mmHg and $62\% \pm 9\%$ vs. $72\% \pm 10\%$, respectively). After treatment with indomethacin, the differences between subjects and controls were not significant [23]. While this study does not suggest that application of NIRS-based monitoring confers an outcome benefit to patients with a PDA, the result of the study does contribute to the understanding of the possible adverse cerebrovascular effects of a PDA.

The current clinical use of cerebral oximetry is commonly justified based on observational data, physiologic rationale, and the non-invasive nature of the monitor [24,25]. The existing clinical studies reporting results of NIRS monitoring are largely observational. However, there are costs associated with additional monitoring, and concerns may reasonably be raised that the evidence does not yet support a change in the standard of care. Findings such as those described above linking prolonged cerebral desaturation to neuroimaging evidence of injury should be considered in the balance, and suggest the importance of further investigations.

Interpreting abnormal cerebral oximetry

Cerebral oximetry in its current configuration reports the percentage of oxygen-saturated hemoglobin in brain tissue. Because most of the hemoglobin is on the venous side of the circulation, it is a reflection of the ratio of oxygen delivery and the metabolic rate of oxygen consumption. Given that most oxygen delivered to the brain is hemoglobin-bound in the arterial blood, this oxygen delivery can be accounted for by few physiologic variables:

$$O_2Del = CBF \times [HbO_2]$$

where CBF is cerebral blood flow and $[HbO_2]$ is the concentration of arterial oxygenated hemoglobin. $[HbO_2]$ is the product of the total hemoglobin and the arterial oxygen saturation ($\%Sat$). CBF is governed by the ratio of cerebral perfusion pressure (CPP) and cerebrovascular resistance, which is itself a function of vessel radius to the fourth power (r^4) and blood viscosity (η).

Simplified, clinically relevant parameters stand out in this equation:

$$O_2Del \propto \frac{CPP \times r^4 \times [Hb] \times \%Sat}{\eta}$$

It is important to note that the above equation is distinct from the equation usually used to quantify oxygen delivery to other organs, as that equation has cardiac output in the place of cerebral blood flow. Blood flow is preferentially diverted to the brain in shock states, and thus cerebral blood flow may be preserved despite a low cardiac output. Heart rate

Table 19.1. Variables affecting cerebral oxygen saturation

Variable	Clinical example
O_2 delivery	
CPP: cerebral perfusion pressure	Patients with hypotension, elevated intracranial pressure, or elevated jugular venous pressure can have inadequate cerebral perfusion pressure.
r^4: resistance vessel radius	Resistance vessels are dilated by hypercarbia and hypoxia. They are restricted by hypocarbia and vasospasm. Blood flow to the brain is profoundly affected by small changes in resistance vessel radius. Cardiopulmonary bypass cannulae can also cause a fixed resistance to the brain vascular circuit.
[Hb]: concentration of hemoglobin	Anemia can be associated with perisurgical patients and with hemodilution at the initiation of cardiopulmonary bypass.
%Sat: arterial oxygen saturation	Cardiopulmonary disease that causes hypoxia can be optimized with lung recruitment and management of the pulmonary-to-systemic blood flow ratio (Q_p/Q_s).
η: viscosity	Hyperviscous blood can be seen in patients with excessive hematocrits, leukemia, and patients with sickle cell disease who are overtransfused. Viscosity due to red cell mass is decreased by increasing serum osmolarity.
O_2 consumption	The cerebral metabolic rate of oxygen consumption is increased by fever, seizure, and arousal. It is decreased by hypothermia, coma, and sedation.

and stroke volume are therefore less important than the cerebral perfusion pressure in considering cerebral desaturation. This distinction also highlights the fact that optimizing cerebral circulation does not necessarily optimize the circulation to other organs, such as the kidney and gut. When a patient has a decrement in cerebral oximetry, the above equation is helpful in determining the root cause (Table 19.1).

Future possibilities with clinical near-infrared spectroscopy
Measures of cerebral blood volume and cerebral blood flow

In addition to measuring oxyhemoglobin saturation, NIRS can also be used to derive the more fundamental hemodynamic parameters of cerebral blood volume and cerebral blood flow by injecting the patient with vascular tracers such as indocyanine green, which has an absorption spectrum in the infrared range [26,27]. Alternatively, blood volume can be calculated with NIRS using oxyhemoglobin as a blood tracer, but this technique requires the induction of fluctuations in arterial oxygen saturation. The oxyhemoglobin tracer method was used to study 27 infants with perinatal asphyxia, and a hyperemic response was described with a characteristic increase in cerebral blood flow and volume post ischemia that was sensitive for poor outcome at 1 year follow-up. These infants also showed blunted responses in the cerebral vasculature to changes in carbon dioxide tension [28]. As perturbations of vasocycling in the cerebrovasculature have been implicated in the development of intraventricular hemorrhage and periventricular leukomalacia, the ability to quantify both the volume and flow of blood in the neonatal brain may open a window toward understanding these mechanisms and their link to neonatal brain injury [29].

Somatic regional oximetry

Attempts have been made to use NIRS to monitor the adequacy of oxygen delivery to the kidney and other organs using NIRS technology. By placing the cerebral oximetry probes of the INVOS monitor over the flank at T_{10}–L_2, the proponents of this practice report rSO_2 readings that are reflective of renal perfusion and metabolism. Somatic and cerebral rSO_2 monitoring was compared in nine patients who had a stage I palliation of hypoplastic left heart syndrome. During cooling, regional cerebral perfusion was used and the cerebral rSO_2 readings were higher than baseline, whereas the somatic rSO_2 was near critical ischemic levels. After bypass, the cerebral rSO_2 readings were significantly lower than pre-bypass levels and the somatic rSO_2 readings were higher than pre-bypass levels. The authors propose a mechanism of elevated cerebrovascular resistance induced by cooling and CPB [30].

Cerebral rSO_2 and somatic rSO_2 were measured during crossclamp of the aorta in another study of 26 patients with coarctation of the aorta. A decrement of oxygenation below the crossclamp was seen in all of the patients, but when stratified by age, neonates ($n = 11$) and infants ($n = 5$) were seen to have much greater reductions in somatic desaturations than were older children ($n = 10$). It was suggested that the older children had more robust collateralization of the post-coarctation vasculature [31].

Critics of the somatic monitoring technique cite a lack of calibration of intersensor spacing and path length factors for the probes used in renal monitoring. However, the potential clinical role of neonatal splanchnic organ monitoring with near-infrared technology is intriguing.

Visible light spectroscopy

Somatic monitoring can also be achieved using visible light spectroscopy (VLS), a new technology that allows real-time early detection of tissue ischemia using visible light in the wavelength range of 475–600 nm [32]. Shorter-wavelength visible light does not penetrate tissue as readily as near-infrared light, so VLS gives an assessment of hemoglobin oxygen saturation in thin, small-volume and shallow-tissue samples, typically mucosal. Conventional pulse oximetry becomes unreliable at extremes of hypoxia, hypothermia, or vasoconstriction, whereas VLS is not affected by these conditions. VLS was used in five children undergoing cardiopulmonary bypass with antegrade cerebral perfusion, a condition which renders pulse oximetry non-functional. In these patients, antegrade perfusion was shown to provide adequate cerebral perfusion by cerebral oximetry monitoring, but VLS monitoring of the esophagus showed inadequate somatic perfusion [33]. There is a potential for mucosal microvascular monitoring of the neonate at risk for necrotizing enterocolitis with VLS.

Autoregulation analysis

Cerebral oximetry has been used to quantify cerebrovascular pressure autoregulation. Cerebrovascular pressure autoregulation is defined as the maintenance of a constant cerebral blood flow in the face of changing cerebral perfusion pressure. This process protects the brain during transient changes in the arterial blood pressure from diminished or excessive blood flow. However, premature infants have been shown to possess an immature cerebrovascular pressure autoregulation mechanism [34]. The limits of autoregulation in the infant brain, and especially the premature infant brain, are not known. Critical illness, especially sepsis and systemic inflammatory responses, further tax the protection of autoregulatory reserve [35–38].

Slow changes in arterial blood pressure cause slow changes in cerebral blood flow when autoregulation is absent (pressure passivity). The waveform analysis that quantifies the relationship between the arterial blood pressure and cerebral blood flow can be performed as a linear correlation of resampled waves (after filtering out high-frequency harmonics) or as a cross-spectral analysis of coherence. Assuming constant oxygen consumption, hemoglobin, and arterial oxygen saturation, the NIRS-derived measure of cerebral oximetry can be used as a surrogate for cerebral blood flow. The linear correlation method was tested in piglets using the INVOS monitor and was found to be sensitive and specific for detecting loss of autoregulation due to hypotension [39].

Clinical work using a cross-spectral analysis of coherence between cerebral oximetry and arterial blood pressure (an index of pressure passivity) suggests that this modality has a potential role in the prevention of postnatally acquired hemorrhage and stroke. Pressure passivity was seen to occur using this method in 87 of 90 premature infants. Prematurity, low birthweight, hypotension, and maternal hemodynamic compromise were all associated with increased time in a pressure-passive state [40]. In another series of 32 very-low-birthweight and premature infants, 47% of the 17 patients who demonstrated pressure passivity developed germinal matrix hemorrhage, periventricular leukomalacia, or both, compared with 13% of the infants with apparently intact autoregulation [41]. A continuous monitor of autoregulation using NIRS has the potential to identify neonates at risk for neurologic injury, but it may also identify arterial blood pressures that allow for improved autoregulatory function.

Summary

NIRS is an important monitoring modality for the critically ill neonate. While still considered in a developmental phase, NIRS-based cerebral oximeters have been approved by the FDA and are widely applied in the perioperative care of children with heart disease. The lack of randomized controlled clinical trials showing a benefit of cerebral oximetry monitoring in patient outcome seems to suggest that the rapid increase in deployment of the monitor is premature. However, a paradigm for evaluating monitoring modalities before introduction into clinical practice has not been established. Most, if not all, of the monitoring devices used in intensive care settings have failed to generate this level of data. Even when a monitor is non-invasive, the insight gained from monitoring impacts clinical decision making, and adds to patient care costs. Antepartum heart-rate monitors and infant cardio-respiratory monitors are two examples of non-invasive modalities that became universally applied without evidence of outcome benefit [42,43]. The pulse oximeter is the staple of anesthetic and intensive care monitoring, and is considered standard of care for all critically ill patients. A recent Cochrane review of the use of perioperative pulse oximetry concluded that available data show that pulse oximetry can detect hypoxemia, but that the use of pulse oximetry has not been shown to have a measurable effect on outcome [44]. Even the use of the pulse oximeter, therefore, is elevated to standard of care on the basis of physiologic principles and observational data alone [45]. Cerebral oximetry is currently on a similar trajectory.

It is probable that NIRS-based monitors have found a more successful market in the congenital cardiac specialty than in the neonatal specialty because of practical considerations. Because the first clinical models are useful as trend-only devices, a baseline setting is required. Surgical patients can provide a baseline setting obtained prior to incision, but neonates in active resuscitation at birth or in a clinically unstable state in the NICU cannot. With recent technical advances, the precision of cerebral oximeters has seen improvement. As these improvements transition from the bench to the marketplace, we can expect to see an amplified role for this modality in the care of critically ill neonates. It remains to be seen if this increased level of monitoring will result in prevention of ischemic and hemorrhagic brain lesions in the premature infant.

References

1. Jobsis FF. Non-invasive, infra-red monitoring of cerebral O2 sufficiency, blood volume, HbO2-Hb shifts and blood flow. *Acta Neurol Scand Suppl* 1977; **64**: 452–3.

2. Brazy JE, Lewis DV, Mitnick MH, *et al.* Noninvasive monitoring of cerebral oxygenation in preterm infants: preliminary observations. *Pediatrics* 1985; **75**: 217–25.

3. Rais-Bahrami K, Rivera O, Short BL. Validation of a noninvasive neonatal optical cerebral oximeter in veno-venous ECMO patients with a cephalad catheter. *J Perinatol* 2006; **26**: 628–35.

4. Yoxall CW, Weindling AM, Dawani NH, *et al.* Measurement of cerebral venous oxyhemoglobin saturation in children by near-infrared spectroscopy and partial jugular venous occlusion. *Pediatr Res* 1995; **38**: 319–23.

5. Greisen G. Is near-infrared spectroscopy living up to its promises? *Semin Fetal Neonatal Med* 2006; **11**: 498–502.

6. Sorensen LC, Greisen G. Precision of measurement of cerebral tissue oxygenation index using near-infrared spectroscopy in preterm neonates. *J Biomed Opt* 2006; **11**: 054005.

7. Daubeney PE, Pilkington SN, Janke E, *et al.* Cerebral oxygenation measured by near-infrared spectroscopy: comparison with jugular bulb oximetry. *Ann Thorac Surg* 1996; **61**: 930–4.

8. Kurth CD, Uher B. Cerebral hemoglobin and optical path length influence near-infrared spectroscopy measurement of cerebral oxygen saturation. *Anesth Analg* 1997; **84**: 1297–305.

9. Nelson LA, McCann JC, Loepke AW, *et al.* Development and validation of a multiwavelength spatial domain near-infrared oximeter to detect cerebral hypoxia–ischemia. *J Biomed Opt* 2006; **11**: 064022.

10. Duncan A, Meek JH, Clemence M, *et al.* Measurement of cranial optical path length as a function of age using phase resolved near infrared spectroscopy. *Pediatr Res* 1996; **39**: 889–94.

11. Rais-Bahrami K, Rivera O, Short BL. Validation of a noninvasive neonatal optical cerebral oximeter in veno-venous ECMO patients with a cephalad catheter. *J Perinatol* 2006; **26**: 628–35.

12. Abdul-Khaliq H, Troitzsch D, Schubert S, *et al.* Cerebral oxygen monitoring during neonatal cardiopulmonary bypass and deep hypothermic circulatory arrest. *Thorac Cardiovasc Surg* 2002; **50**: 77–81.

13. Nollert G, Jonas RA, Reichart B. Optimizing cerebral oxygenation during cardiac surgery: a review of experimental and clinical investigations with near infrared spectrophotometry. *Thorac Cardiovasc Surg* 2000; **48**: 247–53.

14. Abdul-Khaliq H, Troitzsch D, Berger F, *et al.* Regional transcranial oximetry with near infrared spectroscopy (NIRS) in comparison with measuring oxygen saturation in the jugular bulb in infants and children for monitoring cerebral oxygenation. *Biomed Tech (Berl)* 2000; **45**: 328–32.

15. Rais-Bahrami K, Rivera O, Short BL. Validation of a noninvasive neonatal optical cerebral oximeter in veno-venous ECMO patients with a cephalad catheter. *J Perinatol* 2006; **26**: 628–35.

16. Kurth CD, Levy WJ, McCann J. Near-infrared spectroscopy cerebral oxygen saturation thresholds for hypoxia–ischemia in piglets. *J Cereb Blood Flow Metab* 2002; **22**: 335–41.

17. Kurth CD, Steven JM, Nicolson SC. Cerebral oxygenation during pediatric cardiac surgery using deep hypothermic circulatory arrest. *Anesthesiology* 1995; **82**: 74–82.

18. Austin EH, Edmonds HL, Auden SM, *et al.* Benefit of neurophysiologic monitoring for pediatric cardiac surgery. *J Thorac Cardiovasc Surg* 1997; **114**: 707–17.

19. Dent CL, Spaeth JP, Jones BV, *et al.* Brain magnetic resonance imaging abnormalities after the Norwood procedure using regional cerebral perfusion. *J Thorac Cardiovasc Surg* 2006; **131**: 190–7.

20. McQuillen PS, Barkovich AJ, Hamrick SE, *et al.* Temporal and anatomic risk profile of brain injury with neonatal repair of congenital heart defects. *Stroke* 2007; **38**: 736–41.

21. Greeley WJ, Bracey VA, Ungerleider RM, *et al.* Recovery of cerebral metabolism and mitochondrial oxidation state is delayed after hypothermic circulatory arrest. *Circulation* 1991; **84**: III400–6.

22. Greeley WJ, Kern FH, Ungerleider RM, *et al.* The effect of hypothermic cardiopulmonary bypass and total circulatory arrest on cerebral metabolism in neonates, infants, and children. *J Thorac Cardiovasc Surg* 1991; **101**: 783–94.

23. Lemmers PM, Toet MC, van Bel F. Impact of patent ductus arteriosus and subsequent therapy with indomethacin on cerebral oxygenation in preterm infants. *Pediatrics* 2008; **121**: 142–7.

24. Hoffman GM. Neurologic monitoring on cardiopulmonary bypass: what are we obligated to do? *Ann Thorac Surg* 2006; **81**: S2373–80.

25. Andropoulos DB, Stayer SA, Diaz LK, *et al.* Neurological monitoring for congenital heart surgery. *Anesth Analg* 2004; **99**: 1365–75.

26. Leung TS, Aladangady N, Elwell CE, *et al.* A new method for the measurement of cerebral blood volume and total circulating blood volume using near infrared spatially resolved spectroscopy and indocyanine green: application and validation in neonates. *Pediatr Res* 2004; **55**: 134–41.

27. Patel J, Marks K, Roberts I, *et al.* Measurement of cerebral blood flow in newborn infants using near infrared spectroscopy with indocyanine green. *Pediatr Res* 1998; **43**: 34–9.

28. Meek JH, Elwell CE, McCormick DC, *et al.* Abnormal cerebral haemodynamics in perinatally asphyxiated neonates related to outcome. *Arch Dis Child Fetal Neonatal Ed* 1999; **81**: F110–15.

29. von Siebenthal K, Beran J, Wolf M, *et al.* Cyclical fluctuations in blood pressure, heart rate and cerebral blood volume in preterm infants. *Brain Dev* 1999; **21**: 529–34.

30. Hoffman GM, Stuth EA, Jaquiss RD, *et al.* Changes in cerebral and somatic oxygenation during stage 1 palliation of hypoplastic left heart syndrome using continuous regional cerebral perfusion. *J Thorac Cardiovasc Surg* 2004; **127**: 223–33.

31. Berens RJ, Stuth EA, Robertson FA, *et al.* Near infrared spectroscopy monitoring during pediatric aortic coarctation repair. *Paediatr Anaesth* 2006; **16**: 777–81.

32. Benaron DA, Parachikov IH, Friedland S, *et al.* Continuous, noninvasive, and localized microvascular tissue oximetry using visible light spectroscopy. *Anesthesiology* 2004; **100**: 1469–75.

33. Heninger C, Ramamoorthy C, Amir G, *et al.* Esophageal saturation during antegrade cerebral perfusion: a preliminary report using visible light spectroscopy. *Paediatr Anaesth* 2006; **16**: 1133–7.

34. Helou S, Koehler RC, Gleason CA, *et al.* Cerebrovascular autoregulation during fetal development in sheep. *Am J Physiol* 1994; **266**: H1069–74.

35. Dammann O, Leviton A. Maternal intrauterine infection, cytokines, and brain damage in the preterm newborn. *Pediatr Res* 1997; **42**: 1–8.

36. Dammann O, Drescher J, Veelken N. Maternal fever at birth and non-verbal intelligence at age 9 years in preterm infants. *Dev Med Child Neurol* 2003; **45**: 148–51.

37. Leviton A, Paneth N, Reuss ML, *et al.* Maternal infection, fetal inflammatory response, and brain damage in very low birth weight infants. Developmental Epidemiology Network Investigators. *Pediatr Res* 1999; **46**: 566–75.

38. Slater AJ, Berkowitz ID, Wilson DA, *et al.* Role of leukocytes in cerebral autoregulation and hyperemia in bacterial meningitis in rabbits. *Am J Physiol* 1997; **273**: H380–6.

39. Brady KM, Lee JK, Kibler KK, *et al.* Continuous time-domain analysis of cerebrovascular autoregulation using near-infrared spectroscopy. *Stroke* 2007; **38**: 2818–25.

40. Soul JS, Hammer PE, Tsuji M, *et al.* Fluctuating pressure-passivity is common in the cerebral circulation of sick premature infants. *Pediatr Res* 2007; **61**: 467–73.

41. Tsuji M, Saul JP, du Plessis A, *et al.* Cerebral intravascular oxygenation correlates with mean arterial pressure in critically ill premature infants. *Pediatrics* 2000; **106**: 625–32.

42. American College of Obstetricians and Gynecologists. ACOG Practice Bulletin. Clinical management guidelines for obstetrician–gynecologists, number 70, December 2005. Intrapartum fetal heart rate monitoring. *Obstet Gynecol* 2005; **10**: 1453–60.

43. Committee on Fetus and Newborn, American Academy of Pediatrics. Apnea, sudden infant death syndrome, and home monitoring. *Pediatrics* 2003; **111**: 914–17.

44. Pedersen T, Dyrlund Pedersen B, *et al.* Pulse oximetry for perioperative monitoring. *Cochrane Database Syst Rev* 2003; **(3)**: CD002013.

45. Horlocker TT, Brown DR. Evidence-based medicine: haute couture or the emperor's new clothes? *Anesth Analg* 2005; **100**: 1807–10.

Chapter 20

Placental pathology and the etiology of fetal and neonatal brain injury

Theonia K. Boyd and Rebecca N. Baergen

Introduction

In the context of untoward fetal and/or neonatal outcome, the purpose of performing placental pathology is to identify responsible mechanism(s) and their timing with respect to stillbirth or delivery. Placental pathologic correlates of intrauterine stressors resulting in fetal and neonatal brain injury are fairly well defined. The dilemma arises not in identifying placental abnormalities but in their interpretation in the clinical context. This is due primarily to a paucity of prospective studies directly linking specific clinical abnormalities with placental pathology, which are rarely done in humans as they present practical and ethical problems. Also, there are relatively few animal models of induced pregnancy disorders that have analyzed placental correlates. Instead, associations have largely arisen from clinically or pathologically driven retrospective studies. As a result, in an individual case there is room for interpretation with respect to the likelihood of abnormal placental findings in contributing to or causing untoward neurologic outcome. The benefit of gaining a body of experience in examining placentas and recognizing patterns of association narrows an individual pathologist's interpretive variability. Still, there remains scant bedrock of experimental data upon which to build clinicopathologic interpretation. Consensus provides a surrogate mode of demonstrating confidence in placental interpretation, and to this end two coauthors have collaborated in constructing this chapter. The information and opinions expressed herein reflect our collective experience and understanding of the relationship between placental pathology and intrauterine stressors leading to clinically determined fetal and neonatal brain injury. In some instances, our opinions diverge; those passages reflect variance in pathologic interpretation.

Timing intrauterine stress
Meconium

Meconium visually detectable in amniotic fluid is usually (though perhaps at term not always) released in response to fetal stress. It has been stated, but not proven, that meconium is released in small amounts in the last weeks of normal

intrauterine life. If that is true, then there is no convincing correlate in placentas delivered without a history of meconium detected during the intrapartum period. Meconium release is uncommon prior to the third trimester, even in severely stressed fetuses; thus, in second-trimester premature infants the absence of meconium does not necessarily equate to the absence of intrauterine stress.

There is a time lag between the onset of intrauterine stress and meconium release, as evidenced by hyperacute mechanisms of demise (e.g., acute cord prolapse or ruptured vasa previa), when the fetus dies within 15 or 30 minutes of the event onset. In those cases, meconium will not be released prior to demise, despite the fact that the stressor is severe enough to be rapidly fatal. At the other end of the time spectrum, if a fetus is chronically stressed in utero, that is, for many days to weeks, the fetal body may adapt to the stressor so as not to elicit meconium despite a stressor's obvious deleterious effect. The window of intrauterine stress in which meconium is most likely to be seen is between the hyperacute and chronic phases, namely, from intrauterine stressors of a duration between hours and days, if demise does not intervene.

Once meconium is released into the amniotic fluid and comes into contact with amnion epithelium, it can be taken up by macrophages into the extraplacental membranes and chorionic plate. In general, the longer the elapsed time between the onset of meconium release and placental delivery, the deeper the meconium pigment penetrates into the affected tissue layers. There exists one ex vivo study performed to plot the time between application of meconium to delivered placentas, and the appearance of meconium macrophages in the component layers of the extraplacental membranes [1].

Meconium-induced vascular necrosis (Fig. 20.1) is a very important lesion to recognize within the umbilical cord, as it indicates not only prolonged meconium release due to prolonged intrauterine stress, but carries an independent risk of untoward neonatal outcome due to meconium chemical-induced alteration of vascular tone [2–4]. Ex vivo studies have assessed the interval between meconium application to the umbilical cord surface and the histologic appearance of vascular necrosis [5,6]. Although the authors did not address this particular point, it is implicit in these cases not only that meconium release starts many hours prior to delivery, but that there is continued release, or at least that the stressor

Fetal and Neonatal Brain Injury, 4th edition, ed. David K. Stevenson, William E. Benitz, Philip Sunshine, Susan R. Hintz, and Maurice L. Druzin. Published by Cambridge University Press. © Cambridge University Press 2009.

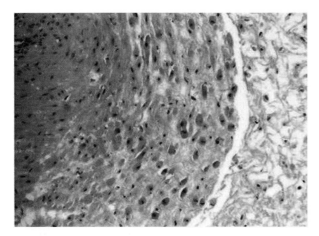

Fig. 20.1. Meconium-induced umbilical vascular necrosis. Outer wall myocytes exhibit pyknosis in the presence of meconium macrophages. *See color plate section.*

eliciting its release persists until the time of delivery. In our experience, this is borne out by clinical and pathologic correlation. Clinically, there is invariably description of abundant meconium, either thick in quality and/or noted to be of prolonged duration prior to delivery. Grossly, the placenta is deeply green or green-brown discolored; umbilical cord discoloration is also present.

On gross placental examination, meconium released shortly prior to delivery will discolor the amniotic membranes and chorionic plate green, perhaps with a patchy distribution, and the discoloration can be wiped from the amnion surface. Often recently released meconium is described clinically as "particulate"; this can also be seen microscopically as entrapped amorphous orange-brown pigment apposed to the amniotic surface. Meconium taken into the tissue, however, remains green even with handling (Fig. 20.2a). Meconium of long-standing duration appears green-brown to brown grossly. This green-brown or brown discoloration may also occur with blood breakdown pigment (biliverdin, hemosiderin), and green discoloration can also be seen sometimes in chorioamnionitis (neutrophil myeloperoxidase): thus green and brown gross discolorations are not restricted to meconium alone.

Microscopically, meconium uptake is seen as an orange-brown, non-refractile macrophage cytoplasmic pigment (Fig. 20.2b). Particulate surface meconium, not yet taken up into tissue macrophages, has the same hue but appears amorphous and globular. However, not all brown-hued cytoplasmic macrophage pigment represents meconium. Sometimes the pigment is related to blood breakdown products; but at times there exists pigment that is not attributable to meconium or bleeding – some authors have suggested this represents lipofuscin, a non-pathologic pigment resulting from the cytoplasmic accumulation of metabolic by-products. In these circumstances, there is no clinical or grossly visible correlate of meconium, and none of the ancillary membrane features that may be associated with meconium discharge (reactive "atypia," amnion necrosis, amnion edema, chorion epithelial necrosis). Utilizing a constellation of findings strengthens the ability to discriminate clinically insignificant macrophage pigment from potentially pathologic meconium.

As a corollary, evidence exists to support the contention that meconium can induce neutrophil chemotaxis via non-infectious, but toxic, chemical components of bile acids [7–9]. Histologically, this may mimic "chorioamnionitis" considered to be of infectious origin. However, in the setting of meconium chemotaxis the fetal inflammatory response is commonly more advanced than the maternal inflammatory response. This view

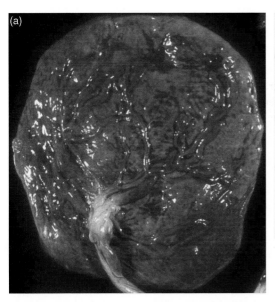

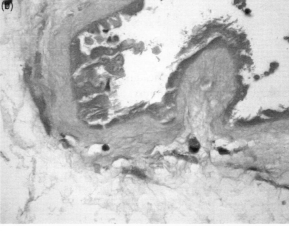

Fig. 20.2. (a) Gross meconium staining: the fetal surface is discolored green to green-brown; the surface typically feels diffluent ("slimy") on palpation. (b) Microscopic meconium uptake into membrane macrophages: through the microscope, meconium appears as a globular or amorphous orange-brown pigment; note the reactive amnion and amnion necrosis due to meconium. *See color plate section.*

is not universally shared among pathologists with placental expertise, however.

There is a general correlation between the thickness of clinically identified meconium and the combination of chronicity and severity of the stressor that elicited its release. Moderate to thick meconium occurs in conditions of overt and/or prolonged intrauterine stress, and according to the clinical literature is associated with an increased risk of adverse outcome [10,11]. Amniotic fluid volume may be one factor that mitigates meconium density; regardless, thick meconium is a marker of non-acute fetal stress.

Microscopically, the density of meconium macrophages reflects meconium thickness, while, as stated above, the depth to which meconium macrophages penetrate reflects the interval between meconium discharge and delivery.

Nucleated red blood cells

In principle, nucleated red blood cells (NRBCs) are not found under normal conditions within the fetal circulation, including that of the placental fetal vascular tree, after the first trimester. In practice, rare NRBCs, either by visual or automated count, may be seen in uncomplicated deliveries. NRBCs represent the immature erythrocyte series (normoblasts) still containing their nuclei. They are normally seen in sites of erythropoiesis, such as the fetal liver and bone marrow, prior to enucleation and release into the peripheral circulation as mature erythrocytes comprised entirely of oxygen-carrying cytoplasm. However, when stimulated, preformed NRBCs are released into the peripheral circulation. These cells have round, dense, hyperchromatic nuclei, and the tinctorial cytoplasmic qualities of their enuclate counterparts (Fig. 20.3). Conditions that stimulate intrauterine release of NRBCs include acute and chronic hypoxic stress, anemia, infection, and maternal diabetes. Initially, preformed normoblasts circulate (normoblastemia), but with prolonged stimulation ever more primitive NRBCs are seen in addition to elevated normoblasts, a likely combination of release and enhanced erythropoiesis. In conditions of prolonged persistent hypoxic stress that

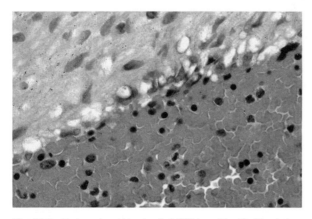

Fig. 20.3. Nucleated red blood cells (NRBCs) are identified by their round hyperchromatic nuclei and pink-red cytoplasm. NRBCs of this proportion indicate non-acute hypoxic stress, in this case from a stillbirth due to umbilical cord hypercoiling. *See color plate section.*

permit intrauterine survival, such as alloimmune hemolytic anemia or chronic fetomaternal hemorrhage, the most primitive nucleated erythrocytes – erythroblasts – are released into the fetal circulation (erythroblastosis). In these circumstances, erythropoiesis is markedly accelerated, often in atypical visceral sites (e.g., kidney, pancreas).

Pure hypoxic stimulation is mediated by the release of erythropoietin. The factors(s) that mediate NRBC release in infection are not well understood. One possible mechanism may be non-specific release of hematopoietic elements in response to cytokine stimulation, perhaps due to immaturity of the fetal immune system and its signals [12]. A second potential mechanism may include a component of hypoxic stimulation in the setting of infection, perhaps mediated by erythropoietin [13,14]; however, these two potential pathways are scantily supported by experimental data.

The timing of NRBC release in response to stimulation has undergone a conceptual shift. Older literature stated that erythropoiesis occurred prior to the appearance of peripherally circulating erythrocytes, meaning the interval between stimulus and release was on the order of days or more. More recent literature indicates that stimulation leads to release of preformed NRBCs, truncating the time interval between stimulus and response. In this latter model, stimulus-driven erythropoiesis occurs only when the stimulus is prolonged. Thus, both acute and chronic modes of hypoxic stress can induce normoblastemia [15,16].

How long after a hypoxic stimulus does it take to detect circulating NRBCs? In our experience, and supported by some literature, NRBCs can begin to be seen within about an hour to a few hours following the onset of hypoxia. With continued intrauterine hypoxic stress, the number of NRBCs will continue to rise, such that at any given time point NRBC values will reflect both the chronicity and severity of the stimulus eliciting their production and/or release. Erythroblastosis, on the other hand, occurs only in conditions of chronic persistent hypoxia, lasting weeks rather than hours or days.

How long after the cessation of a hypoxic stimulus, for example interruption by parturition, does it take for circulating NRBCs to disappear? As a general principle (in one author's experience), the rate of fall approximately mirrors the rate of rise. Thus, a hypoxic stressor of some hours' onset prior to delivery will elicit NRBC release that concomitantly falls also within hours, perhaps up to a day (as opposed to days or weeks) following delivery. In contradistinction, chronic hypoxic stress results in postnatal NRBCs that fall over days to a week or more [17–19]. Persistent elevation of NRBC counts for several days following delivery should also suggest other causes, such as congenital infection or maternal diabetes.

NRBCs are counted in peripheral blood in reference to the normally nucleated peripheral blood cells, the leukocytes (white blood cells, WBCs). This can be done microscopically, as NRBCs are discriminated based upon their nuclear and cytoplasmic morphology from myeloid and lymphoid leukocytes. In the laboratory, NRBCs can also be discriminated from leukocytes by automated separation. In histologic evaluation, and in most laboratory reports, the NRBC count is expressed as a number per 100 WBCs. Some laboratories instead, or also, report an absolute NRBC count, expressed as the number of NRBCs per mm³. In our experience, semi-quantitative counts or estimates of NRBCs per 100 WBCs correlate well with automated counts in initial neonatal laboratory values, if drawn within a short time after delivery. In uncomplicated deliveries, there is excellent correlation between automated absolute NRBC counts and automated counts expressed per 100 WBCs [20]. Absolute counts are preferred if the leukocyte count is abnormally high or low, or rapidly changing. However, counts greater than 2000/mm³ should be considered elevated.

While the majority of the clinical literature supports reliability in using nucleated red blood cell counts and/or clearance times to assess the timing and severity of hypoxic stress in utero [21–25], conflicting results have been reported [26]. The latter may reflect limitations in the use of dichotomous relative NRBC counts (< or > 10 NRBCs per 100 WBCs) rather than continuous absolute NRBC counts (NRBCs per mm³).

Acute blood flow disruption, fetal hemorrhage, and anemia

Acute interruption of maternal or fetal blood flow can occur from obstruction or disruption of blood vessels. Acute interruption of maternal blood flow to the placenta is generally caused by uterine rupture, placental abruption, or maternal circulatory collapse, while interruption of fetal blood flow is usually caused by disruption of large fetal vessels in the placenta or acute cord obstruction.

Traumatic uterine rupture may occur as a result of a motor-vehicle accident, abdominal trauma, or dehiscence of a previous cesarean section scar. Uterine rupture is often associated with life-threatening maternal hemorrhage necessitating hysterectomy, and it may lead to sudden, severe fetal hypoxia sufficient to cause severe neurologic injury or death [27]. Pathologic examination of the uterus can identify the site of the uterine rupture and the associated dissection of blood through the uterine wall. In acute abruption, the placenta separates from the uterus prior to delivery of the infant with loss of blood flow to the placental tissue underlying the abruption. It is estimated that an acute abruption of 50% will lead to fetal demise [28]. Lesser degrees of separation and more chronic abruptions can lead to sublethal injury [29–31]. If cesarean section is performed, direct visualization of placental detachment is possible, and bleeding from the torn decidual vessels will result in a retroplacental hematoma. Gross examination of the delivered placenta will often show compression of the villous tissue underlying the hematoma. Within a few hours, villous stromal hemorrhage with also develop, and over the next few days there are progressive indications of ischemic change in the underlying chorionic villi and eventual infarction [32]. In the following days to weeks, the clot organizes and the villous infarction becomes a firm, tan-white scar. However, many acute abruptions extend over time, and thus the pathologic changes may be of different ages.

Interruption of fetal blood flow most often is caused by trauma. It may occur through any fetal vessel, from the umbilical vessels and their tributaries coursing over the chorionic plate, down to the villous capillaries [33,34]. Interruption of fetal blood flow is usually associated with acute fetal blood loss and anemia, which in turn may lead to hypotension and significant neurologic injury or death. Disruption of larger vessels will result in a large fetal hemorrhage relatively quickly, potentially leading to severe hypovolemia and circulatory collapse, while hemorrhage from small vessels tends to be more chronic but may still be quite significant. The most common etiology of large-vessel hemorrhage is disruption of velamentous or membranous vessels. As these vessels travel in the membranes without the protection of Wharton's jelly, they are quite susceptible to damage. The umbilical cord itself can rupture but this, fortunately, is a rare event. Most cord ruptures are partial but still lead to severe fetal hemorrhage and anemia, with a significant risk of neurologic injury in the infants who survive. The etiologies of cord rupture are very rare but include excessive traction on the cord during delivery from either a short cord [33] or abnormal placental adherence in placenta accreta [31], or from friability of the cord due to aneurysms of the umbilical vessels [34], hemangiomas [34], necrotizing funisitis [35], or meconium-induced myonecrosis [36]. Cord rupture most often occurs at the site of its placental attachment [37]. When fetal vessels or the umbilical cord are disrupted, careful, directed pathologic examination is necessary to document the specific underlying lesion as well as to confirm that the rupture is not a post-delivery event. In some cases, subtlety of findings or lack of clinical correlative information may make diagnosis problematic. However, placental findings indicative of severe fetal anemia are quite straightforward. Since the blood content, and therefore the color, of the villous tissue is generally reflective of the fetal hematocrit, in a significant fetal anemia the placental parenchyma is usually strikingly pale (Fig. 20.4) [38]. On microscopic examination,

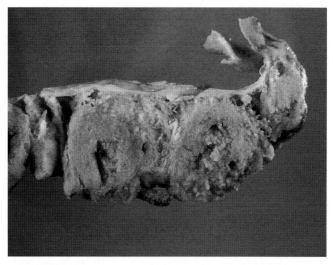

Fig. 20.4. Cut section of a formalin-fixed placenta from a severe fetomaternal hemorrhage. Note the markedly pale parenchymal tissue. *See color plate section.*

one finds a marked increase in fetal nucleated red blood cells and villous edema. The fetal blood vessels may also appear relatively "empty" of blood [31,32].

Fetal hemorrhage from the villous capillaries will cause fetal blood to escape into the intervillous space, resulting in a fetomaternal hemorrhage. This is thought to develop from damage to the trophoblastic cover of the chorionic villi [32], but in most cases there is no history of trauma and the exact cause is obscure. Fetomaternal hemorrhage is seen with increased frequency in the presence of placental choriocarcinomas and large placental chorangiomas [37]. In many cases, there are multiple episodes of bleeding leading to chronic blood loss. Placental findings include evidence of fetal anemia as described above and, in some cases, multiple or large intervillous thrombi. Definitive diagnosis rests on identification of fetal blood in the maternal circulation, most commonly determined by the Kleihauer–Betke test although other tests, such as the Apt test or flow cytometry, are also used. The Kleihauer–Betke test is reported as a percentage of fetal red blood cells in the maternal circulation. Confounding factors in interpretation include a falsely low result when the mother and infant have ABO-incompatible blood types, which causes the fetal blood cells to be quickly cleared from the maternal circulation, or a falsely high result when there is maternal persistence of fetal hemoglobin. Since fetal cells persist in the maternal circulation for up to a month or more, performing the test is useful even if it is not done immediately after delivery. It is strongly recommended that it be performed in any case in which neonatal anemia is diagnosed or there is an unexplained stillbirth.

A specific type of acute exsanguination takes place in monozygotic twins with monochorionic placentas. In these placentas, vascular anastomoses between the two placentas are always present to some degree. In a minority of cases, there is a dominant artery-to-vein anastomosis, causing a chronic shunt of blood from one twin, the donor, to the other twin, the recipient. This is the basis for the twin-to-twin transfusion syndrome, also called chronic twin-to-twin transfusion. The donor twin suffers from lack of growth, anemia, and hypovolemia while the recipient twin suffers from edema, congestion, and hypervolemia. Both are at risk for heart failure, death, and neurologic injury [31,32,38]. However, even when this condition is not present, there is always the potential for acute transfusion of blood from one twin to the other in monochorionic placentas [31]. If one twin dies in utero, the dead twin becomes a "sink" into which the surviving twin bleeds. The surviving twin will be severely anemic and the corresponding placenta will be markedly pale. Depending on the size of the anastomoses, hemorrhage can lead to a variety of outcomes from minimal blood loss to profound neurologic injury or death, all of which will occur within a matter of minutes of death of the co-twin [38]. This type of "acute" transfusion of blood accounts for a significant portion of the increased morbidity and mortality seen in monochorionic twins [32]. The previous theory that embolization of thrombotic material from the dead twin causes damage to the surviving twin makes little sense and has been shown to be untenable [32].

Trauma is an important cause of fetal hemorrhage and may result from fetal blood sampling, cordocentesis, amniocentesis, fetal transfusion, or by direct needle puncture of the fetus during various procedures [31,32]. Blood will often be present in the amniotic fluid, causing a "port wine" discoloration of the fluid. Trauma to the umbilical cord can cause formation of a hematoma, which can be identified as an elongated, fusiform swelling of the cord, with a dark red discoloration and dissection of blood through Wharton's jelly. In very acute injury to fetal vessels, extravasated fresh blood may be visible in the site of the trauma. In subacute injury, there may be hemolysis of the extravasated blood leading to a reddish discoloration of the umbilical cord or fetal surface of the placenta, most prominent in the area of trauma. With remote injury, an organizing blood clot can be visible with hemosiderin deposition that will stain the surface yellow to brown. On microscopic examination, hemosiderin-laden macrophages will be visible, and the presence of an organizing hematoma can provide an estimate of the timing of the traumatic event.

Severe fetal anemia may also occur without trauma or disruption, but it still has the same potential for neurologic injury and death. Other causes include infections, such as parvovirus, which have a predilection for red blood cells, Rh incompatibility (erythroblastosis fetalis), genetic disorders associated with red blood cell destruction, such as hemolytic anemia, or disorders associated with poor production, such as thalassemia. Clinical suspicion and specific diagnostic tests are needed to confirm these conditions in most cases.

Mechanisms of umbilical cord blood-flow compromise

Umbilical cord compression and obstruction

Most types of cord obstruction are associated with compression of the umbilical cord through some type of mechanical force. Compression may be from the fetus itself, as in cord entanglements, membranous vessels, or prolapse, or may be from an abnormal configuration of the cord such as a true knot, abnormal coiling, abnormal length, or a constriction. All have been associated with adverse outcome including fetal demise, neurologic injury, and abnormal developmental outcome [29–32,33,39,40]. Often, structural abnormalities occur together: for example, entanglements and knots are frequently associated with long cords, and excessive coiling is often seen with constrictions. If obstruction is sudden and complete, fetal death will usually result, and in those that do survive, significant neurologic damage is likely [29,32,39,41–44]. The same is true for prolonged partial obstruction. Thus, long-standing conditions such as long cords, hypercoiling, constrictions, and velamentous insertions are significantly more common in infants with cerebral palsy [30,39,43,44]. Experimental studies in lambs have shown that intermittent partial cord occlusion leads to the development of cerebral necrosis and serious neurologic damage [45]. Furthermore, in these conditions, there is often an acute exacerbation of obstruction during delivery: for example, a cord entanglement or knot may tighten during fetal descent in labor or membranous vessels may become compressed after membrane rupture with loss of the cushioning effect of the amniotic fluid. In cord compression, the umbilical vein, being more distensible than the arteries, will be compressed more easily, and Doppler studies have confirmed that cord obstruction and compression lead to impeded venous return from the placenta [41]. Placental venous and capillary congestion will result, and often the fetus can develop some degree of hypovolemia and anemia. In acute compression, placental examination will show marked distension of the umbilical vessels, particularly the vein, tributaries of the umbilical vein in the chorionic plate, and villous capillaries. Direct compression of a portion of the cord by fetal parts or the cervix may also cause some non-specific localized degenerative change of Wharton's jelly or the umbilical vessels.

Chronic cord compression develops from the same type of mechanical forces that lead to acute compression. Except for cord entanglement and prolapse, the cord abnormalities are easily diagnosed by gross examination of the placenta. Chronic obstruction of blood flow through the venous circulation leads to venous stasis in the short term and vascular thrombosis in the long term, which can further embarrass the fetal blood supply. The resultant thrombotic lesions are called fetal thrombotic vasculopathy (see below). Not only have the underlying causes of cord compression been associated with adverse outcome, the resultant thrombotic lesions in the placenta have also been associated with poor outcome including stroke due to thromboembolic phenomenon [29,40,46,47].

Umbilical cord coiling and constriction

The umbilical cord is usually twisted to the left or counter-clockwise, in a ratio of about 7 : 1 [32]. The direction of coiling is not associated with handedness, but right twisting has been associated with placenta previa and perinatal hemorrhage [48]. The direction and amount of coiling is established early in gestation and can be seen by sonography as early as the ninth week. Normally the number of coils in the cord is about 0.2 coils per 1 cm of cord, which is referred to as the coiling index [41]. The origin of umbilical cord coiling has long been debated, but studies suggest that it is due, at least in part, to fetal activity in utero. Thus hypocoiling reflects fetal inactivity, while hypercoiling reflects increased fetal activity, at least to some degree [32]. Absent or minimal coiling is rare, but when present has an ominous prognosis, as it is associated with fetal distress, increased perinatal mortality, fetal demise, fetal anomalies, and chromosomal errors [41,49–51]. Hypercoiling, on the other hand, has been associated with preterm labor, fetal demise, fetal asphyxia, and chronic fetal hypoxia [41,49–51]. It is also seen more frequently in cords with constrictions and those of excessive length, both of which are also associated with adverse outcome [40,41].

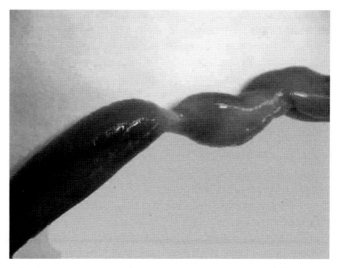

Fig. 20.5. Portion of umbilical cord with constriction in the center of the figure. The cord is discolored green due to long-standing meconium staining.

A significant reduction in the diameter of the umbilical cord is referred to as constriction, stricture, torsion, or coarctation (Fig. 20.5). Constrictions are most commonly found near or at the insertion into the fetal abdomen, and they are seen with increased frequency in long or hypercoiled cords [50]. Obstruction of blood flow occurs by the same mechanism as with excessive coiling, namely, compression of umbilical vessels by the cord itself. Some authors have been skeptical about this lesion, suggesting that it is merely secondary to fetal demise, gradually diminishing Wharton's jelly at the fetal end of the cord [52], or a primary deficiency of Wharton's jelly [53]. However, there is often congestion on one side of the constriction and thrombosis of fetal vessels, which is proof that it is not an artifact at least in those cases. Furthermore, if these were artifacts, they would be seen in the majority, if not all, fetal demises – and that is not the case. Hypercoiling and constriction, like other types of mechanical obstruction, can lead to fetal thrombotic vasculopathy. There have been many publications demonstrating the poor outcome of umbilical cord stricture, including fetal demise, fetal growth restriction, and fetal intolerance to labor [32,41–43].

The excessively long or short cord

The umbilical cord is, on average, 55–61 cm in length at term [54]. The cord lengthens throughout gestation, although growth slows after 28 weeks. At 6 weeks post-conception the cord has an average length of 0.5 cm, by the fourth month it is between 16 and 18 cm, and by the sixth month it is 33–35 cm [32]. It is interesting to note that measurements of cord length can shrink up to 7 cm in the first few hours following delivery. For this reason, and because portions of the cord may be used for laboratory tests or discarded in the delivery room, accurate measurement of the entire length of the cord at the time of birth is optimal. However, attempts to convince delivering physicians of the importance of such measurements have generally failed. For this reason, the diagnosis of a short cord is generally not possible in the pathology laboratory.

As with umbilical cord coiling, cord length has been correlated with fetal activity in utero [32]. This is supported by the fact that short cords are present in conditions where there is intrauterine constraint due to uterine anomalies, amnionic adhesions, or ectopic pregnancies [33], or where there is decreased fetal movement due to neurologic conditions, skeletal dysplasias, or other anomalies [55]. The relationship between long cords and excessive fetal movements is more difficult to assess because of the lack of data on prenatal movements and follow-up on the potential "hyperactivity" in infants with long cords [56,57]. There does appear to be a genetic component as well, since mothers with a history of a long cord are at increased risk of a long cord in subsequent pregnancies [40].

There is no consensus on the minimum length for a diagnosis of an excessively long cord, with definitions ranging from 70 cm to 90 cm. This inconsistency is due in part to the lack of accurate measurement of cord length at the time of delivery such that pathologists are left with a cord length of "at least" a certain measurement rather than the true measurement. A retrospective study of over 38 000 placentas found that excessively long cords occurred in 3.95% of placentas and that right coiling, cord entanglement, hypercoiling, and true knots were more common in long cords [40]. In addition, long cords are associated with histologic findings of villous capillary congestion and fetal thrombotic vasculopathy [40,58] as well as evidence of intrauterine hypoxia such as chorangiosis and increased nucleated red blood cells [40]. It appears that such long or hypercoiled cords have increased resistance to flow, which may lead to greater pressures in the fetal circulation [40,59], and this is supported by the presence of cardiac enlargement and hypertrophy in fetuses with long cords [59]. Fetal growth restriction, intrauterine demise, and neonatal coagulation disorders are all seen with increased frequency in long cords. Furthermore, excessive cord length has been associated with increased morbidity, including cerebral degenerative changes [58], brain imaging abnormalities, neurologic injury, and poor long-term neurologic status [40].

As with long cords, the cut-off for short cords is also not well defined, and figures are reported to be from 32 cm to 40 cm at term. Short cords correlate well with depressed intelligence quotient (IQ) and with a variety of fetal and neonatal problems [60]. The essential question is whether the short cord is due to prenatal problems that caused diminished activity, or whether the problems resulted from perinatal complications from delivery of an infant with a short cord. Extremely short cords, less than 15 cm, are commonly seen in infants with fetal anomalies, particularly abdominal wall defects, and spinal and limb deformities. Short cords can cause problems at delivery as they may prevent descent of the infant and thus lead to abruption, uterine inversion, and even cord rupture. If this occurs, serious neurologic sequelae or death may be the result [32]. These complications may also be seen even when there is a "relative" short cord created by cord entanglement.

Cord entanglement, true knots, and cord prolapse

The umbilical cord may become entangled around any fetal part, but the most common is a nuchal cord, in which the cord is looped around the fetal neck. Entanglements have been found as early as 10 weeks' gestation, and nuchal cords in particular are commonly diagnosed by sonography, but some of these appear to resolve by delivery [35]. Even so, at term, the incidence of nuchal cords is 15–20%. Infrequently, multiple loops of cord may become wrapped around the neck, and up to eight loops have been reported [32]. Cords may encircle the neck in an unlocked or locked pattern, the latter having more severe consequences for fetal outcome [61].

The association of nuchal cords with fetal growth restriction implies that entanglements and their associated cord compression are long-standing prenatal events [62]. Since most cord entanglements are relatively loose, they do not lead to adverse outcome, but they may tighten after membrane rupture when the infant descends down the birth canal. If one looks only at tight entanglements, there is an increase in perinatal complications, low Apgar scores, and fetal demise [39]. Neonates with nuchal cords are also significantly more anemic than controls, presumably because of decreased venous return from compression of the umbilical vein [63]. Rarely, they can be so tight as to lead to hypovolemic shock in the neonate [63]. A correlation between tight nuchal cords and cerebral palsy has also been shown [64].

True knots, like cord entanglements, may be tight or loose. Venous distension distal to the knot and vascular congestion in the placenta is a characteristic finding in tight knots of clinical significance (Fig. 20.6). These are often associated with thrombosis of placental surface veins. The incidence of true knots is reported to be from 0.4% to 1.2% [32], but they are more common with long or hypercoiled cords [31,32,40]. Complex knots and cord entanglements are especially frequent in monoamnionic–monochorionic twins, and cause significant morbidity and mortality [32]. True knots have also been

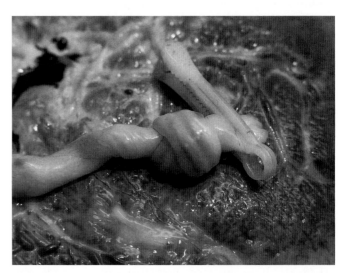

Fig. 20.6. Tight true knot of the umbilical cord. Although congestion was not present on the placental side of the knot grossly, on histologic section the umbilical vein was dilated and early thrombosis was identified.

associated with variable decelerations on fetal heart tracings, fetal distress, fetal hypoxia, long-term neurological damage, and perinatal morbidity [32].

Cord prolapse occurs when the umbilical cord precedes the presenting fetal part during labor and delivery. Here, the cord may be acutely compressed by the fetal head during a vaginal delivery. Prolapse is uncommon, occurring in less than 1% of deliveries, but has significant perinatal mortality, from 10% to 13% [32]. It can also lead to serious neurologic consequences for the fetus [32]. Risk factors include abnormal fetal presentation, preterm labor, multiparity, multiple gestation, low birthweight, obstetric manipulation, polyhydramnios, abruption, placenta previa, and a long cord [65]. Pathologic examination will reveal acute congestion and, rarely, localized damage to the umbilical cord at the site of the compression.

Velamentous vessels

The umbilical cord normally inserts on the placenta near or at the center. In about 7% of term placentas the cord inserts at the margin, and in about 1%, it inserts into the membranes: a velamentous insertion [31,32]. Velamentous vessels are present in velamentous and furcate insertions of the umbilical cord, between accessory lobes and occasionally in marginal cord insertions. These vessels run within the membranes without the protection of Wharton's jelly and are thus susceptible to thrombosis, compression, disruption, or other trauma. This is particularly true in velamentous insertions when the cord inserts far from the placental margin and the vessels have a long membranous course (Fig. 20.7). Velamentous vessels are most vulnerable after membrane rupture, when the protection of the amniotic fluid is lost. Although hemorrhage from ruptured velamentous vessels occurs only in about 1 in 50 velamentous cord insertions, mortality from the subsequent fetal hemorrhage is 58–73% [66]. Velamentous cord insertions are also associated with abnormal fetal heart-rate

tracings, fetal growth restriction, low birthweight, and low Apgar scores [32,67]. Velamentous vessels may also be associated with vasa previa, where the membranous vessels cross the cervical os, preceding the presenting fetal part. These vessels may be compressed during labor and cause fetal distress and hypoxia [68]. If a vaginal delivery is attempted, the membranous vessels will be disrupted and fetal hemorrhage will result. Depending on the extent of the hemorrhage, exsanguination and fetal death may result, or there may be serious neurologic injury in the infants who survive. Examination of the placenta is essential to document the presence of disrupted velamentous vessels and hemorrhage into the surrounding membranes. It is crucial that the suspicion of ruptured velamentous vessels be communicated to the pathologist prior to examination, so that extra care can be taken to preserve these findings.

Fetal vascular thrombosis

Obstruction of blood flow through the cord leads to decreased venous return from the placenta, venous stasis, and subsequent thrombosis in the fetal circulation, which can further embarrass blood supply to the fetus. Thrombosis may occur not only from cord compression or obstruction but also due to a hypercoagulable state, maternal diabetes, infection, and other miscellaneous conditions [69]. There are a number of thrombotic lesions comprising this group, including occlusive and non-occlusive thrombi, mural thrombi, intimal fibrin cushions, avascular villi, and villous stromal karyorrhexis [70]. On microscopic examination, recent thrombi contain fibrin, clot, and extracellular material, which most often does not completely occlude the vascular lumen (Fig. 20.8). Older thrombi are recognizable by the presence of calcification within the vessel wall, indicating duration of many weeks (Fig. 20.9). In mural thrombi or intimal fibrin cushions, fibrin is attached to the endothelium or incorporated into the intima (Fig. 20.10). This is sometimes associated with an increase in

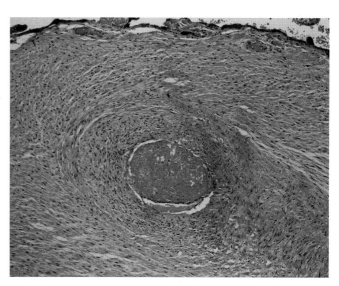

Fig. 20.7. Placenta with a velamentous insertion. Note that the umbilical cord inserts far from the placental margin and numerous membranous vessels are present. In this case, there is no disruption of vessels or hemorrhage in the surrounding membranes. *See color plate section.*

Fig. 20.8. Fetal vessel in a stem villus with a recent, nearly occlusive thrombus. *See color plate section.*

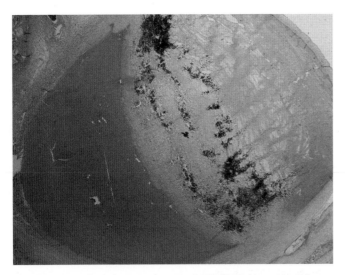

Fig. 20.9. Large fetal chorionic plate vessel with distension and partially occlusive thrombus. Calcification in the thrombus is indicative of chronicity. *See color plate section.*

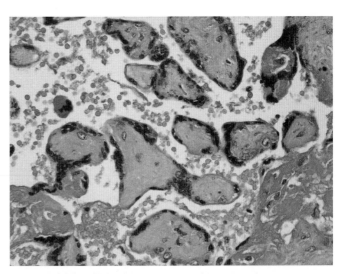

Fig. 20.11. Avascular villi. Focus of villi lacking any villous capillaries and with marked hyalinization of the stroma indicative of upstream fetal vascular thrombosis. *See color plate section.*

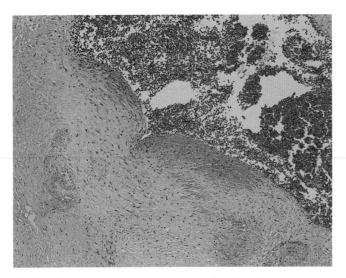

Fig. 20.10. Large fetal chorionic plate vessel with intimal fibrin cushion. Note fibrin deposition in the wall of the vessel in the lower left of the figure and deposition of pale-blue ground substance forming a "cushion." *See color plate section.*

ground substance, forming the appearance of a vascular cushion. Lack of blood flow in the fetal circulation will eventually lead to involution of the "downstream" villi, resulting in the formation of avascular villi, a process also occurring over a period of weeks. Avascular villi contain hyalinized stroma and no fetal vessels, but have a normal-appearing trophoblastic cover (Fig. 20.11). Villous stromal karyorrhexis is most commonly, but not exclusively, found in the smaller villous capillaries [71]. Obstruction of blood flow leads to damage of the vascular wall, necrosis, and extravasation of blood into the stroma. Nuclear debris or karyorrhexis will be present in the villous stroma. This lesion is likely an intermediate lesion in the evolution of avascular villi [70]. Fetal thrombotic vasculopathy, the term applied to regional villous stromal karyorrhexis and/or avascular villi, and fetal vascular thrombosis

in muscularized upstream vessels have been linked to adverse neurologic outcome [71,72].

Amniotic fluid infection

Amniotic fluid infection can elicit both maternal and fetal inflammatory responses. Acute chorioamnionitis, a maternal inflammatory response, is defined histologically as acute inflammatory cells within the fetal membranes: specifically, the amnion and the chorion. Contrary to what is often suggested, the presence of acute inflammatory cells in the membranes is not a normal response to labor or other influences. It is usually, and some believe always, indicative of an ascending bacterial infection, an intrauterine infection. Bacteria ascend from the vagina through the cervix and into the uterine cavity. Whether they gain access to the uterine cavity appears to be due to various host factors in the presence of an intact mucus plug in the cervix, and not due to the presence of ruptured membranes. Indeed, most infections arise in the face of intact membranes, and bacteria have been shown to invade through these layers to infect the amniotic fluid without membrane rupture [36]. Initially, when the bacteria first enter the uterine cavity, the inflammatory response is maternal in origin and is localized to the membranes in the area of the cervical os. If the infection goes unchecked, bacteria will gain access to the amniotic cavity and the fetus will be exposed to bacterial antigens and other products. Once this happens a fetal inflammatory response will ensue. The difference between maternal and fetal response can be seen quite readily through the microscope when one observes from which vessels the inflammatory cells are migrating. Maternal cells migrating from the decidua will be present in the extraplacental membranes and decidua basalis (Fig. 20.12). Maternal cells also migrate from the blood in the intervillous space and can be found under and within the chorionic plate. Fetal inflammatory cells will be seen migrating out of fetal vessels in the umbilical cord (acute

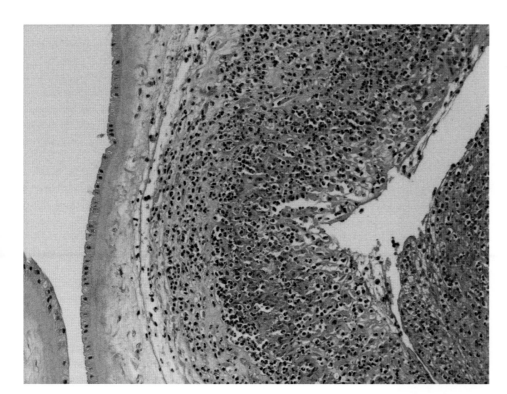

Fig. 20.12. Section of extraplacental membranes with acute chorioamnionitis. Notice infiltration of numerous neutrophils within all layers of the membranes: these are derived from the decidua and thus the maternal circulation. *See color plate section.*

funisitis) and chorionic plate (chorionic plate vasculitis). Inflammation of chorionic vessels can result in endothelial damage and even fetal vascular thrombosis. These events generally occur over a period of days. An alternative perspective suggests that noxious but non-infectious substances such as meconium may elicit a neutrophilic placental inflammatory response (see section on meconium, above).

Ascending infection is a major cause of preterm delivery as well as neonatal morbidity and mortality, and this is mostly due to the elaboration of inflammatory mediators or cytokines by the fetus [36]. The fetal inflammatory response occurs initially, at least, without infection of the fetus. The fetus is exposed to bacterial products and elicits an inflammatory response. This in turn causes the production of numerous cytokines and inflammatory mediators. In preterm infants, cytokines interfere with maturation of oligodendrocytes. In both term and preterm infants, there are many systemic and central nervous system effects caused by cytokines. In particular, the permeability of the blood–brain barrier is altered, vasoactive effects lead to hypoperfusion of the brain, and there are direct toxic effects on brain cells by inflammatory mediators [30,62,63]. Furthermore, if the fetus becomes infected, usually the lungs are initially involved and acute bronchopneumonia develops. This leads to decreased pulmonary function and oxygenation. If the fetus becomes septic, hypotension and decreased vascular perfusion will also occur. Therefore, it is not surprising that the presence of a severe fetal inflammatory response has been linked to adverse neurologic outcome, periventricular leukomalacia, and cerebral palsy [30,71–73].

Mechanisms of chronic diminished placental reserves
Maternal vascular underperfusion

Conditions in this category are secondary to suboptimal uteroplacental underperfusion. Those that are chronic, which are the majority, are at risk for recurrence in future pregnancies unless the underlying disorder is modifiable. The common pathophysiologic pathway is one of maternal vascular disease that reduces spiral arteriolar perfusion, leading to placental ischemic changes and placental and fetal growth restriction; this makes arterioles prone to thrombosis, leading to placental infarction; and this makes arterioles prone to rupture, leading to abruption (Fig. 20.13).

Maternal diseases that fall into this category include chronic hypertension, chronic insulin-dependent diabetes mellitus, pre-eclampsia, certain forms of autoimmunity such as systemic lupus erythematosus, associated lupus-like antibody disorders, connective tissue diseases such as scleroderma, and, rarely, abnormal uterine anatomy with deficient vasculature such as uterine septum. Some authors believe that maternal thrombophilias can also lead to underperfusion, although this view is not universally accepted.

In severely affected pregnancies, the placenta is invariably growth-restricted, and exhibits microscopic features of villous ischemia [74], distal villous hypoplasia, aggregated terminal villi (Fig. 20.14), so-called villous "hypermaturation," increased syncytial knots, intervillous cytotrophoblast/fibrinoid islands, and decidual arteriopathy. Additional features, as noted above,

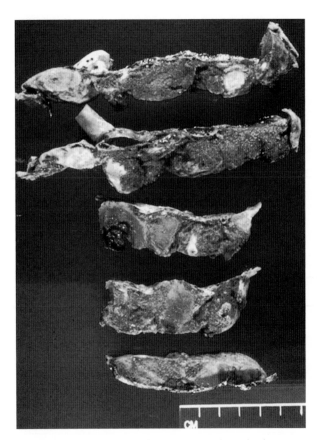

Fig. 20.13. Gross pathology of intrinsic maternal vascular disease leading to chronic maternal vascular underperfusion. Multiple temporally heterogeneous infarcts, with or without placental abruption (present in this case, middle section on left). *See color plate section.*

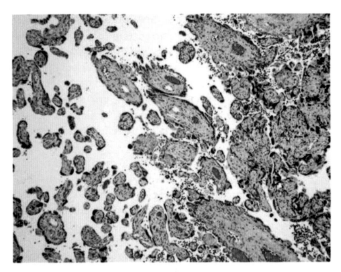

Fig. 20.14. Some of the microscopic features of chronic maternal underperfusion: villous ischemic changes, manifested as distal villous hypoplasia (on left) and villous agglutination (on right). *See color plate section.*

include placental infarction and abruption, which in this may be multifocal and temporally heterogeneous, reflecting the multifocal and progressive nature of maternal vascular abnormalities. The *sine qua non* of vascular disease is the

microscopic phenotype of decidual arteriopathy. In its milder form there is persistence of decidual arteriolar smooth muscle, so-called non-transformation. The more severe form manifests so-called "fibrinoid necrosis," histologically represented by hyalinized eosinophilic arterial walls; if lipid-laden macrophages are also present, then the term "with acute atherosis" is applied (Fig. 20.15). These pathologic vessels are thrombogenic, leading to placental infarction, and prone to rupture, resulting in acute abruption.

Fetuses are commonly growth-restricted. This is due to chronically compromised oxygen and nutrient delivery, a consequence of suboptimal maternal intervillous blood flow. Placental growth restriction, also caused by reduced maternal blood flow, may compound fetal growth restriction via impaired placental-to-fetal blood flow, manifested by abnormal Doppler umbilical arterial studies. Chronically reduced maternal-to-placental blood flow renders the placental fetal vascular tree underdeveloped, with narrow villous caliber and diminished generational branching (distal villous hypoplasia).

The resultant reduction in distal villous fetal vascular caliber and global volume leads to increased placental vascular resistance by Doppler imaging, and, if severe, to reversed diastolic umbilical arterial Doppler flow. While many, perhaps most, live-born fetuses with placental features of underperfusion demonstrate no clinical evidence for neurologic impairment, possibly due to adaptive cerebroprotective mechanisms of persistent hypoxic stress, there are exceptions, particularly in very-low-birthweight infants [75,76].

Other conditions associated with diminished placental reserves, due presumably to maternal immune-mediated mechanisms, including autoantibody and other immune dysregulation, include villitis of unknown etiology (VUE, non-specific chronic villitis) [77], maternal floor infarction (MFI) [78], and a disorder likely related to MFI, massive perivillous fibrin deposition (MPFD) [79]. Indirect evidence for maternal-based pathophysiology in these conditions comes from (1) high recurrence rates in subsequent pregnancies [80] and (2) case reports of recurrent pregnancy loss rescue by immunomodulatory therapy during gestation [81–83].

Villitis of unknown etiology, non-specific chronic villitis (VUE)

Villitis of unknown etiology (VUE) is represented microscopically by maternal T-lymphocyte and histiocyte infiltration into villous stroma. Affected villi exhibit inflammation-induced vascular obliteration; when extensive, the term "obliterative fetal vasculopathy" is used. Extensive villous involvement by VUE with obliterative fetal vasculopathy is associated with growth restriction, stillbirth, and neurologic impairment (Fig. 20.16) [84,85]. As previously mentioned, with severe VUE there is an increased risk of pathologically recurrent placental VUE and untoward pregnancy outcome in future pregnancies. There are no relevant animal models to date.

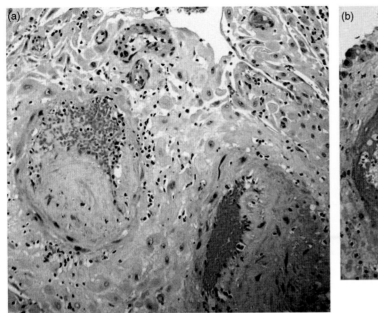
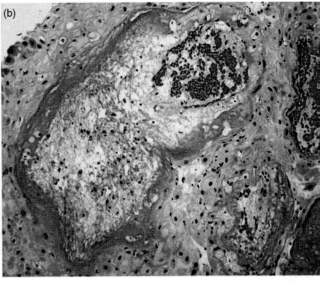

Fig. 20.15. Decidual arteriopathy. (a) Milder phenotype: non-transformation of spiral arterioles. (b) More severe phenotype: fibrinoid necrosis with acute atherosis. *See color plate section.*

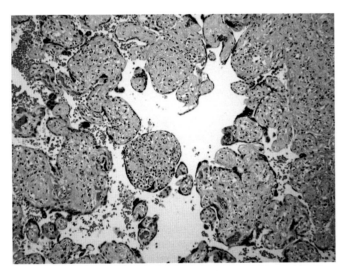

Fig. 20.16. Severe chronic villitis. Widespread obliteration of terminal villous capillaries and distal stem villous vessels (so-called obliterative vasculopathy). *See color plate section.*

Maternal floor infarction (MFI) and massive perivillous fibrin deposition (MPFD)

Maternal floor infarction (MFI) and massive perivillous fibrin deposition (MPFD) are likely variant expressions of pathologically related if not identical phenomena. MFI is characterized by a thick fibrin(oid) rind that coats the basal placenta. Although commonly referred to as fibrin, the component products include not only maternal blood-derived fibrin but also protein-rich extracellular substrate of extravillous trophoblast ("X-cell") derivation, presumably the result of altered metabolism by cytotrophoblast hypoxia. Grossly, regions of firm off-white deposits replace the normally spongy red placenta parenchyma. Microscopically, the maternal intervillous space is packed with eosinophilic proteinaceous material that prohibits blood flow to entrapped villi, leading to ischemic villous damage of affected villi and reduced flow to overlying areas unaffected by the fibrin band. MPFD similarly packs the intervillous space with fibrin(oid), but the distribution is different. There is a regional serpentine involvement that may extend the full thickness of the placental disc (Fig. 20.17). Fetal associations with both MFI and MPFD include recurrent pregnancy loss, prematurity, growth restriction, adverse neurodevelopmental outcome, and stillbirth [86,87]. As with non-specific chronic villitis, animal models have not been identified or constructed for experimental evaluation.

Summary

(1) Numerous mechanisms of intrauterine stress exist capable of leading to fetal morbidity – including neurodisability – and to fetal and neonatal mortality.

(2) Many, but not all, mechanisms of intrauterine stress operative in the last half of gestation are hypoxic and/or infectious in mode.

(3) Most, but not all, mechanisms of intrauterine stress have specific placental correlates – "footprints" of their presence during gestation. The presence and extent of placental pathology depends in part upon timing, as events occurring shortly prior to delivery may not have time to manifest pathologic abnormalities.

(4) Sometimes, the absence of placental footprints in the setting of untoward neonatal outcome is attributable to a mechanism (e.g., head trauma due to external mechanical forces) that has no placental correlates.

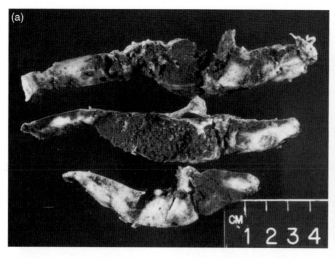 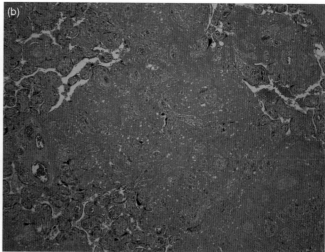

Fig. 20.17. Massive perivillous fibrin deposition (MPFD). (a) Grossly, affected regions appear dense and off-white. (b) Microscopically, affected regions demonstrate intervillous deposition of pink (eosinophilic) material, so-called fibrin(oid). *See color plate section.*

(5) The placenta, therefore, is a critical adjunct in assessing mechanisms and timing of intrauterine stressors. Furthermore, both the presence and absence of findings are relevant to clinicopathologic interpretation.

(6) Pathologic interpretation in a given case is in part evidence-based, but in part must rely on pathology expertise borne of individual experience and inter-observer consensus.

(7) Placental pathology determinants of intrauterine stress, both mechanisms and their timing, are not synonymous with determinants of injury. Except in certain specific circumstances, assessing the extent and timing of injury requires clinical acumen beyond the purview of pathologic evidence and interpretation alone.

References

1. Miller PW, Coen RW, Benirschke K. Dating the time interval from meconium passage to birth. *Obstet Gynecol* 1985; **66**: 459–62.

2. Sepulveda WH, Gonzalez C, Cruz MA, *et al.* Vasoconstrictive effect of bile acids on isolated human placental chorionic veins. *Eur J Obstet Gynecol* 1995; **173**: 1075–8.

3. Holcberg G, Huleihel M, Katz M, *et al.* Vasoconstrictive activity of meconium stained amniotic fluid in the human placental vasculature. *Eur J Obstet Gynecol Reprod Biol* 1999; **87**: 147–50.

4. King EL, Redline RW, Smith SD, *et al.* Myocytes of chorionic vessels from placentas with meconium-associated vascular necrosis exhibit apoptotic markers. *Hum Pathol* 2004; **35**: 412–17.

5. Altshuler G, Hyde S. Meconium-induced vasocontraction: a potential cause of cerebral and other fetal hypoperfusion and of poor pregnancy outcome. *J Child Neurol* 1989; **4**: 137–42.

6. Altshuler G, Arizawa M, Molnar-Nadasy G. Meconium-induced umbilical cord vascular necrosis and ulceration: a potential link between the placenta and poor outcome. *Obstet Gynecol* 1992; **79**: 760–6.

7. De Beaufort AJ, Pelikan DMV, Elferink JGR, *et al.* Effect of interleukin 8 in meconium on in vitro neutrophil chemotaxis. *Lancet* 1998; **352**: 102–5.

8. Burgess AM, Hutchins GM. Inflammation of the lungs, umbilical cord and placenta associated with meconium passage in utero. *Pathol Res Pract* 1996; **192**: 1121–8.

9. Yamada T, Minakami H, Matsubara S, *et al.* Meconium-stained amniotic fluid exhibits chemotactic activity for polymorphonuclear leukocytes in vitro. *J Reprod Immunol* 2000; **46**: 21–30.

10. Locatelli A, Regalia AL, Patregnani C, *et al.* Prognostic value of change in amniotic fluid color curing labor. *Fetal Diagn Ther* 2005; **20**: 5–9.

11. Sheiner E, Hadar A, Shoham-Vardi I. The effect of meconium on perinatal outcome: A prospective analysis. *J Matern Fetal Neonat Med* 2002; **11**: 54–9.

12. Ferber A, Minior VK, Bornstein E, *et al.* Fetal "nonreassuring status" is associated with elevation of nucleated red blood cell counts and interleukin-6. *Am J Obstet Gynecol* 2005; **192**: 1427–9.

13. Ferber A, Fridel Z, Weissmann-Brenner A, *et al.* Are elevated nucleated red blood cell counts an indirect reflection of enhanced erythropoietin activity? *Am J Obstet Gynecol* 2004; **190**: 1473–5.

14. Maier RF, Gunther A, Vogel M, *et al.* Umbilical venous erythropoietin and umbilical arterial pH in relation to morphologic placental abnormalities. *Obstet Gynecol* 1994; **84**: 81–7.

15. Hermansen MC. Nucleated red blood cells in the fetus and newborn. *Arch Dis Child Fetal Neonatal Ed* 2001; **84**: F211–15.

16. Silva AM, Smith RN, Lehmann CU, *et al.* Neonatal nucleated red blood cells and the prediction of cerebral white matter injury in preterm infants. *Obstet Gynecol* 2006; **107**: 550–6.

17. Phelan JP, Korst LM, Ahn MO, *et al.* Neonatal nucleated red blood cell and lymphocyte counts in fetal brain injury. *Obstet Gynecol* 1998; **91**: 485–9.

18. Korst LM, Phelan JP, Ahn MO, *et al.* Nucleated red blood cells: an update in the marker for fetal asphyxia. *Am J Obstet Gynecol* 1996; **175**: 843–6.

19. Phelan JP, Ahn MO, Korst LM, *et al.* Nucleated red blood cells: a marker for fetal asphyxia? *Am J Obstet Gynecol* 1995; **173**: 1380–4.

20. McCarthy JM, Capullari T, Thompson Z, *et al.* Umbilical nucleated red blood cell counts: Normal values and the effect of labor. *J Perinatol* 2006; **26**: 89–92.

21. Manegold G, Meyer-Monard S, Tichelli A, *et al.* Cesarean section due to fetal distress increases the number of stem cells in umbilical cord blood. *Transfusion* 2008; **48**: 871–6.

22. Baschat AA, Gungor S, Kush ML, *et al.* Nucleated red blood cell counts in the first week of life: a critical appraisal of relationships with perinatal outcome in preterm growth-restricted neonates. *Am J Obstet Gynecol* 2007; **197**: 286.e1–8.

23. Buonocore G, Perrone S, Gioia D, *et al.* Nucleated red blood cell count at birth as an index of perinatal brain damage. *Am J Obstet Gynecol* 1999; **181**: 1500–5.

24. Ghosh B, Mittal S, Kumar S, *et al.* Prediction of perinatal asphyxia with nucleated red blood cells in cord blood of newborns. *Int J Gynaecol Obstet* 2003; **81**: 267–71.

25. Hanion-Lundberg KM, Kirby RS, Gandhi S, *et al.* Nucleated red blood cells in cord blood of singleton term neonates. *Am J Obstet Gynecol* 1997; **176**: 1149–54.

26. Hamrick SE, Miller SP, Newton NR, *et al.* Neonatal red blood cell counts: not associated with brain injury or outcome. *Pediatr Neurol* 2003; **29**: 278–83.

27. Phelan JP, Ahn MO, Korst L, *et al.* Intrapartum asphyxial brain injury with absent multiorgan system dysfunction. *J Matern Fetal Med* 1998; **7**: 19–22.

28. Benirschke K. The use of the placenta in the understanding of perinatal injury. In Donn SM, Fisher CW, eds., *Risk Management Techniques in Perinatal and Neonatal Practice.* Armonk, NY: Futura, 1996: 325–45.

29. Grafe MR. The correlation of prenatal brain damage with placental pathology. *J Neuropathol Exp Neurol* 1994; **53**: 407–15.

30. Redline RW, O'Riordan A. Placental lesions associated with cerebral palsy and neurologic impairment following term birth. *Arch Pathol Lab Med* 2000; **124**: 1785–91.

31. Baergen RN. *Manual of Benirschke and Kaufmann's Pathology of the Human Placenta.* New York, NY: Springer, 2005.

32. Benirschke K, Kaufmann P, Baergen RN. *Pathology of the Human Placenta,* 32nd edn. New York, NY: Springer, 2006.

33. Miller ME, Higginbottom M, Smith DA. Short umbilical cord: its origin and relevance. *Pediatrics* 1981; **67**: 618–21.

34. Kumazaki K, Nakayama M, Sumida Y, *et al.* Placental features in preterm infants with periventricular leukomalacia. *Pediatrics* 2002; **109**: 650–5.

35. Chasen ST, Baergen RN. Necrotizing funisitis with intrapartum umbilical cord rupture. *J Perinatol* 1999; **19**: 325–6.

36. Altshuler G, Arizawa M, Molnar-Nadasdy G. Meconium induced umbilical cord vascular necrosis and ulceration: a potential link between the placenta and poor pregnancy outcome. *Obstet Gynecol* 1992; **79**: 760–6.

37. Santamaria M, Benirschke K, Carpenter PM, *et al.* Transplacental hemorrhage associated with placental neoplasms. *Pediatr Pathol* 1987; **7**: 601–15.

38. Karsidag ATK, Kars B, Dansuk R, *et al.* Brain damage to the survivor within 30 minutes of co-twin demise in monochorionic twins. *Fetal Diagn Ther* 2005; **20**: 91–5.

39. Spellancy WN, Gravem H, Fisch RO. The umbilical cord complications of true knots, nuchal coils and cords around the body: a report from the collaborative study of cerebral palsy. *Am J Obstet Gynecol* 1966; **94**: 1136–42.

40. Baergen RN, Malicki D, Behling C, *et al.* Morbidity, mortality, and placental pathology in excessively long umbilical cords: retrospective study. *Pediatr Dev Pathol* 2001; **4**: 144–53.

41. Machin GA, Ackerman J, Gilbert-Barness E. Abnormal umbilical cord coiling is associated with adverse perinatal outcomes. *Pediatr Dev Pathol* 2000; **3**: 462–71.

42. Redline RW. Clinical and pathological umbilical cord abnormalities in fetal thrombotic vasculopathy. *Hum Pathol* 2004; **35**: 1494–8.

43. Peng HQ, Levitin-Smith M, Rochelson B, *et al.* Umbilical cord stricture and overcoiling are common causes of fetal demise. *Pediatr Dev Pathol* 2006; **9**: 14–19.

44. Murphy DJ, MacKenzie IZ. The mortality and morbidity associated with umbilical cord prolapse. *Br J Obstet Gynaecol* 1995; **102**: 826–30.

45. Ikeda T, Murata Y, Quilligan EJ, *et al.* Physiologic and histologic changes in near-term fetal lambs exposed to asphyxia by partial umbilical cord occlusion. *Am J Obstet Gynecol* 1998; **178**: 24–32.

46. Kraus FT, Acheen VI. Fetal thrombotic vasculopathy in the placenta: cerebral thrombi and infarcts, coagulopathies and cerebral palsy. *Hum Pathol* 1999; **30**: 759–69.

47. Heifetz SA. Thrombosis of the umbilical cord: analysis of 52 cases and literature review. *Pediatr Pathol* 1988; **8**: 37–54.

48. Kalish RB, Hunter T, Sharma G, *et al.* Clinical significance of the umbilical cord twist. *Am J Obstet Gynecol* 2003; **189**: 736–9.

49. Strong TH, Elliott JP, Radin TR. Non-coiled umbilical blood vessels: a new marker for the fetus at risk. *Obstet Gynecol* 1993; **81**: 409–11.

50. Benirschke K. Obstetrically important lesions of the umbilical cord. *J Reprod Med* 1994; **39**: 62–72.

51. de Laat MWM, van Alderen ED, Franx A, *et al.* The umbilical coiling index in complicated pregnancy. *Eur J Obstet Gynecol Reprod Biol* 2007; **130**: 66–72.

52. Heifetz SA. The umbilical cord: obstetrically important lesions. *Clin Obstet Gynecol* 1996; **39**: 71–87.

53. Hersh J, Buchino JJ. Umbilical cord torsion/constriction sequence. In Saul RA, ed., *Proceedings of the Greenwood Genetics Conference Vol. 7.* Clinton, SC: Jacobs Press, 1988: 181–2.

54. Gardiner JP. The umbilical cord: normal length; length in cord complications; etiology and frequency of coiling. *Surg Gynecol Obstet* 1922; **34**: 252–6.

55. Snider W. Placental pathology casebook. *J Perinatol* 1997; **17**: 327–9.

56. Naeye RL, Tafari N. Noninfectious disorders of the placenta, fetal membranes and umbilical cord. In Naeye RL, Tafari N, eds., *Risk Factors in Pregnancy and Disease of the Fetus and Newborn.* Baltimore, MD: Williams and Wilkins, 1983: 145–72.

57. Moessinger AC, Blanc WA, Marone PA, *et al.* Umbilical cord length as an index of fetal activity: experimental study and clinical implications. *Pediatr Res* 1982; **16**: 109–12.

58. Boué DR, Stanley C, Baergen RN. Placental pathology casebook. *J Perinatol* 1995; **15**: 429–31.

59. Faye-Petersen O, Baergen RN. Long umbilical cords and pre-viable fetal death. *Pediatr Dev Pathol* 2001; **4**: 414.

60. Gilbert-Barness E, Drut RM, Drut R, *et al.* Developmental abnormalities

resulting in short umbilical cord. *Birth Defects Orig Artic Ser* 1993; **29**: 113–40.

61. Collins JC. Umbilical cord accidents: human studies. *Semin Perinatol* 2002; **26**: 79–82.

62. Soernes T. Umbilical cord encirclements and fetal growth restriction. *Obstet Gynecol* 1995; **86**: 725–8.

63. Vanhaesebrouck P, Vanneste K, de Praeter C, *et al.* Tight nuchal cord and neonatal hypovolemic shock. *Arch Dis Child* 1987; **62**: 1276–7.

64. Nelson KB, Grether JK. Potentially asphyxiating conditions and spastic cerebral palsy in infants of normal birth weight. *Am J Obstet Gynecol* 1998; **179**: 507–13.

65. Lin, MG. Umbilical cord prolapse. *Obstet Gynecol Surv* 2006; **61**: 269–77.

66. Torrey WE. Vasa previa. *Am J Obstet Gynecol* 1952; **63**: 146–52.

67. Heinonen S, Ryynänen M, Kirkinen P, *et al.* Perinatal diagnostic evaluation of velamentous umbilical cord insertion: clinical, Doppler, and ultrasonic findings. *Obstet Gynecol* 1996; **87**: 112–17.

68. Cordero DR, Helfgott AW, Landy HJ, *et al.* A non-hemorrhagic manifestation of *vasa previa*: a clinicopathologic case report. *Obstet Gynecol* 1993; **82**: 698–700.

69. Redline RW, Ariel I, Baergen RN, *et al.* Fetal vascular obstructive lesions: nosology and reproducibility of placental reaction patterns. *Pediatr Dev Pathol* 2004; **7**: 443–52.

70. Sander CM, Gilliland D, Akers C, *et al.* Livebirths with placental hemorrhagic endovasculitis: interlesional relationships and perinatal outcomes. *Arch Pathol Lab Med* 2002; **126**: 157–64.

71. Redline RW. Severe fetal placental vascular lesions in term infants with neurologic impairment. *Am J Obstet Gynecol* 2005; **192**: 452–7.

72. Bejar RF, Wozniak P, Allard M, *et al.* Antenatal origin of neurologic damage in newborn infants. I. Preterm infants. *Am J Obstet Gynecol* 1988; **159**: 357–63.

73. Redline RW, Wilson-Costello D, Borawski E, *et al.* The relationship between placental and other perinatal risk factors for neurologic impairment in very low birth weight children. *Pediatr Res* 2000; **47**: 721–6.

74. Redline RW, Boyd T, Campbell V, *et al.* Maternal vascular underperfusion: nosology and reproducibility of placental reaction patterns. *Pediatr Dev Pathol* 2004; **7**: 237–49.

75. Burke CJ, Tannenberg AE, Payton DJ. Ischaemic cerebral injury, intrauterine growth retardation, and placental infarction. *Dev Med Child Neurol* 1997; **39**: 726–30.

76. Redline RW, Wilson-Costello D, Borawski E, *et al.* Placental lesions associated with neurologic impairment and cerebral palsy in very low-birth-weight infants. *Arch Pathol Lab Med* 1998; **122**: 1091–8.

77. Redline RW. Villitis of unknown etiology: noninfectious chronic villitis in the placenta. *Hum Pathol* 2007; **38**: 1439–46.

78. Bendon RW, Hommel AB. Maternal floor infarction in autoimmune disease: two cases. *Pediatr Pathol Lab Med* 1996; **16**: 293–7.

79. Sebire NJ, Backos M, Goldin RD, *et al.* Placental massive perivillous fibrin deposition associated with antiphospholipid syndrome. *BJOG* 2002; **109**: 570–3.

80. Katzman PJ, Genest DR. Maternal floor infarction and massive previllous fibrin deposition: histological definitions, association with intrauterine fetal growth restriction, and risk of recurrence. *Pediatr Dev Pathol* 2002; **5**: 159–64.

81. Chang P, Miller D, Tsang P, *et al.* Intravenous immunoglobulin in antiphospholipid syndrome and maternal floor infarction when standard treatment fails: a case report. *Am J Perinatol* 2006; **23**: 125–9.

82. Makino A, Suzuki Y, Yamamoto T, *et al.* Use of aspirin and low-molecular-weight heparin to prevent recurrence of maternal floor infarction in women without evidence of antiphospholipid antibody syndrome. *Fetal Diagn Ther* 2004; **19**: 261–5.

83. Chang P, Millar D, Tsang P, *et al.* Intravenous immunoglobulin in antiphospholipid syndrome and maternal floor infarction when standard treatment fails. *Am J Perinatol* 2006; **23**: 125–9.

84. Redline RW, O'Riordan MA. Placental lesions associated with cerebral palsy and neurologic impairment following term birth. *Arch Pathol Lab Med* 2000; **124**: 1785–91.

85. Scher MS, Trucco GS, Beggarly ME, *et al.* Neonates with electrically confirmed seizures and possible placental associations. *Pediatr Neurol* 1998; **19**: 37–41.

86. Adams-Chapman I, Vaucher YE, Bejar RF, *et al.* Maternal floor infarction of the placenta: association with central nervous system injury and adverse neurodevelopmental outcome. *J Perinatol* 2002; **22**: 236–41.

87. Andres RL, Kuyper W, Resnik R, *et al.* The association of maternal floor infarction of the placenta with adverse perinatal outcome. *Am J Obstet Gynecol* 1990; **163**: 935–8.

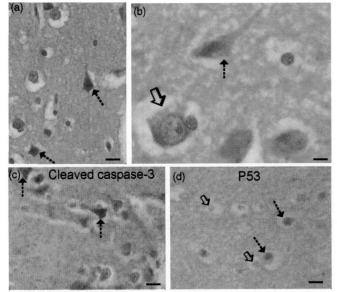

Fig. 2.6. Neuronal cell death in human newborn HIE. (a, b) Hematoxylin staining of neocortex from an infant that survived 3 days after HI due to delivery complications reveals selective degeneration of neurons (hatched arrows) in the form of typical ischemic neuronal death with eosinophilic cytoplasm, shrunken cell body, and condensed nucleus. Other damaged neurons are swollen with a vacuolated cytoplasm (open arrow in b). This pattern of neurodegeneration is much less phenotypically heterogeneous than that seen in neonatal rodent models of HI, but similar to that seen in our piglet model of HI. Scale bars = 33 μm (a), 7 μm (b). (c) Subsets of neocortical neurons (hatched arrows) in human infants with HIE display cleaved caspase-3 throughout the cell. Other cells in the field shown by the cresyl violet counterstaining have no labeling for cleaved caspase-3. Scale bar = 15 μm. (d) Subsets of neocortical neurons (hatched arrows) in human infants with HIE display active p53 within the nucleus. Other cells (open arrow) in the field have no labeling for active p53. Scale bar = 15 μm.

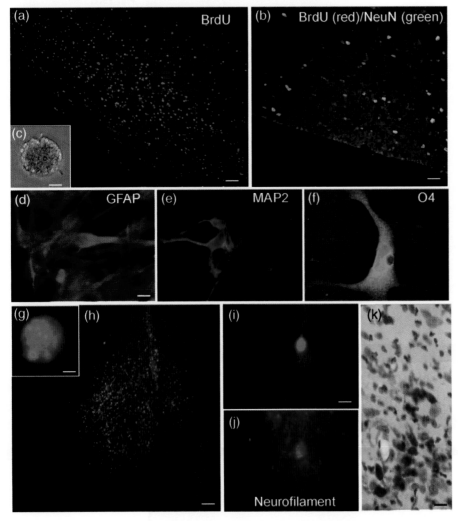

Fig. 2.7. The newborn piglet olfactory bulb (OB) is a rich source of multipotent neural progenitor cells useful for transplantation into damaged newborn brain after HI. (a) The piglet OB core (the ventricular cavity is the black area at left of image) contains numerous newly born cells (green-labeled cells) as identified by BrdU labeling of replicated DNA and antibody detection. Scale bar = 80 μm. (b) The majority of newly born cells (BrdU, red) in the newborn piglet OB core express the neuron-specific nuclear marker NeuN (green), demonstrating that they are newly born neurons. Yellow indicates overlap in two signals. Scale bar = 24 μm. (c) Newborn piglet OB-NSC/NPC neurosphere. OB core cells from newborn piglet can be harvested, cultured, and used to isolate neurosphere-forming cells. Neurospheres can be dissociated into constituent cells and shown by single-cell clonal analysis to be multipotent neural precursor cells. Scale bar = 20 μm. (d–f) Single OB core neurosphere-forming cells can be expanded in vitro to form numerous additional neurospheres with constituent cells that can differentiate into the three primary neural cell types: astrocytes positive for glial fibrillary (GFAP), neurons positive for microtubule-associated protein-2 (MAP2), and oligodendrocytes positive for the cell surface marker O4. Scale bar = 7 μm. (g) Piglet OB-NSC/NPC neurospheres can be stably transfected with a green fluorescent protein (GFP) gene using a lentiviral construct. This cell tagging serves as a reporter for transplanted cells. Scale bar = 20 μm. (h) After transplantation into the newborn piglet with HIE, GFP-OB-NSC/NPC neurospheres disperse entirely into individual green-labeled cells and migrate into damaged areas. Scale bar = 20 μm. (i, j) Subsets of transplanted GFP-labeled cells (green in i) in neocortex and basal ganglia that appear to be differentiating express neuron markers (neurofilament, red in j). Scale bar = 12 μm. (k) Immunoperoxidase detection of GFP using monoclonal antibody can be used as an alternative method to identify transplanted cells in HI piglet brain. These cells (brown-labeled cells) have engrafted, survived, and are differentiating into neurons in striatum. Scale bar = 20 μm.

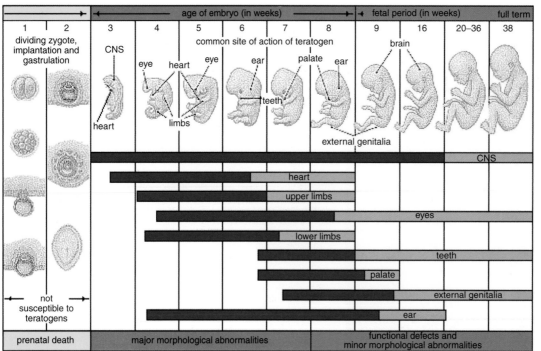

Fig. 10.1. Malformations by organ system as a function of gestational timing. Note that the embryo is not susceptible to teratogenic damage during days 0–10 post-conception. Adapted from: Moore KL, *Before We Were Born: Basic Embryology and Birth Defects*, 2nd edn. Philadelphia, PA: Saunders, 1993. With permission.

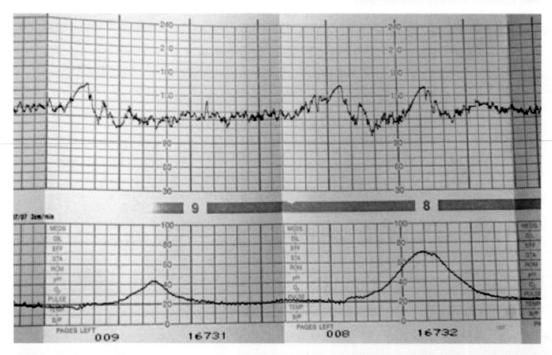

Fig. 15.1. Normal fetal heart-rate tracing. Within a 20-minute window a normal fetal heart-rate baseline is seen with normal (moderate) variability and two accelerations.

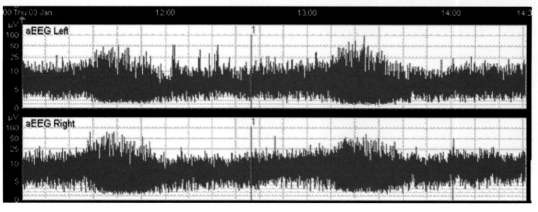

Fig. 17.8. Amplitude-integrated EEG in a healthy term infant. Example shows 3.5-hour recording. Broad portions of band correlate with quiet sleep; narrow portions correlate with active sleep.

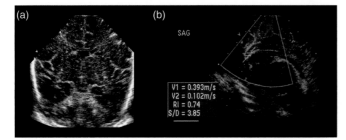

Fig. 18.1. Normal infant and child brain. Ultrasound (US) images of term neonate: (a) coronal US; (b) sagittal US + Doppler with resistive indices (RI).

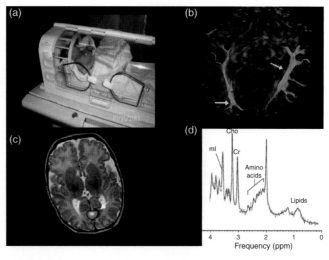

Fig. 18.2. (above) Advanced MRI techniques: (a) MR-compatible incubator; (b) DTI white-matter tractography (arrows); (c) fMRI (primary visual cortex activation: arrow); (d) MR spectroscopy (see text).

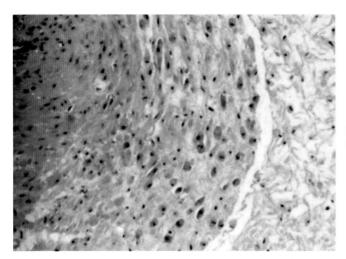

Fig. 20.1. (left) Meconium-induced umbilical vascular necrosis. Outer wall myocytes exhibit pyknosis in the presence of meconium macrophages.

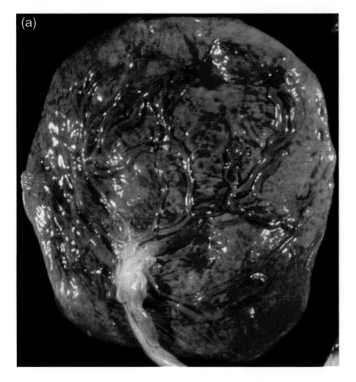

Fig. 20.2. (a) (left) Gross meconium staining: the fetal surface is discolored green to green-brown; the surface typically feels diffluent ("slimy") on palpation. (b) (above) Microscopic meconium uptake into membrane macrophages: through the microscope, meconium appears as a globular or amorphous orange-brown pigment; note the reactive amnion and amnion necrosis due to meconium.

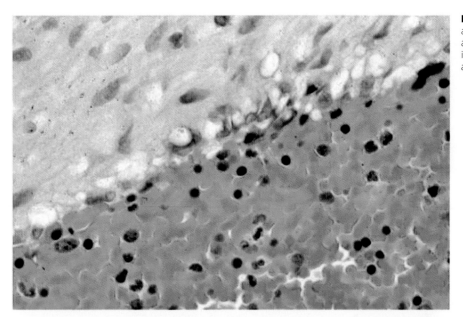

Fig. 20.3. Nucleated red blood cells (NRBCs) are identified by their round hyperchromatic nuclei and pink-red cytoplasm. NRBCs of this proportion indicate non-acute hypoxic stress, in this case from a stillbirth due to umbilical cord hypercoiling.

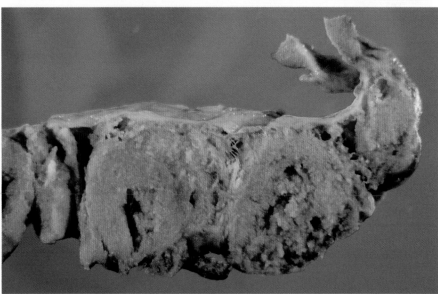

Fig. 20.4. Cut section of a formalin-fixed placenta from a severe fetomaternal hemorrhage. Note the markedly pale parenchymal tissue.

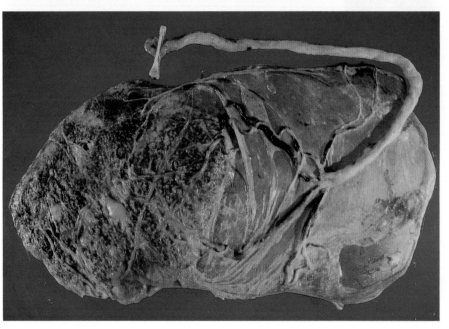

Fig. 20.7. Placenta with a velamentous insertion. Note that the umbilical cord inserts far from the placental margin and numerous membranous vessels are present. In this case, there is no disruption of vessels or hemorrhage in the surrounding membranes.

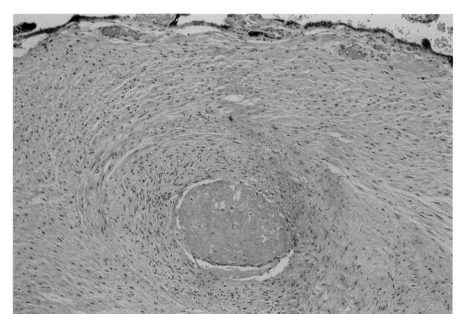

Fig. 20.8. Fetal vessel in a stem villus with a recent, nearly occlusive thrombus.

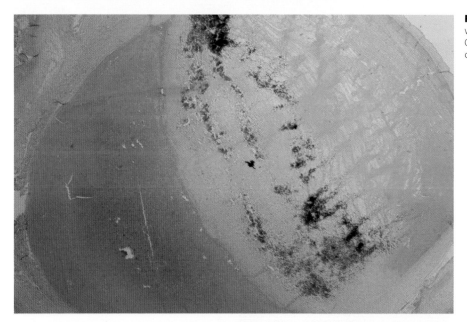

Fig. 20.9. Large fetal chorionic plate vessel with distension and partially occlusive thrombus. Calcification in the thrombus is indicative of chronicity.

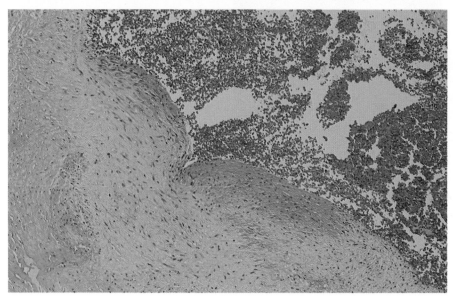

Fig. 20.10. Large fetal chorionic plate vessel with intimal fibrin cushion. Note fibrin deposition in the wall of the vessel in the lower left of the figure and deposition of pale-blue ground substance forming a "cushion."

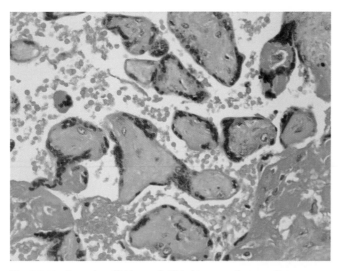

Fig. 20.11. Avascular villi. Focus of villi lacking any villous capillaries and with marked hyalinization of the stroma indicative of upstream fetal vascular thrombosis.

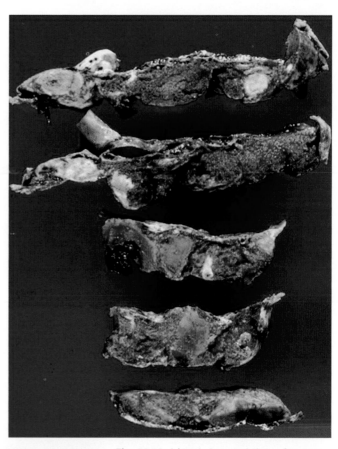

Fig. 20.13. (above) Gross pathology of intrinsic maternal vascular disease leading to chronic maternal vascular underperfusion. Multiple temporally heterogeneous infarcts, with or without placental abruption (present in this case, middle section on left).

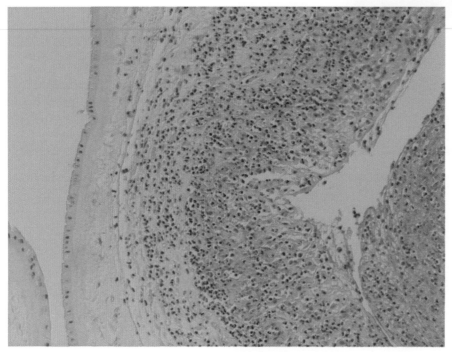

Fig. 20.12. Section of extraplacental membranes with acute chorioamnionitis. Notice infiltration of numerous neutrophils within all layers of the membranes: these are derived from the decidua and thus the maternal circulation.

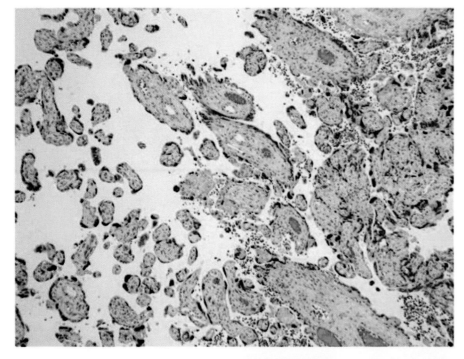

Fig. 20.14. Some of the microscopic features of chronic maternal underperfusion: villous ischemic changes, manifested as distal villous hypoplasia (on left) and villous agglutination (on right).

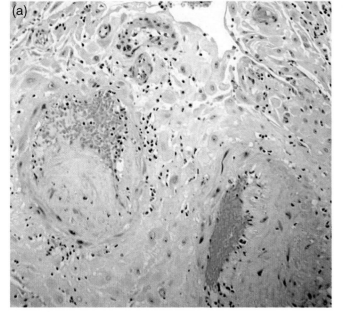

(a)

(b)

Fig. 20.15. (b) Decidual arteriopathy. More severe phenotype: fibrinoid necrosis with acute atherosis.

Fig. 20.15. (a) Decidual arteriopathy. Milder phenotype: non-transformation of spiral arterioles.

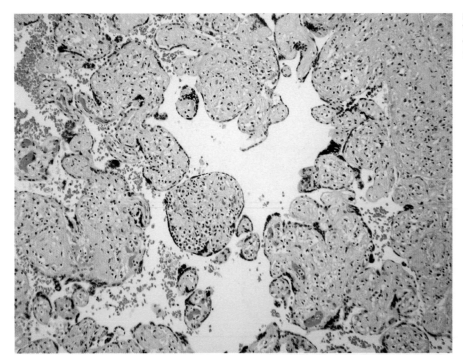

Fig. 20.16. Severe chronic villitis. Widespread obliteration of terminal villous capillaries and distal stem villous vessels (so-called obliterative vasculopathy).

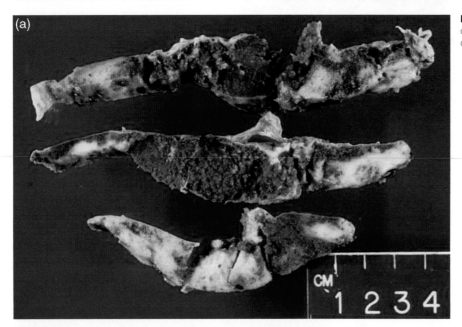

Fig. 20.17. (a) Massive perivillous fibrin deposition (MPFD). Grossly, affected regions appear dense and off-white.

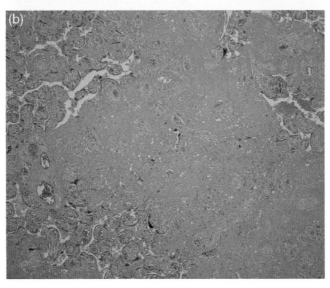

Fig. 20.17. (b) Massive perivillous fibrin deposition (MPFD). Microscopically, affected regions demonstrate intervillous deposition of pink (eosinophilic) material, so-called fibrin(oid).

Correlations of clinical, laboratory, imaging, and placental findings as to the timing of asphyxial events

Philip Sunshine, David K. Stevenson, Ronald J. Wong, and William E. Benitz

Introduction

Following the birth of a depressed newborn, the infant's caretakers are involved in providing appropriate resuscitative techniques, stabilizing the infant's biochemical and physiological abnormalities, and evaluating the infant's response to these measures. The caretakers must also ascertain the cause of the infant's depression, attempt to determine when the event or events leading to the depression occurred, and develop a plan for follow-up evaluation and treatment that will be required. The determination of causation and timing not only has medical–legal implications, but also is becoming extremely important in order to evaluate the types of therapy that may be utilized to mitigate the effects of an asphyxial event. If the infant had suffered significant damage days or weeks prior to birth, then these rescue forms of therapy will have little, if any, beneficial effect on the infant's eventual outcome. In many situations, this determination is very difficult to make, as there may be a myriad of events that could have occurred prior to the time of birth, and overlapping of significant problems makes this exercise an almost impossible task at times.

Identification of the etiology of a cerebral injury is a critical prerequisite to the determination of its timing. For example, lactic acidemia immediately after birth and an elevated serum creatine kinase (CK) level at 24 hours of age in an infant with abnormal intensities of T1- and T2-weighted signals in the basal ganglia on MRI obtained at 2 weeks of age might point to intrapartum timing of an acute hypoxic–ischemic insult. However, these findings would also be consistent with an underlying mitochondrial disease. Distinction between these possibilities would require additional information, such as lactate/pyruvate ratios (normal after an asphyxial insult, elevated in mitochondrial diseases), serial serum CK levels (transiently vs. persistently elevated), or knowledge of the subsequent course (static encephalopathy without recurrent episodes of acidemia vs. progressive encephalopathy or other neurologic findings with recurrent or persistent lactic acidemia). Before attempting to determine the timing of an asphyxial event, all available data should be carefully reviewed to exclude

non-asphyxial etiologies, particularly genetic, metabolic, infectious, and inflammatory disorders as described in other chapters. In many instances, the available data are insufficient, so additional diagnostic studies are required.

When an acute or sentinel event has taken place, such as a readily recognized prolapsed cord, an abruptio placentae, a ruptured uterus, or a disorder leading to acute and profound blood loss in the fetus, the timing of the event can be ascertained with a reasonable degree of accuracy. However, even in these circumstances, the time frame may not be known with certainty, especially if the process has been developing over a period of time. Often, the area of damage to the central nervous system can be found to correlate with this acute event, as it tends to involve the thalamus and the basal ganglia [1,2]. At times, when there is an occult prolapse of the cord, or if the infant is profoundly affected when the mother suffers from an amniotic fluid embolus that has an unusual form of presentation, the timing of an acute event can not be made with precision.

There may also be overlapping of events leading to the infant's problems. Data from laboratory animals have demonstrated that even brief repeated episodes of cord occlusion can not only predispose the fetus to cerebral injury, but can also lead to compromise of the cardiovascular system [3–6]. Thus a fetus with intrauterine compromise may not be able to withstand the stresses of labor, and can develop what would appear to be an acute catastrophic bradycardic episode and therefore complicate an already pre-existing neurological injury.

In addition, many infants who are depressed at birth or who are later found to have suffered neurological or intellectual impairment may have few, if any, indicators as to the cause, severity, or timing of the injury. Because we have limited capabilities of evaluating the neurological well-being of the fetus during the labor process, we use indirect indicators that may be of help in chronicling the sequence of events leading to the birth of a depressed infant. Many of these indicators are encountered in perfectly normal newborns, and the specificity and sensitivity of these findings are often inconclusive. Despite these shortcomings, neonatologists, perinatologists, pediatric neurologists, neuroradiologists, and pathologists are asked to perform retrospective analyses of data collected on the mother, the placenta, and the fetus in an attempt to create a reasonable theory as to the timing and severity of events leading to an infant's problems.

Fetal and Neonatal Brain Injury, 4th edition, ed. David K. Stevenson, William E. Benitz, Philip Sunshine, Susan R. Hintz, and Maurice L. Druzin. Published by Cambridge University Press. © Cambridge University Press 2009.

Table 21.1. Template for timing of neonatal brain injury

Maternal history of fetal activity
Use of biophysical profile
Fetal heart-rate monitoring
Presence of meconium
Neonatal neurological examination
Electroencephalogram
Imaging studies
Ultrasound
CT scan
MRI
Laboratory studies
Cord blood gases and initial postnatal blood gases
Hematological studies
Biochemical evaluations
Examination of the placenta
Neuropathological evaluations
Follow-up evaluations of clinical and laboratory parameters

Notes:
CT, computed tomography; MRI, magnetic resonance imaging.

The approach to such an exercise is outlined in Table 21.1, which can be used as a template for determining the timing. Realizing that many clinical signs may be subjective, one often has to evaluate numerous clues to determine the sequence of events that were involved. In most situations, timing of an injurious event can only be placed within broad periods such as during fetal development, the prelabor period, the intrapartum period, or the postpartum (neonatal) period.

Prepartum evaluation

Currently, most women with high-risk obstetrical problems are readily identified and have frequent and intensive monitoring during their pregnancies. With careful screening that is currently in place in obstetrical practices, many of these women are identified even prior to their pregnancies or in the early part of their gestation. The approach to antepartum evaluation is clearly delineated in Chapter 14. When a low-risk mother develops risk factors during her pregnancy, such as glucose intolerance, pre-eclampsia, decreased intrauterine growth, hydramnios, or post-datism, then she too will be evaluated more intensely and more frequently [7]. Women with a low-risk status will not have these evaluations, and thus subjective signs to alert her caretaker to potential problems become important. The fetus that develops a marked increase in activity, such as writhing movements that do not stop or, as some women describe these, "as if the baby wanted to jump out of the uterus," may be an important sign of a fetus in distress [8]. This is especially true if the writhing movements are followed by a period of fetal inactivity. Similarly, the fetus that has been active and either gradually or suddenly stops moving is another important sign that may be helpful in the

timing of an untoward event [8,9]. Since such findings are found in fetuses with perfectly normal outcomes, they may not be brought to the physician's attention, or are regarded as variations of a normal pregnancy. Nevertheless, these signs should be brought to the attention of the healthcare provider so that further evaluation of the well-being of the fetus can be addressed. Olesen and Svare have developed an algorithm to aid the caregiver in approaching women who note decreased or absent fetal movement [9]. Retrospective analyses of these findings may be helpful in determining the timing of the fetal injury. Similarly, the sudden onset of hydramnios may also be an important sign of fetal compromise.

Recognition of an acute event such as severe abdominal pain, sudden onset of cardiopulmonary insufficiency or arrest in the mother, or acute blood loss associated with vasa previa, abruptio placentae, or placenta previa can also be used to time the onset of an asphyxial event.

Fetal heart-rate monitoring

The specifics of fetal heart-rate monitoring are described in Chapter 15 and will not be addressed in detail here. Schifrin et al. [10] and Phelan and Kim [11] have identified an abnormal fetal heart-rate pattern that is fixed and non-reactive when a women is first admitted to the labor and delivery unit. This pattern is highly suggestive of a neurological injury that occurred prior to the time that labor began. As early as 1985, van der Moer et al. described a fixed fetal heart-rate pattern with normal frequency and without decelerations and accelerations in a fetus who had suffered significant intrauterine brain damage 14 days prior to the time the mother went into labor [12]. Menticoglou and coworkers described two full-term infants with similar courses [13]. Schifrin et al. termed this as a "pattern of autonomic imbalance" [10]. Phelan and Kim described this pattern in 45% of a population of 300 brain-damaged infants, and found it to be associated with a reduction in fetal activity, evidence of meconium-stained skin, and meconium aspiration syndrome [11]. When this heart-rate pattern is found on the mother's admission to the labor unit and does not change, they suggest that this is consistent with a "static encephalopathy that antedated the patient's arrival to the hospital."

If a woman is admitted, is found to have a reactive fetal heart-rate pattern, and then has a sudden and prolonged episode of fetal bradycardia, then it is more likely that an acute intrapartum event has occurred [14].

Other abnormalities that occur during labor, such as decelerations, tachycardias, and their relationship to fetal injury, are discussed in Chapters 13 and 15. Such abnormalities would suggest that, if the fetus is damaged, this damage occurred during the intrapartum period, especially if associated with significant fetal metabolic acidosis [15]. However, the sensitivities and the specificities of the abnormalities to predict outcomes correctly are low [15–17]. The interpretations of these tracings vary from individual to individual [18,19]. Nielsen et al. reported that when four obstetricians examined 50 tracings, agreement was reached in 22% of the cases. Moreover, 2 months later, the same clinicians interpreted 21% of the cases differently than they did during the initial evaluation [19]. In addition, the interpretations are greatly influenced by the interpreter's knowledge of the outcome of the neonate [20]. It has always been a source of amazement to find "experts" point to a specific time on a fetal heart rate tracing and indicate a particular moment when the fetus began to be compromised, and declare that had the infant been delivered within a very short time period, the infant would have been "perfectly normal." While there may be such occurrences, the use of the tracing to identify precise moments of injury to the fetus is speculative at best.

Conversely, significant improvements in the quality of intrapartum assessment can be made with effective educational techniques, and not only would the need for cesarean sections decrease, but the incidence of neonatal encephalopathy could be reduced as well [21–24].

Meconium-stained amniotic fluid

This subject is discussed at length in Chapter 36, and to some extent in Chapter 20. Infants who pass meconium in utero have been thought to have a greater risk of developing respiratory problems than those who do not, but the finding of meconium-stained amniotic fluid in itself, without associated evidence of neurological depression or respiratory insufficiency, does not seem to be associated with significant adverse effects. Nevertheless, there is still a great deal of debate as to whether or not meconium has an adverse effect on the umbilical vasculature or on the lung parenchyma of the fetus. Meconium-stained amniotic fluid is encountered in a large number of deliveries and may be as frequent as 30–40% in post-date pregnancies.

S. H. Clifford was one of the first to note an association of yellow staining of the vernix caseosa, skin, nails, and umbilical cord with an increased rate of neonatal morbidity and mortality [25]. He suggested that the "yellow vernix syndrome" was the result of an episode of fetal asphyxia occurring days to weeks prior to the onset of labor. Similar observations have been made by Phelan and Kim in patients who had persistently non-reactive fetal heart-rate patterns, reduced fetal activity, and passage of "old meconium" at the time the membranes were ruptured [11].

Sienko and Altshuler have demonstrated that meconium itself has vasoconstrictive properties when it is present in amniotic fluid for a period of time [26], and those observations have been substantiated to some degree by Naeye [27]. The length of time that meconium has been present can be ascertained by evaluating the consistency of the meconium, which tends to be thick and tenacious when passed close to the time of delivery, and is thin with particulate matter when passed hours to days previously. However, the infant may have had several episodes of meconium passage, and thus the timing of neurological injury to that of meconium passage is often difficult to make.

In an excellent review of the fetal consequences of amniotic-fluid meconium, Benirschke has delineated the issues that have been raised regarding which of the components of meconium may be ascribed to vascular and/or pulmonary damage [28]. Whether cytokines, bile acids, enzymes, or other factors are involved has remained speculative, and whether the association of meconium aspiration with chorioamnionitis could be a factor is still not completely resolved. He ended his discussion with a quote from Katz and Bowes, stating the topic of meconium will remain a "murky subject for a while" [29].

Seizures

Seizures associated with hypoxic–ischemic encephalopathy (HIE) are associated with an adverse prognostic significance, and increase the risk of neurological sequelae two to five times as compared to those infants without seizures [30]. In most situations, the onset of these seizures occurs within the first 12 hours of life, and they are often refractory to anticonvulsant therapy. The earlier the onset of seizures, usually the worse the outcome [30]. However, neither the time of the onset nor the severity of the seizures has been correlated with the timing of the event that led to the neurological insult affecting the fetus [31]. In some situations, the seizures may have occurred in utero and have not been fully recognized by either the mother or the physician. Such seizures have been reported in asphyxiated fetal lambs, and have resulted in increased heart-rate variability in the brain-damaged animal as well as in the human fetus [32].

More recently, Filan et al. have challenged the concept that the timing of seizures could not be correlated with the time of cerebral injury in utero [33]. Using continuous 12-channel video-EEG monitoring as soon after birth as possible, they noted that the identification of electrographic seizures occurred later than the clinically recognized seizures. They concluded that if the electrographic seizures occurred before 12 hours of age, they were due to prelabor causes, and that onset at 18–20 hours after birth indicated an insult in the peripartum period. They only evaluated nine infants, and it would be of great interest if these initial findings are confirmed.

Electroencephalogram

This aspect of evaluation is discussed in Chapter 17. The electroencephalogram (EEG) is useful in identifying seizures in the neonatal period and is often helpful in determining the severity of the encephalopathy. Takeuchi and Watanabe have described a series of changes that occur in the EEG of asphyxiated term infants that initially demonstrate varying degrees of isoelectric or burst–suppression patterns, and are often followed by increased degrees of discontinuity [34]. In the chronic stages, signs of dysmature and disorganized patterns evolve. There is also a sequence of evolution in the background of the EEG in infants with asphyxia that could be used to time the injury. It would require that the EEG be evaluated very soon after birth and that frequent follow-up studies be performed to evaluate the progress of the patient, the response to antiepileptic medications, if required, and the evolution of the EEG pattern. Similar studies have also been reported in preterm infants by these authors [35].

Using amplitude-integrated EEGs (aEEGs), Toet and co-workers were able to evaluate infants with encephalopathy within 3 and 6 hours after birth and to identify infants who had severe encephalopathic findings that could possibly benefit from interventional therapy, as well as those who had mild changes and would not require such treatment [36].

However, Sarkar et al. found that this technology would not identify all of the infants with severe encephalopathy who could possibly benefit if they were to be treated with hypothermia [37]. Thus the use of aEEGs remains a potential tool in early identification of infants with severe encephalopathy, but the clinical features of the encephalopathy are critical in identifying the infant who would benefit from treatment. These findings would support, to some extent, those reported by Filan et al. [33] (also see Chapters 17 and 43).

Laboratory findings
Lymphocytes and platelets
Hematological abnormalities have been used with increasing frequency to time the injury in affected newborns. Naeye and coworkers have utilized lymphocyte counts and nucleated red blood cell counts to determine the timing of neurological injury [38,39]. These authors have noted that lymphocyte counts increase to levels of greater than $10\,000/mm^3$ within 2 hours of the initiation of the injurious event and return to normal within 14–18 hours even if the hypoxic–ischemic event continues. If the event occurred more than 24 hours prior to birth, the lymphocyte count was not elevated. In the more recent study, Naeye and Lin also showed that if cardiovascular or renal dysfunction was associated with the hypoxic event, the platelet count decreased by 30% at about 30 hours and 50% by 60 hours after the event causing HIE occurred [38]. The use of this low value was especially helpful when an acute intrapartum event occurred.

Nucleated red blood cell count
We have found that elevation of normoblasts or nucleated red blood cells (NRBCs; see Chapter 20) is of great help in identifying those infants who have evidence of intrauterine hypoxia that has been present for a period of time [40–46]. In most situations, if there has been hypoxia in utero, there is a stimulus to produce erythropoietin and increase the number of NRBCs. Based on data from laboratory animals and from human neonates, it has been suggested that it requires at least 48 hours for erythropoietin to increase the number of NRBCs in the circulation. Thus the finding of a markedly elevated NRBC count would be indicative of problems that had been present for at least 48 hours, although the exact duration of insult is often unknown.

In most of these reports, the number of cells and the length of time the count remained elevated were correlated with the

length of time the infant had been in a relatively hypoxic state. Those infants who had suffered an acute injury did not have an elevated count, and Phelan et al. also reported that the infants with chronic rather than acute injuries also had platelet counts of less than 100K within the first 5 days of age [45]. Ferber et al. evaluated 100 low-risk pregnant women who were at term [43]. Twenty-eight patients underwent intrapartum cesarean sections, of which 15 were performed in non-reassuring fetal states. The latter group of infants had elevated NRBCs without elevation of erythropoietin, but had elevated levels of IL-6. These authors suggest that interleukin 6 (IL-6) may have a role in increasing NRBCs in the absence of an elevated erythropoietin response.

Hamrick et al. did not find a correlation of elevated NRBCs with the extent of brain injury or a relationship to outcome [47]. These investigators evaluated infants with encephalopathy, but did not separate those infants who had acute insults from those who may not have been in a relatively hypoxic environment for at least 48 hours. Perri et al. did not find elevated NRBCs in uncomplicated prolonged pregnancies [48], and McCarthy et al. did not find elevated levels in infants with uncomplicated pregnancies delivered either vaginally or by cesarean section [49].

Elevated NRBCs are also seen in response to an acute hypovolemic event such as bleeding from the vasa previa or bleeding from an abruptio placentae, where the outpouring of NRBCs can occur in a matter of hours [38,40]. For a period of time it was thought that this type of response was due to the fetal response of "splenic contraction" and elaboration of immature cells. Studies by Calhoun et al. have shown that active hematopoiesis is not present in the spleen of the mid-gestation of the human fetus [50]. Thus it is conceivable that the NRBCs in circulation most likely come from the liver or the bone marrow, in response to a hypovolemic stimulus.

While it is usual to express the elevation of NRBCs as the number of NRBCs per 100 white blood cells, we prefer to use the total number per cubic millimeter, as one might not appreciate an elevated count in those situations where there is also a leukocytic response. Thus a number greater than 1500 $NRBCs/mm^3$ is abnormal, even in prematurely born infants. Also, the more severe the hypoxic episode that is present, the longer the period of time that the NRBC count remains elevated [45]. Table 21.2 lists the most frequent causes of elevated NRBCs in the circulatory blood volume of neonates.

Biochemical markers of asphyxia
A list of laboratory studies that have been used to assess the severity of HIE is found in Chapter 1 of this text and noted in Volpe's Neurology of the Newborn as well [30]. When these laboratory studies are markedly abnormal, there is good correlation with the severity of the asphyxial episode. Unfortunately, most of these assays are not readily available in many clinical laboratories, and samples have to be sent to specific centers in order to have them assayed. Most laboratories can measure ammonia in blood, and CK and lactate in serum. Even the measurement of brain-specific isozyme of CK

Table 21.2. Causes of elevated nucleated red blood cell (NRBC) counts [38–48]

Chronic intrauterine hypoxia
Prematurity – especially those with IVH
Hemolytic anemia
Rh incompatibility
ABO incompatibility
Homozygous α-thalassemia
Chronic intrauterine anemia
Fetal–maternal bleeding
Twin-to-twin transfusion
Infants of poorly controlled diabetic mothers
Infants with intrauterine growth restriction
Infants of smoking mothers (mildly elevated)
Infants delivered associated with acute blood loss
Placenta abruptio
Vasa previa
Infants with diaphragmatic hernias
Severe placental insufficiency
Recurrent episodes of cord compression
Congenital infections (especially CMV)

Notes:
IVH, intraventricular hemorrhage; CMV, cytomegalovirus.

(CK-BB) may not be available in many clinical laboratories. If CK is to be utilized, it should be measured soon after birth and followed with frequent assays, as it tends to rise and fall rapidly over a 1- to 2-day period [51]. Nagdyman and coworkers demonstrated that CK-BB was found to be elevated 2 hours after birth in infants with moderate or severe HIE, and remained elevated for 12 hours [52].

Measurement of CK-BB in cerebrospinal fluid may be an even better method of detecting asphyxial injury, and abnormalities of this assay seem to correlate better with the severity of short-term outcome following an asphyxial event [53]. Again, this assay is not available in most clinical laboratories. Thus, if an infant is depressed at birth and is found to have a normal or minimally elevated CK, this suggests either that the injury to the infant was mild or that it occurred days prior to the intrapartum period.

Laboratory studies evaluating damage to other organs such as the kidney and liver should also be abnormal in the infant with asphyxia. However, if the asphyxic episode was acute, multiorgan damage may not have occurred, and these laboratory values may be normal. If the infant has suffered from partial prolonged intrapartum damage, elevation of the liver enzymes aspartate aminotransferase (AST) and alanine aminotransferase (ALT) should be found.

These enzymes, as well as lactic dehydrogenase (LDH), have been evaluated primarily in adults following myocardial infarction. There is a temporal pattern of enzyme release, with the ALT and AST rising and falling rapidly over a 2- to 3-day period. The LDH rises slowly during the first day after injury, peaking at 3–4 days and returning to normal levels in 14 days [54]. Such temporal data are not available for liver damage associated with acute hypoxic–ischemic injury in the newborn, and thus often do not have the specificity to aid in the timing of the asphyxial event.

The serum creatinine will also increase over the first 1–2 days of life and remain elevated until renal function improves. The infant's initial serum creatinine measured soon after birth tends to parallel that of the mother's and then will increase if there has been significant renal involvement. If the infant's serum creatinine is found to be elevated soon after birth, is higher than the mother's level, and then begins to decrease, the injury to the infant most likely occurred days prior to the time the infant was born. Also the length of time that the creatinine remains elevated is often, but not always, correlative with the severity of the asphyxial episode. Other markers of renal involvement include hematuria, proteinuria, and elevated urinary β$_2$-microglobulin [55].

Although hypoglycemia can be encountered in infants following an asphyxial event, and its finding should be anticipated as glycogen stores may be depleted, its onset and severity have not been useful in determining the timing of an adverse event.

Newborn neurological evaluations

Infants with severe encephalopathy are obtunded and in coma. They are flaccid, their deep tendon reflexes are depressed or absent, and they often have evidence of autonomic dysfunction. Those with mild encephalopathy have normal or hyperactive tone and reflexes, may be hyperalert, and may have jitteriness, but do not have seizures.

Those with moderate encephalopathy fall between these extremes. They are listless, lethargic but arousable, tend to be hypotonic, but may have absent, normal, or even hypertonic reflexes. They feed poorly, may develop seizures, and have decreased spontaneous motor activity. Some, but not all, infants may pass from one stage to another, with overlapping findings. The detailed clinical features and the time intervals are described in Chapter 16.

It should be noted that those infants who have suffered from intrapartum asphyxial episodes, especially if they have moderate or severe encephalopathy, are hypotonic, which lasts for the first 5–7 days of life. Hypertonicity then becomes apparent during the second week of life. Thus, a newborn who has moderate to severe encephalopathy and has increased tone soon after birth along with somnolence and seizures should be suspected of having suffered an injury prior to the intrapartum period. As noted in Chapter 1, infants may suffer from an intrauterine injury prior to the onset of labor, then have sufficient time to recover, may even appear normal in the immediate newborn period, have relatively normal umbilical cord blood gases, and may even be sent to the normal nursery. However, they may soon develop signs of encephalopathy, often with seizures, and neuroimaging studies obtained at the end of the first week are similar, if not identical, to those of infants who have suffered from an intrapartum event. Perlman noted that in his experience approximately 50% of patients with neonatal encephalopathy exhibit this clinical scenario [56]. Hull and Dodd [57] reported similar experiences in their evaluation of 107 infants and found 43 had courses similar to that described by Perlman [56]. These infants had normal vaginal births. Almost half had no evidence of fetal distress and had good Apgar scores at 5 minutes. Constantinou et al. described 14 infants who were resuscitated after a "near-miss" sudden infant death syndrome (SIDS) [58]. Seven of these infants died without regaining consciousness, and five of the seven remaining infants, who regained consciousness within 1 hour of resuscitation, showed a striking period of appearing almost normal before having neurological deterioration 36–96 hours after resuscitation.

If an infant is found to have arthrogryposis, this problem most likely developed weeks to months prior to birth and had nothing to do with intrapartum difficulties. Significantly increased tone encountered in the newborn period should suggest other diagnoses such as stiff-body syndrome, myotonia congenita, or infants born to mothers who abuse cocaine.

The infant who has marked hypotonia without other findings of asphyxia should be evaluated for syndromes such as Prader–Willi syndrome, Zellweger syndrome, Miller–Dieker syndrome, fragile X syndrome, myotonic dystrophy, and even congenital myasthenia gravis.

The infant with significant cerebral edema will have a full or bulging fontanel, spreading of the cranial sutures, and an enlarging head circumference (see Chapter 16). In most situations cerebral edema is not a prominent feature of HIE in full-term infants [59]. If it is present, it usually requires 16–24 hours to become recognizable clinically, and reaches a maximum pressure at 36–72 hours after the cerebral insult. Therefore, if an infant is born with cerebral edema already clinically evident, it would suggest that the damage had occurred at least 18 hours previously.

Some infants with moderate or severe encephalopathy may also have evidence of severe persistent pulmonary hypertension of the newborn (PPHN). Those infants are extremely difficult to ventilate and may even be candidates for nitric oxide (NO) therapy or even management with ECMO. It generally requires the infant to be in a hypoxic environment for at least 48 hours for pulmonary hypertension to become manifest. Thus the factors responsible for the events causing the pulmonary hypertension could very well be responsible for the central nervous system damage as well (see Chapter 37).

It is also extremely important to evaluate intrauterine growth patterns of depressed newborns and identify those infants with asymmetric growth patterns. In most asymmetrically growth-restricted infants, the head growth is usually protected compared to the infant's weight and length. Thus, if an infant is born with decreased head growth compared to the infant's weight and especially the length, and has neonatal depression or is later found to have cerebral palsy, then one can surmise that the intrauterine event causing this poor head growth occurred long before the onset of labor.

Imaging studies

The ultrasound examination can be used readily in the neonatal period without having to move the infant, and provides important screening information regarding gross structural anomalies, significant hemorrhage, hydrocephalus, and certain cystic changes. Its greatest value is in the preterm infant to detect intraventricular hemorrhage (IVH), to follow the infant for evidence of cystic periventricular leukomalacia (PVL), and to follow the progression of hydrocephalus, should it develop. The ultrasound examination for demonstration of an acute hypoxemic event may not be helpful in evaluating the extent and the timing of the event. The brain may appear normal for the first 12–24 hours, and then changes compatible with cerebral edema develop. There are often differences of opinion when evaluating "slit-like" ventricles in term infants and diffuse increased echogenicity throughout the brain tissue. Studies using Doppler with resistive indices may add some specificity to the physiological timing of the injuries. Low resistive indices are most marked 24–48 hours after the injury. Ultrasound can also detect injury to the thalamus and basal ganglia, especially if accompanied by hemorrhage or hemorrhagic necrosis. Detection of subdural hemorrhage or hematoma is difficult with the ultrasound examination.

The computed tomography (CT) scan has also been useful in detecting various injuries to the central nervous system following asphyxial insult. It is superior to the ultrasound in many aspects, including the detection of focal and multifocal ischemic brain injury, as well as hemorrhagic lesions that accompany or complicate asphyxia.

Magnetic resonance imaging (MRI) is currently becoming the gold standard for fully evaluating the extent and severity of asphyxial injury to the brain [1]. In many, but not all, situations, it is of help in determining the timing of the asphyxial event, even if the study is carried out months to years after the birth of the infant [1,60–65]. It is the study of choice to detect developmental abnormalities, especially disorders of neuronal migration, disorders of myelination, abnormalities of the corpus callosum, and arteriovenous malformations. The MRI is also vastly superior to CT scanning in detecting cerebral infarcts, parasagittal cerebral injury, injury to the thalamus and basal ganglia, and hemorrhagic lesions [61].

Periventricular white-matter injury associated with PVL has been thought to occur only in preterm infants, and it has been suggested that if such findings were encountered in infants born at term, the injury most likely occurred prenatally during the 24th to 34th week of gestation. Such abnormalities have been found in as many as one-half of term infants with HIE [30], but whether the primary insult occurred during the intrapartum period or had been initiated previously is still debatable. Interestingly, Rutherford and coworkers described that the finding of an abnormal signal intensity in the posterior limb of the internal capsule on MRI in term infants with HIE is associated with poor neurological outcome [66]. Whether this finding is associated with capsular white-matter injury only or is associated with thalamic or basal ganglia involvement is unclear at present.

Sie and colleagues studied 104 infants with evidence of bilateral post hypoxic–ischemic brain damage in the chronic phase of this illness [64]. They concluded that the severity of injury was the primary determinant of the location of the lesion rather than the post-conceptual age at which the insult occurred. They describe three specific MR patterns in the infants: (1) PVL, (2) predominant lesion of the basal ganglia and thalamus, in which 95% were preceded by acute profound asphyxia, and (3) multicystic encephalopathy. These lesions were found in both preterm and term infants. Interestingly, these authors found that the "common risk factors in the term infants with PVL patterns were dysmaturity or maternal pre-eclampsia and the majority had multiple risk factors for partial and/or relapsing hypoxia–ischemia."

There appears to be some disagreement in the literature regarding findings on MRI that can, in retrospect, define the timing of injury and specify whether it occurred during the prenatal or the intrapartum period. Because clinically there is overlapping of the causes of HIE, it is no wonder that the MRI may not determine with precision when the injury or injuries have taken place or whether they were confined to a single period of time. As mentioned previously, if the asphyxial event occurred 1–3 days prior to the intrapartum period, the MR findings would often be similar to those recognized as having occurred in the intrapartum period. These issues are discussed at length in Chapter 18.

Nevertheless, it is important to have an MRI study, and if possible a magnetic resonance spectroscopy (MRS) study as well, to detect developmental disorders, to ascertain the areas of involvement of damage associated with HIE, and also to document normal findings. It is important to document a normal MRI in a child who may have been depressed at birth and is later found to have severe mental retardation. The normal MRI would mitigate the diagnosis of an intrapartum event causing the retardation.

Placental pathology

In Chapter 20 the placental features of infants who have suffered from HIE are delineated, and the correlation of findings with the timing of these events is discussed. Unfortunately, much too often the placentas of depressed infants are not retained for examination, or the examination is performed by pathologists who have little interest in this important organ. A great deal of information can be gathered by careful evaluation of the placenta, including the presence and location of meconium in various cells, the presence of thrombosis, edema, or degenerative changes, the presence and concentration of NRBCs, evidence of infection, the presence of chorioamnionitis, and the location of acute and chronic inflammatory cells. If these data are available, timing of the

event or events leading to the infant's difficulties can be determined more readily, especially if they are correlated with clinical, laboratory, and imaging studies.

Neuropathological evaluations

As mentioned in Chapter 1, asphyxial insults that result in central nervous system damage are being recognized in preterm as well as term infants prior to the onset of labor. Sims et al. reported a 17% incidence of central nervous system injury in over 400 stillborn fetuses at the Los Angeles County/ University of Southern California Medical Center [67]. Ellis et al. reported that 25% of infants dying shortly after birth had pathological findings associated with prenatal damage [68]. Similar findings were reported by Squier and Keeling [69]. Gavai et al. described prenatally diagnosed fetal brain injuries following known antenatally acquired injuries [70]. Low found evidence of antepartum injury in 17 of 30 infants who died in the neonatal period with the diagnosis of presumed asphyxia [71]. He also found that 5 of the 30 infants who had intrapartum problems died in the neonatal period. He devised a template to ascertain the timing of neuropathological features that appear following an asphyxial episode. If an infant or fetus dies within the first 18 hours after the asphyxial event, the brain may appear normal, since it requires a minimum of 18 hours before microscopic changes can be recognized. Low also documented a sequence of events leading from neuronal necrosis to microglial response and astrocyte response or hypertrophy over a period of time, and he noted that macroscopic cavitation would appear after 4 days if the necrosis were severe. Table 21.3 outlines the sequence of events that occurred and the interval between the onset of the insult and the neuropathology that ensued.

Conclusion

In many situations it is extremely difficult to ascertain the timing of an intrauterine event or events that cause neurological damage to the developing fetus. Despite the improvement in monitoring of the progress of pregnancies, in identifying and

Table 21.3. Sequence of observed neuropathic features, and the interval between asphyxial insult and neuropathology

| Time | Neuropathology | | | |
	Neuronal necrosis	Microglial response	Astrocyte response	Cavitation
<18 h	0	0	0	0
18–36 h	+	0	0	0
36–72 h	+	+	0	0
73–96 h	+	+	+	0
>96 h	+	+	+	+

Source: Modified from Low [71] with permission.

responding to abnormalities that develop, and in electronic monitoring of fetal heart rate prior to and during labor, the incidence of cerebral palsy and mental retardation has not been significantly altered. While the intrapartum death rate has declined, the complications secondary to these problems have not. When called upon to determine the causation and possible prevention of intrauterine problems, clinicians are often unable to identify the sequence of events that has occurred.

Using retrospective analyses and careful evaluation of subjective and objective parameters, one can often piece together a logical explanation of those adverse events. This is especially true if one carries out a careful analysis of the events of pregnancy, the results of electronic fetal heart-rate monitoring, the condition of the infant at birth, and the biochemical and physiological abnormalities that may be present. Having access to the placenta for histological review is often of great help in identifying various lesions that affect the intrauterine milieu. Serial and continuous EEG evaluation can often help in establishing the timing of events as well as offering appropriate approaches to therapy. Lastly, using imaging studies, especially MRl, abnormalities of the central nervous system, their location, and severity can often determine the timing of adverse events to a reasonable degree. Table 21.4 lists findings that would suggest that antepartum rather than intrapartum events caused the encephalopathic problems in a neonate. These, in conjunction with the recommendations of the American College of Obstetrics and Gynecology (ACOG)/American Academy of Pediatrics (AAP) publication noted in Chapter 1,

Table 21.4. Findings that would suggest an antepartum event causing neonatal encephalopathy

(1) Decreased or absent fetal movement prior to the onset of labor

(2) Non-reassuring fetal heart rate upon admission to the hospital

(3) Lack of significant metabolic acidosis at the time of birth that does not worsen after resuscitation

(4) Normal or near-normal activity at birth and subsequent progression to an encephalopathic state

(5) Presence of persistent pulmonary hypertension

(6) Hyperactivity and hyperreflexia in an obtunded infant

(7) Evidence of a bulging fontanelle within the first day of life

(8) Presence of electroencephalographic seizures within the first 12 h of age

(9) Elevated levels of nucleated red blood cells that remain elevated for 12–24 h

(10) Prolonged period of thrombocytopenia

(11) Lack of documentation of an acute intrapartum event or of a prolonged bradycardic episode

(12) MRI/MRS findings suggestive of a prepartum injury

Notes:
MRI, magnetic resonance imaging; MRS, magnetic resonance spectroscopy.

could lead to a better understanding of the etiology of the infants' difficulties [72].

Until we develop better indicators of intrauterine problems, are able to visualize changes in central nervous system function, and then apply these in a clinical situation that is easy to use and interpret, we are left with many indirect indicators that lack specificity and sensitivity in individual patients.

References

1. Barkovich AJ. MR imaging of the neonatal brain. *Neuroimaging Clin N Am* 2006; **16**: 117–35.

2. Pasternak JF, Gorey MT. The syndrome of acute near-total intrauterine asphyxia in the term infant. *Pediatr Neurol* 1998; **18**: 391–8.

3. Clapp JF, Peress NS, Wesley M, *et al.* Brain damage after intermittent partial cord occlusion in the chronically instrumented fetal lamb. *Am J Obstet Gynecol* 1988; **159**: 504–9.

4. De Haan HH, Gunn AJ, Williams CE, *et al.* Brief repeated umbilical cord occlusions cause sustained cytotoxic cerebral edema and focal infarcts in near-term fetal lambs. *Pediatr Res* 1997; **41**: 96–104.

5. Gunn AJ, Maxwell L, De Haan HH, *et al.* Delayed hypotension and subendocardial injury after repeated umbilical cord occlusion in near-term fetal lambs. *Am J Obstet Gynecol* 2000; **183**: 1564–72.

6. Mallard EC, Williams CE, Johnston BM, *et al.* Repeated episodes of umbilical cord occlusion in fetal sheep lead to preferential damage to the striatum and sensitize the heart to further insults. *Pediatr Res* 1995; **37**: 707–13.

7. Manning FA, Bondaji N, Harman CR, *et al.* Fetal assessment based on fetal biophysical profile scoring. VIII. The incidence of cerebral palsy in tested and untested perinates. *Am J Obstet Gynecol* 1998; **178**: 696–706.

8. Rayburn WF. Clinical implications from monitoring fetal activity. *Am J Obstet Gynecol* 1982; **144**: 967–80.

9. Olesen AG, Svare JA. Decreased fetal movements: background, assessment, and clinical management. *Acta Obstet Gynecol Scand* 2004; **83**: 818–26.

10. Schifrin BS, Hamilton-Rubinstein T, Shields JR. Fetal heart rate patterns and the timing of fetal injury. *J Perinatol* 1994; **14**: 174–81.

11. Phelan JP, Kim JO. Fetal heart rate observations in the brain-damaged infant. *Semin Perinatol* 2000; **24**: 221–9.

12. van der Moer PE, Gerretsen G, Visser GH. Fixed fetal heart rate pattern after intrauterine accidental decerebration. *Obstet Gynecol* 1985; **65**: 125–7.

13. Menticoglou SM, Manning FA, Harman CR, *et al.* Severe fetal brain injury without evident intrapartum asphyxia or trauma. *Obstet Gynecol* 1989; **74**: 457–61.

14. Schifrin BS. The CTG and the timing and mechanism of fetal neurological injuries. *Best Pract Res Clin Obstet Gynaecol* 2004; **18**: 437–56.

15. Low JA, Victory R, Derrick EJ. Predictive value of electronic fetal monitoring for intrapartum fetal asphyxia with metabolic acidosis. *Obstet Gynecol* 1999; **93**: 285–91.

16. American College of Obstetricians and Gynecologists Practice Bulletin. Clinical management guidelines for obstetrician–gynecologists, Number 70, December 2005. Intrapartum fetal heart rate monitoring. *Obstet Gynecol* 2005; **106**: 1453–60.

17. Nelson KB, Dambrosia JM, Ting TY, *et al.* Uncertain value of electronic fetal monitoring in predicting cerebral palsy. *N Engl J Med* 1996; **334**: 613–18.

18. Blix E, Sviggum O, Koss KS, *et al.* Inter-observer variation in assessment of 845 labour admission tests: comparison between midwives and obstetricians in the clinical setting and two experts. *BJOG* 2003; **110**: 1–5.

19. Nielsen PV, Stigsby B, Nickelsen C, *et al.* Intra- and inter-observer variability in the assessment of intrapartum cardiotocograms. *Acta Obstet Gynecol Scand* 1987; **66**: 421–4.

20. Zain HA, Wright JW, Parrish GE, *et al.* Interpreting the fetal heart rate tracing: effect of knowledge of neonatal outcome. *J Reprod Med* 1998; **43**: 367–70.

21. Draycott T, Sibanda T, Owen L, *et al.* Does training in obstetric emergencies improve neonatal outcome? *BJOG* 2006; **113**: 177–82.

22. Keith RD, Beckley S, Garibaldi JM, *et al.* A multicentre comparative study of 17 experts and an intelligent computer system for managing labour using the cardiotocogram. *Br J Obstet Gynaecol* 1995; **102**: 688–700.

23. Parer JT, King T, Flanders S, *et al.* Fetal acidemia and electronic fetal heart rate patterns: is there evidence of an association? *J Matern Fetal Neonatal Med* 2006; **19**: 289–94.

24. Westgate JA, Wibbens B, Bennet L, *et al.* The intrapartum deceleration in center stage: a physiologic approach to the interpretation of fetal heart rate changes in labor. *Am J Obstet Gynecol* 2007; **197**: 236. e1–11.

25. Clifford SH. Clinical significance of yellow staining of the vernix caseosa, skin, nails, and umbilical cord of the newborn. *Arch Dis Child* 1945; **69**: 327–8.

26. Sienko A, Altshuler G. Meconium-induced umbilical vascular necrosis in abortuses and fetuses: a histopathologic study for cytokines. *Obstet Gynecol* 1999; **94**: 415–20.

27. Naeye RL. Can meconium in the amniotic fluid injure the fetal brain? *Obstet Gynecol* 1995; **86**: 720–4.

28. Benirschke K. Fetal consequences of amniotic fluid meconium. *Contemp Obstet Gynecol* 2001; **6**: 76–83.

29. Katz VL, Bowes WA. Meconium aspiration syndrome: reflections on a murky subject. *Am J Obstet Gynecol* 1992; **166**: 171–83.

30. Volpe JJ. Hypoxic–ischemic encephalopathy. In Volpe JJ, ed., *Neurology of the Newborn*, 4th edn. Philadelphia, PA: Saunders, 2001: 217–394.

31. Ahn MO, Korst LM, Phelan JP, *et al.* Does the onset of neonatal seizures correlate with the timing of fetal neurologic injury? *Clin Pediatr (Phila)* 1998; **37**: 673–6.

32. Westgate JA, Bennet L, Gunn AJ. Fetal seizures causing increased heart rate variability during terminal fetal hypoxia. *Am J Obstet Gynecol* 1999; **181**: 765–6.

33. Filan P, Boylan GB, Chorley G, *et al.* The relationship between the onset of electrographic seizure activity after birth and the time of cerebral injury *in utero*. *BJOG* 2005; **112**: 504–7.

34. Takeuchi T, Watanabe K. The EEG evolution and neurological prognosis of neonates with perinatal hypoxia. *Brain Dev* 1989; **11**: 115–20.

35. Watanabe K, Hayakawa F, Okumura A. Neonatal EEG: a powerful tool in the assessment of brain damage in preterm infants. *Brain Dev* 1999; **21**: 361–72.

36. Toet MC, Hellstrom-Westas L, Groenendaal F, *et al.* Amplitude integrated EEG 3 and 6 hours after birth in full term neonates with hypoxic–ischaemic encephalopathy. *Arch Dis Child Fetal Neonatal Ed* 1999; **81**: F19–23.

37. Sarkar S, Barks JD, Donn SM. Should amplitude-integrated electroencephalography be used to identify infants suitable for hypothermic neuroprotection? *J Perinatol* 2008; **28**: 117–22.

38. Naeye RL, Lin HM. Determination of the timing of fetal brain damage from hypoxemia–ischemia. *Am J Obstet Gynecol* 2001; **184**: 217–24.

39. Naeye RL, Localio AR. Determining the time before birth when ischemia and hypoxemia initiated cerebral palsy. *Obstet Gynecol* 1995; **86**: 713–19.

40. Benirschke K. Placenta pathology questions to the perinatologist. *J Perinatol* 1994; **14**: 371–5.

41. Blackwell SC, Hallak M, Hotra JW, *et al.* Timing of fetal nucleated red blood cell count elevation in response to acute hypoxia. *Biol Neonate* 2004; **85**: 217–20.

42. Bracci R, Perrone S, Buonocore G. Red blood cell involvement in fetal/neonatal hypoxia. *Biol Neonate* 2001; **79**: 210–12.

43. Ferber A, Minior VK, Bornstein E, *et al.* Fetal "nonreassuring status" is associated with elevation of nucleated red blood cell counts and interleukin-6. *Am J Obstet Gynecol* 2005; **192**: 1427–9.

44. Ghosh B, Mittal S, Kumar S, *et al.* Prediction of perinatal asphyxia with nucleated red blood cells in cord blood of newborns. *Int J Gynaecol Obstet* 2003; **81**: 267–71.

45. Phelan JP, Kirkendall C, Korst LM, *et al.* Nucleated red blood cell and platelet counts in asphyxiated neonates sufficient to result in permanent neurologic impairment. *J Matern Fetal Neonatal Med* 2007; **20**: 377–80.

46. Soothill PW, Nicolaides KH, Campbell S. Prenatal asphyxia, hyperlacticaemia, hypoglycaemia, and erythroblastosis in growth retarded fetuses. *Br Med J* 1987; **294**: 1051–3.

47. Hamrick SE, Miller SP, Newton NR, *et al.* Nucleated red blood cell counts: not associated with brain injury or outcome. *Pediatr Neurol* 2003; **29**: 278–83.

48. Perri T, Ferber A, Digli A, *et al.* Nucleated red blood cells in uncomplicated prolonged pregnancy. *Obstet Gynecol* 2004; **104**: 372–6.

49. McCarthy JM, Capullari T, Thompson Z, *et al.* Umbilical cord nucleated red blood cell counts: normal values and the effect of labor. *J Perinatol* 2006; **26**: 89–92.

50. Calhoun DA, Li Y, Braylan RC, *et al.* Assessment of the contribution of the spleen to granulocytopoiesis and erythropoiesis of the mid-gestation human fetus. *Early Hum Dev* 1996; **46**: 217–27.

51. Lackmann GM, Tollner U. The predictive value of elevation in specific serum enzymes for subsequent development of hypoxic–ischemic encephalopathy or intraventricular hemorrhage in full-term and premature asphyxiated newborns. *Neuropediatrics* 1995; **26**: 192–8.

52. Nagdyman N, Komen W, Ko HK, *et al.* Early biochemical indicators of hypoxic–ischemic encephalopathy after birth asphyxia. *Pediatr Res* 2001; **49**: 502–6.

53. De Praeter C, Vanhaesebrouck P, Govaert P, *et al.* Creatine kinase isoenzyme BB concentrations in the cerebrospinal fluid of newborns: relationship to short-term outcome. *Pediatrics* 1991; **88**: 1204–10.

54. Pincus MR, Zimmerman AJ, Henry JB. Clinical enzymology. In Henry JB, ed., *Clinical Diagnosis and Management by Laboratory Methods*. Philadelphia, PA: Saunders, 1996: 268–95.

55. Tack ED, Perlman JM, Robson AM. Renal injury in sick newborn infants: a prospective evaluation using urinary beta 2-microglobulin concentrations. *Pediatrics* 1988; **81**: 432–40.

56. Perlman JM. Intrapartum asphyxia and cerebral palsy: is there a link? *Clin Perinatol* 2006; **33**: 335–53.

57. Hull J, Dodd K. What is birth asphyxia? *Br J Obstet Gynaecol* 1991; **98**: 953–5.

58. Constantinou JE, Gillis J, Ouvrier RA, *et al.* Hypoxic–ischaemic encephalopathy after near miss sudden infant death syndrome. *Arch Dis Child* 1989; **64**: 703–8.

59. Lupton BA, Hill A, Roland EH, *et al.* Brain swelling in the asphyxiated term newborn: pathogenesis and outcome. *Pediatrics* 1988; **82**: 139–46.

60. Barkovich AJ, Westmark KD, Bedi HS, *et al.* Proton spectroscopy and diffusion imaging on the first day of life after perinatal asphyxia: preliminary report. *AJNR Am J Neuroradiol* 2001; **22**: 1786–94.

61. Barnes PD. Neuroimaging and the timing of fetal and neonatal brain injury. *J Perinatol* 2001; **21**: 44–60.

62. Cowan F, Rutherford M, Groenendaal F, *et al.* Origin and timing of brain lesions in term infants with neonatal encephalopathy. *Lancet* 2003; **361**: 736–42.

63. Rutherford M, Srinivasan L, Dyet L, *et al.* Magnetic resonance imaging in perinatal brain injury: clinical presentation, lesions and outcome. *Pediatr Radiol* 2006; **36**: 582–92.

64. Sie LT, van der Knaap MS, Oosting J, *et al.* MR patterns of hypoxic–ischemic brain damage after prenatal, perinatal or postnatal asphyxia. *Neuropediatrics* 2000; **31**: 128–36.

65. Soul JS, Robertson RL, Tzika AA, *et al.* Time course of changes in diffusion-weighted magnetic resonance imaging in a case of neonatal encephalopathy with defined onset and duration of hypoxic–ischemic insult. *Pediatrics* 2001; **108**: 1211–14.

66. Rutherford MA, Pennock JM, Counsell SJ, *et al.* Abnormal magnetic resonance signal in the internal capsule predicts poor neurodevelopmental outcome in infants with hypoxic–ischemic encephalopathy. *Pediatrics* 1998; **102**: 323–8.

67. Sims ME, Turkel SB, Halterman G, *et al.* Brain injury and intrauterine death. *Am J Obstet Gynecol* 1985; **151**: 721–3.

68. Ellis WG, Goetzman BW, Lindenberg JA. Neuropathologic documentation of prenatal brain damage. *Am J Dis Child* 1988; **142**: 858–66.

69. Squier M, Keeling JW. The incidence of prenatal brain injury. *Neuropathol Appl Neurobiol* 1991; **17**: 29–38.

70. Gavai M, Hargitai B, Varadi V, *et al.* Prenatally diagnosed fetal brain injuries with known antenatal etiologies. *Fetal Diagn Ther* 2008; **23**: 18–22.

71. Low JA. Relationship of fetal asphyxia to neuropathology and deficits in children. *Clin Invest Med* 1993; **16**: 133–40.

72. American College of Obstetricians and Gynecologists/American Academy of Pediatrics. *Neonatal Encephalopathy and Cerebral Palsy: Defining the Pathogenesis and Pathophysiology.* Washington, DC: ACOG, 2003.

Specific conditions associated with fetal and neonatal brain injury
Congenital malformations of the brain

Jin S. Hahn and Ronald J. Lemire

Introduction

This chapter focuses on some of the more common brain malformations that are encountered early in life. Tremendous advances in neuroimaging with MRI in the past two decades have significantly improved our ability to diagnose brain malformations. In conjunction, there have been rapid advances in neurobiology that have led to better understanding of how the brain develops and what disturbances to the development lead to malformation. Each year more and more genes responsible for malformations are being discovered. Furthermore, modern fetal ultrasonography and more recently fetal MRI have increased the ability to detect a large variety of central nervous system malformations in utero. Prenatal detection and anatomic diagnosis of the malformations will better allow the medical caregivers to provide prognosis and management counseling.

Normal brain development

A brief overview of normal embryonic and fetal brain development will help to clarify the timing and etiology of brain malformations. Normal human brain development occurs in a highly defined spatial and temporal sequence of events in utero (Table 22.1). The temporal sequence consists of several overlapping phases. During the *induction* phase, signals sent to the ectoderm cause it to develop into neural tissue. The neural plate, a sheet of cells that will ultimately develop into the nervous system, develops by the 17th to 20th day of gestation. *Neurulation* occurs next, where the neural plate begins to fold into the neural tube, a process that begins by the 21st day. Toward the rostral end, cephalic enlargement and vesicle formation start to occur by day 23. By day 27, the ends of the neural tube, the neuropores, close.

After 3 weeks of gestation, at the cephalic end the brain has developed into the three primary vesicles: prosencephalon, mesencephalon, and rhombencephalon. By the end of the sixth week, these vesicles will develop further into five vesicles: telencephalon, diencephalon, mesencephalon, metencephalon, and myelencephalon. By the fifth week *ventral induction* (or

patterning) causes the telencephalic vesicle to bifurcate (or cleave) into the two hemispheres.

Cell proliferation and *neuronal generation* peak between the second and the fifth month. During this phase neuronal precursor cells in the germinal layer of the ventricular zone undergo rapid proliferation, resulting in a large number of neurons that will migrate to the cortex.

Cell migration occurs between the sixth and the 20th weeks. Cells that will become neurons exit the cell cycle and move out through the ventricular and subventricular zone along the fibers of radial glial cells. In the neocortex, there is an inside-out migration pattern. Newer neurons migrate past older neurons to occupy the more exterior layer.

Cell process and synapse formation begins around the fifth month, peaks around the seventh month of gestation, and continues after birth. During this phase neuronal processes must extend locally, and at times long distances, to find their targets in other neurons. Neurons also undergo differentiation into specific neuronal subtypes.

Etiologies and timing of malformations

Various disturbances in any of the developmental stages described above will result in specific brain malformation, depending on the timing and nature of the perturbation. A useful concept in assessing the timing of human brain malformation is that of a "termination period," a point in time beyond which a specific malformation cannot occur. For example, in humans the ventral patterning process that leads to the bifurcation of the cerebral hemispheres from the telencephalon occurs by the fifth week of gestation. Holoprosencephaly is thought to arise when there is failure of ventral patterning, and therefore suspected genetic mutations or teratogenic agents acting at a later time would not likely be the cause for this anomaly.

The general principle underlying brain malformations is that the same anomaly may arise from genetic or environmental causes. Genetic etiologies include chromosomal abnormalities as well as gene mutations. Some complex malformations can be due to multiple unrelated genes. Exogenous or environmental etiologies include congenital infections (especially rubella, toxoplasmosis, and cytomegalovirus), radiation, chemical agents, drugs, vitamin deficiency or excess, and nutritional deficiencies. Ischemia occurring at various stages of development can also lead to several different types of malformation.

Fetal and Neonatal Brain Injury, 4th edition, ed. David K. Stevenson, William E. Benitz, Philip Sunshine, Susan R. Hintz, and Maurice L. Druzin. Published by Cambridge University Press. © Cambridge University Press 2009.

Table 22.1. Selected features in the development of the human embryonic brain

Stage	Age (days)	Features of brain development
7–8	16–18	Neural plate/groove
9	20	Neural folds, three rhombomeres
10	22	Optic primordium; fusion of rhombencephalic folds; cranial flexure
11	24	Rostral neuropore closes; acousticofacial complex; optic vesicle; primordium of corpus striatum
12	26	Caudal neuropore closes; hindbrain roof thins; cerebellar plate
13	28	Three divisions of trigeminal nerve; pontine flexure; olfactory placode
14	32	Oculomotor nerve; hypothalamic sulcus; roots of CN5–10 formed
15	33	Cerebral vesicles appear; striatal ridge; CN4 decussate
16	37	Infundibulum; subthalamic nucleus
17	41	Frontal and parietal lobe areas; choroid fissure closes; posterior commissure
18	44	Choroid plexus in fourth ventricle; superior and inferior colliculi; caudate nucleus
19	48	Choroid plexus in lateral ventricle; putamen; occipital pole area present; first fibers in internal capsule
20	50	Tentorium begins laterally; nerve fiber layer in retina
21	52	Choroid plexus in third ventricle
22	54	Anlage of dentate nucleus; superior colliculus
23	56	Temporal pole area present

Disorders of neural tube formation and related events

Neural tube defects

The neurulation process completes with the closure of the neural tube between the third and fourth week of gestation. Failure of the closure of the neural tube at either end causes neural tube defects (NTDs). Rostral non-closure results in anencephaly, and caudal non-closure results in myelomeningocele. Until recently the prevalence of NTDs has averaged about 1/1000 deliveries, but a wide geographical variation exists [1]. The highest rates have been found in Ireland (4.6–6.7/1000), south Wales (3.55), and Scotland (2.59). Low prevalence rates occurred in Columbia (0.1), Norway (0.2), and France (0.5). Prenatal screening with serum α-fetoprotein (AFP) and ultrasounds are used to detect NTDs early.

Anencephaly

Anencephaly is one of the most severe malformations of the brain and arises from failure of closure of the rostral neuropore. This results in a large defect of the cranial vault, meninges, and scalp. The cerebral hemispheres are absent or rudimentary, and tissue is softened with blood infiltration.

The brainstem has variable preservation of nuclei. Some infants with anencephaly are born alive, but usually expire within several days. Prenatal screening with maternal serum AFP and fetal ultrasound enable relatively straightforward detection of anencephaly. Ultrasound detection of anencephaly is possible from 12 weeks gestation.

The prevalence of anencephaly is approximately 1/2000 live births and the recurrence risk is approximately 4%. Some studies show as much as a 100-fold increase in risk of recurrence among mothers who have had a previous child with this condition.

Encephalocele

Encephaloceles occur when there is herniation of intracranial structures through a midline defect in the skull to form a sac covered by intact skin. When the prolapse involves meninges only the term meningocele is used. When neural tissue is present, it is called encephalocele. Most commonly encephaloceles are located in the occipital region at or below the inion (Fig. 22.1). They may also be found in the frontal or nasofrontal location. In the United States, the frontal to occipital ratio is 1 : 6. Compared to anencephaly, which occurs during primary neurulation (neural tube formation), encephaloceles occur later (after 4 weeks). The prevalence is between 1/2000 and 1/5000 live births [2].

Children with *occipital encephalocele* are at risk for visual problems, microcephaly, mental retardation, and seizures. The nature and severity of disabilities depends on location and the amount of cerebral tissue involved in the defect. When the ventricular systems are involved or there are associated anomalies, such as aqueductal stenosis or Dandy–Walker malformation, hydrocephalus may be a complication.

Anterior encephaloceles may be visible, located around the root of the nose or in the superior medial aspect of the orbital cavity. *Basal encephaloceles* are not visible and are often located in the orbit, nasal fossae, or sphenoid sinuses. These types of encephaloceles are less common than the occipital encephaloceles, and may have a more favorable neurodevelopmental prognosis.

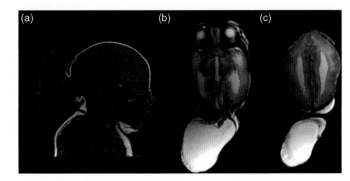

Fig. 22.1. MRI of a term newborn with occipital encephalocele. (a) Sagittal T1-weighted image shows herniation of brain tissue through the defect in the skull posteriorly. (b,c) Axial T2-weighted images demonstrate the large encephalocele and cobblestone lissencephaly in the cerebral cortex. The corpus callosum is also dysplastic in appearance. This child was diagnosed with Walker–Warburg syndrome with congenital muscular dystrophy.

Myelomeningocele

Although myelomeningoceles are not a brain malformation per se, they represent a neural tube defect due to a failure of closure of the caudal neuropore (which normally occurs by the 26th day). They are almost always associated with brain malformations such as Chiari II malformation and hydrocephalus. Pathology shows failure of closure of the posterior vertebral arches (spina bifida) most commonly in the lumbosacral region, and protrusion of dura and leptomeninges through the spinal defect. In addition, myelomeningoceles entail protrusion of nerve roots and malformed spinal cord. Clinically the affected children have lower motor neuron paralysis of the lower limbs, cutaneous sensory deficits below the level of the lesion, and bowel and bladder dysfunction.

Maternal serum AFP level is elevated in myelomeningoceles, and this provides a method of screening for open NTDs. Ultrasound can detect spina bifida from 16–20 weeks of gestation.

Chiari II malformation

Chiari II malformation (Arnold–Chiari malformation) consists of caudal displacement of the posterior lobe of the cerebellar vermis into the foramen magnum and upper cervical spinal canal, beaked tectum, fusion of the colliculi, kinking of the medulla, and small, shallow posterior fossa. Associated spinal cord abnormalities include myelomeningocele, hydromyelia, syringomyelia, and diastematomyelia.

Hydrocephalus is a major complication of Chiari II malformation, and postnatally about 80% of these infants require a ventriculoperitoneal shunt to decrease intracranial pressure and provide a route for adequate CSF drainage. Some patients require surgical bony decompression of suboccipital bones and high cervical laminectomies if they develop apnea, cranial nerve palsies, and dysphagia.

There is nearly a constant association of hydrocephalus in patients with myelomeningocele and Chiari II malformation. Several hypotheses have been advanced regarding the pathogenesis of Chiari II, but none has been universally accepted, as they do not adequately explain all of the findings. There is also a temporal dissociation of the onset of myelomeningocele (before 26 days) and Chiari II, which occurs later.

Disorders of ventral patterning (prosencephalic cleavage)
Holoprosencephaly

Holoprosencephaly (HPE) is a complex brain malformation characterized by failure of the forebrain to bifurcate into two hemispheres. This ventral patterning process is normally complete by the fifth week of gestation [3]. It is the most common developmental defect of the forebrain and midface in humans, occurring in 1/250 pregnancies [4]. Because only 3% of fetuses with HPE survive to delivery [5], the live birth prevalence is only about 1/10 000 [6–8].

Holoprosencephaly has traditionally been classified according to DeMyer's classification into three grades of severity: alobar, semilobar, and lobar. In addition to these classic forms, there is another milder subtype of HPE, called middle interhemispheric variant (MIH) or syntelencephaly [9,10]. The sine qua non feature of HPE is an incomplete separation of the cerebral hemispheres. In the most severe form, *alobar* HPE, there is complete or nearly complete lack of separation of the cerebral hemispheres with a single midline forebrain ventricle (monoventricle), which often communicates with a dorsal cyst (Fig. 22.2). The interhemispheric fissure and corpus callosum are completely absent. The thalami and basal ganglia are often fused in appearance. In *semilobar* HPE, there is a failure of separation of the anterior hemispheres, while some portions of the posterior hemispheres show separation. The frontal horns of the lateral ventricle are absent, but posterior horns are present (Fig. 22.3). The corpus callosum is absent anteriorly, but the splenium of the corpus callosum is present. In *lobar* HPE, the mildest form, the cerebral hemispheres are fairly well separated, while only the most rostral/ventral aspects are non-separated. The splenium and body of the corpus callosum are present, although the genu may be poorly developed. Rudimentary formation of the frontal horns may be present. In contrast to "classic" HPE, in the middle interhemispheric variant of HPE (*MIH*) there is failure of separation of the posterior frontal and parietal lobes while the poles of the frontal and occipital lobes are well separated [9,10].

Patients with HPE have various midline craniofacial and facial malformations, and the severity in general correlates with the severity of the brain malformation. Very severe abnormalities, such as cyclopia, ethmocephaly (a proboscis between severely hypoteloric eyes), and cebocephaly (hypotelorism with a single nostril), are rare (~ 2%) [11]. Severe defects, including midline cleft lip (premaxillary agenesis) and cleft palate and flat nose, are seen in 16%. Moderate defects, including midface hypoplasia and moderate hypotelorism, occur in 14%. Mild malformations, including single maxillary central incisors and iris colobomas, are seen in 36%.

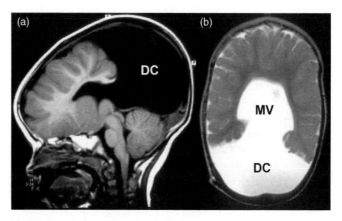

Fig. 22.2. MRI of a child with alobar holoprosencephaly. (a) Sagittal T1-weighted and (b) axial T2-weighted images show failure of separation of the two hemispheres and thalami, a monoventricle (MV), and a large dorsal cyst (DC) that communicates with the MV.

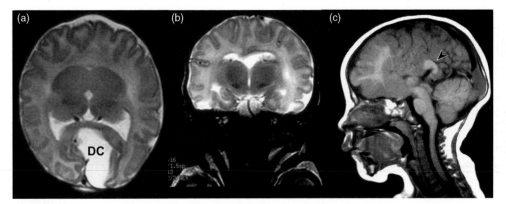

Fig. 22.3. MRI of a child with semilobar holoprosencephaly. (a) Axial T2-weighted image shows posterior portions of the hemispheres are well separated, but the anterior cerebral hemispheres are not cleaved. A dorsal cyst (DC) is present. The posterior horns of the lateral ventricles are well formed. The frontal horns are poorly developed (b) and posteriorly there is a monoventricle demonstrated on a coronal T2-weighted image. (c) A sagittal T1-weighted image of another patient demonstrates that the splenium of corpus callosum is formed (arrowhead), but the genu and body are not developed (arrowhead). This latter finding is highly suggestive of semilobar or lobar HPE.

Children with HPE experience many medical and neurological problems including mental retardation, epilepsy, weakness, spasticity, dystonia, choreoathetosis, and endocrine disorders, particularly diabetes insipidus [11,12]. Developmental disability affects virtually all patients with HPE. The degree of disability and neurological problems generally correlates with the severity of the brain malformation. Abnormalities of tone and movement are present in all forms of HPE [11–13]. The pituitary gland may be absent, dysplastic, or heterotopic. Diabetes insipidus, owing to posterior pituitary dysfunction, is a common problem in HPE. Anterior pituitary dysfunctions, such as growth hormone deficiency, hypocortisolism, and hypothyroidism, are also seen, but less frequently.

HPE is etiologically heterogeneous, and both environmental and genetic causes have been identified. *Chromosomal anomalies* including trisomies (13 and 18), duplications, deletions (e.g., 18p), and ring arrangements have played an important role in HPE. About 40% of live births with HPE have a chromosomal anomaly, and trisomy 13 accounts for over half of these cases [6]. Of infants born with trisomy 13, 70% have holoprosencephaly [14]. The prognosis in HPE is much worse for those with cytogenetic abnormalities, with only 2% surviving beyond 1 year, compared to 30–54% for those without cytogenetic anomalies [6]. Familial HPE also occurs, with both autosomal dominant and autosomal recessive inheritance.

Several multiple-malformation syndromes have been associated with HPE, with as many as 25% of HPE cases having a recognizable monogenic syndrome [6,15]. These include pseudotrisomy 13, Pallister–Hall, Meckel, and velocardiofacial syndromes. In addition, there is an increased incidence of HPE (∼ 5%) in patients with Smith–Lemli–Opitz syndrome, in which affected children have a defect in 7-dehydrocholesterol reductase, the enzyme that catalyzes the final step of cholesterol biosynthesis. Defective cholesterol synthesis may have a role in the pathogenesis of HPE through the sonic hedgehog (SHH) signaling pathway, since cholesterol is required for activation of SHH.

Mutations in several genes have been associated with HPE in humans: *SHH*, *PATCHED1* (*PTCH*), *TGIF*, *TDGF1*, *ZIC2*, *SIX3*, *GLI2*, *FAST1*, and *DISPATCHEDA* [16]. Two of these genes (*SHH* and *PTCH*) encode members of the sonic hedgehog signaling pathway, which regulates ventral development in both the forebrain and spinal cord. Human mutations have been discovered in *SHH* [17], which encodes a secreted signaling ligand localized at early stages to ventral domains in the developing neural tube, and *PATCHED1* (*PTCH*) [18], which encodes a receptor for *SHH*. The currently known mutations have been identified in only 15–20% of the HPE cases in a cohort with normal karyotypes [16].

Maternal diabetes, including gestational diabetes, is a well-established risk factor [19]. A diabetic mother's risk of having a child with HPE is approximately 1%, a greater than 100-fold increase over that of the general population. Prenatal exposures to alcohol, antiepileptic medications, retinoic acid, and cytomegalovirus infection have also been reported in cases of HPE.

Absence of septum pellucidum and septo-optic dysplasia

Absence of septum pellucidum (ASP) is associated with various congenital brain malformations including holoprosencephaly (HPE), septo-optic dysplasia (SOD), schizencephaly, and agenesis of the corpus callosum. One study of fetal ultrasounds indicated that the two most common conditions associated with ASP were HPE (including the MIH variant) and hydrocephalus that causes a disruption of the septum pellucidum [20]. When seen in isolation with an intact corpus callosum (Fig. 22.4), it may indicate a syndrome of SOD. SOD is a midline anomaly characterized by a triad of (1) ASP, (2) optic nerve hypoplasia, and (3) pituitary dysfunction. SOD has a wide range of clinical presentation, including decreased visual acuity, endocrine dysfunctions, cholestatis, and mental retardation/developmental delay [20]. SOD may also be associated with cortical malformations, HPE, callosal agenesis, and schizencephaly. In some patients with SOD, mutations of homeobox gene, *HESX1*, have been noted.

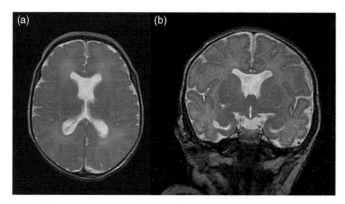

Fig. 22.4. (a) Axial T2-weighted and (b) coronal T2-weighted MR images of a term infant with isolated absence of septum pellucidum. The corpus callosum was intact.

Disorders of cell proliferation and neuronal generation

Microcephaly and microencephaly

Microcephaly is a term that applies to heads in which the circumference is smaller than 2 standard deviations (SD) below the mean for age and sex, although some studies have used smaller than 3 SD. The measurement should be corrected for prematurity and intrauterine growth retardation. *Microcephaly* (small skull) goes hand in hand with *microencephaly* (small brain) and can be associated with mental retardation.

In primary microcephaly, no other malformations are present. It may be familial or associated with a specific genetic syndrome (microcephaly vera). In autosomal recessive primary microcephaly (MCPH) individuals are born with a small brain, which subsequently grows but always remains relatively small, while the rest of the body grows normally [21]. MCPH is thought to be a disorder of neuronal proliferation (mitosis), resulting in a reduced number of neurons. Several genes have been identified for this disorder, including *ASPM* and *MICROCEPHALIN*.

Secondary microcephaly results from a large number of insults that affect the fetus in utero or in infancy during periods of rapid brain growth (first 2 years of life). Chromosomal and gene aberrations are often associated with small brains. Environmental factors include prenatal radiation (during the first two trimesters), drugs, other chemicals, and congenital infections including rubella, cytomegalovirus, toxoplasmosis, and type 2 HSV. In utero ischemia to the developing brain can also lead to secondary microcephaly.

Megalencephaly

The terms *megalencephaly* and *macrencephaly* are synonymous and imply large brains, in contrast to the term *macrocephaly*, which denotes a large head from various causes (e.g., hydrocephalus). In megalencephaly there is diffuse neuroepithelial proliferation and an increased number of cells in the brain. To standardize the definition, the head circumference must be over 2.5 SD above the mean corrected for age and sex.

Megalencephaly may be primary. Familial megalencephaly has an autosomal dominant inheritance, and affected individuals have normal or near-normal intelligence. There are a number of syndromes associated with megalencephaly including Soto syndrome (cerebral gigantism), fragile-X syndrome, autism, and various neurocutaneous disorders. Numerous storage diseases, such as Tay–Sachs disease, Canavan disease, and Alexander disease, are associated with megalencephaly, which is not usually present at birth but develops during infancy and beyond.

The clinical manifestations depend on the etiology. Familial megalencephalies can be associated with learning disabilities, neurological abnormalities, and epilepsy.

Hemimegalencephaly

Hemimegalencephaly (HME) is a rare malformation of cortical development where there is unilateral enlargement of one side of the brain. It may affect one hemisphere or some of its lobes with macroscopic enlargement due to abnormal proliferation of anomalous cells. Clinical manifestation of HME is dominated by refractory epilepsy, but also includes developmental delay and hemiparesis [22]. HME can occur alone or in association with neurocutaneous disorders, such as linear sebaceous nevus syndrome, hypomelanosis of Ito, and neurofibromatosis. Surgical hemispherectomy is the most effective treatment for medically refractory epilepsy.

Disorders of neuronal migration

Neuronal migration is characterized by an inside-out migrating pattern into six distinct layers in which the successive waves of newer post-mitotic neurons in the ventricular zone migrate past the older neurons to occupy a more exterior layer in the neocortex [21]. Neuronal migration begins at day 40–41 of gestation. Disturbances in the migration process will cause failure of neurons to reach their intended destination in the cerebral cortex and lead to disorganization of the cortical cytoarchitecture. This abnormality may be focal or diffuse.

Failure of neurons to leave the ventricular zone would result in periventricular heterotopias. Failure to complete their migration in the cortex would cause lissencephaly. Finally, failure of a subpopulation of neurons to complete their migration while others finish their migration could result in nodular or band heterotopias [23]. A revised classification of the cortical malformations based on genetic knowledge and developmental stages has been published by Barkovich and coworkers [24].

Lissencephaly/agyria and pachygyria

Lissencephaly is defined as a smooth brain without gyri. Pachygyria describes a reduced number of broad and flat gyri, shallow sulci, and fewer than normal foldings of the cortex. Both lissencephaly and pachygyria may be seen in the same brain. Affected infants have failure to thrive, microcephaly, marked developmental delay, and severe epilepsy.

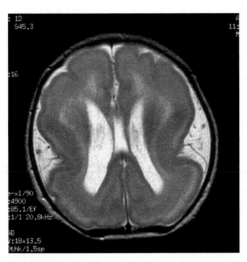

Fig. 22.5. Nine-day-old male infant with type 1 lissencephaly. Axial T2-weighted MR image shows smooth cortical surface (agyria/lissencephaly) that is prominent posteriorly. Frontal pachygyria is present. The Sylvian fissure is poorly formed.

Type 1 lissencephaly

The brain is small in type 1 lissencephaly, with only the primary and sometimes a few secondary gyri (Fig. 22.5). There is lack of opercularization, resuling in abnormal Sylvian fissure formation. The cortex is thick with white matter forming a thin rim along the ventricles. The most common genetic cause is a mutation of the *LIS1* gene. In Miller–Dieker syndrome, there are also dysmorphic facial features and deletion of 17p13.3, a region that includes the *LIS1* gene. A mutation in doublecortin gene, *DCX*, also causes lissencephaly in males. For a review see Kerjan and Gleeson [25].

Cobblestone lissencephaly (type 2)

Type 2 lissencephaly is also known as "cobblestone lissencephaly," because the smooth cortex has a granular surface and is covered with meninges that are thickened [23]. Abnormal migration of neurons through the defective glia limitans and into the leptomeningeal space results in disruption of cortical organization. This is seen in a group of rare autosomal recessive disorders characterized by congenital muscular dystrophy, severe brain malformations, and ocular abnormalities. Walker–Warburg syndrome, which is the most severe phenotype of the cobblestone lissencephaly (Fig. 22.1), can result from mutations in Fukutin (*FCMD*), Fukutin-related protein (*FKRP*), *POMT1*, or *POMT2* [21]. Fukuyama congenital muscular dystrophy resulting from different *FCMD* mutations also is associated with cobblestone lissencephaly.

Heterotopias

Heterotopia is a term used to describe ectopic neurons in white matter or neuronal malorientation. Periventricular heterotopias are abnormal collections of neurons in the subependymal region. They may be clinically silent or associated with epilepsy and neurodevelopmental dysfunction. Bilateral periventricular nodular heterotopia (BPNH) is an X-linked dominant disorder that is caused by a mutation in the filamin gene, *FLNA*.

Subcortical band heterotopias are also known as laminar heterotopias or "double cortex." Most of the cases in females are due to a mutation in the doublecortin gene, *DCX*, which in males causes type 1 lissencephaly.

Abnormal cortical organization or late migration

Polymicrogyria

Polymicrogyria is characterized by abundance of small gyral convolutions. The etiology is not well understood. It may be a genetic neuronal migration disorder or due to midcortical ischemic laminar necrosis affecting primarily the fifth cortical layer. The onset of the disorder is after 20 weeks (fifth month of gestation). It may be associated with genetic and chromosomal disorders. *Bilateral perisylvian syndrome* (or anterior operculum syndrome) consists of bilateral opercular abnormalities that include polymicrogyria visible on MRI. Patients have dysarthria, dysphagia, and pseudobulbar palsy.

Schizencephaly

Schizencephaly is characterized by unilateral or bilateral clefts within the cerebral hemispheres in which the borders of the cleft are surrounded by abnormal gray matter, particularly *microgyria*. Because this disorder is thought to be due to an ischemic lesion of the cerebrum in the first trimester it is discussed below in the section on encephaloclastic lesions.

Cortical dysplasia and microdysgenesis

Cortical microdysgeneses are microscopic abnormalities of cortical arrangement that may lead to epilepsy and other neurodevelopmental syndromes. Focal cortical dysplasias are larger than microdysgenesis and can usually be detected by high-resolution MRI. Resection of the dysplasias in affected patients may lead to significant improvement in seizure control.

Tuberous sclerosis complex

Tuberous sclerosis complex (TSC) is an autosomal dominant disorder characterized by cortical tubers, subependymal nodules, and retinal hamartomas. Children often develop epilepsy and neurodevelopmental delay, and may also have involvement of other organs (cardiac rhabdomyomas and renal angiomyolipomas and cysts). *TSC1* (hamartin) and *TSC2* (tuberin) are causative genes for TSC. The diagnosis can be made clinically, based on neurocutaneous features (hypopigmented macules, facial angiofibromas, or shagreen patch), neuroimaging findings, and clinical picture. Prenatal diagnosis is sometimes made on fetal MRI when there is a high index of suspicion for this disorder. Mothers carrying a child with TSC are often referred to a prenatal diagnostic center because of detection of a cardiac tumor (usually rhabdomyomas) on fetal ultrasound. When images of the fetal brain are carefully examined, subependymal nodules can be seen.

Combined and overlapping cerebral malformations

Agenesis of the corpus callosum

The corpus callosum is a fiber tract bridge that connects neurons between the two hemispheres. Its function is to coordinate communication of information between the left and right cerebral hemispheres. The corpus callosum begins to develop from the lamina reunions of His between 6 and 8 weeks of gestation. The last of the commissural fibers cross at 18–20 weeks [26].

Agenesis of the corpus callosum (ACC) can result from many causes, including infections, inherited errors of metabolism, and genetic syndromes. ACC occurs in over 50 congenital syndromes [27], and may also be associated with specific chromosomal abnormalities such as trisomy 8 and 18. The prevalence of ACC is between 0.1% and 0.7% in the general population and 2.3% in the developmentally disabled population [26].

The agenesis may be complete or partial. When partial, the defect is usually in the posterior portion of the corpus callosum. When the agenesis is complete the cingulate gyrus fails to form and a radial orientation of the mesial gyri is seen on sagittal MRI (Fig. 22.6). The enlargement of the occipital horns of the lateral ventricles associated with ACC is known as *colpocephaly*. Although the lateral ventricles in colpocephaly appear enlarged (ventriculomegaly), they should not be mistaken for hydrocephalus. "True" callosal agenesis should be distinguished from secondary agenesis, which is associated with major brain malformation of the embryonic forebrain such as holoprosencephaly [23].

Isolated ACC may be inherited, but no single gene defect has been identified. Children with isolated ACC may appear and function normally. However, as they grow older, they often function in the low borderline to normal range. With testing, difficulties in higher cortical function, language, perception, behavior, and integration of hemispheric functions

may be demonstrated. Some patients have mental retardation, cerebral palsy, and epilepsy. ACC may be associated with several other CNS malformations. The most common co-existing malformations include Dandy–Walker malformation, interhemispheric cysts, hydrocephalus, midline lipoma of the corpus callosum, and Chiari II malformation. Cortical anomalies associated with ACC include heterotopias, microgyria, and pachygyria. When there are other CNS malformations associated with ACC, the outcomes are often less favorable than in the isolated type.

MRI is the neuroimaging technique of choice because the brain can be imaged in three orthogonal planes. This provides a better assessment of the extent of corpus callosal hypogenesis. In fetal MRI, direct visualization of the corpus callosum is possible by 20 weeks of gestation. Mothers with suspected ACC are often referred for fetal MRI because of lack of visualization of the cavum septum pellucidum on fetal ultrasound. The fetal MRI offers the ability to assess for associated CNS anomalies, and in one study using fetal MRI additional anomalies were seen in over half of cases [26]. The additional malformations included diffuse or focal cortical malformations, delayed sulcal development, dysplastic deep gray nuclei, and brainstem anomalies.

Aicardi syndrome

Aicardi syndrome (AS) is a complex disorder defined as a triad of abnormalities: (1) total or partial agenesis of the corpus callosum, (2) chorioretinal "lacunae," and (3) infantile spasms (Fig. 22.7) [28]. Other associated findings include eye defects (colobomas of the optic disc), cortical polymicrogyria, periventricular heterotopia, cysts of the choroid plexus and/or the pineal or periventricular interhemispheric regions. Other brain abnormalities, such as intracranial cysts or tumors, represent a specific malformation complex of AS. It is an X-linked dominant disorder that affects and is lethal in males with only a single X chromosome.

Recognition of this complex on fetal MRI is sometimes possible due to the associated brain and eye malformation. This is important, since AS carries a much more severe prognosis than that of isolated ACC.

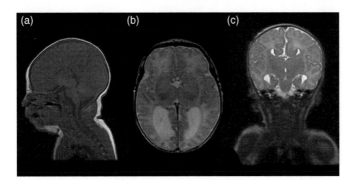

Fig. 22.6. MRI of a term newborn with isolated agenesis of corpus callosum. (a) Sagittal T1-weighted image shows absence of corpus callosum and cingulate gyrus. There is radial orientation of the mesial gyri. (b) T2-weighted axial image shows dilated posterior horn of the lateral ventricles, colpocephaly. (c) T2-weighted coronal image shows absence of callosal fibers across midline, and continuity of the third ventricle with the interhemispheric fissure superiorly.

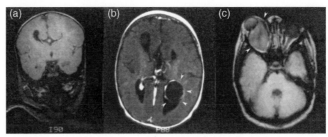

Fig. 22.7. MR images of an infant girl with Aicardi syndrome demonstrates absence of corpus callosum on (a) T1-weighted coronal and (b) axial images. The arrowheads on panel B outline an intraventricular cystic mass. (c) A retro-orbital mass (optic nerve coloboma) is noted (arrowheads) in the axial image through the orbits.

Encephaloclastic lesions

A number of conditions can lead to destruction of the fetal brain that in turn will develop into a congenital brain malformation. These conditions include maternal hypoxia, congenital infections, toxins, and pregnancies at risk of brain damage [29]. Examples of cerebrovascular causes of ischemia to the brain include cord accidents, twin-to-twin transfusion, embolic events, and cocaine exposure. During fetal neuroimaging, one usually observes the fetal responses to those injuries that are chronic in nature. A mild form of a chronic response may be slight ventriculomegaly with irregular ventricular wall, or nodular and irregular germinal matrix [29]. White-matter gliosis and ependymal abrasions are not visible on fetal MRI, but can be found on autopsy. A more severe response may result in parenchymal cystic cavities or hydranencephaly. Calcifications and malformation of the cortex are most likely seen in congenital infections, but can also be seen in antenatal hypoxic–ischemic injury.

Hydranencephaly

Hydranencephaly is considered to be an encephaloclastic lesion of the brain, in which most of the cortical plate and hemispheric white matter has been damaged or resorbed. The cerebral hemispheres are replaced by thin-walled sacs containing CSF (Fig. 22.8). Remnants of a thin cortical rim may be present. The thalami, brainstem, and cerebellum are usually relatively preserved [30]. The meninges are intact and the skull appears normal. The presence of the falx is important in distinguishing hydranencephaly from alobar holoprosencephaly.

Hydranencephaly develops as a result of an in utero destructive process of a brain that has been previously normally formed. The insult to the brain occurs at a time when the brain reacts by liquefaction necrosis (20th to 27th week) [31]. This insult could result from ischemia, hemorrhage, infection, or vasculopathies. Infectious causes such as toxoplasmosis, syphilis, mucormycosis, cytomegalovirus, and herpes simplex have been found in some cases. The vascular insult must occur within a relatively narrow window of time to produce hydranencephaly. Similar injuries after 27 weeks tend to cause multicystic encephalomalacia with astroglial reaction.

Since the injury occurs late in gestation, the infants can appear completely normal at birth. Transillumination of the head results in a striking positive sign. Newborns may develop epilepsy, extensor rigidity, and respiratory failure. The outcome is unfavorable, with global delays, but some children may live many years with these deficits.

Schizencephaly

Schizencephaly is a brain malformation that is characterized by infolding of the cortical gray matter along a hemispheric cleft near the primary cerebral fissures. The cleft traverses the full thickness of the hemisphere, connecting the ventricle to the subarachnoid space. The clefts are often bilateral. Schizencephalies are classified as closed-lip or separated-lip, depending on whether or not there is an open gap between the edges of the cleft (Fig. 22.9). Frequently the patients with schizencephaly have severe retardation and refractory epilepsy, language delay, and motor dysfunction.

Typically, schizencephaly is thought to be a sporadic occurrence, accompanying an insult to the brain, often following hypoperfusion or disruption of blood flow in the developing fetus, thought to occur before 26 weeks of gestation. Because of limited astroglial response in early fetal life, the necrotic tissue becomes reabsorbed and leaves fluid-filled cavities. Genetic factors are likely to play a role in some cases of schizencephaly. A small percentage of cases of schizencephaly occur in familial clusters [32]. Familial and sporadic cases of schizencephaly have been associated with mutations in the homeobox gene *EMX2* [33].

Porencephaly

Porencephaly is a term used for cavities within the cerebral hemispheres that communicate with the subarachnoid space (external porencephaly), the ventricle (internal porencephaly),

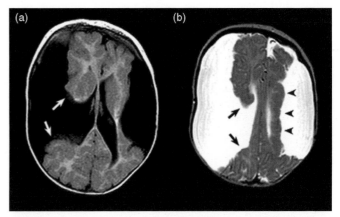

Fig. 22.9. (a) Axial fluid inversion recovery and (b) T2-weighted MR images obtained at 7 months of an infant who at birth had a hamartomatous umbilical cord mass containing multiple vessels. The cord mass is presumed to have caused hypoperfusion. The images show separated-lip schizencephaly in the right hemisphere with a cleft that is lined by gray matter (arrows). The cleft communicates with the right lateral ventricle. The cortex around the cleft appears dysplastic. In the left hemisphere, the cleft does not communicate with the lateral ventricle (b). The cortex lining the cleft appears polymicrogyric (arrowheads).

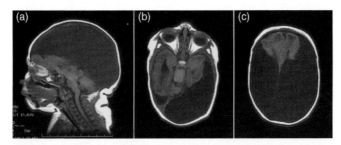

Fig. 22.8. T1-weighted MR images of 1-day-old newborn female with hydranencephaly and history of twin-to-twin transfusion syndrome. Mid-sagittal image shows that most of the cerebral hemispheres are replaced by a large CSF-containing sac. (a) There is preservation of brainstem, cerebellum, and inferior frontal lobes. The cranial vault is intact. (b) Low axial image shows relative preservation of the temporal lobes, with enlargement of the temporal horns. (c) High axial image shows preservation of part of the frontal lobes and presence of a falx.

neither (central porencephaly), or both. There is an overlap between porencephaly, hydranencephaly, and schizencephaly. At times porencephaly and schizencephaly can co-exist in the same brain. Porencephaly can be due to a developmental defect or acquired lesions, including in utero infarction of tissue. Injury occurring during late second trimester (24–26 weeks) leads to encephaloclastic porencephalies with smooth walls but lacking gray-matter-lined clefts. Injury during the third trimester is likely to result in encephalomalacia with shaggy-walled cavities and astroglial reaction [30]. Children with these lesions may have hemiparesis, focal seizures, or mental retardation.

Defects of midbrain and hindbrain organization and patterning
Dandy–Walker malformation

The classic Dandy–Walker malformation (DWM) includes three features: (1) cerebellar vermis agenesis (complete or partial), (2) cystic dilation of the posterior fossa communicating with the fourth ventricle, and (3) abnormally high tentorium with enlargement of the posterior fossa (Fig. 22.10) [34]. The mechanisms of DWM are poorly understood, but it is thought to occur due to a disturbance in development of the cerebellum and the opening of the fourth ventricle associated with the presence of a posterior fossa cyst. Pathologically, DWM is sometimes but not always associated with atresia of the foramina of Luschka or Magendie. The incidence is 1 in 25 000–30 000 births.

Children with DWM often have motor delay, hypotonia, and mental deficiency [34]. Clinical presentation also depends on the severity of the associated hydrocephalus and other brain malformations that occur in over half of the patients. These anomalies include microcephaly, encephalocele, syringomyelia, gyral malformation, and ACC. Total or partial absence of the corpus callosum is seen is 60%. They may also have a variety of extracerebral anomalies.

DWM may be seen in genetic disorders (e.g., Meckel syndrome), chromosomal disorders, or sporadic defects (e.g.,

holoprosencephaly). Other causal associations include environmental toxins (e.g., rubella, alcohol), or multifactorial etiology (e.g., congenital heart defect, neural tube defects). Some cases of DWM have been linked to heterozygous loss of ZIC1 and ZIC4 genes in individuals with a 3q2 deletion [35].

Cerebellar vermis hypoplasia (Dandy–Walker variant)

The Dandy–Walker variant consists of (1) variable hypoplasia of the cerebellar vermis and (2) absence of elevated tentorium and enlargement of the posterior fossa. The severity of the neurodevelopmental problems associated with the Dandy–Walker variant may be less severe than those of DWM, but outcome depends on the presence or absence of associated anomalies [36]. Mega-cisterna magna consists of a large cisterna magna without cerebellar abnormalities, and it seems to carry a more benign prognosis.

Joubert syndrome

Joubert syndrome (JS) is an autosomal recessive disorder characterized by the "molar tooth" malformation, which is a complex brainstem malformation of hypoplasia of the vermis, thickened and elongated superior cerebellar peduncles, and a deepened interpeduncular fossa that is apparent on axial MRI (Fig. 22.11) [37]. JS presents with neonatal hypotonia and neonatal tachypnea/apnea. As children get older they may have psychomotor retardation, ataxia, nystagmus, and oculomotor apraxia.

Molar tooth malformation has been reported in several distinct syndromes that are known collectively as JS-related disorders. The phenotype includes the neurological features of JS plus variable multiorgan involvement (primarily retinal dystrophy and nephronophthisis). To date, three genes have been identified in JS-related disorders, AHI1, NPHP1, and CEP290 [21]. The locus for classic JS phenotype of cerebellar and midbrain–hindbrain junction involvement is mapped to 9q34.3 (JBTS1) but the gene has not been cloned.

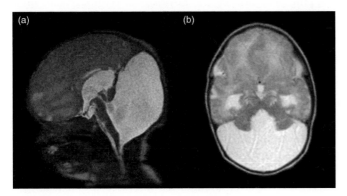

Fig. 22.10. (a) Mid-sagittal and (b) axial MR images of Dandy–Walker malformation with agenesis of the vermis, elevated tentorium, and enlargement of the posterior fossa with a fluid-filled cyst that communicates with the fourth ventricle. The brainstem also appears dysplatic and the anterior hemispheres are not separated, indicating co-existing holoprosencephaly.

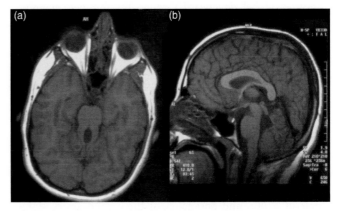

Fig. 22.11. Eighteen-year-old female with Joubert syndrome. (a) Axial T1-weighted MR image at the level of midbrain shows typical "molar tooth" anomaly of the midbrain and cerebellar peduncles. (b) Mid-sagittal T1-weighted image shows expansion of the fourth ventricle.

Hydrocephalus

Hydrocephalus has been defined in many ways, and clinicians are familiar with the terms *communicating* versus *non-communicating* (depending on whether the cerebrospinal fluid flow is contiguous from the ventricular system to the subarachnoid spaces). When cerebral hypoplasia or atrophy is present with enlarged ventricles, the term "hydrocephalus ex vacuo" is often used. When hydrocephalus results in ventricular enlargement there is centifugal atrophy of the white matter and thinning of the cortical mantle. In infancy clinical manifestations of hydrocephalus include macrocephaly, accelerated rate of head growth, bulging fontanel, separated cranial sutures, and downward deviation of eyes ("setting sun" sign). The infants may display irritability, lethargy, vomiting, and papilledema. After closure of sutures the intracranial pressure may increase rapidly.

Communicating hydrocephalus

In communicating hydrocephalus there is free communication between the cerebral ventricles and the lumbar subarachnoid space. The problem arises from impaired CSF reabsorption due to arachnoiditis or defective reabsorption into cerebral venous sinuses. Etiologies include earlier meningitis or other meningeal inflammation, meningeal infiltration, prior subarachnoid hemorrhage, intraventricular hemorrhage, and sino-venous thrombosis.

Non-communicating hydrocephalus

In non-communicating (obstructive) hydrocephalus there is a block in the flow of CSF within the ventricular system or at the exit foramina. CSF accumulates proximal to the block and causes dilation of the proximal ventricles. This type tends to produce higher intracranial pressure and a more acute clinical picture than communicating hydrocephalus.

Common causes of non-communicating hydrocephalus include aqueductal stenosis, congenital malformation, congenital infections (toxoplasmosis and cytomegalovirus), ependymitis, intraventricular hemorrhage, compression, Dandy–Walker malformation, Chiari II malformation (medulla and cerebellar tonsils displaced downward through the foramen magnum), and neoplasm or other mass obstructing the flow of CSF.

Genetic forms of hydrocephalus exist. The X-linked recessive form of inherited hydrocephalus is often accompanied by aqueductal stenosis; it results from mutations in the *L1CAM* gene [38]. Affected males demonstrate enlargement of the lateral and third ventricles.

Vascular malformations

Malformations involving blood vessels include arteriovenous malformations, malformations of the vein of Galen, hemangioblastoma of the cerebellum, congenital aneurysms of the circle of Willis, and anomalies of the carotid artery system. Of these the vein of Galen malformations are most likely to present in the newborn period. The other vascular malformations will not be discussed here.

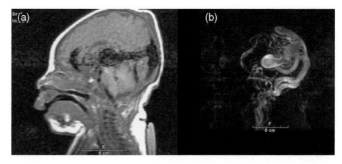

Fig. 22.12. One-day-old boy with vein of Galen malformation. (a) Sagittal T1-weighted MR image shows a dilated, round, Galenic varix communicating posteriorly through the falx to the venous sinuses. (b) 2D phase-contrast MR venogram shows the large midline Galenic varix and vein draining into dilated venous sinuses.

Vein of Galen malformations

In this malformation, the vein of Galen is dilated and branches of the posterior cerebral, superior cerebellar, and middle cerebral arteries communicate with it (Fig. 22.12). When the vein of Galen enlarges it can compress the quadrigeminal plate and aqueduct, causing hydrocephalus. Because of the arterial–venous shunting to the malformation, bypassing the capillary network, ischemic damage can occur to cerebral tissue.

In the neonatal period infants with cyanosis and respiratory distress who are in congestive heart failure can have blood abnormally shunted to the venous system by this malformation. This steal phenomenon may cause cerebral ischemia. Intracranial bruits, seizures, and intracranial hemorrhage may also be present. In contrast, those cases presenting during infancy usually have progressive hydrocephalus along with intracranial bruits and seizures. Upgaze paralysis is frequent, and proptosis may be found. Subarachnoid hemorrhage occurs in one-third of cases.

Cranial ultrasound with Doppler studies in the newborn period can be diagnostic. MRI with magnetic resonance angiogram and venogram will delineate the extent of the malformation. Prenatal detection with fetal ultrasound and MRI has also been reported. These are usually treated with endovascular techniques (embolization) by an interventional radiologist or clipping of feeders by a neurosurgeon. Hydrocephalus often requires ventriculoperitoneal shunting [39].

Diagnostic approaches

Modern fetal ultrasonography has facilitated the ability to detect a large variety of central nervous system malformations in utero. The widespread use of fetal ultrasonography makes it also more likely that severe malformations will be detected early (by 20 weeks of gestation) and that appropriate counseling can be given to the parents about the management of the pregnancy. In addition, when anomalies of the CNS are detected by fetal ultrasound, the increased use of fetal MRI to get better resolution has increased our ability to provide a more accurate diagnosis of the malformation [40,41]. Fetal MRI is becoming an increasingly important tool in diagnosis and management.

There are limitations to the resolution, however, even with fetal MRI. While it is relatively easy to detect overt anomalies, such as severe hydrocephalus, agenesis of corpus callosum, alobar or semilobar holoprosencephaly, anencephaly, and spina bifida, it is challenging at times to detect subtle lesions such as microdysgenesis, heterotopias, and gyral malformations. This is particularly true because the imaging is done on immature fetal brains, which are small, have poor gray–white matter signal contrast, and often have smooth-appearing cortical surfaces.

Neuroimaging studies after birth depend on the extent of prenatal imaging studies. If there were abnormalities detected in the CNS on fetal US or MRI, then another MRI after birth may be indicated. This is not always the case: for example, in a neonate who has had isolated ACC diagnosed prenatally with fetal MRI and who is otherwise doing well in the newborn period, postnatal MRI can be deferred. If there are neurologic symptoms and signs, it may be worthwhile repeating the MRI, since more subtle lesions that are associated with ACC may be easier to detect in a postnatal MRI. If the newborn has not had any prenatal studies, there are often other clinical indications as to why the neuroimaging study is being done. MRI is favored over CT because of its higher resolution, as well as its ability to scan in three orthogonal planes.

After a neuroanatomic diagnosis is made on the neuroimaging studies, it is important to determine if the child has a genetic syndrome. Careful investigation for extracerebral malformations should be undertaken as well as a genetic evaluation. Consultation with neurologists, geneticists, ophthalmologists, and other specialists should be considered. High-resolution chromosomes are also often carried out.

This chapter has highlighted several brain malformations, many of which have a genetic basis. With certain malformations, gene mutational analysis is appropriate. However, many of the malformations may be due to environmental causes. Thus it is important to ascertain a careful history of any complications during the pregnancy (drug exposure, infections, trauma, bleeding) and to try to correlate the timing of those events, if any, to the stage of embryonic/fetal brain development. A careful evaluation of the placenta and cord may also provide clues to in utero encephaloclastic lesions.

Providing prognostic evaluation prenatally can be quite challenging. This is in part due to the lower resolution of neuroimaging studies in fetuses. In addition, there is a paucity of long-term outcome studies in infants with many of the disorders that we detect in utero. The outcomes for many disorders, such as ACC, can be quite varied. Therefore, it is difficult to give a precise prognosis to expectant parents. After the birth, having postnatal MRI study information and clinical examination enables clinicians to provide a more specific diagnosis and precise prognosis.

References

1. Elwood JM, Little J, Elwood JH. *Epidemiology and Control of Neural Tube Defects.* Oxford: Oxford University Press, 1992.

2. Warkany J, Lemire RJ, Cohen MM. *Mental Retardation and Congenital Malformations of the Central Nervous System.* Chicago, IL: Yearbook, 1981.

3. Golden JA. Towards a greater understanding of the pathogenesis of holoprosencephaly. *Brain Dev* 1999; **21**: 513–21.

4. Matsunaga E, Shiota K. Holoprosencephaly in human embryos: epidemiologic studies of 150 cases. *Teratology* 1977; **16**: 261–72.

5. Cohen MM. Perspectives on holoprosencephaly: Part III. Spectra, distinctions, continuities, and discontinuities. *Am J Med Genet* 1989; **34**: 271–88.

6. Croen LA, Shaw GM, Lammer EJ. Holoprosencephaly: epidemiologic and clinical characteristics of a California population. *Am J Med Genet* 1996; **64**: 465–72.

7. Rasmussen SA, Moore CA, Khoury MJ, *et al.* Descriptive epidemiology of holoprosencephaly and arhinencephaly in metropolitan Atlanta, 1968–1992. *Am J Med Genet* 1996; **66**: 320–33.

8. Bullen PJ, Rankin JM, Robson SC. Investigation of the epidemiology and prenatal diagnosis of holoprosencephaly in the North of England. *Am J Obstet Gynecol* 2001; **184**: 1256–62.

9. Barkovich AJ, Quint DJ. Middle interhemispheric fusion: an unusual variant of holoprosencephaly. *AJNR Am J Neuroradiol* 1993; **14**: 431–40.

10. Simon EM, Hevner RF, Pinter JD, *et al.* The middle interhemispheric variant of holoprosencephaly. *AJNR Am J Neuroradiol* 2002; **23**: 151–5.

11. Plawner LL, Delgado MR, Miller VS, *et al.* Neuroanatomy of holoprosencephaly as predictor of function: beyond the face predicting the brain. *Neurology* 2002; **59**: 1058–66.

12. Barr M, Cohen MM. Holoprosencephaly survival and performance. *Am J Med Genet* 1999; **89**: 116–20.

13. Lewis AJ, Simon EM, Barkovich AJ, *et al.* Middle interhemispheric variant of holoprosencephaly: a distinct cliniconeuroradiologic subtype. *Neurology* 2002; **59**: 1860–5.

14. Taylor AI. Autosomal trisomy syndromes: a detailed study of 27 cases of Edwards' syndrome and 27 cases of Patau's syndrome. *J Med Genet* 1968; **5**: 227–52.

15. Olsen CL, Hughes JP, Youngblood LG, *et al.* Epidemiology of holoprosencephaly and phenotypic characteristics of affected children: New York State, 1984–1989. *Am J Med Genet* 1997; **73**: 217–26.

16. Ming JE, Muenke M. Multiple hits during early embryonic development: digenic diseases and holoprosencephaly. *Am J Hum Genet* 2002; **71**: 1017–32.

17. Roessler E, Belloni E, Gaudenz K, *et al.* Mutations in the human Sonic Hedgehog gene cause holoprosencephaly. *Nat Genet* 1996; **14**: 357–60.

18. Ming JE, Kaupas ME, Roessler E, *et al.* Mutations in PATCHED-1, the receptor for SONIC HEDGEHOG, are associated with holoprosencephaly. *Hum Genet* 2002; **110**: 297–301.

19. Barr M, Jr., Hanson JW, Currey K, *et al.* Holoprosencephaly in infants of diabetic mothers. *J Pediatr* 1983; **102**: 565–8.

20. Malinger G, Lev D, Kidron D, *et al.* Differential diagnosis in fetuses with absent septum pellucidum. *Ultrasound Obstet Gynecol* 2005; **25**: 42–9.

21. Carmichael J, Woods C. Genetic defects of human brain development. *Curr Neurol Neurosci Rep* 2006; **6**: 437–46.

22. Di Rocco C, Battaglia D, Pietrini D, *et al.* Hemimegalencephaly: clinical

implications and surgical treatment. *Childs Nerv Syst* 2006; **22**: 852–66.

23. Verity C, Firth H, ffrench-Constant C. Congenital abnormalities of the central nervous system. *J Neurol Neurosurg Psychiatry* 2003; **74**: i3–8.

24. Barkovich AJ, Kuzniecky RI, Jackson GD, *et al.* A developmental and genetic classification for malformations of cortical development. *Neurology* 2005; **65**: 1873–87.

25. Kerjan G, Gleeson JG. Genetic mechanisms underlying abnormal neuronal migration in classical lissencephaly. *Trends Genet* 2007; **23**: 623–30.

26. Glenn OA, Goldstein RB, Li KC, *et al.* Fetal magnetic resonance imaging in the evaluation of fetuses referred for sonographically suspected abnormalities of the corpus callosum. *J Ultrasound Med* 2005; **24**: 791–804.

27. Richards LJ, Plachez C, Ren T. Mechanisms regulating the development of the corpus callosum and its agenesis in mouse and human. *Clin Genet* 2004; **66**: 276–89.

28. Aicardi J. Aicardi syndrome. *Brain Dev* 2005; **27**: 164–71.

29. Girard N, Chaumoitre K, Confort-Gouny S, *et al.* Magnetic resonance imaging and the detection of fetal brain anomalies, injury, and physiologic adaptations. *Curr Opin Obstet Gynecol* 2006; **18**: 164–76.

30. Barkovich AJ. *Pediatric Neuroimaging.* 3rd edn. Philadelphia, PA: Lippincott Williams & Wilkins, 2000.

31. Volpe JJ. *Neurology of the Newborn*, 4th edn. Philadelphia, PA: Saunders, 2001.

32. Haverkamp F, Zerres K, Ostertun B, *et al.* Familial schizencephaly: further delineation of a rare disorder. *J Med Genet* 1995; **32**: 242–4.

33. Brunelli S, Faiella A, Capra V, *et al.* Germline mutations in the homeobox gene EMX2 in patients with severe schizencephaly. *Nat Genet* 1996; **12**: 94–6.

34. Adamsbaum C, Moutard ML, Andre C, *et al.* MRI of the fetal posterior fossa. *Pediatr Radiol* 2005; **35**: 124–40.

35. Grinberg I, Northrup H, Ardinger H, *et al.* Heterozygous deletion of the linked genes ZIC1 and ZIC4 is involved in Dandy–Walker malformation. *Nat Genet* 2004; **36**: 1053–5.

36. Ecker JL, Shipp TD, Bromley B, *et al.* The sonographic diagnosis of Dandy–Walker and Dandy–Walker variant: associated findings and outcomes. *Prenat Diagn* 2000; **20**: 328–32.

37. Louie CM, Gleeson JG. Genetic basis of Joubert syndrome and related disorders of cerebellar development. *Hum Mol Genet* 2005; **14**: R235–42.

38. Kanemura Y, Okamoto N, Sakamoto H, *et al.* Molecular mechanisms and neuroimaging criteria for severe L1 syndrome with X-linked hydrocephalus. *J Neurosurg* 2006; **105**: 403–12.

39. Alvarez H, Garcia Monaco R, Rodesch G, *et al.* Vein of Galen aneurysmal malformations. *Neuroimaging Clin N Am* 2007; **17**: 189–206.

40. Glenn OA, Barkovich AJ. Magnetic resonance imaging of the fetal brain and spine: an increasingly important tool in prenatal diagnosis, part 1. *AJNR Am J Neuroradiol* 2006; **27**: 1604–11.

41. Glenn OA, Barkovich J. Magnetic resonance imaging of the fetal brain and spine: an increasingly important tool in prenatal diagnosis: part 2. *AJNR Am J Neuroradiol* 2006; **27**: 1807–14.

Chapter 23

Neurogenetic disorders of the brain

Jonathan A. Bernstein and Louanne Hudgins

Introduction

A number of genetic disorders share clinical features with fetal and neonatal brain injury. Although these conditions are individually rare, collectively they should be expected encounters in the neonatal intensive care setting. This chapter aims to familiarize the reader with select inherited conditions that may clinically mimic neonatal brain injury. The majority of genetic conditions with clinical resemblance to neonatal brain injury discussed here present with hypotonia. Other syndromes can result in central nervous system hemorrhage, findings similar to congenital infection, hydrocephalus, and central hypoventilation.

Conditions included in this chapter do not ordinarily present with malformations or minor anomalies. Such conditions should be readily distinguishable from the sequelae of fetal and neonatal injury. Several inborn errors of metabolism have clinical findings similar to hypoxic–ischemic encephalopathy (HIE). These disorders are reviewed in Chapter 34.

The following discussion of inherited disorders with features similar to those of fetal and neonatal brain injury begins with an overview of the clinical genetics evaluation and its rationale. Subsequently, the chapter is organized by clinical presentation: hypotonia, apparent congenital infection, intracranial hemorrhage, hydrocephalus, and central hypoventilation. Information regarding clinical findings, diagnostic approach, and management is provided. A brief overview of management is also provided. References are included for additional reading.

The clinical genetics evaluation

The goal of the clinical genetics evaluation in the setting of suspected brain injury is to determine a specific diagnosis. Identifying the genetic etiology of a patient's condition enables the care team to better provide guidance regarding prognosis and recurrence risk. Additionally, a specific genetic diagnosis can have important implications for therapy.

In evaluating a patient for a genetic disorder the clinician should draw upon history, physical examination, clinical imaging, diagnostic procedures, and laboratory testing as indicated. Evaluating a case from a genetics perspective should additionally include review of family history in the form of a three-generation pedigree. This portion of the family history allows the identification of consanguinity as well as evidence of a specific mode of inheritance. Such information can significantly impact the differential diagnosis for a patient.

Determination of a diagnosis by molecular DNA studies is by its nature a greater part of genetic medicine than of other specialties. The *GeneTests* online resource available at www.genetests.org includes a database of laboratories able to perform the molecular and biochemical tests mentioned in this chapter and many others [1]. The accompanying *GeneReviews* site hosts regularly updated review articles on many of the conditions discussed in this chapter.

Conditions presenting with hypotonia
General approach

Low muscle tone in the newborn period can result from an inborn or acquired defect at any or multiple levels of the neuraxis from brain to spine to neuromuscular junction to muscle. Hypotonia as a manifestation of vascular accident, infection, or other acquired cause is addressed elsewhere in this volume. The diagnostic approach to the infant with a suspected genetic disorder can be stepwise or, alternatively, multiple investigations can be pursued in parallel. Efforts should be made to perform less invasive testing before undertaking procedures such as muscle or nerve biopsy, nerve conduction studies, or electromyogram, unless dictated otherwise by clinical decision-making or genetic-counseling imperatives.

Elements of the prenatal history relevant to the investigation of neonatal hypotonia include fetal movement, positioning, and amniotic fluid levels. History should also include first- and/or second-trimester biochemical and ultrasound screening as well as diagnostic testing by amniocentesis or chorionic villus sampling, if performed.

Physical exam findings helpful in the diagnosis of the hypotonic infant include involvement of facial musculature, presence and quality of deep tendon reflexes, as well as the presence or absence and location of contractures and flexion creases. Hypotonia with increased reflexes suggests cortical or upper motor neuron disease. Hypotonia accompanied by weakness or decreased reflexes is consistent with lower motor neuron or muscular disease. Congenital contractures or decreased evidence of flexion creases, which form by 11–12 weeks of

Fetal and Neonatal Brain Injury, 4th edition, ed. David K. Stevenson, William E. Benitz, Philip Sunshine, Susan R. Hintz, and Maurice L. Druzin. Published by Cambridge University Press. © Cambridge University Press 2009.

Table 23.1. Approach to neonatal hypotonia

	Condition	Characteristic clinical features	Inheritance	Initial diagnostics
Tier 1				
	Prader–Willi syndrome	Absence of respiratory distress, cryptorchidism in males	AD	Methylation studies or SNRPN expression assay
	Spinal muscular atrophy I	Tongue fasiculations, arreflexia	AR	PCR for recurrent deletion
	Myotonic dystrophy type 1	Positive maternal history	AD	PCR or Southern blot for trinucleotide repeat expansion
	MECP2-related encephalopathy	Poor head growth, central hypoventilation	XD	DNA sequencing
Tier 2				
	Pompe disease	Cardiomegaly, elevated CK	AR	Fibroblast enzyme assay
	Syndromic congenital muscular dystrophies	Structural brain anomalies, elevated CK, eye anomalies	AR	DNA sequencing or muscle biopsy
Tier 3				
	Congential myopathies	Often non-progressive	Varies	Muscle biopsy
	Non-syndromic congenital muscular dystrophies	Elevated CK	Varies	Muscle biopsy
	Congenital myasthenia	Fatiguability	Varies	Electromyography
	Congenital neuropathies	Arreflexia	Varies	Nerve conduction studies

Notes:
AD, autosomal dominant; AR, autosomal recessive; XD, X-linked dominant.

gestation, provide evidence of decreased movement in utero [2]. The presence of organomegaly should increase suspicion of storage disease.

Eye examination, preferably performed by a pediatric ophthalmologist, can be useful in examining for anterior chamber defects, cataracts and retinal anomalies. Radiologic evaluation should include ultrasound and preferably magnetic resonance imaging to define brain anatomy. Ideally, these studies should be reviewed by a pediatric neuroradiologist with experience in evaluating congenital malformations. Abnormalities of the central nervous system can be seen in several of the conditions described in this chapter, but specific brain malformation syndromes such as holoprosencephaly and neuronal migration defects are covered elsewhere in this volume.

Measurement of serum creatine kinase (CK) can be useful in identifying muscular disease. Laboratory screening for inborn errors of metabolism should also be considered in the evaluation of infantile hypotonia, as discussed in Chapter 34. Multiorgan dysfunction can be suggestive of metabolic disease. When sufficient clinical information has been gathered to narrow the differential diagnosis, molecular DNA studies or biochemical assays can be selected to confirm a diagnosis.

The following sections describe selected inherited conditions known to present in infancy with moderate to severe hypotonia. Conditions that can be diagnosed by less invasive methods are presented first, followed by those requiring more invasive testing such as muscle or nerve biopsy and nerve conduction studies or electromyogram. An overview of conditions presented can be found in Table 23.1. This table presents the disorders in three diagnostic tiers. Disorders in tier 1 can generally be diagnosed without invasive testing, disorders in tier 2 can sometimes be diagnosed without invasive testing, and disorders in tier 3 generally require biopsy or neurophysiologic studies.

Prader–Willi syndrome

Prader–Willi syndrome (PWS) is a genetically complex disorder resulting from loss of paternal gene expression from an imprinted region on chromosome 15q11. For recent review see Cassidy & Schwartz [3]. Incidence is estimated to be approximately 1 in 25 000 [4,5]. Although most commonly associated with the features of compulsive eating, obesity, and behavioral difficulties that develop in childhood, manifestations of PWS are frequently evident at birth. Newborns with PWS often feed poorly and are hypotonic; there can be a history of decreased movement prenatally. Neonatal respiratory distress is generally not observed as a result of PWS. Physical findings of PWS evident in the newborn period include characteristic facial features such as bitemporal narrowing, "almond-shaped" eyes, and downturned mouth. Cryptorchidism is almost universal among affected males.

A number of diagnostic studies can be pursued in the evaluation of suspected PWS. Currently, the most sensitive tests are DNA methylation studies and *SNRPN* expression. More than 99% of affected patients demonstrate an exclusively maternal methylation pattern at 15q11, which can arise by multiple mechanisms including chromosomal deletions, translocations, uniparental disomy, and imprinting center defects.

Management of infants with PWS requires an interdisciplinary approach and should be coordinated by a clinical geneticist or other practitioner familiar with the condition. In early infancy feeding difficulties are the most common management issue, and can necessitate gastrostomy tube placement. Detailed recommendations regarding the management of individuals with PWS have been published [6].

Spinal muscular atrophy (SMA I type)

Spinal muscular atrophy (SMA) is an autosomal recessive condition that can present at any time between the prenatal period and adulthood. For review see Monani [7] and Prior & Russman [8]. The overall incidence in the United States is estimated at approximately 1 in 10 000 births. SMA results from homozygous loss of function of the *SMN1* gene. Weakness develops due to the progressive loss of lower motor neurons. The prenatal form of disease features congenital contractures as the result of decreased movement in utero. SMA I presents between birth and 6 months of age, most commonly with hypotonia and weakness. Reflexes are generally absent or diminished, and tongue fasiculations are often present. Mild contractures are seen at the knees more commonly than at the elbows. In severe cases difficulty with feeding and respiration will develop.

Molecular diagnosis of SMA includes PCR or Southern blot studies of the *SMN1* gene to detect a recurrent intragenic deletion responsible for approximately 95% of cases. *SMN1* sequencing is also available on a clinical basis and is useful when the diagnosis of SMA is suspected but a deletion is found on only one allele.

Predicted life expectancy for infants diagnosed with SMA I is less than 2 years. However, long-term survival has been observed and is much more common when assisted ventilation is elected. Management in the newborn period is interdisciplinary and focuses on feeding and respiration.

Myotonic dystrophy type 1

Myotonic dystrophy type 1 is an autosomal dominant condition resulting from trinucleotide expansion within the *DM1* gene. For review see Scriver [9] and Bird [10]. It most commonly presents in adulthood, with myotonia and weakness of distal leg muscles. The adult-onset form of disease is associated with between 100 and 1000 repeats in *DM1* (the normal allele contains between 5 and 34 repeats). Congenital myotonic dystrophy has been observed in infants with especially large intragenic expansions. The incidence of myotonic dystrophy varies widely according to the population studied; 1 in 8000 is a frequently cited estimate [11]. Features of congenital myotonic dystrophy include hypotonia, clubfeet, and respiratory insufficiency. Facial muscles are affected, which results in a tented appearance to the upper lip. MRI findings including cortical atrophy and ventriculomegaly can mimic HIE. Subcortical white-matter lesions can also be seen [12]. The majority of infants with congenital myotonic dystrophy type 1 experience developmental delay/intellectual disability, in contrast to later-onset forms of the disease. There is an increased risk of cardiac conduction defects in all forms of myotonic dystrophy.

Trinucleotide repeats in *DM1* are known to expand in succeeding generations. For reasons that are incompletely understood, expansions within *DM1* more commonly enlarge in the maternal germline. As the expansions in congenital myotonic dystrophy are large, mothers of congenitally affected infants often manifest the condition. Maternal symptomatology can be mild, and it includes myopathic facies, cataracts, and myotonia.

Molecular diagnosis of myotonic dystrophy is widely available on a clinical basis. Polymerase chain reaction or Southern blot methods are used to determine *DM1* allele size, and these are predicted to detect all cases. Serum CK may be mildly elevated in myotonic dystrophy. Electromyogram is less useful in demonstrating electrical myotonia in infants than in older patients. Muscle biopsy may demonstrate characteristic changes, but molecular diagnosis is preferable as it is less invasive and more sensitive and specific.

Management of infants with myotonic dystrophy is supportive. An interdisciplinary approach is recommended to maximize developmental progress and overall health status. Notably, patients with neonatal presentation can demonstrate significant improvement in motor function during childhood. However, they remain at risk for longer-term complications.

MECP2-related congenital encephalopathy

The *MECP2* gene encoding methyl CpG binding protein 2 is known for its causative role in Rett syndrome, an X-linked progressive developmental disorder affecting girls. For many years Rett syndrome was felt to be lethal in males, as it was diagnosed exclusively in females. However, in recent years the availability of molecular testing facilitated recognition that loss of *MECP2* function in males can result in a severe congenital encephalopathy [13]. To date, 17 infants have been reported with this condition [14]. The diagnosis was considered in the majority of patients identified to date because they were siblings of girls with Rett syndrome. Therefore the condition may be significantly under-recognized.

The diagnosis of *MECP2*-related congenital encephalopathy should be considered in male infants with severe neurologic impairment. In this condition, hypotonia is frequently noted in the first days of life, although it may not be as prominent as in other conditions described in this chapter. Other recurring features of this congenital encephalopathy are microcephaly or poor head growth, difficulty with suck and swallow, gastroesophageal reflux, and episodic apnea or central hypoventilation. With time, seizures and movement disorders often become evident.

DNA sequence analysis of *MECP2* is clinically available in several laboratories and is the only means of definitively diagnosing a related congenital encephalopathy. Electroencephalogram demonstrating generalized slowing or seizure activity may be supportive of the diagnosis. Apparent brain atrophy has been observed on magnetic resonance imaging in a minority of cases.

Management of infants with congenital encephalopathy is supportive. The condition is associated with profound developmental delay and a severely shortened lifespan. Diagnosis of the condition can be beneficial for both prognosis and estimation of recurrence risk.

Pompe disease (infantile type)

Pompe disease is an autosomal recessive glycogen storage condition resulting from deficiency of the enzyme acid α-glucosidase. For review see Tinkle and Leslie [15]. Most commonly it manifests with weakness and cardiomyopathy. The age at presentation can range from the prenatal period to adulthood. Overall incidence in the United States is estimated at approximately 1 in 40 000 births [16]. As evident in a recently reported large case series [17], the infantile form of Pompe disease classically presents in the first months of life with delayed motor development secondary to weakness and cardiomyopathy. However, symptoms may be evident at birth. Classically, the cardiac silhouette is enlarged on chest x-ray, and a shortened PR interval is seen on electrocardiogram. Moderate elevation of serum CK is a common feature of infantile Pompe disease.

The diagnostic standard for Pompe disease is assay of acid α-glucosidase performed on cultured fibroblasts. A leukocyte enzyme activity is also available, but may be less sensitive and specific. Sequencing of the *GAA* gene encoding acid α-glucosidase is available clinically; sensitivity varies, based on a patient's ethnic background. The diagnosis can also be suggested by muscle biopsy demonstrating lysosomal glycogen accumulation.

The management of Pompe disease has changed dramatically in recent years with the development of enzyme replacement therapy (ERT). ERT currently requires weekly infusions. Response to therapy is variable, but can be dramatic in some cases. In some patients the duration of response to therapy is limited by the development of neutralizing antibodies. Guidelines for the management of Pompe disease were recently published [18]. Interdisciplinary care includes attention to nutrition and feeding, cardiac disease, and motor development.

Congenital myopathies

Congenital disorders of muscle are referred to as myopathies when there appears to be a primary defect in muscle fiber assembly. The term dystrophy refers to the degeneration of existing muscle fibers due to an intrinsic defect. As these conditions are increasingly understood on a molecular basis, the distinction between myopathy and dystrophy is sometimes blurred. In recent years several conditions historically recognized as myopathies or dystrophies have been found to be allelic. This section provides an overview of the congenital myopathies. Congenital muscular dystrophies are addressed in the next section.

A large clinically, histopathologically, and genetically diverse group of disorders is collectively referred to as the congenital myopathies. For recent review see Goebel [19]. These disorders can demonstrate autosomal dominant, recessive, and X-linked inheritance. Major histopathologic categories include nemaline myopathy, central core disease, and myotubular myopathy. The neonatal presentation of congenital myopathies can feature hypotonia, decreased or absent reflexes, contractures, and respiratory insufficiency. Facial muscles are generally affected. There can be a history of decreased movement in utero. Although symptoms can be severe, they are generally non-progressive. Cardiomyopathy can occur in the congenital myopathies.

In contrast to the congenital muscular dystrophies, it is unusual to detect significant elevation of serum CK in a congenital myopathy. Muscle biopsy is the primary method for diagnosis. The pathologic findings in a congenital myopathy may not be evident on routine light-microscopic examination. Therefore it is recommended that investigation of this family of disorders be pursued with the assistance of a pathologist with special expertise in the area. This collaboration should ideally begin prior to biopsy to be sure appropriate tissue is obtained for evaluation. Although diagnostic, histopathologic categorization of a congenital myopathy is not always predictive of its underlying genetic defect or prognosis.

Among the congenital myopathies that may present in the newborn period, X-linked myotublar myopathy has several features that may aid in diagnosis. By nature of its inheritance this condition affects male infants. A family history of affected maternal male relatives is present in approximately one-third of cases. Affected infants tend to be relatively long and macrocephalic for gestational age. Long fingers and toes, as well as cryptorchidism, may also be noted. DNA analysis of the *MTM1* gene is available clinically. Causative mutations are identified in 60–90% of cases. Molecular testing is more likely to be positive in more severe disease.

Specific therapy is not currently available for the congenital myopathies. Therefore treatment is supportive.

Congenital muscular dystrophies

The congenital muscular dystrophies (CMD) are a genetically diverse group of conditions that characteristically present at birth with elevation of serum CK due to muscle breakdown and associated weakness and hypotonia. For recent reviews see Gordon *et al.* [20] and Mendell *et al.* [21]. With rare exceptions they are inherited in an autosomal recessive manner. Estimates of the combined incidence of all forms of congenital muscular dystrophy are imprecise, but are reported as approximately 1 in 20 000 [22].

Syndromic and non-syndromic forms of CMD are recognized. In syndromic disease (e.g., Walker–Warburg syndrome, Fukuyama CMD, muscle–eye–brain disease), there are characteristically anomalies of brain and eye development in addition to muscular pathology. Eye anomalies in syndromic CMD include anterior chamber defects such as Peters anomaly, cataracts, and retinal degeneration. The characteristic brain appearance in syndromic congenital muscular dystrophies is "cobblestone lissencephaly." Significant cognitive and motor developmental impairment is associated with the syndromic CMD, although the degree of disability varies widely between the disorders in this group.

In general the cognitive difficulties seen in syndromic CMD are not present in non-syndromic forms. However, brain malformations and developmental delay have been observed, highlighting limitations of the current nomenclature. As in syndromic CMD, motor function can be severely impacted in non-syndromic disease. Consequently, complications of disease include contractures and respiratory insufficiency. Creatine kinase is not consistently elevated in some forms of non-syndromic CMD.

Ophthalmologic evaluation and head imaging are potentially useful in the evaluation of any infant with an undiagnosed neuromuscular condition. They are specifically indicated in the evaluation of suspected CMD, in order to distinguish syndromic from non-syndromic forms.

Molecular DNA diagnosis for syndromic and some forms of non-syndromic CMD is available on a clinical basis. As the eye findings and brain malformations of syndromic disease are distinctive, selection of genes for DNA analysis is more straightforward in these conditions. Although non-syndromic disease can be highly suspected on the basis of hypotonia, weakness, and elevated CK, muscle biopsy is generally necessary to define the subtype of disease.

The management of patients with CMD is supportive, as specific therapy is not available.

Congenital neuropathies

Congenital neuropathies presenting in the newborn period represent the severest manifestations of hereditary nerve dysfunction. They have been reported only rarely. Congenital neuropathies presenting in the neonatal period are characterized by extremely slow conduction. Clinical manifestations include hypotonia, arreflexia, ptosis, difficulty with suck and swallow, and respiratory insufficiency. Increased CSF protein has been noted in a minority of cases. Although controversy exists in the literature regarding the appropriate nomenclature for these conditions they are frequently referred to as Dejerine–Sottas syndrome (DSS) [23]. Both autosomal dominant and autosomal recessive inheritance of this phenotype has been described.

Dominant mutations in a number of genes, including *PMP22*, *MPZ*, and *PRX*, have been reported to result in the DSS phenotype. Dominant and recessive mutations in *EGR2* have also been observed. Some authors distinguish DSS from congenital hypomyelinating neuropathy (CHN) on the basis of histologic features seen on nerve biopsy. However, as findings historically described as DSS or CHN can result from allelic mutations, the distinction is not consistently observed.

DNA analysis of *PMP22*, *MPZ*, *PRX*, and *EGR2* is available on a clinical basis. However, based on reported case series, the yield of DNA sequencing in cases demonstrating neonatal onset appears low [24]. Presently, the diagnosis of a congenital neuropathy is best established by nerve conduction studies and biopsy.

Congenital myasthenia

Congenital myasthenia can result from inherited defects in a number of components of the neuromuscular junction. Most commonly autosomal recessive inheritance is observed, although dominant forms have been documented. This family of conditions most commonly presents in the first year of life, although prenatal and neonatal onset has been described. For recent reviews see Abicht & Lochmüller [25] and Harper [26]. Collectively, the congenital myasthenias are very rare, but estimates of incidence are uncertain. As is the case for many of the disorders covered in this section, prenatal onset of symptoms can lead to presentation with arthrogryposis rather than hypotonia or weakness. Clinical features that may be useful in distinguishing myasthenia from other neuromuscular conditions include fatigability and eyelid ptosis. Additionally, congenital myasthenias often worsen with fever or infection.

The clinical symptoms of congenital myasthenia are very similar to those of myasthenia gravis and seronegative myasthenia gravis; however, these conditions have not been observed in the first year of life. Transient neonatal myasthenia as the result of placental transfer of maternal antibody may closely mimic congenital myasthenia, but should be distinguishable by the presence of antibodies in maternal or infant serum.

Electromyography can be useful in establishing the diagnosis of myasthenia. Repeated muscle stimulation demonstrates a characteristically decreasing response over time. Presently, molecular DNA diagnostics are available on a clinical basis for the evaluation of seven components of the neuromuscular junction. Mutations in the *CHRNE* gene are responsible for approximately 60% of cases in persons of Caucasian descent. However, prenatal and neonatal presentation has been observed more commonly with mutations in *RAPSN* and *CHAT* [25].

Therapy for infants with congenital myasthenia should be directed by or in consultation with a pediatric neurologist familiar with these conditions. In many cases pharmacologic therapy with acetylcholinesterase inhibitors or other agents can be helpful. However, in other cases symptoms may be unchanged or worsen with treatment. Identification of the causative mutation(s) may aid in the choice of therapeutic agents. As respiratory status can deteriorate acutely in congenital myasthenia, apnea monitors and CPR training of caretakers may be indicated. As symptoms can worsen during acute illness, patients should be managed closely during such periods.

Apparent TORCH infection

Congenital infection with a TORCH agent (toxoplasmosis, rubella, cytomegalovirus, herpes simplex virus, and others) is often considered in the evaluation of the ill-appearing newborn. These infections are discussed in detail in Chapter 32. A group of genetic disorders collectively referred to as Aicardi–Goutières syndrome can mimic several features of these conditions, particularly thrombocytopenia, hepatitis, intracranial calcifications, chorioretinitis, and meningoencephalitis.

Aicardi–Goutières syndrome

Aicardi–Goutières syndrome (AGS) is an autosomal recessive condition that can clinically resemble toxoplasmosis and cytomegalovirus (CMV) infection. For recent review see Aicardi & Crow [27] and Rice *et al.* [28]. AGS is a very rare but likely underdiagnosed condition. Less than 100 cases have been published. Mutations in at least four genes *TREX1*, *RNASEH2A*, *RNASEH2B*, and *RNASEH2C*, can result in the AGS phenotype, which includes basal ganglia calcifications, leukodystrophy, recurrent fevers, and a chronic cerebrospinal fluid lymphocytosis. Neurologic findings include hypotonia, dystonia, and occasionally seizures. Vasculitic skin lesions with associated swelling of the fingers and toes are less frequently observed. The majority of cases of AGS present with developmental delay and/or loss of previously acquired milestones, abnormal neurologic findings, and recurrent fevers after several months of normal development. However, central nervous system calcifications have been observed prenatally, as have microcephaly and intrauterine growth restriction at birth, and neurologic findings in the first week of life. Therefore, the diagnosis of AGS should be considered when evidence of congenital infection is present but diagnostic studies are negative.

Molecular DNA testing has recently become available on a clinical basis for AGS, including sequencing of *TREX1*, *RNASEH2A*, *RNASEH2B*, and *RNASEH2C*. *TREX1* mutations are responsible for the majority of cases reported to date. In addition to CSF lymphocytosis, mentioned above, elevated interferon α levels are supportive of the diagnosis of AGS. It is important to rule out prenatal infections such as CMV, toxoplasmosis, rubella, and herpes simplex virus (HSV), as well as other genetic conditions which can result in leukodystrophy, in evaluating for AGS.

The outcome of AGS diagnosed in early infancy is severe. Treatment is supportive.

Bleeding

The primary considerations in the evaluation of unexplained bleeding in the newborn are infectious and hematologic disorders. Although frequently genetic in origin, disorders of platelet function and the coagulation cascade are outside the scope of this chapter. Glutaric acidemia, discussed elsewhere in this volume, is rarely symptomatic in the newborn period. However, it can predispose to subdural hemorrhage due to macrocephaly and extra-axial hydrocephalus. Bleeding in early infancy has also been described in congenital disorders of glycosylation [29].

Hereditary hemorrhagic telangiectasia

Hereditary hemorrhagic telangiectasia (HHT) is an autosomal dominant condition featuring multiple arteriovenous malformations (AVMs). For recent review see Guttmacher & McDonald [30]. Estimated incidence has been reported as approximately 1 in 10 000 [31]. Although the condition most commonly presents in mid-childhood or adulthood, with recurrent epistaxis and multiple mucocutaneous telangiectasias, presentation in the newborn with catastrophic central nervous system bleeding is documented [32]. HHT is known

to result from mutations in *endoglin* and *ACVRL1*. A third locus is under investigation. In the vast majority of cases HHT is inherited from a parent, and therefore assessment of family history is important in determining this diagnosis in an infant. Minimally affected parents may only report a history of epistaxis after specific questioning.

Clinical criteria for the diagnosis of HHT have been published [33]. In older children and adults the diagnosis should be considered in the presence of recurrent epistaxis associated with mucocutaneous telangiectasias or arteriovenous malformations. DNA sequencing of *endoglin* and *ACVRL1* is available on a clinical basis. Mutations in one of these two genes can be identified in 60–80% of cases.

Detailed age-specific protocols for the identification, monitoring, and management of AVMs in patients with HHT have been developed [30,34]. Components of the initial evaluation of the newly diagnosed infant include pulse oximetry, head MRI, and hepatic ultrasound to screen for AVMs.

Hydrocephalus

Hydrocephalus and ventriculomegaly are frequently encountered in the neonatal intensive care setting. Hydrocephalus can result from excessive CSF production, obstruction of CSF flow, or decreased CSF absorption. Frequently recognized causes include intraventricular bleeds, hypoxic injury, and congenital brain malformations. As discussed below, hydrocephalus can also result from metabolic disease and mutations in the X-linked gene *L1CAM*.

Cobalamin disorders and MTHFR deficiency

Hydrocephalus and ventriculomegaly have also been reported in a number of inborn errors of metabolism involving vitamin B_{12} and folate metabolism: cblC disease, cblD disease, and homozygous methylene tetrahydrofolate reductase (MTHFR) deficiency [35,36]. Preliminary screening for these conditions can be accomplished by measurement of a total plasma homocysteine level. They are currently included in the list of disorders evaluated for in some, but not all, tandem mass-spectrometry-based newborn screening programs in the United States.

X-linked hydrocephalus with stenosis of the aqueduct of Sylvius (HSAS)

An X-linked recessive form of inherited hydrocephalus, often accompanied by aqueductal stenosis, results from mutations in the *L1CAM* gene. Affected males characteristically demonstrate enlargement of the lateral and third ventricles. Approximately one-half of affected males demonstrate persistently adducted thumbs. Other frequent features include spasticity and severe developmental disability. Notably, hydrocephalus can occur without aqueductal stenosis. In recent years it has been recognized that HSAS is one of several phenotypes resulting from *L1CAM* mutations. Collectively, they are referred to as L1 syndrome. For review see Schrander-Stumpel *et al.* [37]. In some individuals only spastic paraplegia and mild developmental difficulties are observed. The incidence of

HSAS has been estimated at approximately 1 in 30 000 births [38]. *L1CAM* mutations are believed to explain up to 10% of cases of non-syndromic hydrocephalus in males.

The diagnosis of HSAS has traditionally been based on clinical findings, including family history of affected male maternal relatives, hydrocephalus, adducted thumbs, and spasticity. The finding on MRI of absent pyramids is felt to be highly specific for HSAS and other forms of L1 syndrome [39]. *L1CAM* DNA sequencing and deletion/duplication analysis is available in several laboratories on a clinical basis. However, the sensitivity of molecular testing has not been precisely determined.

Management of L1 syndrome is symptomatic. Recommended participants in the care team include pediatrician, neurologist, neurosurgeon, developmental specialist, and geneticist.

Central hypoventilation

Hypoventilation and apnea are frequently encountered in hospitalized infants. Recognized causes include prematurity, infection, and neuromuscular disease. In the absence of another recognizable cause persistent hypoventilation, especially during sleep, should raise the possibility of congenital central hypoventilation syndrome. As noted above, central hypoventilation has also been reported in *MECP2*-related congenital encephalopathy.

Congenital central hypoventilation syndrome

Congenital central hypoventilation syndrome (CCHS) is an autosomal dominant condition resulting from disruption of the *PHOX2B* gene. For review see Weese-Mayer *et al.* [40]. The majority of CCHS cases occur as the result of trinucleotide expansion within *PHOX2B* leading to polyalanine repeats. Precise estimates of incidence are not available, but several cases are diagnosed each month in the United States [40]. Infants with CCHS typically maintain adequate ventilation while awake, but hypoventilate when asleep despite a normal respiratory rate. In severely affected infants hypoventilation can occur during wakefulness. At the other end of the spectrum, a number of individuals have been diagnosed later in childhood or adulthood with milder hypoventilation. CCHS is believed to be the result of autonomic nervous system dysfunction, as abnormal regulation of heart rate and blood pressure has been observed in affected individuals. CCHS has also been described as a disorder of neural crest development, as Hirschsprung's disease, and tumors of neural crest origin are seen with increased frequency. Mild facial dysmorphism has also been reported in individuals with CCHS [41]. Affected individuals have been found to have relatively broad and flat facies.

PCR-based molecular testing for *PHOX2B* expansions is clinically available and is diagnostic in over 90% of cases. Other *PHOX2B* mutations have been found in the remainder of confirmed cases [42]. Sequence variants in a number of other genes have been reported in patients with features of CCHS, but the role of other genes in this condition is currently debated.

The primary focus of treatment in CCHS is the provision of adequate respiratory support to avoid hypoventilation. Thorough cardiac evaluation is also recommended for children diagnosed with CCHS. Individuals with large polyalanine repeats or mutations not involving trinucleotide expansion are at greater risk of neural-crest-derived tumors such as neuroblastoma [43]. Screening for this condition is recommended in this population. Trinucleotide expansion length of 27 or greater repeats, and mutations not involving expansions, also confer an increased risk of Hirschsprung's disease; therefore screening is recommended in these cases [42].

Conclusion

The possibility of a genetic etiology to the apparent sequelae of fetal and neonatal brain injury should be kept in mind when evaluating the infant presenting with hypotonia, congenital infection, intracranial hemorrhage, hydrocephalus, and central hypoventilation. More common causes of these signs and symptoms can be difficult to distinguish from rarer hereditary etiologies. Obtaining a detailed family history is essential in evaluating the newborn for the possibility of a genetic disorder. In cases where a specific genetic diagnosis is not determined, but continues to be suspected, follow-up evaluation with a clinical geneticist is worthwhile. This provides the best chance of ultimately identifying a diagnosis with potentially significant impact on medical management and estimates of recurrence risk. Prenatal genetic counseling should be routinely recommended to the families of children with significant congenital illness of unclear origin as well as those of known genetic cause.

References

1. GeneTests: Medical Genetics Information Resource. 1993–2008. www.genetests.org. Accessed February 1, 2008.

2. Jones KL, Smith DW. *Smith's Recognizable Patterns of Human Malformation*, 6th edn. Philadelphia, PA: Elsevier Saunders, 2006.

3. Cassidy SB, Schwartz S. Prader–Willi syndrome. *GeneReviews* 2008. www.ncbi.nlm.nih.gov/bookshelf/br.fcgi?book=gene&part=pws. Accessed October, 2008.

4. Smith A, Egan J, Ridley G, *et al.* Birth prevalence of Prader–Willi syndrome in Australia. *Arch Dis Child* 2003; **88**: 263–4.

5. Vogels A, Van Den Ende J, Keymolen K, *et al.* Minimum prevalence, birth incidence and cause of death for Prader–Willi syndrome in Flanders. *Eur J Hum Genet* 2004; **12**: 238–40.

6. Cassidy SB, McCandless SE. Prader–Willi syndrome. In Cassidy SB, Allanson JE, eds., *Management of Genetic Syndromes*, 2nd edn. Hoboken, NJ: Wiley-Liss, 2005: 429–448.

7. Monani UR. Spinal muscular atrophy: a deficiency in a ubiquitous protein; a motor neuron-specific disease. *Neuron* 2005; **48**: 885–96.

8. Prior TW, Russman BS. Spinal muscular atrophy. *GeneReviews* 2006.

www.ncbi.nlm.nih.gov/bookshelf/br.
fcgi?book=gene&partid=1352. Accessed
February, 2008.

9. Scriver CR. *The Metabolic and Molecular
Bases of Inherited Disease*, 8th edn.
New York, NY: McGraw-Hill, 2001.

10. Bird TD. Myotonic dystrophy type 1.
GeneReviews 2007. www.ncbi.nlm.nih.
gov/bookshelf/br.fcgi?book=gene&
partid=1165#myotonic-d. Accessed
February, 2008.

11. Harper PS. *Myotonic Dystrophy*, 2nd
edn. Philadelphia, PA: Saunders, 1989.

12. Bachmann G, Damian MS, Koch M,
et al. The clinical and genetic correlates
of MRI findings in myotonic dystrophy.
Neuroradiology 1996; **38**: 629–35.

13. Wan M, Lee SS, Zhang X, *et al.* Rett
syndrome and beyond: recurrent
spontaneous and familial MECP2
mutations at CpG hotspots. *Am J Hum
Genet* 1999; **65**: 1520–9.

14. Schule B, Armstrong D, Vogel H, *et al.*
Severe congenital encephalopathy
caused by MECP2 null mutations in
males: central hypoxia and reduced
neuronal dendritic structures. *Clin Genet*
2008; **74**: 116–26.

15. Tinkle BT, Leslie N. Glycogen storage
disease type II (Pompe disease).
GeneReviews 2007. www.ncbi.nlm.nih.
gov/bookshelf/br.fcgi?book=gene&
partid=1261#gsd2. Accessed February,
2008.

16. Martiniuk F, Chen A, Mack A, *et al.*
Carrier frequency for glycogen storage
disease type II in New York and estimates
of affected individuals born with the
disease. *Am J Med Genet* 1998; **79**: 69–72.

17. Kishnani PS, Hwu WL, Mandel H, *et al.*
A retrospective, multinational,
multicenter study on the natural history
of infantile-onset Pompe disease.
J Pediatrics 2006; **148**: 671–6.

18. Kishnani PS, Steiner RD, Bali D,
et al. Pompe disease diagnosis and
management guideline. *Genet Med*
2006; **8**: 267–88.

19. Goebel HH. Congenital myopathies
in the new millennium. *J Child Neurol*
2005; **20**: 94–101.

20. Gordon E, Hoffman EP, Pegoraro E.
Congenital muscular dystrophy
overview, *GeneReviews* 2006. www.ncbi.
nlm.nih.gov/bookshelf/br.fcgi?book=
gene&partid=1291#cmd-overview.
Accessed February, 2008.

21. Mendell JR, Boue DR, Martin PT. The
congenital muscular dystrophies: recent
advances and molecular insights.
Pediatr Dev Pathol 2006; **9**: 427–43.

22. Mostacciuolo ML, Miorin M, Martinello
F, *et al.* Genetic epidemiology of
congenital muscular dystrophy in a
sample from north-east Italy. *Hum
Genet* 1996; **97**: 277–9.

23. Plante-Bordeneuve V, Said G. Dejerine–
Sottas disease and hereditary
demyelinating polyneuropathy of
infancy. *Muscle Nerve* 2002; **26**: 608–21.

24. Plante-Bordeneuve V, Parman Y,
Guiochon-Mantel A, *et al.* The range of
chronic demyelinating neuropathy of
infancy: a clinico-pathological and
genetic study of 15 unrelated cases.
J Neurol 2001; **248**: 795–803.

25. Abicht A, Lochmüller H. Congenital
myasthenic syndromes. *GeneReviews*
2006. www.ncbi.nlm.nih.gov/bookshelf/
br.fcgi?book=gene&partid=1168#cms.
Accessed February, 2008.

26. Harper CM. Congenital myasthenic
syndromes. *Semin Neurol* 2004; **24**: 111–23.

27. Aicardi J, Crow YJ. Aicardi–Goutières
syndrome. *GeneReviews* 2005.
www.ncbi.nlm.nih.gov/bookshelf/br.
fcgi?book=gene&partid=1475#ags.
Accessed February, 2008.

28. Rice G, Patrick T, Parmar R, *et al.*
Clinical and molecular phenotype of
Aicardi–Goutières syndrome. *Am J Hum
Genet* 2007; **81**: 713–25.

29. Cohn RD, Eklund E, Bergner AL, *et al.*
Intracranial hemorrhage as the initial
manifestation of a congenital disorder
of glycosylation. *Pediatrics* 2006; **118**:
e514–21.

30. Guttmacher AE, McDonald J.
Hereditary hemorrhagic telangiectasia.
GeneReviews 2005. www.ncbi.nlm.nih.
gov/bookshelf/br.fcgi?book=gene&
partid=1351#hht. Accessed February,
2008.

31. Marchuk DA, Guttmacher AE, Penner
JA, *et al.* Report on the workshop on
Hereditary Hemorrhagic Telangiectasia,
July 10–11, 1997. *Am J Med Genet* 1998;
76: 269–73.

32. Morgan T, McDonald J, Anderson C,
et al. Intracranial hemorrhage in
infants and children with hereditary
hemorrhagic telangiectasia (Osler–
Weber–Rendu syndrome). *Pediatrics*
2002; **109**: E12.

33. Shovlin CL, Guttmacher AE, Buscarini
E, *et al.* Diagnostic criteria for hereditary
hemorrhagic telangiectasia (Rendu–
Osler–Weber syndrome). *Am J Med
Genet* 2000; **91**: 66–7.

34. Porteous ME, Berg JN. Hereditary
hemorrhagic telangiectasia. In Cassidy SB,
Allanson JE, eds., *Management of
Genetic Syndromes*, 2nd edn. Hoboken,
NJ: Wiley-Liss, 2005: 279–90.

35. Longo D, Fariello G, Dionisi-Vici C,
et al. MRI and 1H-MRS findings in
early-onset cobalamin C/D defect.
Neuropediatrics 2005; **36**: 366–72.

36. Baethmann M, Wendel U,
Hoffmann GF, *et al.* Hydrocephalus
internus in two patients with 5,10-
methylenetetrahydrofolate reductase
deficiency. *Neuropediatrics* 2000; **31**:
314–17.

37. Schrander-Stumpel C, Vos YJ. L1
Syndrome. *GeneReviews* 2006. www.
ncbi.nlm.nih.gov/bookshelf/br.fcgi?
book=gene&partid=1484#l1cam.
Accessed February, 2008.

38. Halliday J, Chow CW, Wallace D, *et al.*
X linked hydrocephalus: a survey of
a 20 year period in Victoria, Australia.
J Med Genet 1986; **23**: 23–31.

39. Chow CW, Halliday JL, Anderson RM,
et al. Congenital absence of pyramids
and its significance in genetic
diseases. *Acta Neuropathol* 1985;
65: 313–17.

40. Weese-Mayer DE, Marazita ML,
Berry-Kravis EM. Congenital central
hypoventilation syndrome. *GeneReviews*
2007. www.ncbi.nlm.nih.gov/bookshelf/
br.fcgi?book=gene&partid=1427#ondine.
Accessed February, 2008.

41. Todd ES, Weinberg SM, Berry-Kravis
EM, *et al.* Facial phenotype in children
and young adults with PHOX2B-
determined congenital central
hypoventilation syndrome: quantitative
pattern of dysmorphology. *Pediatr Res*
2006; **59**: 39–45.

42. Berry-Kravis EM, Zhou L, Rand CM,
et al. Congenital central hypoventilation
syndrome: PHOX2B mutations and
phenotype. *Am J Respir Crit Care Med*
2006; **174**: 1139–44.

43. Trochet D, O'Brien LM, Gozal D, *et al.*
PHOX2B genotype allows for prediction
of tumor risk in congenital central
hypoventilation syndrome. *Am J Hum
Genet* 2005; **76**: 421–6.

Hemorrhagic lesions
of the central nervous system

Linda S. de Vries

Intracranial hemorrhage in preterm infants

During the last decade, attention has increasingly been drawn to ischemic damage occurring in the periventricular white matter (PWMI, periventricular white-matter injury), compared to the early days of neonatal imaging, when the focus was on intracranial hemorrhage (ICH). This is due to improvements in neonatal brain imaging, from only having access to cranial ultrasound (US) and computed tomography (CT) in the early 1980s, to increased use of magnetic resonance imaging (MRI) at present. The majority of the neonatal MRI studies have focused on lesions in the white matter, especially the more subtle lesions, which can now be clearly visualized; this was not so easy, and certainly more subjective, when imaging was restricted to cranial ultrasound. With better ultrasound equipment and more detailed examinations, using more acoustic windows than the anterior fontanel, for example the mastoid window and the posterior fontanel, hemorrhagic lesions of the cerebellum have increasingly been recognized, especially in the very immature and extremely low-birthweight infant. Germinal matrix hemorrhage–intraventricular hemorrhage (GMH–IVH) is still common, and especially the severe hemorrhages can lead to adverse neurologic sequelae.

Neuropathology and pathogenesis of GMH–IVH

The germinal matrix area is highly vascularized and is described as an "immature vascular rete," as the vessels within the germinal matrix are primitive and can not be classified as arterioles, venules, or capillaries. It is a transient structure, and is initially the site where neuroblast and glioblast mitotic activity occurs, before cells migrate to other parts of the cerebrum. Once cell division and migration is complete, the germinal matrix progressively decreases in size, with regression being almost complete by term. The germinal matrix area is most abundant over the head and body of the caudate nucleus, but is also seen in the roof of the temporal horn until approximately 33–34 weeks of gestation. MRI has recently

confirmed the abundance of the germinal matrix. More than a third of cases from a large autopsy series from New Jersey with a germinal matrix hemorrhage had involvement of the temporal or occipital germinal matrix [1]. The arterial supply of the germinal matrix is from the recurrent artery of Heubner (a branch of the anterior cerebral artery), as well as terminal branches of the lateral striate arteries. Venous drainage of the deep white matter occurs through a fan-shaped leash of short and long medullary veins through which blood flows into the germinal matrix and subsequently into the terminal vein which lies below the germinal matrix. This has led to the understanding of a unilateral parenchymal hemorrhage, which is now considered to be due to venous infarction or to a reperfusion injury following an ischemic insult [2–4].

It is most often considered that hemorrhage arises from the thin-walled veins [5,6], although Pape and Wigglesworth suggested from their injection studies that capillary bleeding was more common than terminal vein rupture [7]. Ment *et al.* have suggested that the germinal matrix vessels change significantly over the first days of life to greater continuity of the basement membrane [8]. This rapid maturation, presumably as a result of early birth, may be one of the reasons why GMH–IVH usually occurs during the first few days of life.

Risk factors for GMH–IVH

In the *prenatal* period, histologic signs of amniotic infection have been noted to increase the risk of GMH–IVH [9]. A correlation was shown between raised blood cytokine concentrations and altered hemodynamic function [10].

There is no evidence that cesarean section protects the premature infant against GMH–IVH. In a recent hospital-based study in preterm infants with a birthweight of ≤ 1250 g no beneficial effect was shown of an elective cesarean section on either reduced mortality or neurodisability at 2 years of age [11]. Breech delivery is in some studies associated with a higher risk of large GMH–IVH, but this effect was lost in a multivariate analysis [12]. In another study, a positive effect was shown for the most immature infants, with a gestation < 27 weeks [9]. A reduced mortality, but not a reduced risk of a GMH–IVH, was recently reported in a Swedish population-based study for preterm infants with a gestation of 25–36 weeks [13].

The importance of delayed cord clamping was suggested by Mercer *et al.*, showing a reduction in GMH–IVH, with five

Fetal and Neonatal Brain Injury, 4th edition, ed. David K. Stevenson, William E. Benitz, Philip Sunshine, Susan R. Hintz, and Maurice L. Druzin. Published by Cambridge University Press. © Cambridge University Press 2009.

(14%) in the delayed clamping group versus 13 (36%) in the non-delayed group ($p = 0.03$) [14]. The impact of delayed cord clamping on IVH was evaluated adjusting for gestational age and cesarean section. The final model indicated that the IVH rate was more than three times higher in the immediate cord clamping group (OR 3.5, 95% CI 1.1–11.1). In a systematic review by Rabe *et al.* there were no significant differences for infant deaths, but a significant difference in the incidence of IVH was reported by seven of the ten published studies ($p = 0.002$) [15].

It has also been suggested that infants born outside a perinatal center and transported in have a higher incidence of GMH–IVH [9,16,17]. Data from the NEOPAIN trial did show that outborn babies were more likely to have severe IVH ($p = 0.0005$) and this increased risk persisted after controlling for severity of illness, but when adjustments were made for use of antenatal steroids the effect of birth center was no longer significant [17].

Cardiovascular and respiratory problems have always been considered to play a major role in the development of a GMH–IVH in the immediate *neonatal* period. Fluctuations of the intravascular pressure or blood flow may lead to rupture of the "immature vascular rete" in the germinal matrix, and occurrence of a hemorrhage is known to occur during reperfusion following a period of hypotension [18]. Early assessment of the flow in the superior vena cava, within the first few hours after birth, showed that a low flow preceded a GMH-IVH [19]. Although the possible lack of cerebral autoregulation, rendering the cerebral circulation "pressure-passive," is still considered important, it is not present in all preterm infants [20]. Continuous monitoring with near-infrared spectroscopy (NIRS) may be a useful tool in the identification of infants at risk [21]. Respiratory risk factors can occur with complications during mechanical ventilation, such as vasodilation secondary to hypercapnia, for instance following a pneumothorax [22]. Improvements in ventilatory techniques, and increased use of non-ventilatory support such as CPAP and even BIPAP, are likely to further reduce the incidence of GMH-IVH.

A *reduced risk* of GMH-IVH was found with maternal pre-eclampsia, which appears to be due to enhanced in utero maturation of the fetus, associated with a reduced risk of postnatal development of respiratory distress [12].

Incidence of GMH–IVH

The incidence of GMH–IVH is directly related to the maturity of the infant. Initial studies in the late 1970s and early 1980s showed an incidence as high as 40–50% in those weighing < 1500 g, but these numbers came down to 20% in the 1990s according to some studies – though not according to others [16,23,26]. The average incidence of a unilateral parenchymal hemorrhage varies from 3% to 11%, with the lowest incidence coming from a French population-based study [27,29]. No decrease in this type of lesion was seen by Hamrick *et al.*, in contrast to the decrease they reported in cystic white-matter disease [30].

Diagnosis of GMH–IVH

Even though MRI is increasingly being used, GMH–IVH is still more likely to be diagnosed during routine bedside ultrasonography. Performing ultrasound as part of the admission procedure, and several times during the first week, will allow the most accurate timing and identification of antenatal onset of the lesion. Almost all hemorrhages will have developed by the end of the first week after birth, and many within the first hours after birth. Only about 10% of GMH–IVH occurs beyond the end of the first week, in contrast to white-matter injury, where late onset is not uncommon [31]. Progression from a small GMH–IVH to a parenchymal hemorrhage can occur, and this is most likely related to impaired venous drainage of the medullary veins in the white matter with obstruction at the site of the germinal matrix [27]. Sequential imaging over the first few days has helped in the past to identify the most common risk factors.

Clinical diagnosis does not play a major role, as most of the GMH–IVH will be silent. Three clinical syndromes have been described in the past [32], the first being associated with a *catastrophic* deterioration, with a sudden deterioration of the clinical state of the infant, such as a sudden fall in blood pressure and/or metabolic acidosis. It is, however, more common to find a sudden fall in hemoglobin without a clear change in the condition of the child. The second clinical syndrome is the *saltatory* one, with a more gradual onset, presenting with a change in general movements. Most commonly the *silent*, asymptomatic syndrome is seen, and this can even occur in infants who show a parenchymal hemorrhage on a routine repeat ultrasound examination.

The classification system suggested by Volpe is suitable to describe early and late ultrasound appearances (Table 24.1) [32]. The use of grade IV is avoided, and a separate description of the size, site, and appearance of a parenchymal lesion is preferred. Making a distinction between a small hemorrhage restricted to the germinal matrix and a GMH with some blood ruptured through the ependyma into the ventricular lumen is not always possible. The use of the posterior fontanel as an alternative acoustic window has been advocated by Correa *et al.*, showing improvement in the diagnosis of a small IVH [33]. GMHs at sites, other than at the head of the caudate nucleus, such as the roof of the temporal horn, often remain undiagnosed unless an MRI is also performed [34].

Table 24.1. Ultrasound description of GMH–IVH, adapted from Volpe [32]

Description	Generic term
Grade I: Germinal matrix hemorrhage	GMH–IVH
Grade II: Intraventricular hemorrhage without ventricular dilatation	GMH–IVH
Grade III: Intraventricular hemorrhage with acute ventricular dilatation (clot fills > 50% of the ventricle)	GMH–IVH and ventriculomegaly
Intraparenchymal lesion – describe size, location	IPL

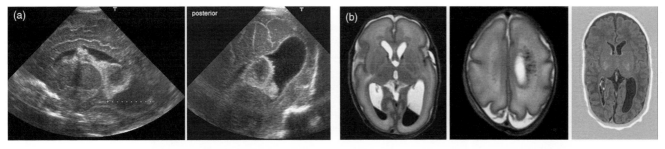

Fig. 24.1. (a) Cranial ultrasound of a preterm infant born at 29 weeks gestational age, parasagittal views, taken through the anterior (left) and posterior (right) fontanelle, showing a large intraventricular clot and a severely dilated occipital horn. (b) MRI of the same child, T2-weighted spin-echo sequence, taken at 2 weeks of age, shows associated punctate lesions in the white matter. The inversion recovery sequence taken at term-equivalent age still shows a dilated occipital horn and poor myelination of the posterior limb of the internal capsule, especially on the left.

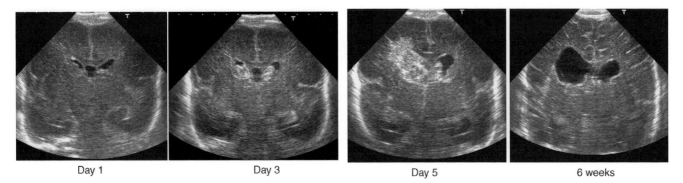

| Day 1 | Day 3 | Day 5 | 6 weeks |

Fig. 24.2. Cranial ultrasound of a preterm infant, born at 27 weeks gestational age, coronal views, taken on days 1, 3, 5, and at 6 weeks, showing a normal scan on day 1, a bilateral intraventricular hemorrhage on day 3, a parenchymal hemorrhage and large IVH on the right on day 5, and evolution into a single porencephalic cyst 6 weeks later.

A large IVH can be confidently diagnosed with US, although associated white-matter damage may be more reliably diagnosed with early MRI (Fig. 24.1). Distinction of a large, bulky choroid plexus, which is common in very immature infants, from a large IVH is not always easy, and sequential examinations and an examination through the posterior fontanel may aid in making this distinction. Blood can acutely dilate the ventricle or can lead to posthemorrhagic ventricular dilation (PHVD) a few weeks later, and the larger the amount of blood, the more likely this will subsequently occur. Blood will rapidly spread through the foramen of Monro into the third ventricle, the aqueduct of Sylvius, the fourth ventricle, and the foramina of Magendie and Luschka, to eventually spread into the posterior fossa. Clot formation can occur at any level, and can lead to outflow obstruction, but it is most commonly seen at the level of the aqueduct, or more diffusely in the posterior fossa. Depending on the degree of blood and the site of obstruction, PHVD can be rapidly progressive and non-communicating, usually due to obstruction at the level of the aqueduct of Sylvius, or be more gradual in onset, communicating, and considered to be due to obliterative arachnoiditis.

A unilateral parenchymal hemorrhage accounts for 3–15% of all GMH–IVH [28,29]. It is usually unilateral, triangular in shape, with the apex at the outer border of the lateral ventricle, and associated with a moderate to large ipsilateral GMH–IVH.

It has been thought in the past that parenchymal hemorrhage was due to direct extension of hemorrhage into the periventricular white matter, but this is no longer considered to be the most likely explanation for this type of parenchymal lesion. Most would now agree that this type of lesion is caused by the presence of GMH–IVH, which can lead to impaired venous drainage and subsequent venous infarction of the medullary veins of the white matter. This sequence of events can sometimes be followed by sequential ultrasound examinations, changing from a normal image to a stage of simple GMH–IVH and involvement of the parenchyma on the following day (Fig. 24.2). While this type of lesion used to be globular and would usually communicate with the lateral ventricle, with subsequent evolution into a porencephalic cyst, more recently the pattern has been shown to be more variable, with a more discrete parenchymal lesion that does not necessarily communicate with the lateral ventricle and can evolve into a few small cysts in the white matter that may resolve with eventual ex vacuo dilation on the affected side. These white-matter cysts can be mistaken for unilateral cystic leukomalacia, but seeing the evolution of this unilateral lesion with sequential ultrasound examinations would not favor a diagnosis of leukomalacia, which is almost invariably bilateral and not often associated with a large IVH (Fig. 24.3). MRI performed later in infancy or early childhood will also help to make a distinction between the two conditions, showing more focal injury in

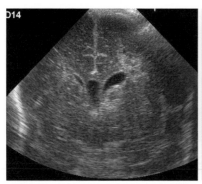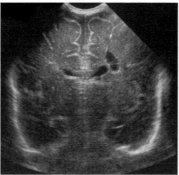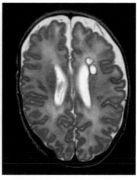

Fig. 24.3. Cranial ultrasound of a preterm infant born at 29 weeks gestational age, coronal view, resolving left-sided hemorrhage on day 14 (left). Ultrasound taken at term-equivalent age (middle) showed cystic evolution, confirmed with MRI (T2 spin-echo sequence) (right). Also note the enlarged subarachnoid space. Outcome at 24 months was within the normal range (BSID-II; MDI 91; PDI 100).

those with a parenchymal hemorrhage. Detailed studies by Dudink et al. have made it possible to identify the veins that were involved in the parenchymal injury [35]. A recent proposal was made by Bassan et al. to grade the severity of this parenchymal lesion [36], taking the extent of the lesion, the presence of a contralateral parenchymal lesion, and also the presence of a midline shift due to this lesion into account. The grading system also helped in the prediction of neurodevelopmental outcome at 2 years of age [37].

Intracerebellar hemorrhage

Intracerebellar hemorrhage is increasingly recognized together with a GMH–IVH. This type of lesion is especially common in those with a birthweight < 750 g and a gestational age below 27 weeks [38,39]. Twenty-five of the 35 infants examined by Limperopoulos et al. had a unilateral hemispheric hemorrhage [39]. Of the 35 infants, 27 also had supratentorial lesions. Apnea, bradycardia, and a falling hematocrit may be associated with this type of lesion. Ultrasonography can be diagnostic when the lesion is large or when care is taken to use the posterolateral fontanel as the acoustic window [38]. MRI will give better definition of the extent of the lesion. Follow-up at a mean age of 32 months showed neurologic abnormalities in 66% of the isolated cerebellar hemorrhagic injury cases compared with 5% of the control preterm infants [40]. Infants with isolated cerebellar hemorrhagic injury versus controls had severe motor disabilities (48% vs. 0%), deficits in expressive language (42% vs. 0%), delayed receptive language (37% vs. 0%), and cognitive deficits (40% vs. 0%). Preterm infants with cerebellar hemorrhagic injury and supratentorial parenchymal injury were not at overall greater risk for neurodevelopmental disabilities, although neuromotor impairment was more severe. Cerebellar atrophy without apparent cerebellar hemorrhage has also been reported as a common sequel of severe immaturity [41–43]. Srinivasan et al. [44] showed reduced cerebellar volume only in preterm infants at term-equivalent age in association with supratentorial pathology such as hemorrhagic parenchymal infarction, intraventricular hemorrhage with dilation, and periventricular leukomalacia (PVL).

Management of GMH–IVH

Once the diagnosis of a GMH–IVH is made, immediate clinical management will not be different from that of other at-risk preterm infants. Optimization of any coagulopathy, minimal handling, prevention of fluctuations in blood pressure or CO_2 levels, and prevention of breathing against the ventilator may be used in an effort to prevent extension of the initial hemorrhage [45–47]. Continuous aEEG registration may detect subclinical seizures, which may require treatment [48].

Repeat US scans are indicated for timely diagnosis of the development of PHVD, which is usually seen within 10–14 days following the occurrence of the hemorrhage. PHVD can progress either slowly or rapidly. In the majority of cases (65%) slowly progressive PHVD is followed by spontaneous arrest. In the remaining 30–35% of infants with PHVD, ventricular size increases rapidly over the course of days to weeks [49].

Increase in ventricular size, as assessed with repeated US examinations, will precede any clinical symptoms, such as a rapid increase in head circumference (> 2 cm/week), diastasis of the sutures, a full fontanel, vomiting, irritability, bradycardias, and apneas, by several weeks, due to the large extracerebral space and the high water content of the white matter. Sunsetting will only be seen at a late stage. There is no agreement as to whether treating progressive PHVD before the occurrence of any clinical symptoms is beneficial to the child. Measurements are usually taken in the coronal view at the foramen of Monro, using the "ventricular width," according to Levene and Starte [50]. The "ventricular index" is the distance between the midline and the lateral border of the ventricle. Most intervention studies have taken the 97th percentile + 4 mm as a starting point for randomization. Another useful measurement is the so-called "anterior horn width," taken just anterior to the thalamic notch [51]. This anterior horn width measurement does not change much with increasing maturation and should be < 3 mm, with measurements > 6 mm suggesting PHVD. Measuring the occipital horn in a sagittal plane can also be useful, as there can be a discrepancy between dilation of the anterior and posterior horn. Although the best angle may be more variable in the sagittal plane, any measurement of the occipital horn ≥ 25 mm also does suggest severe PHVD. Assessing the shape of the lateral ventricles may be useful, when making a distinction between pressure-driven PHVD and ex vacuo dilation following white-matter injury. Measuring the cerebrospinal fluid pressure may also aid in making a distinction, but reliable measurements can be hard to obtain [52].

Adverse short-term effects on the central nervous system have been shown using different techniques, including evoked potentials, aEEG, Doppler ultrasonography, and NIRS [53,54]. Cerebrospinal fluid measurements of cytokines, non-protein-bound iron, hypoxanthine, and sFas were all noted to be raised in infants with PHVD, and especially so in those with associated periventricular leukomalacia [55,58]. In spite of all these data, there is no direct evidence that early drainage of CSF alters the natural and long-term outcome of children with PHVD. In the two largest RCTs so far, randomization was done once the 97th percentile + 4 mm line was crossed, and 60% of the infants in both arms subsequently required shunt placement [59]. The RCT for DRIFT (drainage intervention fibrinolytic therapy) also used this measurement as an entry point for the study [60]. The initial data were promising, with shunt requirement in 22%, but the RCT was stopped early due to a high risk (33%) of rebleeding in the DRIFT group, without an apparent positive effect on the need for a ventriculoperitoneal shunt [61]. In two retrospective observational studies, a significant reduction in the need for shunt placement was noted when intervention was started before this line was crossed and when the threshold for inserting a subcutaneous reservoir was low [62,63]. Whether earlier and more active intervention is effective is now being studied in a prospective RCT.

Outcome following GMH–IVH

Most studies of infants with mild grades of GMH–IVH (hemorrhage restricted to the germinal matrix or small amount of ventricular blood) suggest that these infants were performing as well in cognitive and motor developmental outcome as preterm infants with no GMH–IVH, although a lower score was found with regard to their visual–motor integration [64]. Recent neonatal 3D-volumetric imaging studies, however, have shown reduced gray-matter volumes at term-equivalent age associated with a reduced MDI on the BSID-II, but this was only seen in the most immature infants, with gestation below 30 weeks [65,67]. Whether associated mild white-matter abnormalities were present, and could have played a role, is not discussed in these studies. This association was previously suggested by Kuban et al. [68].

The term *ventriculomegaly* (VM) has been used for infants with ventricular enlargement following a GMH–IVH, but also for those without apparent preceding hemorrhage, in whom it is more likely to be due to white-matter loss. It is therefore preferable to use VM for those without an apparent preceding large GMH–IVH, and to use the term *posthemorrhagic ventricular dilation* (PHVD) when ventricular enlargement follows

a large hemorrhage [68,69]. Having access to sequential ultrasound examinations, and looking at the shape of the ventricles, will enable us in most cases to make this important distinction.

The risk of a poor outcome has been reported to increase significantly with the presence of PHVD following a large GMH–IVH (40–60%), and even further in those who require shunt insertion (75–88%) [59,70,71]. In the cohort from Sweden, associated problems (cerebral visual impairment, epilepsy, and especially cognitive problems) were very common [71]. In a retrospective hospital-based population study, outcome was considerably better than reported previously, with cerebral palsy occurring in only 7.4% of the infants with a large IVH (grade III according to Papile) compared to 37 (48.7%) of the 76 infants with a parenchymal hemorrhage ($p < 0.001$). The mean developmental quotient (DQ) in the grade III group was 99, and in the grade IV group 95 at 24 months corrected age [63]. Whether this better outcome was related to earlier treatment of PHVD, or due to a cohort with more localized lesions and of higher gestational age, needs to be determined, and a prospective study is now under way. Magnetic resonance imaging (at approximately 8.5 years) in children with arrested or shunted hydrocephalus has revealed persistence of enlarged lateral ventricles, enlarged occipital horns, hypoplastic corpus callosum, and atrophy or dysplasia of the cerebral cortex. When preterm infants with no hydrocephalus are compared to those with arrested hydrocephalus, shunted hydrocephalus, and a term comparison group, the children with shunted hydrocephalus have the lowest verbal and perceptual IQ scores. Visual–spatial–motor scores are lower in the shunted compared to the arrested hydrocephalus group, and even lower in the arrested compared to the no hydrocephalus group. Tests of academic skills (arithmetic, science, writing) also demonstrate poorer performance in children with shunted hydrocephalus as compared to those with arrested hydrocephalus.

While the infants without apparent parenchymal involvement are more likely to develop diplegia, those with a venous infarction are more at risk of developing a hemiplegia. Outcome with intraparenchymal hemorrhage (IPH) varies, and depends on the extent and site of the lesion [37,72]. A recent scoring system reported by Bassan et al. showed an association between a higher score, based on the presence of a more extensive lesion, a midline shift, or bilateral parenchymal involvement, and mortality and outcome at 2 years of age [37]. This supported studies published in the 1980s showing that extensive lesions are associated with a higher mortality rate (81% vs. 37%), major motor deficits (100% vs. 80%), and more cognitive delays (86% vs. 53%) in comparison to a more localized IPH [73]. Long-term outcome into adolescence showed that most of the 14 cases with parenchymal hemorrhage and porencephaly were ambulatory, required learning assistance in school, and had social challenges [74].

Early prediction of development of a hemiplegia is now possible, using MRI at 40–42 weeks. Myelination of the posterior limb of the internal capsule (PLIC) should be present at term-equivalent age. In infants who go on to develop a hemiplegia, asymmetry and even lack of myelination of the PLIC was noted in those who subsequently developed a hemiplegia [75,76]. Using diffusion tensor imaging, visualization of the tracts may be possible at an earlier stage, but data are only available in preterm children studied in childhood, looking at thalamocortical connectivity [77,78].

Prevention of GMH–IVH in preterm infants

The incidence of GMH–IVH has decreased over time in most studies. Both prenatal and postnatal pharmacologic prophylaxis has been used to reduce the incidence of GMH–IVH. Many different drugs have been used, such as phenobarbital, tranexamic acid, pancuronium, etamsylate, vitamin E, and indomethacin. Only a few of these will be discussed here in more detail.

Antenatal prevention

Antenatal steroids
Administration of antenatal corticosteroids has been shown in several studies to be the most important protective factor against the development of GMH–IVH [13,79]. A systematic review of 21 randomized controlled trials, involving over 4000 babies, has shown that corticosteroid administration is associated with a significant reduction in the risk of GMH–IVH (OR 0.54, 95% CI 0.43–0.69) and with a strong trend towards improving long-term neurologic outcome in survivors (OR 0.64, 95% CI 0.14–2.98) [80]. The effect of steroid administration could be due to a reduction in risk and severity of respiratory distress syndrome, postnatal stabilization of blood pressure, or maybe even a direct cerebral protective effect. Repeated courses of antenatal corticosteroids are not recommended, as a negative effect on brain growth has been shown [81]. Bethamethasone instead of dexamethasone is recommended, as the latter was associated with an increased incidence of PVL [82].

Magnesium sulfate
Antenatal administration of magnesium sulfate was not associated with a reduction in the incidence of either a small or a large GMH–IVH in two recent large randomized multicenter studies [83,84].

Vitamin K
Vitamin K was used antenatally to prevent neonatal GMH–IVH, as vitamin-K-dependent factors are deficient in preterm infants. The initial reports were promising [85,86]. A recent systematic review compared five randomized studies involving 420 women to evaluate the role of vitamin K, given to women in labor or very likely to deliver a premature infant, in the prevention of GMH–IVH, and was not able to show a beneficial effect [87].

Postnatal prevention

Phenobarbital
The rationale for phenobarbital use was sedation of the preterm infant to prevent the fluctuations of blood pressure that occur with clinical care of high-risk infants. Phenobarbital was the first drug used postnatally in the prevention of GMH–IVH. A meta-analysis of 10 trials was unable to show a reduction in the incidence of GMH–IVH (typical relative risk 1.04, 95% CI 0.87–1.25), or in its severity (typical RR for severe IVH 0.91, 95% CI 0.66–1.24) [88]. There was a consistent trend in the trials towards increased use of mechanical ventilation in the phenobarbital-treated group, which was supported by the meta-analysis (typical RR 1.18, 95% CI 1.06–1.32).

Indomethacin
A meta-analysis on the postnatal use of indomethacin in the prevention of GMH–IVH and subsequent brain injury [89] showed a significant reduction in the incidence of GMH–IVH of all grades in indomethacin-treated groups (RR 0.88, 95% CI 0.80–0.96). When only more severe degrees of hemorrhage were reported (Papile grade 3 and 4) this effect was still present (RR 0.66, 95% CI 0.53–0.82).

Outcome measures of death or severe neurosensory impairment were reported in four studies, but no significant effect of indomethacin could be found (RR 1.02, 95% CI 0.90–1.15) [89,90]. A recent post-hoc analysis of the orginal indomethacin trial suggested that boys exposed to indomethacin had significantly better outcome in verbal test scores than girls, suggesting a gender-specific effect [91].

Ibuprofen
Ibuprofen is used as an alternative to indomethacin in the medical management of patent ductus arteriosus, and it acts in a similar manner by prostaglandin synthase inhibition. A recent RCT has evaluated whether ibuprofen when given shortly after birth to a group of premature infants (< 28 weeks' gestation) reduces the incidence of GMH–IVH [92]. Ibuprofen did not reduce the incidence of any degree of GMH–IVH when compared to controls (OR 0.96, 95% CI 0.48–2.03) or more severe GMH–IVH (grade 2–4) (OR 0.87, 95% CI 0.25–3.05) compared with controls.

General measures
Paying closer attention to blood pressure, gentle handling, synchronous ventilation, and less severe respiratory distress syndrome due to antenatal and postnatal surfactant therapy was associated with a reduction in GMH–IVH [93]. Data from the Canadian network also showed that the incidence and severity of GMH–IVH is affected by NICU characteristics. A high patient volume and a high neonatologist/staff ratio was associated with a lower rate of severe IVH [94].

Intracranial hemorrhage in term infants
Intraventricular hemorrhage
Intraventricular hemorrhage (IVH) is an uncommon problem in full-term as compared to preterm neonates. Origins of the IVH can be the germinal matrix, choroid plexus, or parenchyma. In term infants only remnants of the germinal matrix

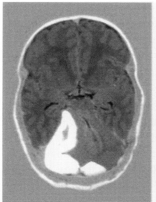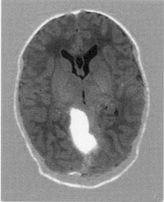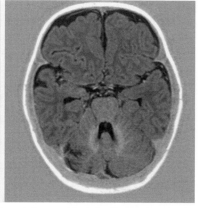

Fig. 24.4. Term infant, admitted because of PHVD. MRI on day 26 shows a large infratentorial subdural hemorrhage, with a shift and possibly involvement of the right cerebellar hemisphere. A repeat scan at 3 months (right) shows loss of volume and loss of tissue of the right cerebellar hemisphere.

remain. The incidence of germinal matrix hemorrhage is therefore low, and infants are often asymptomatic. The mechanism of IVH in term infants has been attributed to trauma at birth (precipitous delivery) or hypoxia; however, no etiology is detected in many cases. Recently, thalamic hemorrhage in term infants has been shown to be associated with cerebrosinovenous thrombosis [95]. The pathogenesis of thalamic hemorrhage is a hemorrhagic venous infarction of the large venous channels that are in close proximity to the ventricular walls. In the majority of infants none of the previously associated risk factors for thalamic hemorrhage, such as coagulation disorders or hypoxic–ischemic birth injury, was noted.

Predisposing factors noted by Roland *et al.* [96] included sepsis, cyanotic heart disease, and polycythemia. Symptomatology (irritability, seizures, apnea, bulging fontanel) occurred later than that seen in infants with IVH from choroid plexus or germinal matrix hemorrhage.

Management of IVH in term infants is supportive. Prognosis depends on the location and extent of the underlying insult. As a rule, among infants for whom no etiology of the IVH is detected, outcome appears to be good. In infants with IVH secondary to a GMH–IVH, prognosis is also good. Neurodevelopmental sequelae are seen in infants with IVH with parenchymal involvement [97]. When bilateral thalamic hemorrhage is associated with birth asphyxia, mortality is high and sequelae in survivors are high. Thalamic hemorrhage with IVH seen in infants with an uneventful birth history is associated with a greater risk for cerebral palsy than IVH from other sites.

Subdural hemorrhage

Subdural and subarachnoid hemorrhage are probably underdiagnosed, as they are difficult to recognize using cranial ultrasound. Subdural hemorrhage usually occurs secondary to birth trauma. These hemorrhages are relatively uncommon today because of improvements in obstetric care. Vaginal breech deliveries are for instance no longer commonly performed, after recent multicenter randomized studies [98]. Occipital diastasis can occur during a vaginal breech delivery

with excessive extension of the neck of the infant. The pathogenesis is secondary to mechanical injury to the cranium associated with instrumental delivery with forceps or ventouse extraction of the head, abnormal presentation (face or brow), precipitous delivery, and a large infant resulting in a difficult delivery [94,99,100]. There are shearing forces on the tentorium and the deep venous system. Children are usually born at term, and present with a full fontanel, lethargy, apneas, and/or seizures. Hydrocephalus can develop due to outflow obstruction and may require temporary external drainage, sometimes followed by permanent drainage, due to difficulties of CSF reabsorption at the level of the arachnoid granulations. Secondary cerebral infarction has also been reported and has been related to prolonged arterial compression [101]. The majority of the subdural hemorrhages are infratentorial (Fig. 24.4), but a supratentorial location can also be noted and is then sometimes associated with a lobar hemorrhage, which can be large and associated with a shift of the midline, requiring neurosurgical intervention. Short-term outcome in children with an isolated infratentorial subdural hemorrhage, but also in those with a lobar hemorrhage, has often been reported to be more favorable than expected, but the groups are usually small [100,102].

Subgaleal hemorrhage

Subgaleal hemorrhage is a rare and potentially fatal condition of the neonate often associated with instrumental delivery. It is caused by rupture of the emissary veins, which are connections between the dural sinuses and the scalp veins. Blood accumulates between the epicranial aponeurosis of the scalp and the periosteum. Most cases of subgaleal hemorrhage reported have been associated with the use of the vacuum extractor. The incidence of subgaleal hemorrhage is estimated to be 4–6 per 10 000 spontaneous vaginal deliveries and 46–59 per 10 000 vacuum-assisted deliveries [103,104]. The children will present with diffuse swelling of the head and evidence of hypovolemic shock. In a study by Kilani and Wetmore, associated intracranial hemorrhage was present in half of the 34 infants studied, and four (11.8 %) infants died [105].

In another study of 42 infants, 31% had a poor outcome (five died, four had epilepsy, three had severe auditory dysfunction, two had cerebral palsy, and one had renal vein thrombosis) [106]. The group with the poor outcome included significantly more patients who had been transferred from other hospitals ($p < 0.001$). Those with a poor outcome had significantly more hypotension ($p < 0.001$) and seizures ($p < 0.05$). Prompt and aggressive administration of blood products and treatment of associated coagulopathy are recommended to improve outcome.

Intracranial hemorrhage associated with other specific conditions in term infants
Neonatal alloimmune thrombocytopenia

In neonatal alloimmune thrombocytopenia (NAITP), fetal and neonatal thrombocytopenia results from the formation of a maternal antiplatelet antibody to a paternally derived platelet antigen, usually platelet surface antigen (PLAI), expressed on the surface of the fetal platelets. NAITP occurs in 1/2000 to 1/5000 fetuses, and up to 30% of infants with this condition have ICH secondary to thrombocytopenia. ICH occurs in as many as 10–30% of the infants with alloimmune thrombocytopenia, 25–50% of which occur in utero [107]. NAITP has an estimated mortality rate of 15%, with ICH accounting for most deaths. Fetal and neonatal platelet counts less than 20×10^9 are common even before 24 weeks' gestation [108]. Management in the antenatal period includes administration of intravenous gammaglobulin to the mother with or without corticosteroids prior to delivery. Transfusion of matched compatible platelets to the fetus may safeguard against ICH during the birthing process. Abdominal delivery is suggested if cordocentesis reveals fetal thrombocytopenia. After birth, transfusion with antigen-negative platelets (maternal platelets) is recommended. Hemispheric porencephalic cyst, following a hemorrhage which is most commonly located within a temporal lobe, is usually present at birth, but extra-axial hemorrhages, intraventricular hemorrhage, acute parenchymal hemorrhage, and neuronal migrational disorder have also been reported [107].

Extracorporeal membrane oxygenation (ECMO)

ECMO is the treatment of choice in infants with persistent pulmonary hypertension and cardiorespiratory failure unresponsive to inhaled nitric oxide. In term infants, ICH following ECMO occurs in 10–13% of infants [109,110]. The lesions are hemorrhagic, with ischemia (60%) or hemorrhage alone (40%). The pathogenesis of ICH following ECMO is multifactorial, and it has been attributed to reperfusion injury, hemodynamic and cerebrovascular instability, systemic heparinization, and increased central venous pressure. Initially, gestational age (GA) < 34 weeks, acidosis, sepsis, coagulopathy, and treatment with epinephrine are major independent factors associated with ICH in neonates treated with ECMO [109]. More recent data have shown that postconceptional age (PCA) shows a strong univariate correlation with decreasing ICH: 26% of patients ≤ 32 weeks' PCA developed ICH, compared with 6% of patients of 38 weeks' PCA ($p = 0.004$) [109]. In ECMO-treated infants, the combination of a normal bedside US and an EEG without marked abnormalities is highly predictive of normal post-ECMO CT and MRI neuroimaging studies [111]. Among 183 ECMO survivors, 85 infants had neuroimaging abnormalities. Survivors with non-hemorrhagic abnormalities had a higher risk of delayed development than did those with isolated hemorrhagic abnormalities (39% vs. 21%) [112]. Attempts at decreasing risk of ICH with ECMO include venovenous (VV) ECMO, in which integrity of blood flow to the brain is maintained and cannulation and sacrifice of only the internal jugular vein occur.

References

1. Paneth N, Rudelli R, Kazam E, *et al. Brain Damage in the Preterm Infant.* Clinics in Developmental Medicine 131. London: MacKeith Press, 1994.

2. Takashima S, Takashi M, Ando Y. Pathogenesis of periventricular white matter haemorrhage in preterm infants. *Brain Dev* 1986; **8**: 25–30.

3. Gould SJ, Howard S, Hope PL, *et al.* Periventricular intraparenchymal cerebral haemorrhage in preterm infants: the role of venous infarction. *J Pathol* 1987; **151**: 197–202.

4. Volpe JJ. Intraventricular hemorrhage in the premature infant: current concepts. Part I. *Ann Neurol* 1989; **25**: 3–11.

5. Moody DM, Brown WR, Challa VR, *et al.* Alkaline phosphatase histochemical staining in the study of germinal matrix hemorrhage and brain vascular morphology in a very-low-birth-weight neonate. *Pediatr Res* 1994; **35**: 424–30.

6. Ghazi-Birry HS, Brown WR, Moody DM, *et al.* Human germinal matrix: venous origin of hemorrhage and vascular characteristics. *AJNR Am J Neuroradiol* 1997; **18**: 219–29.

7. Pape KE, Wigglesworth JS. *Haemorrhage, Ischaemia and Perinatal Brain.* Clinics in Developmental Medicine 69/70. London: SIMP/Heinemann, 1979: 133–48.

8. Ment LR, Stewart WB, Ardito TA, *et al.* Germinal matrix microvascular maturation correlates inversely with the risk period for neonatal intraventricular hemorrhage. *Brain Res Dev Brain Res* 1995; **84**: 142–9.

9. Thorp JA, Jones PG, Clark RH, *et al.* Perinatal factors associated with severe intracranial hemorrhage. *Am J Obstet Gynecol* 2001; **185**: 859–62.

10. Yanowitz TD, Jordan JA, Gilmour CH, *et al.* Hemodynamic disturbances in premature infants born after chorioamnionitis: association with cord blood cytokine concentrations. *Pediatr Res* 2002; **51**: 310–6.

11. Haque KN, Hayes AM, Ahmed Z, *et al.* Caesarean or vaginal delivery for preterm very-low-birth weight ($\leq 1,250$ g) infant: experience from a district general hospital in UK. *Arch Gynecol Obstet* 2008; **277**: 207–12.

12. Shankaran S, Bauer CR, Bain R, *et al.* Prenatal and perinatal risk and protective factors for neonatal intracranial hemorrhage. *Arch Pediatr Adolesc Med* 1996; **150**: 491–7.

13. Herbst A, Källén K. Influence of mode of delivery on neonatal mortality and

morbidity in spontaneous preterm breech delivery. *Eur J Obstet Gynecol Reprod Biol* 2007; **133**: 25–9.

14. Mercer JS, Vohr BR, McGrath MM, *et al.* Delayed cord clamping in very preterm infants reduces the incidence of intraventricular hemorrhage and late-onset sepsis: a randomized, controlled trial. *Pediatrics* 2006; **117**: 1235–42.

15. Rabe H, Reynolds G, Diaz-Rossello J. A systematic review and meta-analysis of a brief delay in clamping the umbilical cord of preterm infants. *Neonatology* 2008; **93**: 138–44.

16. Heuchan AM, Evans N, Henderson Smart DJ. Perinatal risk factors for major intraventricular haemorrhage in the Australian and New Zealand Neonatal Network, 1995–97. *Arch Dis Child Fetal Neonatal Ed* 2002; **86**: F86–90.

17. Palmer KG, Kronsberg SS, Barton BA, *et al.* Effect of inborn versus outborn delivery on clinical outcomes in ventilated preterm neonates: secondary results from the NEOPAIN trial. *J Perinatol* 2005; **25**: 270–5.

18. Watkins AM, West CR, Cooke RWI. Blood pressure and cerebral haemorrhage and ischaemia in very low birthweight infants. *Early Hum Dev* 1989; **19**: 103–10.

19. Osborn DA, Evans N, Kluckow M. Hemodynamic and antecedent risk factors of early and late periventricular/ intraventricular hemorrhage in premature infants. *Pediatrics* 2003; **112**: 33–9.

20. Tsuji M, Saul P, du Plessis A, *et al.* Cerebral intravascular oxygenation correlates with mean arterial pressure in critically ill premature infants. *Pediatrics* 2000; **106**: 625–32.

21. Soul JS, Hammer PE, Tsuji M, *et al.* Fluctuating pressure-passivity is common in the cerebral circulation of sick premature infants. *Pediatr Res* 2007; **61**: 467–73.

22. Fabres J, Carlo WA, Phillips V, *et al.* Both extremes of arterial carbon dioxide pressure and the magnitude of fluctuations in arterial carbon dioxide pressure are associated with severe intraventricular hemorrhage in preterm infants. *Pediatrics* 2007; **119**: 299–305.

23. Burstein J, Papile L, Burstein R. Intraventricular hemorrhage in premature newborns: a prospective study with CT. *AJR Am J Roentgenol* 1979; **132**: 631–5.

24. Dolfin T, Skidmore MB, Fong KW, *et al.* Incidence, severity and timing of subependymal and intraventricular hemorrhages in preterm infants born in a perinatal unit as detected by serial real-time ultrasound. *Pediatrics* 1983; **71**: 541–6.

25. Batton DG, Holtrop P, Dewitte D, *et al.* Current gestational age-related incidence of major intraventricular hemorrhage. *J Pediatr* 1994; **125**: 623–5.

26. Gleissner M, Jorch G, Avenarius S. Risk factors for intraventricular hemorrhage in a birth cohort of 3721 premature infants. *J Perinat Med* 2000; **28**: 104–10.

27. de Vries LS, Rademaker KJ, Roelants-van Rijn AM, *et al.* Unilateral haemorrhagic parenchymal infarction in the preterm infant. *Eur J Pediatr Neurol* 2001; **5**: 139–149.

28. Lemons JA, Bauer CR, Oh W, *et al.* Very low birthweight outcomes of the National Institute of Child Health and Human Development neonatal research network, January 1995 through December 1996. NICD Neonatal Research Network. *Pediatrics* 2001; **107**: E1.

29. Larroque B, Marret S, Ancel PY, *et al.* White matter damage and intraventricular hemorrhage in very preterm infants: the EPIPAGE study. *J Pediatr* 2003; **143**: 477–83.

30. Hamrick SE, Miller SP, Leonard C, *et al.* Trends in severe brain injury and neurodevelopmental outcome in premature newborn infants: the role of cystic periventricular leukomalacia. *J Pediatr* 2004; **145**: 593–9.

31. Andre P, Thebaud B, Delavaucoupet J, *et al.* Late-onset cystic periventricular leukomalacia in premature infants: a threat until term. *Am J Perinatol* 2001; **18**: 79–86.

32. Volpe JJ. *Neonatal Neurology*, 4th edn. Philadelphia, PA: Saunders, 2001.

33. Correa F, Enríquez G, Rosselló J, *et al.* Posterior fontanelle sonography: an acoustic window into the neonatal brain. *AJNR Am J Neuroradiol* 2004; **25**: 1274–82.

34. Maalouf EF, Duggan PJ, Counsell SJ, *et al.* Comparison of findings on cranial ultrasound and magnetic resonance imaging in preterm infants. *Pediatrics* 2001; **107**: 719–27.

35. Dudink J, Lequin M, Weisglas-Kuperus N, *et al.* Venous subtypes of preterm periventricular haemorrhagic infarction. *Arch Dis Child Fetal Neonatal Ed* 2007; **93**: F201–6.

36. Bassan H, Benson CB, Limperopoulos C, *et al.* Ultrasonographic features and severity scoring of periventricular hemorrhagic infarction in relation to risk factors and outcome. *Pediatrics* 2006; **117**: 2111–18.

37. Bassan H, Limperopoulos C, Visconti K, *et al.* Neurodevelopmental outcome in survivors of periventricular hemorrhagic infarction. *Pediatrics* 2007; **120**: 785–92.

38. Merrill JD, Piecuch RE, Fell SC, *et al.* A new pattern of cerebellar hemorrhages in preterm infants. *Pediatrics* 1998; **102**: E62.

39. Limperopoulos C, Benson CB, Bassan H, *et al.* Cerebellar hemorrhage in the preterm infant: ultrasonographic findings and risk factors. *Pediatrics* 2005; **116**: 717–24.

40. Limperopoulos C, Bassan H, Gauvreau K, *et al.* Does cerebellar injury in premature infants contribute to the high prevalence of long-term cognitive, learning, and behavioral disability in survivors? *Pediatrics* 2007; **120**: 584–93.

41. Bodensteiner JB, Johnsen SD. Cerebellar injury in the extremely premature infant: a newly recognized but relatively common outcome. *J Child Neurol* 2005; **20**: 139–42.

42. Messerschmidt A, Fuiko R, Prayer D, *et al.* Disrupted cerebellar development in preterm infants is associated with impaired neurodevelopmental outcome. *Eur J Pediatr* 2008; **167**: 1141–7.

43. Messerschmidt A, Brugger PC, Boltshauser E, *et al.* Disruption of cerebellar development: potential complication of extreme prematurity. *AJNR Am J Neuroradiol* 2005; **26**: 1659–67.

44. Srinivasan L, Allsop J, Counsell SJ, *et al.* Smaller cerebellar volumes in very preterm infants at term-equivalent age are associated with the presence of supratentorial lesions. *AJNR Am J Neuroradiol* 2006; **27**: 573–9.

45. Bada HS, Korones SB, Perry EH, *et al.* Frequent handling in the neonatal intensive care unit and intraventricular hemorrhage. *J Pediatr* 1990; **117**: 126–31.

46. Bejar R, Saugstad OD, James H, *et al.* Increased hypoxanthine concentrations in cerebrospinal fluid of infants with hydrocephalus. *J Pediatr* 1983; **103**: 44–8.

47. Dasgupta SJ, Gill AB. Hypotension in the very low birth weight infant: the old, the new and the uncertain. *Arch Dis Child Fetal Neonatal Ed* 2003; **88**: F450–4.

48. Olischar M, Klebermass K, Waldhoer T, et al. Background patterns and sleep–wake cycles on amplitude-integrated electroencephalography in preterms younger than 30 weeks gestational age with peri-/intraventricular haemorrhage. *Acta Paediatr* 2007; **96**: 1743–50.

49. Murphy BP, Inder TE, Rooks V, et al. Posthaemorrhagic ventricular dilatation in the premature infant: natural history and predictors of outcome. *Arch Dis Child Fetal Neonatal Ed* 2002; **87**: F37–41.

50. Levene MI, Starte DR. A longitudinal study of posthaemorrhagic ventricular dilatation in the newborn. *Arch Dis Child* 1981; **56**: 905–10.

51. Davies MW, Swaminathan M, Chuang SI, et al. Reference ranges for the linear dimensions of the intracranial ventricles in preterm neonates. *Arch Dis Child Fetal Neonatol Ed* 2000; **82**: F219–23.

52. Kaiser A, Whitelaw A. Cerebrospinal fluid pressure during posthaemorrhagic ventricular dilatation in newborn. *Arch Dis Child* 1985; **60**: 920–4.

53. Soul JS, Eichenwald E, Walter G, et al. CSF removal in infantile posthemorrhagic hydrocephalus results in significant improvement in cerebral hemodynamics. *Pediatr Res* 2004; **55**: 872–6.

54. van Alfen-van der Velden AA, Hopman JC, Klaessens JH, et al. Cerebral hemodynamics and oxygenation after serial CSF drainage in infants with PHVD. *Brain Dev* 2007; **29**: 623–9.

55. Sävman K, Blennow M, Hagberg H, et al. Cytokine response in cerebrospinal fluid from preterm infants with posthaemorrhagic ventricular dilatation. *Acta Paediatr* 2002; **91**: 1357–63.

56. Felderhoff-Mueser U, Buhrer C, Groneck P, et al. Soluble Fas (CD95/Apo-1), soluble Fas ligand and activated caspase 3 in the cerebrospinal fluid of infants with posthemorrhagic and nonhemorrhagic hydrocephalus. *Pediatr Res* 2003; **54**: 659–64.

57. Heep A, Stoffel-Wagner B, Bartmann P, et al. Vascular endothelial growth factor and transforming growth factor-β1 are highly expressed in the cerebrospinal fluid of premature infants with posthemorrhagic hydrocephalus. *Pediatr Res* 2004; **56**: 768–74.

58. Schmitz T, Heep A, Groenendaal F, et al. Interleukin-1β, interleukin-18, and interferon-γ expression in the cerebrospinal fluid of premature infants with posthemorrhagic hydrocephalus–

markers of white matter damage? *Pediatr Res* 2007; **61**: 722–6.

59. Ventriculomegaly Trial Group. Randomized trial of early tapping in neonatal posthaemorrhagic ventricular dilatation: results at 30 months. *Arch Dis Child Fetal Neonatal Ed* 1994; **70**: F129–36.

60. Whitelaw A, Pople I, Cherian S, et al. Phase 1 trial of prevention of hydrocephalus after intraventricular hemorrhage in newborn infants by drainage, irrigation and fibrinolytic therapy. *Pediatrics* 2003; **111**: 759–65.

61. Whitelaw A, Evans D, Carter M, et al. Randomized clinical trial of prevention of hydrocephalus after intraventricular hemorrhage in preterm infants: brain-washing versus tapping fluid. *Pediatrics* 2007; **119**: e1071–8.

62. de Vries LS, Liem KD, van Dijk K, et al. Early versus late treatment of posthaemorrhagic ventricular dilatation: results of a retrospective study from five neonatal intensive care units in the Netherlands. *Acta Paediatrica* 2002; **91**: 212–17.

63. Brouwer AJ, Groenendaal F, van Haastert IC, et al. Neurodevelopmental outcome of preterm infants with severe intraventricular hemorrhage and therapy for post-hemorrhagic ventricular dilatation. *J Pediatr* 2008; **152**: 648–54.

64. Vohr BR, Garcia-Coll C, Flanagan P, et al. Effects of intraventricular hemorrhage and socioeconomic status on perceptual, cognitive, and neurologic status of low birth weight infants at 5 years of age. *J Pediatr* 1992; **121**: 280–5.

65. Vasileiadis GT, Gelman N, Han VK, et al. Uncomplicated intraventricular hemorrhage is followed by reduced cortical volume at near-term age. *Pediatrics* 2004; **114**: e367–72.

66. Patra K, Wilson-Costello D, Taylor HG, et al. Grades I–II intraventricular hemorrhage in extremely low birth weight infants: effects on neurodevelopment. *J Pediatr* 2006; **149**: 169–73.

67. Vavasseur C, Slevin M, Donoghue V, et al. Effect of low grade intraventricular hemorrhage on developmental outcome of preterm infants. *J Pediatr* 2007; **151**: e6–7.

68. Kuban K, Sanocka U, Leviton A, et al. White matter disorders of prematurity: association with intraventricular hemorrhage and ventriculomegaly. The Developmental Epidemiology Network. *J Pediatr* 1999; **134**: 539–46.

69. Ment LR, Vohr B, Allan W, et al. The etiology and outcome of ventriculomegaly at term in very low birth weight infants. *Pediatrics* 1999; **104**: 243–8.

70. Fernell E, Hagberg G, Hagberg B. Infantile hydrocephalus in preterm, low-birth-weight infants: a nationwide Swedish cohort study 1979–1988. *Acta Paediatr* 1993; **82**: 45–8.

71. Persson EK, Hagberg G, Uvebrant P. Disabilities in children with hydrocephalus: a population-based study of children aged between four and twelve years. *Neuropediatrics* 2006; **37**: 330–6.

72. Rademaker KJ, Groenendaal F, Jansen GH, et al. Unilateral haemorrhagic parenchymal lesions in the preterm infant: shape, site and prognosis. *Acta Paediatr* 1994; **83**: 602–28.

73. Guzzetta F, Shackleford GD, Volpe S, et al. Periventricular echodensities in the newborn period: critical determinant of neurologic outcome. *Pediatrics* 1986; **78**: 955–1006.

74. Sherlock RL, Synnes AR, Grunau RE, et al. Long-term outcome after neonatal intraparenchymal echodensities with porencephaly. *Arch Dis Child Fetal Neonatal Ed* 2008; **93**: F127–31.

75. De Vries LS, Groenendaal F, Eken P, et al. Asymmetrical myelination of the posterior limb of the internal capsule: an early predictor of hemiplegia. *Neuropediatrics* 1999; **30**: 314–19.

76. Cowan FM, de Vries LS. The internal capsule in neonatal imaging. *Semin Fetal Neonatal Med* 2005; **10**: 461–74.

77. Counsell SJ, Dyet LE, Larkman DJ, et al. Thalamo-cortical connectivity in children born preterm mapped using probabilistic magnetic resonance tractography. *Neuroimage* 2007; **34**: 896–904.

78. Staudt M, Braun C, Gerloff C, et al. Developing somatosensory projections bypass periventricular brain lesions. *Neurology* 2006; **67**: 522–5.

79. Crowley P. Prophylactic corticosteroids for preterm delivery. *Cochrane Database Syst Rev* 2000; (2): CD000065.

80. Roberts D, Dalziel S. Antenatal corticosteroids for accelerating fetal lung maturation for women at risk of preterm birth. *Cochrane Database Syst Rev* 2006; (3): CD004454.

81. Modi N, Lewis H, Al-Naqeeb N, et al. The effects of repeated antenatal glucocorticoid therapy on the brain. *Pediatr Res* 2001; **50**: 581–5.

82. Baud O, Foix-L'Helias L, Kaminski M, et al. Antenatal glucocorticoid treatment and cystic periventricular leukomalacia in very premature infants. *N Engl J Med* 1999; **341**: 1190–6.

83. Crowther CA, Hiller JE, Doyle LW, et al. Effect of magnesium sulfate given for neuroprotection before preterm birth. *JAMA* 2003; **290**: 2669–76.

84. Rouse DJ, Hirtz DG, Thom E, et al. A randomized controlled trial of magnesium sulfate for the prevention of cerebral palsy. *N Engl J Med* 2008; **359**: 895–905.

85. Morales WJ, Angel JL, O'Brien WF, et al. The use of antenatal vitamin K in the prevention of early neonatal intraventricular hemorrhage. *Am J Obstet Gynecol* 1988; **159**: 774–9.

86. Pomerance JJ, Teal JG, Gogolok JF, et al. Maternally administered antenatal vitamin K1: effect on neonatal prothrombin activity, partial thromboplastic time, and intraventricular hemorrhage. *Obstet Gynecol* 1987; **70**: 235–41.

87. Crowther CA, Henderson-Smart DJ. Vitamin K prior to birth for preventing neonatal periventricular hemorrhage. *Cochrane Database Syst Rev* 2001; (1): CD000229.

88. Whitelaw A, Odd D. Postnatal phenobarbital for the prevention of intraventricular hemorrhage in preterm infants. *Cochrane Database Syst Rev* 2007; (4): CD001691.

89. Fowlie PW, Davis PG. Prophylactic indomethacin for preterm infants: a systematic review and meta-analysis. *Arch Dis Child Fetal Neonatal Ed* 2003; **88**: F464–6.

90. Schmidt B, Davis P, Moddeman D, et al. Trial of indomethacin prophylaxis in preterm investigators: long-term effects of indomethacin prophylaxis in extremely-low-birth-weight infants. *N Eng J Med* 2001; **344**: 1966–72.

91. Ment LR, Peterson BS, Meltzer JA, et al. A functional magnetic resonance imaging study of the long-term influences of early indomethacin exposure on language processing in the brains of prematurely born children. *Pediatrics* 2006; **118**: 961–70.

92. Dani C, Bertini G, Pezzati M, et al. Prophylactic ibuprofen for the prevention of intraventricular hemorrhage among preterm infants: a multicenter, randomized study. *Pediatrics* 2005; **115**: 1529–35.

93. Wells JT, Ment LR. Prevention of intraventricular haemorrhage in preterm infants. *Early Hum Dev* 1995; **42**: 209–33.

94. Synnes AR, Macnab YC, Qiu Z, et al. Neonatal intensive care unit characteristics affect the incidence of severe intraventricular hemorrhage. *Med Care* 2006; **44**: 754–9.

95. Wu YW, Hamrick SEG, Miller SP, et al. Intraventricular hemorrhage in term neonates caused by sinovenous thrombosis. *Ann Neurol* 2003; **54**: 123–6.

96. Roland EH, Flodmark O, Hill A. Thalamic hemorrhagic with intraventricular hemorrhage in the full term newborn. *Pediatrics* 1990; **85**: 737–42.

97. Jocelyn LJ, Casiro OG. Neurodevelopmental outcome of term infants with intraventricular hemorrhage. *Am J Dis Child* 1992; **146**: 194–7.

98. Hofmeyr GJ, Hannah ME. Planned caesarean section for term breech delivery. *Cochrane Database Syst Rev* 2003; (3): CD000166.

99. Volpe JJ. Intracranial hemorrhage: subdural, primary subarachnoid, intracerebellar, intraventricular (term infant), and miscellaneous. In Volpe JJ, ed., *Neurology of the Newborn*. Philadelphia, PA: Saunders. 2001: 397–427.

100. Hanigan WC, Powell FC, Miller TC, et al. Symptomatic intracranial hemorrhage in full-term infants. *Childs Nerv Syst* 1995; **11**: 698–707.

101. Govaert P, Vanhaesebrouck P, de Praeter C. Traumatic neonatal intracranial bleeding and stroke. *Arch Dis Child* 1992; **67**: 840–5.

102. Chamnanvanakij S, Rollins N, Perlman JM. Subdural hematoma in term infants. *Pediatr Neurol* 2002; **26**: 301–14.

103. Uchil D, Arulkumaran S. Neonatal subgaleal hemorrhage and its relationship to delivery by vacuum extraction. *Obstet Gynecol Surv* 2003; **58**: 687–93.

104. Chadwick LM, Pemberton PJ, Kurinczuk JJ. Neonatal subgaleal haematoma: associated risk factors, complications and outcome. *J Paediatr Child Health* 1996; **32**: 228–32.

105. Kilani RA, Wetmore J. Neonatal subgaleal hematoma: presentation and outcome. Radiological findings and factors associated with mortality. *Am J Perinatol* 2006; **23**: 41–8.

106. Chang HY, Peng CC, Kao HA, et al. Neonatal subgaleal hemorrhage: clinical presentation, treatment, and predictors of poor prognosis. *Pediatr Int* 2007; **49**: 903–7.

107. Dale ST, Coleman LT. Neonatal alloimmune thrombocytopenia: antenatal and postnatal imaging findings in the pediatric brain. *AJNR Am J Neuroradiol* 2002; **23**: 1457–65.

108. Bussel JB, Zavusky MR, Berkowitz RL, et al. Fetal alloimmune thrombocytopenia. *N Engl J Med* 1997; **337**: 22–6.

109. Hardart GE, Fackler JC. Predictors of intracranial hemorrhage during neonatal extracorporeal membrane oxygenation. *J Pediatr* 1999; **134**: 156–9.

110. Hardart GE, Hardart MKM, Arnold JH. Intracranial hemorrhage in premature neonates treated with extracorporeal membrane oxygenation correlates with conceptional age. *J Pediatr* 2004; **145**: 184–9.

111. Gannon CM, Kornhauser MS, Gross GW, et al. When combined, early bedside head ultrasound and electroencephalography predict abnormal computerized tomography or magnetic resonance brain images obtained after extracorporeal membrane oxygenation treatment. *J Perinatol* 2001; **21**: 451–5.

112. Bulas DI, Glass P, O'Donnell RM, et al. Neonates treated with ECMO: predictive value of early CT and US neuroimaging findings on short-term neurodevelopmental outcome. *Radiology* 1995; **195**: 407–12.

Chapter 25

Neonatal stroke

Hannah C. Glass and Donna M. Ferriero

Introduction

Perinatal stroke is increasingly recognized as an important cause of neurological morbidity including cerebral palsy, epilepsy, and behavioral disorders, as well as impaired visual function and language development [1–8]. The estimated incidence of perinatal stroke is approximately 1/4000 [9].

Perinatal stroke can be classified by blood supply (venous vs. arterial), age at stroke (fetal vs. neonatal), age at diagnosis (neonatal symptomatic vs. presumed perinatal/neonatal asymptomatic), or type of stroke (ischemic vs. hemorrhagic). Investigators have used a variety of terms, including "perinatal stroke," "arterial ischemic stroke," and "perinatal arterial stroke" to describe the conditions. A recent workshop of the National Institute of Child Health and Human Development and the National Institute of Neurological Disorders and Stroke focused on refining the terminology. *Ischemic perinatal stroke* (IPS), now the term of choice, is defined as "a group of heterogeneous conditions in which there is focal disruption of cerebral blood flow secondary to arterial or cerebral venous thrombosis or embolization, between 20 weeks of fetal life through the 28th postnatal day, confirmed by neuroimaging or neuropathologic studies."[10] The group further divided IPS into three categories based on the timing of diagnosis: (1) *fetal ischemic stroke*, diagnosed prior to birth using fetal imaging or following stillbirth on the basis of neuropathologic examination, (2) *neonatal ischemic stroke*, diagnosed after birth and $\leq$ 28th postnatal day (including preterm infants), and (3) *presumed perinatal ischemic stroke* (PPIS), diagnosed in children > 28 days of age in whom the ischemic event is presumed to have occurred between the 20th week of fetal life and the 28th postnatal day [10]. This terminology does not take into account venous thrombosis without ischemic infarction, or purely hemorrhagic conditions. Hemorrhagic perinatal stroke is less well characterized, and there is no consensus on terminology or classification.

Epidemiology

Perinatal stroke accounts for approximately 25% of arterial and 50% of cerebral sinovenous thrombosis (CSVT) in the pediatric population [4]. The incidence of neonatal stroke is estimated between 1/2300 and 1/5000 [9,11–13]. Approximately 2/3 of children with motor impairment due to perinatal stroke present after 3 months of age [14]. There are no apparent differences by infant sex or racial group, though data are somewhat inconsistent between study cohorts [9,12,13].

Clinical manifestations

The clinical manifestations of perinatal stroke depend on the timing of presentation (fetal, neonatal, or during infancy and childhood) and the extent of the brain involvement.

Fetal ischemic stroke

Fetal ischemic stroke is diagnosed prior to birth using ultrasound and/or magnetic resonance imaging (MRI) or following stillbirth on the basis of neuropathologic examination. Though typically asymptomatic to the mother and child before delivery, there is a high rate of pregnancy termination, preterm delivery, and neonatal complications including hypotonia and seizures [15].

Neonatal ischemic stroke

Neonatal ischemic stroke includes both arterial stroke and CSVT diagnosed after birth and before or on the 28th postnatal day. This category includes the special case of infants with ischemic stroke who were born prematurely.

Neonatal arterial stroke

Term newborn infants with arterial stroke most commonly present with persistent focal seizures in the first hours of life [16,17].

Infants may otherwise appear well, or have subtle motor asymmetry, generalized hypotonia, or, especially in the setting of concurrent global hypoxic–ischemic brain injury, signs of encephalopathy including depressed level of alertness, apnea, and altered feeding [3,18]. Motor asymmetry, if present, is typically subtle, though the infant's general movements are frequently abnormal [19].

Arterial infarcts are slightly more common in the left hemisphere than in the right hemisphere (Fig. 25.1). The stroke may involve small- or large-artery territory, and multiple infarcts are present in up to 20% of cases [4].

Neonatal cerebral sinovenous sinus thrombosis

Cerebral sinovenous thrombosis (CSVT) typically presents in the first weeks of life with non-specific signs and symptoms

Fetal and Neonatal Brain Injury, 4th edition, ed. David K. Stevenson, William E. Benitz, Philip Sunshine, Susan R. Hintz, and Maurice L. Druzin. Published by Cambridge University Press. © Cambridge University Press 2009.

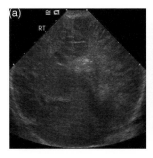
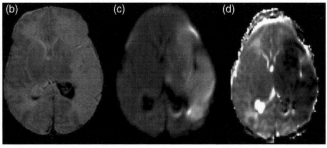

Fig. 25.1. Neonatal ischemic arterial stroke in a 2-day term infant with seizures at 36 hours of life. (a) High-resolution ultrasound through the anterior fontanel showing echogenic left thalamus, basal ganglia, and hemispheric white matter with mild mass effect effacing the left ventricle in keeping with left middle cerebral territory infarct. MRI showing (b) T2 prolongation and (c, d) reduced diffusion in the entire left middle cerebral area territory including cortex, basal ganglia, and caudate.

including encephalopathy, apnea, and seizures. Infants with CSVT frequently have comorbid risk factors, including dehydration, cardiac defects, sepsis, or meningitis, and extracorporeal life-support requirement [20–23].

Computed tomography, or magnetic resonance or conventional angiographic venography, may show that one or more venous structures is involved, most often the sagittal, transverse, and straight sinuses [20,23]. Common sequelae include venous infarction with parenchymal and intraventricular hemorrhage [20,24,25].

Neonatal ischemic stroke in the preterm infant

Increased use of imaging in premature infants has led to greater recognition of arterial stroke prior to term-equivalent post-menstrual age. The clinical presentation in premature infants is very different from that of term infants, with less than one-third presenting with seizures or apnea. Premature infants with stroke are most often identified during routine cranial ultrasound monitoring, with the diagnosis later confirmed using MRI [26]. As with term gestation infants, arterial stroke in premature newborns is more often unilateral, in the middle cerebral artery territory distribution and left-sided. Lenticulostriate distribution is common, especially in infants born at 28–32 weeks' gestation [27]. Twin-to-twin transfusion syndrome, fetal heart rate abnormalities, and hypoglycemia appear to be risk factors for preterm arterial stroke [28].

Presumed perinatal ischemic stroke

Presumed perinatal ischemic stroke (PPIS) is diagnosed in a child > 28 days with a normal neonatal period who presents with non-acute neurological signs or symptoms (typically pathological hand preference, hemiplegia, or seizures in the first 4–12 months of life) referable to focal, remote (gliosis, encephalomalacia, and/or atrophy and absent restricted diffusion) infarct(s) on neuroimaging [10,29]. PPIS may be due to either arterial or venous infarction, but excludes global injuries such as periventricular leukomalacia and basal ganglia or watershed injury due to hypoxic–ischemic injury [29–31].

Hemorrhagic stroke

Perinatal hemorrhagic stroke has received little attention, although, according to a recent population-based study, the

population incidence (6.2/100 000) is similar to the incidence of subarachnoid hemorrhage in adults [32]. In this same study, neonates with hemorrhagic stroke presented with encephalopathy or seizures, and strokes were typically unilateral and in the frontal or parietal lobes. Fetal distress and post-term delivery > 41 weeks were both independently associated with neonatal hemorrhage. Type IV collagen α1 mutation is a risk factor for intracerebral hemorrhage and may play a role in porencephaly due to in utero hemorrhagic stroke, though the relationship with neonatal hemorrhagic stroke in humans is unclear [33–35].

Risk factors

The etiology and pathogenesis of perinatal stroke are not well understood. Multiple potential risk factors have been recognized through case series and reports, as well as population-based epidemiological studies. Frequently, multiple concurrent risk factors are present and, in one study, the presence of multiple risk factors before delivery significantly increased the risk of perinatal stroke [12]. It is important to note that the majority of infants with one or more risk factors for stroke are entirely normal, and that, conversely, in many cases, no risk factor for the stroke is identified.

Maternal factors

Maternal acquired and inherited thrombophilias are an important risk factor for perinatal stroke. Pregnancy itself is a physiologic prothrombotic and proinflammatory state for the mother and her child [36]. Antiphospholipid antibodies (lupus anticoagulant and cardiolipin antibody) present in women with systemic lupus erythematosis or other autoimmune disorders increase the risk for fetal loss and for ischemic perinatal stroke [37–39]. Inherited thrombophilias may be present in either the mother or her child with perinatal stroke, and are further discussed under infant factors.

Hypertensive disorders of pregnancy, and specifically eclampsia and pre-eclampsia, are associated with a higher risk of neonatal stroke [12,40]. The pathophysiology may be related to a high frequency of factor V Leiden mutation in women with pre-eclampsia and with HELLP (hemolytic anemia, elevated liver enzymes, and low platelet count) syndrome [41].

Further maternal risk factors for perinatal stroke include a history of infertility and primiparity [12], whereas obesity, older maternal age, family history of thromboemboblic events, surgery, dehydration, shock, and prolonged bed rest are all risk factors for maternal thrombosis [42]. Maternal cocaine use is a rare but important cause of ischemic perinatal stroke [43,44].

Antepartum and intrapartum factors

Independent risk factors that may occur during pregnancy and delivery include oligohydramnios, cord abnormality, chorioamnionitis, and prolonged rupture of membranes [12].

Infant factors

A number of systemic illnesses or conditions may increase the risk of stroke in the newborn infant. Several prothrombotic disorders have been reported in infants with stroke, including protein S, protein C, and antithrombin III deficiencies, elevated lipoprotein(a), antiphospholipid antibodies, factor V G1691A, prothrombin G20210A, MTHFR mutations, and elevated homocysteine [39,45–50]. However, many of these prothrombotic disorders are seen with high frequency in the general population and, conversely, some infants with stroke have no detectable abnormality [51]. Therefore, the exact role of thrombophilia in the pathophysiology of perinatal stroke remains uncertain. Meningitis/encephalitis, polycythemia, congenital heart disease, and extracorporeal membrane oxygenation have all been reported in infants with stroke [52–56].

Evaluation

History and physical examination

The history and physical examination are important in the initial evaluation of an infant with suspected stroke (Table 25.1). Detailed family history, as well as evaluation of maternal medical conditions and events during pregnancy and delivery, may reveal one or more risk factors for perinatal stroke. The initial infant examination is often normal, though there may be subtle signs of hemiparesis or abnormal general movements.

Neuroimaging

Magnetic resonance imaging (MRI) is the study of choice for the diagnosis and evaluation of perinatal stroke. Cranial ultrasound with transcranial Doppler may detect obliteration of normal gyral patterns, echogenicity in an arterial territory distribution, mass effect, or decrease in cerebral artery flow velocities in the affected hemisphere [57,58]. However, cranial ultrasound is less sensitive than other imaging modalities and should be supplemented with computed tomography (CT), or preferably MRI, when available [59,60]. CT has the advantage of being readily available, and it can often be performed without sedation. However, it provides less detailed anatomy than MRI and exposes the infant to ionizing radiation.

Restricted water motion on diffusion-weighted imaging (DWI) sequences is apparent shortly after the injury but becomes falsely negative (pseudonormalizes) by approximately 7 days [61,62]. Conventional T1- and T2-weighted sequences

Table 25.1. Evaluation and investigation of perinatal stroke

Investigation	Comment
History	
Family	Careful history may reveal one or more risk factors for perinatal stroke
Maternal	
Pregnancy	
Delivery	
Imaging	
Magnetic resonance imaging (MRI)	MRI with diffusion weighted imaging is the imaging study of choice
Computed tomography	
Cranial ultrasound	
Laboratory evaluation	
Complete blood count with differential	Thrombophilia evaluation can be performed in the mother and child in the acute and convalescent periods
Prothrombin time with international normalized ratio (PT/INR)	
Partial thromboplastin time (PTT)	
Serum electrolytes and glucose	
Protein S/C and antithrombin III activity	
Activated protein C resistance	
Lipoprotein(a)	
Homocysteine	
Factor V Leiden	
Prothrombin 20210A	
Antiphospholipid antibody testing	
Other	
Electroencephalogram	Further evaluation can be tailored to the nature and timing of the insult
Cardiac echocardiogram	

may be normal in the first 48 hours, making 2–5 days of life an ideal time to image the infant with stroke. In cases of suspected CSVT, vascular imaging (magnetic resonance venography, MRV) with or without gadolinium contrast is essential to accurately diagnose and follow venous thrombosis [23,63].

In cases of presumed perinatal ischemic stroke, conventional T1- and T2-weighted images may reveal signs of remote infarct, including absent restricted diffusion, cystic encephalomalacia, gliosis, focal ventricular dilation, and Wallerian degeneration of the descending corticospinal tracts (Figs. 25.2, 25.3) [29,30,64,65].

Electroencephalography

Recurrent focal seizure is the most common initial presentation of neonatal stroke [17]. An electroencephalogram (EEG)

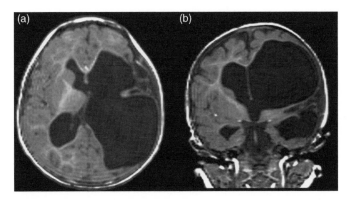

Fig. 25.2. Chronic T1 appearance of the infarct seen in Fig. 25.1. (a) Axial and (b) coronal images show a large porencephalic cyst that encompasses the left middle cerebral artery territory and causes mass effect with midline shift and expansion of the left hemicalvarium.

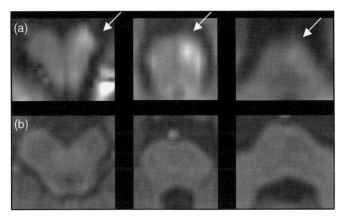

Fig. 25.3. (a) Acute appearance of diffusion-weighted imaging and (b) chronic T1 changes in midbrain and pons of the patient seen in Figs. 25.1 and 25.2. Note that the areas of reduced diffusion (arrows) show later Wallerian degeneration on the T1 images.

is essential to evaluate for subclinical seizures (especially after administration of antiseizure medication, which may lead to electroclinical dissociation) and to identify background abnormalities, which indicate poor neuromotor prognosis [3,66]. EEG abnormalities, including focal attenuation, epileptiform discharges, and/or focal seizures, are typically transient and present only during the first days to weeks after the injury [67].

Laboratory studies

Initial laboratory evaluation should include studies that are routinely performed in an infant with seizures or encephalopathy, such as complete blood count with differential electrolytes (including calcium and magnesium), glucose levels, prothrombin time with international normalized ratio, partial thromboplastin, as well as cultures for infection. Once ischemic stroke is confirmed by imaging, the infant and mother can be investigated for thrombophilia, both in the acute period and again at 3 months, though the results are unlikely to change management [68]. Transthoracic echocardiogram should be performed in infants with abnormal cardiac examination or suspected embolic infarct to exclude underlying cardiac disease.

Management

During the acute phase of perinatal stroke, excellent supportive care is important to minimize secondary brain injury. While there are no data from human neonatal trials, animal and adult studies support active maintenance of physiologic homeostasis, including temperature and blood glucose levels [69,70]. Expert opinion supports aggressive treatment of clinical and electrographic seizures that are frequent and/or prolonged [71].

The value of antithrombotic therapy in neonates with ischemic stroke is uncertain, and guidelines or recommendations are based on clinical experience in older populations, observational or case studies, and clinical consensus. Guidelines by the American College of Chest Physicians recommend 3 months of anticoagulation with unfractionated or low-molecular-weight heparin for infants with cardioembolic arterial stroke or CSVT and without large-territory involvement or hemorrhage [72]. Antithrombotic therapy is not suggested for non-cardioembolic neonatal arterial stroke. For infants with CSVT who are not treated with antithrombotic therapy, imaging should be repeated at 1 week to look for propagation of the thrombosis. Infants with CSVT who are treated with antithrombotic therapy should be imaged again at 3 months to ensure complete recanalization of the venous sinuses [72]. In the Canadian Registry of perinatal stroke, 25–30% of neonates with arterial stroke or CSVT were treated with antithrombotic therapy [4,23]. There were no cases of death or neurologic complication due to hemorrhage, but the impact of treatment on outcome is unknown.

Chronic treatment for cerebral palsy due to perinatal stroke diagnosed either in the neonatal period or retrospectively involves traditional rehabilitation with passive stretching, splinting, and casting, as well as medical or surgical treatment for spasticity including baclofen, tendon release surgery, or botulinum toxin A [73]. Constraint-induced movement therapy (CIMT), which involves restraint of the non-affected limb and frequent repetition of manual therapeutic tasks with the affected limb, is a promising treatment approach for children with hemiplegic cerebral palsy. Emerging evidence from studies using functional MRI suggests changes in cortical activation with CIMT [74,75]; however, a recent Cochrane review concluded that there is only limited evidence of the clinical effect and suggested further trials to evaluate the efficacy of CIMT for hemiplegic children [76]. Children should also be monitored through school age to look for subtle signs of cognitive impairment, and referred for psychoeducational testing as needed.

Outcome

Neurodevelopmental outcome following perinatal stroke is extremely variable between studies due to a variety of factors including heterogeneity of the injury, variable duration of follow-up, and differences in outcome measures. Most studies suggest high risk for neurodevelopmental disability (including cerebral palsy, epilepsy, and behavioral disorders, as well as impaired visual function and language development) [1–8,77,78]. In one population-based study, 68% of children who presented in the neonatal period and 94% of children with delayed presentation were diagnosed with one or more disability [8].

In spite of high rates of neurological disabilities, many studies show that children who survive perinatal stroke have good functional outcome. This result may be due in part to high plasticity in the developing brain. Recent studies using functional MRI (fMRI) show bilateral or right-sided activation of language-area homologues in children with a history of left-hemisphere perinatal stroke [79,80].

Neuromotor outcome

Perinatal stroke is a common cause of hemiplegic cerebral palsy. Functional motor impairment is present in up to 30–40% of children examined after 12 months of age, and 30% have some asymmetry of tone without definite hemiplegia [1,3,8]. The risk of motor impairment is approximately twice as high in children who present after the neonatal period, which is not surprising, since many of these children are diagnosed following evaluation of pathologic handedness or evolving cerebral palsy [8,29]. In spite of the high frequency of motor abnormalities, the great majority of children with neonatal ischemic stroke achieve independent walking, especially in cases of unilateral infarct [75,79].

Predicting neuromotor outcome based on early clinical, EEG, and imaging features is important for providing prognostic information to families and facilitating rehabilitation. Furthermore, accurate early tools for predicting outcome may ultimately aid in selecting patients for therapeutic interventions. Stroke size and location are helpful in predicting neuromotor outcome. Infants with larger stroke size have a higher risk of hemiplegia, especially when there is injury to the motor cortex, basal ganglia, *and* posterior limb of the internal capsule [1,3,8]. Children with injury to only cortex, basal ganglia, or posterior limb of the internal capsule have a good chance of normal neuromotor outcome [1,3]. Neuromotor outcome is also highly correlated with the length and volume of diffusion change along the descending corticospinal tracts [65,82]. Early abnormal electroencephalogram background may also be helpful in predicting hemiparesis outcome, with 93% sensitivity and 100% specificity in one study [1].

Neonatal seizures and epilepsy

The incidence of epilepsy after perinatal stroke is variable, and probably depends not only on the nature of the lesion but also on the timing and duration of follow-up. Published rates of epilepsy after age 6 months range widely, from 0% to 67% [6,8,83–85]. In a recent study of 64 children with neonatal stroke and at least 6 months' follow-up, 67% developed seizures after age 6 months (median age 16 months), but most

were seizure-free with or without medication and only 11% of children had one or more seizures per month [85].

Neurobehavioral outcome

Cognitive outcome in children with perinatal arterial stroke or sinovenous thrombosis is variable, but often impaired. Some studies report "language delay" in up to 25–30% of children [8,29]. In a study of preschool children, average scores on the Mental Developmental Index of the Bayley Scales of Infant Development (whose normative mean is 100 and standard deviation 15) at age 24 months were in the low 90s (range 50s–120s) [5]. In school-age children, language development and intelligence quotient were lower in infants with unilateral hemispheric neonatal stroke than in with age-matched peers [86,87]. Interestingly, the side of the lesion (right vs. left hemisphere) did not appear to be an important factor in language development, whereas presence of seizures beyond the neonatal period was associated with worse outcome [87].

Behavioral abnormality was diagnosed by a physician in 11% of children who presented in the neonatal period and 35% of children with delayed presentation in one population-based study [8]. However, another study, using the Achenbach Child Behavior Checklist, found no evidence of clinically significant behavioral or emotional problems and no significant difference from controls after adjusting for intelligence quotient.

Visual function

Impairment of acuity, visual fields, or stereopsis was present in approximately 30% of school-age children with a history of perinatal stroke [2]. In this study, there was no relationship between lesions of the optic radiations or visual cortex and visual impairment, but larger middle cerebral artery lesions were more often associated with visual findings. Children presenting with congenital hemiplegia had a higher incidence of visual field defects [88,89].

Stroke recurrence

The rate of stroke recurrence following perinatal stroke is much lower than for childhood or adult stroke, which suggests that long-term prophylaxis is probably unwarranted in most cases. There were no recurrences in a population-based study that identified 40 children with perinatal stroke [8]. Most of the symptomatic recurrences (including extracerebral venous thrombosis) seen in a prospective cohort of 215 occurred in the context of congenital or acquired systemic illness [45].

Modeling stroke

Although mechanisms of ischemic injury in the developing nervous system have been studied in sheep and rodent models for over 20 years, it is only recently that animal models recapitulating stroke have been established [90–93]. It is clear from these newer models that mechanisms of neonatal stroke differ both from adult stroke and from global hypoxia–ischemia. For example, the blood–brain barrier breaks down early after injury in the mature brain, but in the transient ischemia–reperfusion model in the newborn rat the blood–brain barrier remains intact for over 48 hours [95]. This finding will influence the development of therapies, since the ability to cross the blood–brain barrier will greatly affect efficacy of a drug. In addition, although necrosis is a prominent feature of adult stroke, especially in the core of the lesion, in the newborn animal the core undergoes apoptotic cell death [95]. Again, these findings will influence the development of therapies, since cell injury may be reversible in larger areas of the newborn brain, and the cell death cascade is very different in apoptotic cell death (see Chapter 3 for mechanisms of ischemic injury). Although therapeutic hypothermia is moving toward standard of care for global hypoxia–ischemia, it is yet to be studied adequately in the setting of ischemia–reperfusion injury as seen in neonatal stroke.

References

1. Mercuri E, Barnett A, Rutherford M, *et al.* Neonatal cerebral infarction and neuromotor outcome at school age. *Pediatrics* 2004; **113**: 95–100.

2. Mercuri E, Anker S, Guzzetta A, *et al.* Neonatal cerebral infarction and visual function at school age. *Arch Dis Child Fetal Neonatal Ed* 2003; **88**: F487–91.

3. Mercuri E, Rutherford M, Cowan F, *et al.* Early prognostic indicators of outcome in infants with neonatal cerebral infarction: a clinical, electroencephalogram, and magnetic resonance imaging study. *Pediatrics* 1999; **103**: 39–46.

4. deVeber GA, MacGregor D, Curtis R, *et al.* Neurologic outcome in survivors of childhood arterial ischemic stroke and sinovenous thrombosis. *J Child Neurol* 2000; **15**: 316–24.

5. McLinden A, Baird AD, Westmacott R, *et al.* Early cognitive outcome after neonatal stroke. *J Child Neurol* 2007; **22**: 1111–16.

6. Sran SK, Baumann RJ. Outcome of neonatal strokes. *Am J Dis Child* 1988; **142**: 1086–8.

7. Sreenan C, Bhargava R, Robertson CM. Cerebral infarction in the term newborn: clinical presentation and long-term outcome. *J Pediatr* 2000; **137**: 351–5.

8. Lee J, Croen LA, Lindan C, *et al.* Predictors of outcome in perinatal arterial stroke: a population-based study. *Ann Neurol* 2005; **58**: 303–8.

9. Lynch JK, Nelson KB. Epidemiology of perinatal stroke. *Curr Opin Pediatr* 2001; **13**: 499–505.

10. Raju TN, Nelson KB, Ferriero D, *et al.* Ischemic perinatal stroke: summary of a workshop sponsored by the National Institute of Child Health and Human Development and the National Institute of Neurological Disorders and Stroke. *Pediatrics* 2007; **120**: 609–16.

11. Schulzke S, Weber P, Luetschg J, *et al.* Incidence and diagnosis of unilateral arterial cerebral infarction in newborn infants. *J Perinat Med* 2005; **33**: 170–5.

12. Lee J, Croen LA, Backstrand KH, *et al.* Maternal and infant characteristics associated with perinatal arterial stroke in the infant. *JAMA* 2005; **293**: 723–9.

13. Laugesaar R, Kolk A, Tomberg T, *et al.* Acutely and retrospectively diagnosed perinatal stroke: a population-based study. *Stroke* 2007; **38**: 2234–40.

14. Wu YW, March WM, Croen LA, *et al.* Perinatal stroke in children with motor impairment: a population-based study. *Pediatrics* 2004; **114**: 612–19.

15. Ozduman K, Pober BR, Barnes P, *et al.* Fetal stroke. *Pediatr Neurol* 2004; **30**: 151–62.

16. Levy SR, Abroms IF, Marshall PC, *et al.* Seizures and cerebral infarction in the full-term newborn. *Ann Neurol* 1985; **17**: 366–70.

17. Clancy R, Malin S, Laraque D, *et al.* Focal motor seizures heralding stroke in full-term neonates. *Am J Dis Child* 1985; **139**: 601–6.

18. Ramaswamy V, Miller SP, Barkovich AJ, *et al.* Perinatal stroke in term infants with neonatal encephalopathy. *Neurology* 2004; **62**: 2088–91.

19. Guzzetta A, Mercuri E, Rapisardi G, *et al.* General movements detect early signs of hemiplegia in term infants with neonatal cerebral infarction. *Neuropediatrics* 2003; **34**: 61–6.

20. Fitzgerald KC, Williams LS, Garg BP, *et al.* Cerebral sinovenous thrombosis in the neonate. *Arch Neurol* 2006; **63**: 405–9.

21. Wu YW, Miller SP, Chin K, *et al.* Multiple risk factors in neonatal sinovenous thrombosis. *Neurology* 2002; **59**: 438–40.

22. Fitzgerald KC, Golomb MR. Neonatal arterial ischemic stroke and sinovenous thrombosis associated with meningitis. *J Child Neurol* 2007; **22**: 818–22.

23. deVeber G, Andrew M, Adams C, *et al.* Cerebral sinovenous thrombosis in children. *N Engl J Med* 2001; **345**: 417–23.

24. Roland EH, Flodmark O, Hill A. Thalamic hemorrhage with intraventricular hemorrhage in the full-term newborn. *Pediatrics* 1990; **85**: 737–42.

25. Wu YW, Hamrick SE, Miller SP, *et al.* Intraventricular hemorrhage in term neonates caused by sinovenous thrombosis. *Ann Neurol* 2003; **54**: 123–6.

26. Benders MJ, Groenendaal F, Uiterwaal CS, *et al.* Maternal and infant characteristics associated with perinatal arterial stroke in the preterm infant. *Stroke* 2007; **38**: 1759–65.

27. de Vries LS, Groenendaal F, Eken P, *et al.* Infarcts in the vascular distribution of the middle cerebral artery in preterm and fullterm infants. *Neuropediatrics* 1997; **28**: 88–96.

28. Groenendaal F, Benders MJ, de Vries LS. Pre-Wallerian degeneration in the neonatal brain following perinatal cerebral hypoxia–ischemia demonstrated with MRI. *Semin Perinatol* 2006; **30**: 146–50.

29. Golomb MR, MacGregor DL, Domi T, *et al.* Presumed pre- or perinatal arterial ischemic stroke: risk factors and outcomes. *Ann Neurol* 2001; **50**: 163–8.

30. Takanashi J, Barkovich AJ, Ferriero DM, *et al.* Widening spectrum of congenital hemiplegia: periventricular venous infarction in term neonates. *Neurology* 2003; **61**: 531–3.

31. Takanashi J, Tada H, Barkovich AJ, *et al.* Magnetic resonance imaging confirms periventricular venous infarction in a term-born child with congenital hemiplegia. *Dev Med Child Neurol* 2005; **47**: 706–8.

32. Armstrong-Wells J, Johnston CS, Wu YW, *et al.* Prevalence and predictors of perinatal hemorrhagic stroke. *Pediatrics* (in press).

33. Gould DB, Phalan FC, Breedveld GJ, *et al.* Mutations in Col4a1 cause perinatal cerebral hemorrhage and porencephaly. *Science* 2005; **308**: 1167–71.

34. Breedveld G, de Coo IF, Lequin MH, *et al.* Novel mutations in three families confirm a major role of COL4A1 in hereditary porencephaly. *J Med Genet* 2006; **43**: 490–5.

35. Gould DB, Phalan FC, van Mil SE, *et al.* Role of COL4A1 in small-vessel disease and hemorrhagic stroke. *N Engl J Med* 2006; **354**: 1489–96.

36. Arkel YS, Ku DH. Thrombophilia and pregnancy: review of the literature and some original data. *Clin Appl Thromb Hemost* 2001; **7**: 259–68.

37. Silver RK, MacGregor SN, Pasternak JF, *et al.* Fetal stroke associated with elevated maternal anticardiolipin antibodies. *Obstet Gynecol* 1992; **80**: 497–9.

38. Akanli LF, Trasi SS, Thuraisamy K, *et al.* Neonatal middle cerebral artery infarction: association with elevated maternal anticardiolipin antibodies. *Am J Perinatol* 1998; **15**: 399–402.

39. Gunther G, Junker R, Strater R, *et al.* Symptomatic ischemic stroke in full-term neonates: role of acquired and genetic prothrombotic risk factors. *Stroke* 2000; **31**: 2437–41.

40. Ballem P. Acquired thrombophilia in pregnancy. *Semin Thromb Hemost* 1998; **24**: 41–7.

41. Rigo J, Nagy B, Fintor L, *et al.* Maternal and neonatal outcome of preeclamptic pregnancies: the potential roles of factor V Leiden mutation and 5,10 methylenetetrahydrofolate reductase. *Hypertens Pregnancy* 2000; **19**: 163–72.

42. Hague WM, Dekker GA. Risk factors for thrombosis in pregnancy. *Best Pract Res Clin Haematol* 2003; **16**: 197–210.

43. Chasnoff IJ, Bussey ME, Savich R, *et al.* Perinatal cerebral infarction and maternal cocaine use. *J Pediatr* 1986; **108**: 456–9.

44. Heier LA, Carpanzano CR, Mast J, *et al.* Maternal cocaine abuse: the spectrum of radiologic abnormalities in the neonatal CNS. *AJNR Am J Neuroradiol* 1991; **12**: 951–6.

45. Kurnik K, Kosch A, Strater R, *et al.* Recurrent thromboembolism in infants and children suffering from symptomatic neonatal arterial stroke: a prospective follow-up study. *Stroke* 2003; **34**: 2887–92.

46. Brenner B, Fishman A, Goldsher D, *et al.* Cerebral thrombosis in a newborn with a congenital deficiency of antithrombin III. *Am J Hematol* 1988; **27**: 209–11.

47. Hogeveen M, Blom HJ, Van Amerongen M, *et al.* Hyperhomocysteinemia as risk factor for ischemic and hemorrhagic stroke in newborn infants. *J Pediatr* 2002; **141**: 429–31.

48. Garoufi AJ, Prassouli AA, Attilakos AV, *et al.* Homozygous MTHFR C677T gene mutation and recurrent stroke in an infant. *Pediatr Neurol* 2006; **35**: 49–51.

49. Curry CJ, Bhullar S, Holmes J, *et al.* Risk factors for perinatal arterial stroke: a study of 60 mother–child pairs. *Pediatr Neurol* 2007; **37**: 99–107.

50. Lynch JK, Han CJ, Nee LE, *et al.* Prothrombotic factors in children with stroke or porencephaly. *Pediatrics* 2005; **116**: 447–53.

51. Miller SP, Wu YW, Lee J, *et al.* Candidate gene polymorphisms do not differ between newborns with stroke and normal controls. *Stroke* 2006; **37**: 2678–83.

52. Ment LR, Ehrenkranz RA, Duncan CC. Bacterial meningitis as an etiology of perinatal cerebral infarction. *Pediatr Neurol* 1986; **2**: 276–9.

53. Amit M, Camfield PR. Neonatal polycythemia causing multiple cerebral infarcts. *Arch Neurol* 1980; **37**: 109–10.

54. Konishi Y, Kuriyama M, Sudo M, *et al.* Superior sagittal sinus thrombosis in neonates. *Pediatr Neurol* 1987; **3**: 222–5.

55. Jarjour IT, Ahdab-Barmada M. Cerebrovascular lesions in infants and children dying after extracorporeal membrane oxygenation. *Pediatr Neurol* 1994; **10**: 13–19.

56. Pellicer A, Cabanas F, Garcia-Alix A, *et al.* Stroke in neonates with cardiac right-to-left shunt. *Brain Dev* 1992; **14**: 381–5.

57. Hernanz-Schulman M, Cohen W, Genieser NB. Sonography of cerebral infarction in infancy. *AJR Am J Roentgenol* 1988; **150**: 897–902.

58. Messer J, Haddad J, Casanova R. Transcranial Doppler evaluation of cerebral infarction in the neonate. *Neuropediatrics* 1991; **22**: 147–51.

59. Golomb MR, Dick PT, MacGregor DL, *et al.* Cranial ultrasonography has a low sensitivity for detecting arterial ischemic stroke in term neonates. *J Child Neurol* 2003; **18**: 98–103.

60. Cowan F, Mercuri E, Groenendaal F, *et al.* Does cranial ultrasound imaging identify arterial cerebral infarction in term neonates? *Arch Dis Child Fetal Neonatal Ed* 2005; **90**: F252–6.

61. Mader I, Schoning M, Klose U, *et al.* Neonatal cerebral infarction diagnosed by diffusion-weighted MRI: pseudonormalization occurs early. *Stroke* 2002; **33**: 1142–5.

62. Kuker W, Mohrle S, Mader I, *et al.* MRI for the management of neonatal cerebral infarctions: importance of timing. *Childs Nerv Syst* 2004; **20**: 742–8.

63. Shroff M, deVeber G. Sinovenous thrombosis in children. *Neuroimaging Clin N Am* 2003; **13**: 115–38.

64. De Vries LS, Van der Grond J, Van Haastert IC, *et al.* Prediction of outcome in new-born infants with arterial ischaemic stroke using diffusion-weighted magnetic resonance imaging. *Neuropediatrics* 2005; **36**: 12–20.

65. Kirton A, Deveber G, Pontigon AM, *et al.* Presumed perinatal ischemic stroke: vascular classification predicts outcomes. *Ann Neurol* 2008; **63**: 436–43.

66. Weiner SP, Painter MJ, Geva D, *et al.* Neonatal seizures: electroclinical dissociation. *Pediatr Neurol* 1991; **7**: 363–8.

67. Scher MS, Wiznitzer M, Bangert BA. Cerebral infarctions in the fetus and neonate: maternal–placental–fetal considerations. *Clin Perinatol* 2002; **29**: 693–724, vi–vii.

68. Chalmers EA. Perinatal stroke: risk factors and management. *Br J Haematol* 2005; **130**: 333–43.

69. Baird TA, Parsons MW, Phanh T, *et al.* Persistent poststroke hyperglycemia is independently associated with infarct expansion and worse clinical outcome. *Stroke* 2003; **34**: 2208–14.

70. Vannucci RC, Mujsce DJ. Effect of glucose on perinatal hypoxic–ischemic brain damage. *Biol Neonate* 1992; **62**: 215–24.

71. Clancy RR. Prolonged electro-encephalogram monitoring for seizures and their treatment. *Clin Perinatol* 2006; **33**: 649–65, vi.

72. Monagle P, Chan A, Massicotte P, *et al.* Antithrombotic therapy in children: the Seventh ACCP Conference on Antithrombotic and Thrombolytic Therapy. *Chest* 2004; **126**: 645S–687S.

73. Jones MW, Morgan E, Shelton JE. Primary care of the child with cerebral palsy: a review of systems (part II). *J Pediatr Health Care* 2007; **21**: 226–37.

74. Juenger H, Linder-Lucht M, Walther M, *et al.* Cortical neuromodulation by constraint-induced movement therapy in congenital hemiparesis: an FMRI study. *Neuropediatrics* 2007; **38**: 130–6.

75. Sutcliffe TL, Gaetz WC, Logan WJ, *et al.* Cortical reorganization after modified constraint-induced movement therapy in pediatric hemiplegic cerebral palsy. *J Child Neurol* 2007; **22**: 1281–7.

76. Hoare BJ, Wasiak J, Imms C, *et al.* Constraint-induced movement therapy in the treatment of the upper limb in children with hemiplegic cerebral palsy.

Cochrane Database Syst Rev 2007; (2): CD004149.

77. Trauner DA, Chase C, Walker P, *et al.* Neurologic profiles of infants and children after perinatal stroke. *Pediatr Neurol* 1993; **9**: 383–6.

78. Wulfeck BB, Trauner DA, Tallal PA. Neurologic, cognitive, and linguistic features of infants after early stroke. *Pediatr Neurol* 1991; **7**: 266–9.

79. Tillema JM, Byars AW, Jacola LM, *et al.* Cortical reorganization of language functioning following perinatal left MCA stroke. *Brain Lang* 2008; **105**: 99–111.

80. Jacola LM, Schapiro MB, Schmithorst VJ, *et al.* Functional magnetic resonance imaging reveals atypical language organization in children following perinatal left middle cerebral artery stroke. *Neuropediatrics* 2006; **37**: 46–52.

81. Golomb MR, deVeber GA, MacGregor DL, *et al.* Independent walking after neonatal arterial ischemic stroke and sinovenous thrombosis. *J Child Neurol* 2003; **18**: 530–6.

82. Kirton A, Shroff M, Visvanathan T, *et al.* Quantified corticospinal tract diffusion restriction predicts neonatal stroke outcome. *Stroke* 2007; **38**: 974–80.

83. Koelfen W, Freund M, Varnholt V. Neonatal stroke involving the middle cerebral artery in term infants: clinical presentation, EEG and imaging studies, and outcome. *Dev Med Child Neurol* 1995; **37**: 204–12.

84. Estan J, Hope P. Unilateral neonatal cerebral infarction in full term infants. *Arch Dis Child Fetal Neonatal Ed* 1997; **76**: F88–93.

85. Golomb MR, Garg BP, Carvalho KS, *et al.* Perinatal stroke and the risk of developing childhood epilepsy. *J Pediatr* 2007; **151**: 409–13.e2.

86. Trauner DA, Nass R, Ballantyne A. Behavioural profiles of children and adolescents after pre- or perinatal unilateral brain damage. *Brain* 2001; **124**: 995–1002.

87. Hetherington R, Tuff L, Anderson P, *et al.* Short-term intellectual outcome after arterial ischemic stroke and sinovenous thrombosis in childhood and infancy. *J Child Neurol* 2005; **20**: 553–9.

88. Mercuri E, Spano M, Bruccini G, *et al.* Visual outcome in children with congenital hemiplegia: correlation with MRI findings. *Neuropediatrics* 1996; **27**: 184–8.

89. Guzzetta A, Fazzi B, Mercuri E, *et al.* Visual function in children with hemiplegia in the first years of life. *Dev Med Child Neurol* 2001; **43**: 321–9.

90. Wen TC, Rogido M, Gressens P, *et al.* A reproducible experimental model of focal cerebral ischemia in the neonatal rat. *Brain Res Brain Res Protoc* 2004; **13**: 76–83.

91. Derugin N, Ferriero DM, Vexler ZS. Neonatal reversible focal cerebral ischemia: a new model. *Neurosci Res* 1998; **32**: 349–53.

92. Renolleau S, Aggoun-Zouaoui D, Ben-Ari Y, *et al.* A model of transient unilateral focal ischemia with reperfusion in the P7 neonatal rat: morphological changes indicative of apoptosis. *Stroke* 1998; **29**: 1454–61.

93. Wen TC, Rogido M, Genetta T, *et al.* Permanent focal cerebral ischemia activates erythropoietin receptor in the neonatal rat brain. *Neurosci Lett* 2004; **355**: 165–8.

94. Wendland M, Manabat C, Fox CK, *et al.* The blood–brain barrier is more preserved in neonatal versus adult rats following transient focal cerebral ischemia. *J Cereb Blood Flow Metab* 2003; **23**: 169.

95. Manabat C, Han BH, Wendland M, *et al.* Reperfusion differentially induces caspase-3 activation in ischemic core and penumbra after stroke in immature brain. *Stroke* 200; **34**: 207–13.

Chapter 26

Hypoglycemia in the neonate

Satish C. Kalhan, Robert Schwartz, and Marvin Cornblath

Introduction

The mammalian fetus, in utero, is entirely dependent upon the mother for a continuous supply of glucose and other nutrients. Data from a number of studies in humans and animals have shown that under physiological circumstances there is no measurable production of glucose by the fetus, and that the entire glucose pool in the fetal compartment is derived from the mother [1,2]. The transition from the intrauterine environment to an independent extrauterine life is associated with a number of metabolic and hormonal responses, which allow the vast majority of neonates to adapt to the extrauterine environment without any problem. Among the key events involved in this adaptation is the initiation of systemic glucose production, both from glycogenolysis and gluconeogenesis, in the period immediately after birth [1,2]. Failure to adapt, as a consequence of alterations in maternal metabolism such as in diabetes in pregnancy, or as a consequence of metabolic problems in the neonate, may result in perturbations in glucose homeostasis leading to low blood glucose concentrations or hypoglycemia. It should be underscored that, during the initial period after birth, there is a decline in plasma glucose concentration from the cord blood levels in all infants, followed by an increase to a steady-state concentration. Although in the majority of infants this decrease in blood glucose concentration may be transient and inconsequential, in others it may be profound or persistent and lead to clinically serious problems involving significant neurological injury.

Definition

Several different approaches have been used to define clinically significant hypoglycemia in the newborn infant [3–8]. These have been based upon (1) clinical signs, (2) statistical analysis of glucose concentrations measured in large groups of infants, i.e., glucose levels more than 2 SD below the mean, (3) acute changes in metabolic and endocrine responses and neurological function, and (4) long-term neurological outcome. None of these methods has been entirely satisfactory. The first, based upon clinical manifestations, is confounded by the fact that similar clinical signs can occur with a number of clinical problems in the newborn infant, and they are not correlated with plasma glucose concentration. The second approach is an artificial statistical analysis without any relation to biology, and assumes that a plasma glucose level below a certain statistically defined value is likely to cause harm or requires intervention [3,5–7]. The approach relating endocrine and hormone responses is not easy to establish in the newborn infant because of ethical considerations. The currently established definitions are based on very few data [9]. The data correlating long-term neurological sequelae are also confounded because of the lack of suitable normal controls, the small number of infants followed, and failure to consider the impact of other associated clinical problems [10,11]. Finally, all of these approaches assume the relation between plasma glucose concentration and clinical manifestations or cellular metabolic changes as a threshold effect, i.e., below a given glucose concentration, brain injury would occur. However, from a physiological perspective this is not likely.

Because of these problems with definition, Cornblath *et al.* have suggested the use of "operational thresholds" or levels of plasma glucose concentration at which clinical intervention may be considered [12]. These values were suggested based upon the contemporary physiological and clinical data. During the first 24 hours of age, in both term and premature infants, a plasma glucose concentration less than 45 mg/dL (2.5 mmol/L) may be considered to be "hypoglycemia." This definition provides an indication to raise and sustain the plasma glucose levels to above 45–50 mg/dL (2.5–2.78 mmol/L). These glucose levels are similar to the fetal plasma glucose concentration in utero. Beyond 24 hours of age, the threshold value of plasma glucose concentration may be increased to 45–50 mg/dL (2.5–2.78 mmol/L). Values below this range are an indication to clinically intervene; however, they do not necessarily imply pathological neuroglucopenia or potential risk for neurologic damage.

In clinically symptomatic infants, a plasma glucose concentration of 45 mg/dL (2.5 mmol/L) or less should be considered as the threshold for intervention. In asymptomatic babies and those at risk for hypoglycemia, irrespective of gestational or postnatal age, a plasma glucose concentration less than 36 mg/dL (2.0 mmol/L) should be considered as the threshold value. Since exclusively breastfed babies maintain lower plasma glucose concentrations and higher concentrations of ketone bodies than formula-fed infants, the above

Fetal and Neonatal Brain Injury, 4th edition, ed. David K. Stevenson, William E. Benitz, Philip Sunshine, Susan R. Hintz, and Maurice L. Druzin. Published by Cambridge University Press. © Cambridge University Press 2009.

threshold values may not be applicable to them [3,13]. These infants may well tolerate lower plasma glucose levels without any significant clinical manifestation or sequelae.

There are no recent data to support the adoption of different threshold values for preterm infants. Infants on parenteral nutrition often have higher plasma insulin secretion due to the β-cell stimulatory effect of administered glucose and amino acids. The higher insulin levels will also result in suppression of lipolysis and therefore lower concentration of alternative fuels, i.e., ketones and fatty acids.

Hypoglycemia and the brain

The relationship between low plasma glucose concentration and clinical brain injury has been difficult to discern, especially in newborn infants, because of a number of confounding factors, in particular acute or chronic hypoxemia in at-risk infants. The data from studies in animals have demonstrated that severe persistent hypoglycemia (severe enough to result in isoelectric EEG) certainly causes neuronal loss or damage. These studies, although extremely important for understanding the mechanism of hypoglycemia-induced neuronal injury, are not easily translated into clinical practice. This is because of the "protective" counter-regulatory responses in vivo leading to availability of the alternative fuels, i.e., ketones and lactate, for the energy metabolism of brain and thus possibly attenuating the effects of hypoglycemia. In addition, various confounding variables, both intrinsic, such as hypoxemia and other clinical disorders, and extrinsic, such as therapeutic interventions, make the clinical data, in spite of various statistical adjustments, extremely difficult to evaluate.

Cerebral glucose and oxygen uptake

The brain, along with the renal medulla and red and white blood cells, is the primary consumer of glucose in the body. Of these, the brain is quantitatively the major organ utilizing glucose in vivo. Detailed analyses of oxygen and glucose consumption by the brain under basal conditions in healthy infants have not been undertaken. Previous data had examined the arteriovenous differences and calculated the rate of glucose consumption by Fick's principle in anesthetized and unanesthetized children (summarized by Kalhan and Kiliç [14]). The estimated rate of glucose consumption by brain at 5 months of age (range 11 days–12 months, $n = 12$) was 27.2 µmol/100 g brain weight per minute. This rate of glucose consumption, if completely oxidized, was higher than the corresponding rate of oxygen consumption by the brain [15,16]. Although similar data are not available for the neonate, Kalhan and Kiliç estimated that based upon the brain weight (~ 399 g) and body weight (3.2 kg) of a full-term neonate, the estimated glucose consumption by the brain would correspond to ~ 8 mg/kg body weight per minute, a rate very similar to the endogenous rate of production of glucose [1,2].

The local cerebral metabolic rate of glucose (LCMRglc) has been quantified using $2-[^{18}F]$fluoro-2-deoxy-D-glucose (FDG) in combination with positron emission tomography (PET) [17,18]. FDG, like glucose, is transported across the blood–brain barrier by glucose transporters, and is taken up by the neurons and phosphorylated by hexokinase. However, unlike glucose, phosphorylated deoxyglucose (and FDG) is not metabolized further along the glycolytic pathway, and is trapped in the tissue. Thus, these studies quantify only the tissue uptake of glucose rather than the rate of metabolism or glycolysis by the organ or tissue. The estimated rates of glucose consumption by this technique are lower than those by the Fick principle [14–16]. The reasons for the discrepancy are not easily evident. Nevertheless, PET scanning provides a non-invasive method to examine the effects of altered metabolism. Kinnala and colleagues quantified the LCMRglc in eight infants after their hypoglycemia had been appropriately corrected [18]. At the time of PET study, the infants were 5.3 ± 6.2 days (mean $\pm$ SD) of age and their plasma glucose concentration was 4.3 ± 1.1 mmol/L. Their data were compared with eight control infants of comparable gestational age who were at risk for hypoxic–ischemic brain injury and were older at the time of study (30.8 ± 20.7 days). The post-conceptional age-adjusted LCMRglc for the whole brain was not different between the hypoglycemic (5.33 ± 0.60 µmol/100 g brain weight/min) and the controls (6.71 ± 0.60 µmol/100 g brain weight/min). The average MRglc in the cerebellum, frontal, temporal, and occipital cortex did not differ amongst the groups. This was not surprising, because unless a pathological lesion with an altered rate of glucose metabolism had occurred as a consequence of hypoglycemic encephalopathy, no change in the metabolic rate of glucose should be expected following recovery from hypoglycemia when the patients are normoglycemic.

Studies in animals

Siesjo and associates have studied the effects of hypoglycemia alone on the electroencephalogram (EEG), brain energy metabolism, neurophysiology, and neuropathology in adult rats. Their elegant model was controlled for hypotension, anoxia, ischemia, and acidosis [19,20]. Their studies clearly indicated that both profound (EEG isoelectric, glucose 18 mg/dL: 1.0 mmol/L) and prolonged (~ 30 min) hypoglycemia were necessary to demonstrate cell necrosis in the brain. Hypoglycemic neuronal damage required that cellular energy states be perturbed, suggesting that cell necrosis was the consequence of energy failure and membrane depolarization. The energy failure was characterized by decreases in concentrations of phosphocreatine and adenosine phosphates; and membrane depolarization by an influx of calcium and an efflux of potassium, with an ensuing acceleration of proteolytic and lipolytic reactions.

The distribution of the hypoglycemic neuronal necrosis was unique, differed from that in ischemia or seizures, and suggested the involvement of a fluid-borne extracellular toxin as well. This could be an excitatory amino acid, such as glutamate or aspartate. These accelerated cell death by causing a dendrosomatic lesion attributed to calcium influx. Hypoglycemia in the newborn rat is also associated with increased activation of the cerebral N-methyl-D-aspartate (NMDA) receptor ion channel by glutamate [21]. In the neonatal pig, a prolonged period of profound hypoglycemia (10 mg/dL) and the presence of an isoelectric EEG (as in the adult rat) was necessary before there was glutamate release (an early marker of activation of the NMDA receptor ion channel) [22].

Vannucci and his collaborators have investigated the effects of hypoglycemia alone or in association with either hypoxemia (8% oxygen) or anoxia (100% nitrogen) in neonatal rats and puppies [23–25]. In contrast to the adult rat, newborn animals tolerated as long as 60–120 minutes of blood glucose concentrations under 18 mg/dL (1.0 mmol/L) without changes in behavior or untoward pathologic or pathophysiologic consequences. If then exposed to anoxia (100% nitrogen), hypoglycemic rats died sooner than normoglycemic rats (5 vs. 25 minutes). However, if they were given glucose prior to exposure to anoxia, no significant differences in survival times were noted [24].

In contrast, 3- to 7-day-old dogs, after similar periods of hypoglycemia (18 mg/dL: 1 mmol/L), showed identical rates of demise and changes in acid–base parameters, PCO_2, heart rate, and blood pressure as normoglycemic controls following asphyxiation. Again, this indicates the resistance of the neonatal animal to low levels of plasma glucose. However, a recent study by Kim *et al.* in newborn rats showed more cellular injury in animals rendered hypoglycemic for 4 hours at age 7 days when compared with those aged 21 days, and that A_1 adenosine receptor activation contributed to the damage [26]. Other studies in newborn piglets indicate that hypoglycemia (10–18 mg/dL: 0.55–1.0 mmol/L) promotes increases in cerebral adenosine concentrations which contribute to pial dilation and parenchymal hyperemia with local cerebral blood flow increase of $\sim 36\%$ [27].

Studies in human neonates

A number of investigators have reported morphological changes in the brain as a result of hypoglycemia, using computed tomography and magnetic resonance imaging. These data are limited because only the symptomatic subjects were examined and only a few cases are reported [28–33]. Additionally, imaging studies were done at varying ages in a pathologically heterogeneous population, with the goal to relate the observed changes with the neurological consequences. Because several studies were done in small-for-gestational-age infants, the impact of chronic hypoxemia on the observed changes cannot be easily separated. The published case reports on 23 subjects have been reviewed by Alkalay *et al.* [32]. The neurological findings included dilation of the ventricle, cerebral edema, areas of restricted diffusion, and loss of gray–white matter differentiation. However, a consistent involvement of the occipital lobes or parieto-occipital cortex was reported in a majority (82%) of infants. These neuroimaging data are consistent with pathological studies of occipital lobe involvement reported by Anderson *et al.* and by Banker [34,35]. The reason for the vulnerability of the occipital cortex to hypoglycemic injury is not clear; it may be related to developmental changes in local blood flow in response to hypoglycemia.

Finally, it is important to underscore that no clinical correlates of these hypoglycemia-related occipital cortex insults or injuries have been reported thus far. Only future studies in a large group of patients will help identify specific neurological lesions associated with hypoglycemia. Such specificity will go a long way in helping resolve the controversy regarding the long-term neurodevelopmental outcomes of hypoglycemia in the newborn.

Neurodevelopmental outcome

A number of studies [36–38] have examined the long-term neurological consequences of neonatal hypoglycemia (analyzed by Sinclair [39]). All of these studies are difficult to compare because of (1) lack of a consistent definition of hypoglycemia, (2) inconsistent clinical interventions within and between the studies, (3) duration of follow-up, (4) retrospective nature of analysis, (5) inadequate or no control group, and (6) impact of other variables such as prematurity and intrauterine growth restriction. Nevertheless, these studies suggest that symptomatic hypoglycemia may be associated with long-term neurodevelopmental consequences, and that asymptomatic transient hypoglycemia does not appear to be associated with significant morbidity.

Lucas *et al.* enlarged the area of uncertainty in a retrospective analysis of their data of over 600 infants of less than 1800 g birthweight, who were participants in a well-designed prospective nutritional intervention trial [10]. They examined the relationship between the frequency of low blood glucose concentration over several days and neurological outcome at 18 months. They suggested that a blood glucose concentration less than 2.6 mmol/L (~ 47 mg/dL), regardless of symptoms, observed 3–7 times (i.e., over 3–7 days), was associated with adverse neurological outcome. It is important to note that their data do not imply that the babies were continuously hypoglycemic over 3–7 days but that they had recorded that many low blood glucose levels. In addition, low blood glucose levels were recorded on separate, not necessarily consecutive, days. The broad significance of these data remains unclear. In a follow-up report in response to a letter to the editor [11], the authors indicated that a clinically significant reduction in math and motor skills (approximately 0.5 SD reduction) was the only abnormality observed at 7.5–8 years of age. Whether the lack of persistence of neurological disability is due to plasticity and adaptation of the developing brain or due to inability to do precise developmental evaluation of younger infants remains unclear.

A study of small-for-gestational-age infants has documented a strong correlation between recurrent episodes of hypoglycemia and neurodevelopmental and physical growth deficits at 5 years of age [40]. Again, the hypoglycemia occurred on a background of intrauterine growth restriction, and therefore the outcome is confounded by the impact of intrauterine milieu.

Clinical considerations

The clinical presentations of significant hypoglycemia are never specific, especially in the neonate, and include a wide range of local or generalized manifestations common in sick infants.

Episodes of changes in levels of consciousness, tremors, cyanosis, seizures, apnea, irregular respirations, irritability, apathy, limpness, hypothermia, difficulty in feeding, exaggerated Moro reflex, high-pitched cry, and coma have all been attributed to or have resulted from significant hypoglycemia. On occasion, vomiting, tachypnea, bradycardia, and "eye-rolling" have also been associated with hypoglycemia. Some infants with hypoglycemia are asymptomatic for unexplained reasons. Alternative substrates such as lactate, ketones, glycerol, and selected amino acids may support brain metabolism and prevent clinical manifestations in these neonates.

The possible causes of hypoglycemia are listed in Table 26.1. From a clinical perspective, the causes of neonatal hypoglycemia are divided into those causing transient hypoglycemia and those causing persistent or recurrent hypoglycemia. Transient hypoglycemia, often short-lived, is related to intrapartum and perinatal issues. Persistent or recurrent hypoglycemia is caused by metabolic or endocrine disorders. The long-term outcome of these infants is related to that of the primary metabolic disorder. The management and routine monitoring of the neonate at risk are shown in Tables 26.2 and 26.3

Therapy

Preventive interventions that have been recommended include the early use of oral feedings [41], parenteral fluids, and nutrient supplementation [42].

Once the diagnosis of hypoglycemia has been established by a reliable laboratory determination, therapy should be initiated promptly. In the asymptomatic infant during the first hours after birth, an oral feed of mixed nutrient (formula) may be given, and another plasma glucose measurement obtained within 30–60 minutes after the feed. If this is still low, parenteral glucose therapy may be indicated. In the symptomatic infant, a blood sample can be obtained for a glucose determination when the parenteral glucose is started. If this initial plasma glucose value is significantly low and symptoms disappear following the restoration of normoglycemia, the diagnosis of symptomatic hypoglycemia has been established.

Parenteral glucose should be given as an initial minibolus of glucose 0.25 g/kg (1 mL/kg of 25% glucose in water or 2.5 mL/kg of 10% glucose in water) intravenously [43], followed immediately by a continuous infusion of glucose at the rate of 6–8 mg/kg body weight per minute. For a term infant weighing 3000 g body weight, it corresponds to 80–110 mL/kg per day of 10–12.5% dextrose solution. Plasma glucose concentrations should be measured frequently to determine the effectiveness of the therapy. If levels of plasma glucose cannot be maintained over 45–50 mg/dL (2.5–2.78 mmol/L), the rate of infusion of glucose should be increased as necessary to achieve normoglycemia.

Oral feedings can be introduced as soon as possible after clinical manifestations subside. If the rate of glucose infusion

Table 26.1. Causes of neonatal hypoglycemia

(I) Transient hypoglycemia

  (A) Associated with changes in maternal metabolism

    (1) Intrapartum administration of glucose

    (2) Drug treatment

      (a) Terbutaline, ritodrine, propranolol

      (b) Oral hypoglycemic agents

    (3) Diabetes in pregnancy: infant of diabetic mother

  (B) Associated with neonatal problems

    (1) Idiopathic condition or failure to adapt

    (2) Intrauterine growth restriction

    (3) Birth asphyxia

    (4) Infection

    (5) Hypothermia

    (6) Hyperviscosity

    (7) Erythroblastosis fetalis

    (8) Other

      (a) Iatrogenic causes

      (b) Congenital cardiac malformations

(II) Persistent or recurrent hypoglycemia

  (A) Hyperinsulinism

    (1) β-cell hyperplasia, nesidioblastosis–adenoma spectrum, sulfonylurea receptor defect

    (2) Beckwith–Wiedemann Syndrome

  (B) Endocrine disorders

    (1) Pituitary insufficiency

    (2) Cortisol deficiency

    (3) Congenital glucagon deficiency

    (4) Epinephrine deficiency

  (C) Inborn errors of metabolism

    (1) Carbohydrate metabolism

      (a) Galactosemia

      (b) Hepatic glycogen storage diseases

      (c) Fructose intolerance

    (2) Amino acid metabolism

      (a) Maple syrup urine disease

      (b) Propionic acidemia

      (c) Methylmalonic acidemia

      (d) Hereditary tyrosinemia

      (e) 3-hydroxy, 3-methyl glutaric acidemia

      (f) Ethylmalonic-adipic aciduria

      (g) Glutaric acidemia type II

    (3) Fatty acid metabolism

      (a) Defects in carnitine metabolism

      (b) Acyl-coenzyme dehydrogenase

  (D) Neurohypoglycemia (hypoglycorrhachia) due to defective glucose transport

Table 26.2. Management of the neonate at risk

Clinical management of neonatal hypoglycemia is based on four basic principles
(1) Monitoring infants at highest risk
(2) Confirming that the plasma glucose concentration is low and is responsible for the clinical manifestations
(3) Demonstrating that all of the symptoms have responded following appropriate glucose therapy
(4) Observing and documenting all of these events

Table 26.3. Routine monitoring for infants at the highest risk for developing significant hypoglycemia

(1) LGA as well as all infants of insulin-dependent and gestational diabetic mothers and obese mothers
(2) SGA, including the smaller of discordant twins
(3) Apgar scores < 5 at 5 min or later as well as those who require significant resuscitation
(4) Significant hypoxia and/or perinatal distress
(5) ELBW infants (< 1250 g)
(6) Severe erythroblastosis
(7) Infants of mothers on tocolytic therapies, oral hypoglycemic agents, β-adrenergic blockers, etc.

Notes:
In these high-risk infants, routine screening should be done on admission to the nursery or at 2–2.5 h of age and then before feedings. Certainly, any infant with the clinical manifestations noted above should be screened for hypoglycemia.
LGA, large for gestational age; SGA, small for gestational age; ELBW, extremely low birthweight.

exceeds 10–12 mg/kg body weight per minute for a prolonged period, the infant may have a persistent type of hypoglycemia.

When normoglycemia has been established, the rate of infusion of parenteral glucose can be decreased gradually over 4–6 hours, while oral feedings are taken.

Persistence of the clinical manifestations after normalization of the plasma glucose concentration indicates that the hypoglycemia may have been associated with or secondary to other primary abnormalities. A systematic clinical and laboratory diagnostic evaluation to determine the primary disease is important, since hypoglycemia may be secondary to a variety of neonatal conditions that in themselves may be life-threatening or debilitating.

Transient hyperinsulinemia occurs in newborn infants of diabetic mothers [44], or as a consequence of intrapartum maternal hyperglycemia caused by administration of glucose or some pharmacologic agents or tocolytic drugs. Rigorous control of maternal metabolism during pregnancy and during labor has reduced the incidence of hypoglycemia in infants of diabetic mothers. Recurrent or persistent (> 7 days) hypoglycemia, although rare, is associated with high mortality and morbidity. A definite pathophysiologic classification can often be determined, even though specific molecular defects for every type are still not known. A detailed discussion of these syndromes, as well as the hereditary defects in carbohydrate,

amino acid, and/or fatty acid metabolism, has been published elsewhere [45,46]. This category of neonatal hypoglycemia may be suspected as either requiring infusions of large amounts of glucose (> 12–16 mg/kg body weight/min) to maintain normoglycemia or low blood glucose levels persisting or recurring beyond the first 7–14 days of life.

If persistent or recurrent hypoglycemia is anticipated or suspected, a diagnostic blood sample should be taken for the determination of plasma glucose, insulin, and β-hydroxybutyrate concentrations prior to initiating therapy. Analyses for growth hormone, adrenocorticotropic hormone (ACTH), cortisol, thyroxine (T_4), glucagon, somatomedins (insulin-like growth factors (IGF) 1 and 2 and their binding proteins), as well as for other substrates, such as lactate, pyruvate, uric acid, and quantitative amino acids (especially glutamine and alanine), are also indicated. These blood samples, if obtained before and after glucagon administration at the time when the patient is hypoglycemic, are often diagnostic [46].

Hyperinsulinemic (organic) hypoglycemia

The concept of hyperinsulinemic hypoglycemia is not new. Subtotal pancreatectomy, introduced by Graham and Hartmann [47], had been utilized in infants who could not be managed by the contemporary therapies. The major advance in diagnosis occurred in 1960 when Yalow and Berson [48] described the radioimmunoassay of insulin, allowing for micro- and then rapid analysis (within hours to days) of plasma insulin concentrations in infants. The simultaneous analysis of plasma glucose and insulin has permitted rapid diagnosis and early definitive therapy. Recent studies also indicate that hyperinsulinemia, especially with diffuse islet-cell abnormalities, is inherited as an autosomal recessive [49,50]. The gene locus for this rare autosomal recessive "disease" of persistent hyperinsulinemic hypoglycemia of infancy has been identified at the region of chromosome 11p between markers D11S1334 and D11S899 [49–51]. The β-cell sulfonylurea receptor (SUR) has been cloned [53]. Furthermore, individuals with hyperinsulinemic hypoglycemia were found to have two separate SUR gene site mutations [49,52]. In addition, functional candidate genes are being investigated in an autosomal dominant form of this disorder. Glaser [51] has reported on the etiology as well as the molecular biology of this disorder. The diagnosis of primary hyperinsulinemia can even be made in utero, by analyzing insulin concentrations in amniotic fluid in subsequent pregnancies, and this permits treatment to begin soon after birth [54].

Medical therapy has been most effective with diazoxide, which inhibits insulin secretion [55]. Pharmacologic agents such as somatostatin and/or glucagon have permitted preoperative stabilization but have not usually provided long-term effective therapy. Octreotide (a long-acting somatostatin preparation) has been used with mixed success in conjunction with frequent feedings and raw cornstarch at night for long-term therapy to avoid pancreatectomy and the potential of subsequent diabetes mellitus [51,56].

Surgical outcome improved with preservation of the spleen to avoid delayed major infections but was not consistently successful with subtotal pancreatectomy. As a result, Harken *et al.* strongly recommended near-total (95–99%) or total pancreatectomy [57]. Over time, this form of aggressive therapy has become accepted at early stages (weeks) after diagnosis and failed medical therapy.

A detailed report of the clinical features of 52 neonates with hyperinsulinism was presented by de Lonlay-Debeney *et al.* [58,59]. Their studies were unique because of preoperative pancreatic vein catheterization with insulin measurements and intraoperative histologic studies. Surgical resection was partial pancreatectomy for focal lesions but near-total resection for diffuse lesions. To date, the outcome for patients with focal lesions was satisfactory, i.e., normal parameters of glucose metabolism. In contrast, patients with diffuse pancreatic lesions had a variety of defects in glucose metabolism (hypoglycemia or hyperglycemia) in the year after surgery. The neurologic outcome of these plus 48 patients was reported in 2001 [60]. These data show that, in spite of early and aggressive treatment, psychomotor retardation and epilepsy were often seen in patients with neonatal onset of hyperinsulinemic hypoglycemia. Moreover, these findings also support the possibility that the fetus could have been damaged in utero.

The frequency of hyperinsulinemic hypoglycemia is unknown. Birth weights have been normal, but are usually increased. Both sexes are affected, and familial occurrence has been reported on a number of occasions [61]. Aggressive, early medical or surgical intervention does not assure a successful outcome [62]. Of 12 infants who were operated on between 5 and 18 days after birth, 10 were reported with normal mental status. However, five had seizures, one was retarded, and another died. This limited outcome may relate to the severity and duration of the hypoglycemia or to other congenital metabolic factors. However, the data, at present, do not show a clear relationship between the duration or severity of hypoglycemia, type of underlying pathology, type of therapy, and outcome.

Summary

Significantly low blood glucose concentration is a frequent observation in the healthy newborn infant during transition to extrauterine life. While the majority of these hypoglycemic episodes are transient, in some infants hypoglycemia can be severe and persistent. Transient hypoglycemia has not been associated with any long-term neurological consequences. In contrast, recurrent or persistent symptomatic hypoglycemia can result in neuronal injury and long-term morbidity. An expeditious recognition of hypoglycemia and prudent clinical interventions may help prevent several of these consequences of brain injury. Newer non-invasive techniques will help assess the magnitude of brain injury and relate it to later morbidity.

References

1. Kalhan SC. Metabolism of glucose and methods of investigation in the fetus and newborn. In Polin RA, Fox WW, Abman SH, eds., *Fetal and Neonatal Physiology*, 3rd edn. Philadelphia, PA: Saunders, 2003: 449–64.

2. Kalhan SC, Parimi P. Disorders of carbohydrate metabolism. In Fanaroff AA, Martin RJ, eds., *Neonatal–Perinatal Medicine: Diseases of the Fetus and Infant*, 8th edn. St. Louis, MO: Mosby–Year Book, 2005: 1467–90.

3. Cornblath M, Hawdon JM, Williams AF, *et al.* Controversies regarding definition of neonatal hypoglycemia: suggested operational thresholds. *Pediatrics* 2000; **105**: 1141–5.

4. Cornblath M, Ichord R. Hypoglycemia in the neonate. *Semin Perinatol* 2000; **24**: 136–49.

5. World Health Organization. *Hypoglycaemia of the Newborn: Review of the Literature.* Geneva: World Health Organization, 1997. who.int/reproductive-health/docs/ hypoglycaemia_newborn.htm. Accessed October, 2008.

6. Cornblath M. Neonatal hypoglycemia 30 years later: does it injure the brain? Historical summary and present challenges. *Acta Paediatr Jpn* 1996; **1**: S7–11.

7. Stanley CA, Anday EK, Baker L, *et al.* Metabolic fuel and hormone responses to fasting in newborn infants. *Pediatrics* 1979; **64**: 613–19.

8. Koh THHG, Aynsley-Green A, Tarbit M, *et al.* Neural dysfunction during hypoglycaemia. *Arch Dis Child* 1988; **63**: 1353–8.

9. Sinclair JC. Approaches to the definition of neonatal hypoglycemia. *Acta Paediatr Jpn* 1997; **39**: S17–20.

10. Lucas A, Morley R, Cole JJ. Adverse neurodevelopmental outcome of moderate neonatal hypoglycemia. *BMJ* 1988; **297**: 1304–8.

11. Cornblath M, Schwartz R. Outcome of neonatal hypoglycaemia: complete data are needed. *BMJ* 1999; **318**: 194–5.

12. Cornblath M, Schwartz R, Aynsley-Green A, *et al.* Hypoglycemia in infancy: the need for a rational definition. A Ciba Foundation discussion meeting. *Pediatrics* 1990; **95**: 834–7.

13. Kalhan S, Peter-Wohl S. Hypoglycemia: what is it for the neonate? *Am J Perinatol* 2000; **17**: 11–18.

14. Kalhan S, Kiliç Ì. Carbohydrate as nutrient in the infant and child: range of acceptable intake. *Eur J Clin Nutr* 1999; **53**: S94–100.

15. Settergren G, Lindblad BS, Persson B. Cerebral blood flow and exchange of oxygen, glucose, ketone bodies, lactate, pyruvate and amino acids in infants. *Acta Paediatr Scand* 1976; **65**: 343–53.

16. Settergren G, Lindblad BS, Persson B. Cerebral blood flow and exchange of oxygen, glucose, ketone bodies, lactate, pyruvate and amino acids in anesthetized children. *Acta Paediatr Scand* 1980; **69**: 457–45.

17. Kinnala A, Korvenranta H, Parkkola R. Newer techniques to study neonatal hypoglycemia. *Semin Perinatol* 2000; **24**: 116–19.

18. Kinnala A, Nuutila P, Ruotsalainen U, *et al.* Cerebral metabolic rate for glucose after neonatal hypoglycaemia. *Early Hum Dev* 1997; **49**: 63–72.

19. Auer RN, Siesjo BK. Biological differences between ischemia, hypoglycemia and epilepsy. *Ann Neurol* 1988; **24**: 699–708.

20. Siesjo BK. Hypoglycemia, brain metabolism and brain damage. *Diabetes Metab Rev* 1988; **4**: 113–44.

21. McGowan JE, Haynew-Laing AG, Mishra OP, et al. The effect of acute hypoglycemia on the cerebral NMDA receptor in newborn piglets. *Pediatr Res* 1995; **670**: 283–8.

22. Ichord RN, Northington FJ, Van Wylen DG, et al. Brain O_2 consumption and glutamate release during hypoglycemic coma in piglets are temperature sensitive. *Am J Physiol* 1999; **276**: H2053–62.

23. Vannucci RC, Vannucci SJ. Glucose metabolism in the developing brain. *Semin Perinatol* 2000; **24**: 107–15.

24. Vannucci RC, Vannucci SJ. Cerebral carbohydrate metabolism during hypoglycemia and anoxia in newborn rats. *Ann Neurol* 1978; **4**: 73–9.

25. Vannucci RC, Nardis EE, Vannucci SJ, et al. Cerebral carbohydrate and energy metabolism during hypoglycemia in newborn dogs. *Am J Physiol* 1981; **240**: R192–9.

26. Kim M, Yu ZX, Fredholm BB, et al. Susceptibility of the developing brain to acute hypoglycemia involving A_1 adenosine receptor activation. *Am J Physiol Endocrinol Metab* 2005; **289**: E562–9.

27. Ruth VJ, Park TS, Gonzales ER, et al. Adenosine and cerebrovascular hyperemia during insulin-induced hypoglycemia in newborn piglet. *Am J Physiol* 1993; **265**: H1762–8.

28. Filan PM, Inder TE, Cameron FJ, et al. Neonatal hypoglycemia and occipital cerebral injury. *J Pediatr* 2006; **148**: 552–5.

29. Traill Z, Squier M, Anslow P. Brain imaging in neonatal hypoglycaemia. *Arch Dis Child Fetal Neonatal Ed* 1998; **79**: F145–7.

30. Barkovich AJ, Ali FA, Rowley HA, et al. Imaging patterns of neonatal hypoglycemia. *AJNR Am J Neuroradiol* 1998; **19**: 523–8.

31. Kinnala A, Rikalainen H, Lapinleimu H, et al. Cerebral magnetic resonance imaging and ultrasonography findings after neonatal hypoglycemia. *Pediatrics* 1999; **103**: 724–9.

32. Alkalay AL, Flores-Sarnat L, Sarnat HB, et al. Brain imaging findings in neonatal hypoglycemia: case report and review of 23 cases. *Clin Pediatr* 2005; **44**: 783–90.

33. Aslan Y, Dinc H. Findings of neonatal hypoglycemia. *AJNR Am J Neuroradiol* 1997; **18**: 994–5.

34. Anderson JM, Milner RDG, Strich SJ. Effects of neonatal hypoglycaemia on the nervous system: a pathological study.

J Neurol Neurosurg Psychiatr 1967; **30**: 295–10.

35. Banker BQ. The neuropathological effects of anoxia and hypoglycaemia in the newborn. *Dev Med Child Neurol* 1967; **9**: 544–50.

36. Griffiths AD. Association of hypoglycaemia with symptoms in the newborn. *Arch Dis Child* 1968; **43**: 688–94.

37. Koivisto M, Blanco-Sequerios M, Krause U. Neonatal symptomatic and asymptomatic hypoglycaemia: a follow-up study of 151 children. *Dev Med Child Neurol* 1971; **14**: 603–14.

38. Pildes RS, Cornblath M, Warren L, et al. A prospective controlled study of neonatal hypoglycemia. *Pediatrics* 1974; **54**: 5–14.

39. Sinclair JC, Bracken MB. *Effective Care of the Newborn Infant. Part 111. Diseases, Abnormal Glucose Homeostasis.* Oxford: Oxford University Press, 1992.

40. Duvanel CB, Fawer CL, Cotting J, et al. Long-term effects of neonatal hypoglycemia on brain growth and psychomotor development in small-for-gestational-age preterm infants. *J Pediatr* 1999; **134**: 492–8.

41. Smallpeice V, Davies PA. Immediate feeding of premature infants with undiluted breast milk. *Lancet* 1964; **2**: 1349–52.

42. Sann L, Mousson B, Rousson M, et al. Prevention of neonatal hypoglycaemia by oral lipid supplementation in low birth weight infants. *Eur J Pediatr* 1988; **147**: 158–61.

43. Lilien LD, Pildes RS, Srinivasan G, et al. Treatment of neonatal hypoglycemia with minibolus and intravenous glucose infusion. *J Pediatr* 1980; **97**: 295–8.

44. Schwartz R, Teramo KA. Effects of diabetic pregnancy on the fetus and newborn. *Semin Perinatol* 2000; **24**: 120–35.

45. Cornblath M, Schwartz R. *Disorders of Carbohydrate Metabolism in Infancy*, 3rd edn. Cambridge, MA: Blackwell, 1991.

46. Cornblath M, Poth M. Hypoglycemia. In Kaplan S, ed., *Clinical Pediatric and Adolescent Endocrinology*. Philadelphia, PA: Saunders, 1982: 157–70.

47. Graham EA, Hartmann AF. Subtotal resection of the pancreas for hypoglycemia. *Surg Gynecol Obstet* 1934; **59**: 474–9.

48. Yalow RS, Berson SA. Immunoassay of endogenous plasma insulin in man. *J Clin Invest* 1960; **39**: 1157–75.

49. Glaser B, Chin KC, Anker R, et al. Familial hyperinsulinism maps to chromosome 11p14–15.1. *Nat Genet* 1994; **7**: 185–8.

50. Thomas PM, Cote GJ, Hallman DM, et al. Homozygosity mapping to chromosome 11p, of the gene for familial persistent hyperinsulinemic hypoglycemia of infancy. *Am J Hum Genet* 1995; **56**: 416–21.

51. Glaser B. Hyperinsulinism of the newborn. *Semin Perinatol* 2000; **24**: 150–63.

52. Thomas PM, Cote GJ, Wahlick N, et al. Mutations in the sulfonylurea receptor gene in familial persistent hyperinsulinemic hypoglycemia in infancy. *Science* 1995; **268**: 426–9.

53. Aguilar-Bryan L, Nichols CG, Wechsler SW, et al. Cloning of the β cell high affinity sulfonylurea receptor: a regulator of insulin secretion. *Science* 1995; **268**: 423–6.

54. Aparicio L, Carpenter MW, Schwartz R, et al. Prenatal diagnosis of familial neonatal hyperinsulinemia. *Acta Paediatr Scand* 1993; **82**: 683–6.

55. Wolff FW, Parmeley WW. Aetiological factors in benzothiadiazine hyperglycemia. *Lancet* 1963; **2**: 69.

56. Glaser B, Hirsch HJ, Landau H. Persistent hyperinsulinemic hypoglycemia of infancy: long-term octreotide treatment without pancreatectomy. *J Pediatr* 1993; **12**: 644–50.

57. Harken AH, Filler RM, AvRuskin TW, et al. The role of "total" pancreatectomy in the treatment of unremitting hypoglycemia of infancy. *J Pediatr Surg* 1971; **6**: 284–9.

58. de Lonlay-Debeney P, Poggi-Travert F, Fournet JC, et al. Clinical features of 52 neonates with hyperinsulinism. *N Engl J Med* 1999; **340**: 1169–75.

59. Delonlay P, Simon A, Galmiche-Rolland L, et al. Neonatal hyperinsulinism: clinicopathologic correlation. *Hum Pathol* 2007; **38**: 387–99.

60. Menni F, de Lonlay P, Sevin C, et al. Neurologic outcomes of 90 neonates and infants with persistent hyperinsulinemic hypoglycemia. *Pediatrics* 2001; **108**: 476–9.

61. Thornton PS, Sumner AE, Ruchalli ED, et al. Familial and sporadic hyperinsulinism: histopathologic findings and segregation analysis support a single autosomal recessive disorder. *J Pediatr* 1991; **119**: 721–4.

62. Horev Z, Ipp M, Levey P, et al. Familial hyperinsulinism: successful conservative management. *J Pediatr* 1991; **119**: 717–20.

Hyperbilirubinemia and kernicterus

David K. Stevenson, Ronald J. Wong, and Phyllis A. Dennery

Introduction

The term *kernicterus* was originally used to describe the deposition of bilirubin in the basal ganglia. It was first described in 1903 by Schmorl [1]. More recently, the term has also been used in reference to the chronic and permanent clinical sequelae of bilirubin toxicity [2]. For the acute manifestations of bilirubin toxicity, the term *acute bilirubin encephalopathy* or ABE has been adopted. Another acronym, BIND, has been adopted to describe any bilirubin-induced neurologic dysfunction [3]. Although technically the diagnosis of kernicterus can only be confirmed at autopsy, brain magnetic resonance imaging (MRI) studies may now aid in the confirmation of the diagnosis in a living child with severe jaundice. The MRI signature for kernicterus includes high signal intensity on T1-weighted (T1W) images in the globus pallidus, internal capsule, thalamus, and hippocampi (Fig. 27.1). The associated T2W images have abnormal increased signal in the globus pallidus and thalamus in the same regions as the high signal on the T1W images (Fig. 27.2). Loss of demarcation between globus pallidus, internal capsule, and the anterior thalamus was the major finding [4,5]. The source of these abnormal signals has not been definitively identified, and therefore the MRI findings should not be considered diagnostic in themselves, but only consistent with the diagnosis of kernicterus in the context of severe neonatal jaundice and the acute and chronic clinical features of bilirubin toxicity (Table 27.1).

Neonatal jaundice and neurotoxicity

Most often a benign condition, a majority of term neonates develop neonatal jaundice, which is a consequence of relatively increased bilirubin production (two- to threefold higher in a neonate compared to an adult) and limited ability to conjugate bilirubin in the transitional time after birth. Compared to healthy term infants, polycythemic infants or those with hemolysis can produce significant amounts of bilirubin [6]. By convention, a serum or plasma bilirubin concentration higher than the 95th percentile or high-risk zone on the hour-specific bilirubin nomogram [3] is considered pathologic. Moreover, there is not any "safe" level of bilirubin that can be universally

agreed upon, because the level at which neurotoxicity develops and the conditions under which toxicity manifests remain incompletely understood. Importantly, BIND or bilirubin toxicity, including ABE and kernicterus, does not occur in the absence of hyperbilirubinemia. Among the survivors, the acute and chronic features of ABE and kernicterus, respectively, are listed in Table 27.1. Importantly, each infant may not have all of the features of the syndrome, and the permanent injuries may vary in severity and include subtle neurologic deficits, suggesting that there may be a spectrum of injuries caused specifically by bilirubin.

The topic of bilirubin neurotoxicity has also been reviewed by Volpe [7]. That bilirubin is toxic is undisputed, and a variety of cellular toxic effects of bilirubin have been described [8–13]. From a clinical perspective, there are a variety of factors that influence empirically the neurotoxic effects of bilirubin. However, the exact mechanism(s) by which bilirubin injures the brain, and in particular what contributes to injury in an individual infant, is poorly understood.

Most of the experimental work on bilirubin toxicity has been done in vitro. In such systems the binding of bilirubin to albumin is a critical phenomenon for understanding bilirubin toxicity [14–16]. However, its relevance to toxicity in intact animals or humans remains uncertain or is not known in most cases [17]. Nothing is known with certainty with respect to where bilirubin acts and how it acts. Overall, the in vitro studies of bilirubin toxicity are inconclusive, and extrapolation to in vivo conditions is uncertain because of confounding uncontrolled factors. Additionally, data suggest a beneficial antioxidant role of bilirubin [18,19], although it is not clear whether this is of physiologic relevance in neonates. Conjugating capacity (hence the ability to excrete bilirubin) probably varies significantly in the general population and is further influenced by genetic conditions like Gilbert syndrome, which is associated with a mildly decreased uridine diphosphate glucuronosyltransferase (UGT) activity, attributed to an expansion of thymine–adenine (TA) repeats in the promoter region of the *UGT1A1* gene, the principal gene encoding UGT [20–22]. There may also be racial variation in the number of TA repeats, thus suggesting a reason for differences in bilirubin metabolism between certain ethnic groups [23]. Recently, a DNA sequence variant (Gly71Arg) has also been associated with decreased UGT activity and neonatal hyperbilirubinemia in Asians [24]. Even more interesting is the potential for gene

Fetal and Neonatal Brain Injury, 4th edition, ed. David K. Stevenson, William E. Benitz, Philip Sunshine, Susan R. Hintz, and Maurice L. Druzin. Published by Cambridge University Press. © Cambridge University Press 2009.

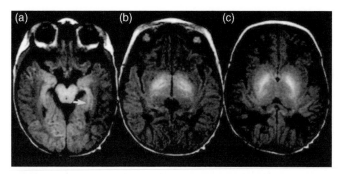

Fig. 27.1. Series of three axial T1-weighted (T1W) images showing the following anatomy: (a) the hippocampus and temporal lobe; (b) the basal ganglia and subthalamus; and (c) the lenticular nuclei and thalamus. The major abnormality on these T1W images was the abnormal high signal intensity seen in the hippocampus in the medial temporal lobe (arrow, a). This was confirmed on sagittal images. This abnormally high signal intensity was also noted in the globus pallidus but not the putamen (b, c). The thalamus was less involved, but some increased signal intensity was present in the ventroposterolateral nucleus. The findings were bilateral and symmetrical in these structures and typical of regions of the brain damaged in kernicterus. Reproduced with permission of the AAP from *Pediatrics* 1994; **93**: 1003–6 [4].

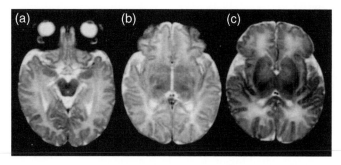

Fig. 27.2. T2-weighted images at the same anatomical levels as the T1-weighted (T1W) images shown in Fig. 27.1. Findings on these images are more subtle than the T1W abnormalities and are characterized by increased signal intensity in the same regions: the globus pallidus and anterior thalamus are best seen in image (c). The basal ganglia abnormality is seen primarily as a loss of demarcation between the globus pallidus, internal capsule, and thalamus. The increased signal in the hippocampi is also subtle and best seen in image (a) as an area of increased signal intensity paralleling the temporal horn medially. Reproduced with permission of the AAP from *Pediatrics* 1994; **93**: 1003–6 [4].

Table 27.1. Clinical features of bilirubin toxicity

Acute bilirubin encephalopathy (ABE)	
Early phase	Lethargy
(Reversible)	Hypotonia
	Poor sucking
Intermediate phase	Moderate stupor
(Reversible)	Irritability
	Hypertonia, manifested by backward arching of the neck (retrocollis) and trunk (opisthotonos)
	Fever
	High-pitched cry
Advanced phase	Pronounced retrocollis–opisthotonos
(Probably irreversible)	Shrill cry
	No feeding
	Apnea
	Fever
	Deep stupor to coma
	Sometimes seizures and death
Chronic bilirubin encephalopathy or kernicterus	
(Irreversible)	Severe form of athetoid cerebral palsy
	Auditory dysfunction
	Dental-enamel dysplasia
	Paralysis of upward gaze
	Sometimes intellectual and other handicaps

interaction suggested in a number of reports on glucose-6-phosphate dehydrogenase (G6PD) deficiency and Gilbert syndrome [20,25,26]. Besides genetic differences in conjugating capacity, genetic differences in the capacity to produce bilirubin attributed to polymorphisms (GT expansions) in the heme oxygenase 1 (HO-1) gene promoter [27–30], and genetic differences in the transporters (organic anion transporter protein 2) involved in bilirubin uptake from circulation [31,32], also may contribute to individual differences in transitional hyperbilirubinemia.

One of the major risk factors for severe neonatal hyperbilirubinemia and bilirubin toxicity is severe hemolysis [33]. Under such conditions (Rh disease), a serum or plasma bilirubin level of 20 mg/dL or greater has been empirically associated with a risk for neonatal brain injury or death. Thus "vigintiphobia" has a historical and not a scientific basis, but extrapolation to other hyperbilirubinemic conditions besides Rh disease is not clear [34,35]. One historical exception to the

role of hemolysis in severe hyperbilirubinemia is the clinical experience reported by Silverman *et al.* in 1956 [36] with premature infants treated with sulfisoxazole. This tragedy suggested that great caution should be exercised in using any new drug in a neonate. In fact, all drugs considered for use in neonates should be tested for their capacities to displace bilirubin from albumin, in order to avoid history repeating itself. Practically, the prediction of severe jaundice, or more accurately the lack of it, is now possible by combining an hour-specific bilirubin level with an estimate of the degree of bilirubin production with carboxyhemoglobin (COHb) or end-tidal breath carbon monoxide (CO) or ETCO analyses [37].

Prediction of hyperbilirubinemia

With early discharge, it is often difficult to observe infants long enough to detect pathologic hyperbilirubinemia. Although not perfect, hour-specific bilirubin levels can assist in the prediction of which infants might develop severe neonatal jaundice, or be less likely to develop it, according to predetermined thresholds [3]. An hour-specific bilirubin level represents the interaction of increased bilirubin load and the ability to excrete the load. Hemolysis can be diagnosed sensitively by estimating bilirubin production non-invasively. Measurements of CO or COHb, corrected for ambient CO (ETCOc or COHbc, respectively) are useful techniques that have been used experimentally to estimate hemolysis and the potential for hemolytic jaundice [38]. These early detection tools may help in deciding which infants should be observed more frequently and treated, because jaundice associated with hemolysis represents one of the most common serious threats. The importance of identifying increased bilirubin production as a contributing cause of neonatal jaundice cannot be over-emphasized. Empirically, the rate of rise of the bilirubin level serves as a surrogate for this bilirubin load phenomenon. The risk of injury associated with hyperbilirubinemia is dependent upon how much bilirubin gets into tissues. This varies with the capacity to keep bilirubin in circulation (mainly deter-mined by the albumin concentration) [14,39], the amount of bilirubin produced over time relative to what can be elimin-ated, and the metabolic state of the infant [11,40]. Thus the bilirubin level by itself may not always reflect the magnitude of risk, but the higher the bilirubin level associated with increased production of the pigment, the higher the risk. An estimate of the magnitude of the bilirubin load using an index of bilirubin production, like ETCOc or COHbc, combined with an hour-specific bilirubin level provides even more infor-mation about the nature of the infant's transitional hyperbili-rubinemia. Such a diagnostic approach could allow clinicians to make better judgments about which infants could be dis-charged early, which should be followed more closely over the first week of life, and which might require therapy, includ-ing home phototherapy. With the burden still on physicians to exclude hemolytic disease for compliance with the 2004 American Academy of Pediatrics (AAP) clinical practice guideline for management of hyperbilirubinemia in the new-born infant $\geq$ 35 weeks' gestation [2], infants who are dis-charged before 48 hours should probably have more than a direct Coombs test in order to determine if they have

hemolysis. A positive direct Coombs test does not make this diagnosis. Only 50% of infants with a positive Coombs test actually hemolyze, and up to 25% of those with an ABO blood type incompatibility with their mother and lacking a positive Coombs test will have evidence of hemolysis based on a more sensitive test, the ETCOc [41].

Management of neonatal hyperbilirubinemia

Neonatal hyperbilirubinemia was reviewed in 2001 [42]. Moreover, the AAP has attempted to address the management of hyperbilirubinemia in the healthy term newborn (Fig. 27.3) [2]. However, the latter practice parameter now does apply to term infants with a variety of complicating conditions, and to near-term (35–37 weeks' gestation) infants or preterm infants. These guidelines should not be characterized as stand-ards, as they have important limitations. Nonetheless, they should be followed with the exclusion of infants of less than 35 weeks' gestation. When newborn infants are discharged before the total serum bilirubin (TSB) level is likely to have peaked, the medical responsibility for follow-up of the infant cannot be shifted to the parents without clear recommenda-tions for follow-up by a physician or an appropriately trained individual [2].

The practice in many communities suggests that some lower-risk infants with serum or plasma total bilirubin levels above 20 mg/dL (depending upon the postnatal age in hours) may be managed without exchange transfusion, but according to the new guideline all should be treated with intensive phototherapy; and if the TSB level is 25 mg/dL or higher, it should be considered a medical emergency and the infant

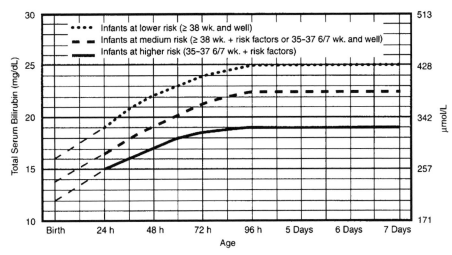

• The dashed lines for the first 24 hours indicate uncertainty due to a wide range of clinical circumstances and a range of responses to phototherapy.
• Immediate exchange transfusion is recommended if infant shows signs of acute bilirubin encephalopathy (hypertonia, arching, retrocollis, opisthotonos, fever, high pitched cry) or if TSB is ≥5 mg/dL (85 µmol/L) above these lines.
• Risk factors – isoimmune hemolytic disease, G6PD deficiency, asphyxia, significant lethargy, temperature instability, sepsis, acidosis.
• Measure serum albumin and calculate B/A ratio (See legend)
• Use total bilirubin. Do not subtract direct reacting or conjugated bilirubin
• If infant is well and 35–37 6/7 wk (median risk) can individualize TSB levels for exchange based on actual gestational age.

Fig. 27.3. Guidelines for exchange transfusion in infants of 35 or more weeks' gestation. Note that these suggested levels represent a consensus of most of the committee but are based on limited evidence, and the levels shown are approximations. During birth hospitalization, exchange transfusion is recommended if the TSB rises to these levels despite intensive phototherapy. For readmitted infants, if the TSB level is above the exchange level, repeat TSB measurement every 2–3 hours and consider exchange if the TSB remains above the levels indicated after intensive phototherapy for 6 hours. Reproduced with permission of the AAP from *Pediatrics* 2004; **114:** 297–316 [2].

should be admitted to the hospital pediatrics service for intensive phototherapy while preparation for an exchange transfusion is undertaken [2]. Immediate exchange transfusion is recommended if the infant shows signs of bilirubin encephalopathy or if the TSB is ≥ 5 mg/dL above the hour-specific lines for the various risk categories. The many other nomograms for guiding the decision making of practitioners with respect to the treatment of hyperbilirubinemia also should not be considered irrefutable standards, but rather recommendations for practice that need to be adapted and modified on an individual basis. Furthermore, there is no absolute standard level at which phototherapy should be applied, although the AAP recommendations are reasonable in this regard. In premature infants, some investigators have recommended the use of phototherapy at very low bilirubin levels, because kernicterus has been diagnosed in such infants at bilirubin levels between 5 and 8 mg/dL [43]. Common sense usually weighs heavily in the decision to start phototherapy in an effort to avoid exchange transfusion – a procedure that carries a small but definite risk. Another factor that needs to be considered is the duration of exposure to high bilirubin levels, and this may also influence the decision to intervene earlier or more aggressively in a context where a level remains high despite intensive phototherapy.

In the presence of hemolysis, a total bilirubin level of 20 mg/dL or greater has been associated with an increased risk of neonatal brain injury or death. Therefore, exchange transfusion should be seriously considered in the infant under such circumstances, and particularly if the bilirubin level does not decrease rapidly under intensive phototherapy. An infant with jaundice associated with breastfeeding is a typical example. Such infants should not have markedly increased bilirubin production. However, despite the assumed benign nature of jaundice associated with breastfeeding, some practitioners would recommend exchange transfusion for any infant with a total bilirubin level greater than 25 mg/dL that does not respond to intensive phototherapy. Moreover, exchange transfusion might be considered at a lower level if the infant were preterm or sick in any way, in particular if the infant were asphyxiated or infected or had cardiorespiratory or metabolic instability. Infants with bilirubin levels greater than 30 mg/dL should definitely be exchanged if technically possible. Occasionally, an exchange might reasonably be avoided if the bilirubin level dropped dramatically below 25 mg/dL under intense phototherapy while preparing for the exchange. The use of drugs capable of displacing bilirubin from albumin in general should be avoided in the newborn. The use of intralipid as a continuous infusion at a rate to prevent central fatty acid deficiency is not dangerous, because free fatty acid albumin ratios are not elevated into the range at which displacement of bilirubin from albumin would be expected.

Breastfeeding of any infant with a propensity for increased bilirubin production (e.g., bruising, hematoma, prematurity) represents an increased risk for hyperbilirubinemia and warrants close follow-up of the infant throughout the first week and into the second week of life. Early discharge of an infant from the hospital requires that a practitioner follow the AAP practice guideline [2].

Reemergence of kernicterus

In the 1980s and 1990s, kernicterus had become a rare occurrence. However, with discharge from the hospital occurring sooner after birth, the peak of neonatal hyperbilirubinemia more often occurs outside the hospital, observed by parents and not by physicians or other trained personnel. Thus there has been a re-emergence of reported kernicterus in the USA and possibly elsewhere [4,44–48].

There are some particular clinical problems that get practitioners into trouble more often than others. Most of them can be related to the early discharge of infants from the hospital. One example is the breastfeeding infant with increased bilirubin production. The source of the increased bilirubin production may be unrecognized hemolytic disease or simply bruising or hematoma formation. The increased bilirubin production, combined with a lack of a decrease in the enterohepatic circulation, may contribute to a very rapid early rise in the TSB level over the first several days of life, which can be missed if the infant is discharged before the time of peak hyperbilirubinemia at approximately 3–4 days. The peak may also be later, as is often the case when increased bilirubin production is a major factor contributing to jaundice, or when a conjugating defect is present, such as in a certain proportion of Asians [41,49]. Even a large premature or near-term infant who is breastfeeding, and does not have an obvious complication predisposing to increased bilirubin production, may have more difficulty in lowering the bilirubin level and should be followed closely throughout the first 2 weeks of life. Currently, term newborns are rarely seen by a practitioner in this period once discharged from the hospital. This is not a good practice. In hemolytic disease, late anemia is a complication that should also not be overlooked once hyperbilirubinemia has been successfully managed. Such anemia may be so severe as to require transfusion by the second to fourth week of life. An estimate of bilirubin production will help in the recognition of this problem in the absence of hyperbilirubinemia.

In summary, bilirubin toxicity, manifested as either ABE or kernicterus, is a real entity that has been more frequently reported in the last decade due to relaxed vigilance in the treatment of neonatal hyperbilirubinemia. It is most often preventable by the use of predictive tools, and aggressive intervention when appropriate.

References

1. Schmorl G. Zur kenntis des icterus neonatorum. *Verh Dtsch Ges Pathol* 1903; **6**: 109.

2. American Academy of Pediatrics. Management of hyperbilirubinemia in the newborn infant 35 or more weeks of gestation. *Pediatrics* 2004; **114**: 297–316.

3. Bhutani VK, Johnson L, Sivieri EM. Predictive ability of a predischarge hour-specific serum bilirubin for subsequent significant hyperbilirubinemia in healthy

term and near-term newborns. *Pediatrics* 1999; **103**: 6–14.

4. Penn AA, Enzmann DR, Hahn JS, *et al.* Kernicterus in a full term infant. *Pediatrics* 1994; **93**: 1003–6.

5. Govaert P, Lequin M, Swarte R, *et al.* Changes in globus pallidus with (pre) term kernicterus. *Pediatrics* 2003; **112**: 1256–63.

6. Stevenson DK, Bartoletti AL, Ostrander CR, *et al.* Pulmonary excretion of carbon monoxide in the human newborn infant as an index of bilirubin production: III. Measurement of pulmonary excretion of carbon monoxide after the first postnatal week in premature infants. *Pediatrics* 1979; **64**: 598–600.

7. Volpe JJ. Bilirubin and brain injury. In Volpe JJ, ed., *Neurology of the Newborn*, 2nd edn. Philadelphia, PA: Saunders, 2000: 490–514.

8. Amato M. Mechanisms of bilirubin toxicity. *Eur J Pediatr* 1995; **154**: S54–9.

9. Amit Y, Chan G, Fedunec S, *et al.* Bilirubin toxicity in a neuroblastoma cell line N-115: I. Effects on Na+K+ATPase, [3H]-thymidine uptake, L-[35S]-methionine incorporation, and mitochondrial function. *Pediatr Res* 1989; **25**: 364–8.

10. Wennberg RP. Cellular basis of bilirubin toxicity. *NY State J Med* 1991; **91**: 493–6.

11. Wennberg RP, Gospe SM, Rhine WD, *et al.* Brainstem bilirubin toxicity in the newborn primate may be promoted and reversed by modulating PCO_2. *Pediatr Res* 1993; **34**: 6–9.

12. Hanko E, Hansen TW, Almaas R, *et al.* Bilirubin induces apoptosis and necrosis in human NT2-N neurons. *Pediatr Res* 2005; **57**: 179–84.

13. Brito MA, Silva RF, Brites D. Bilirubin induces loss of membrane lipids and exposure of phosphatidylserine in human erythrocytes. *Cell Biol Toxicol* 2002; **18**: 181–92.

14. Ahlfors CE. Measurement of plasma unbound unconjugated bilirubin. *Anal Biochem* 2000; **279**: 130–5.

15. Ahlfors CE. Unbound bilirubin associated with kernicterus: a historical approach. *J Pediatr* 2000; **137**: 540–4.

16. Ahlfors CE, Wennberg RP. Bilirubin-albumin binding and neonatal jaundice. *Semin Perinatol* 2004; **28**: 334–9.

17. Levine RL, Fredericks WR, Rapoport SI. Clearance of bilirubin from rat brain after reversible osmotic opening of the blood–brain barrier. *Pediatr Res* 1985; **19**: 1040–3.

18. Dennery PA, McDonagh AF, Spitz DR, *et al.* Hyperbilirubinemia results in reduced oxidative injury in neonatal Gunn rats exposed to hyperoxia. *Free Radic Biol Med* 1995; **19**: 395–404.

19. Stocker R, Yamamoto Y, McDonagh AF, *et al.* Bilirubin is an antioxidant of possible physiological importance. *Science* 1987; **235**: 1043–6.

20. Kaplan M, Renbaum P, Levy-Lahad E, *et al.* Gilbert syndrome and glucose-6-phosphate dehydrogenase deficiency: a dose-dependent genetic interaction crucial to neonatal hyperbilirubinemia. *Proc Natl Acad Sci USA* 1997; **94**: 12128–32.

21. Kaplan M, Hammerman C, Rubaltelli FF, *et al.* Hemolysis and bilirubin conjugation in association with UDP-glucuronosyltransferase 1A1 promoter polymorphism. *Hepatology* 2002; **35**: 905–11.

22. Berardi A, Lugli L, Ferrari F, *et al.* Kernicterus associated with hereditary spherocytosis and UGT1A1 promoter polymorphism. *Biol Neonate* 2006; **90**: 243–6.

23. Beutler E, Gelbart T, Demina A. Racial variability in the UDP-glucuronosyltransferase 1 (UGT1A1) promoter: a balanced polymorphism for regulation of bilirubin metabolism? *Proc Natl Acad Sci USA* 1998; **95**: 8170–4.

24. Akaba K, Kimura T, Sasaki A, *et al.* Neonatal hyperbilirubinemia and mutation of the bilirubin uridine diphosphate-glucuronosyltransferase gene: a common missense mutation among Japanese, Koreans and Chinese. *Biochem Mol Biol Int* 1998; **46**: 21–6.

25. Kaplan M, Hammerman C, Renbaum P, *et al.* Differing pathogenesis of perinatal bilirubinemia in glucose-6-phosphate dehydrogenase-deficient versus normal neonates. *Pediatr Res* 2001; **50**: 532–7.

26. Kaplan M, Renbaum P, Vreman HJ, *et al.* (TA)n UGT 1A1 promoter polymorphism: a crucial factor in the pathophysiology of jaundice in G-6-PD deficient neonates. *Pediatr Res* 2007; **61**: 727–31.

27. Denschlag D, Marculescu R, Unfried G, *et al.* The size of a microsatellite polymorphism of the haem oxygenase 1 gene is associated with idiopathic recurrent miscarriage. *Mol Hum Reprod* 2004; **10**: 211–14.

28. Yamada N, Yamaya M, Okinaga S, *et al.* Microsatellite polymorphism in the heme oxygenase-1 gene promoter is associated with susceptibility to emphysema. *Am J Hum Genet* 2000; **66**: 187–95.

29. Exner M, Minar E, Wagner O, *et al.* The role of heme oxygenase-1 promoter polymorphisms in human disease. *Free Radic Biol Med* 2004; **37**: 1097–104.

30. Takeda M, Kikuchi M, Ubalee R, *et al.* Microsatellite polymorphism in the heme oxygenase-1 gene promoter is associated with susceptibility to cerebral malaria in Myanmar. *Jpn J Infect Dis* 2005; **58**: 268–71.

31. Watchko JF, Daood MJ, Hansen TW. Brain bilirubin content is increased in P-glycoprotein-deficient transgenic null mutant mice. *Pediatr Res* 1998; **44**: 763–6.

32. Huang MJ, Kua KE, Teng HC, *et al.* Risk factors for severe hyperbilirubinemia in neonates. *Pediatr Res* 2004; **56**: 682–9.

33. Mollison PL, Cutbush M. Haemolytic disease of the newborn. In Gairdner D, ed., *Recent Advances in Pediatrics*. New York, NY: Blakinston, 1954: 110.

34. Watchko JF, Oski FA. Bilirubin 20 mg/dL = vigintiphobia. *Pediatrics* 1983; **71**: 660–3.

35. Watchko JF. Vigintiphobia revisited. *Pediatrics* 2005; **115**: 1747–53.

36. Andersen DH, Blanc WA, Crozier DN, *et al.* A difference in mortality rate and incidence of kernicterus among premature infants allotted to two prophylactic antibacterial regimens. *Pediatrics* 1956; **18**: 614–25.

37. Stevenson DK, Fanaroff AA, Maisels MJ, *et al.* Prediction of hyperbilirubinemia in near-term and term infants. *Pediatrics* 2001; **108**: 31–9.

38. Vreman HJ, Stevenson DK, Oh W, *et al.* Semiportable electrochemical instrument for determining carbon monoxide in breath. *Clin Chem* 1994; **40**: 1927–33.

39. Brodersen R, Stern L. Deposition of bilirubin acid in the central nervous system: a hypothesis for the development of kernicterus. *Acta Paediatr Scand* 1990; **79**: 12–19.

40. Bratlid D, Cashore WJ, Oh W. Effect of acidosis on bilirubin deposition in rat brain. *Pediatrics* 1984; **73**: 431–4.

41. Stevenson DK, Vreman HJ, Oh W, *et al.* Bilirubin production in healthy term

infants as measured by carbon monoxide in breath. *Clin Chem* 1994; **40**: 1934–9.

42. Dennery PA, Seidman DS, Stevenson DK. Neonatal hyperbilirubinemia. *N Engl J Med* 2001; **344**: 581–90.

43. Gartner LM, Snyder RN, Chabon RS, *et al.* Kernicterus: high incidence in premature infants with low serum bilirubin concentrations. *Pediatrics* 1970; **45**: 906–17.

44. Maisels MJ, Newman TB. Kernicterus in otherwise healthy, breast-fed term newborns. *Pediatrics* 1995; **96**: 730–3.

45. Newman TB, Maisels MJ. Less aggressive treatment of neonatal jaundice and reports of kernicterus: lessons about practice guidelines. *Pediatrics* 2000; **105**: 242–5.

46. Perlman JM, Rogers BB, Burns D. Kernicteric findings at autopsy in two sick near term infants. *Pediatrics* 1997; **99**: 612–15.

47. Ebbesen F. Recurrence of kernicterus in term and near-term infants in Denmark. *Acta Paediatr* 2000; **89**: 1213–17.

48. Ebbesen F, Andersson C, Verder H, *et al.* Extreme hyperbilirubinaemia in term and near-term infants in Denmark. *Acta Paediatr* 2005; **94**: 59–64.

49. Fischer AF, Nakamura H, Uetani Y, *et al.* Comparison of bilirubin production in Japanese and Caucasian infants. *J Pediatr Gastroenterol Nutr* 1988; 7: 27–9.

Chapter 28

Polycythemia and fetal–maternal bleeding

Ted S. Rosenkrantz, Shikha Sarkar, and William Oh

Introduction

Since the third edition, this chapter has been expanded to cover both polycythemia and fetomaternal hemorrhage, a topic that is not extensively or comprehensively discussed in most commonly used textbooks. In the former the hematocrit and blood volume are generally increased, while in the latter both are generally very low. In both conditions, however, there is concern about inadequate organ blood flow, oxygenation delivery, and potential for hypoxic injury, especially in the brain. A large body of definitive information on polycythemia is available that allows conclusions to be made as to management and patient outcome. However, the area of fetomaternal hemorrhage has not been as comprehensively investigated and relies mostly on small clinical series and case reports. There are no controlled basic or clinical trials, which hampers our understanding of pathophysiology as well as therapeutic modalities. This leaves us with gaps in our knowledge of this important topic. What is presented here is the most current body of information and recommendations for diagnosis, treatment, and reported outcomes.

Polycythemia

Polycythemia and hyperviscosity were first associated with adverse neurologic events and sequelae in a series of case reports. The first case often referenced was published by Wood in 1952, and this was followed by a small series of infants with polycythemia and hyperviscosity who displayed multiple problems, including cerebral dysfunction [1–5]. Since those early reports it has become clear that polycythemia has multiple etiologies which influence whether and which problems may be associated with it in the newborn period. In addition, more recent animal and human studies have clarified the relationship between polycythemia and alterations in function of various organs [6–33].

Definition

Polycythemia is usually defined in the literature as a hematocrit value $\geq 65\%$ when the blood sample is obtained from a free-flowing, large venous blood vessel such as the inferior

vena cava (umbilical vein sample) spun in a centrifuge [34]. Sampling from small vessels with low flow or capillary samples will produce higher values. In addition, hematocrits calculated by a Coulter counter will yield comparatively lower values [35–37]. Independent of sample site or measurement technique, the hematocrit increases over the first 2–4 hours of life, gradually returning to the birth value by 12–24 hours of age [34,38,39].

Incidence

The incidence of polycythemia varies by definition, altitude of the population, pregnancy risk factors, and techniques involved in the delivery of the fetus, and timing and sampling sites of blood samples. Studies by Wirth *et al.* have demonstrated that higher altitude is associated with a higher incidence of polycythemia in the general newborn population. At sea level the incidence is 1–2%, while at 1600 feet (430 m), it has been documented to be 5% [40,41].

Causes of polycythemia

A number of fetal and birth complications are known to increase the hematocrit. These problems can usually be attributed to acute or chronic fetal hypoxia, or placental transfusion due to delayed clamping of the umbilical cord (Table 28.1) [2,6,41–54].

Effects of increased hematocrit on organ blood flow and function

Using in vitro techniques, increases in hematocrit are associated with increases in whole-blood viscosity [55,56]. This observation led many to believe that very high hematocrit levels would be associated with decreased organ blood flow, particularly in the brain. It has been hypothesized that this reduction in blood flow would lead to organ hypoxia and damage. A detailed examination of the data from several sources will clarify the relationship between hematocrit, blood viscosity, organ blood flow, and oxygenation.

Viscosity

Fluids can be categorized as Newtonian and non-Newtonian [57,58]. Blood is a non-homogeneous, non-Newtonian fluid. This means that there is not a reciprocal relationship between shear stress and shear rate as with Newtonian fluids such as water [57–59]. There are numerous factors that affect

Fetal and Neonatal Brain Injury, 4th edition, ed. David K. Stevenson, William E. Benitz, Philip Sunshine, Susan R. Hintz, and Maurice L. Druzin. Published by Cambridge University Press. © Cambridge University Press 2009.

Table 28.1. Polycythemia: etiologies and high-risk groups

Delayed cord clamping
Acute hypoxia
Meconium-stained infants
Post-term infants
Chronic hypoxia
Placental insufficiency
Infants of diabetic mothers
Large-for-gestational age infants
Twin-to-twin transfusion
Other
Trisomy 21
Beckwith–Wiedemann syndrome
Fetal/neonatal hyperthyroidism

whole-blood viscosity, including pH, plasma protein concentration, red cell deformity, white blood cell, fibrinogen, and platelet concentration, blood vessel diameter, and blood velocity [14,56,60–66]. However, in the newborn, the single most important factor is red cell concentration or hematocrit. When measured in vitro by a Wells viscometer, blood viscosity will increase as hematocrit increases [60]. In the newborn the increase becomes exponential at hematocrit values $\geq 65\%$. However, in small tubes and the capillaries, blood viscosity becomes similar to the viscosity of the plasma, independent of the hematocrit [58,59,67,68]. This suggests that changes in organ blood flow are not likely to be affected by hematocrit alone or blood viscosity as determined by in vitro techniques.

Relationship between polycythemia, blood viscosity, and organ oxygenation

Based on the stipulation that polycythemia is associated with an increase in blood viscosity that results in decreased blood flow, many individuals have assumed that polycythemia and hyperviscosity result in organ – particularly brain – ischemia and hypoxia. However, a series of experiments performed between 1980 and 1995 have now clarified the changes in blood flow, oxygen delivery, and utilization of the brain of the newborn with polycythemia.

Since Wood's first report, it has been assumed that infants with polycythemia had a reduction of brain blood flow due to sludging of red blood cells within the small blood vessels and capillaries of the brain. Utilizing Doppler techniques, we demonstrated that infants with polycythemia did have a reduction in brain blood flow that returned to normal baseline values following a partial exchange transfusion to reduce the hematocrit [9]. In order to understand the factors that were responsible for the reduction of brain blood flow, our group studied a series of newborn lambs in which hematocrit, whole-blood viscosity, and arterial oxygen content were independently varied [19]. The data demonstrated that the changes in brain blood flow were due to changes in oxygen content, which change in parallel with the changes in the hematocrit in the newborn. This is a normal physiologic response. Viscosity did not influence brain blood flow in this study. This finding has been confirmed by others [69]. Additional studies found that the usual reciprocal relationship between arterial oxygen content and brain blood flow which results in a consistent delivery of oxygen to the brain existed in conditions of increased hematocrit [18,20,70,71]. Further, brain uptake of oxygen was unaffected by polycythemia. These data strongly suggest that the elevated hematocrit alone cannot account for the neurologic abnormalities observed in infants with polycythemia and hyperviscosity.

Blood flow and functional changes in other organs related to increases in hematocrit

As noted, there are numerous signs and symptoms attributed to polycythemia. These are listed in Table 28.2. Cardiac output, as reflected clinically by heart rate, is decreased [7,9,72,73]. Systemic oxygen delivery is normal, due to the reciprocal relationship between increased arterial oxygen content and cardiac output. Systemic blood pressure is not affected by polycythemia. The respiratory distress and cyanosis that occur are likely due to decreased pulmonary blood flow [10,21,74]. Decreased pulmonary blood flow and increased pulmonary vascular resistance associated with shunting have been documented in human and animal investigations. Feeding intolerance, as evidenced by poor suck and oral feeding, is probably due to neurologic dysfunction [75]. On the other hand there is an increased risk of lower gastrointestinal dysfunction, including ileus and necrotizing enterocolitis [7,10,23,24,76–79]. Nowicki *et al.* have documented changes in gastrointestinal blood flow and oxygen delivery and utilization in the unfed and fed state [7]. A study by Black *et al.* has suggested that partial exchange transfusion may contribute significantly to the development of necrotizing enterocolitis [24]. Renal function is compromised, as evidenced by a decreased renal plasma flow and glomerular filtration rate, and decreased urine output in those infants with normovolemic polycythemia [13].

Table 28.2. Signs and symptoms associated with polycythemia

Cyanosis
Plethora
Tremulousness/jitteriness
Seizures
Respiratory distress
Cardiomegaly
Lethargy
Poor suck and feeding
Hyperbilirubinemia
Thrombocytopenia
Hypoglycemia
Hypocalcemia

Newborn infants with polycythemia are at increased risk for hypoglycemia [26,27]. It is not clear whether this is due to decreased gluconeogenesis or increased glucose utilization. Of concern is the finding that cerebral glucose delivery and uptake at whole-blood or plasma glucose concentrations are somewhat greater than concentrations that are generally accepted as normal [71]. This is due to the fact that glucose only exists in the plasma fraction of the blood. This fraction is reduced in polycythemia. Therefore the glucose-carrying capacity of the blood is reduced. When taken in combination with the decreased cerebral blood and plasma flow, cerebral glucose delivery, the limiting determinant of cerebral glucose uptake, reaches its lower limit for normal cerebral glucose uptake at higher concentrations of glucose compared to normal infants. This may have some implication for impaired cerebral function in infants with polycythemia.

Effects of polycythemia on neurologic function

Information about neurologic function is limited by study design and selection process for subjects. A number of studies have examined neurologic function in the newborn period, while others have concentrated on long-term development outcome. Of those examining symptomatic newborns, only two studies have been prospective and randomized. To date, there are no controlled randomized studies of asymptomatic polycythemic infants to determine their long-term neurologic outcome with reference to treatment. However, as cited in the discussion below, some of the studies, such as those by Bada et al. [75] and Høst and Ulrich [79], included asymptomatic infants as well as those exhibiting signs and symptoms that are associated with polycythemia.

Symptomatic infants
Problems in the newborn period
Symptoms associated with polycythemia are listed in Table 28.2 [5,76,77,80]. The first controlled study of symptomatic infants and the effects of a partial exchange transfusion to reduce the hematocrit were reported by Goldberg et al. [77]. Prechtl and Brazelton examinations were initially abnormal in the polycythemic population compared to control infants. Normalization of these examinations in the polycythemic infants who received therapy to reduce the hematocrit was not accelerated. Van der Elst et al. performed a study of similar design in which the Brazelton score alone was used to evaluate the infants [78]. While the polycythemic infants were different from control infants, again, therapy to reduce the hematocrit did not alter outcome in the newborn period.

There have been some studies that have specifically examined the outcome of small-for-gestational-age infants. As a group, the small-for-gestational-age infants have an increased incidence of polycythemia and an outcome that is inferior to those infants who have normal intrauterine growth [52,81]. Polycythemia, likely a compensatory mechanism for chronic hypoxia, does not appear to be an independent factor in the outcome of this group of infants [53,75].

Long-term sequelae
Goldberg et al. were able to re-examine a subset of the original study population at 8 months of age [77]. Abnormalities were found in 67% of the infants treated with partial exchange transfusion, 50% of the untreated infants, and 17% of the control infants. These findings are in contrast to those of van der Elst et al., who found that all of the infants had normal neurologic examinations [78]. There were no differences in the developmental scores of the three groups.

Black et al. have performed two studies to determine the long-term outcome of infants with polycythemia. In the first study 111 infants with polycythemia and 110 control infants were studied [80]. The infants with polycythemia were not randomized as to observation or treatment. Follow-up examinations were performed between 1 and 3 years of age. Control infants had fewer abnormalities compared to the polycythemia group. The polycythemic infants were characterized by a 25% incidence of motor abnormalities, especially spastic diplegia. Forty percent had some type of handicap. However, there were no differences in outcome when the two subsets of polycythemic infants (observed vs. treated) were compared.

In 1985 Black and colleagues published data on a group of 93 infants with polycythemia who were randomized to treatment or observation [82]. The total population included infants who were symptomatic and asymptomatic in the newborn period. At 1 year 59% of the infants were available for follow-up, and no differences between the groups were found. At 2 years 61% of the original group was examined, and the treated group had fewer abnormalities. This same group was called back again at school age (7 years of age) [83]. At that time only 49 of the original 93 infants were available for evaluation. Significant differences between the control and polycythemic infants persisted. However, the observed and treated polycythemic groups were virtually identical.

Høst and Ulrich revealed the outcome of 635 infants as part of a public health project [79]. Screening in the newborn period revealed that 117 (18%) had venous hematocrit > 60%, 30 (4.7%) had hematocrit > 65%, and seven had hematocrit greater than 70%. Only 13 had any symptomatology that could be ascribed to polycythemia. None received an exchange transfusion to reduce the hematocrit. Over 80% of the infants were available for follow-up at age 6 years. Of those restudied, 104 of 113 polycythemic infants were normal. The remainder had minor problems, such as febrile convulsions, that could not be attributed to polycythemia in the newborn period.

Lastly, Bada et al. examined a group of infants with asymptomatic and symptomatic polycythemia and a control group of infants [75]. Follow-up at 30 months of age revealed no differences between the three groups of infants. However, when multivariant analysis was performed using multiple perinatal factors, it became clear that these other perinatal risk factors were highly related to outcome in all groups of infants, and polycythemia fell out as a non-significant factor.

When the results of these studies are taken together with our current knowledge of adaptive fetal physiology, several conclusions can be made. First, polycythemia appears to be an adaptive mechanism for chronic and acute fetal hypoxia. Hypoxia alone is known to be responsible for irreversible brain injury. Second, exchange transfusion does not appear to have an appreciable influence on the long-term neurologic function of infants with elevated hematocrits at birth, although the polycythemia is clearly a marker for increased risk of cerebral dysfunction. The demographic data from the studies of Black *et al.* and Bada *et al.* clearly indicate that these infants, particularly those who are symptomatic in the newborn period and in later life, are those infants that experience an adverse fetal environment [75,82,83]. Therefore it would appear that the events, particularly hypoxic–ischemic events, that result in an increase in hematocrit are likely to be responsible for the observed cerebral dysfunction. This would explain the failure of postnatal reduction of the hematocrit to alter the long-term prognosis.

Asymptomatic infants

There are still institutions that screen either all or high-risk infants for polycythemia. There are no large population studies of the long-term outcome of this type of population. Based on the findings in the studies cited in the preceding section, as well as a meta-analysis by Dempsey and Barrington [84], these infants may be at some non-quantifiable increased risk for long-term sequelae; however, current data strongly suggest that there is no evidence that an exchange transfusion to reduce the hematocrit will change the outcome, as these sequelae appear to be due to other adverse perinatal events. Based on the data from well-designed trials, the American Academy of Pediatrics Committee of the Fetus and Newborn made the following statement: "The accepted treatment of polycythemia is partial exchange transfusion. However, there is no evidence that exchange transfusion affects long-term outcome. Universal screening for polycythemia fails to meet the methodology and treatment criteria and also, possibly the natural criterion." [85]

Recommendations for therapy

Partial exchange transfusion may be of benefit for those infants who exhibit signs and symptoms or complications that have been demonstrated to be related to physiologic abnormalities caused by polycythemia. Such manifestations or clinical conditions include respiratory distress with cyanosis, renal failure, and hypoglycemia. Before considering therapy, the infant should be evaluated for other temporal and clinical events which may, in fact, be responsible for the problems observed. A partial exchange transfusion should not be done in the hope of correcting neurologic abnormalities in the immediate newborn period or preventing future neurologic dysfunction.

As there are no adequate scientific data to demonstrate any benefit for polycythemic infants who are asymptomatic in the newborn period, simple observation alone would seem prudent. In situations when there are subtle signs and symptoms, or in the presence of an extremely high hematocrit (e.g., >70%), the decision to perform a partial exchange transfusion may be initiated on individual clinical judgment based on the level of hematocrit, certainty of interpreting clinical symptoms, and the potential risk of the treatment (partial exchange transfusion). For those who develop neurologic abnormalities at a later time, the events during the prenatal and perinatal period should be examined carefully to verify an etiology, other than polycythemia, that might explain the cerebral dysfunction.

Summary

Since the last version of this chapter there has not been further original work on polycythemia, hyperviscosity and outcome [86]. The new meta-analyses and the statement from the American Academy of Pediatrics concur with our thoughts on this topic [84–86]. That is, there are no data to support a direct relationship between polycythemia and neurologic dysfunction. Polycythemia appears to be a marker for adverse prenatal and perinatal events that are known to cause mild to catastrophic neurologic injury. Postnatal exchange transfusion has not been shown to be of long-term benefit to infants who are symptomatic in the newborn period. There are no data to support the efficacy of this therapy in the infant with an elevated hematocrit who is otherwise normal.

Fetomaternal hemorrhage

Fetal cells very commonly cross the placental barrier before delivery, during labor, and after delivery. The volume of fetal cells entering the maternal circulation is generally quite small (0.01–0.1 mL) [87]. When the mother is Rh-negative and the fetus is Rh-positive, this may lead to maternal antibody production and hemolysis in the fetus. This is a preventable problem with the availability of Rhogram®.

The focus of this review is the passage of a large volume of fetal cells into the maternal circulation (massive fetomaternal hemorrhage, FMH), which results in either acute anemia and hypovolemia or chronic and progressive anemia in the fetus. An acute FMH is frequently associated with a sudden deterioration in fetal well-being. A more chronic hemorrhage generally allows the fetus to compensate unless the hemoglobin concentration becomes so low that the fetus develops hydrops fetalis. A catastrophic outcome secondary to FMH can be prevented if the hemorrhage is detected in a timely fashion so that appropriate intervention can take place that prevents fetal hypoxia. What follows is a discussion of the incidence, presentation, potential interventions, and outcomes of pregnancies complicated by FMH.

Incidence

Although 50–75% of pregnancies are associated with some degree of FMH, volumes of transfer are usually small, from 0.01 to 0.1 mL. Massive FMH is defined as the presence of 20–60 mL or more of fetal blood in the maternal circulation. FMH of this size is reported to occur 1 to 6/1000 births [88–90]. Large hemorrhages with clinical impact on the fetus and newborn are so uncommon that most of the information is based on case reports and a few small series [88–92]. Most of these data are retrospective. Lastly, the diagnosis may be affected by the method used to detect fetal cells in the maternal circulation.

Etiology

FMH has been associated with a maternal history of vaginal bleeding, abdominal trauma, placenta previa, placental abruption, and cord compression [88,93]. There are contradictory reports regarding the mode of delivery. Ness *et al.* reported a higher incidence with cesarean section, and Salim *et al.* reported no difference for a large FMH between cesarean section and vaginal deliveries [90,94]. Emergency cesarean, cord around the neck, and low birthweight were associated with larger FMH [90]. Large FMH have also been described with external cephalic version, with anterior placenta, and with placental tumors such as chorioangiomata and choriocarcinoma [95–99]. Lastly, there is only speculation on the pathophysiology of how fetal cells enter the maternal circulation and what is responsible for the large, clinically important hemorrhages.

Diagnosis

The diagnosis of FMH is made by detecting fetal RBCs in maternal blood. The Kleihauer–Betke test (KB) has been used as the standard since it was described in 1957 [100]. The principle of the KB test is that fetal hemoglobin (HbF) is resistant to elution by an acidic buffer whereas the adult hemoglobin (HbA) is eluted by the acid buffer. When the blood film is fixed and stained, the fetal cells containing HbF are stained and the maternal cells appear as "ghost cells."

The extent of the FMH can only be estimated accurately if done before delivery, as postpartum estimates may be falsely elevated from extra fetal blood extravasated into the maternal circulation with delivery of the placenta. There may also be false-positive results in mothers with increased fetal hemoglobin synthesis such as sickle cell disease, thalassemia, and hereditary persistence of HbF.

Using the KB test and basic physiologic principles, FMH can be calculated using the following formula [101]:

$$\text{Fetal blood volume} = \frac{\text{Maternal blood volume} \times \text{Maternal HCT} \times \text{\%fetal cells (KB)}}{\text{Newborn HCT}}$$

This is based on the assumption that maternal blood volume is 5000 mL, maternal hematocrit (HCT) is 35%, and newborn HCT is 50%.

Flow cytometry is a new technology also available for the estimation of FMH [102]. It has been shown to be accurate, more sensitive, and reproducible [103]. It is a more specialized test that is more expensive and not done routinely in all hospitals. It has been useful in Rh-incompatible pregnancies to decide accurate dosage of anti-D immunoglobulin. It is also useful in clarifying KB test results when there is a known maternal excess of fetal hemoglobin such as hereditary

persistence of Hemoglobin F (HPHF) and the KB test would overestimate the FMH [104].

Clinical presentation

Presentation of the fetus or newborn depends on the amount and timing of the FMH [93]. The most common presentation appears to be an acute event. In this situation a large FMH is associated with decreased fetal movement or loss of fetal movements and sinusoidal fetal heart-rate pattern. FMH has been associated with 3–14% of all stillbirths, and should be suspected in unexplained stillbirth and anemia [93,105]. Giacoia reviewed these variables to see if there was a correlation to the amount of hemorrhage [89]. One hundred thirty-four cases were evaluated, and 17 had absent fetal movements for 1–7 days. A sinusoidal heart-rate pattern was found in 21% and decreased fetal movements in 40%. No difference was found between cases with FMH less than 200 mL or more than 200 mL. Others have found that the absolute blood flow velocity of the middle cerebral artery in the fetus may also aid in the diagnosis of fetal anemia [106].

Infants born after an acute hemorrhage are often tachycardic and tachypneic. The newborn's hemoglobin can be as low as 4–6 g/dL [92]. In cases of acute massive FMH, the newborn presents with hypovolemic shock, acidosis, respiratory distress, persistent pulmonary hypertension, hypoxic ischemic encephalopathy, and multiorgan failure.

If the FMH is a slow, chronic process the newborn may present with pallor but is otherwise hemodynamically stable as there has been time for the fetus to compensate. If the hemoglobin reaches very low levels, then the fetus will develop hydrops fetalis. There have been reports of fetal transfusion in instances when the fetus is still very premature. The correction of fetal anemia leads to resolution of the hydrops and allows continuation of the pregnancy [107].

Treatment

Newborn infants with a significant hemorrhage require rapid assessment and treatment. Treatment of an acute hemorrhage consists of volume replacement with crystalloid and packed RBC under close monitoring. These infants will also need assessment and treatment for metabolic acidosis, respiratory distress, and ongoing hypotension. Evaluation and therapy for possible hypoxic–ischemic encephalopathy and seizures is also required. For infants with chronic anemia and symptoms of hydrops, exchange transfusion is a more appropriate means of correcting the anemia, as these infants will have a normal blood volume. These infants will often need additional therapy for respiratory distress and congestive heart failure.

Outcomes

In the study by Giacoia, six infants survived, five were stillborn, and five died in the neonatal period [89]. Kecskes found that only the postnatal presentation and an initial hemoglobin of < 4 g/dL were associated with a poor outcome [108]. Other case reports with reviews of the literature have shown good outcomes with very low hematocrits. Rubod *et al.* studied the long-term prognosis for infants after massive fetomaternal hemorrhage and concluded that FMH ≥ 20 mL/kg significantly increased the risk of death and preterm delivery, but long-term follow up in survivors was not associated with neurologic sequelae [88]. However a detailed review of documented cases of FMH reveals that a significant number of survivors develop cerebral changes including in intraventricular hemorrhage, cerebral infarction, ventriculomegaly, periventricular leukomalacia, and cerebral atrophy. There are also some infants with initial normal neurological examinations and imaging studies who eventually developed cerebral palsy [89,109]. Therefore the ultimate outcome may be dependent on multiple factors, including the size of the hemorrhage and the time between hemorrhage and delivery, as well as on recognition of the anemia and hypotension and timely therapy [108].

Conclusion

Massive FMH is not as uncommon as previously believed. It is an important cause of fetal morbidity and mortality in low-risk pregnancies. KB test and flow cytometry are the two diagnostic tools available to establish the diagnosis. Outcomes appear to be related to the degree of fetal/neonatal anemia, a high index of suspicion leading to prompt obstetrical diagnosis and intervention, and rapid evaluation and treatment of the newborn. In all cases of unexplained fetal death a KB test should be performed.

References

1. Wood JL. Plethora in the newborn infant associated with cyanosis and convulsions. *J Pediatr* 1952; **54**: 143–51.

2. Michael A, Mauer AM. Maternal–fetal transfusion as a cause of plethora in the neonatal period. *Pediatrics* 1961; **28**: 458–61.

3. Minkowski A. Acute cardiac failure in connection with neonatal polycythemia in monovular twins and single newborn infants. *Biol Neonate* 1962; **4**: 61–74.

4. Danks DM, Stevens LH. Neonatal respiratory distress associated with a high haematocrit reading. *Lancet* 1964; **2**: 499–500.

5. Gross CP, Hathaway WE, McCaughey HR. Hyperviscosity in the neonate. *J Pediatr* 1973; **82**: 1004–12.

6. Oh W, Oh MA, Lind J. Renal function and blood volume in newborn infants related to placental transfusion. *Acta Paediatr Scand* 1966; **56**: 197–210.

7. Nowicki P, Oh W, Yao A, et al. Effect of polycythemia on gastrointestinal blood flow and oxygenation in piglets. *Am J Physiol* 1984; **247**: G220–5.

8. Surjadhana A, Rouleau J, Boerboom L, et al. Myocardial blood flow and its distribution in anesthetized polycythemic dogs. *Circ Res* 1978; **43**: 619–31.

9. Rosenkrantz TS, Oh W. Cerebral blood flow velocity in infants with polycythemia and hyperviscosity: effects of partial exchange transfusion with plasmanate. *J Pediatr* 1982; **101**: 94–8.

10. Fouron JC, Hebert F. The circulatory effects of hematocrit variations in normovolemic newborn lambs. *J Pediatr* 1973; **82**: 995–1003.

11. Gatti RA, Muster AJ, Cole RB, et al. Neonatal polycythemia with transient cyanosis and cardiorespiratory abnormalities. *J Pediatr* 1966; **69**: 1063–72.

12. Kotagal VR, Keenan WJ, Reuter JH, et al. Regional blood flow in polycythemia and hypervolemia. *Pediatr Res* 1977; **11**: 394.

13. Kotagal VR, Kleinman LI. Effect of acute polycythemia on newborn renal hemodynamics and function. *Pediatr Res* 1982; **16**: 148–51.

14. Bergqvist G, Zetterman R. Blood viscosity and peripheral circulation in newborn infants. *Acta Paediatr Scand* 1974; **63**: 865–8.

15. Linderkamp O, Strohhacker I, Versmold HT, et al. Peripheral circulation in the newborn: interaction of peripheral blood flow, blood pressure, blood volume and blood viscosity. *J Pediatr* 1978; **129**: 73–81.

16. Gustafsson L, Applegren L, Myrvold HE. The effect of polycythemia on blood flow in working and non-working skeletal muscle. *Acta Physiol Scand* 1980; **109**: 143–8.

17. Waffarn F, Cole CD, Huxtable RF. Effects of polycythemia on cutaneous blood flow and transcutaneous PO2 and PCO2 in the hyperviscosity neonate. *Pediatrics* 1984; **74**: 389–94.

18. Jones MD, Traystman RJ, Simmons MA, et al. Effects of changes in arterial O$_2$ content on cerebral blood flow in the lamb. *Am J Physiol* 1981; **240**: H209–15.

19. Rosenkrantz TS, Stonestreet BS, Hansen NB, et al. Cerebral blood flow in the newborn lamb with polycythemia and hyperviscosity. *J Pediatr* 1984; **104**: 276–80.

20. Rosenkrantz TS, Philipps AF, Skrzypczak PS, et al. Cerebral metabolism in the newborn lamb with polycythemia. *Pediatr Res* 1988; **23**: 329–33.

21. Oh W, Wallgren G, Hanson JS, et al. The effects of placental transfusion on respiratory mechanics of normal term newborn infants. *Pediatrics* 1967; **40**: 6–12.

22. Hakanson DO, Oh W. Necrotizing enterocolitis and hyperviscosity in the newborn infant. *J Pediatr* 1977; **90**: 458–61.

23. LeBlanc MH, D'Cruz C, Pate K. Necrotizing enterocolitis can be caused by polycythemic hyperviscosity in the newborn dog. *J Pediatr* 1984; **105**: 804–9.

24. Black VD, Rumack CM, Lubchenco LO, et al. Gastrointestinal injury in polycythemic term infants. *Pediatrics* 1985; **76**: 225–31.

25. Herson VC, Raye JR, Rowe JC, et al. Acute renal failure associated with polycythemia in a neonate. *J Pediatr* 1982; **100**: 137–9.

26. Leake RD, Chan GM, Zakauddin S, et al. Glucose perturbation in experimental hyperviscosity. *Pediatr Res* 1980; **14**: 1320–3.

27. Creswell JS, Warburton D, Susa JB, et al. Hyperviscosity in the newborn lamb produces perturbation in glucose homeostasis. *Pediatrics* 1981; **15**: 1348–50.

28. Rivers RPA. Coagulation changes associated with a high haematocrit in the newborn infant. *Acta Paediatr Scand* 1975; **64**: 449–56.

29. Katz J, Rodriquez E, Mandani G, et al. Normal coagulation findings, thrombocytopenia, and peripheral hemoconcentration in neonatal polycythemia. *J Pediatr* 1982; **101**: 99–102.

30. Henriksson P. Hyperviscosity of the blood and haemostasis in the newborn infant. *Acta Paediatr Scand* 1979; **68**: 701–4.

31. Shaikh BS, Erslev AJ. Thrombocytopenia in polycythemic mice. *J Lab Clin Med* 1978; **92**: 765–71.

32. Jackson CW, Smith PJ, Edwards CC, *et al.* Relationship between packed cell volume platelets and platelet survival in red blood cell-hypertransfused mice. *J Lab Clin Med* 1979; **94**: 500–9.

33. Meberg A. Transitory thrombocytopenia in newborn mice after intrauterine hypoxia. *Pediatr Res* 1980; **14**: 1071–3.

34. Rosenkrantz TS, Oh W. Neonatal polycythemia and hyperviscosity. In Milunsky A, Friedman EA, Gluck L, eds., *Advances in Perinatal Medicine*, Vol. 5. New York, NY: Plenum, 1986: 93–123.

35. Cornbleet J. Spurious results from automated hematology cell counters. *Lab Med* 1983; **14**: 509–14.

36. Penn D, Williams PR, Dutcher TF, *et al.* Comparison of hematocrit determination by microhematocrit electronic particle counter. *Am J Clin Pathol* 1979; **72**: 71–4.

37. Pearson TC, Guthrie L. Trapped plasma in the microhematocrit. *Am J Clin Pathol* 1982; **78**: 770–2.

38. Oh W, Lind J. Venous and capillary hematocrit in newborn infants and placental transfusion. *Acta Paediatr Scand* 1966; **55**: 38–40.

39. Shohat M, Reisner SH, Mimouni F, *et al.* Neonatal polycythemia II. Definition related to time of sampling. *Pediatrics* 1984; **73**: 11–13.

40. Wirth FH, Goldberg KE, Lubchenco LO. Neonatal hyperviscosity I. Incidence. *Pediatrics* 1979; **63**: 833–6.

41. Stevens K, Wirth FH. Incidence of neonatal hyperviscosity at sea level. *J Pediatr* 1980; **97**: 118–19.

42. Oh W, Blankenship W, Lind J. Further study of neonatal blood volume in relation to placental transfusion. *Ann Paediatr* 1966; **207**: 147–59.

43. Yao AC, Moinian M, Lind J. Distribution of blood between infants and placenta after birth. *Lancet* 1969; **2**: 871–3.

44. Linderkamp O. Placental transfusion: determinants and effects. *Clin Perinatol* 1981; **9**: 559–92.

45. Saigal S, Usher RH. Symptomatic neonatal plethora. *Biol Neonate* 1977; **32**: 62–72.

46. Philip AGS, Yee AB, Rosy M, *et al.* Placental transfusion as an intrauterine phenomenon in deliveries complicated by fetal distress. *Br Med J* 1969; **2**: 11–13.

47. Flod NE, Ackerman BD. Perinatal asphyxia and residual placenta blood volume. *Acta Paediatr Scand* 1971; **60**: 433–6.

48. Yao AC, Lind J. Effect of gravity on placental transfusion. *Lancet* 1969; **2**: 505–8.

49. Oh W, Omori K, Emmanouilides GC, *et al.* Placenta to lamb fetus transfusion *in utero* during acute hypoxia. *Am J Obstet Gynecol* 1975; **122**: 316–21.

50. Sacks MO. Occurrence of anemia and polycythemia in phenotypically dissimilar single ovum human twins. *Pediatrics* 1959; **24**: 604–8.

51. Schwartz JL, Maniscalco WM, Lane AT, *et al.* Twin transfusion syndrome causing cutaneous erythropoiesis. *Pediatrics* 1984; **74**: 527–9.

52. Humbert JR, Abelson H, Hathaway WE, *et al.* Polycythemia in small for gestational age infants. *J Pediatr* 1969; **75**: 812–19.

53. Widness JA, Garcia JA, Oh W, *et al.* Cord serum erythropoietin values and disappearance rates after birth in polycythemic newborns. *Pediatr Res* 1982; **16**: 218A.

54. Philipps AF, Dubin JW, Matty PJ, *et al.* Arterial hypoxemia and hyperinsulinemia in the chronically hyperglycemic fetal lamb. *Pediatr Res* 1982; **16**: 653–8.

55. Wells RE, Penton R, Merrill EW. Measurements of viscosity of biologic fluids by core plate viscometer. *J Lab Clin Med* 1961; **57**: 646–56.

56. Linderkamp O, Versmold HT, Riegel KP, *et al.* Contributions of red cells and plasma to blood viscosity in preterm and full-term infants and adults. *Pediatrics* 1984; **74**: 45–51.

57. Poiseuille JLM. Recherches expérimentales sur le mouvement des liquides dans les tubes de très petits diameters. *C R Acad Sci* 1840; **11**: 961–1041.

58. van der Elst CW, Malan AF, de Heese HV. Blood viscosity in modern medicine. *S Afr Med J* 1977; **52**: 526–8.

59. Dintenfass L. Blood viscosity, internal fluidity of the red cell, dynamic coagulation and the critical capillary radius as factors in the physiology and pathology of circulation and microcirculation. *Med J Aust* 1968; **1**: 688–96.

60. Wells RE, Merrill EW. Influence of flow properties of blood upon viscosity–hematocrit relationships. *J Clin Invest* 1962; **41**: 1591–8.

61. Bergqvist G. Viscosity of the blood in the newborn infants. *Acta Paediatr Scand* 1974; **63**: 858–64.

62. Wells R. Syndromes of hyperviscosity. *N Engl J Med* 1970; **283**: 183–6.

63. Smith CM, Prasler WJ, Tukey DP, *et al.* Fetal red cells are more deformable than adult red cells. *Blood* 1981; **58**: 35a.

64. Lichtman MA. Cellular deformability during maturation of the myeloblast: possible role in marrow egress. *N Engl J Med* 1970; **283**: 943–8.

65. Lichtman MA. Rheology of leukocytes, leukocyte suspensions, and blood in leukemia. *J Clin Invest* 1973; **52**: 350.

66. Miller ME. Developmental maturation of human neutrophil motility and its relationship to membrane deformability. In Bellanti UA, Dayton DH, eds., *The Phagocytic Cell in Host Resistance*. New York, NY: Raven Press, 1975: 295.

67. Burton AC. Role of geometry, of size and shape, in the microcirculation. *Fed Proc* 1966; **25**: 1753–60.

68. Fahraeus R, Lindqvist T. The viscosity of the blood in narrow capillary tubes. *Am J Physiol* 1931; **96**: 561–8.

69. Goldstein M, Stonestreet BS, Brann BS, *et al.* Cerebral cortical blood flow and oxygen metabolism in normocythemic hyperviscous newborn piglets. *Pediatr Res* 1988; **24**: 486–9.

70. Massik J, Tang YL, Hudak ML, *et al.* Effect of hematocrit on cerebral blood flow with induced polycythemia. *J Appl Physiol* 1987; **62**: 1090–6.

71. Rosenkrantz TS, Philipps AF, Knox I, *et al.* Regulation of cerebral glucose metabolism in normal and polycythemic newborns. *J Cereb Blood Flow Metab* 1992; **12**: 856–65.

72. LeBlanc MH, Kotagal UR, Kleinman LI. Physiological effects of hypervolemic polycythemia in newborn dogs. *J Appl Physiol* 1982; **53**: 865–72.

73. Murphy DJ, Reller MD, Meyer RA, *et al.* Effects of neonatal polycythemia and partial exchange transfusion on cardiac function: an echocardiographic study. *Pediatrics* 1985; **76**: 909–13.

74. Brashear RE. Effects of acute plasma for blood exchange in experimental polycythemia. *Respiration* 1980; **40**: 297–306.

75. Bada HS, Korones SB, Pourcyrous M, *et al.* Asymptomatic syndrome of polycythemic hyperviscosity: effect of partial plasma exchange transfusion. *J Pediatr* 1992; **120**: 579–85.

76. Ramamurthy RS, Brans YW. Neonatal polycythemia. I. Criteria for diagnosis and treatment. *Pediatrics* 1981; **68**: 168–74.

77. Goldberg K, Wirth FH, Hathaway WE, *et al.* Neonatal hyperviscosity. II. Effect of partial plasma exchange transfusion. *Pediatrics* 1982; **69**: 419–25.

78. van der Elst CW, Molteno CD, Malan AF, *et al.* The management of polycythemia in the newborn infant. *Early Hum Dev* 1980; **4**: 393–403.

79. Høst A, Ulrich M. Late prognosis in untreated neonatal polycythemia with minor or no symptoms. *Acta Paediatr Scand* 1982; **71**: 629–33.

80. Black VD, Lubchenco LD, Luckey DW, *et al.* Developmental and neurologic sequelae of neonatal hyperviscosity syndrome. *Pediatrics* 1982; **69**: 426–31.

81. Hakanson DO, Oh W. Hyperviscosity in the small-for-gestational age infant. *Biol Neonate* 1980; **37**: 109–12.

82. Black VD, Lubchenco LO, Koops BL, *et al.* Neonatal hyperviscosity: randomized study of effect of partial plasma exchange on long-term outcome. *Pediatrics* 1985; **75**: 1048–53.

83. Black VD, Camp BW, Lubchenco LO, *et al.* Neonatal hyperviscosity is associated with lower achievement and IQ scores at school age. *Pediatr Res* 1988; **23**: 442A.

84. Dempsey EM, Barrington K. Short and long term outomes following partial exchange transfusion in the polycythemic newborn: a systematic review. *Arch Dis Child Fetal Neonatal Ed* 2006; **91**: F2–6.

85. American Academy of Pediatrics Committee on the Fetus and Newborn. Routine evaluation of blood pressure, hematocrit and glucose in newborns. *Pediatrics* 1993; **92**: 474–6.

86. Rosenkrantz TS. Polycythemia and hyperviscosity in the newborn. *Semin Thromb Hemost* 2003; **29**: 515–27.

87. Scott JR, Warenski JC. Tests to detect and quantitate fetomaternal bleeding. *Clin Obstet Gynecol* 1982; **25**: 277–82.

88. Rubod C, Deruelle P, Le Goueff F, *et al.* Long-term prognosis for infants after massive fetomaternal hemorrhage. *Obstet Gynecol* 2007; **110**: 256–60.

89. Giacoia GP. Severe fetomaternal hemorrhage: a review. *Obstet Gynecol Surv* 1997; **52**: 372–80.

90. Salim R, Ben-Shlomo I, Nachum Z, *et al.* The incidence of large fetomaternal hemorrhage and Kleihauer–Betke test. *Obstet Gynecol* 2005; **105**: 1039–44.

91. Sebring E, Polesky H. Fetomaternal hemorrhage: incidence, risk factors, time of occurrence, and clinical effects. *Transfusion* 1990; **30**: 344–57.

92. Kosasa T, Ebesugawa I, Nakayama R, *et al.* Massive fetomaternal hemorrhage preceded by decreased fetal movement and a nonreactive fetal heart rate pattern. *Obstet Gynecol* 1993; **82**: 711–14.

93. Markham LA, Charsha DS, Peelmuter B. Case report of massive fetomaternal hemorrhage and a guideline for acute neonatal management. *Adv Neonatal Care* 2006; **6**: 197–207.

94. Ness PM, Baldwin ML, Niebyl JR. Clinical high risk designation does not predict excess fetal–maternal hemorrhage. *Am J Obstet Gynecol* 1987; **156**: 154–8.

95. Bänninger V, Schmid J. External cephalic version close to term in the management of breech presentation. *Z Geburtshilfe Perinatol* 1977; **181**: 189–92.

96. Blom AH, Gevers RH. Een patient met diffuse chorangiomatosis placenta. *Ned Tijdschr Geneeskd* 1974; **118**: 7–10.

97. Blackburn GK. Massive fetomaternal hemorrhage due to choriocarcinoma of the uterus. *J Pediatr* 1976; **89**: 680–1.

98. Shankar M, Gough GW, Chakravarti S, *et al.* Massive feto-maternal haemorrhage with good perinatal outcome following failed external cephalic version. *Fetal Diagn Ther* 2004; **19**: 68–71.

99. Lam CM, Wong SF, Lee DW, *et al.* Massive feto-maternal hemorrhage: an early presentation of women with gestational choriocarcinoma. *Acta Obstet Gynecol Scand* 2002; **81**: 573–6.

100. Kleihauer E, Betke K. Practical use of the demonstration of cells containing hemoglobin F in fixed blood smears [in German]. *Izv Mikrobiol Inst* 1960; **1**: 92–295.

101. Cunningham FG, Gant NF, Leveno KJ, *et al.* Diseases and injuries of the fetus and newborn. In *Williams Obstetrics*, 21st edn. New York, NY: McGraw-Hill, 2001; 1039–91.

102. Bromilow IM, Duguid JK. Measurement of feto-maternal haemorrhage: a comparative study of three Kleihauer techniques and two flow cytometry methods. *Clin Lab Haematol* 1997; **19**: 137–42.

103. Fong EA, Davies JI, Grey DE, *et al.* Detection of massive transplacental haemorrhage by flow cytometry. *Clin Lab Haematol* 2000; **22**: 325–7.

104. Kush ML, Muench MV, Harman CR, *et al.* Persistent fetal hemoglobin in maternal circulation complicating the diagnosis of fetomaternal hemorrhage. *Obstet Gynecol* 2005; **105**: 872–4.

105. Laube DW, Schauberger CW. Fetomaternal bleeding as a cause for unexplained fetal death. *Obstet Gynecol* 1982; **60**: 649–51.

106. Malcus P, Bjorklund LJ, Lilja M, *et al.* Massive feto-maternal hemorrhage: diagnosis by cardiotocography, Doppler ultrasonography and ST waveform analysis of fetal electrocardiography. *Fetal Diagn Ther* 2006; **21**: 8–12.

107. Rubod C, Houfflin V, Belot F, *et al.* Successful *in utero* treatment of chronic and massive fetomaternal hemorrhage with fetal hydrops. *Fetal Diagn Ther* 2006; **21**: 410–13.

108. Kecskes Z. Large fetomaternal hemorrhage: clinical presentation and outcome. *J Matern Fetal Neonatal Med* 2003; **13**: 128–32.

109. Parveen V, Patole SK, Whitehall JS. Massive fetomaternal hemorrhage with persistent pulmonary hypertension in a neonate. *Indian Pediatr* 2002; **39**: 385–8.

Chapter 29

Hydrops fetalis

David P. Carlton

Introduction

Hydrops fetalis is the presence of excess body water in the fetus resulting in skin edema coupled with effusions in the pleural, peritoneal, or pericardial space. Because most pregnancies in the United States include routine fetal assessment by ultrasound, most cases of hydrops will be recognized before birth. An associated abnormality can be diagnosed either ante- or postnatally in the majority of patients who have hydrops. The prognosis for survival is generally poor. Over 50% of fetuses diagnosed with hydrops die in utero, and of those that survive to delivery, over half will die postnatally despite aggressive support [1,2].

Immune hydrops

Immune hydrops is a late manifestation of the anemia that results from fetal erythrocyte destruction by transplacentally acquired maternal antibodies to fetal red-cell antigens. The severity of anemia necessary to disturb total body water is unpredictable, but a hematocrit of less than 20% is commonly associated with hydrops [3]. Fetuses with an immune basis for their hydrops who are not treated with intrauterine red-cell transfusion face a significant risk of in utero death.

Historically, the most common antigen causing an antibody-mediated hemolytic anemia was the Rh D. Anemia as a function of sensitization to the D antigen is infrequent today because of the routine use of Rh immunoglobulin in the management of women who are Rh-D-negative [4,5]. Sensitization to other red-cell antigens, including Kell, e, and c also causes fetal hemolytic anemia and results in immune hydrops [6].

Non-immune hydrops

Non-immune hydrops occurs in approximately 1/2000–4000 deliveries and is a more frequent category of hydrops than immune hydrops [7]. Observational studies suggest that postnatal mortality averages ∼50%, but the risk of death in a patient with non-immune hydrops is influenced significantly by the presence of accompanying disorders [1,8–10].

Approximately 60–80% of the cases of non-immune hydrops in the United States occur in association with an identifiable disorder. Well over 100 different diagnoses have been linked to non-immune hydrops, but in only a limited number of these conditions are there pathophysiological links between the associated disorder and the development of hydrops [11]. In 20–40% of patients who have non-immune hydrops, an associated condition will not be found despite a thorough investigation [1,9,12]. These patients are considered to have "idiopathic" non-immune hydrops (Table 29.1).

Proposed mechanisms of edema formation in patients with hydrops

The net flux of liquid into the interstitial space governs whether edema formation occurs. Excess fluid will leave the circulation and enter the interstitial space if vascular surface area is increased, endothelial barrier integrity is compromised, hydrostatic pressure difference between the vascular and interstitial spaces is increased, or protein oncotic pressure difference between the vascular and interstitial spaces is decreased [13]. Fluid clearance from the interstitial space is impaired when lymphatic drainage is impeded.

Processes that increase right atrial and central venous pressures are common in hydropic infants and will result in an increase in upstream microvascular hydrostatic pressure and thus an increase in transvascular fluid filtration into the interstitium. Simultaneously, this same elevation in central venous pressure will also impede lymphatic return of interstitial fluid back into the central circulation. Even minimal increases in lymphatic outflow pressure impair lymphatic drainage [14,15]. Because central venous pressure is the relevant outflow pressure for lymphatic drainage in the fetus, even small increases in central venous pressure may reduce the effectiveness of interstitial fluid clearance. Thus, in conditions that increase central venous pressure, hydrops may be caused, or at least aggravated, by two distinct mechanisms: increased transvascular fluid entry and impaired fluid clearance.

Tachyarrhythmias or myocardial dysfunction may also be associated with an elevated central venous pressure. For instance, myocardial dysfunction is the presumed basis for hydrops in fetuses who have an elevation in umbilical venous pressure [16,17]. Packed red-cell transfusion in anemic fetuses reduces umbilical venous pressure, presumably by improving cardiac function, and thus prevents hydrops formation. Even in hydropic fetuses that are not anemic, there is evidence of myocardial dysfunction and elevated umbilical venous

Fetal and Neonatal Brain Injury, 4th edition, ed. David K. Stevenson, William E. Benitz, Philip Sunshine, Susan R. Hintz, and Maurice L. Druzin. Published by Cambridge University Press. © Cambridge University Press 2009.

Table 29.1. Conditions associated with non-immune hydrops

Idiopathic
Non-immune anemias
Homozygous α-thalassemia (Hb Bart's hydrops)
Erythrocyte enzyme abnormalities
Fetal hemorrhage
Fetal–maternal hemorrhage
Twin-to-twin transfusion sequence (donor or recipient)
Parvovirus infection
Red-cell aplasia
Chromosomal/syndromic/genetic abnormalities
Trisomy 21, 18, 13
Turner syndrome
Chromosomal deletions/rearrangements
Noonan syndrome
Myotonic dystrophy
Tuberous sclerosis
Cardiovascular abnormalities
Arrhythmias (congenital heart block and supraventricular tachyarrhythmias)
Structural heart disease
Chest masses
Congenital cystic adenomatoid malformation
Congenital lymphangiectasis
Sequestration
Bronchogenic cyst
Gastrointestinal abnormalities
Diaphragmatic hernia
Meconium peritonitis
Intestinal atresia
Urinary tract abnormalities
Kidney dysplasia
Urinary tract malformations and obstructions
Intracranial abnormalities
Developmental brain malformations
Intracranial hemorrhage
Arterial or venous intracranial malformations
Encephalocele
Lymphatic and vascular abnormalities
Intravascular thrombosis
Chylothorax
Cystic hygroma
Placental or umbilical cord abnormalities
Chorioangioma
Fetal tumors
Rhabdomyosarcoma
Sacrococcygeal teratoma
Neuroblastoma
Hemangioendothelioma
Hepatoblastoma
Infections
Parvovirus B19
TORCH (*Toxoplasma*, syphilis, rubella, cytomegalovirus, herpes simplex) infections
Enteroviruses
Metabolic abnormalities
Storage diseases
Skeletal dysplasias
Maternal-specific associations
Antepartum indomethacin
Diabetes mellitus

pressure, although in many of these fetuses the etiology of myocardial dysfunction is obscure [16,17].

Another mechanism that has been proposed to account for hydrops is an increase in endothelial permeability. At least in infants with Rh hemolytic anemia, transvascular albumin flux measurements are similar regardless of the presence of hydrops, which suggests that there is no impairment of vascular integrity [18]. Similarly, tachyarrhythmias increase central venous pressure and total body water, but vascular permeability is unaffected [19]. Thus, there is insufficient evidence at this time to confirm or refute the notion that increased vascular permeability is one of the pathophysiological mechanisms underlying the formation of hydrops.

Another possible explanation for hydrops is hypoalbuminemia. Indeed, information from infants with Rh hemolytic disease and hydrops suggests that serum albumin concentration correlates with the degree of body water [18]. Likewise, pericardial fluid accumulation is related to the presence of hypoalbuminemia, not myocardial dysfunction [20]. On the other hand, observations from infants who are born with inherited abnormalities of serum proteins suggest that hypoproteinemia alone does not consistently result in hydrops. Patients who have congenital nephrotic syndrome or analbuminemia do not have hydrops in utero or at the time of birth, although they may become edematous postnatally [21,22]. Similarly, in fetal lambs made hypoproteinemic, total body water is relatively unaffected [23]. Taken together, the experimental evidence linking hypoproteinemia as an essential component in the pathophysiology of hydrops remains controversial.

Neurologic injury associated with hydrops

Neurologic injury in patients who have hydrops may occur under several different settings. First, obvious abnormalities of the central nervous system such as porencephaly, absence of the corpus callosum, and encephalocele have all been identified as primary lesions that at times are associated with hydrops [24].

Second, occult neurological injury may be present in patients who have no obvious cause of their hydrops. The neuropathological changes of antenatal anoxia have been observed in patients who died with idiopathic non-immune hydrops, suggesting that some types of neurologic injury may be present, but undiagnosed, in otherwise "idiopathic" cases of non-immune hydrops [25]. The possibility that asphyxia plays a causative role in some cases of hydrops is underscored by the disturbances in total body water seen in fetal animal experiments of umbilical cord occlusion [26–28]. Short periods of cord occlusion sufficient to cause hypotension, acidemia, and cerebral hypoperfusion, but not death, result in hydrops within days, and the excess body water may persist for as long as 6 weeks post-occlusion [26–28]. There is a marked reduction in brain growth and structural maturation, and microscopically there is neuronal loss in the basal ganglia, hippocampus, and brainstem [28,29].

Third, and perhaps most common, is the brain injury that is associated with the underlying disorder that accompanies the hydrops. Genetic and chromosomal syndromes, congenital infections, and metabolic diseases are examples of disorders that are seen in conjunction with hydrops and that often have abnormal neurologic sequelae as a feature of their symptom complex. Other brain injury syndromes are more directly linked to hydrops. For instance, the presence of severe platelet alloimmunization has been linked to intracranial hemorrhage in utero and resultant fetal anemia which then causes hydrops; intracranial hemorrhage in the absence of thrombocytopenia has also been associated with hydrops [30,31]. An anecdotal report has linked maternal parvovirus infection, a common infectious agent linked to fetal anemia and non-immune hydrops, to stroke and seizures in the fetus [32].

Antenatal management

Antenatal management of the hydropic fetus is focused initially on diagnosing associated conditions, because therapeutic options are limited in most cases. Obtaining the appropriate samples for genetic analysis, infectious agents, and anatomic screening are but a few examples of the diagnostic categories that will be investigated by the obstetrical staff. Of the therapeutic interventions available, intravascular infusion of packed red blood cells is the most consistently successful strategy available to treat hydrops, but its usefulness is limited, of course, to fetuses that have anemia [33,34]. Successful treatment of fetal supraventricular tachycardia, evacuation of pleural fluid collections, and fetal surgical repair of lesions such as congenital cystic adenomatoid malformation or sacrococcygeal teratoma has resulted in the resolution of hydrops, but of these, treatment of supraventricular tachycardia is the most widely available and well-accepted [35–37].

Management of the hydropic fetus around the time of birth

Although the most appropriate time for delivery of a hydropic fetus cannot be discerned from the available observational studies, delivery at a more immature gestational age does not appear to confer a survival advantage [1,8,38]. Timing of delivery should be based on several factors, including the degree of fetal lung development and maturation, general fetal health, and progression of hydrops as an indication of fetal deterioration. Antenatal steroids should be administered to accelerate fetal lung maturation if they are otherwise indicated. Although there is no information available to allow for firm recommendations as to mode of delivery, most hydropic fetuses are delivered by cesarean section. Regardless of mode of delivery, fetuses that have non-immune hydrops often have some degree of birth depression, and for this reason delivery should occur at a tertiary neonatal center [39]. Tracheal intubation is almost always needed in patients who have significant hydrops, and edema of the face and oropharynx can make this procedure difficult even for experienced clinicians [1]. Diminished thoracic compliance often requires drainage of the pleural and peritoneal spaces in the delivery room to improve gas exchange. Pleural effusions are more common in patients who die soon after birth than in patients who survive, presumably as a result of effusion-induced pulmonary hypoplasia [1,8].

Postnatal diagnostic studies

The choice of diagnostic studies postnatally should be guided by history and neonatal examination, but in a significant proportion of patients who have had a thorough fetal evaluation, no associated disorder will be discovered postnatally [11,40,41]. Diagnostic studies should include chromosomal assessment, as well as other studies to exclude genetic syndromes. Echocardiography should be performed to evaluate whether structural heart disease is present and to assess myocardial function. Electrocardiography will be necessary if a rhythm disturbance is suspected. Imaging studies are often necessary, and these may include plain film radiography of the chest and abdomen or ultrasonography of the head and abdomen. These investigations will sometimes reveal occult abnormalities that will help clarify whether a genetic syndrome is present. Subspecialty consultation with an expert in clinical genetics may be helpful if further evaluation of the patient is necessary.

Pathological examination of the placenta is important, and plans to preserve the placenta for subsequent evaluation should be considered, because some conditions associated with hydrops are readily diagnosed by placental examination but are difficult to diagnose in the newborn in the absence of invasive procedures. For example, a few of the inborn errors of metabolism that are associated with hydrops have characteristic pathological features on placental examination [42].

Postnatal management

If the patient survives the initial resuscitative period, numerous life-threatening complications may occur, including infection, airleak syndromes, and hypotension. All of these complications may result in direct or indirect neurological injury, predominantly because they cause or aggravate cardiorespiratory instability. Cardiorespiratory instability may result in ischemia and hypoxemia, and thus increase the risk for neurological injury in a manner similar to other conditions in high-risk patients in the newborn intensive care unit who suffer from physiological instability.

Respiratory failure is common, not infrequently requiring aggressive conventional mechanical ventilation or high-frequency ventilation [43]. Extracorporeal membrane oxygenation (ECMO) has been used successfully in hydropic infants, but selection of patients who are likely to have good outcome from treatment with ECMO remains problematic because lung growth sufficient to provide for adequate gas exchange may not occur during the period of ECMO treatment [44]. Although there is no information regarding surfactant content or function in newborn infants who have hydrops, if exogenous surfactant replacement is otherwise indicated in a non-hydropic infant of similar gestational age, surfactant should be administered.

Cardiovascular instability is frequent, and will be exacerbated if high mean airway pressure is necessary to provide adequate gas exchange. Fluid infusions are often needed to help maintain circulating volume, and vasopressors may be required to treat hypotension and myocardial depression. In patients with structural heart disease, therapy is directed towards correcting the abnormal physiology, as it would be in a non-hydropic infant who has a similar lesion. Prostaglandin E_1 infusion should be used to maintain ductal patency if otherwise indicated.

Intravenous fluids should be administered, keeping in mind the goal of promoting sodium and water loss during the first week after birth. Serum electrolytes and body weight measurements should be used to help guide fluid therapy. After the initial period of fluid stabilization, parenteral nutrition will be necessary. The goal of intravenous nutrition should be to provide targeted calorie and nutrient requirements while limiting fluid administration to the greatest extent possible, at least until body edema has resolved. Patients who have hydrops will often lose 20–30% of birthweight during the first 2 weeks after birth before the nadir of postnatal weight is reached, but clinical examination should guide this assessment [1].

If significant asphyxia complicates the hospital course, coagulopathy is common, and prothrombin and partial thromboplastin times should be measured. Treatment for clinically important coagulopathy consists of the administration of fresh frozen plasma or, if indicated, cryoprecipitate.

Most patients who have non-immune hydrops will be hypoproteinemic and hypoalbuminemic. Diminished serum protein concentration at the time of birth increases the risk of early death [1]. Although there is no evidence to suggest that outcome is improved by the infusion of colloid solutions, infusion of 5% or 25% albumin is a common therapeutic maneuver. Whether maintaining serum albumin in the range usually found in non-hydropic infants improves outcome is unclear.

Many of the comments above regarding postnatal management of patients with hydrops apply to those who have either immune or non-immune hydrops. However, additional management issues are relevant for the infant who has immune hydrops, specifically if hemolysis continues to complicate the postnatal course. Intravenous immune globulin

decreases the rate of erythrocyte destruction and reduces the likelihood that exchange transfusion will be necessary. Intravenous immune globulin can be administered at 0.5 g/kg body weight, and may have to be repeated within 24–48 hours after the initial infusion [45,46]. Other complications encountered in patients with immune hydrops include thrombocytopenia and hypoglycemia, either of which may lead to neurologic injury.

Outcome of hydropic infants

In selected patients who have non-immune hydrops, the electroencephalogram (EEG) can show marked abnormalities, including burst–suppression, abnormal background patterns, multifocal sharp waves, and seizure activity [47]. Patients who have significant abnormalities on EEG also show severe abnormalities neuropathologically, at least some which appear to be antenatal in origin. Of interest, cranial ultrasound examination fails to demonstrate anatomic abnormalities in the majority of these patients. In a series of patients with hydrops who died in utero or shortly after birth, neuropathological findings of antenatal hypoxic–ischemic injury were found in over 50% of the patients [48].

Only limited information is available documenting the long-term neurological outcome of hydropic infants. In patients who receive intrauterine transfusions for severe Rh hemolytic disease, neurologic outcome appears to be independent of the presence of hydrops at initial fetal presentation [33,34]. Of course, in this population survival of hydropic infants is reduced compared to non-hydropic infants, thus introducing selection bias as a contributor to the apparent equivalence in outcome. In fetuses with immune hydrops, 90–95% will have normal neurological exam and 80–85% will have a normal developmental outcome at follow-up between 6 months and 6 years [33,34]. These outcomes compare favorably with other high-risk infants managed in the neonatal intensive care unit. As might be expected, perinatal asphyxia is related significantly to abnormal neurologic outcome [34]. Because hydropic infants who are anemic do not tolerate the hypoxemia that accompanies vaginal delivery, cesarean section is frequently the most prudent route of delivery [49]. The long-term neurologic outcome for patients with non-immune hydrops is limited, but observational data would suggest a normal neurologic outcome in 65–85% [8,38,50,51].

Summary

Many patients who have hydrops will die soon after delivery because of pulmonary hypoplasia and the inability to establish adequate gas exchange. Of those patients that survive the immediate postnatal period, many will succumb to the underlying condition associated with their hydrops. In patients who have non-immune hydrops and who survive to discharge, neurologic outcome is not routinely dismal, despite the difficulty encountered during their hospital course. The risk of neurologic impairment appears to increase in association with birth at earlier gestational ages, and with underlying disorders in which neurologic dysfunction is an expected feature.

References

1. Carlton DP, McGillivray BC, Schreiber MD. Nonimmune hydrops fetalis: a multidisciplinary approach. *Clin Perinatol* 1989; **16**: 839–51.

2. Ismail KM, Martin WL, Ghosh S, *et al.* Etiology and outcome of hydrops fetalis. *J Matern Fetal Med* 2001; **10**: 175–81.

3. Nicolaides KH, Soothill PW, Clewell WH, *et al.* Fetal haemoglobin measurement in the assessment of red cell isoimmunisation. *Lancet* 1988; **1**: 1073–5.

4. Adams MM, Marks JS, Gustafson J, *et al.* Rh hemolytic disease of the newborn: using incidence observations to evaluate the use of Rh immune globulin. *Am J Public Health* 1981; **71**: 1031–5.

5. Clarke CA, Mollison PL, Whitfield AG. Deaths from rhesus haemolytic disease in England and Wales in 1982 and 1983. *Br Med J* 1985; **291**: 17–19.

6. Wenk RE, Goldstein P, Felix JK. Kell alloimmunization, hemolytic disease of the newborn, and perinatal management. *Obstet Gynecol* 1985; **66**: 473–6.

7. Maidman JE, Yeager C, Anderson V, *et al.* Prenatal diagnosis and management of nonimmunologic hydrops fetalis. *Obstet Gynecol* 1980; **56**: 571–6.

8. Nakayama H, Kukita J, Hikino S, *et al.* Long-term outcome of 51 liveborn neonates with non-immune hydrops fetalis. *Acta Paediatr* 1999; **88**: 24–8.

9. Abrams ME, Meredith KS, Kinnard P, *et al.* Hydrops fetalis: a retrospective review of cases reported to a large national database and identification of risk factors associated with death. *Pediatrics* 2007; **120**: 84–9.

10. Huang HR, Tsay PK, Chiang MC, *et al.* Prognostic factors and clinical features in liveborn neonates with hydrops fetalis. *Am J Perinatol* 2007; **24**: 33–8.

11. Jones DC. Non-immune fetal hydrops: diagnosis and obstetrical management. *Semin Perinatol* 1995; **19**: 447–61.

12. Holzgreve W, Holzgreve B, Curry CJ. Non-immune hydrops fetalis: diagnosis and management. *Semin Perinatol* 1985; **9**: 52–67.

13. Apkon M. Pathophysiology of hydrops fetalis. *Semin Perinatol* 1995; **19**: 437–46.

14. Brace RA. Effects of outflow pressure on fetal lymph flow. *Am J Obstet Gynecol* 1989; **160**: 494–7.

15. Gest AL, Bair DK, Vander Straten MC. The effect of outflow pressure upon thoracic duct lymph flow rate in fetal sheep. *Pediatr Res* 1992; **32**: 585–8.

16. Johnson P, Sharland G, Allan LD, *et al.* Umbilical venous pressure in non-immune hydrops fetalis: correlation with cardiac size. *Am J Obstet Gynecol* 1992; **167**: 1309–13.

17. Weiner CP. Umbilical pressure measurement in the evaluation of non-immune hydrops fetalis. *Am J Obstet Gynecol* 1993; **168**: 817–23.

18. Phibbs RH, Johnson P, Tooley WH. Cardiorespiratory status of erythroblastotic newborn infants. II. Blood volume, hematocrit, and serum albumin concentration in relation to hydrops fetalis. *Pediatrics* 1974; **53**: 13–23.

19. Gest AL, Hansen TN, Moise AA, *et al.* Atrial tachycardia causes hydrops in fetal lambs. *Am J Physiol* 1990; **258**: H1159–63.

20. DeVore GR, Acherman RJ, Cabal LA, *et al.* Hypoalbuminemia: the etiology of antenatally diagnosed pericardial effusion in rhesus-hemolytic anemia. *Am J Obstet Gynecol* 1982; **142**: 1056–7.

21. Cormode EJ, Lyster DM, Israels S. Analbuminemia in a neonate. *J Pediatr* 1975; **86**: 862–7.

22. Hallman N, Norio R, Rapola J. Congenital nephrotic syndrome. *Nephron* 1973; **11**: 101–10.

23. Moise AA, Gest AL, Weickmann PH, *et al.* Reduction in plasma protein does not affect body water content in fetal sheep. *Pediatr Res* 1991; **29**: 623–6.

24. Hutchison AA, Drew JH, Yu VY, *et al.* Non-immunologic hydrops fetalis: a review of 61 cases. *Obstet Gynecol* 1982; **59**: 347–52.

25. Kobori JA, Urich H. Intrauterine anoxic brain damage in non-immune hydrops fetalis. *Biol Neonate* 1986; **49**: 311–17.

26. Lumbers ER, Gunn AJ, Zhang DY, *et al.* Non-immune hydrops fetalis and activation of the renin–angiotensin system after asphyxia in preterm fetal sheep. *Am J Physiol Regul Integr Comp Physiol* 2001; **280**: R1045–51.

27. O'Connell AE, Boyce AC, Lumbers ER, *et al.* The effects of asphyxia on renal function in fetal sheep at midgestation. *J Physiol* 2003; **552**: 933–43.

28. O'Connell AE, Boyce AC, Kumarasamy V, *et al.* Long-term effects of a midgestational asphyxial episode in the ovine fetus. *Anat Rec A Discov Mol Cell Evol Biol* 2006; **288**: 1112–20.

29. George S, Gunn AJ, Westgate JA, *et al.* Fetal heart rate variability and brain stem injury after asphyxia in preterm fetal sheep. *Am J Physiol Regul Integr Comp Physiol* 2004; **287**: R925–33.

30. Bose C. Hydrops fetalis and *in utero* intracranial hemorrhage. *J Pediatr* 1978; **93**: 1023–4.

31. Stanworth SJ, Hackett GA, Williamson LM. Fetomaternal alloimmune thrombocytopenia presenting antenatally as hydrops fetalis. *Prenat Diagn* 2001; **21**: 423–4.

32. Craze JL, Salisbury AJ, Pike MG. Prenatal stroke associated with maternal parvovirus infection. *Dev Med Child Neurol* 1996; **38**: 84–5.

33. Doyle LW, Kelly EA, Rickards AL, *et al.* Sensorineural outcome at 2 years for survivors of erythroblastosis treated with fetal intravascular transfusions. *Obstet Gynecol* 1993; **81**: 931–5.

34. Janssens HM, de Haan MJ, van Kamp IL, *et al.* Outcome for children treated with fetal intravascular transfusions because of severe blood group antagonism. *J Pediatr* 1997; **131**: 373–80.

35. Ahmad FK, Sherman SJ, Hagglund KH, *et al.* Isolated unilateral fetal pleural effusion: the role of sonographic surveillance and *in utero* therapy. *Fetal Diagn Ther* 1996; **11**: 383–9.

36. Bullard KM, Harrison MR. Before the horse is out of the barn: fetal surgery for hydrops. *Semin Perinatol* 1995; **19**: 462–73.

37. Simpson LL. Fetal supraventricular tachycardias: diagnosis and management. *Semin Perinatol* 2000; **24**: 360–72.

38. Haverkamp F, Noeker M, Gerresheim G, *et al.* Good prognosis for psychomotor development in survivors with nonimmune hydrops fetalis. *BJOG* 2000; **107**: 282–4.

39. McMahan MJ, Donovan EF. The delivery room resuscitation of the hydropic neonate. *Semin Perinatol* 1995; **19**: 474–82.

40. Poeschmann RP, Verheijen RH, Van Dongen PW. Differential diagnosis and causes of nonimmunological hydrops fetalis: a review. *Obstet Gynecol Surv* 1991; **46**: 223–31.

41. Steiner RD. Hydrops fetalis: role of the geneticist. *Semin Perinatol* 1995; **19**: 516–24.

42. Beck M, Bender SW, Reiter HL, *et al.* Neuraminidase deficiency presenting as non-immune hydrops fetalis. *Eur J Pediatr* 1984; **143**: 135–9.

43. Wy CA, Sajous CH, Loberiza F, et al. Outcome of infants with a diagnosis of hydrops fetalis in the 1990s. *Am J Perinatol* 1999; **16**: 561–7.

44. Bealer JF, Mantor PC, Wehling L, et al. Extracorporeal life support for nonimmune hydrops fetalis. *J Pediatr Surg* 1997; **32**: 1645–7.

45. Alpay F, Sarici SU, Okutan V, et al. High-dose intravenous immunoglobulin therapy in neonatal immune haemolytic jaundice. *Acta Paediatr* 1999; **88**: 216–19.

46. Rubo J, Albrecht K, Lasch P, et al. High-dose intravenous immune globulin therapy for hyperbilirubinemia caused by Rh hemolytic disease. *J Pediatr* 1992; **121**: 93–7.

47. Laneri GG, Claassen DL, Scher MS. Brain lesions of fetal onset in encephalopathic infants with nonimmune hydrops fetalis. *Pediatr Neurol* 1994; **11**: 18–22.

48. Larroche JC, Aubry MC, Narcy F. Intrauterine brain damage in nonimmune hydrops fetalis. *Biol Neonate* 1992; **61**: 273–80.

49. Phibbs RH, Johnson P, Kitterman JA, et al. Cardiorespiratory status of erythroblastotic infants. 1. Relationship of gestational age, severity of hemolytic diseases, and birth asphyxia to idiopathic respiratory distress syndrome and survival. *Pediatrics* 1972; **49**: 5–14.

50. Dembinski J, Haverkamp F, Maara H, et al. Neurodevelopmental outcome after intrauterine red cell transfusion for parvovirus B19-induced fetal hydrops. *BJOG* 2002; **109**: 1232–4.

51. Nagel HT, de Haan TR, Vandenbussche FP, et al. Long-term outcome after fetal transfusion for hydrops associated with parvovirus B19 infection. *Obstet Gynecol* 2007; **109**: 42–7.

Chapter 30

Bacterial sepsis in the neonate

Hayley A. Gans

Introduction

Bacterial sepsis in the neonate is a significant cause of morbidity and mortality. More than half of all admissions to a neonatal intensive care unit (NICU) are for infants with or who are at risk of developing sepsis. Diagnosis is challenging since clinical signs are non-specific, supportive rapid screening laboratory assays lack good positive predictive value (PPV), and the entity carries a high mortality rate. As a result, a conservative approach to these patients has evolved, with many infants who are not septic receiving antibiotics. This chapter will discuss the epidemiology, diagnosis, treatment, and prevention of neonatal sepsis.

Meningitis accompanies sepsis in approximately one-quarter of cases of neonatal disease, and thus the two processes share a common etiology and pathogenesis. This chapter will cover only bacterial sepsis of the term infant, since meningitis is covered elsewhere (Chapter 31). Further, prematurity and residence in an intensive care unit are independent risk factors for bacterial sepsis that differ from sepsis in the term infant, and these will not be considered here. In addition, the emphasis of this chapter will be on early-onset neonatal disease, with less of a concentration on late-onset sepsis.

Epidemiology

Although the ability to diagnose bacterial sepsis has improved, septicemia remains a frequent cause of neonatal morbidity and mortality. The first records of positive blood cultures were reported from Yale in 1928 [1]. Since then, the predominant bacterial organisms that cause sepsis in the neonate continue to change [1–4]. The cause of these variations is complex and often unidentified, but recent patterns will most strongly reflect the use of intrapartum antibiotic prophylaxis (IAP) among other influences [2,3,5–10].

Two distinct patterns of neonatal sepsis have been described, differentiated by time of disease onset, predominant organism, and associated risk factors [3,5,10–15]. Early-onset disease (EOD) is defined as occurring ≤ 7 days postnatally with a strong association with obstetrical complications or risk factors. Therefore, disease is caused by microorganisms that colonize the maternal genital tract [12,14]. Some argue for a further stratification into "very-early" onset, within 48 hours of birth, since the pathophysiology may be different. It is believed that this group acquires infection in utero at a particularly susceptible stage, accounting for the very high mortality in these infants. Acquisition in utero can be through ascending spread from the lower genital tract or through transplacental transmission after maternal bacteremia [14,16]. In contrast, infants with EOD acquire the infecting organism at the time of delivery, resulting in a lower case-fatality rate [16].

Late-onset disease (LOD) presents > 7 days of life, in infants lacking a history of obstetrical risk factors, and involves organisms that could be acquired perinatally as well as postnatally [14,17]. Therefore these infections are acquired through passage in the birth canal, horizontally in the hospital, or in the community [14].

The incidence of neonatal sepsis has been difficult to gauge, since sepsis is a clinical diagnosis and some septic episodes are culture-negative. In the age of IAP, culture-negative sepsis rates will rise, making incidence rates more difficult to evaluate. In addition, as the number of preterm infants rises, the rates of sepsis have been influenced by this population's unique susceptibility to infection. Later reports have included many of these infants in studies, and thus determining rates for term infants has been more difficult. Despite these challenges, there are several reports attempting to characterize the incidence of neonatal sepsis (Fig. 30.1) [1,3–5,12,13,16, 18–20]. The longest-running record, dating to the 1960s, shows incidence rates of EOD at 1/1000 live births in the United States, with rates peaking at 3.89/1000 live births in 1978 [1], followed by a subsequent decline and stabilization throughout the 1980s to a rate of approximately 2.2–2.8/1000 live births [1,4]. Enhanced surveillance since the 1990s has provided varying rates, with reports of 7.1–19/1000 live births, with trends in the early and late 1990s indicating no overall changes in the incidence of EOD despite advances in prevention practices [3,18]. Recent reports concentrating on EOD have shown a dramatic decline in neonatal sepsis, owing to the decreased rates attributable to group B *Streptococcus* (GBS) infection, with rates from other organisms remaining unchanged or increasing [2,3,5,10,13,18,19].

There are discrepant reports for LOD rates, but these appear to be unchanged overall, with some reports showing

Fetal and Neonatal Brain Injury, 4th edition, ed. David K. Stevenson, William E. Benitz, Philip Sunshine, Susan R. Hintz, and Maurice L. Druzin. Published by Cambridge University Press. © Cambridge University Press 2009.

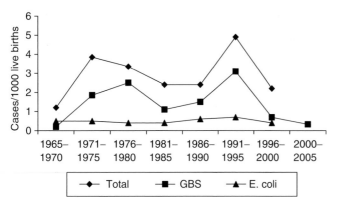

Fig. 30.1. Sepsis rates for early-onset neonatal disease in the United States from 1965 to 2005. Adapted from references 1, 2, 3, 4, 9.

Table 30.1. Maternal risk factors associated with early-onset neonatal sepsis in term infants for all pathogens and specific to Group B streptococcal disease

	Risk of proven sepsis
All neonatal pathogens	
Maternal fever ≥ 38 °C (100.4 °F)	↑ 1–4 times
Prolonged rupture of membranes > 18 h	1%
Chorioamnionitis	3–20%
Vaginal exams ≥ 6	↑ 3 times
Maternal urinary tract infection	Unknown
Group B *Streptococcus* (GBS)	
GBS bacteriuria	Unknown
Previous infant with invasive GBS disease	Additive with fever ↑ 5 times
Maternal colonization with GBS	1–2%

Source: Adapted from [10,12,14,25,35].

increased rates secondary to *Escherichia coli* (*E. coli*) [2,3]. Current reports show overall rates of neonatal sepsis of 0.8–8.2/1000 live term births in developed countries [2,3,5, 13,18]. EOD has an annual incidence of 0.3–7.2/1000 live births [2,3,5,13,18], and LOD, 1.9–8.23/1000 live births [2,3]. The incidence rates for the major individual organisms are described below.

Risk factors and pathogenesis

A neonate's susceptibility to infection is multifactorial. Unique to the neonatal host are deficiencies in various arms of the immune system and circumstances where exposure to a large number of organisms occurs. Susceptibility to infections in the neonate also arises when there are interruptions in the natural barriers of the body, which occur frequently in the birthing process.

Immunologic limitations have been documented in both innate immunity, including cellular defenses (such as eosinophils, neutrophils, platelets, and monocytes) and adaptive immunity, involving both cell-mediated immunity and humoral responses [21,22]. Antigen presentation by dendritic cells and activity of natural killer cells have also been shown to be deficient in the neonate, and in neonatal sepsis in particular [23]. In addition, the lack of opsonizing antibody to encapsulated bacteria confers a susceptibility to many of the bacteria in the maternal genital tract to which the neonate is exposed [24].

Obstetrical factors for the term infant can be used to determine risks for early-onset, but not late-onset, neonatal sepsis (Table 30.1). These risk factors have been most extensively studied for GBS and not for non-GBS sepsis, and differences do exist. Particularly, 80% of GBS disease is seen in infants born > 37 weeks, while only 40% of non-GBS sepsis is reported under these circumstances. Thus, preterm delivery is a strong risk factor for non-GBS neonatal sepsis [10,15].

Documented obstetrical risk factors that all organisms share include prolonged rupture of membranes > 18 hours [25], with the longer time between rupture of membranes and delivery increasing the exposure of the fetus. Some organisms, such as *Listeria monocytogenes* and *Treponema pallidum*, can cause infection despite the barrier of the placenta and amniotic fluid, with inoculation occurring via maternal bacteremia [12].

Maternal fever is also associated with neonatal sepsis, with the degree of fever reflecting strongly on the risk to the infant [10,16]. Studies have shown that maternal fever alone predicts approximately 26% of term infants with proven EOD and who were asymptomatic at birth [26]. For GBS, EOD is 10-fold higher in the presence of maternal fever [27]. Additional risk factors for GBS infection include a pregnancy complicated by GBS bacteriuria, history of a previous infant with invasive GBS disease, young maternal age, African-American race, Hispanic ethnicity, and frequent vaginal examinations during labor [15,28,29].

Risk factors for LOD have been rarely reported. One recent study has identified IAP exposure, with a nearly twofold higher risk for developing sepsis compared to control patients [30].

Etiology

Overall there is only a small group of organisms accounting for the majority of neonatal sepsis, with a very large and varied group of organisms accounting for the minority of cases [16]. Before the introduction of antibiotics, the predominant organisms causing neonatal sepsis were Gram-positive, with group A β-hemolytic *Streptococcus* (*Streptococcus pyogenes*) the major etiologic entity. This was replaced by the intestinal Gram-negative bacilli, particularly *E. coli*, after the introduction of sulfonamides in the early 1940s [1]. *Staphylococcus aureus* (*S. aureus*) was observed to be a major pathogen from 1950 to 1963, but for reasons that are not clear has diminished in importance since this time [1,4]. Recent reports of increasing rates of *S. aureus* infections in NICUs, with a particular focus on methicillin-resistant *S. aureus* (MRSA) have been almost exclusively in the preterm infant or resident of a NICU [31,32]. This is true also of the rising prevalence of commensal organisms as a cause of neonatal sepsis, such as coagulase-negative *S. aureus*, and thus neither will be covered further here [3].

Even in early reports, GBS held its place as a major contributor to neonatal sepsis, and was a leader in early fulminant disease (Figure 30.1). Over time, the predominance of GBS has risen to assume the lead in causing Gram-positive septicemia in EOD since the 1970s, with a peak incidence in the 1990s before prevention methods were put into place [1–5,10,13,14]. GBS previously accounted for 25–35% of sepsis overall, with 80% occurring in the first 48 hours of life, resulting in 55% of EOD. Recent reports show a dramatic decline in overall numbers of EOD by about 80%, secondary to decreases in GBS. Rates of EOD caused by GBS now parallel infections caused by *E. coli*, which traditionally ranked second. *E. coli* causes 27% of sepsis overall, and traditionally caused 13% of EOD, but 31% of LOD [1–4]. Rates of *E. coli* have been reported to have declined, remained unchanged, or increased since the introduction of intrapartum antibiotics, depending on the study, but these changes do not appear to be dramatic [2,5,7]. *Klebsiella pneumoniae* and *Enterobacter cloacae* are seen in about 15% of cases of septicemia, with less frequent reports of other organisms, such as *Listeria monocytogenes*, *Haemophilus* spp., *Pseudomonas* spp., *Streptococcus pneumoniae*, viridans *Streptococcus*, enterococcal Group D *Streptococcus* (enterococcus), and *Staphylococcus* spp. Some of the latter organisms have a strong association with prematurity or an underlying condition or procedure. The important individual organisms are discussed separately below.

Clinical presentation

The spectrum of clinical signs in neonates that develop sepsis is varied, and symptoms are non-specific. During delivery, signs of fetal distress, such as tachycardia and low Apgar scores, have been associated with sepsis, but both lack specificity [33,34].

Subtle signs of infection include poor feeding and decreased responsiveness, with more prominent symptoms being temperature instability, apnea, respiratory distress, jaundice, lethargy, vomiting, and diarrhea [35]. Though a serious bacterial infection is rare in asymptomatic neonates [36], infants who are bacteremic may have no symptoms initially, but deteriorate rapidly [17,37]. Due to the non-specific and subtle presenting clinical signs of septic neonates, clinical symptoms cannot be used alone to identify high-risk infants.

Concerns regarding an increase in asymptomatic neonates who become septic have arisen with the institution of guidelines for the prevention of GBS sepsis and rise of IAP in at-risk mothers. Ottolini *et al.* studied 20 554 newborns, with a group of 1665 asymptomatic at-risk infants [38]. In this group, 1.0% developed clinical signs of early-onset sepsis within 48 hours of delivery, but none had a positive blood culture and complete blood count (CBC) parameters did not add value to clinical findings. All septic infants in this study were symptomatic within 48 hours of birth, with the majority symptomatic before this time. Ninety-one percent of infants had more than one sign or symptom of sepsis and 71% had three or more, indicting that vigilance within the first 48 hours is the most sensitive tool for determining septic newborns. The frequency of signs and symptoms of sepsis in this study is shown in Table 30.2.

Table 30.2. Frequency of signs of sepsis in neonates

Signs	Frequency (%)
Tachypnea	58.0
Cyanosis	25.0
Lethargy	20.0
Apnea/bradycardia	20.0
Hypoglycemia	8.4
Fever	7.0
Hypothermia	3.5

Source: Adapted from [38].

Focal infections, such as meningitis, are more commonly seen in LOD, and thus symptoms particular to the area of infection may be present [12].

Diagnosis

The optimal workup of a newborn with suspected sepsis is not well defined. Presenting clinical signs are often non-specific, and thus differentiating truly infected infants from infants symptomatic as a result of non-infectious causes is challenging. In addition, many septic infants will show rapid clinical deterioration relatively late, making clinical parameters less useful for treating sepsis early. The importance of initiating prompt antimicrobial therapy to reduce the high mortality rate, and for improving long-term outcomes, makes identifying the septic infant early essential. In addition, standard culturing procedures do not offer a timely method to differentiate septic neonates, and may not prove helpful if IAP was used.

Given the inherent difficulty in determining which infants are at risk for developing sepsis, infants with signs consistent with sepsis of any pattern historically have received therapy to reduce the potential morbidity and mortality. It is estimated that 11–23 infants are treated for every documented case of neonatal sepsis, accounting for the treatment of 4.4–10.5% of all infants born in the United States [39,40]. This overutilization of antibiotics results in most infants receiving antibiotics unnecessarily, putting these infants at risk for complications of therapy and contributing to the development of multiple-drug-resistant bacteria.

Efforts have been made to develop rapid diagnostic methods for the early detection of infants who will progress to sepsis, and for identifying those infants who are symptomatic for non-infectious reasons. In the latter group, the goal is to safely allow for the discontinuation of antibiotics. Ideally, the development of a rapid test would also aid in guiding the initiation of therapy on only those infants in whom it is necessary [39]. Adjunctive tests have been evaluated, including markers such as C-reactive protein (CRP), interleukin 6 (IL-6), interleukin 8 (IL-8), procalcitonin (PCT), tumor necrosis factor α (TNF-α), neutrophil CD-11b, granulocyte colony-stimulating factor (G-CSF), neutrophil surface antigen CD64, and hematologic abnormalities, such as an elevated immature-to-mature neutrophil ratio.

Cultures are the gold standard for the definitive diagnosis of neonatal sepsis. All infants suspected of sepsis should have a blood culture drawn prior to the initiation of antibiotics. Venous puncture is the preferred method for obtaining blood for culture [41]. The optimal number of blood cultures is under debate. Some suggest obtaining blood from two sites in order to increase the yield of a positive result, especially when a small bacterial load is expected, as in the case of infants born to mothers who received IAP [42]. In addition, this may help clarify when a contaminating organism is isolated. However, the density of bacteria may be higher in neonates and the bacteremia more continuous than in older patients, and thus a single blood culture may be adequate [43].

Approximately 92% of true pathogens are isolated from blood culture within 36 hours and 98% within 48 hours [44]. The negative predictive value for infection with a definite bacterial pathogen negative blood culture is 99.7% at 36 hours and 99.8% at 48 hours [45]. This high bacterial isolation rate would support the discontinuation of antibiotics in the asymptomatic term neonate who is undergoing a suspected sepsis rule-out. It will be important to determine if this remains the case in the era of increased use of IAP.

Obtaining cultures of the cerebrospinal fluid (CSF) and urine has been debated. The necessity of doing a lumbar puncture in a neonate suspected of sepsis is covered in Chapter 31. Urine cultures have been shown to be important in LOD [46], but the data are variable for EOD. Given that neonatal urine tract infections are thought to be a result of hematogenous spread of the organism and not direct inoculum into the urinary tract, the low yield of urine cultures in the evaluation of infants with suspected sepsis – only about 0.1–1% – warrants eliminating urine cultures from the workup in the first 24 hours of life [47]. There does not appear to be any additional information obtained from the culturing of non-sterile surface sites [48].

In an attempt to develop a rapid diagnostic test to distinguish between infants suspected of and infants with sepsis, many researchers have looked to blood test assays. One study evaluated multiple rapid tests and their utility in diagnosing neonatal bacteremia in cases of suspected sepsis [49]. The results showed the non-specific nature of an elevated white blood cell (WBC) count, since it was positive in 71% of culture-proven bacteremia, but also 42% of infants with negative blood cultures. Immature-to-total neutrophil ratios were not elevated in the majority of infants with negative blood cultures, but it was also negative in 29% of infants with positive blood cultures.

CRP, an acute-phase reaction to inflammation or tissue necrosis, is thought to be a good predictor of bacterial sepsis in the neonate [50], with its predictability peaking at 24–48 hours after presentation with infection [51]. The majority of the highest titers have been documented in response to bacterial illnesses, with moderate elevations tending to be more non-specific. Levels decline rapidly once the ongoing process resolves, and thus serial titers are a helpful measure of disease activity [52]. Authors have shown that the negative predictive

value (NPV) of a negative CRP after 24 hours is approximately 85–99% predictive of not having a bacterial process, and thus a negative CRP may warrant the discontinuation of antibiotics [39,51]. Unfortunately, the PPV is not high enough right after delivery, approximately 89–93%, in proven EOD, given that other processes, such as the stresses of delivery (prolonged rupture of membranes, low Apgar score) correlate with a non-specific rise of CRP for approximately 3 days [51,53,54]. Thus, CRP cannot be used to guide the initiation of therapy to only infants who are truly infected and in the early stages of sepsis, but has value in discontinuing therapy in neonates undergoing a sepsis evaluation if levels remain low.

The poor PPV of CRP has led to evaluations of other cytokines, independently or in combination with CRP, to increase the sensitivity of rapid determination of infants at risk for sepsis, since many of these cytokines may become abnormal prior to elevations in CRP. Many cytokines have been evaluated from multiple sources, and in many different settings, and thus the results vary depending on the study [54–58]. IL-6, the major inducer of CRP, has been one target of investigation [53,54]. While not performing better than CRP as a single marker of infection, IL-6 did have high NPV. In addition, the combination of IL-6 and CRP performed better than each parameter alone as a negative predictive guide, with a value of 90% even early in the first 24 hours after delivery. IL-8 has also been studied in combination with CRP since it is an early proinflammatory marker [59]. Franz et al. showed that using high thresholds for both IL-8 and CRP (> 70 pg/mL and > 10 mg/L, respectively) achieved a sensitivity of 96–100%, but a PPV of only 65–77% for determining neonatal bacterial sepsis [59]. By restricting therapy to infants in this group only, there was a 60% reduction in antimicrobial use and only 23% of infants were treated unnecessarily. Once again, there was a good NPV of having two negative tests 24 hours apart.

PCT and TNF-α have also been targeted as proinflammatory markers [56,58]. While some discrepancy in results exists, Kocabas et al. demonstrated that with high cutoff values, PCT and TNF-α had the best PPV and NPV compared with other markers studied, including CRP [56]. PPVs were 97% and 96%, and NPVs were 97% and 100% for TNF-α and PCT, respectively. The levels of these cytokines declined over the first 7 days of treatment in neonates that recovered, and stayed elevated in those neonates who died, indicating the potential value of these markers for determining response to therapy.

Neutrophil CD11b, a surface marker activated early in a host's innate immune response to invading microbes, is elevated in infants with proven and suspected sepsis, and remains low in infants with symptoms caused by non-infectious disorders [60,61]. Once again, if CD11b is determined to be helpful in the diagnosis of neonatal bacterial sepsis, it will most likely be in concert with the other markers, especially CRP. Weirich et al. showed that, while CD11b was elevated in infants with proven viral illnesses and symptoms indistinguishable from bacterial sepsis, the CRP never rose in these infants [61], and Nupponen et al. showed that, used in combination with IL-8, most proven and suspected bacterial illnesses were determined very early in the workup of symptomatic neonates [60].

Both G-CSF and intercellular adhesion molecule 1 (ICAM-1) have been studied, and have been shown to have some promise for the early detection of neonatal sepsis. They lack reliable PPV and sensitivity, but again have good NPV [62,63].

Many of these assays are not readily accessible or results rapidly available to be useful clinically. Continuing the quest to determine the best diagnostic assay or profile has brought neutrophil surface antigen CD64 under investigation, since levels have the potential to be rapidly determined using flow cytometry, using very small blood volumes, and levels can be quantified precisely [55]. Studies have shown the high sensitivity of this marker (95–96%) in septic neonates, and a good NPV of 93–97%, but again it requires further evaluation for broader applicability [57].

None of the studied methods has improved upon the PPV of using risk factors and clinical signs consistent with infection, low absolute neutrophil count, and immature-to-total neutrophil ratio ≥ 0.25 to determine infants with sepsis, even in the age of IAP, as revealed by a large outcome study of 2785 infants [36]. In this study, the majority of infants that had either culture-proven or suspected sepsis were identified as "at risk for infection" using obstetrical risk factors including maternal chorioamnionitis, prolonged rupture of membranes (> 18 h), maternal fever (> 38 °C), GBS carriage, foul-smelling amniotic fluid, and prematurity. The rest of the infants were identified through screening, CBC, and clinical presentations. Eighty percent of these infants were symptomatic within 12 hours of birth. All of the infants, including the 20% that were asymptomatic at the time of evaluation, had significantly lower absolute neutrophil counts than the infants without sepsis, and all received antibiotics by 12 hours of age. The infants whose mothers had received IAP were more likely to be asymptomatic, less likely to be critically ill or to be infected, and had better outcomes compared with infants whose mothers did not receive IAP.

Treatment

Empiric treatment with broad-spectrum antibiotics guided by the knowledge of etiologic organisms and their susceptibility patterns is the standard of care in neonatal sepsis. The goal of any antibiotic therapy is the elimination of the bacteria as quickly as possible, reducing the source for the host inflammatory process that is responsible for the clinical signs related to sepsis. In addition, it is important to avoid hematogenous dissemination of the infecting organism to secondary sites. Ampicillin is most commonly chosen for its coverage of GBS, Group D non-enterococcal *Streptococcus*, *L. monocytogenes*, *Enterococcus*, and other anaerobes. In addition, an aminoglycoside is added for appropriate coverage of Gram-negative organisms and for synergy with ampicillin for treatment of *Enterococcus*, GBS, and *L. monocytogenes* [64,65]. The choice of initial antibiotic therapy will require close monitoring in the

age of growing IAP and the potential for emerging microbial resistance. A number of reports have tried to address the issue of changing patterns of antibiotic susceptibility in the era of IAP [2,6,9]. Most studies have not documented increased antibiotic resistance among term infants with sepsis, but have shown an increased incidence of resistant *E. coli* sepsis in preterm infants, particularly after prolonged antepartum exposures. Antibiotic treatment can be narrowed in culture-proven sepsis once susceptibility of the organism is known.

Despite appropriate antibiotic treatment, the mortality rate for neonates remains high. Therefore, there is interest in adjunctive therapy targeted at areas of immune immaturity in the neonate. Given the success of intravenous immuno-globulin (IVIG) in the prevention of bacterial infections in primary agammaglobulinemia, studies have been tried in neonatal sepsis. A meta-analysis reviewed three studies, all of which showed a sixfold decrease in acute mortality in the infants treated with one dose of 500–750 mg/kg of IVIG, but long-term mortality and morbidity must still be evaluated [66].

Granulocyte–macrophage colony-stimulating factor (GM-CSF) has been evaluated to target neonatal neutropenia, which is associated with increased morbidity and mortality when present during bacterial sepsis [67]. Studies have documented the safety of both G-CSF and GM-CSF in neonates, and a recent randomized controlled trial showed a significant increase in neutrophil count in the GM-CSF-treated infants [68–70]. The mortality rate in this study was decreased by 20% in the infants receiving GM-CSF. Though promising for improving outcome of neonatal sepsis, there is concern about the long-term toxicity on the developing bone marrow of the neonate, and further efficacy studies in larger cohorts are still required before GM-CSF is used as standard adjunctive therapy for neonatal sepsis.

Outcome

There is a clear association between sepsis and mortality, with a less well-defined causal relationship with long-term morbidity. Mortality from sepsis accounts for approximately 16% of neonatal deaths, but reports on early-onset mortality rates attributable to sepsis range from 15% to 50% [16,21]. Mortality in the first few days after birth was highest, and is not dependent on the causative agent. LOD carries a much lower case-mortality rate of approximately 17–22%, and is more dependent on the etiologic organism, with *E. coli* carrying the highest rates of mortality, followed by *S. aureus* and GBS [16].

Over time a dramatic decrease in mortality has been demonstrated, most closely associated with changes in mortality due to GBS sepsis. In the 1930s, mortality rates as high as 80% were demonstrated, with a continued decline to present levels, which appear to have plateaued [21]. Mortality from GBS sepsis peaked at 47% in 1974, reaching a nadir of 18% in 1978. Mortality from other entities remained appreciably unchanged during the same period despite the use of appropriate antimicrobial therapy [1]. The cases of GBS reported in the later series also document a falling rate of fulminant disease. Using a National Hospital Discharge survey, Lukacs *et al.* reported a decline in mortality rates for term infants with neonatal sepsis from 19/1000 live births in 1990 to 14/1000 live births in 2001, a decline of 23% [18]. The decline in neonatal mortality secondary to sepsis is multifactorial, related to prevention, early detection, advanced supportive care, and antimicrobial therapy [4].

With declining mortality rates, and increasing numbers of survivors of neonatal sepsis, defining the morbidity in these survivors is becoming increasingly important. Most of the documented adverse outcomes, particularly neurologic deficits, are seen in neonates that had meningitis as part of their sepsis [71], and there are clear orthopedic deformities as a result of neonatal osteomyelitis [72]. These infants, however, are neurologically intact. Bennet *et al.* reviewed the outcomes of survivors of neonatal sepsis from 1969 to 1983, including premature and term neonates, and showed that approximately 8% of septic neonates that survived without meningitis or osteomyelitis had long-term sequelae [73]. These infants account for 40% of the infants that developed sequelae and 50% of those with severe developmental delay. Other complications were deafness, hydrocephalus, and mild developmental delay. The hearing impairment observed was associated with Gram-negative sepsis, but it could not be determined if it was as a result of treatment with an aminoglycoside, sepsis alone, or both. All of the infants that developed sequelae were those with obstetrical and neonatal risk factors, and thus identifying these infants and utilizing preventive measures should impact not only survival, but also long-term outcome. Unfortunately, the same does not hold true for meningitis. Alfven *et al.* studied 90 infants with neonatal sepsis and also reported that most survivors of sepsis without meningitis that developed long-term sequelae had other underlying conditions, such as prematurity, and maternal preconditions such as diabetes. Most other survivors were noted to have normal growth and development at the time of follow-up 2–6 years later [74].

The role of bacterial sepsis as an independent factor in the poor outcomes and long-term morbidity in infants with other neonatal complications, such as perinatal asphyxia, preterm labor, and prematurity, cannot be easily determined and has not been reported [75].

Investigators have also studied the role of intrauterine exposure to infection and inflammation, even in uninfected neonates, in long-term neurologic outcomes, particularly cerebral palsy. While associations are strongest for preterm infants, there are some increased risks for the term infant reported [76]. Changing epidemiology would be expected with the increased use of intrapartum antibiotics, but this has not been addressed.

Prevention

Prevention measures have been targeted almost exclusively at GBS sepsis, and these are covered in more detail below. In theory, these strategies have the potential efficacy for preventing non-GBS sepsis, but this has not been well studied.

Schuchat *et al.* showed in a multicenter study that prevention was 63% effective in the prevention of non-GBS EOD [15]. Currently the first-line agents for IAP are penicillin and ampicillin, which are less effective against the second leading cause of EOD, *E. coli*. Whether the impact would be greater on non-GBS EOD with different chemoprophylaxis is yet to be studied.

Global approaches to the prevention of neonatal sepsis are challenging, since there is a variety of pathogens causing disease, and thus pathogen-specific approaches will not be broadly applicable. One renewed area of interest is in disinfection of the birth canal during labor and/or of the newborn at birth with topical microbicides that have broad antimicrobial activity. Studies in the developing world have shown promise, while others have not shown a benefit [77,78]. The fear of increased bacterial resistance with the use of IAP has prompted interest in pursuing this preventive strategy, which has the potential to cover multiple pathogens and has the benefit of ease of implementation.

Specific organisms

The major organisms associated with bacterial sepsis will be covered in more detail, but an exhaustive review of all etiologic agents of neonatal sepsis is beyond the scope of this chapter. Given the importance of GBS in neonatal sepsis and mortality, it will be discussed in more detail than other organisms, which will be reviewed for the qualities that are unique to them and deserve mention beyond the general discussion above.

Group B *Streptococcus*

The organism

GBS emerged as a leading cause of neonatal infections and mortality in the 1970s, and remains an important cause of disease in the term and preterm infant [17,79]. The organism is a Gram-positive coccus and is found as a colonizer of the female genital and rectal areas. The organism gains access to these secondary sites of colonization from the gastrointestinal tract, which serves as the most likely human reservoir [80]. Approximately 10–35% of women are asymptomatic carriers of GBS. The colonization rate of infants exposed to maternal sources of GBS is about 50%, but 98% of these infants are asymptomatic. Eighty percent of the remaining 1–2% of exposed infants will develop EOD presenting as sepsis, pneumonia, or meningitis. The majority of these infants are symptomatic within 2 days of birth, with the rest presenting within the first week [79,80].

Approximately nine serotypes of GBS have been identified, with serotype III causing approximately 36% of EOD, 90% of early-onset meningitis, and 71% of LOD (regardless of site of infection), despite a smaller representation in maternal colonization rates [17,81]. Recently serotype V has been increasing as an important isolate in neonatal disease, accounting for about 14% of GBS EOD [82]. In EOD without meningitis the non-III GBS serotypes are evenly distributed, with non-typable strains accounting for approximately 2–10% of disease [81].

The capsular polysaccharide (CPS) antigens are major virulence factors of GBS, and immunity is known to be a type-specific anticapsular antibody that promotes opsonization of homologous GBS strains in concert with the complement system. The concentration of CPS-specific antibody that is protective is not known and may depend on serotype and bacterial inoculum, as well as the maturity of the immune system [83]. The lack of passive antibodies at protective levels may partially explain the virulence of GBS serotype III in EOD disease with meningitis and LOD.

Epidemiology

The exact incidence of GBS disease is hard to determine. Published reports are variable, reflecting reporting practices based on high-risk groups and single institutions, and may not correctly reflect disease incidence in a larger population. GBS was an infrequently reported pathogen in neonatal sepsis until the 1970s, when it became dominant in EOD, resulting in 7500 cases and over 1000 deaths annually [1]. Studies over a 10-year period from 1989 to 1999 in the United States report an incidence of 1.4–3.2/1000 births for EOD and 0.24–0.5/1000 births for LOD [84]. After GBS incidence rose, prevention strategies were shown to be efficacious in preventing EOD by interrupting transmission vertically between mothers and their newborns [85]. Reports from the Centers for Disease Control and Prevention (CDC) surveillance showed a decline in the incidence of GBS EOD by 43% in some sites for the years 1993–95, but no changes were found at other locations [86]. In this evaluation, there were clear differences in rates when race was considered, with African-American rates the highest, and this has been substantiated in other studies [87]. During the same period the incidence for LOD remained unchanged. This trend, therefore, most likely represents practices that interrupt intrapartum transmission of GBS, including practice guidelines and enhanced detection techniques, rather than decreasing GBS carriage rates. This led to further attempts at prevention, and initial guidelines were issued in 1996, with revisions in 2002 [88,89]. After the implementation of these guidelines, studies showed declining incidence rates in EOD by 80% in GBS EOD, bringing the incidence from 1.7/1000 live births in 1993 to 0.34/1000 live births in 2004 (Fig. 30.2) [90]. The greatest change was seen in the mid-1990s, but active surveillance by the CDC showed a continued decline of 33% during 2003–2005 for GBS EOD, while LOD rates were unchanged [91]. Annual cases for early-onset GBS disease were 131–202 over the study period, with an incidence of 0.33/1000 live births, and LOD accounting for 0.12/1000 live births annually. The race discrepancy was again noted, with rates in African-American infants increasing by 70%. Whether there will continue to be a decline in rates of EOD from GBS is unknown.

Recurrent disease occurs in only a small percentage (0.4–0.9%) of appropriately treated infants that survive their initial GBS infection [92]. Though GBS is strongly associated with disease in preterm infants, the majority of cases (up to 82%) are still seen in term infants [28].

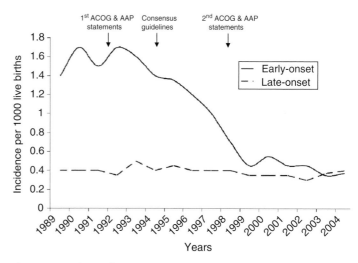

Fig. 30.2. Incidence of early- and late-onset Group B streptococcal disease and impact of preventive strategies from 1998 to 2004.

Pathogenesis

The pathogenesis of very-early-onset GBS disease is hypothesized to occur through ascending spread of the organism into amniotic fluid from which the fetus aspirates [80]. This results in exposure to a larger inoculum of organisms than could be achieved through other routes. GBS has been shown to cross intact membranes [93]. EOD is thought to represent acquisition of the organism at the time of delivery. LOD is less well understood, with only a portion of cases reflecting colonization at the time of delivery, since only 50% of infants with LOD are born to mothers with positive cultures for GBS, with nosocomial and community acquisition thought to account for the remainder of cases [17,94,95].

Risk factors

The major risk factors associated with GBS EOD are outlined above and in Table 30.1. The risk of disease is associated with infant exposure to a high inoculum of organisms and a relatively immunocompromised host. An infant will be at an increased risk for colonization with GBS if the mother is heavily colonized, or if obstetrical manipulations allow for bacterial replication [96]. African-American women have higher rates of heavy colonization with GBS, which may account for the higher rates of neonatal disease [97].

Clinical presentation

The clinical presentations of GBS disease are non-specific and include sepsis, meningitis, pneumonia, and less frequently cellulitis, omphalitis, osteomyelitis, and septic arthritis. Bacteremia with or without pneumonia accounts for 89% of disease in infants under 90 days, with meningitis only complicating 10% of these cases [86]. Septicemia accounts for 25–40% of presentations, and pneumonia for 35–55% [17].

Infants presenting with sepsis represent the full range of the spectrum of disease, including multiorgan failure, acidemia, and hypotension requiring full life-support measures, as well as interventions to correct metabolic abnormalities. Respiratory findings were prominent in the majority of EOD (80%), but poor feeding, lethargy, hypothermia or fever, abdominal distension, pallor, tachycardia, and jaundice have all been described [17].

Severe pulmonary hypertension can adversely affect the clinical course and outcome of these infants, and is thought to be secondary to cardiolipin and phosphatidylglycerol, which are elaborated by the bacteria [98]. Many of these infants require treatment with inhaled nitric oxide (iNO), extracorporeal membrane oxygenation (ECMO), or both.

Diagnosis

The only definitive diagnostic test for GBS sepsis is a positive culture. Culture results are obviously not available at the time of presentation, and all symptomatic neonates require a full septic evaluation and initiation of broad-spectrum antibiotics, usually with ampicillin and an aminoglycoside. These can be narrowed once culture results and sensitivities of the organism are determined (see below).

The evaluation and management of high-risk infants born to women with risk factors, particularly if they have received IAP, present particular difficulties and are controversial. This is particularly true if the infant is asymptomatic, as some infants that are bacteremic may be asymptomatic at birth, and partial treatment afforded by antibiotics given to the mother may mask early signs [99]. Guidelines have been created in some institutions (Fig. 30.3) that include obtaining a blood culture and CBC in infants that have one or more risk factors for sepsis. Empiric antibiotics are initiated if the total WBC count is below 5000/mm^3 or an immature-to-total neutrophils ratio (I/T ratio) is above 0.2. These are discontinued at 48 hours if blood cultures remain negative [44].

Treatment

Antibiotics are the hallmark of treatment for all forms of GBS sepsis, with the drug of choice being penicillin at 2 000 000 units/kg per day. There have been no clinical isolates of GBS showing resistance to penicillin or ampicillin, though the latter has a slightly broader spectrum and thus, when GBS has been confirmed, it is often recommended that penicillin be used when possible. These organisms are also sensitive to cephalosporins, vancomycin, and semisynthetic penicillins at variable activities. Erythromycin resistance is reported in 7–25% of isolates, and resistance to clindamycin in 4–15%. There is evidence of synergy with an aminoglycoside. The duration of treatment of bacteremia without meningitis is 10–14 days [17,100].

Outcome

Initial reports of GBS sepsis in the neonate documented mortality rates of approximately 50% [17], but this dropped quickly in the 1980s to 15% and further to present levels of about 4–6% [86].

Morbidity has been more difficult to define, but reports from the 1970s showed profound neurologic sequelae if meningitis was documented [17], and more recent reports of infants treated with ECMO have shown some long-term neurologic

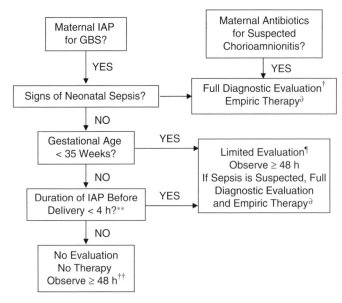

* If no maternal intrapartum prophylaxis (IAP) for GBS was administered despite an indication being present, data are insufficient on which to recommend a single management strategy.
† Includes complete blood cell (CBC) count and differential, blood culture, and chest radiograph if respiratory abnormalities are present. When signs of sepsis are present, a lumbar puncture, if feasible, should be performed.
∂ Duration of therapy varies depending on results of blood culture, cerebrospinal fluid (CSF) findings, if obtained, and the clinical course of the infant. If laboratory results and clinical course do not indicate bacterial infection, duration may be as short as 48 h.
¶ CBC with differential and blood culture.
** Applies only to penicillin, ampicillin, or cefazolin and assumes recommended dosing regimens.
†† A healthy-appearing infant who was ≥ 38 weeks' gestation at delivery and whose mother received ≥ 4 h of IAP before delivery may be discharged home after 24 h if other discharge criteria have been met and a person able to comply fully with instructions for home observation will be present. If any one of these conditions is not met, the infant should be observed in the hospital for at least 48 h and until criteria for discharge are achieved.

Fig. 30.3. Sample algorithm for management of a newborn whose mother received intrapartum antimicrobial agents for prevention of early-onset Group B streptococcal disease or suspected chorioamnionitis. This represents one approach only, and is not definitive or the only algorithm that has been developed. From [89].

impairments [101]. Newer evaluations are needed for infants that survive GBS sepsis in the age of intensive supportive care.

Prevention

With the increase in GBS incidence and the decline in mortality, efforts have now turned to prevention. The strategies for the prevention of GBS transmission from mother to fetus have evolved over the past 25 years, but it was not until the CDC, American College of Obstetricians and Gynecologists (ACOG), and the American Academy of Pediatrics (AAP) reached a consensus that prevention made sense and was economically affordable that practices started changing [88,102,103]. Since GBS disease in the neonate is rapidly progressive and often evident shortly after birth, and antenatal

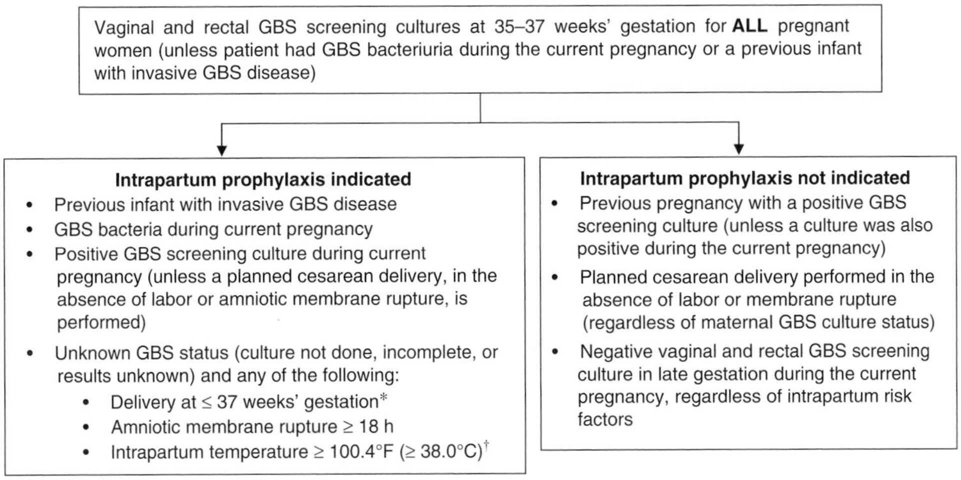

Vaginal and rectal GBS screening cultures at 35–37 weeks' gestation for **ALL** pregnant women (unless patient had GBS bacteriuria during the current pregnancy or a previous infant with invasive GBS disease)

Intrapartum prophylaxis indicated
- Previous infant with invasive GBS disease
- GBS bacteria during current pregnancy
- Positive GBS screening culture during current pregnancy (unless a planned cesarean delivery, in the absence of labor or amniotic membrane rupture, is performed)
- Unknown GBS status (culture not done, incomplete, or results unknown) and any of the following:
  - Delivery at ≤ 37 weeks' gestation*
  - Amniotic membrane rupture ≥ 18 h
  - Intrapartum temperature ≥ 100.4°F (≥ 38.0°C)†

Intrapartum prophylaxis not indicated
- Previous pregnancy with a positive GBS screening culture (unless a culture was also positive during the current pregnancy)
- Planned cesarean delivery performed in the absence of labor or membrane rupture (regardless of maternal GBS culture status)
- Negative vaginal and rectal GBS screening culture in late gestation during the current pregnancy, regardless of intrapartum risk factors

* If onset of labor or rupture of amniotic membranes occurs at < 37 weeks' gestation and there is a significant risk for preterm delivery (as assessed by the clinician), a suggested algorithm for GBS prophylaxis management is provided

† If amnionitis is suspected, broad-spectrum antibiotic therapy that includes an agent known to be active against GBS should replace GBS prophylaxis.

Fig. 30.4. Indications for intrapartum antibiotic prophylaxis to prevent Group B streptococcal disease under a universal prenatal screening strategy based on combined vaginal and rectal cultures collected at 35–37 weeks' gestation from all pregnant women. From [89].

antibiotics are effective in preventing the majority of EOD, the burden of prevention has fallen on those caring for pregnant women. Two strategic guidelines are in use to address this dilemma, with different efficacy and risk factors associated with each. ACOG first published guidelines in 1992, and supported a risk-based strategy, while the AAP published a screening-based approach. Confusion persisted for a number of years as to the best strategy to use, and in 1996–97 all three bodies reissued consensus statements. After this time, all institutions that offered obstetrical services must either adapt a screening-based or a risk-based approach to GBS prevention, but it was not clear which was superior, if either. In 2002, a report comparing the rates of GBS EOD showed that the use of screening strategies prevented 50% more neonatal disease than risk-based protocols, calling into question the recommendation for endorsing both strategies as equivalent [27]. These findings led to the new prenatal GBS prevention guidelines put forth in 2002, which recommended antenatal screening of all pregnant women (Fig. 30.4) [89]. The screening-based approach allows for the potential use of antibiotics early in delivery (as opposed to the alternative of waiting 18 hours after ruptured membranes or until a fever develops in the mother), and in mothers who may still colonize their infants despite the lack of symptoms. Reviews of maternal and infant records of infants with EOD show that 50–70% of these infants were born to mothers who lack risk factors [28,104]. One of these studies reported that up to 79% of EOD could be prevented by the screening-based approach [104]. Consequently, the risk-based strategy has been abandoned, and is now used only when screening has not been done.

Despite the better performance of the screening strategies, methods for GBS detection are not sensitive enough to abandon the importance of intrapartum risk factors, since GBS

EOD continues to occur in institutions relying on screening-based strategies [105].

Screening-based approaches provide IAP to all women with positive cultures for GBS performed late in gestation and all women without cultures that are delivering < 37 weeks' gestation. Risk-based approaches provide IAP to women with the following risk factors: delivery < 37 weeks' gestation, prolonged rupture of membranes ≥ 18 hours, intrapartum temperature ≥ 38 °C. Both strategies provide IAP to women with GBS bacteriuria, and to women who previously delivered an infant with GBS disease.

There is also evidence to suggest that at least 4 hours of intrapartum antibiotics is better than shorter courses: up to 40% of infants born to colonized mothers were still colonized if antibiotics were given within 1 hour of delivery, but only 1% of infants were colonized if the mothers received ampicillin > 4 hours before delivery [106].

Others have advocated more selective use of intrapartum chemoprophylaxis (SIC) [107,108]. By restricting intrapartum prophylaxis to GBS-colonized women with additional intrapartum risk factors, it was predicted that approximately 60% of the cases could be prevented while exposing fewer than 5% of women to antibiotics, with the remaining cases being of lesser severity because of the absence of risk factors.

Some of the issues raised above are addressed by combining this strategy with the use of intramuscular penicillin in neonates of colonized mothers without risk factors (selective neonatal chemoprophylaxis or SNC). The use of penicillin in neonates has been shown to reduce the rate of EOD GBS without an increase in incidence of LOD [109]. Some authors advocate combining SIC with SNC [108]. In their proposal all prenatal cultures would be obtained at 35 weeks' gestation, and risk factors extended to include all women without prenatal care and delivering prematurely. In addition, any woman with a febrile course consistent with chorioamnionitis would receive full treatment with ampicillin and an aminoglycoside, and not just prophylaxis. Further, all asymptomatic infants born to GBS-colonized women would be given penicillin. This approach would be expected to protect those infants born to colonized mothers that are symptomatic at the time of delivery. Infants more likely to be infected with GBS at the time of delivery are more likely to be born to colonized mothers without risk factors, and therefore should be protected by SNC. This would be expected to decrease the incidence of GBS EOD by approximately 75–90% and limit the exposure to penicillin to < 10%. There is still concern about the use of this strategy, particularly with the postpartum use of penicillin in neonates [110].

It is clear that the use of prevention strategies reduces the incidence of EOD. The CDC surveyed hospitals in eight states, and reported that the proportion of hospitals with formal intrapartum GBS prevention policies increased to 59% in 1997 [86]. Even limited compliance with any prevention strategy that resulted in a reduction in EOD GBS was shown to be cost-effective [111]. It is important to note that despite best practices and the institution of appropriate IAP, GBS disease is not likely to be eliminated without the development of other strategies.

The impact of IAP on LOD has been evaluated in one study, which showed that in a small cohort of infants, cases of LOD were 14% more likely to occur in infants exposed to IAP than in unexposed infants. In addition, the bacterial isolates of the exposed infants were more likely to be resistant to ampicillin, but not to other antibiotics [30]. Clearly this is an area that deserves further study.

Chemoprophylaxis

Chemoprophylaxis during pregnancy, prior to onset of labor, has been studied as a way of preventing neonatal GBS disease. Most studies show that there is no impact on maternal carriage despite a reduction in the colonization of neonates and thus invasive GBS disease [112]. The administration of antepartum chemoprophylaxis to all GBS carriers has potential for approximately 10 deaths annually from anaphylaxis [113], and a proportion of women and fetuses suffering less severe reactions [114]. In addition, the use of antepartum chemoprophylaxis challenges the pediatrician to understand how to treat the neonates born to mothers who have been treated with antibiotics [115].

Challenges for the use of IAP include adherence to the recommendation for administration of antibiotics at least 4 hours prior to delivery. As many as 50% of woman who are GBS carriers do not receive the antibiotics as recommended due to the rapidity of labor and delivery [116]. The use of intrapartum antibiotics is also plagued with the potential emergence of resistant microbes, including non-GBS organisms. Towers et al. showed that, while the incidence of GBS in their institution declined over an 8-year study period as a result of increasing intrapartum ampicillin use, there was also

a coincident rise in EOD caused by non-GBS organisms [114]. The majority of these cases were in infants whose mothers had been given intrapartum ampicillin, and 87% of the bacteria were ampicillin-resistant. The conclusion was drawn that the use of penicillin, with a more narrow spectrum, would be more prudent in this setting. These findings have not been supported by more recent studies that have sought to define the situation in more detail. In these early studies the bulk of this disease was found in preterm rather than term infants [15].

The influence of IAP alone on these trends is not clear, since bacterial resistance is seen as a general pattern outside of neonatal sepsis. Recent studies support no link between the increased use of IAP and emerging resistant GBS or non-GBS bacteria, except in preterm, low-weight neonates [6,9]. Further, there seems to be a trend towards decreasing non-GBS EOD by both Gram-positive and in some studies Gram-negative bacteria. It is probable that the phenomenon now highlighted is that the remaining cases of EOD reflect pathogens that are not susceptible to the current IAP, and thus these strains are causing a higher proportion of cases without an overall change in incidence [6].

In an attempt to define if differences exist in neonatal bacterial colonization, Jaureguy et al. studied stool pathogens of 3-day-old neonates exposed to IAP compared with unexposed infants [117]. No differences were seen with the colonization of resistant organisms, but infants receiving IAP had lower rates of anaerobic colonizers, such as Clostridium.

Immunoprophylaxis

Despite the successes of prevention strategies on reduced incidence of GBS sepsis, there continue to be challenges in implementation of the guidelines and concerns related to adverse outcomes. In addition, the prevention strategies are not expected to prevent LOD, GBS-related stillbirths, or prematurity, and so recent developments are focusing on vaccines. Vaccines are expected to be effective by providing a boost in the maternal anticapsular antibody titers so that higher levels are transferred transplacentally to the neonate. The hope is to overcome the neonatal susceptibility to GBS disease that is believed to arise from deficiencies in protective levels of maternal anticapsular antibodies, particularly to serotype III [81].

The initial attempts at producing an effective vaccine concentrated on GBS serotype III, but it was not until the polysaccharide was conjugated to tetanus toxoid that promising results were observed [118]. In addition, the initial target populations for these vaccines were pregnant women in their second trimester, but this proved to be very controversial. Therefore the focus for vaccine-induced immunity to GBS has shifted to women in the child-bearing age prior to pregnancies, and also to children. The immunity for a conjugate vaccine is expected to be lasting, and vaccinating the latter two populations would offer protection even to newborns born years after effective immunization.

One goal of GBS vaccination is to achieve decreases in mucosal colonization as well as protective antibody titers. Given the multitude of serotypes causing GBS disease, a multivalent vaccine will be the only viable strategy to potential disease elimination, although great accomplishments can be expected using vaccines targeted at GBS serotype III since it is the major cause of EOD associated with meningitis and LOD. Other GBS serotypes have been tested for immunogenicity, but a multivalent candidate vaccine has not yet been fully developed [119,120].

One approach focuses on the development of a recombinant vaccine that contains the pili that afford the bacteria ability for enhanced colonization and infection. Animal studies have been successful, paving the way for phase I clinical trials. If successful, this vaccine would reduce bacterial colonization at the mucosal level and induce both humoral and mucosal immunity [121,122].

Overall, while promising in early studies, all the proposed vaccines in development face obstacles to starting phase III clinical trials. Among the challenges is the need for large-scale trials, and the use of intrapartum prophylaxis has created a necessity for immunologic correlates, which have not yet been identified. Most important are the issues regarding the use of vaccines in pregnant women.

Escherichia coli

E. coli is the second most important pathogen in neonatal sepsis, and the primary Gram-negative coliform causing disease [1,16]. The antigenic structure of *E. coli* is very complex, and a great genetic diversity exists in the strains that colonize humans. Despite the large number of different colonizing strains, there is a strikingly small number of strains that cause disease [123]. One of the capsular antigens of *E. coli*, the K1 antigen, is related to invasive disease and is uniquely associated with neonatal meningitis. Approximately 80% of *E. coli* meningitis in neonates is caused by K1 strains, and though this association is not as strong with bacteremia, K1 strains have been cultured from the blood of infants with sepsis without meningitis [124]. There is also a higher rate of morbidity and mortality associated with sepsis and meningitis caused by the K1 strains compared with disease caused by non-K1 strains. The increased morbidity and mortality are related to the concentration and persistence of the capsular polysaccharides of these K1 strains in blood and CSF [125].

Pili on the surface of *E. coli* K1 strains are important for mucosal colonization, but a shift to a non-piliated form where the capsular protein becomes important is the form of the bacterium that is found in the blood stream of animal models. The importance of these phase shifts in the *E. coli* K1 strain's ability to avoid immune recognition by the host defenses is considered an important virulence factor [126].

The pathogenesis of fetal colonization is similar to that of GBS and other organisms that are acquired from the maternal birth canal either prior to or at the time of delivery (see above). Though *E. coli* only causes approximately 13% of EOD, it is responsible for 31% of LOD, for reasons that are not clearly understood [1,4]. Sarff *et al.* and McCracken *et al.* showed high rates of carriage of K1 strains of *E. coli* in hospital personnel, and subsequent acquisition of identical strains in the neonates they cared for [124,125]. In addition, there was acquisition of these strains in neonates born to mothers that were not colonized with these strains. Cook *et al.* examined other virulence factors of *E. coli* strains associated with neonatal sepsis, documenting unique adherence phenotypes that enhance the virulence of these strains [127]. These properties are related to those seen in other extra-intestinal *E. coli* infections.

The epidemiology of *E. coli* disease is outlined above. Unique to *E. coli* sepsis are higher rates of morbidity, longer hospital stays, and increased need for mechanical ventilation compared with GBS EOD. In addition, *E. coli* EOD carries higher mortality rates, despite appropriate treatment [128]. Further, changing patterns of *E. coli* LOD will need to be monitored, as one study documented an increase in both term and preterm *E. coli* LOD since 1997, the cause of which is yet unidentified [2]. In addition, multiple studies have identified prematurity as an increased risk for *E. coli* sepsis in any period after birth, while term *E. coli* EOD appears to be declining, and there appears to be protection associated with longer exposure (≥ 4 h) of IAP [20,129].

Treatment for *E. coli* bacteremia without meningitis is dictated by the susceptibility to antibiotics of the isolate. Treatment with ampicillin in susceptible strains alone or in combination with an aminoglycoside is appropriate therapy. The use of broader regimens, particularly cephalosporins, should be carefully considered and used only if deemed necessary, since there is concern for the emergence of cephalosporin-resistant strains of *Enterobacter cloacae*, *Klebsiella*, and *Serratia* species in the institutions where these infants reside. The duration of therapy for uncomplicated disease is usually 10–14 days.

Streptococcus pyogenes (group A β-hemolytic Streptococcus)

Streptococcus pyogenes has been a historically important cause of neonatal sepsis from the sixteenth century, and was the predominant organism causing disease from 1930 to 1940 [1], but incidence dropped off markedly in the antibiotic era [130]. There has been a recent increase in group A β-hemolytic *Streptococcus* (GAS) disease rates in children and adults, and, while still rare, increased reports of GAS disease in neonates from sporadic disease and associated with outbreaks have been published [131,132]. Surveillance will indicate if this trend continues, and the impact on neonatal disease, but given the continued susceptibility of GAS to intrapartum penicillin and ampicillin, IAP is thought to represent a viable prevention strategy for this pathogen.

GAS has been cultured from the anus and vagina of pregnant women, the umbilical stumps of neonates, and the hands and nasopharynx of neonates, mothers, and nursery personnel. Transmission is thought to be at the time of delivery and postnatally. Most colonized infants are asymptomatic, but rare cases of invasive disease, such as sepsis and meningitis, have been documented. In the past, most disease presented as indolent omphalitis [130]. This is in contrast to more recent reports of neonates with a severe EOD associated with high mortality rates, pointing to the possibility of a resurgence of disease with a more aggressive course similar to GBS EOD [133,134]. If there appears to be a true increased incidence of such disease then preventive measures such as those utilized to decrease the incidence of GBS may become increasingly important.

No strains of GAS have emerged that are resistant to penicillin, and this remains the drug of choice for treatment [135]. In the era of new more invasive neonatal sepsis caused by GAS, adjunctive therapies with clindamycin and IVIG may be warranted, but studies in neonates are lacking at the present time [136,137].

Enterococcal group D *Streptococci*

The incidence of enterococcal group D *Streptococci* (*Enterococcus*) as a cause of neonatal sepsis rose in the 1980s and 1990s from approximately 0.12/1000 live births to 0.8/1000 live births in one study and three-fold in another [138,139]. Eliminating prematurity as a risk factor, EOD was not associated with obstetrical complications, and very few term infants were noted to have LOD, and these were associated with complicated postnatal courses with invasive procedures. Further, the increased incidence was not a result of the use of broader-spectrum antibiotics, which were not in common use at the reporting institutions. Since the increased cases were late, occurring in hospitalized neonates, they were thought to represent longer survival of mostly preterm infants in NICUs [138,139].

The organism is a Gram-positive organism that has been known as a human pathogen for approximately 100 years [140]. The two important species that cause disease in humans are *Enterococcus faecalis* and *E. faecium* [139].

The clinical signs again are often subtle and non-specific. The major signs of enterococcal sepsis include respiratory distress and apnea, but rarely are chest x-rays positive. Temperature instability and hypothermia are also present in 15–60% of infants. Diarrhea was the second most frequent symptom encountered in EOD, and rarely does meningitis complicate EOD. About 40% of infants with EOD can be expected to be asymptomatic at birth, and they are often screened only because of maternal risk factors [138,139].

Enterococci are moderately resistant to ampicillin and penicillin, and highly resistant to all cephalosporins. Optimal therapy includes both a penicillin and an aminoglycoside for synergy, or vancomycin. There are concerns that neonatal enterococcal infections will continue to rise and be more difficult to treat, given the appearance of strains that are vancomycin-resistant in the United States. The hospital survival rates of infants with vancomycin-resistant enterococcus (VRE) are significantly worse than those of infants with susceptible strains [138]. Outcomes for *Enteroccocus* sepsis appear to be good, with quick clinical improvements, but long-term studies are lacking. Case-fatality rates are low – approximately 5.5–10% – and appear to relate to underlying conditions [138,139].

Summary

The changing prevalence of organisms responsible for neonatal sepsis, and the potential for emerging resistance in these organisms, underscores the necessity for close vigilance and surveillance of this disease. Many advances have been made in the prevention and treatment of neonatal bacterial sepsis, but mortality and morbidity remain high. By adapting more stringent prevention guidelines and developing better diagnostic and treatment strategies, there is hope that dramatic improvement will occur in both the mortality rates and the incidence of morbidity in the survivors. Ideally, the future focus will be on the development of other prevention strategies such as vaccines and local antiseptics that could have broader and more dramatic influences on neonatal sepsis.

References

1. Freedman RM, Ingram DL, Gross I, *et al.* A half century of neonatal sepsis at Yale: 1928 to 1978. *Am J Dis Child* 1981; **135**: 140–4.

2. Bizzarro MJ, Dembry LM, Baltimore RS, *et al.* Changing patterns in neonatal *Escherichia coli* sepsis and ampicillin resistance in the era of intrapartum antibiotic prophylaxis. *Pediatrics* 2008; **121**: 689–96.

3. Bizzarro MJ, Raskind C, Baltimore RS, *et al.* Seventy-five years of neonatal sepsis at Yale: 1928–2003. *Pediatrics* 2005; **116**: 595–602.

4. Gladstone IM, Ehrenkranz RA, Edberg SC, *et al.* A ten-year review of neonatal sepsis and comparison with the previous fifty-year experience. *Pediatr Infect Dis J* 1990; **9**: 819–25.

5. Baltimore RS, Huie SM, Meek JI, *et al.* Early-onset neonatal sepsis in the era of group B streptococcal prevention. *Pediatrics* 2001; **108**: 1094–8.

6. Chen KT, Puopolo KM, Eichenwald EC, *et al.* No increase in rates of early-onset neonatal sepsis by antibiotic-resistant group B *Streptococcus* in the era of intrapartum antibiotic prophylaxis. *Am J Obstet Gynecol* 2005; **192**: 1167–71.

7. Daley AJ, Isaacs D. Ten-year study on the effect of intrapartum antibiotic prophylaxis on early onset group B streptococcal and *Escherichia coli* neonatal sepsis in Australasia. *Pediatr Infect Dis J* 2004; **23**: 630–4.

8. Edwards RK, Jamie WE, Sterner D, *et al.* Intrapartum antibiotic prophylaxis and early-onset neonatal sepsis patterns. *Infect Dis Obstet Gynecol* 2003; **11**: 221–6.

9. Moore MR, Schrag SJ, Schuchat A. Effects of intrapartum antimicrobial prophylaxis for prevention of group-B-streptococcal disease on the incidence and ecology of early-onset neonatal sepsis. *Lancet Infect Dis* 2003; **3**: 201–13.

10. Schrag SJ, Stoll BJ. Early-onset neonatal sepsis in the era of widespread intrapartum chemoprophylaxis. *Pediatr Infect Dis J* 2006; **25**: 939–40.

11. Baker CJ, Halsey NA, Schuchat A. 1997 AAP guidelines for prevention of early-onset group B streptococcal disease. *Pediatrics* 1999; **103**: 701.

12. Eichenwald EC. Perinatally transmitted neonatal bacterial infections. *Infect Dis Clin North Am* 1997; **11**: 223–39.

13. Hyde TB, Hilger TM, Reingold A, *et al.* Trends in incidence and antimicrobial resistance of early-onset sepsis: population-based surveillance in San Francisco and Atlanta. *Pediatrics* 2002; **110**: 690–5.

14. Schrag S, Schuchat A. Prevention of neonatal sepsis. *Clin Perinatol* 2005; **32**: 601–15.

15. Schuchat A, Zywicki SS, Dinsmoor MJ, *et al.* Risk factors and opportunities for prevention of early-onset neonatal sepsis: a multicenter case–control study. *Pediatrics* 2000; **105**: 21–6.

16. Vesikari T, Janas M, Gronroos P, *et al.* Neonatal septicaemia. *Arch Dis Child* 1985; **60**: 542–6.

17. Edwards MS, Nizet V, Baker CJ. Group B streptococcal infections. In Remington JS, Klein JO, Wilson CB, *et al.*, eds., *Infectious Diseases of the Fetus and Newborn Infant*, 6th edn. Philadelphia, PA: Elsevier Saunders, 2006: 404–64.

18. Lukacs SL, Schoendorf KC. *National Estimates of Newborn Sepsis Rates in the United States, 1990–2001.* Salt Lake City, UT: Society for Pediatric and Perinatal Epidemiologic Research, 2004.

19. Lukacs SL, Schoendorf KC, Schuchat A. Trends in sepsis-related neonatal mortality in the United States, 1985–1998. *Pediatr Infect Dis J* 2004; **23**: 599–603.

20. Schrag SJ, Hadler JL, Arnold KE, *et al.* Risk factors for invasive, early-onset *Escherichia coli* infections in the era of widespread intrapartum antibiotic use. *Pediatrics* 2006; **118**: 570–6.

21. Arachaisri T, Ballow M. Developmental immunology of the newborn. *Immunol Allergy Clin North Am* 1999; **19**: 253–79.

22. Lewis DB, Wilson CB. Developmental immunology and role of the host defenses in neonatal susceptibility to infection. In: Remington JS, Klein JO, Wilson CB, *et al.*, *Infectious Diseases of the Fetus and Newborn Infant*, 6th edn. Philadelphia, PA: Elsevier Saunders, 2006: 88–210.

23. Georgeson GD, Szony BJ, Streitman K, *et al.* Natural killer cell cytotoxicity is deficient in newborns with sepsis and recurrent infections. *Eur J Pediatr* 2001; **160**: 478–82.

24. Wilson DC, Edgar JD. Predictors of bacterial infection in neonates. *J Pediatr* 1997; **130**: 166.

25. Herbst A, Kallen K. Time between membrane rupture and delivery and septicemia in term neonates. *Obstet Gynecol* 2007; **110**: 612–18.

26. Chen KT, Ringer S, Cohen AP, *et al.* The role of intrapartum fever in identifying asymptomatic term neonates with early-onset neonatal sepsis. *J Perinatol* 2002; **22**: 653–7.

27. Schrag SJ, Zell ER, Lynfield R, *et al.* A population-based comparison of strategies to prevent early-onset group B streptococcal disease in neonates. *N Engl J Med* 2002; **347**: 233–9.

28. Towers CV, Suriano K, Asrat T. The capture rate of at-risk term newborns for early-onset group B streptococcal sepsis determined by a risk factor approach. *Am J Obstet Gynecol* 1999; **181**: 1243–9.

29. Yancey MK, Duff P, Kubilis P, *et al.* Risk factors for neonatal sepsis. *Obstet Gynecol* 1996; **87**: 188–94.

30. Glasgow TS, Young PC, Wallin J, *et al.* Association of intrapartum antibiotic exposure and late-onset serious bacterial infections in infants. *Pediatrics* 2005; **116**: 696–702.

31. Denniston S, Riordan FA. *Staphylococcus aureus* bacteraemia in children and neonates: a 10 year retrospective review. *J Infect* 2006; **53**: 387–93.

32. Hakim H, Mylotte JM, Faden H. Morbidity and mortality of staphylococcal bacteremia in children. *Am J Infect Control* 2007; **35**: 102–5.

33. Schiano MA, Hauth JC, Gilstrap LC. Second-stage fetal tachycardia and neonatal infection. *Am J Obstet Gynecol* 1984; **148**: 779–81.

34. Soman M, Green B, Daling J. Risk factors for early neonatal sepsis. *Am J Epidemiol* 1985; **121**: 712–19.

35. Gerdes JS. Diagnosis and management of bacterial infections in the neonate. *Pediatr Clin North Am* 2004; **51**: 939–59.

36. Escobar GJ, Li DK, Armstrong MA, *et al.* Neonatal sepsis workups in infants ≥ 2000 grams at birth: a population-based study. *Pediatrics* 2000; **106**: 256–63.

37. Baker CJ. Group B streptococcal infections. *Clin Perinatol* 1997; **24**: 59–70.

38. Ottolini MC, Lundgren K, Mirkinson LJ, *et al.* Utility of complete blood count and blood culture screening to diagnose neonatal sepsis in the asymptomatic at risk newborn. *Pediatr Infect Dis J* 2003; **22**: 430–4.

39. Bomela HN, Ballot DE, Cory BJ, *et al.* Use of C-reactive protein to guide duration of empiric antibiotic therapy in suspected early neonatal sepsis. *Pediatr Infect Dis J* 2000; **19**: 531–5.

40. Townsend TR, Shapiro M, Rosner B, *et al.* Use of antimicrobial drugs in general hospitals. I. Description of population and definition of methods. *J Infect Dis* 1979; **139**: 688–97.

41. Paerregaard A, Bruun B, Andersen GE, *et al.* No advantage of capillary blood compared with venous blood for culture in neonates. *Pediatr Infect Dis J* 1989; **8**: 659–60.

42. Wiswell TE, Hachey WE. Multiple site blood cultures in the initial evaluation for neonatal sepsis during the first week of life. *Pediatr Infect Dis J* 1991; **10**: 365–9.

43. Sarkar S, Bhagat I, DeCristofaro JD, *et al.* A study of the role of multiple site blood cultures in the evaluation of neonatal sepsis. *J Perinatol* 2006; **26**: 18–22.

44. Jardine L, Davies MW, Faoagali J. Incubation time required for neonatal blood cultures to become positive. *J Paediatr Child Health* 2006; **42**: 797–802.

45. Kumar Y, Qunibi M, Neal TJ, *et al.* Time to positivity of neonatal blood cultures. *Arch Dis Child Fetal Neonatal Ed* 2001; **85**: F182–6.

46. Visser VE, Hall RT. Urine culture in the evaluation of suspected neonatal sepsis. *J Pediatr* 1979; **94**: 635–8.

47. DiGeronimo RJ. Lack of efficacy of the urine culture as part of the initial workup of suspected neonatal sepsis. *Pediatr Infect Dis J* 1992; **11**: 764–6.

48. Evans ME, Schaffner W, Federspiel CF, *et al.* Sensitivity, specificity, and predictive value of body surface cultures in a neonatal intensive care unit. *JAMA* 1988; **259**: 248–52.

49. Kite P, Millar MR, Gorham P, *et al.* Comparison of five tests used in diagnosis of neonatal bacteraemia. *Arch Dis Child* 1988; **63**: 639–43.

50. Schouten-Van Meeteren NY, Rietveld A, Moolenaar AJ, *et al.* Influence of perinatal conditions on C-reactive protein production. *J Pediatr* 1992; **120**: 621–4.

51. Benitz WE, Han MY, Madan A, *et al.* Serial serum C-reactive protein levels in the diagnosis of neonatal infection. *Pediatrics* 1998; **102**: E41.

52. Jaye DL, Waites KB. Clinical applications of C-reactive protein in

pediatrics. *Pediatr Infect Dis J* 1997; **16**: 735–47.

53. Chiesa C, Signore F, Assumma M, *et al.* Serial measurements of C-reactive protein and interleukin-6 in the immediate postnatal period: reference intervals and analysis of maternal and perinatal confounders. *Clin Chem* 2001; **47**: 1016–22.

54. Laborada G, Rego M, Jain A, *et al.* Diagnostic value of cytokines and C-reactive protein in the first 24 hours of neonatal sepsis. *Am J Perinatol* 2003; **20**: 491–501.

55. Bhandari V, Wang C, Rinder C, *et al.* Hematologic profile of sepsis in neonates: neutrophil CD64 as a diagnostic marker. *Pediatrics* 2008; **121**: 129–34.

56. Kocabas E, Sarikcioglu A, Aksaray N, *et al.* Role of procalcitonin, C-reactive protein, interleukin-6, interleukin-8 and tumor necrosis factor-alpha in the diagnosis of neonatal sepsis. *Turk J Pediatr* 2007; **49**: 7–20.

57. Ng PC, Li G, Chui KM, *et al.* Neutrophil CD64 is a sensitive diagnostic marker for early-onset neonatal infection. *Pediatr Res* 2004; **56**: 796–803.

58. Santana Reyes C, Garcia-Munoz F, Reyes D, *et al.* Role of cytokines (interleukin-1β, 6, 8, tumour necrosis factor-α, and soluble receptor of interleukin-2) and C-reactive protein in the diagnosis of neonatal sepsis. *Acta Paediatr* 2003; **92**: 221–7.

59. Franz AR, Steinbach G, Kron M, *et al.* Reduction of unnecessary antibiotic therapy in newborn infants using interleukin-8 and C-reactive protein as markers of bacterial infections. *Pediatrics* 1999; **104**: 447–53.

60. Nupponen I, Andersson S, Jarvenpaa AL, *et al.* Neutrophil CD11b expression and circulating interleukin-8 as diagnostic markers for early-onset neonatal sepsis. *Pediatrics* 2001; **108**: E12.

61. Weirich E, Rabin RL, Maldonado Y, *et al.* Neutrophil CD11b expression as a diagnostic marker for early-onset neonatal infection. *J Pediatr* 1998; **132**: 445–51.

62. Edgar JD, Wilson DC, McMillan SA, *et al.* Predictive value of soluble immunological mediators in neonatal infection. *Clin Sci (Lond)* 1994; **87**: 165–71.

63. Kennon C, Overturf G, Bessman S, *et al.* Granulocyte colony-stimulating factor as a marker for bacterial infection in neonates. *J Pediatr* 1996; **128**: 765–9.

64. Starr SE. Antimicrobial therapy of bacterial sepsis in the newborn infant. *J Pediatr* 1985; **106**: 1043–8.

65. Backes RJ, Rouse MS, Henry NK, *et al.* Activity of penicillin combined with an aminoglycoside against group B streptococci in vitro and in experimental endocarditis. *J Antimicrob Chemother* 1986; **18**: 491–8.

66. Jenson HB, Pollock BH. Meta-analyses of the effectiveness of intravenous immune globulin for prevention and treatment of neonatal sepsis. *Pediatrics* 1997; **99**: E2.

67. Manroe BL, Rosenfeld CR, Weinberg AG, *et al.* The differential leukocyte count in the assessment and outcome of early-onset neonatal group B streptococcal disease. *J Pediatr* 1977; **91**: 632–7.

68. Schibler KR, Osborne KA, Leung LY, *et al.* A randomized, placebo-controlled trial of granulocyte colony-stimulating factor administration to newborn infants with neutropenia and clinical signs of early-onset sepsis. *Pediatrics* 1998; **102**: 6–13.

69. Gillan ER, Christensen RD, Suen Y, *et al.* A randomized, placebo-controlled trial of recombinant human granulocyte colony-stimulating factor administration in newborn infants with presumed sepsis: significant induction of peripheral and bone marrow neutrophilia. *Blood* 1994; **84**: 1427–33.

70. Bilgin K, Yaramis A, Haspolat K, *et al.* A randomized trial of granulocyte–macrophage colony-stimulating factor in neonates with sepsis and neutropenia. *Pediatrics* 2001; **107**: 36–41.

71. Bennet R, Eriksson M, Zetterstrom R. Neonatal septicemia: comparison of onset and risk factors during three consecutive 5-year periods. *Acta Paediatr Scand* 1987; **76**: 361–2.

72. Mok PM, Reilly BJ, Ash JM. Osteomyelitis in the neonate: clinical aspects and the role of radiography and scintigraphy in diagnosis and management. *Radiology* 1982; **145**: 677–82.

73. Bennet R, Bergdahl S, Eriksson M, *et al.* The outcome of neonatal septicemia during fifteen years. *Acta Paediatr Scand* 1989; **78**: 40–3.

74. Alfven G, Bergqvist G, Bolme P, *et al.* Longterm follow-up of neonatal septicemia. *Acta Paediatr Scand* 1978; **67**: 769–73.

75. Sehdev HM, Stamilio DM, Macones GA, *et al.* Predictive factors for neonatal

morbidity in neonates with an umbilical arterial cord pH less than 7.00. *Am J Obstet Gynecol* 1997; **177**: 1030–4.

76. Wu YW. Systematic review of chorioamnionitis and cerebral palsy. *Ment Retard Dev Disabil Res Rev* 2002; **8**: 25–9.

77. Stray-Pedersen B, Bergan T, Hafstad A, *et al.* Vaginal disinfection with chlorhexidine during childbirth. *Int J Antimicrob Agents* 1999; **12**: 245–51.

78. Taha TE, Biggar RJ, Broadhead RL, *et al.* Effect of cleansing the birth canal with antiseptic solution on maternal and newborn morbidity and mortality in Malawi: clinical trial. *BMJ* 1997; **315**: 216–20.

79. Schuchat A. Group B streptococcal disease: from trials and tribulations to triumph and trepidation. *Clin Infect Dis* 2001; **33**: 751–6.

80. Schuchat A. Epidemiology of group B streptococcal disease in the United States: shifting paradigms. *Clin Microbiol Rev* 1998; **11**: 497–513.

81. Davies HD, Adair C, McGeer A, *et al.* Antibodies to capsular polysaccharides of group B *Streptococcus* in pregnant Canadian women: relationship to colonization status and infection in the neonate. *J Infect Dis* 2001; **184**: 285–91.

82. Blumberg HM, Stephens DS, Modansky M, *et al.* Invasive group B streptococcal disease: the emergence of serotype V. *J Infect Dis* 1996; **173**: 365–73.

83. Klegerman ME, Boyer KM, Papierniak CK, *et al.* Estimation of the protective level of human IgG antibody to the type-specific polysaccharide of group B *Streptococcus* type Ia. *J Infect Dis* 1983; **148**: 648–55.

84. Schuchat A, Deaver-Robinson K, Plikaytis BD, *et al.* Multistate case–control study of maternal risk factors for neonatal group B streptococcal disease. The Active Surveillance Study Group. *Pediatr Infect Dis J* 1994; **13**: 623–9.

85. Boyer KM, Gotoff SP. Prevention of early-onset neonatal group B streptococcal disease with selective intrapartum chemoprophylaxis. *N Engl J Med* 1986; **314**: 1665–9.

86. Centers for Disease Control and Prevention. Decreasing incidence of perinatal Group B streptococcal disease: United States, 1993–1995. *MMWR Morb Mortal Wkly Rep* 1997; **46**: 473–7.

87. Whitney CG, Plikaytis BD, Gozansky WS, *et al.* Prevention practices for

perinatal group B streptococcal disease: a multi-state surveillance analysis. Neonatal Group B Streptococcal Disease Study Group. *Obstet Gynecol* 1997; **89**: 28–32.

88. Centers for Disease Control and Prevention. Prevention of perinatal group B streptococcal disease: a public health perspective. *MMWR Recomm Rep* 1996; **45**: 1–24.

89. Schrag S, Gorwitz R, Fultz-Butts K, *et al.* Prevention of perinatal group B streptococcal disease. Revised guidelines from CDC. *MMWR Recomm Rep* 2002; **51**: 1–22.

90. Centers for Disease Control and Prevention. Diminishing racial disparities in early-onset neonatal group B streptococcal disease: United States, 2000–2003. *MMWR Morb Mortal Wkly Rep* 2004; **53**: 502–5.

91. Centers for Disease Control and Prevention. Perinatal group B streptococcal disease after universal screening recommendations: United States, 2003–2005. *MMWR Morb Mortal Wkly Rep* 2007; **56**: 701–5.

92. Ekelund K, Konradsen HB. Invasive group B streptococcal disease in infants: a 19-year nationwide study. Serotype distribution, incidence and recurrent infection. *Epidemiol Infect* 2004; **132**: 1083–90.

93. Katz V, Bowes WA, Jr. Perinatal group B streptococcal infections across intact amniotic membranes. *J Reprod Med* 1988; **33**: 445–9.

94. Dillon HC, Khare S, Gray BM. Group B streptococcal carriage and disease: a 6-year prospective study. *J Pediatr* 1987; **110**: 31–6.

95. Trager JD, Martin JM, Barbadora K, *et al.* Probable community acquisition of group B *Streptococcus* in an infant with late-onset disease: demonstration using field inversion gel electrophoresis. *Arch Pediatr Adolesc Med* 1996; **150**: 766–8.

96. Ancona RJ, Ferrieri P, Williams PP. Maternal factors that enhance the acquisition of group-B streptococci by newborn infants. *J Med Microbiol* 1980; **13**: 273–80.

97. Regan JA, Klebanoff MA, Nugent RP. The epidemiology of group B streptococcal colonization in pregnancy. Vaginal Infections and Prematurity Study Group. *Obstet Gynecol* 1991; **77**: 604–10.

98. Curtis J, Kim G, Wehr NB, *et al.* Group B streptococcal phospholipid causes pulmonary hypertension. *Proc Natl Acad Sci USA* 2003; **100**: 5087–90.

99. Centers for Disease Control and Prevention. Hospital-based policies for prevention of perinatal Group B streptococcal disease: United States, 1999. *MMWR Morb Mortal Wkly Rep* 2000; **49**: 936–40.

100. Fernandez M, Hickman ME, Baker CJ. Antimicrobial susceptibilities of group B streptococci isolated between 1992 and 1996 from patients with bacteremia or meningitis. *Antimicrob Agents Chemother* 1998; **42**: 1517–19.

101. Glass P, Wagner AE, Papero PH, *et al.* Neurodevelopmental status at age five years of neonates treated with extracorporeal membrane oxygenation. *J Pediatr* 1995; **127**: 447–57.

102. Committee on Obstetric Practice, American College of Obstetrics and Gynecologists. Prevention of early-onset group B streptococcal disease in newborns. *Int J Gynaecol Obstet* 1996; **54**: 197–205.

103. American Academy of Pediatrics Committee on Infectious Diseases and Committee on Fetus and Newborn. Revised guidelines for prevention of early-onset group B streptococcal (GBS) infection. *Pediatrics* 1997; **99**: 489–96.

104. Rosenstein NE, Schuchat A. Opportunities for prevention of perinatal group B streptococcal disease: a multistate surveillance analysis. The Neonatal Group B Streptococcal Disease Study Group. *Obstet Gynecol* 1997; **90**: 901–6.

105. Puopolo KM, Madoff LC, Eichenwald EC. Early-onset group B streptococcal disease in the era of maternal screening. *Pediatrics* 2005; **115**: 1240–6.

106. deCueto M, Sanchez M, Sampedro A, *et al.* Relationship between timing of intrapartum ampicillin administration and its effectiveness in preventing vertical transmission of group B streptococci. *Obstet Gynecol* 1998; **91**: 112–14.

107. American Academy of Pediatrics Committee on Infectious Diseases and Committee on Fetus and Newborn. Guidelines for prevention of group B streptococcal (GBS) infection by chemoprophylaxis. *Pediatrics* 1992; **90**: 775–8.

108. Gotoff SP, Boyer KM. Prevention of early-onset neonatal group B streptococcal disease. *Pediatrics* 1997; **99**: 866–9.

109. Siegel JD, Cushion NB. Prevention of early-onset group B streptococcal disease: another look at single-dose

penicillin at birth. *Obstet Gynecol* 1996; **87**: 692–8.

110. Benitz WE. The neonatal group B streptococcal debate. *Pediatrics* 1998; **101**: 494–6.

111. Lieu TA, Mohle-Boetani JC, Ray GT, *et al.* Neonatal group B streptococcal infection in a managed care population. *Obstet Gynecol* 1998; **92**: 21–7.

112. Yow MD, Mason EO, Leeds LJ, *et al.* Ampicillin prevents intrapartum transmission of group B streptococcus. *JAMA* 1979; **241**: 1245–7.

113. Heim K, Alge A, Marth C. Anaphylactic reaction to ampicillin and severe complication in the fetus. *Lancet* 1991; **337**: 859–60.

114. Towers CV, Carr MH, Padilla G, *et al.* Potential consequences of widespread antepartal use of ampicillin. *Am J Obstet Gynecol* 1998; **179**: 879–83.

115. Pylipow M, Gaddis M, Kinney JS. Selective intrapartum prophylaxis for group B streptococcus colonization: management and outcome of newborns. *Pediatrics* 1994; **93**: 631–5.

116. Davis RL, Hasselquist MB, Cardenas V, *et al.* Introduction of the new Centers for Disease Control and Prevention group B streptococcal prevention guideline at a large West Coast health maintenance organization. *Am J Obstet Gynecol* 2001; **184**: 603–10.

117. Jaureguy F, Carton M, Panel P, *et al.* Effects of intrapartum penicillin prophylaxis on intestinal bacterial colonization in infants. *J Clin Microbiol* 2004; **42**: 5184–8.

118. Kasper DL, Paoletti LC, Wessels MR, *et al.* Immune response to type III group B streptococcal polysaccharide-tetanus toxoid conjugate vaccine. *J Clin Invest* 1996; **98**: 2308–14.

119. Baker CJ, Paoletti LC, Rench MA, *et al.* Immune response of healthy women to 2 different group B streptococcal type V capsular polysaccharide–protein conjugate vaccines. *J Infect Dis* 2004; **189**: 1103–12.

120. Guttormsen HK, Liu Y, Paoletti LC. Functional activity of antisera to group B streptococcal conjugate vaccines measured with an opsonophagocytosis assay and HL-60 effector cells. *Hum Vaccin* 2008; **4**: 370–4.

121. Buccato S, Maione D, Rinaudo CD, *et al.* Use of *Lactococcus lactis* expressing pili from group B *Streptococcus* as a broad-coverage vaccine against streptococcal disease. *J Infect Dis* 2006; **194**: 331–40.

122. Rosini R, Rinaudo CD, Soriani M, *et al.* Identification of novel genomic islands coding for antigenic pilus-like structures in *Streptococcus agalactiae*. *Mol Microbiol* 2006; **61**: 126–41.

123. Bingen E, Picard B, Brahimi N, *et al.* Phylogenetic analysis of *Escherichia coli* strains causing neonatal meningitis suggests horizontal gene transfer from a predominant pool of highly virulent B2 group strains. *J Infect Dis* 1998; **177**: 642–50.

124. Sarff LD, McCracken GH, Schiffer MS, *et al.* Epidemiology of *Escherichia coli* K1 in healthy and diseased newborns. *Lancet* 1975; **1**: 1099–104.

125. McCracken GH, Jr., Sarff LD, Glode MP, *et al.* Relation between *Escherichia coli* K1 capsular polysaccharide antigen and clinical outcome in neonatal meningitis. *Lancet* 1974; **2**: 246–50.

126. Guerina NG, Kessler TW, Guerina VJ, *et al.* The role of pili and capsule in the pathogenesis of neonatal infection with *Escherichia coli* K1. *J Infect Dis* 1983; **148**: 395–405.

127. Cook SW, Hammill HA, Hull RA. Virulence factors of *Escherichia coli* isolated from female reproductive tract infections and neonatal sepsis. *Infect Dis Obstet Gynecol* 2001; **9**: 203–7.

128. Mayor-Lynn K, Gonzalez-Quintero VH, O'Sullivan MJ, *et al.* Comparison of early-onset neonatal sepsis caused by *Escherichia coli* and group B *Streptococcus*. *Am J Obstet Gynecol* 2005; **192**: 1437–9.

129. Alarcon A, Pena P, Salas S, *et al.* Neonatal early onset *Escherichia coli* sepsis: trends in incidence and antimicrobial resistance in the era of intrapartum antimicrobial prophylaxis. *Pediatr Infect Dis J* 2004; **23**: 295–9.

130. Charles D, Larsen B. Streptococcal puerperal sepsis and obstetric infections: a historical perspective. *Rev Infect Dis* 1986; **8**: 411–22.

131. Chuang I, Van Beneden C, Beall B, *et al.* Population-based surveillance for postpartum invasive group A *Streptococcus* infections, 1995–2000. *Clin Infect Dis* 2002; **35**: 665–70.

132. Miyairi I, Berlingieri D, Protic J, *et al.* Neonatal invasive group A streptococcal disease: case report and review of the literature. *Pediatr Infect Dis J* 2004; **23**: 161–5.

133. Greenberg D, Leibovitz E, Shinnwell ES, *et al.* Neonatal sepsis caused by *Streptococcus pyogenes*: resurgence of an old etiology? *Pediatr Infect Dis J* 1999; **18**: 479–81.

134. Macris MH, Hartman N, Murray B, *et al.* Studies of the continuing susceptibility of group A streptococcal strains to penicillin during eight decades. *Pediatr Infect Dis J* 1998; **17**: 377–81.

135. Kaplan EL, Johnson DR, Del Rosario MC, *et al.* Susceptibility of group A beta-hemolytic streptococci to thirteen antibiotics: examination of 301 strains isolated in the United States between 1994 and 1997. *Pediatr Infect Dis J* 1999; **18**: 1069–72.

136. Zimbelman J, Palmer A, Todd J. Improved outcome of clindamycin compared with beta-lactam antibiotic treatment for invasive *Streptococcus pyogenes* infection. *Pediatr Infect Dis J* 1999; **18**: 1096–100.

137. Norrby-Teglund A, Ihendyane N, Kansal R, *et al.* Relative neutralizing activity in polyspecific IgM, IgA, and IgG preparations against group A streptococcal superantigens. *Clin Infect Dis* 2000; **31**: 1175–82.

138. Dobson SR, Baker CJ. Enterococcal sepsis in neonates: features by age at onset and occurrence of focal infection. *Pediatrics* 1990; **85**: 165–71.

139. McNeeley DF, Saint-Louis F, Noel GJ. Neonatal enterococcal bacteremia: an increasingly frequent event with potentially untreatable pathogens. *Pediatr Infect Dis J* 1996; **15**: 800–5.

140. Murray BE. The life and times of the *Enterococcus*. *Clin Microbiol Rev* 1990; **3**: 46–65.

Neonatal bacterial meningitis

Alistair G. S. Philip

Introduction

The term *meningitis* refers to inflammation of the leptomeninges covering the brain. Bacterial infection of the meninges usually produces a suppurative process or "purulent meningitis." However, it is probably more correct in the newborn infant to consider the condition as bacterial *meningoencephalitis*, since it is common to have involvement of the cerebral hemispheres as well as involvement of the meninges.

From the clinician's perspective it has been traditional to think of neonatal sepsis (septicemia) and meningitis together, because the clinical manifestations may be indistinguishable. For many years, the proportion of cases of neonatal sepsis that also had documented meningitis was considered to be one-quarter to one-third. For instance, in 1986 it was estimated that one case of neonatal meningitis occurs for every four cases of sepsis [1]. Indeed, this was my personal experience in Vermont between 1975 and 1980, when 12 of 41 cases (29%) with neonatal sepsis in the first week after birth had associated meningitis [2]. However, in the early 1990s the proportion of cases decreased to as low as 5% [3]. This may be less true in other countries, with 32 of 229 (14%) noted in Israel, 107 of 577 (18.5%) in Panama, and 14 of 84 (17.8%) in Kenya [4–6]. It is also noteworthy that with meningitis due to Group B *Streptococcus* (GBS), the proportion of cases may relate to the time of onset of the disease. For instance, if GBS sepsis was detected within 12 hours of birth, the proportion with meningitis was 6%, whereas it was 53% if over 7 days of age, in a recent study from the Netherlands [7].

Incidence

The incidence of neonatal bacterial meningitis will vary from one center to the next, but national studies have shown the incidence to be quite similar (Table 31.1). In the Netherlands [8] the incidence in 1976–82 was 0.23/1000 live births, and in England and Wales the incidence in 1985–87 was 0.32/1000 live births and did not change significantly when re-evaluated in 1996–97 [9]. Twenty years ago the lowest incidence, of 0.16–0.17/1000 live births, was reported from Australia, where rates have since fallen to even lower levels [10–12]. We are now in an era of widespread intrapartum chemoprophylaxis to prevent GBS infection, and this seems to have resulted in a decrease in meningitis incidence in several countries [13]. In a review of early-onset infection from Australia and New Zealand (Australasia), the incidence of early-onset GBS meningitis fell from 0.24/1000 in 1993 to 0.03/1000 in 2002, whereas the incidence of meningitis due to *Escherichia coli* did not change [14]. On the other hand, data from the Netherlands documented a sharp reduction in early-onset GBS sepsis, from 0.54/1000 in 1997–98 to 0.36/1000 in 1999–2001, but GBS meningitis rates were 0.14 and 0.17/1000 live births respectively for these two time periods [7].

A further indication that the incidence may be falling is the fact that, compared to the latter half of the twentieth century, there have been few reports concerning neonatal meningitis so far in the twenty-first century. The incidence of sepsis and meningitis is higher in neonates of low birthweight ($< 2500\,\mathrm{g}$) and especially very low birthweight (VLBW: $< 1500\,\mathrm{g}$) [14–17]. There is also a slight male preponderance in most reports.

Need for lumbar puncture

It is unusual to encounter meningitis in the first 24 hours after delivery, and because of this many clinicians elect not to perform a lumbar puncture at that time, particularly when evaluation for sepsis/meningitis is being performed only for risk factors (e.g., prolonged rupture of membranes, maternal fever, etc.) [3].

This issue remains controversial, but in places with a higher incidence of neonatal meningitis it would seem prudent to perform lumbar puncture whenever meningitis is suspected [18]. Where there is a low incidence of meningitis, there are differences of opinion about the best approach to adopt in the term infant, but there is also no uniformity of opinion regarding the VLBW infant. This is because the procedure itself may cause disruption of normal physiology, may produce a "traumatic tap," or may be unsuccessful [19].

Some authors have documented an extremely low yield from cerebrospinal fluid (CSF) obtained very early, particularly when performed for features of respiratory distress syndrome, and it may add little to blood culture alone. However, one study documented that 28% of infants (12 of 43) with meningitis had a negative blood culture, including seven of the eight infants whose mothers received prenatal antibiotics. With an increasing number of women receiving prenatal antibiotics to prevent GBS infection, this raises some concern,

Fetal and Neonatal Brain Injury, 4th edition, ed. David K. Stevenson, William E. Benitz, Philip Sunshine, Susan R. Hintz, and Maurice L. Druzin. Published by Cambridge University Press. © Cambridge University Press 2009.

Table 31.1. Incidence of neonatal bacterial meningitis

Authors	Country	Years	Rate per 1000 live births
Mulder and Zanen 1984 [8]	Netherlands	1976–82	0.23
Tessin et al. 1990 [16]	Sweden	1975–86	0.40
De Louvois et al. 2005 [9]	England and Wales	1985–87	0.32
Francis and Gilbert 1992 [11]	Australia	1987–89	0.17
Greenberg et al. 1997 [4]	Southern Israel	1986–94	0.45
Isaacs et al. 1999 [10]	Australia	1991–97	0.16
De Louvois et al. 2005 [9]	England and Wales	1996–97	0.31
Gordon and Isaacs 2006 [12]	Australia and New Zealand	1992–2002	0.10

but there may be alternative strategies that can be adopted (see Diagnosis, below). A 5-year analysis of neonatal bacterial sepsis also stressed the possible interference of intrapartum maternal antibiotics in obtaining positive blood cultures, but recorded only five cases of bacterial meningitis and 209 cases of septicemia [20].

Johnson et al. (in 1997) looked at 24 452 term newborns from 1987 to 1993 [21]. Of the infants evaluated for infection based on risk factors, 3423 (14%) were asymptomatic. Among this group, 17 (0.5%) were bacteremic, but none had meningitis. An additional 1712 (7%) were evaluated for signs of sepsis, 55 of whom (3.2%) were bacteremic, with 11 cases of meningitis (10 of whom had positive blood cultures). They concluded that lumbar puncture is unnecessary in asymptomatic term newborns – a position affirmed by Pong and Bradley in their review [22].

I agree with this approach and, even in the presence of signs of sepsis, would recommend a selective policy on the first day, taking specific signs and markedly abnormal laboratory values into consideration (see Diagnosis, below). After the first day, evaluation for sepsis/meningitis should include a lumbar puncture, in most cases. Particularly when neonates with nonspecific illnesses are seen in an outpatient setting, the need to consider meningitis has been emphasized [23].

It is also important to note that a lumbar puncture may be indicated even more in VLBW infants. In a large experience from the NICHD Neonatal Research Network, one-third of VLBW infants had meningitis in the absence of a positive blood culture [24].

Case fatality

Despite a decrease in meningitis relative to sepsis, the case-fatality rate has remained extremely high until recently. The rate in England and Wales among 450 cases seen in 1985–87 was 20% [9]. Case-fatality rates are usually higher in neonates

with Gram-negative infections, with a rate of 32% in England and Wales and a threefold increase compared to Gram-positive infections in another study [9,25].

On the other hand, a 21-year experience in Dallas, Texas, indicated a case-fatality rate with Gram-negative bacillary meningitis of 17% for the years 1969–89 [26]. It should also be noted that 61% of the survivors in Dallas had long-term sequelae. Even with Gram-positive meningitis the outcome frequently involves impairment. For instance, Edwards et al. evaluated 38 survivors of GBS meningitis at over 3 years of age [27]. Only 50% were functioning normally. In a more recent study from Toronto, Canada, the case-fatality rate was 13% in 101 infants with definitive bacterial meningitis born between 1979 and 1998, and an additional 17% had moderate or severe disability at 1 year of age [28]. The best outcome was reported from Greece for the years 1983–97, where 70 of 72 term infants with Gram-negative bacterial meningitis survived to discharge and survivors had a low incidence of neurologic sequelae [29]. Experience in England and Wales also suggests a marked decrease in case fatality in more recent years (8% in 1996–97) [30], but with continued high rates of disability [9]. Case-fatality rate was also markedly reduced (to 8%) in southern Taiwan in 1994–2001, compared to 17% in 1986–93 [31]. The most recent data from other countries (less well developed) continue to show high case-fatality rates of 30–40%, with a high incidence of neurologic sequelae in survivors [32,33]. It has also been observed that case-fatality rates are higher in VLBW infants [13,24].

Thus it is clear that neonatal meningitis remains an important cause of mortality and morbidity. Early diagnosis and treatment remain desirable goals, but prevention may be even more desirable. These areas will be discussed later.

Etiology

Prior to the mid-1970s, *Escherichia coli* was the leading cause of neonatal bacterial meningitis in most developed countries. Even in the period 1975–83, *E. coli* was the leading cause of neonatal meningitis in England and Wales [34], and the same was true in the Netherlands from 1976 to 1982. However, as long ago as the early 1970s, GBS accounted for 31% of 131 cases of neonatal meningitis and *E. coli* for 38% in the Neonatal Meningitis Co-operative Study. Since the late 1970s, GBS, also known as *Streptococcus agalactiae*, has assumed the dominant role in most countries reporting on the causative organisms of neonatal meningitis. However, Gram-negative bacteria (*Klebsiella* spp. and *E. coli*) continue to predominate in some developing countries [4,5,15,35], although GBS may be increasing [4,33]. Experience from Dallas during 1987–94 indicated that GBS accounted for 52% and *E. coli* for only 9% of 74 cases of neonatal bacterial meningitis (Trujillo and McCracken, personal communication). On the other hand, in Toronto, Canada, between 1979 and 1998 GBS decreased from 59% to 42% and *E. coli* increased from 22% to 27% [28]. A further decrease in GBS meningitis, but not *E.coli* meningitis, has been seen in Australasia in recent years, presumably related to increased use of intrapartum antibiotics [14].

Meningitis due to GBS is usually associated with late-onset infection, generally considered to be more than 5 days after birth, in contrast to the clinical picture of sepsis and pneumonia associated with early-onset GBS infection, although cases of early-onset meningitis certainly occur. In a recent report from Italy, among 30 infants with early-onset GBS infection, only two had culture-proven meningitis, whereas meningitis was documented in 12 of 26 with late-onset GBS disease [36]. Similarly, babies infected with *Listeria monocytogenes*, particularly serotype IVb, are more likely to have meningitis as the most frequent clinical manifestation with late-onset infection [37]. Although *L. monocytogenes* is not as prevalent in the USA, it has been an important organism in some countries and has been implicated in epidemics in North America [38]. In a report from Kuwait, *L. monocytogenes* was the commonest organism isolated in 45 neonates with bacterial meningitis, accounting for 31% of the total, compared to 15% for GBS and 11% for *E. coli* [39].

Meningitis due to GBS is most frequently due to serotype III, even with early-onset meningitis. In contrast to a broad distribution of serotypes in neonatal early-onset sepsis, over 85% of early-onset ($n = 46$) and late-onset ($n = 121$) meningitis cases were due to serotype III by Baker in 1979 [40]. Rather similar findings were reported by Carstensen *et al.* when describing a national study from Denmark [41], when 77% of early-onset ($n = 13$) and 100% of late-onset ($n = 18$) meningitis cases were type III infections. Experience from the Netherlands showed 57% of GBS meningitis to be the result of type III [8]. Recently, serotype V has been implicated more, and it has been shown that the biotype may be an important factor, as a result of the loss of catabolic function [42]. Of 15 biotypes, B1 to B6 were 13 times more likely to invade the central nervous system of the neonate than B7 to B15. Among 42 GBS strains associated with neonatal meningitis, 86% were identified as B1 to B6 [42]. Cases of neonatal meningitis attributed to *E. coli* are predominantly the result of those carrying the K1 capsular antigen. Most reports indicate that 75% of strains of *E. coli* causing neonatal meningitis are K1 strains, and Mulder *et al.* had 88% K1 strains [43].

In at least one country (Serbia), recent experience (1991–2000) indicates that *Klebsiella* species account for more cases of neonatal meningitis than either *E. coli* or GBS [44]. There are many other organisms that have been implicated in neonatal meningitis, most of which are relatively uncommon (for extensive lists, with references, see Davies & Rudd, and Pong & Bradley [22,45]). It should be noted that the fourth commonest organism in England and Wales was *Streptococcus pneumoniae* (or pneumococcus), which was almost as common as *L. monocytogenes* [34]. *Neisseria meningitidis*, which is a frequent etiologic agent in older infants and children, is an uncommon cause of neonatal meningitis, but cases continue to be reported [46]. *Hemophilus influenzae*, which was a common causative organism of meningitis in infancy until recently, has also been an uncommon etiologic agent in the neonate and is usually non-typable (not type b), even in years prior to the introduction of *H. influenzae* type b

vaccine. In the VLBW infant the organisms noted above may still be implicated, but infection with coagulase-negative staphylococci (especially *Staphylococcus epidermidis*) is more common [47].

Some organisms have a penchant for causing more difficulty than others. Important among them is *Citrobacter diversus*, which seems to predispose to the development of brain abscess (or abscesses) [48], for reasons that are not completely clear.

Pathophysiology and pathology
Bacteremia and susceptibility
Although some cases of neonatal meningitis are encountered without accompanying bacteremia, the most likely route of spread is via bloodstream infection. Indeed, it has been suggested that the magnitude of bacteremia is associated with the occurrence of Gram-negative meningitis. Thus, those factors that predispose to neonatal sepsis (septicemia) may also be considered as risk factors for meningitis.

Infection may be acquired from the mother or may be acquired after birth. Bacteria may also possibly gain access to the meninges by direct spread from the oropharynx. Prenatal risk factors include prolonged rupture of the fetal membranes, particularly if there is evidence of chorioamnionitis, and preterm labor without apparent explanation. Much research has linked amniotic fluid infection to preterm labor [49]. Male infants seem to be more susceptible to infection than female, with a higher incidence in almost every series. VLBW infants are at particularly high risk (see Introduction, above) and an increased risk for GBS infection has been reported in twins [50], although this may be related to the higher incidence of preterm delivery with multiple births. An additional high-risk group is infants with galactosemia, who are particularly susceptible to infection with *E. coli* [51].

The characteristics of some bacteria seem to be associated with an increased propensity to cause neonatal meningitis [52]. The capsular polysaccharide of GBS type III, *E. coli* K1, and *L. monocytogenes* serotype IVb all contain sialic acid in high concentration. All these organisms have been closely linked to meningitis. The ability of bacteria to interact with neutrophils may also affect virulence. It has been shown that impaired interaction with neutrophils is characteristic of virulent clones of *E. coli*, more likely to produce invasive infection [53].

The hospital environment can be particularly hostile for VLBW infants, who may require prolonged intubation with endotracheal tubes or prolonged catheterization of major blood vessels. Central venous catheters, in particular, seem to predispose to bacteremia, with the possibility of meningitis as a consequence.

Anatomical pathology
Because meningitis is now relatively infrequent, it is necessary to rely on older information for a description of the morphological inflammatory response [54]. Initially (during the first

Table 31.2. Neuropathological features of neonatal bacterial meningitis

Acute[a]	Chronic
Arachnoiditis	Cerebral cortical atrophy
Cerebral edema	Developmental defects
Cerebral abscess	Hydrocephalus
Encephalopathy	Multicystic encephalomalacia
Infarction	Organizational defects
Vasculitis	Subdural effusion
Ventriculitis	White-matter atrophy

Note:
[a]May be visible on ultrasonography [74].

week) polymorphonuclear leukocytes (PMNs) aggregate in a meshwork of fibrin over the outer part of the arachnoid membrane. This exudate may occur over the cerebral hemispheres, but is also found at the base of the brain. Later (second and third week) PMNs decrease, while histiocytes and macrophages increase [54].

Pathologically, changes in blood vessels are very common, with inflammatory infiltrates leading to thromboses of arachnoidal or subependymal veins. There may be severe congestion or hemorrhagic encephalopathy of the brain substance. This may lead to necrosis of nerve cells and leukomalacia. Additional findings that may help to explain the sequelae among survivors of bacterial meningitis are segmental arteritis of meningeal and perforating branches of the carotid artery, compression or collapse of surface veins by purulent meningeal exudate and by cerebral edema, and phlebitis of cortical veins [55]. The major neuropathological features of neonatal bacterial meningitis are summarized in Table 31.2.

Cytokines and chemokines

In recent years, there has been an increased awareness that outcome may be related to circulating humoral factors as well as direct bacterial invasion of the meninges [56]. These humoral factors are called cytokines and chemokines. Levels of the proinflammatory cytokines interleukin 1β and tumor necrosis factor α (cachectin) were detected in the CSF of most neonates with Gram-negative bacterial meningitis, and peak concentrations of interleukin-1β correlated with outcome. While some cytokines may produce adverse effects, others have been shown to have beneficial effects (e.g., interleukin 10, which is an anti-inflammatory cytokine) and could prove useful as adjunctive therapy [56].

Blood–brain barrier

Another factor that normally plays a role in protection against the spread of bacterial infection is the blood–brain barrier. The permeability of the blood–brain barrier has been shown to increase in stressed neonates and those with bacterial meningitis, when compared to "healthy" infants or neonates with aseptic meningitis [57]. The brain is normally protected from undesirable fluctuations of humoral factors by the blood–CSF–brain barrier, which primarily exists at the arachnoid

membranes, the choroid plexus, and the endothelial cells of brain capillaries. The endothelial cells produce continuous tight junctions in the walls of capillaries, which act as the barrier, but can be disrupted by hyperosmotic solutions.

The ability of lipopolysaccharide derived from *E. coli* O111 B4 to disrupt the blood–brain barrier has been shown in newborn piglets during experimental neonatal meningitis [58]. Disruption was demonstrated by leakage of sodium fluorescein from blood vessels within about 1 hour of intracisternal injection of lipopolysaccharide. *E. coli* was chosen because this organism remains a frequent cause of meningitis in human newborns. The authors postulated that "the products of Gram-negative organisms could adhere to the adventitial surface of cerebral capillaries, resulting directly in separation of the tight junctions between endothelial cells and a marked increase in pinocytotic activity within the endothelium" [58]. This model could prove useful for studying both pathogenesis of neonatal meningitis and also its therapy.

Disruption of the blood–brain barrier with exudation of albumin across the leaky junctions may lead to cerebral edema, with increased intracranial pressure and altered cerebral blood flow. These in turn can produce cranial nerve injury, seizures, and hypoxic–ischemic injury.

There is also evidence to suggest that genetic factors may contribute to bacterial penetration of the blood–brain barrier. This transcellular penetration (transcytosis) has been demonstrated for GBS, *E. coli* K1, *L. monocytogenes*, *Citrobacter freundii*, and *Streptococcus pneumoniae* [59].

Diagnosis
Clinical features

Bell and McGuinness have noted that there were only occasional publications on neonatal bacterial meningitis in the first half of the twentieth century [55], with authors stressing the rareness of the condition and the difficulty of clinical diagnosis until the advanced stages were reached. However, during the second half of the twentieth century, many cases were encountered and diagnosed, probably as a result of increased awareness, and there was a voluminous literature on the subject. Now, in the twenty-first century, the condition is becoming relatively rare again, but those clinical features that initiate investigation for sepsis continue to be those that should also raise the possibility of meningitis. These clinical manifestations include lethargy, abdominal distension, respiratory distress, temperature instability, irritability, apnea, or cyanotic spells [26,60]. When these features cannot be explained by other diagnoses, it is important to evaluate the baby for infection, including a lumbar puncture to obtain cerebrospinal fluid.

Late signs of bacterial meningitis are a bulging anterior fontanel and seizures, although in some reports seizures were surprisingly common [26,28,29]. Nuchal rigidity is almost never seen in the neonate [29]. If investigation of meningitis is not performed until these late signs are seen, serious mortality and morbidity are likely to result [30]. Unfortunately, in many cases of later onset, this is the situation that prevails.

Table 31.3. Findings in the cerebrospinal fluid (CSF) of non-infected term neonates

Features	Bonadio et al. [123]	Ahmed et al. [124]
Number of infants	35	108
Age at evaluation	0–4 weeks	0–30 days
White blood cells		
Mean	11/mm³ (11 × 10⁶/L)	7.3/mm³ (7.3 × 10⁶/L)
Range	0–35/mm³ (0–35 × 10⁶/L)	0–130/mm³ (0–130 × 10⁶/L) (only 3 with > 20/mm³)
Protein – mean	84 mg/dL (0.84 G/L)	64 mg/dL (0.64 G/L)
Glucose – mean	47 mg/dL (2.6 mmol/L)	51 mg/dL (2.8 mmol/L)

Cerebrospinal fluid

In contrast to older infants and children, CSF obtained early in the course of meningitis may not demonstrate specific cellular changes in the neonate. The interpretation of CSF changes is compounded by the presence of up to 25–30 white blood cells per cubic millimeter (WBC/mm³) in neonates without infection (Table 31.3), and by the difficulties in obtaining CSF uncontaminated with blood. In one study, 21 samples from 39 neonates with meningitis on CSF culture could be evaluated with cell counts. Only 12 of 21 had more than 25 WBC/mm³, illustrating the importance of sending the fluid for culture in every case where lumbar puncture is performed. It also illustrates that, when infection is suspected, antibiotics should be initiated promptly after specimens for culture have been sent. Decisions about discontinuing antibiotics can be made 48–72 hours later.

Culture of CSF remains the "gold standard" as far as diagnosis of bacterial meningitis in the neonate is concerned. Higher WBC counts may be seen with Gram-negative rods than with Gram-positive cocci, although CSF protein and glucose usually are not different [61]. As just mentioned, it is possible to have a lack of pleocytosis, but to have a positive culture (presumably early in the course of the illness). A recent study showed that 10% of infants with meningitis had less than 4 WBC/mm³ in the CSF, leading to the suggestion that no single value in the CSF can reliably exclude the presence of meningitis in the neonate [62]. For this reason, CSF should always be sent for culture. A case has also been made for repeating lumbar punctures when bacteremia is documented, since pleocytosis developed in several infants whose CSF was initially normal [63]. In cases of meningitis which grow Gram-negative organisms, it is common for the CSF to remain culture-positive for several days [26]. This seems to be less true with Gram-positive organisms, but whenever persistently positive cultures occur, it suggests that ventriculitis may be present.

The technique of performing a lumbar puncture (or spinal tap) is important. Care needs to be taken to avoid excessive flexion of the trunk or neck, since this may produce hypoxemia. Although intuitively local anesthesia might seem to lessen physiologic instability, this was not observed in a controlled trial [64]. On the other hand, it seems important to use needles with stylets, since needles without stylets carry the risk of introducing epithelial cells into the spinal canal, with subsequent development of epidermoid tumors [65]. Short needles for this purpose are available, and they allow considerable stability during manipulation.

Examination of CSF microscopically may reveal a specific organism more rapidly than waiting for culture. In one large cooperative study, smear with Gram's stain correctly identified 80% of organisms prior to culture results [66].

Although it was suggested in older children that CSF C-reactive protein (CRP) levels might help to make a rapid diagnosis of bacterial meningitis, CRP in CSF was not shown to be helpful in neonates [67].

It is also possible to detect bacterial antigen in CSF using either countercurrent immunoelectrophoresis or latex particle agglutination (LPA). The latter is quicker and simpler and has proved quite useful in type III GBS meningitis. Although there is an LPA test for E. coli K1 antigen, which cross-reacts with Neisseria meningitidis group B, this has not been shown to be particularly reliable or useful.

Other laboratory evaluations

Additional help in evaluating infants with suspected sepsis and/or meningitis comes from blood leukocyte counts and CRP measurements. As with any severe infection, total leukocyte counts are frequently low (below 5.0×10^9/L), with increased ratios of immature to total neutrophils [68]. Important observations on the usefulness of serum CRP determinations in bacterial meningitis were published over 30 years ago [69]. The most uniform pattern of high serum CRP values in neonates was seen with cases of E. coli meningitis. Marked increases in serum CRP were noted in four cases of neonatal meningitis reported by Sabel and Wadsworth, with three cases seen on the first day after delivery [70]. Although serum CRP may not always be elevated at the initial evaluation for suspected sepsis/meningitis [68,71], it increases reliably in cases of meningitis, sometimes to very high levels within 24–48 hours [68,72]. Pourcyrous et al. documented increased levels of CRP in 11 of 13 (85%) neonates with meningitis at initial evaluation [71]. By 12 hours later, all 13 had elevated levels. Consequently, CRP determinations may be particularly helpful if a decision has been made to defer performing a lumbar puncture in an unstable infant. If the serum CRP remains normal, meningitis is virtually eliminated, but if it increases substantially (above 4 mg/dL) lumbar puncture should be performed. This number proved useful in infants over 2 months of age, who had been ill for more than 12 hours and had fever [73]. When CRP was less than 2 mg/dL, all had confirmed or probable viral infection, whereas above 4 mg/dL 79% had bacterial infection [73].

Imaging studies

The most useful technique for imaging the brain in cases of bacterial meningitis is probably ultrasonography. This is because it can be accomplished at the bedside (through the anterior fontanel) and considerable experience has accumulated with this technique in the last 25 years [74,75]. In recent years magnetic resonance imaging has proved valuable. In particular, diffusion tensor imaging (DTI) has documented meningeal inflammation by revealing increased fractional anisotropy in cases of neonatal bacterial meningitis, which decreased with antibiotic treatment [76]. Computed tomography may also provide better delineation than ultrasonography [22].

In a series of infants from Toronto, a constellation of abnormalities was documented by ultrasonography in the great majority (25 of 34) with pyogenic meningitis [74]. Abnormalities included ventriculomegaly, echogenic sulci, subdural effusion, ventriculitis, infarction, cerebritis, cerebral edema, and porencephalic cysts [74].

As noted earlier, brain abscess (or abscesses) may be seen more commonly in association with meningitis due to *Citrobacter diversus*, and imaging studies are particularly valuable in this context [48].

Antibody to common bacteria

Susceptibility to infection is related to the presence (or absence) of antibody. This has been most strikingly demonstrated with regard to Group B streptococcal infection. Vogel *et al.* documented the lack of sero-specific antibody in neonates who acquired GBS infection [77]. The increased susceptibility of VLBW infants is probably related (in part) to decreased transfer of antibody from mother to baby, since transfer of immunoglobulin G occurs predominantly after 32 weeks' gestation [78]. Only immunoglobulin G usually traverses the placenta. Transfer of IgG seems to be by an active, rather than passive, process.

Since meningitis is a serious infection, it would be suspected that survivors would have a significant antibody response. It is therefore interesting to learn that the patterns of response in survivors of type III GBS meningitis were quite variable [79]. In five of ten infants, specific immunoglobulin M antibody failed to develop at a mean of 3.8 weeks after diagnosis, increased after another 4–8 weeks, and declined to baseline again another 2–4 months later. This inability to sustain an antibody response is akin to the comparatively low response of mothers to unconjugated GBS vaccine [80].

The prominence of *E. coli* in neonatal infection has been attributed to the fact that antibody to this and other Gram-negative organisms is predominantly found in the immunoglobulin M fraction, which does not cross the placenta. However, it has been documented that selective transport of anti-*E. coli* antibody in the immunoglobulin G fraction can provide some protection, even in very preterm infants [81].

Complications

There are several acute complications that have been reported in association with bacterial meningitis in the neonate. The most frequently reported are ventriculitis, hydrocephalus, and cerebral abscess, but more recently cerebral infarction

has been noted in infants with meningitis [82]. Although frequently recognized in older infants, very few cases of inappropriate secretion of antidiuretic hormone have been documented in the neonate. Diabetes insipidus has been associated with GBS sepsis/meningitis and was presumed to be related to brain edema, inflammation, and vasculitis leading to infarction [83]. In a few instances, the inflammatory process and ischemic change may lead to liquefaction of the brain. The author has encountered three such cases, one with GBS and one each with *Streptococcus pneumoniae* and *E. coli* (unpublished) [68].

Because ventriculitis was so commonly encountered with Gram-negative organisms, the first Neonatal Meningitis Co-operative Study Group used intrathecal antibiotics and the second used intraventricular gentamicin [66,84]. The results of these interventions were no better (and possibly worse) than intravenous antibiotics alone, so that intrathecal or intraventricular therapy is not considered necessary or particularly beneficial. It may be possible to detect ventriculitis using cephalic ultrasound [75].

Hydrocephalus seems to be the result of outflow obstruction secondary to high CSF protein levels. Earlier treatment may possibly minimize this problem, but when it develops (possibly in one-third) it usually requires ventriculoperitoneal shunt repair.

As noted earlier, cerebral abscesses seem to be particularly common in association with neonatal meningitis caused by *Citrobacter diversus* [48]. The diagnosis has become easier to make because of newer imaging techniques. Cranial ultrasonography, in particular, allows the imaging to be performed at the bedside, although MRI may provide better images. Other organisms that have been associated with neonatal brain abscesses are *Proteus* and *Enterobacter* species. In one series, among 30 cases of brain abscess, 27 were caused by *Proteus* species infections [85]. Many of them were enormous and easily detected with ultrasonography or computed tomography scans. In only 20 cases did meningitis precede the brain abscess. *Enterobacter sakazakii* also has been reported to produce brain abscess, because it seems to have neurotropic qualities [86].

Ment *et al.* performed cranial computed tomographic scans on all eight neonates with bacterial meningitis admitted during a 36-month period [82]. Six had large areas of infarction related to major arterial vascular distributions. They suggested that computed tomographic scans be done on all neonates with bacterial meningitis, although magnetic resonance imaging might now be considered. Long-term complications (such as deafness) are discussed in the subsection on neurological sequelae in the outcome section, below.

Treatment and management

Although antibiotic therapy is often referred to as "specific treatment," it should be remembered that antibiotics are used to suppress bacterial growth, so that the baby's defense mechanisms have time to respond. There are many instances where appropriate antibiotic therapy is used, with a sensitive organism, but the baby with sepsis and/or meningitis has been overwhelmed by the infection and died. Nevertheless, the judicious use of antibiotics may minimize the emergence of resistant organisms [87].

In addition, as mentioned earlier, there may be other humoral factors (e.g., cytokines) that produce undesirable effects. With Gram-negative enteric organisms there is frequently release of endotoxin and with GBS, "endotoxin-like effects" have been described [56]. The presence of endotoxin was found in the CSF of all infants with Gram-negative bacterial meningitis who died, but was also frequently found in those with an abnormal or normal outcome [88].

Thus, although antibiotic therapy is very important for the eradication of bacteria, other adjunctive measures may be almost as important in determining survival and in minimizing the long-term sequelae. The two major supportive measures that are used are assisted ventilation (for those infants who develop respiratory failure) and cardiovascular support. It is common with severe infections to have shock, and the use of volume (colloid or crystalloid) replacement, as well as pressor agents (such as dopamine) to support blood pressure, may be life-saving. It is also important to recognize (and aggressively treat) seizure activity. In this situation, assisted ventilation may be particularly valuable and there may be benefits from moderate hyperventilation, which may decrease increased intracranial pressure. Extreme hypocarbia ($PCO_2 < 20$ mmHg) may substantially decrease cerebral blood flow and should probably be avoided.

Choice of antibiotics

The recommendations made by an American Academy of Pediatrics Task Force regarding antibiotic therapy for neonatal meningitis still seem to be valid [1]. Initial antibiotic therapy in the first week after birth seems to be fairly well agreed upon in most developed countries and consists of ampicillin and an aminoglycoside (usually gentamicin). This combination has stood the test of time (somewhat remarkably) and seems to be effective for the most common etiologic bacteria, although this may be changing and the combination of ampicillin and cefotaxime has been suggested more recently [88,89]. In a retrospective review from Sweden, covering the years 1975–86, of the 365 pathogens isolated from blood and/or CSF, 91% were sensitive to either ampicillin or aminoglycosides or both [90]. Treatment failed in six of 34 patients with neonatal meningitis, but the failure was not related to ampicillin or aminoglycoside resistance [90]. Ampicillin resistance occurred most frequently with late-onset infections in VLBW and low-birthweight infants. Currently, initial antibiotic therapy after the first week usually includes anti-staphylococcal coverage in such infants.

It is often stated that aminoglycosides do not penetrate well into CSF, but in the presence of inflamed meninges the penetration may be better. Certainly, intrathecal administration combined with intravenous gentamicin seemed to offer no advantage over intravenous therapy alone [66]. Nevertheless, one disadvantage of aminoglycosides is that levels may

need to be monitored to avoid toxicity, although data about nephrotoxicity and ototoxicity in neonates are limited. Much of what is written concerns potentially toxic concentrations rather than documented permanent sequelae [91].

While there seems to be reasonable unanimity of opinion about ampicillin–aminoglycoside in the first week after birth, this is not the case beyond that age. Another Swedish study has documented (in infants up to 1 year) that ampicillin plus gentamicin is inadequate empiric therapy for meningitis [92]. The combination of ampicillin and ceftazidime has proved superior, and cefotaxime has also shown more effective coverage [89]. However, when cefotaxime is incorporated into empiric therapy, it has been shown to increase bacterial resistance [93].

In older infants and children, both cefuroxime and ceftriaxone proved efficacious, with ceftriaxone perhaps superior [94]. However, the prolonged excretion time for ceftriaxone makes it difficult to know what should be its dosing frequency in the neonate.

Prior to the introduction of the cephalosporins, another antibiotic that was deemed to be of considerable value was chloramphenicol. In contrast to the cephalosporins, use of chloramphenicol necessitates the determination of levels to accomplish therapeutic, but non-toxic, levels [95]. This is certainly a disadvantage, but does not exclude chloramphenicol from the therapeutic armamentarium, if sensitivities suggest that it may be the antibiotic of choice. In addition, chloramphenicol is comparatively inexpensive, especially when compared to the cephalosporins. Although frequently used in England and Wales in the mid-1980s, chloramphenicol use there decreased from 50% to less than 5% in the late 1990s [30]. The cost factor may make chloramphenicol particularly valuable in developing countries.

With late-onset infection in VLBW infants, there is the strong possibility of staphylococcal infection. There are now many methicillin-resistant strains of *Staphylococcus aureus*, and most hospital-acquired strains of *S. epidermidis* are resistant to the penicillins. With these organisms, it may be possible to use nafcillin or oxacillin [88], but it is frequently necessary to use vancomycin, and in the sick infant beyond the first week it is probably wise to initiate antibiotic treatment with vancomycin and a cephalosporin, although few data are available concerning their use in neonatal meningitis [96]. Vancomycin levels need to be monitored.

Since there is considerable variation from one country to another (and even within countries), it is important to keep track locally of the most frequent organisms causing sepsis and meningitis and to know local antibiotic sensitivities. The more frequently used antibiotics are displayed in Table 31.4. Successful treatment of Gram-negative bacterial meningitis in term neonates was reported quite recently using cefotaxime and amikacin [29].

Special mention was made earlier of *Citrobacter diversus* and its propensity to lead to brain abscesses. One report describes the poor response to third-generation cephalosporins, aminoglycosides, and trimethoprim–sulfamethoxazole, but the

Table 31.4. Antibiotics commonly used in neonatal meningitis and their dosage[a]

	< 1 week	> 1 week	Frequency
Penicillin G	100 000 units	200 000 units	b.i.d./q.i.d.
Ampicillin	200 mg	300 mg	b.i.d./q.i.d.
Gentamicin[b]	4 mg load, then	3 mg	Daily
Cefotaxime	100 mg	150 mg	b.i.d./t.i.d.
Vancomycin[b]	30 mg	45 mg	b.i.d./t.i.d.
Chloramphenicol[b]	25 mg	50 mg	Daily/b.i.d.
Nafcillin	50 mg	100 mg	b.i.d./q.i.d.

Notes:
[a]All as per kg per day.
[b]Serum levels need to be monitored.

successful treatment of *C. diversus* meningitis complicated by brain abscesses using imipenem–cilastatin [97]. On the other hand, a favorable outcome has been reported with protracted courses of more traditional antibiotics [98].

Duration of antibiotics

Since there is reasonable consensus regarding which antibiotics to use in the first week, one might imagine that duration of therapy would also be agreed upon. Unfortunately, although many authors have firm opinions about duration of therapy for neonatal bacterial meningitis, there are very few data upon which to base those opinions. In older infants and children there has been re-evaluation of the duration of therapy for sepsis/meningitis. In particular, the "7–10–14-day rule" has been called in question [99]. To quote Radetsky, "The numerology of infectious disease has never been investigated. Even in the absence of specific data certain numbers have an unaccountable power to satisfy and reassure, and they are the numbers that are preferentially chosen. For the duration of antimicrobial therapy 7, 10, 14 and 21 days have consistently appeared . . . The numbers 7, 10, and 14 are enshrined in the treatment recommendations for meningitis in all current textbooks" [99].

In older infants and children, serum CRP levels have been shown to be helpful in following the course of illness. Peltola *et al.* in Finland documented that, in uncomplicated cases of bacterial meningitis, CRP levels returned to normal within 7 days. Secondary elevations of CRP may indicate complications such as subdural effusion [100]. Further experience from Peltola's group documented the value of CRP in helping to determine the duration of antibiotic therapy. Although the mean duration was 10 days, it varied from 5.5 to 34 days and antibiotic therapy was not discontinued unless CRP values had normalized [100].

The ability of serum CRP to distinguish complicated cases from uncomplicated cases of bacterial meningitis in infants and children was also reported from France [101]. They were able to shorten the duration of antibiotic therapy in the majority of these children to 4–5 days for 21 of 24 with meningococcal meningitis, and to 7 days for 16 of 22 with *Haemophilus*

influenzae meningitis and four of six with pneumococcal meningitis, without an increase in neurological sequelae.

Data in neonates are quite limited, but in the early experience of Sabel and Hanson relapse of meningitis was only encountered (in three cases) when the CRP remained elevated at the time of discontinuance of antibiotics [69]. In my reported experience and unpublished observations serum CRP was elevated in neonatal meningitis for a minimum of 5 days and not infrequently for more than 10 days [67]. It therefore seems reasonable to discontinue antibiotics within 2–3 days of the CRP level returning to normal (less than 1.0 mg/dL or 10 mg/L). Saez-Llorens and McCracken have supported this position [88]. While acknowledging traditional and commonly recommended durations of therapy (quite prolonged), their recommendation was that "duration of antibiotics should be individualized, on the basis of clinical, laboratory and bacteriologic responses. Normalization of the acute-phase reaction (i.e. ESR [erythrocyte sedimentation rate] and CRP) can be considered one index for when antimicrobial therapy could be safely stopped" [88].

Peak levels of CRP with neonatal meningitis are frequently in excess of 10 mg/dL (100 mg/L) and almost always greater than 7.0 mg/dL [68–70]. It is not completely clear whether extremely high levels of CRP (e.g., over 20 mg/dL) can predict an adverse neurological outcome, although limited experience suggests this [68].

Corticosteroids

The role of corticosteroids in the management of neonatal meningitis is not well defined. Even in infants and children, the benefits of dexamethasone are debated. The arguments for and against have been summarized by Prober [102]. It seems reasonably clear that dexamethasone administered before antibiotics are given is beneficial in meningitis due to *Haemophilus influenzae* type b, but the picture is not clear with other organisms, particularly when dexamethasone is given after antibiotics have been started. The rationale for use of corticosteroids is to decrease meningeal inflammation and swelling and to decrease concentrations of potentially harmful cytokines. To date, there is limited experience in neonates. Daoud *et al.* in Jordan performed a randomized controlled trial of dexamethasone use in 52 cases of neonatal bacterial meningitis, the majority being due to *Klebsiella pneumoniae*, and showed no benefit [103]. Of 27 in the dexamethasone group, six died and six had permanent neurological deficit. The control group had 25 neonates, with seven deaths and seven neurologically impaired [103].

Other anti-inflammatory therapy

While there are limited data concerning corticosteroids in neonates, even less is known about most other anti-inflammatory agents that could be used in human bacterial meningitis. Various animal studies have dealt with indomethacin, anticytokine antibodies or inhibitors, anti-endothelium leukocyte adhesion agents, etc. [88].

Table 31.5. Outcome in neonatal bacterial meningitis

Authors	Country	Year	Number	Case fatality (%)	Neurological sequelae (%)[a]	Predominant bacteria
Mulder and Zanen 1984 [8]	Netherlands	1976–82	380	27	N/A	*Escherichia coli*
Bennet *et al.* 1989 [105]	Sweden (Stockholm)	1969–83	60	28	40	*Staphylococcus aureus*[b]
DeLouvois *et al.* 2005 [9]	England and Wales	1985–87	280	25	20	GBS, *Escherichia coli*
Francis and Gilbert 1992 [11]	Australia	1987–89	116	26	23	GBS, *Escherichia coli*
Unhanand *et al.* 1993 [26]	USA (Dallas)	1969–89	98	17	61	*Escherichia coli*
Daoud *et al.* 1996 [32]	Jordan	1992–94	53	32	39	*Klebsiella pneumoniae*
Klinger *et al.* 2000 [28]	Canada (Toronto)	1979–98	101	13	26	GBS
Dellagrammaticas *et al.* 2000 [29]	Greece (Athens)	1983–97	72	3	8	*Escherichia coli*
De Louvois *et al.* 2005 [9]	England and Wales	1996–97	166	7	23	GBS

Notes:
N/A, not available; GBS, Group B β-hemolytic *Streptococcus*.
[a]Percent of survivors.
[b]Cases of sepsis, N/A for meningitis.

Table 31.6. Outcome in infants with group B β-hemolytic *Streptococcus* (GBS) meningitis

Authors	Age at diagnosis	Case-fatality	Number of survivors	Major neurological sequelae[a]	Age at follow-up
Edwards *et al.* [27]	0–3 months	38%	38	11 (29%)	3.3–9.0 years
Harvey *et al.* [30]	0–28 days	25%	65	12 (18%)	5 years
Klinger *et al.* [28]	1–28 days	13%[b]	50	15 (30%)	1–19 years

Notes:
[a]Percentages of survivors.
[b]Based on all cases, not just GBS.

Outcome
Case fatality

It was mentioned in the introduction that case-fatality (mortality) rates are high in almost every series dealing with neonatal bacterial meningitis, although recent experience provides a more optimistic view [28–30].

The national studies from the Netherlands, from England and Wales in the 1980s, and from Australia had case-fatality rates of 27%, 20%, and 26% respectively, and more recent experience from Dallas documented a case-fatality rate of 17% [8,9,11,26]. My own limited experience in Maine in the late 1980s and early 1990s, with 18 cases, was associated with a case-fatality rate of 25% within 1 week of diagnosis and 28% if one late death (5 months later, following cerebral infarction) was included [3]. Age at diagnosis may also be important, with higher case-fatality rates at younger ages. Mulder *et al.* documented case-fatality rates of 77% at 0–2 days, 28% at 3–6 days, and 15% at 7–27 days in cases of neonatal meningitis caused by *E. coli* [43]. Different rates may also be seen with different strains of *E. coli*. The *E. coli* K1 strains produced a 31% case-fatality rate in one study, versus 0% with non-K1 strains [104]. In addition, case-fatality rates are usually higher in VLBW infants and those with a high CSF protein [13,24,27].

More recently, data from England and Wales documented a case-fatality rate in 1996–97 of only 8% [9,30]. Experience in Toronto, Canada, for 1979–98 revealed a case-fatality rate of 13% and in Athens, Greece, the rate was only 3% for Gram-negative bacterial meningitis in term infants during the period 1983–97 [28,29]. These data are summarized in Table 31.5.

Neurological sequelae

The high percentage of major neurological sequelae in survivors was emphasized in a series of papers in the mid-1980s dealing with GBS meningitis [27]. With case-fatality rates varying between 26% and 38%, major neurological sequelae were found in 15–29% of the survivors (Table 31.6). Edwards *et al.* summarized the long-term sequelae of several groups reporting on GBS meningitis [27]. Of a total of 218, the case-fatality rate was 26% and, of the 152 survivors, 17% had major neurodevelopmental sequelae, 16% had mild/moderate sequelae, and 67% were considered normal. More recent experience is quite similar [9,28].

In their review in 1982, Bell and McGuinness noted that sequelae had been reported in 31–56% of survivors in different reports [55]. Almost identical figures were reported from Stockholm, Sweden, for 5-year periods from 1969 to 1983, with sequelae from neonatal meningitis noted in 31–53% of survivors, and case-fatality rates of 23–35% [105]. The highest rate of sequelae accompanied the lowest case-fatality rate. The most recent data from England and Wales document

Table 31.7. Factors associated with poor outcome in neonatal bacterial meningitis

Very low birthweight (< 1500 g)
Coma (or semi-coma)
Decreased perfusion
Need for inotropes to maintain blood pressure
Seizures (> 12 hours duration)
Peripheral wbc count < 5000/mm^3 (< 5.0 × 10^9/L)
Absolute neutrophil count < 1000/mm^3 (< 1.0 × 10^9/L)
CSF protein > 300 mg/dL (> 3 g/L)
Delay in achieving sterile CSF
Abnormal EEG reading (moderate to severe)

a decrease in acute mortality to 6.6% in 1996–97, but serious disability remained at 23% [9].

The most common severe sequelae include "hydrocephalus, seizures, mental retardation, hyperactivity and cranial nerve or long tract signs. Localized deficits include hearing loss, optic atrophy and hypothalamic injury manifested by endocrine deficiencies, diabetes insipidus, precocious puberty or abnormalities of temperature regulation" [55]. In addition, spastic paresis (hemiplegia or quadriplegia) is frequently mentioned [27,106].

In the large experience with Gram-negative enteric bacillary meningitis reported by Unhanand et al., hydrocephalus, seizure disorder, cerebral palsy, developmental delay, and hearing loss were seen in 28%, 28%, 19%, 25%, and 16% respectively in 32 term infants and 36%, 36%, 45%, 55%, and 18% respectively in 11 preterm infants who survived [26]. On the other hand, more recently, Dellagrammaticas et al. reported in term babies both a high survival rate and a low incidence of sequelae, with persisting seizures, spastic paralysis, developmental delay, and hearing deficit in 4%, 3%, 4%, and 6% respectively [29]. Delay in achieving sterile CSF may increase the frequency of sequelae [29].

Table 31.7 shows the factors that are associated with poor outcome in bacterial meningitis. Clinical manifestations on admission that were predictive of a poor outcome (death or severe impairment) in the study of Edwards et al. were presence of coma or semi-coma, decreased perfusion, total peripheral WBC count < 5.0 × 10^9/L, absolute neutrophil count < 1.0 × 10^9/L or CSF protein > 3 g/L [27]. The study by Klinger et al. showed that the best predictors of an adverse outcome were quite similar [28]. Both at 12 hours and 96 hours after admission, seizures, coma, use of inotropes to maintain blood pressure and leukopenia (< 5.0 × 10^9/L) were predictive of a poor outcome. Of 101 infants (born in the years 1979–98) with bacterial meningitis, 13 died and 17 others had moderate to severe disability at 1 year of age [23]. Among 50 infants with GBS meningitis, 15 (30%) had an adverse outcome.

Although not routinely obtained in neonatal meningitis, an additional predictor of outcome is the neonatal electroencephalogram (EEG). When interpretation is normal or only mildly abnormal, the outcome is usually good. An adverse outcome has been associated with moderate to marked abnormality. Repeating the EEG may improve the accuracy of prediction [107].

Klein et al. suggested that a cautiously optimistic note be struck with parents when discussing the long-term complications of meningitis, since "there is a tendency for even major neurologic defects to resolve unpredictably with time" [1].

Prevention

Before discussing the potential for preventing specific kinds of meningitis, it should be remembered that general infection control measures (especially careful hand washing) may be particularly important in preventing the spread of infection.

Attempts to prevent neonatal bacterial meningitis have largely dealt with those organisms that are frequently implicated. There are two major strategies that have been employed. The first is chemoprophylaxis and the second is immunoprophylaxis. Both strategies have been used to prevent neonatal sepsis and meningitis, rather than specifically preventing meningitis. In keeping with the important role it plays in many countries, GBS infection has received the most attention.

Neonatal approach

Both chemo- and immunoprophylaxis have been evaluated from the maternal or neonatal approach. While there has been some success using the maternal approach, using only the neonatal approach has been contradictory or disappointing. For instance, prophylactic administration of penicillin to neonates seemed to be beneficial in reducing GBS infection in some centers, but not in others [108,109]. There was also the possibility that one problem (early-onset GBS infection) might be exchanged for another (late-onset GBS or Gram-negative bacterial infection). Similarly, the use of prophylactic intravenous immunoglobulin in VLBW infants seemed beneficial in one large ($n = 588$) study, but not in an even larger ($n = 2416$) study [110,111]. Different preparations were used in the two studies, which may explain the differences. Another large study ($n = 753$), using the same preparation as Fanaroff et al., also failed to find a protective effect in early-onset or late-onset infection [111,112]. It has been documented that considerable variability of availability of specific antibody to the common pathogens occurs within different lots of immunoglobulin [113]. Greater success seems likely if preparations with species-specific antibody can be administered.

Maternal approach

The use of maternal chemoprophylaxis has proved to be much more striking. In the study of Boyer and Gotoff, bacteremia was seen in none of 85 babies born to ampicillin-treated women, versus five of 79 babies born to untreated mothers [114]. Although this strategy does not prevent transmission of infection in all cases, in the early 1990s a consensus developed that women at high risk (rupture of membranes longer than

18 hours, preterm labor, or maternal fever possibly caused by choriamnionitis) should be screened and treated [115].

This led to the publication by the Centers for Disease Control and Prevention (CDC) in 1996 of new guidelines for the prevention of GBS infection, which resulted in a substantial change in obstetrical practice in North America, with approximately 25% of women receiving intrapartum antibiotics (penicillin or ampicillin) [116]. This resulted in a marked decrease in the incidence of early-onset GBS infection, with a 65% decrease from 1.7 cases per 1000 live births in 1993 to 0.6/1000 live births in 1998. Only 6% with early-onset GBS infection had meningitis [117]. This contrasts with a study from Finland, where 17% had meningitis in 1985–94 [118]. After changing the strategy in the USA to concentrate on routine maternal screening (the "era of widespread intrapartum chemoprophylaxis" mentioned earlier) [13], there has been a further reduction to 0.37 cases per 1000 live births [119]. Other countries have also adopted a more aggressive approach to prevention of GBS infection. Using a risk-based strategy in the Netherlands, early-onset GBS sepsis declined, but the incidence of GBS meningitis did not [7]. To date, this increased use of intrapartum antibiotics has not changed antibiotic sensitivity patterns substantially, although it has created some difficulty in deciding which neonates should be treated after delivery [120].

With regard to maternal immunoprophylaxis, there is variable enthusiasm. While intuitively it would seem that this might be the most effective strategy, there are several possible drawbacks. One significant disadvantage is that, since transfer of antibody from mother to infant occurs primarily after 32 weeks' gestation, the group of infants at greatest risk might not be protected. Another disadvantage (to date) is that the response of women to a polysaccharide vaccine of GBS has been disappointing [80]. Of 35 women with low or unprotected antibody levels before immunization, only 20 (57%) responded to the vaccine in a study published in 1988 [80]. This study used type III capsular polysaccharide vaccine. While it is true that this serotype accounts for the majority of cases of neonatal meningitis, it would be preferable to have a polyvalent vaccine with increased immunogenicity. The many problems in finding and distributing a suitable vaccine have been discussed [121]. One approach that has shown promise is to increase the immunogenicity of vaccines by conjugating (coupling) them to tetanus toxoid or other agents. Polyvalent conjugate vaccines for GBS infection have been tested, show promise with several different strains, and may soon be commercially available [122]. For other organisms, particularly *E. coli*, the ability to provide protection by maternal immunization seems a daunting prospect.

Conclusion

Despite the fact that the incidence of neonatal bacterial meningitis may be falling, there is little room for complacency. This is a disease with high case-fatality rates, although these have fallen in some recent reports, and very high morbidity rates. The neurological sequelae can be quite devastating in some cases, and a completely normal outcome can be anticipated in only half of the survivors. It is therefore important to consider the possibility of sepsis/meningitis in any sick neonate, so that treatment can be initiated as early as possible. However, prevention is even more desirable, and continued efforts in this direction must remain a high priority.

References

1. Klein JO, Feigin RD, McCracken GH. Report on the task force on diagnosis and management of meningitis. *Pediatrics* 1986; **78**: 959–82.

2. Philip AGS. *Neonatal Sepsis and Meningitis,* Appendix. Boston, MA: GK. Hall, 1985.

3. Philip AGS. The changing face of neonatal infection: experience at a regional medical center. *Pediatr Infect Dis J* 1994; **13**: 1098–102.

4. Greenberg D, Shinwell ES, Yagupsky P, *et al.* A prospective study of neonatal sepsis and meningitis in southern Israel. *Pediatr Infect Dis J* 1997; **16**: 768–73.

5. Moreno MT, Vargas S, Poveda R, *et al.* Neonatal sepsis and meningitis in a developing Latin American country. *Pediatr Infect Dis J* 1994; **13**: 516–20.

6. Laving AM, Musoke RN, Wasunno AO, *et al.* Neonatal bacterial meningitis at the newborn unit of Kenyatta National Hospital. *East Afr Med J* 2003; **80**: 456–62.

7. Trijbels-Smeulders M, de Jonge GA, Pasker-de Jonge PC, *et al.* Epidemiology of neonatal group B streptococcal disease in the Netherlands before and after introduction of guidelines for prevention. *Arch Dis Child Fetal Neonatal Ed* 2007; **92**: F271–6.

8. Mulder CJJ, Zanen HC. A study of 280 cases of neonatal meningitis in the Netherlands. *J Infect* 1984; **9**: 177–84.

9. De Louvois J, Halket S, Harvey D. Neonatal meningitis in England and Wales: sequelae at 5 years of age. *Eur J Pediatr* 2005; **164**: 730–4.

10. Isaacs D, Royle JA. Intrapartum antibiotics and early onset neonatal sepsis caused by group B *Streptococcus* and by other organisms in Australia. Australasian Study Group for Neonatal Infections. *Pediatr Infect Dis J* 1999; **18**: 524–8.

11. Francis BM, Gilbert GL. Survey of neonatal meningitis in Australia: 1987–1989. *Med J Aust* 1992; **156**: 240–3.

12. Gordon A, Isaacs D. Late onset neonatal Gram-negative bacillary infection in Australia and New Zealand, 1992–2002. *Pediatr Infect Dis J* 2006; **25**: 25–9.

13. Schrag SJ, Stoll BJ. Early-onset neonatal sepsis in the era of widespread intrapartum chemoprophylaxis. *Pediatr Infect Dis J* 2006; **25**: 939–40.

14. May M, Daley AJ, Donarth S, *et al.* Early onset neonatal meningitis in Australia and New Zealand, 1992–2002. *Arch Dis Child Fetal Neonatal Ed* 2005; **90**: F324–7.

15. Longe AC, Omene JA, Okolo AA. Neonatal meningitis in Nigerian infants. *Acta Paediatr Scand* 1984; **73**: 477–81.

16. Tessin I, Trollfors B, Thiringer K. Incidence and etiology of neonatal septicemia and meningitis in western Sweden 1975–1986. *Acta Paediatr Scand* 1990; **79**: 1023–30.

17. Hristeva L, Booy R, Bowler I, *et al.* Prospective surveillance of neonatal meningitis. *Arch Dis Child* 1993; **69**: 14–18.

18. Shiva F, Mosaffa N, Khabbaz R, *et al.* Lumbar puncture in neonates under and over 72 hours of age. *J Coll Physicians Surg Pak* 2006; **16**: 525–8.

19. Weiss MG, Ionides SP, Anderson CL. Meningitis in premature infants with respiratory distress: role of admission lumbar puncture. *J Pediatr* 1991; **119**: 973–5.

20. Sanghvi KP, Tudehope DI. Neonatal bacterial sepsis in a neonatal intensive care unit: a 5 year analysis. *J Paediatr Child Health* 1996; **32**: 333–8.

21. Johnson CE, Whitwell JK, Pethe K, *et al.* Term newborns who are at risk for sepsis: are lumbar punctures necessary? *Pediatrics* 1997; **99**: E10.

22. Pong A, Bradley JS. Bacterial meningitis and the newborn infant. *Infect Dis Clin North Am* 1999; **13**: 711–33.

23. Albanyan EA, Baker CJ. Is lumbar puncture necessary to exclude meningitis in neonates and young infants: lessons from the group B streptococcus cellulitis–adenitis syndrome. *Pediatrics* 1998; **102**: 985–6.

24. Stoll BJ, Hansen N, Fanaroff AA, *et al.* To tap or not to tap: high likelihood of meningitis without sepsis among very low birth weight infants. *Pediatrics* 2004; **113**: 1181–6.

25. Franco SM, Cornelius VE, Andrews BF. Long-term outcome of neonatal meningitis. *Am J Dis Child* 1992; **146**: 567–71.

26. Unhanand M, Mustafa MM, McCracken GH Jr, *et al.* Gram-negative enteric bacillary meningitis: a twenty-one-year experience. *J Pediatr* 1993; **122**: 15–21.

27. Edwards MS, Rench MA, Haffar AAM, *et al.* Long-term sequelae of group B streptococcal meningitis in infants. *J Pediatr* 1985; **106**: 717–22.

28. Klinger G, Chin CN, Beyene J, *et al.* Predicting the outcome of neonatal bacterial meningitis. *Pediatrics* 2000; **106**: 477–82.

29. Dellagrammaticas HD, Christodoulou C, Megaloyanni E, *et al.* Treatment of gram-negative bacterial meningitis in term neonates with third generation cephalosporins plus amikacin. *Biol Neonate* 2000; **77**: 139–46.

30. Harvey D, Holt DE, Bedford H. Bacterial meningitis in the newborn: a prospective study of mortality and morbidity. *Semin Perinatol* 1999; **23**: 218–25.

31. Chang CJ, Chang WN, Huang LT, *et al.* Neonatal bacterial meningitis in southern Taiwan. *Pediatr Neurol* 2003; **29**: 288–94.

32. Daoud AS, al-Sheyyab M, Abu-Ekteish F, *et al.* Neonatal meningitis in northern Jordan. *J Trop Pediatr* 1996; **42**: 267–70.

33. Molyneux E, Walsh A, Phiri A, *et al.* Acute bacterial meningitis in children admitted to the Queen Elizabeth Central Hospital, Blantyre, Malawi in 1996–97. *Trop Med Int Health* 1998; **3**: 610–18.

34. Synnott MB, Morse DL, Hall SM. Neonatal meningitis in England and Wales: a review of routine national data. *Arch Dis Child* 1994; **71**: F75–80.

35. Gebremariam A. Neonatal meningitis in Addis Ababa: a 10 year review. *Ann Trop Paediatr* 1998; **18**: 279–83.

36. Berardi A, Lugli L, Baronciani D, *et al.* Group B streptococcal infections in a northern region of Italy. *Pediatrics* 2007; **120**: e487–93.

37. Mulder CJJ, Zanen HC. Listeria monocytogenes neonatal meningitis in the Netherlands. *Eur J Pediatr* 1986; **145**: 60–2.

38. Linnan MJ, Mascola L, Lou XD, *et al.* Epidemic listeriosis associated with Mexican-style cheese. *N Engl J Med* 1988; **319**: 823–8.

39. Zaki M, Daoud AS, al Saleh Q, *et al.* Bacterial meningitis in the newborn: a Kuwaiti experience. *J Trop Pediatr* 1990; **36**: 62–5.

40. Baker CJ. Group B streptococcal infections in neonates. *Pediatr Rev* 1979; **1**: 5–15.

41. Carstensen H, Henrichsen J, Jepsen OB. A national survey of severe group B streptococcal infections in neonates and young infants in Denmark, 1978–83. *Acta Paediatr Scand* 1985; **74**: 934–41.

42. Domelier AS, van der Mee-Marquet N, Grandet A, *et al.* Loss of catabolic function in *Streptococcus agalactiae* strains and its association with neonatal meningitis. *J Clin Microbiol* 2006; **44**: 3245–50.

43. Mulder CJJ, van Alphen L, Zanen HC. Neonatal meningitis caused by *Escherichia coli* in the Netherlands. *J Infect Dis* 1984; **150**: 935–40.

44. Ignjatovic M. Bacterial causes of meningitis in newborns [in Serbian]. *Srp Arh Calok Lek* 2001; **129**: 36–41.

45. Davies PA, Rudd PT. *Neonatal Meningitis.* Clinics in Developmental Medicine 132. London: MacKeith Press, 1994.

46. Arango CA, Rathore MH. Neonatal meningococcal meningitis: case reports and review of literature. *Pediatr Infect Dis J* 1996; **15**: 1134–6.

47. Doctor BA, Newman N, Minich NM, *et al.* Clinical outcomes of neonatal meningitis in very-low birth-weight infants. *Clin Pediatr* 2001; **40**: 473–80.

48. Tse G, Silver M, Whyte H, *et al.* Neonatal meningitis and multiple brain abscesses due to *Citrobacter diversus*. *Pediatr Pathol Lab Med* 1997; **17**: 977–82.

49. Goldenberg RL, Hauth JC, Andrews WW. Intrauterine infection and preterm delivery. *N Engl J Med* 2000; **342**: 1500–7.

50. Edwards MS, Jackson CV, Baker CJ. Increased risk of group B streptococcal disease in twins. *JAMA* 1981; **245**: 2044–6.

51. Levy HL, Sepe SJ, Shih VE, *et al.* Sepsis due to *Escherichia coli* in neonates with galactosemia. *N Engl J Med* 1977; **297**: 823–5.

52. Bingen E, Bonacorsi S, Brahimi N, *et al.* Virulence patterns of *Escherichia coli* K1 strains associated with neonatal meningitis. *J Clin Microbiol* 1997; **35**: 2981–2.

53. Öhman L, Tullus K, Katouli M, *et al.* Correlation between susceptibility of infants to infection and interaction with neurotrophils of *Escherichia coli* strains, causing neonatal and infantile septicemia. *J Infect Dis* 1995; **171**: 128–33.

54. Berman P, Banker B. Neonatal meningitis: a clinical and pathological study of 29 cases. *Pediatrics* 1966; **38**: 6–24.

55. Bell WE, McGuinness GA. Suppurative central nervous system infections in the neonate. *Semin Perinatol* 1982; **6**: 1–24.

56. Polin RA, Harris MC. Neonatal bacterial meningitis. *Semin Neonatol* 2001; **6**: 157–72.

57. Anagnostakis D, Messaritakis J, Damianos D, *et al.* Blood–brain barrier permeability in "healthy," infected and stressed neonates. *J Pediatr* 1992; **121**: 291–4.

58. Temesvari P, Abraham CS, Speer CP, *et al. Escherichia coli* O111 B4 lipopolysaccharide given intracisternally induces blood–brain barrier opening during experimental neonatal meningitis in piglets. *Pediatr Res* 1993; **34**: 182–6.

59. Huang S, Stins MF, Kim KS. Bacterial penetration across the blood–brain barrier during the development of neonatal meningitis. *Microbes Infect* 2000; **2**: 1237–44.

60. Chang Chien HY, Chiu NC, Li WC, *et al.* Characteristics of neonatal

bacterial meningitis in a teaching hospital in Taiwan from 1984–1997. *J Microbiol Immunol Infect* 2000; **33**: 100–4.

61. Smith PB, Cotton CM, Garges HP, *et al.* A comparison of neonatal Gram-negative rod and Gram-positive cocci meningitis. *J Perinatol* 2006; **26**: 111–14.

62. Garges HP, Moody MA, Cotten CM, *et al.* Neonatal meningitis: what is the correlation among cerebrospinal fluid cultures, blood cultures and cerebrospinal fluid parameters? *Pediatrics* 2006; **117**: 1094–100.

63. Sarman G, Moise AA, Edwards MS. Meningeal inflammation in neonatal Gram-negative bacteremia. *Pediatr Infect Dis J* 1995; **14**: 701–4.

64. Porter FL, Miller JP, Cole FS, *et al.* A controlled clinical trial of local anesthesia for lumbar puncture in newborns. *Pediatrics* 1991; **88**: 663–9.

65. Halcrow SJ, Crawford PJ, Craft AW. Epidermoid spinal cord tumour after lumbar puncture. *Arch Dis Child* 1985; **60**: 978–9.

66. McCracken GH, Mize SG. A controlled study of intrathecal antibiotic therapy in gram negative enteric meningitis of infancy: report of the Neonatal Meningitis Co-operative Study Group. *J Pediatr* 1976; **89**: 66–72.

67. Philip AGS, Baker CJ. Cerebrospinal fluid C-reactive protein in neonatal meningitis. *J Pediatr* 1983; **102**: 715–17.

68. Philip AGS. Response of C-reactive protein in neonatal group B streptococcal infection. *Pediatr Infect Dis J* 1985; **4**: 145–8.

69. Sabel KG, Hanson LA. The clinical usefulness of C-reactive protein (CRP) determinations in bacterial meningitis and septicemia in infancy. *Acta Paediatr Scand* 1974; **63**: 381–8.

70. Sabel KG, Wadsworth C. C-reactive protein (CRP) in early diagnosis of neonatal septicemia. *Acta Paediatr Scand* 1979; **68**: 825–31.

71. Pourcyrous M, Bada HS, Korones SB, *et al.* Significance of serial C-reactive protein responses in neonatal infection and other disorders. *Pediatrics* 1993; **92**: 431–5.

72. Andersen J, Christensen R, Hartel J. Clinical features and epidemiology of septicemia and meningitis in neonates due to *Streptococcus agalactiae* in Copenhagen County, Denmark: a 10 year survey from 1992 to 2001. *Acta Paediatr* 2004; **93**: 1334–9.

73. Putto A, Ruuskanen O, Meurman O, *et al.* C-reactive protein in the evaluation of febrile illness. *Arch Dis Child* 1986; **61**: 24–9.

74. Raju VSN, Rao MN, Rao VSRM. Cranial sonography in pyogenic meningitis in neonates and infants. *J Trop Pediatr* 1995; **41**: 68–73.

75. Hill A, Shackelford GD, Volpe JJ. Ventriculitis with neonatal bacterial meningitis: identification by real-time ultrasound. *J Pediatr* 1981; **99**: 133–6.

76. Trivedi R, Malik GK, Gupta RK, *et al.* Increased anisotropy in neonatal meningitis: an indicator of meningeal inflammation. *Neuroradiology* 2007; **49**: 767–75.

77. Vogel LC, Boyer KM, Gadzala CA, *et al.* Prevalence of type-specific group B streptococcal antibody in pregnant women. *J Pediatr* 1980; **96**: 1047–51.

78. Sidiropoulos D, Hermann U, Morell A, *et al.* Transplacental passage of intravenous immunoglobulin in the last trimester of pregnancy. *J Pediatr* 1986; **109**: 505–8.

79. Edwards MS, Hall MA, Rench MA, *et al.* Patterns of immune response among survivors of group B streptococcal meningitis. *J Infect Dis* 1990; **161**: 65–70.

80. Baker CJ, Rench MA, Edwards MS, *et al.* Immunization of pregnant women with a polysaccharide vaccine of group B *Streptococcus. N Engl J Med* 1988; **319**: 1180–5.

81. Sennhauser FH, Balloch A, MacDonald RA, *et al.* Materno-fetal transfer of IgG anti-*Escherichia coli* antibodies with enhanced avidity and opsonic activity in very premature neonates. *Pediatr Res* 1990; **27**: 365–71.

82. Ment LR, Ehrenkranz RA, Duncan CC. Bacterial meningitis as an etiology of perinatal cerebral infarction. *Pediatr Neurol* 1986; **2**: 276–9.

83. Cohen C, Rice EN, Thomas DE, *et al.* Diabetes insipidus as a hallmark neuroendocrine complication of neonatal meningitis. *Curr Opin Pediatr* 1998; **10**: 449–52.

84. McCracken GH, Mize SG, Threlkeld N. Intraventricular gentamicin therapy in gram-negative bacillary meningitis of infancy: report of the Second Neonatal Meningitis Co-operative Study Group. *Lancet* 1980; **i**: 787–91.

85. Renier D, Flandin C, Hirsch E, *et al.* Brain abscesses in neonates: a study of 30 cases. *J Neurosurg* 1988; **69**: 877–82.

86. Burdette JH, Santos C. *Enterobacter sakazakii* brain abscess in the neonate: the importance of neuroradiologic imaging. *Pediatr Radiol* 2000; **30**: 33–4.

87. Isaacs D. Unnatural selection: reducing antibiotic resistance in neonatal units. *Arch Dis Child Fetal Neonatal Ed* 2006; **91**: F72–4.

88. Saez-Llorens X, McCracken GH. Antimicrobial and anti-inflammatory treatment of bacterial meningitis. *Infect Dis Clin North Am* 1999; **13**: 619–36.

89. Heath PT, Nik Yussoff NK, Baker CJ. Neonatal meningitis. *Arch Dis Child Fetal Neonatal Ed* 2003; **88**: F137–8.

90. Tessin I, Trollfors B, Thiringer K, *et al.* Ampicillin–aminoglycoside combination as initial treatment for neonatal septicaemia or meningitis: a retrospective evaluation of 12 years experience. *Acta Paediatr Scand* 1991; **80**: 911–16.

91. Adelman RD, Wirth F, Rubio T. A controlled study of the nephrotoxicity of mezlocillin and gentamicin plus ampicillin in the neonate. *J Pediatr* 1987; **111**: 888–93.

92. Tullus K, Olsson-Liljequist B, Lundstrom G, *et al.* Antibiotic susceptibility of 629 bacterial blood and CSF isolates from Swedish infants and the therapeutic implications. *Acta Paediatr Scand* 1991; **80**: 205–12.

93. Quinn JP, Rodvold KA. Antibiotic policies in neonatal intensive-care units. *Lancet* 2000; **355**: 946–7.

94. Lebel MH, Hoy MJ, McCracken GH. Comparative efficacy of ceftriaxone and cefuroxime for treatment of bacterial meningitis. *J Pediatr* 1989; **114**: 1049–54.

95. Black SB, Levine P, Shinefield HR. The necessity for monitoring chloramphenicol levels when treating neonatal meningitis. *J Pediatr* 1978; **92**: 235–6.

96. Ahmed A. A critical evaluation of vancomycin for treatment of bacterial meningitis. *Pediatr Infect Dis J* 1997; **16**: 895–3.

97. Haimi-Cohen Y, Amir J, Weinstock A, *et al.* The use of imipenem–cilastatin in neonatal meningitis caused by *Citrobacter diversus. Acta Paediatr Int J Paediatr* 1993; **82**: 530–2.

98. Leggiadro RJ. Favorable outcome possible in *Citrobacter* brain abscess. *Pediatr Infect Dis J* 1996; **15**: 557.

99. Radetsky M. Duration of treatment in bacterial meningitis: a historical inquiry. *Pediatr Infect Dis J* 1990; **9**: 2–9.

100. Peltola H, Luhtala K, Valmari P. C-reactive protein as a detector of organic complications during recovery from childhood purulent meningitis. *J Pediatr* 1984; **104**: 869–72.

101. Astruc J, Taillebois L, Rodière F, *et al.* Raccourcissement du traitement antibiotiques des méningites bactériennes de l'enfant: interêt de la surveillance de la C-réactive protéine. *Arch Franc Pédiatr* 1990; **47**: 637–40.

102. Prober CG. The role of steroids in the management of children with bacterial meningitis. *Pediatrics* 1995; **95**: 29–31.

103. Daoud AS, Batieha A, Al-Sheyyab M, *et al.* Lack of effectiveness of dexamethasone in neonatal bacterial meningitis. *Eur J Pediatr* 1999; **158**: 230–3.

104. McCracken GH, Sarff LD, Glode MP, *et al.* Relation between *Escherichia coli* K1 capsular polysaccharide antigen and clinical outcome in neonatal meningitis. *Lancet* 1974; **ii**: 246–50.

105. Bennet R, Bergdahl S, Eriksson M, *et al.* The outcome of neonatal septicemia during fifteen years. *Acta Paediatr Scand* 1989; **78**: 40–3.

106. Moffett KS, Berkowitz FE. Quadriplegia complicating *Escherichia coli* meningitis in a newborn infant: case report and review of 22 cases of spinal cord dysfunction in patients with acute bacterial meningitis. *Clin Infect Dis* 1997; **25**: 211–14.

107. Klinger G, Chin CN, Otsobu H, *et al.* Prognostic value of EEG in neonatal bacterial meningitis. *Pediatr Neurol* 2001; **24**: 28–31.

108. Siegel JD, McCracken GH, Threlkeld N, *et al.* Single-dose penicillin prophylaxis of neonatal group

B streptococcal disease: conclusion of a 41 month controlled trial. *Lancet* 1982; **i**: 1426–30.

109. Pyati SP, Pildes RS, Jacobs NM, *et al.* Penicillin in infants weighing two kilograms or less with early-onset group B streptococcal disease. *N Engl J Med* 1983; **308**: 1383–9.

110. Baker CJ, Melish ME, Hall RT, *et al.* Intravenous immune globulin for the prevention of nosocomial infection in low-birth-weight neonates. *N Engl J Med* 1992; **327**: 213–19.

111. Fanaroff AA, Korones SB, Wright LL, *et al.* A controlled trial of intravenous immune globulin to reduce nosocomial infections in very-low-birth-weight infants. National Institute of Child Health and Human Development Neonatal Research Network. *N Engl J Med* 1994; **330**: 1107–13.

112. Weisman LE, Stoll BJ, Kueser TJ, *et al.* Intravenous immune globulin prophylaxis of late-onset sepsis in premature neonates. *J Pediatr* 1994; **125**: 922–30.

113. Weisman LE, Cruess DF, Fischer GW. Opsonic activity of commercially available standard intravenous immunoglobulin preparations. *Pediatr Infect Dis J* 1994; **13**: 1122–5.

114. Boyer KM, Gotoff SP. Prevention of early-onset neonatal group B streptococcal disease with selective intrapartum chemoprophylaxis. *N Engl J Med* 1986; **314**: 1665–9.

115. Ascher DP, Becker JA, Yoder BA, *et al.* Failure of intrapartum antibiotics to prevent culture-proved neonatal group B streptococcal sepsis. *J Perinatol* 1992; **13**: 212–16.

116. Centers for Disease Control and Prevention. Prevention of perinatal group B streptococcal disease: a public health perspective. *MMWR Recomm Rep* 1996; **45**: 1–24.

117. Schrag SJ, Zywicki S, Farley MM, *et al.* Group B streptococcal disease in the era of intrapartum antibiotic prophylaxis. *N Engl J Med* 2000; **342**: 15–20.

118. Kalliola S, Vuopio-Varkilla J, Takala AK, *et al.* Neonatal group B streptococcal disease in Finland: a ten-year nationwide study. *Pediatr Infect Dis J* 1999; **18**: 806–10.

119. Puopolo KM, Madoff LC, Eichenwald EC. Early-onset group B streptococcal disease in the era of maternal screening. *Pediatrics* 2005; **115**: 1240–6.

120. Philip AGS, Mills PC. Use of C-reactive protein in minimizing antibiotic exposure: experience with infants initially admitted to a well-baby nursery. *Pediatrics* 2000; **106**: e4.

121. Paoletti LC, Madoff LC. Vaccines to prevent neonatal GBS infection. *Semin Neonatol* 2002; **7**: 315–23.

122. Baker CJ, Paoletti LC, Rench MA, *et al.* Immune response of healthy women to two different group B streptococcal type V capsular polysaccharide–protein conjugate vaccines. *J Infect Dis* 2004; **189**: 1103–12.

123. Bonadio WA, Stanco L, Bruce R, *et al.* Reference values of normal cerebrospinal fluid composition in infants ages 0 to 8 weeks. *Pediatr Infect Dis J* 1992; **11**: 589–91.

124. Ahmed A, Hickey SM, Ehrett S, *et al.* Cerebrospinal fluid values in the term neonate. *Pediatr Infect Dis J* 1996; **15**: 298–303.

Neurological sequelae of congenital perinatal infection

Rima Hanna-Wakim, Andrea Enright, and Kathleen Gutierrez

Introduction

Maternal infections, contracted during pregnancy, may be without fetal consequence or they may have serious adverse effects on the fetus. These adverse effects may include fetal death, stillbirth, intrauterine growth restriction, or congenital infection. Congenitally infected neonates may be symptomatic or asymptomatic at birth. Those who are symptomatic at birth generally have significant long-term sequelae. Those who are asymptomatic at birth may never manifest evidence of damage or they may develop clinically evident sequelae later in life. The overwhelming morbidity attributable to congenital infections is borne by this latter group.

The following chapter will discuss the neurologic consequences of congenital infections. The specific infectious agents that will be discussed are often referred to as the TORCH agents: T represents the parasite *Toxoplasma gondii*; O represents other agents such as varicella-zoster virus (VZV), human immunodeficiency virus (HIV), and *Treponema pallidum* (syphilis); R represents rubella virus; C represents cytomegalovirus (CMV); and H represents herpes simplex virus (HSV). With the exception of HSV, the major clinical impact of these agents results from exposure in utero. Morbidity and mortality attributable to neonatal HSV infection usually result from infection contracted at delivery.

Perinatal HIV infection is discussed in Chapter 33.

Toxoplasmosis

The etiologic agent of toxoplasmosis, *Toxoplasma gondii*, was first demonstrated in the brain of a newborn infant with encephalomyelitis in 1939 [1]. The incidence of congenital toxoplasmosis in the USA is estimated to range from 1/1000 to 1/10 000 live births [2–6]. *Toxoplasma* infection in pregnancy is usually asymptomatic, but occasionally women develop non-specific symptoms and signs of malaise, fever, myalgias, and lymphadenopathy [6]. Among immunocompetent women, transmission to the fetus is limited almost solely to those who contract primary infection during gestation. There are some case reports describing congenital toxoplasmosis in infants born to immunocompetent women who had

toxoplasma infection 2–3 months prior to conception [7–12]. Most cases of vertical transmission resulting from reactivation of previous maternal infection have occurred in women with immunodeficiency from acquired immune deficiency syndrome (AIDS), neoplasm, or autoimmune disease [3,4].

The risk of fetal infection increases as pregnancy progresses [3]. Increasing placental blood flow with advancing gestation may explain the increased transplacental transmission [4]. The transmission rate may be as low as 5% if maternal infection occurs before 16 weeks' gestation and as high as 75–80% if maternal infection occurs near term [3]. Fortunately, the severity of neonatal disease decreases with advancing gestational age [3,4]. Thus, although transmission of toxoplasmosis to the fetus is greatest late in pregnancy, manifestations resulting from infection are uncommon.

Several studies suggest that the incidence and severity of neonatal infection may be reduced if mothers who acquire toxoplasmosis during pregnancy receive antiparasitic therapy [13]. In one study of 1270 women with proven toxoplasmosis during pregnancy, fetal transmission was reduced to 7%. Most (81%) of the infected newborns had subclinical disease if mothers were treated with spiramycin or pyrimethamine/-sulfadiazine/folinic acid during pregnancy. Thus treatment appeared to decrease both the incidence and the severity of congenital toxoplasmosis. Although a second study failed to demonstrate a decrease in transplacental transmission of *T. gondii* by prenatal treatment, it did confirm that the severity of neonatal illness was significantly decreased by prenatal treatment [14]. Recently, the SYROCOT (Systematic Review on Congenital Toxoplasmosis) study group published a meta-analysis using individual patients' data from 26 cohorts. They found weak evidence that treatment started within 3 weeks of maternal seroconversion reduced maternal–child transmission compared to treatment started after more than 8 weeks. Also, they did not find any evidence that prenatal treatment significantly reduced the risk of clinical manifestations before 1 year of age [15]. There is still a need for large randomized controlled clinical trials to evaluate the efficacy of prenatal treatment.

The clinical spectrum of congenital toxoplasmosis is broad [3,4]. Although the majority of infants infected in utero with *T. gondii* are asymptomatic at birth, approximately 90% of infected infants will manifest sequelae at a later age, particularly ophthalmologic and intellectual impairment [3–5, 13,14,16].

Fetal and Neonatal Brain Injury, 4th edition, ed. David K. Stevenson, William E. Benitz, Philip Sunshine, Susan R. Hintz, and Maurice L. Druzin. Published by Cambridge University Press. © Cambridge University Press 2009.

Outcome in infants asymptomatic at birth

Congenital toxoplasmosis is not as prevalent as congenital CMV, but it is potentially more dangerous for the individual. Although about 85% of infants with congenital toxoplasmosis appear normal at birth, subclinical infection with *T. gondii* is more frequently associated with impaired intellectual performance and chorioretinitis than subclinical infection with CMV [2–4,16–18]. Nearly all children with subclinical congenital toxoplasma infection will develop adverse sequelae later in life [3]. An estimated 85% of untreated infants with congenital toxoplasmosis will suffer at least one episode of chorioretinitis, developmental delay will be evident in 20–75%, and hearing loss will occur in 10–30% [2–4,16–18]. These sequelae of congenital infection may not become clinically apparent until 6–18 years of age [3,16].

Outcome in infants symptomatic at birth

Only about 15% of neonates congenitally infected with *T. gondii* are symptomatic at birth [3]. Their infection is rarely fulminant but it is often severe. Symptoms and signs of generalized infection are prominent, and signs of central nervous system involvement are invariably present [3]. The "classic triad" in these symptomatic neonates is hydrocephalus, chorioretinitis, and diffuse intracranial calcifications. The most frequent extraneural signs associated with symptomatic congenital toxoplasmosis include hepatosplenomegaly, fever, anemia, and jaundice [3]. The mortality rate of symptomatic infants is 10–15%. Approximately 85% of untreated survivors develop mental retardation, 75% develop convulsions, spasticity, and palsies, and 50% develop severe visual impairment [2]. Deafness, a prominent sequela of congenital viral infections (e.g., CMV and rubella), occurs less frequently after congenital toxoplasmosis. The approximate incidence of hearing loss is 0–30% [2,4,19–21]. Microcephaly, also commonly seen in other congenital infections, is less common in congenital toxoplasmosis, the highest reported incidence being less than 25% [20,21]. When microcephaly does occur it is a predictor of poor outcome. Other factors associated with poor prognosis in congenital toxoplasmosis include neonatal hypothermia, apnea, bradycardia, prolonged hypoxemia, cerebrospinal fluid (CSF) protein > 1 g/dL, delayed treatment, and brain atrophy on computed tomography (CT) scan which persists for months after ventriculoperitoneal shunt placement [3,20,21].

Good outcomes have occurred in children with significant central nervous system (CNS) involvement at birth treated with antiparasitic drugs for 1 year. The US National Collaborative Chicago-based, Congenital Toxoplasmosis Treatment Trial Study (NCCTS) is a prospective longitudinal study evaluating long-term outcomes of infants with congenital toxoplasmosis treated for 1 year with pyrimethamine, sulfadiazine, and leucovorin [20,21]. The group recently published the results of their study conducted between 1981 and 2004 [21]. Their study group included 120 infants who were routinely evaluated at diagnosis (near the time of birth), and at

frequent intervals therafter (at 1, 3.5, 5, 7.5, 10, 15, and 20 years). Treatment of infants who had moderate to severe neurologic disease at birth resulted in normal neurologic and/or cognitive outcomes in more than 72% of the patients. None of the patients had sensorineural hearing loss. Ninety percent of infants without substantial neurologic disease and 64% of those with moderate to severe disease at birth did not develop new eye lesions. Almost all of the outcomes in the NCCTS were better and more favorable than outcomes reported for children who were untreated or treated only for 1 month in earlier decades [21].

Disseminated calcifications at birth do not necessarily reflect poor prognosis; following treatment, normal development can occur despite these findings [3]. Intracranial calcifications may diminish or completely resolve with 1 year of therapy. In one study, intracranial calcifications were demonstrated in 40 of 56 newborns with congenital toxoplasmosis [22]. Following 1 year of therapy with pyrimethamine, sulfadiazine, and leucovorin, 75% had decreased or undetectable calcifications.

Screening and prenatal diagnosis

Since the majority of infants with subclinical congenital toxoplasmosis ultimately develop sequelae, identification and treatment of all infected newborns should decrease long-term morbidity. Massachusetts and New Hampshire have screened newborns for congenital toxoplasmosis since 1986 and 1988, respectively. All 50 infected neonates identified by screening had normal newborn exams [5]. However, on the basis of detailed perinatal evaluations conducted shortly after serologic diagnosis, 19% had ocular disease (4% active chorioretinitis, 15% uninflamed retinal scars), 20% had intracranial calcifications found on CT, 25% had increased protein in CSF, and 2% had ventriculomegaly. All infants were treated for 1 year with pyrimethamine, sulfadiazine, and folinic acid. Only one of 46 infants had persistent neurologic deficits. None of nine infants with macular lesions at birth had progressive ocular disease. However, 10% developed new ocular lesions.

The recent NCCTS study demonstrated that treatment during the first year of life with pyrimethamine and sulfadiazine results in better outcomes in general compared to no treatment or short-term treatment [21]. Thus, treatment for 1 year with pyrimethamine, sulfadiazine, and folinic acid seems to benefit both symptomatic and asymptomatic neonates with congenital toxoplasmosis. Currently, 1 year of therapy is recommended.

In order to maximize the benefits of prenatal and postnatal therapy, infected neonates must be identified. In France, where the toxoplasmosis seronegative rate among women of child-bearing age is low, monthly serologic screening is performed for all seronegative pregnant women [3]. If seroconversion is documented, prompt therapy is given to the mother during pregnancy and to the neonate from birth. In the USA there has been much debate over systematic universal screening for toxoplasmosis in pregnant women [3]. The seronegative prevalence in the USA is much higher than in

Europe; thus, more US women would need routine screening. In addition, the sensitivity, specificity, positive and negative predictive values vary with each serologic test and are less reliable if run outside of reference laboratories [3,23].

An alternative to screening pregnant women is to screen neonates at birth for serologic evidence of congenital infection. Due to limitations in the immunoglobulin (IgM) assays, newborn screens employing these assays only diagnose 70–80% of congenital infections [3,23]. The 20–30% false-negative rate of neonatal screens may be unacceptably high. In a European study of various prenatal and postnatal screening tests, the sensitivity of IgM testing of neonatal blood was 43%; IgA testing of neonatal blood was 66% sensitive [23]. Sensitivity increased to 70% if results of IgM and IgA testing on neonatal blood were combined. Moreover, maternal prenatal treatment with antiparasitic drugs significantly decreased the incidence of positive serologic diagnosis. The 85% positive rate for specific IgM in neonatal blood dropped to 25% in those neonates whose mothers were treated prenatally. The lack of accuracy of neonatal IgM and IgA tests to diagnose congenital toxoplasmosis was also demonstrated in other studies [24]. Fetal infection may be detected through amniocentesis or cordocentesis [3,23,25]. Polymerase chain reaction (PCR) on amniotic fluid is superior to cordocentesis with fetal blood serologic evaluation. PCR of amniotic fluid has a sensitivity of 80–90% and a specificity of 96–100% [3,23,25].

Recommendations

Infants with congenital *T. gondii* infection must be recognized as being at high risk for the development of ophthalmologic and intellectual impairment. Serial ophthalmologic and intellectual assessments must be performed until the child is at least 18 years of age because onset of sequelae can be delayed.

Normal developmental, ophthalmologic, and neurologic outcomes have been observed in up to 70% of treated infants, despite the presence of systemic disease, hydrocephalus, microcephaly, multiple intracranial calcifications, and extensive macular involvement evident at birth [3,4,20,21]. Since delays in diagnosis and therapy are associated with worse outcomes, prompt diagnosis and treatment are important [3,4,20,21].

Prevention is possible [3,4,23]. Primary prevention to decrease infection of susceptible pregnant women should focus on hygiene: avoiding consumption of raw meat, avoiding potentially contaminated material (cat feces, litter boxes, soil when gardening), and washing fruits and vegetables before consumption. Secondary prevention involves identifying seroconversion in pregnant women and instituting prenatal therapy to reduce transmission and decrease the severity of infection in the fetus. Tertiary prevention includes neonatal evaluation, antiparasitic treatment, and long-term follow-up of congenitally infected infants. Evaluations should include general physical, neurologic, audiologic, and developmental exams, head CT, serologic tests, complete blood counts, liver function tests, cerebrospinal evaluation, and close monitoring for drug toxicity while on therapy.

Cytomegalovirus

CMV is the most common cause of congenital infection; the incidence ranges from 0.2% to 2.2% of all live births (average, 1%) [26]. Congenital CMV infection may result from maternal primary infection, reactivation of a prior latent infection, or, rarely, from reinfection with a new CMV strain. Since most congenital CMV infections result from maternal reactivated infections, it is fortunate that maternal immunity attenuates the severity of neonatal illness. More than 90% of neonates with congenital CMV infection are asymptomatic at birth [26]. Approximately 10–15% of these asymptomatic infants develop late-onset sequelae, including sensorineural hearing loss, microcephaly, motor defects, chorioretinitis, and learning and behavioral abnormalities [26–39]. In contrast, most congenitally infected neonates who are symptomatic at birth manifest severe developmental deficits and mental retardation [29,40–44]. With a few rare exceptions, most cases of symptomatic congenital CMV infection result from a primary maternal infection [26,27]. Primary infections early in pregnancy (before the 27th week of gestation) are more likely to be associated with a poor outcome than those occurring later in gestation [26,27,33].

Outcome in infants asymptomatic at birth

Most neonates with congenital CMV infections are asymptomatic at birth. These infants are likely to be detected only if routine viral cultures of newborns are performed within the first few weeks of life. Several prospective studies assessing the possible long-term effects of these "silent" congenital CMV infections have been conducted [28,30,31,34–36,38,39,45–47]. The most common sequelae of asymptomatic congenital CMV infection are sensorineural hearing loss that may not be present or detected at birth, and possible intellectual impairment. The incidence of sensorineural hearing loss in older children with asymptomatic congenital CMV ranges from 7% to 15% [38,45,48,49]. Chorioretinitis may develop later in life in children with asymptomatic congenital CMV infection [26].

Congenital CMV infection is estimated to be responsible for one-third of all cases of sensorineural hearing loss in children [38]. A large prospective study of 307 asymptomatic congenitally infected children and 277 controls found a 7% incidence of sensorineural hearing loss in infected children and no hearing loss in the matched controls [38]. Of those children with sensorineural hearing loss, 50% had bilateral disease; 23% suffered from profound bilateral sensorineural hearing loss. In this study none of the children with sensorineural hearing loss had other risk factors for hearing impairment. Since CMV hearing impairment often presents after the newborn period, is progressive, and can fluctuate, researchers estimate that two-thirds of sensorineural hearing loss from asymptomatic congenital CMV infection may be missed by universal newborn hearing screens [38,49]. These researchers argue that in order to identify all those at risk for hearing impairment in childhood, universal newborn hearing screening must be accompanied by universal newborn CMV screening. A recent study demonstrated an association between

CMV virus burden and hearing loss. Children with asymptomatic congenital CMV infection who developed hearing loss had increased amounts of CMV DNA detected in urine and blood compared to children who did not develop hearing loss [50].

The impact of hearing impairment on intellectual development has confounded the evaluation of intellectual function in congenitally infected infants. Several studies have attempted to evaluate the possible intellectual consequences of asymptomatic congenital CMV infection. Interpretation of the results of some of the studies is hampered by relatively short periods of follow-up, lack of appropriately matched controls, and failure to control for hearing loss. One well-designed study evaluated the intellectual development of 18 prospectively followed school-aged children with asymptomatic congenital CMV infection and normal hearing [39]. The results of testing these children were compared with the results from 18 controls matched for age, sex, race, school grade, and socioeconomic status. All children were evaluated between 6.5 and 12.5 years of age using the Wechsler Intelligence Scale for Children – Revised, the Kaufman Assessment Battery for Children, and the Wide Range Achievement Test. No differences between the infected and uninfected children on intelligence scores or subscales, achievement scores, or incidence of learning disabilities were observed. These researchers concluded that children with asymptomatic CMV infection and normal hearing have normal intellectual development. However, the small sample size of this study prohibits a definite conclusion regarding the independent effects of congenital CMV infection on intellectual impairment.

Expression of adverse consequences of asymptomatic CMV infections appears to be influenced by socioeconomic conditions. One study predicted increased school failure rate in infected children of lower socioeconomic class but not in those infected children from middle and higher socioeconomic classes [36]. Future studies must attempt to control for other relevant factors contributing to intellectual development.

Outcome in infants symptomatic at birth

Most neonates who are symptomatic at birth as a result of congenital CMV have been infected as a result of a primary maternal gestational infection [26,51]. The clinical abnormalities found most frequently in neonates with symptomatic congenital CMV are listed in Table 32.1 [26]. Cerebral abnormalities reported in association with congenital CMV infection include microcephaly, microgyria, periventricular calcifications, migrational abnormalities, disturbed myelination, spongiosus of the brain, encephalomalacia, calcification of the cerebral arteries, parietal lobe cysts, cerebral cortical immaturity, cerebellar hypoplasia, paraventricular cysts, intraventricular strands, and dolichocephaly [26,28,29,41–44,52,53]. CMV has been isolated from CSF by PCR in six of ten patients with symptomatic congenital infection [54]. Follow-up was available for five of those patients with a positive CSF CMV PCR: all five had developmental delay. Postmortem examination of brains from infants who have died with severe congenital CMV infection have noted decreased brain weight, subependymal cysts, deformed cerebellum, irregular gyri, thickened leptomeninges,

Table 32.1. Clinical manifestations of symptomatic congenital cytomegalovirus infection

Petechiae	++++
Thrombocytopenia	++++
Hepatosplenomegaly	+++
Jaundice with direct hyperbilirubinemia	+++
Microcephaly	+++
Small for gestational age	++
Prematurity	++
Inguinal hernia	++
Chorioretinitis	+

Notes:
++++ 75–100% incidence; +++ 50–75%; ++ 25–50%; + 0–25%.
Source: Adapted from [28,29,40–43].

cortical and cerebellar neuronal migration abnormalities, and paraventricular bands of necrosis and calcification [26,43]. CSF β_2-microglobulin was elevated in newborns with symptomatic congenital CMV infection, and it correlated with the neuroimaging abnormalities [55].

Fortunately, fewer than 10% of neonates congenitally infected with CMV manifest overt signs of disease at birth. The long-term prognosis of symptomatic infants is usually poor [40,42–49,51–54,56]. CNS sequelae include microcephaly, mental retardation and developmental delays, learning and behavioral disorders, seizures, neuromuscular disorders including facial asymmetry, spasticity, quadriparesis, diplegia, hemiatrophy, and hemiparesis [26,54,57]. Defects in hearing and vision are also common after symptomatic congenital CMV infection.

One of the earlier prospective studies of symptomatic neonates was published in 1980 [42]. In that study, 34 patients who had clinically evident disease at birth were followed for a mean duration of 4 years. Twenty-nine percent of the patients died and more than 90% of the survivors developed CNS or auditory handicaps; 70% had microcephaly, 61% mental retardation, 35% neuromuscular disorders, 30% hearing loss, and 22% chorioretinitis or optic atrophy. Although the extent of disease apparent at birth was not entirely predictive of CNS sequelae, all children with IQs < 50 or neuromuscular disorders were clearly abnormal by 1 year of age. Other studies have documented similarly poor outcomes. In a long-term follow-up of 17 children with symptomatic congenital CMV followed for a mean of 5.5 years, 75% met criteria for mental retardation [40]. In this study, three children with normal hearing and IQ scores still exhibited deficits in expressive language. It is possible that these young children would manifest more severe deficits at later ages.

The Houston CMV longitudinal study followed 41 children with symptomatic congenital CMV infection; the median age at follow-up was 5.7 years [57]. Microcephaly at birth (present in 19.5% of the study population) was the most specific predictor of mental retardation and major motor disability [57]. Although the estimated risk of permanent neurologic sequelae after a symptomatic congenital CMV infection is high, in a given case the development may be more favorable than expected [56].

Another long-term prospective follow-up study evaluated the predictors of hearing loss in children with symptomatic congenital CMV infection [58]. Hearing outcome was followed in 180 children, and 48% of the children had hearing loss on follow-up. Of these children, 70% had hearing loss at birth or in the neonatal period. The presence of disseminated disease at birth was predictive for the development of hearing loss. Microcephaly and other neurologic findings were not predictive of hearing loss [58].

Recommendations

Congenital CMV infection should be considered in any newborn with unexplained prematurity, growth restriction, hepatomegaly, splenomegaly, jaundice, microcephaly, chorioretinitis, or petechiae. This diagnosis can be confirmed by isolating the virus from a urine or salivary culture obtained during the first 3 weeks of life. CMV isolated after the first few weeks of life with a documented negative culture in the neonatal period represents perinatal CMV infection.

Neuroimaging by CT scan or magnetic resonance imaging (MRI) has been shown to be useful in identifying infants at risk for CNS sequelae of congenital CMV infection [44,53]. In a study of 56 infants with symptomatic congenital CMV, 70% had CT abnormalities [44]. Of those with CT abnormalities, 60% had IQ scores less than 70; half of the IQ scores were below 50. In contrast, none of the 17 symptomatic infants with normal CT scans had severe mental retardation. In this study, clinical and laboratory data were not able to predict the neurologic sequelae. Microcephaly, seizures, lethargy, and poor suck did not predict CT scan abnormality. Intracranial calcification was the most common abnormality found in 77% of abnormal scans. White-matter abnormalities were also identified, with MRI more sensitive than CT in a small number of patients [53].

The effectiveness of antiviral therapy for treatment of infants with congenital CMV infection continues to be studied. The Collaborative Antiviral Study Group (CASG) conducted a phase III randomized controlled study evaluating the effect of intravenous ganciclovir therapy on hearing in newborns with symptomatic congenital CMV infection involving the CNS [59]. Ganciclovir treatment, at a dose of 6 mg/kg intravenously every 12 hours for 6 weeks, prevented hearing deterioration at 6 months in the treated group compared to the placebo group. This study did not include infants without CNS involvement. Approximately 63% of the ganciclovir-treated infants developed significant neutropenia during therapy [59].

The CASG is evaluating valganciclovir, the oral bioavailable prodrug of ganciclovir. An initial phase I/II pharmacokinetic study of liquid valganciclovir versus intravenous ganciclovir has been completed and a phase III study of the drug has recently been initiated [60]. Information regarding clinical trials of antiviral therapy for treatment of congenital CMV infection is available at www.casg.uab.edu.

Until more data are available about the efficacy and safety of ganciclovir/valganciclovir, the decision to treat newborns with congenital CMV infection must be individualized. Discussion with the parents should include the uncertainty regarding the effects of treatment on prevention of hearing loss, the long duration of therapy, the need for intravenous access, and the side effects of ganciclovir.

It is important to identify all infants with congenital CMV infection as early as possible. Early identification will permit frequent audiometric and intellectual examinations over the first several years of the child's life. In order to maximize a child's full potential, defects, including those in hearing and language, should be corrected as soon as possible.

Rubella

Rubella is an RNA virus, classified as a togavirus, unrelated to any other human viral pathogen [61,62]. Before the introduction of childhood immunization for rubella in the late 1960s, rubella virus caused major epidemics once or twice every decade in the USA [62]. During rubella epidemics, many infected individuals were asymptomatic while others had classic infection with diffuse exanthem, low-grade fevers, lymphadenopathy, and arthritis/arthralgia [62]. As most children in the USA are now immunized during the second year of life, widespread epidemics of rubella have disappeared. However, outbreaks of rubella and congenital rubella syndrome have occurred in the USA in the late 1980s and early 1990s [63–65]. Most outbreaks have been attributed to a failure to vaccinate susceptible individuals in colleges, prisons, and religious communities [63–65]. In October 2004, the Centers for Disease Control and Prevention (CDC) convened an independent panel of internationally recognized authorities on public health, infectious disease, and immunization that concluded that rubella and congenital rubella syndrome are no longer endemic in the United States [66]. Congenital rubella syndrome was reported in infants born to mothers who immigrated to the United States from countries without rubella control programs [67]. Since 2001, only five infants with congenital rubella syndrome were reported [68].

In many developing countries, congenital rubella syndrome continues to be a problem, with an estimate of more than 100 000 new cases of congenital rubella syndrome annually [69,70].

The transmission of rubella to the fetus

Rubella produces viremia in the susceptible host during primary infection [62]. In pregnant women, this viremic phase often results in placental infection with or without subsequent infection of the fetus [62]. The risk of fetal infection depends on gestational age at the time of maternal infection [61,62,71,72]. The risk of fetal infection is highest in the first trimester, declines during the second trimester, and then increases again during the end of the third trimester [61,62,71,72]. Specifically, the risk of fetal infection is 80–90% during the first 12 weeks of gestation, drops to 25% by 23–26 weeks, and then increases to 60–100% near term [61,62,71,72].

Clinical manifestations of intrauterine rubella infection and the risk of neurologic sequelae

Isolation of virus from the oropharynx of infants with suspected intrauterine rubella is the most reliable method of proving congenital infection [61,62]. Infants with congenital rubella shed virus from this site for 6 months or longer after birth [61,62]. The virus can also be found in the stool, urine, and CSF [61,62]. Although efforts have been made to develop a rubella-specific IgM antibody assay for the diagnosis of congenital rubella infection, many infants with infection proven by culture do not have detectable rubella-specific IgM antibodies using optimal serologic methodology [61,62,73]. The lack of detectable antibodies in infants with congenital rubella syndrome may reflect infection at a time of fetal immune system immaturity in early gestation [73]. Infection before 20–22 weeks may not produce a detectable humoral response despite active viral replication and infection of fetal tissues [62]. A few studies have evaluated the use of reverse transcriptase PCR to detect rubella virus RNA in amniotic fluid, chorionic villus samples, and fetal blood, and this appears to offer a reliable method of diagnosis [74,75].

Fewer than 10% of infants with intrauterine rubella infection have obvious signs of congenital rubella infection at birth [61,62]. The likelihood of clinical manifestations of intrauterine rubella infection is inversely related to fetal age at the time of maternal infection [71,76]. The estimated risk of defects is 85% following maternal rubella infection at 8 weeks, 52% at 9–12 weeks, and 16% at 13–20 weeks' gestation [77]. Maternal infection after 20 weeks' gestation can cause fetal infection but these infants are asymptomatic in the newborn period and the risk of late-onset sequelae is low [62,71,76]. Infants infected with rubella virus at the earliest stages of development are more likely to have cardiac defects (patent ductus arteriosus, pulmonary artery stenosis) in addition to the hearing and ocular abnormalities that are characteristic of later in utero infection.

Neurologic manifestations of congenital rubella syndrome include meningoencephalitis, microcephaly, mental and motor retardation, behavioral difficulties, psychiatric disorders, sensorineural hearing loss, and, rarely, late-onset progressive rubella panencephalitis [61,62,71,72,76,78,79]. Meningoencephalitis occurs in 10–20% of infected neonates who are symptomatic at birth [62]. In these cases, CSF analysis reveals elevated protein concentrations with or without a pleocytosis [62]. Extensive meningoencephalitis is one cause of early postnatal death from congenital rubella.

The risk of microcephaly depends on the gestational age at infection. Microcephaly occurs in 60% of fetuses infected before 13 weeks' gestation. In contrast, less than 10% of infants infected after 20 weeks' gestation are microcephalic [71]. Infants with congenital rubella who are microcephalic can be expected to have additional neurologic impairment [79]. Acquired microcephaly has also been documented in congenital rubella syndrome. Chang et al. described five neonates with confirmed congenital rubella syndrome [80]. Despite having normal head size at birth, head ultrasonography revealed linear and punctuate hyperechogenicities and occasional subependymal cysts. These non-specific findings of CNS damage were markers for later neurologic sequelae: by 27 months of age, all five had documented microcephaly and profound global developmental delay [80]. In another study, white-matter hyperintensities were noted on MRI scans performed on 11 adults with a history of congenital rubella syndrome and schizophrenia-like symptoms [81]. These hyperintensities were not found in any of 19 controls with schizophrenia who had no evidence of congenital infection.

A few children with congenital rubella developed a syndrome of progressive rubella panencephalitis similar to subacute sclerosing panencephalitis caused by the measles virus [78,81]. These children manifest progressive neurologic deterioration after 10 years of age. Neurologic manifestations have included progressive mental retardation, motor incoordination, and cerebellar signs, including nystagmus, ataxia, and choreoathetoid movements. Elevated rubella-specific IgG was demonstrated in the CSF and rubella virus was recovered from brain biopsy in one case [78]. Autopsies revealed diffuse white-matter involvement, microglial nodules, panencephalitis, reactive gliosis, ventricular enlargement, and brain atrophy [78,82].

Neurologic sequelae of congenital rubella are often subtle and include hearing deficits, language delays, psychomotor retardation, and behavioral/psychiatric disturbances. The progressive nature of intrauterine rubella infection was demonstrated in a group of non-retarded children who were followed for 9–12 years [83]. With increasing age, an increase in the percentage of the population with hearing loss, motor incoordination, and behavioral disturbances was observed. At last follow-up, 86% of the children had hearing deficits, 52% had learning problems, 48% had behavioral problems, and 61% had poor balance and/or muscle weakness. Fifty-year follow-up of cohorts from congenital rubella epidemics in Australia and the USA have been reported [84,85]. In the Australian cohort of 40 individuals, long-term outcomes were considered to be "good" [84]. Although 100% had hearing deficits, most of which were profound, and 50% had visual deficits, over 50% were employed. In contrast, in the New York cohort one-third had normal lives, one-third were semi-independent, and one-third were institutionalized [85].

Behavioral and psychiatric disorders are often found at later ages in children with congenital rubella syndrome. Chess et al. described the psychiatric and behavioral consequences of congenital rubella among 243 preschoolers examined at 2.5–5 years of age; 205 children of this cohort were re-examined at 8–9 years of age [86]. Between 25% and 40% of the children were mentally retarded, 15–20% had diagnoses of reactive or other behavior disorders, and approximately 6% were autistic. In another psychiatric outcome study, the Diagnostic Interview Schedule for Children was administered to 70 young adults with a history of congenital rubella syndrome and 164 controls [87]. Those with congenital rubella syndrome were 5–16 times more likely than age-matched controls to have non-affective psychiatric disorders defined as delusions and/or hallucinations [87]. Conclusions from these studies are tentative, because the impact of multiple handicaps in hearing, visual, and other neurologic domains have not been clearly separated from the direct impact of viral infection on behavior and psychiatric well-being.

Recommendations

The evaluation of a pregnancy potentially complicated by rubella remains a difficult diagnostic problem. The interval required to isolate the virus limits the utility of tissue culture as a diagnostic method [61,62]. If the pregnant woman has not had a previous rubella titer, it is often impossible to determine whether seroconversion has occurred because rubella antibodies are present within a few days of onset of infection [61,62]. The detection of rubella-specific IgM antibodies can be helpful, but the method can yield false-positive results and the absence of an IgM response does not exclude recent rubella infection [61,62]. A high titer of rubella antibodies in a single serum sample does not establish a diagnosis of recent infection since many individuals maintain persistently high rubella titers [61,62]. PCR has been performed on amniotic fluid, chorionic villi samples, and fetal blood for detection of in utero rubella infection, and use of PCR as a diagnostic tool appears very promising [74,75,88].

If a pregnant woman is exposed to rubella and her immune status is not known, she should be tested for rubella antibodies immediately [61,62]. A positive rubella titer at the time of exposure eliminates any concern. If the titer is negative, it should be repeated at 2 and 6 weeks after exposure to be certain that subclinical infection has not occurred [61,62]. Transplacental transmission of the virus is possible if seroconversion is demonstrated, whether or not the pregnant woman has had symptoms [61,62].

The risk of congenital rubella can be eliminated by an effective vaccination program. The rubella vaccination program has reduced the annual number of cases of rubella by 99% since the prevaccine era [64,68,70,79,89,90]. However, localized rubella outbreaks continue to occur. Most outbreaks of congenital rubella syndrome can be attributed to multiple missed opportunities to vaccinate susceptible women of child-bearing age [63–65]. Immunization coverage rates of 80–90% are needed to prevent rubella transmission in a community [64]. Susceptible young women should be encouraged to receive rubella vaccine. While pregnancy is a contraindication to rubella immunization, inadvertent rubella vaccination during pregnancy has not been associated with congenital rubella syndrome [61,62,91,92]. Long-term medical, neurologic, psychiatric, ophthalmologic, audiologic, and developmental evaluations are required for infants with congenital rubella.

Congenital syphilis

In the USA, the late 1980s and early 1990s were marked by a resurgence in the number of congenital infections caused by *Treponema pallidum*, the etiologic agent of syphilis [93,94]. Factors believed to contribute to this increased frequency of

infection include patterns of substance abuse (especially crack cocaine), HIV infection, and changing patterns of sexual activity [95]. In addition, modification of the Centers for Disease Control and Prevention (CDC) case definition of congenital syphilis facilitated the identification and reporting of cases to the CDC [96,97]. Fortunately, the rate of congenital syphilis in the USA has declined steadily since 1992 [98–100].

The risk of syphilis transmission to the fetus varies with the stage of maternal illness [101–103]. In early, untreated primary maternal infection, transmission rates range from 70% to 100%. In early latent infection (infection of less than 1 year's duration) the risk of fetal infection is 40%. Once a mother has late latent infection, fetal transmission rates drop to 10%, due in part to low levels of spirochetemia and treponemal proliferation.

There are substantial problems in the diagnosis of congenital syphilis and the evaluation of neurosyphilis in infants [104–108]. *T. pallidum* cannot be cultured from clinical specimens except by inoculation into rabbits, a process that is time-consuming, costly, and impractical [101,104,109]. In addition, *T. pallidum* is often present in low numbers in clinical specimens. Thus, the value of histologic documentation of infection by dark-field microscopy or antigen detection is limited [101,104,109]. Thus, most cases of congenital syphilis are not established by definitive diagnosis, but rather by presumptive diagnosis based on various clinical and laboratory evaluations [97,101,103,108–110]. Unfortunately, there is no gold standard for diagnosis. Presumptive diagnosis relies on non-treponemal titers: rapid plasma reagin (RPR) card test or Venereal Disease Research Laboratory (VDRL) titers. However, transplacentally acquired maternal antibodies complicate the serologic evaluation of exposed infants. Moreover, an infected infant may have a titer four times higher than his/her mother, a lower titer than his/her mother, or a negative titer despite active infection [103].

Clinical diagnosis of congenital syphilis is also challenging, since approximately two-thirds of infants are asymptomatic at birth [101,103]. Sequelae from these asymptomatic infections frequently develop at later ages. When symptoms appear within the first 2 years of life, they are designated early congenital syphilis; those developing thereafter are designated late congenital syphilis [101,107]. Manifestations of syphilitic infections may include stillbirth, prematurity, intrauterine growth restriction, hepatosplenomegaly, generalized lymphadenopathy, rhinitis ("snuffles"), dermatologic abnormalities, renal disease, hyperbilirubinemia, and CNS abnormalities [101,102,111]. In order to prevent morbidity from congenital syphilis, it is important to identify and treat both asymptomatic and symptomatic newborns.

Early congenital syphilis

Older literature suggested that more than 60% of neonates with congenital syphilis had abnormal findings on CSF examinations [112]. However, this high rate of abnormality was based on considering CSF abnormal if it contained ≥ 5 white blood cells/mm^3 and had a protein content > 45 mg/dL [112]. These definitions of abnormal CSF may not be appropriate for newborn infants [101,113–115]. A study of 78 newborn infants born to mothers with serologic evidence of syphilis found only one neonate with a positive CSF VDRL titer [106]. None of the 78 infants had more than 32 white blood cells/mm^3 or a CSF protein greater than 170 mg/dL [106]. Another study evaluated the CSF of 19 infants born to mothers with untreated early syphilis using the rabbit infectivity test, PCR, and immunoblot IgM assays in addition to CSF cell count, protein, and VDRL titer [104]. Eighty-six percent of symptomatic infants with congenital syphilis in this study had evidence of CNS disease. In contrast, only one of 12 asymptomatic newborns had laboratory evidence of CNS disease. The authors concluded that CNS invasion by *T. pallidum* is common in symptomatic congenital syphilis and uncommon in asymptomatic disease. A recent study by Michelow *et al.* evaluated CNS involvement in 76 infants with untreated congenital syphilis using rabbit-infectivity testing of the CSF along with syphilis IgM immunoblotting and PCR on blood and CSF specimens [108]. Spirochetes were detected in the CSF in 17 out of the 76 infants. CNS infection was best predicted by IgM immunoblotting of serum or PCR assay of serum or blood [108].

Sequelae from neurosyphilis include hydrocephalus, cranial nerve palsies, gradual decline in intelligence quotients, mental retardation, seizures, strokes, deafness, blindness, general paresis, and behavioral/learning difficulties [101,102]. Neurologic manifestations of congenital syphilis that are evident during the first 2 years of life are infrequent [106]. When reported, the most common clinical types of CNS involvement with early congenital syphilis are acute leptomeningitis and chronic meningovascular syphilis [101]. Leptomeningitis usually becomes evident between 3 and 6 months of age. It is clinically indistinguishable from other bacterial causes of meningitis. The CSF typically contains 100–200 mononuclear cells/mm^3, has an increased protein concentration, and a positive serologic test for syphilis. This form of neurosyphilis responds to penicillin therapy [101,102].

Chronic meningovascular syphilis tends to follow a protracted and progressive course starting late in the first year of life. It usually results in communicating hydrocephalus and cranial nerve palsies [101]. Cerebral infarctions from syphilitic endarteritis may also result in a variety of cerebrovascular syndromes, with paresis and seizures being the most consistent features [101]. Unfortunately, these later forms of neurosyphilis often do not respond to penicillin treatment [101,102].

Neurologic involvement in late congenital syphilis is infrequent [106,116,117]. Interestingly, deafness, a common sequela of other congenital infections, occurs in only 3% of children with congenital syphilis [101].

Recommendations

Congenital syphilis is a devastating disease if not treated. Identification of infected mothers and neonates must be

Table 32.2. Criteria for evaluation of infants for congenital syphilis

Infants born to seropositive women who meet the following criteria should be thoroughly evaluated
Mother with untreated syphilis
Mother treated for syphilis during pregnancy with a non-penicillin regimen (e.g., erythromycin)
Mother treated for syphilis less than 1 month before delivery
Mother treated for syphilis during pregnancy with the appropriate penicillin regimen but non-treponemal antibody titers did not decrease sufficiently after therapy (fourfold decline) to indicate an adequate response to treatment
Mother did not have syphilis treatment well documented
Mother was treated appropriately before pregnancy but did not have adequate serologic follow-up to assure response to therapy and to rule out reinfection

Source: Adapted from [101,103,104,109].

optimized. Serologic screening for gestational infection should be conducted early in pregnancy, during the third trimester (especially for high-risk women), and at delivery [96,97, 101,109,118]. Even with adherence to these guidelines, some infants with congenital syphilis may be missed, probably because the maternal infection occurred immediately prior to delivery, providing insufficient time for an antibody response to develop, or the mothers received no treatment or inadequate treatment for syphilis [101,109,119]. Thus, in areas where the infection is prevalent, retesting of infants presenting during the first weeks of life with symptoms or signs compatible with congenital syphilis may be prudent [101,119]. Screening should be with a non-treponemal test: VDRL or RPR. RPR is preferred in pregnancy by some experts [101]. If the non-treponemal test is positive, one of the treponemal-specific tests should be performed to confirm maternal infection: either microhemagglutination *Treponema pallidum* (MHA-TP) or fluorescent treponemal antibody absorption (FTA-ABS) may be used. Maternal treatment history must be reviewed in detail if both non-treponemal and treponemal tests are positive. In addition, any mother with positive syphilis serology needs HIV testing, because 15% of adults with syphilis are co-infected with HIV [102].

The diagnosis of congenital syphilis should be considered in any neonate born to a mother with a reactive serologic test for syphilis. All infants should have a physical exam and non-treponemal antibody titer obtained [96,97,101,105,109,111,118,120]. For accurate comparison, the non-treponemal test used must be the same for the infant and mother. Testing of cord blood is inadequate for screening because it can be contaminated by maternal blood and can yield false-positive results [110]. Criteria for further evaluation of neonates are listed in Table 32.2. Evaluation for congenital syphilis should also be considered for stillbirths occurring after 20 weeks' gestation and in neonates with unexplained prematurity or low birthweight, bullous skin lesions, maculopapular rashes, rhinitis, skeletal lesions, jaundice, hepatosplenomegaly, or lymphadenopathy [96,97,101,105,109,111,118,120].

Complete diagnostic evaluation of infants includes physical exam, non-treponemal titers, long-bone x-rays, and CSF analysis [96,97,101,104,105,107,109,111,115,118,120]. X-rays are suggested because 6–20% of asymptomatic infants will have detectable abnormalities [101,102,111]. CSF evaluation is still recommended by most experts, despite the low sensitivity with older CSF tests and debate over normal ranges for neonates [96,97,101,108,109,111]. Finally, if possible, the placenta and umbilical cord should undergo histologic examination [97,110].

Symptomatic infants may require additional testing, including liver function tests, complete blood counts with platelets, chest x-rays, auditory brainstem response tests, and ophthalmology exams [97,101,109,110]. CSF analysis should include cell counts, concentrations of glucose and protein, and a VDRL titer. The CSF VDRL titer is highly specific for neurosyphilis, but has a sensitivity of only 22–69% [104,120]. PCR analysis of the CSF has 90% correlation with the rabbit-infectivity test [104]. PCR for *T. pallidum* DNA in the CSF is 75% sensitive and 96–100% specific [104]. Thus, if available, PCR should also be performed on CSF fluid.

Ten days of parenteral aqueous crystalline penicillin G or penicillin G procaine is recommended for the treatment of symptomatic congenital syphilis in infants ≤ 4 weeks of age. Aqueous crystalline penicillin G or penicillin G procaine are recommended because they provide adequate treatment for possible neurosyphilis; benzathine penicillin does not. This treatment regimen is considered prudent even if tests for neurosyphilis are negative, because these tests may be falsely negative. Treatment is also indicated for asymptomatic infants born to women with untreated syphilis, inadequate treatment, treatment with a non-penicillin regimen, and inadequate documentation of treatment. In addition, treatment should be given to asymptomatic infants born to women treated within 1 month of delivery even if an appropriate regimen was given [97,101,109,110].

Treatment of asymptomatic infants born to a mother who received appropriate treatment without adequate titer decline is controversial [97,101,103,106,107,109–112,118]. The controversy stems from the inability definitely to exclude neurosyphilis or congenital syphilis in at-risk infants. In addition, in late latent maternal infection, non-treponemal titers decline slowly and may remain stably positive at low titers (≤ 1 : 4) [101,103]. Thus, in some pregnant women, appropriate treatment may fail to produce a fourfold titer decline [101,103]. Debate continues on how to manage infants in this scenario. Some advocate close observation and follow-up if the complete evaluation is negative [101,109]. Others would treat these infants with a single dose of benzathine penicillin [101,103,109–111,121]. Consultation with local infectious disease experts is recommended.

To date, though serology may be less reliable in HIV-infected women, there is no indication to alter maternal treatment or neonatal evaluation and treatment when caring for HIV-infected pregnant women and their children [97,101,110]. Recommendations are changing constantly, and consultation with local infectious disease experts is recommended.

All infants with suspected or proven congenital syphilis, whether or not CNS involvement is confirmed, must undergo careful long-term evaluations of mental and motor function, hearing, and vision [97,101,109,110]. In addition, serologic tests should be monitored until they become non-reactive [97,101,105,109,110]. In the absence of fetal infection, the VDRL titer should be decreasing by 3–4 months of age. VDRL is undetectable in most infants by 6 months [97,101,105,109,110]. If the infant was congenitally infected, adequate treatment should result in a decreasing VDRL, with disappearance by 6 months of age [97,101,105,109,110]. Treponemal-specific antibodies (e.g., FTA-ABS) may be detectable up to 15 months of age in uninfected neonates due to persistence of transplacental antibodies [97,101,105,109,110]. If antibodies persist beyond these limits, the infant should be reassessed and treated. In 85% of infected individuals, treponemal antibodies persist for life; therefore, these tests should not be monitored during follow-up assessments of congenitally infected children [101,103,110]. If the CSF VDRL was originally positive, it should be repeated at 6 months of age. If it remains positive and CSF abnormalities persist by 2 years, retreatment is indicated [101,103,105,109,110].

Varicella-zoster virus

Primary infection with VZV causes varicella (chickenpox), and reactivation of latent VZV infection results in herpes zoster (shingles). Although pregnant women occasionally develop varicella, this virus is an unusual cause of intrauterine or perinatal infection because more than 90% of women of child-bearing age who live in temperate climates have had varicella in childhood [122]. The current rate of pregnancies complicated by varicella is estimated at 0.4–0.7/1000 pregnancies [122–125]. VZV may be transmitted across the placenta, resulting in congenital or neonatal varicella infection [122].

Congenital varicella syndrome was first described in 1947 [126]. Infants with congenital varicella syndrome have characteristic cicatricial cutaneous scars, limb atrophy, rudimentary digits, chorioretinitis, and microcephaly [123,126–132]. In 1987, Alkalay *et al.* proposed three diagnostic criteria for congenital varicella syndrome, which included a documented maternal varicella infection in pregnancy, congenital cutaneous lesions in a dermatomal distribution, and evidence of congenital infection by immunologic proof (VZV-specific IgM at delivery) or zoster in infancy accompanied by a rise in VZV antibody titers (Table 32.3) [132]. In their study, 77% of the 22 infants fulfilling the diagnostic criteria for congenital varicella syndrome had abnormalities that included hypoplasia of upper or lower extremities (80%), limb paresis (65%), hydrocephalus/cortical atrophy (35%), seizures (24%), Horner's syndrome (24%), mental retardation (18%), and auditory palsy (6%). The region of neurologic involvement correlated well with the anatomic distribution of dermatomal disease.

The series of Enders *et al.* of 1373 pregnant women with varicella during pregnancy is the largest experience to date [130]. Nine cases of congenital varicella and an additional 10 cases of zoster in infancy occurred in offspring of these women.

Table 32.3. Proposed diagnostic criteria for congenital varicella syndrome

(1) Documented maternal varicella infection in pregnancy
(2) Congenital cutaneous lesions in a dermatomal distribution
(3) Evidence of congenital infection by either:
(a) Immunologic proof of in utero varicella infection (VZV-specific IgM at delivery) or
(b) Zoster in infancy accompanied by a rise in VZV antibody titers

Notes:
VZV, varicella-zoster virus; IgM, immunoglobulin M.
Source: Adapted from Alkalay et al. [132].

Table 32.4. Neurologic abnormalities in congenital varicella syndrome

Limb paresis
Hypoplasia of extremities (usually ipsilateral and distal to cutaneous abnormalities)
Seizures
Horner's syndrome
Mental retardation
Auditory nerve palsy
Hydrocephalus
Microcephaly
Cortical atrophy
Central nervous system structural anomalies (prosencephalic cysts, glial fiber proliferation)
Encephalitis
Autonomic dysfunction
Ocular disease (chorioretinitis, microphthalmia, endophthalmitis, optic atrophy, cataracts)
Gastrointestinal dysmotility
Genitourinary dysfunction

Source: Adapted from [122,126–128,130–132,134,139].

The overall risk of congenital varicella syndrome was 1%. This risk increased to 2% if maternal infection occurred between 13 and 20 weeks' gestation. In previous smaller studies the risk of congenital varicella syndrome ranged from 0% to 9% [123,127,129,130].

In a prospective study in the United States, researchers followed a cohort of 347 pregnant women who developed varicella infection during pregnancy; there was one case of congenital varicella syndrome, one case of fetal death at 20 weeks, and one case of fetal hydrops at 17 weeks. The mother of the infant with congenital varicella syndrome had varicella at 24 weeks of gestation; the infant had skin, eye and central nervous system involvement [125].

Neurologic damage is an important consequence of congenital varicella syndrome [123,128–135]. Table 32.4 lists the various neurologic abnormalities that have been reported. Varicella is a neurotropic virus. Autopsies of neonates with congenital varicella syndrome have demonstrated VZV virus in the cerebrum and spinal cord by dot-blot and Southern blot hybridization [136]. Postmortem evaluations of suspected and confirmed congenital varicella syndrome cases report cortical and cerebellar necrosis, severe encephalopathy involving gray and white matter, and spinal cord disease including myelopathy, anterior horn cell loss, and gray-matter gliosis [123,131,136–138].

Maternal varicella during the few days before and after pregnancy can result in transplacental infection or exposure to the virus during delivery [139]. This perinatal infection is not associated with congenital malformations but can be the cause of severe neonatal morbidity and mortality. Infants whose mothers develop varicella more than a week before delivery can be expected to escape infection or to have an uncomplicated illness, probably because the interval between the onset of maternal infection and birth provides sufficient time for transplacental transmission of VZV antibodies [140]. In contrast, maternal chickenpox developing 5 days before or within 2 days following delivery poses a substantial risk to the newborn. The attack rate for perinatal infection under these circumstances is approximately 20%, and the incidence of fatal infection is about 30%. Nosocomial exposure of high-risk infants can also result in neonatal varicella [141].

Infants who contract perinatal VZV during this high-risk period are typically well for the first 5–10 days of life. Infection is recognized thereafter with the typical cutaneous exanthema. The diagnosis is usually obvious, because of the characteristic vesicular lesions and the recognition of recent maternal varicella. Progressive cutaneous infection is associated with life-threatening illness due to VZV pneumonia, encephalitis, hepatitis, and bleeding diathesis. Encephalitis is suggested by the occurrence of seizures accompanied by CSF and electroencephalogram abnormalities. Because of the limited number of infants with perinatal VZV infection that have been reported, the risk of neurologic involvement has not been established.

Herpes zoster, due to the reactivation of latent VZV, occurs during pregnancy but has not been associated with the classic features of congenital varicella syndrome. Enders et al. followed 366 women with zoster during pregnancy; none of these women had an affected newborn [130]. Other studies also document the absence of fetal/neonatal sequelae in cases of herpes zoster infection during pregnancy [122,132]. The lack of neonatal disease may be explained by the absence of viremia during herpes zoster infection in otherwise healthy pregnant women. Infants whose mothers develop varicella-zoster late in pregnancy or immediately postpartum are not at risk for serious illness because these infants are protected by transplacentally acquired VZV antibodies.

In March 1995 the Food and Drug Administration approved licensure of a live attenuated vaccine for varicella [142,143]. This vaccine is not approved for pregnant women or women who might conceive within 1–3 months following vaccination. The company manufacturing the vaccine and the CDC have established a pregnancy registry to follow pregnant women inadvertently vaccinated with varicella-zoster virus-containing vaccines: www.merckpregnancyregistries.com/varivax.html [144]. No cases of live births with congenital varicella syndrome have occurred in the pregnancies reported to this registry to date [145].

Recommendations

If a pregnant woman is known to be susceptible to VZV infection, she should be offered varicella-zoster immune globulin (VariZIG) or intravenous immune globulin (IVIG) prophylaxis within 96 hours of exposure in order to modify the severity of her infection [146,147]. It is possible, although not proven, that varicella-zoster immune globulin (VZIG) may reduce the risk of congenital varicella infection. In the study by Enders *et al.* none of the 97 women who received VZIG had an infant with congenital varicella syndrome [130,148]. The production of VZIG was discontinued in 2006. The only varicella-zoster immune globulin currently available in the USA is VariZIG, which at this time is available under an investigational new drug application only.

VariZIG or IVIG should be given to infants born to mothers whose onset of varicella is between 5 days before and 2 days after delivery [146–148]. These infants also should be treated with intravenous acyclovir. Although controlled clinical evaluations of acyclovir treatment of infants with perinatal varicella are lacking, the drug prevents progressive VZV infection among other immunodeficient patients.

No intervention is required for infants who are exposed to maternal varicella-zoster. These infants will have transplacentally acquired VZV antibodies and can be expected to be free of infection or to develop mild varicella.

Women who contract varicella during pregnancy should have ultrasounds performed at 20–22 weeks' gestation to look for abnormalities associated with congenital varicella syndrome (limb hypoplasia, microcephaly, intrauterine growth restriction, etc.) [132,136,149]. Studies have examined the potential utility of a variety of VZV-specific immunologic studies from blood obtained by cordocentesis from fetuses exposed in utero to maternal VZV infection [136,137]. The potential value of viral culture and PCR from amniotic fluid of pregnancies complicated by varicella has also been assessed [130,137]. To date, the data do not support the routine use of any of these diagnostic methods.

Herpes simplex virus

The incidence of neonatal HSV infection is estimated to range from 1/3000 to 1/20 000 live births [150,151]. Neonatal herpes has four disease manifestations: disease limited to the skin, eye, and mouth (SEM), isolated CNS disease, disseminated disease, and, rarely, congenital disease due to intrauterine infection [150,151]. Approximately 35% of neonatal infections primarily involve the CNS [150,151].

Transmission of HSV to the fetus and newborn

Neonatal infection with HSV can be caused by either HSV-1 or HSV-2, but two-thirds of these infections result from HSV-2 [150,151]. More than 85% of neonates with HSV infection contract the virus during labor and delivery from infected maternal secretions [150,151]. More than 70% of infected neonates are born to women who are asymptomatic during labor and delivery and have no prior history of genital herpes [152,153]. Intrapartum asymptomatic HSV excretion by the mother may represent a primary infection or reactivation of latent virus from a previous genital HSV infection [154]. In a study of almost 16 000 women prospectively cultured for HSV at delivery, 56 (0.35%) were found to have asymptomatic HSV excretion [154]. Based on serologic evaluation, one-third of these women had primary genital infections and two-thirds had recurrent infections. The attack rate among infants born to mothers with primary genital herpes at delivery is estimated to be 33–50% [151]. Fortunately, the attack rate for HSV infection among infants whose mothers are experiencing recurrent HSV at delivery is substantially lower: 0–5% [151,154]. The difference in neonatal infection rates following primary versus recurrent maternal infection is due to many factors, including concentration of virus, site of viral excretion (cervix vs. labia), and presence of transplacentally acquired protective antibodies in infants born to mothers with recurrent infection [150,151,154].

Postnatal exposure to HSV accounts for approximately 10% of neonatal infections [150,151]. These infections result from close contact with individuals who have active HSV-1 infection. These infections may be symptomatic or asymptomatic. Nosocomial transmission of HSV from infant to infant, apparently by personnel or fomites, has also occurred in neonatal nurseries [150].

Fewer than 5% of neonatal HSV infections are congenital [150,155]. The risk factors for HSV infection before birth have not been determined. Affected infants have been born to mothers with symptomatic and asymptomatic, primary and recurrent HSV infections during pregnancy [150,151,155,156]. HSV-2 is responsible for most intrauterine infections [155].

Clinical manifestations and consequences of perinatal and intrauterine HSV infections

Although the rate and severity of neurologic abnormalities vary, SEM, isolated CNS, disseminated disease, and intrauterine infection have all been associated with neurologic deficits at follow-up.

Approximately 40% of perinatal HSV infections are classified as SEM [150,151]. This mucocutaneous form of infection is characterized by vesicular lesions of the skin and mucosal surfaces with or without ocular disease. It is crucial to identify herpetic mucocutaneous lesions as soon as possible because, without proper identification and treatment, SEM disease will progress to the disseminated or CNS forms of neonatal herpes in more than 75% of cases [150]. In addition, during the pre-antiviral drug era, neurologic sequelae occurred in more than 25% of infants with localized SEM disease [150]. In contrast, with timely acyclovir treatment, the chance that the infant will escape neurologic sequelae exceeds 90% [157]. Nonetheless, even with appropriate therapy for limited mucocutaneous disease, 5–10% will have evidence of neurologic impairment at follow-up [157]. One predictor of neurologic morbidity appears to be the frequency of mucocutaneous recurrences during the first 6 months of life [158].

Thirty-five percent of neonatal herpes cases have isolated CNS involvement [151]. Herpes encephalitis usually occurs in infants who are about 2 weeks old (range 1–6 weeks). At presentation, some infants have active or resolving mucocutaneous lesions, but the majority do not. Only 60% of infants with CNS herpes have cutaneous lesions documented at any time during the course of their illness [150]. The signs of neonatal HSV encephalitis include fever or temperature instability, lethargy, poor feeding, bulging fontanel, pyramidal tract signs, tremors, and seizures [150,151]. The seizures often begin as focal, unilateral tonic–clonic movements that become generalized. Apnea is common. The CSF can be normal at the onset of symptoms but usually shows a mild lymphocytic pleocytosis (20–100 cells/mm^3) and elevated protein; the glucose may be normal or slightly low. Serial evaluations of the CSF usually show progressive abnormalities with substantial increase in protein (up to 1 g/dL) and inflammatory cells [150,151]. The electroencephalogram is usually diffusely abnormal. CT brain scans may be normal or show diffuse enhancement. MRI is superior to CT in demonstrating subtle abnormalities early in infection. Cultures of the CSF for HSV have a low yield: less than one-third are positive [150]. PCR of CSF is the preferred method to diagnose HSV meningoencephalitis [150,151,159]. The sensitivity of PCR on the CSF is 75–100%, with a specificity of 70–100% [159]. Although antiviral treatment of infants with herpes encephalitis reduces the mortality rate, very few survivors escape serious neurologic sequelae [157,158]. At follow-up, over 60% have neurologic deficits, including persistent seizures, spasticity, chorioretinitis, blindness, learning disabilities, and developmental delays [157,158]. HSV-1 CNS infection may have a better prognosis than CNS disease caused by HSV-2 [158].

Disseminated disease represents 25% of cases of neonatal HSV infection [151]. Infants with disseminated herpes usually present during the first 2 weeks of life with fever and signs indistinguishable from bacterial sepsis [150]. Disseminated HSV is often fulminant and associated with severe hepatitis, coagulopathy, pneumonitis, and possible concomitant encephalitis [150]. Unfortunately, infants with disseminated disease often lack cutaneous symptoms at presentation; 20% never develop mucocutaneous lesions [150]. Disseminated neonatal herpes has a mortality rate of greater than 80% if untreated [150]. The mortality rate is approximately 30% even with appropriate antiviral therapy [157]. Infants who have had CNS infection in the course of their disseminated disease usually have neurologic sequelae if they survive. Despite the severity of the acute illness, up to 80% of treated survivors are developmentally normal at follow-up [157].

In utero infection accounts for less than 5% of neonatal HSV [151]. The consequences of in utero infection are devastating. Infants with intrauterine infection have skin vesicles or scars at birth, chorioretinitis in the first week of life, microphthalmia, and abnormal head CT [155]. In 13 infants infected in utero, all had multisystem disease [155]. Four died; six had severe neurologic sequelae, including hydranencephaly, brain atrophy, seizures, and severe developmental delay [155]. Antiviral therapy does not reverse CNS damage sustained in utero [150,155].

Table 32.5. Predictors of mortality with neonatal herpes simplex virus (HSV) infection based on signs at presentation

Coma or semicomatose state
Disseminated intravascular coagulation
Prematurity
Disseminated disease due to HSV-1

Notes:
Mortality was the same in those with central nervous system disease from HSV-1 and HSV-2.
Source: Adapted from Whitley et al. [158] with permission.

Table 32.6. Predictors of morbidity from neonatal herpes infection

Infection with HSV-2
Seizures
Extent of disease at presentation (disseminated, CNS, or SEM)
For SEM only, ≥ 3 mucocutaneous recurrences in 6 months after therapy

Notes:
HSV, herpes simplex virus; CNS, central nervous system; SEM, skin, eyes, and mouth.
Source: Adapted from Whitley et al. [158] with permission.

Table 32.7. Mortality and morbidity in neonatal herpes

Diagnosis	Untreated mortality	Treated mortality	Treated morbidity
Disseminated	80%	50–60%	40%
CNS disease	50%	14%	55–65%
SEM disease	—	0%	5–10%

Notes:
CNS, central nervous system; SEM, skin, eyes, and mouth (mucocutaneous only).
Source: Adapted from [150,151,158].

Predictors of mortality and morbidity from neonatal HSV infections are outlined in Tables 32.5 and 32.6 [158]. Morbidity is defined as developmental delay of greater than 6 months, blindness, microcephaly, spastic quadriplegia, and/or seizures. The presence of seizures prior to the initiation of antiviral therapy significantly influences the incidence of neurologic deficits in survivors. Ninety-three percent of survivors with seizures have neurologic deficits, compared with a 34% incidence of neurologic impairment in the absence of seizures [158]. The highest morbidity occurs in neonates with CNS disease, followed by those infants with disseminated disease (Table 32.7) [158]. Only a small percentage of those with SEM have neurologic sequelae [158].

Recommendations
Prevention
Since most neonatal disease is acquired from maternal genital infection at the time of delivery, the first problem is to identify women with active genital HSV at the onset of labor. If the mother has genital lesions or prodromal symptoms consistent with genital HSV, cesarean delivery is recommended to avoid infant exposure [160,161]. Although some reports suggest that the benefits of cesarean section are more likely to be realized if cesarean section is performed within 4–6 hours of membrane

rupture, the American College of Obstetricians and Gynecologists (ACOG) recommends cesarean section regardless of the duration of membrane rupture [150,151,160].

Approximately 0.5–1% of women with a past history of recurrent genital herpes will have HSV excretion without any lesions at the time of delivery [150,151,154]. Unfortunately, these women cannot be identified by antepartum screening cultures [162,163]. Cesarean delivery for every woman with a past history of genital herpes is not reasonable and not recommended by ACOG [160]. Women who have had symptomatic primary genital herpes late in pregnancy may constitute a special subpopulation at greater risk of high-titer asymptomatic shedding; special consideration for cesarean section in these cases may be necessary [164].

Since most mothers of infants with neonatal herpes have no history of genital herpes, the infant's risk of HSV exposure will not be known. Maternal history of genital infection caused by HSV may be negative because the prior HSV-2 infection was asymptomatic or because the mother had primary genital HSV late in gestation that was not diagnosed or was asymptomatic.

Diagnosis and treatment

Direct immunofluorescence, PCR, and viral cultures provide the only means of confirming the diagnosis of HSV in the symptomatic infant [150,151,159,165,166]. Serologic tests are not helpful because the majority of newborn infants have passive HSV antibodies due to transplacental acquisition [150,151]. Furthermore, absence of HSV antibodies does not rule out herpes, because the infant may have acquired the infection as a result of primary maternal HSV or from a non-maternal source [150,151]. In addition, some infected neonates have delayed or no serologic response to infection. Currently, there is no reliable method for detection of HSV IgM.

Since the maternal history of herpes is not a reliable clue, infants with neonatal herpes will only be recognized if viral diagnostic procedures are included in the evaluation of infants with suspicious mucocutaneous lesions, non-bacterial sepsis, or unexplained seizures. Timely antiviral therapy may result in increased survival and improved long-term outcome for neonates infected with HSV [158].

High-dose parenteral acyclovir therapy (60 mg/kg per day) is now recommended for the treatment of neonatal herpes. SEM disease should be treated for 14 days and CNS and disseminated disease for 21 days [151]. Survival appears to be improved with this high-dose regimen. The National Institute of Allergy and Infectious Diseases Collaborative Antiviral Study Group evaluated high-dose acyclovir in an open label study comparing high-dose acyclovir (60 mg/kg per day) with lower-dose acyclovir (30–45 mg/kg per day) [167]. The survival rate for patients with disseminated or CNS HSV disease treated with the high-dose regimen was higher than observed in previous studies with lower-dose acyclovir [150,167]. There was no significant difference in morbidity at 12 months of follow-up between high-dose and lower-dose acyclovir in all the disease categories [150,167].

The efficacy of long-term suppressive acyclovir after initial therapy has yet to be elucidated [168]. Any infant who has had neonatal HSV should have continued evaluation of developmental milestones through childhood, with appropriate referrals to speech, occupational, and physical therapy as needed.

References

1. Wolf A, Cowen D, Paige BH. Toxoplasmic encephalomyelitis. III. A new case of granulomatous encephalomyelitis due to a protozoa. *Am J Pathol* 1939; **15**: 657–94.

2. Wong SY, Remington JS. Toxoplasmosis in pregnancy. *Clin Infect Dis* 1994; **18**: 853–62.

3. Remington JS, McLeod R, Thulliez P, *et al.* Toxoplasmosis. In Remington JS, Klein JO, eds., *Infectious Diseases of the Fetus and Newborn Infant*, 6th edn. Philadelphia, PA: Elsevier Saunders, 2006: 947–1091.

4. Lynfield R, Guerina NG. Toxoplasmosis. *Pediatr Rev* 1997; **18**: 75–83.

5. Guerina NG, Hsu HW, Meissner HC, *et al.* Neonatal serologic screening and early treatment for congenital *Toxoplasma gondii* infection. The New England Regional Toxoplasma Working Group. *N Engl J Med* 1994; **330**: 1858–63.

6. American Academy of Pediatrics. *Toxoplasma gondii* infections (toxoplasmosis). In Pickering LK, Baker CJ, Long SS, *et al.*, eds. *Red Book: 2006 Report of the Committee on Infectious Diseases*, 27th edn. Elk Grove Village, IL: American Academy of Pediatrics, 2006: 666–71.

7. Marty P, Le Fichoux Y, Deville A, *et al.* [Congenital toxoplasmosis and preconceptional maternal ganglionic toxoplasmosis]. *Presse Med* 1991; **20**: 387.

8. Gavinet MF, Robert F, Firtion G, *et al.* Congenital toxoplasmosis due to maternal reinfection during pregnancy. *J Clin Microbiol* 1997; **35**: 1276–7.

9. Hennequin C, Dureau P, N'Guyen L, *et al.* Congenital toxoplasmosis acquired from an immune woman. *Pediatr Infect Dis J* 1997; **16**: 75–7.

10. Vogel N, Kirisits M, Michael E, *et al.* Congenital toxoplasmosis transmitted from an immunologically competent mother infected before conception. *Clin Infect Dis* 1996; **23**: 1055–60.

11. Boumahni B, Randrianivo H, Flodrops H, *et al.* [Maternal toxoplasmosis before conception and chorioretinitis in twin sisters]. *J Gynecol Obstet Biol Reprod (Paris)* 2004; **33**: 248–50.

12. Chemla C, Villena I, Aubert D, *et al.* Preconception seroconversion and maternal seronegativity at delivery do not rule out the risk of congenital toxoplasmosis. *Clin Diagn Lab Immunol* 2002; **9**: 489–90.

13. Hohlfeld P, Daffos F, Thulliez P, *et al.* Fetal toxoplasmosis: outcome of pregnancy and infant follow-up after in utero treatment. *J Pediatr* 1989; **115**: 765–9.

14. Foulon W, Villena I, Stray-Pedersen B, *et al.* Treatment of toxoplasmosis during pregnancy: a multicenter study of impact on fetal transmission and children's sequelae at age 1 year. *Am J Obstet Gynecol* 1999; **180**: 410–15.

15. Thiebaut R, Leproust S, Chene G, *et al.* Effectiveness of prenatal treatment for congenital toxoplasmosis: a meta-analysis of individual patients' data. *Lancet* 2007; **369**: 115–22.

16. Koppe JG, Loewer-Sieger DH, de Roever-Bonnet H. Results of 20-year follow-up of congenital toxoplasmosis. *Lancet* 1986; **1**: 254–6.

17. Stagno S, Reynolds DW, Amos CS, *et al.* Auditory and visual defects resulting from

symptomatic and subclinical congenital cytomegaloviral and toxoplasma infections. *Pediatrics* 1977; **59**: 669–78.

18. Wilson CB, Remington JS, Stagno S, *et al.* Development of adverse sequelae in children born with subclinical congenital *Toxoplasma* infection. *Pediatrics* 1980; **66**: 767–74.

19. Roizen N, Swisher CN, Stein MA, *et al.* Neurologic and developmental outcome in treated congenital toxoplasmosis. *Pediatrics* 1995; **95**: 11–20.

20. McAuley J, Boyer KM, Patel D, *et al.* Early and longitudinal evaluations of treated infants and children and untreated historical patients with congenital toxoplasmosis: the Chicago Collaborative Treatment Trial. *Clin Infect Dis* 1994; **18**: 38–72.

21. McLeod R, Boyer K, Karrison T, *et al.* Outcome of treatment for congenital toxoplasmosis, 1981–2004: the National Collaborative Chicago-based, Congenital Toxoplasmosis Study. *Clin Infect Dis* 2006; **42**: 1383–94.

22. Patel DV, Holfels EM, Vogel NP, *et al.* Resolution of intracranial calcifications in infants with treated congenital toxoplasmosis. *Radiology* 1996; **199**: 433–40.

23. Naessens A, Jenum PA, Pollak A, *et al.* Diagnosis of congenital toxoplasmosis in the neonatal period: a multicenter evaluation. *J Pediatr* 1999; **135**: 714–19.

24. Gilbert RE, Thalib L, Tan HK, *et al.* Screening for congenital toxoplasmosis: accuracy of immunoglobulin M and immunoglobulin A tests after birth. *J Med Screen* 2007; **14**: 8–13.

25. Foulon W, Pinon JM, Stray-Pedersen B, *et al.* Prenatal diagnosis of congenital toxoplasmosis: a multicenter evaluation of different diagnostic parameters. *Am J Obstet Gynecol* 1999; **181**: 843–7.

26. Stagno S, Britt W. Cytomegalovirus infections. In Remington JS, Klein JO, eds., *Infectious Diseases of the Fetus and Newborn Infant*, 6th edn. Philadelphia, PA: Elsevier Saunders, 2006: 739–81.

27. Stagno S, Reynolds DW, Huang ES, *et al.* Congenital cytomegalovirus infection. *N Engl J Med* 1977; **296**: 1254–8.

28. Stagno S, Pass RF, Alford CA. Perinatal infections and maldevelopment. *Birth Defects Orig Artic Ser* 1981; **17**: 31–50.

29. Saigal S, Lunyk O, Larke RP, *et al.* The outcome in children with congenital cytomegalovirus infection: a longitudinal follow-up study. *Am J Dis Child* 1982; **136**: 896–901.

30. Reynolds DW, Stagno S, Stubbs KG, *et al.* Inapparent congenital cytomegalovirus infection with elevated cord IgM levels: casual relation with auditory and mental deficiency. *N Engl J Med* 1974; **290**: 291–6.

31. Preece PM, Pearl KN, Peckham CS. Congenital cytomegalovirus infection. *Arch Dis Child* 1984; **59**: 1120–6.

32. Noyola DE, Demmler GJ, Williamson WD, *et al.* Cytomegalovirus urinary excretion and long term outcome in children with congenital cytomegalovirus infection. Congenital CMV Longitudinal Study Group. *Pediatr Infect Dis J* 2000; **19**: 505–10.

33. Monif GR, Egan EA, Held B, *et al.* The correlation of maternal cytomegalovirus infection during varying stages in gestation with neonatal involvement. *J Pediatr* 1972; **80**: 17–20.

34. Kumar ML, Nankervis GA, Gold E. Inapparent congenital cytomegalovirus infection: a follow-up study. *N Engl J Med* 1973; **288**: 1370–2.

35. Ivarsson SA, Lernmark B, Svanberg L. Ten-year clinical, developmental, and intellectual follow-up of children with congenital cytomegalovirus infection without neurologic symptoms at one year of age. *Pediatrics* 1997; **99**: 800–3.

36. Hanshaw JB, Scheiner AP, Moxley AW, *et al.* School failure and deafness after "silent" congenital cytomegalovirus infection. *N Engl J Med* 1976; **295**: 468–70.

37. Halwachs-Baumann G, Genser B, Danda M, *et al.* Screening and diagnosis of congenital cytomegalovirus infection: a 5-y study. *Scand J Infect Dis* 2000; **32**: 137–42.

38. Fowler KB, McCollister FP, Dahle AJ, *et al.* Progressive and fluctuating sensorineural hearing loss in children with asymptomatic congenital cytomegalovirus infection. *J Pediatr* 1997; **130**: 624–30.

39. Conboy TJ, Pass RF, Stagno S, *et al.* Intellectual development in school-aged children with asymptomatic congenital cytomegalovirus infection. *Pediatrics* 1986; **77**: 801–6.

40. Williamson WD, Desmond MM, LaFevers N, *et al.* Symptomatic congenital cytomegalovirus: disorders of language, learning, and hearing. *Am J Dis Child* 1982; **136**: 902–5.

41. Whitley RJ, Cloud G, Gruber W, *et al.* Ganciclovir treatment of symptomatic congenital cytomegalovirus infection: results of a phase II study. National

Institute of Allergy and Infectious Diseases Collaborative Antiviral Study Group. *J Infect Dis* 1997; **175**: 1080–6.

42. Pass RF, Stagno S, Myers GJ, *et al.* Outcome of symptomatic congenital cytomegalovirus infection: results of long-term longitudinal follow-up. *Pediatrics* 1980; **66**: 758–62.

43. McCracken GH, Shinefield HM, Cobb K, *et al.* Congenital cytomegalic inclusion disease: a longitudinal study of 20 patients. *Am J Dis Child* 1969; **117**: 522–39.

44. Boppana SB, Fowler KB, Vaid Y, *et al.* Neuroradiographic findings in the newborn period and long-term outcome in children with symptomatic congenital cytomegalovirus infection. *Pediatrics* 1997; **99**: 409–14.

45. Williamson WD, Demmler GJ, Percy AK, *et al.* Progressive hearing loss in infants with asymptomatic congenital cytomegalovirus infection. *Pediatrics* 1992; **90**: 862–6.

46. Kumar ML, Nankervis GA, Jacobs IB, *et al.* Congenital and postnatally acquired cytomegalovirus infections: long-term follow-up. *J Pediatr* 1984; **104**: 674–9.

47. Melish ME, Hanshaw JB. Congenital cytomegalovirus infection: developmental progress of infants detected by routine screening. *Am J Dis Child* 1973; **126**: 190–4.

48. Fowler KB, Dahle AJ, Boppana SB, *et al.* Newborn hearing screening: will children with hearing loss caused by congenital cytomegalovirus infection be missed? *J Pediatr* 1999; **135**: 60–4.

49. Hicks T, Fowler K, Richardson M, *et al.* Congenital cytomegalovirus infection and neonatal auditory screening. *J Pediatr* 1993; **123**: 779–82.

50. Boppana SB, Fowler KB, Pass RF, *et al.* Congenital cytomegalovirus infection: association between virus burden in infancy and hearing loss. *J Pediatr* 2005; **146**: 817–23.

51. Stagno S, Pass RF, Cloud G, *et al.* Primary cytomegalovirus infection in pregnancy: incidence, transmission to fetus, and clinical outcome. *JAMA* 1986; **256**: 1904–8.

52. Butt W, Mackay RJ, de Crespigny LC, *et al.* Intracranial lesions of congenital cytomegalovirus infection detected by ultrasound scanning. *Pediatrics* 1984; **73**: 611–14.

53. Steinlin MI, Nadal D, Eich GF, *et al.* Late intrauterine cytomegalovirus infection: clinical and neuroimaging findings. *Pediatr Neurol* 1996; **15**: 249–53.

54. Troendle Atkins J, Demmler GJ, Williamson WD, *et al.* Polymerase chain reaction to detect cytomegalovirus DNA in the cerebrospinal fluid of neonates with congenital infection. *J Infect Dis* 1994; **169**: 1334–7.

55. Alarcon A, Garcia-Alix A, Cabanas F, *et al.* Beta$_2$-microglobulin concentrations in cerebrospinal fluid correlate with neuroimaging findings in newborns with symptomatic congenital cytomegalovirus infection. *Eur J Pediatr* 2006; **165**: 636–45.

56. Ahlfors K, Ivarsson SA, Harris S, *et al.* Congenital cytomegalovirus infection and disease in Sweden and the relative importance of primary and secondary maternal infections: preliminary findings from a prospective study. *Scand J Infect Dis* 1984; **16**: 129–37.

57. Noyola DE, Demmler GJ, Nelson CT, *et al.* Early predictors of neurodevelopmental outcome in symptomatic congenital cytomegalovirus infection. *J Pediatr* 2001; **138**: 325–31.

58. Rivera LB, Boppana SB, Fowler KB, *et al.* Predictors of hearing loss in children with symptomatic congenital cytomegalovirus infection. *Pediatrics* 2002; **110**: 762–7.

59. Kimberlin DW, Lin CY, Sanchez PJ, *et al.* Effect of ganciclovir therapy on hearing in symptomatic congenital cytomegalovirus disease involving the central nervous system: a randomized, controlled trial. *J Pediatr* 2003; **143**: 16–25.

60. Acosta EP, Brundage RC, King JR, *et al.* Ganciclovir population pharmacokinetics in neonates following intravenous administration of ganciclovir and oral administration of a liquid valganciclovir formulation. *Clin Pharmacol Ther* 2007; **81**: 867–72.

61. American Academy of Pediatrics. Rubella. In Pickering LK, Baker CJ, Long SS, *et al.*, eds., *Red Book: 2006 Report of the Committee on Infectious Diseases*, 27th edn. Elk Grove Village, IL: American Academy of Pediatrics, 2006: 574–9.

62. Cooper L, Alford C. Rubella. In Remington JS, Klein JO, eds., *Infectious Diseases of the Fetus and Newborn Infant*, 6th edn. Philadelphia, PA: Elsevier Saunders, 2006: 893–926.

63. Centers for Disease Control. Increase in rubella and congenital rubella syndrome: United States, 1988–1990. *MMWR Morb Mortal Wkly Rep* 1991; **40**: 93–9.

64. Centers for Disease Control and Prevention. Measles, rubella, and congenital rubella syndrome: United States and Mexico, 1997–1999. *MMWR Morb Mortal Wkly Rep* 2000; **49**: 1048–50, 1059.

65. Centers for Disease Control and Prevention. Rubella and congenital rubella syndrome: United States, 1994–1997. *MMWR Morb Mortal Wkly Rep* 1997; **46**: 350–4.

66. Achievements in public health: elimination of rubella and congenital rubella syndrome: US, 1969–2004. *Ann Pharmacother* 2005; **39**: 1151–2.

67. Centers for Disease Control and Prevention. Brief report. Imported case of congenital rubella syndrome: New Hampshire, 2005. *MMWR Morb Mortal Wkly Rep* 2005; **54**: 1160–1.

68. Reef SE, Redd SB, Abernathy E, *et al.* The epidemiological profile of rubella and congenital rubella syndrome in the United States, 1998–2004: the evidence for absence of endemic transmission. *Clin Infect Dis* 2006; **43**: S126–32.

69. Robertson SE, Featherstone DA, Gacic-Dobo M, *et al.* Rubella and congenital rubella syndrome: global update. *Rev Panam Salud Publica* 2003; **14**: 306–15.

70. Banatvala JE. Rubella: could do better. *Lancet* 1998; **351**: 849–50.

71. Miller E, Cradock-Watson JE, Pollock TM. Consequences of confirmed maternal rubella at successive stages of pregnancy. *Lancet* 1982; **2**: 781–4.

72. Frey TK. Neurological aspects of rubella virus infection. *Intervirology* 1997; **40**: 167–75.

73. Meitsch K, Enders G, Wolinsky JS, *et al.* The role of rubella-immunoblot and rubella-peptide-EIA for the diagnosis of the congenital rubella syndrome during the prenatal and newborn periods. *J Med Virol* 1997; **51**: 280–3.

74. Muller CP, Kremer JR, Best JM, *et al.* Reducing global disease burden of measles and rubella: report of the WHO Steering Committee on research related to measles and rubella vaccines and vaccination, 2005. *Vaccine* 2007; **25**: 1–9.

75. Mace M, Cointe D, Six C, *et al.* Diagnostic value of reverse transcription-PCR of amniotic fluid for prenatal diagnosis of congenital rubella infection in pregnant women with confirmed primary rubella infection. *J Clin Microbiol* 2004; **42**: 4818–20.

76. Ueda K, Nishida Y, Oshima K, *et al.* Congenital rubella syndrome: correlation of gestational age at time of maternal rubella with type of defect. *J Pediatr* 1979; **94**: 763–5.

77. Peckham CS. Clinical and laboratory study of children exposed in utero to maternal rubella. *Arch Dis Child* 1972; **47**: 571–7.

78. Weil ML, Itabashi H, Cremer NE, *et al.* Chronic progressive panencephalitis due to rubella virus simulating subacute sclerosing panencephalitis. *N Engl J Med* 1975; **292**: 994–8.

79. Macfarlane DW, Boyd RD, Dodrill CB, *et al.* Intrauterine rubella, head size, and intellect. *Pediatrics* 1975; **55**: 797–801.

80. Chang YC, Huang CC, Liu CC. Frequency of linear hyperechogenicity over the basal ganglia in young infants with congenital rubella syndrome. *Clin Infect Dis* 1996; **22**: 569–71.

81. Lane B, Sullivan EV, Lim KO, *et al.* White matter MR hyperintensities in adult patients with congenital rubella. *AJNR Am J Neuroradiol* 1996; **17**: 99–103.

82. Townsend JJ, Baringer JR, Wolinsky JS, *et al.* Progressive rubella panencephalitis: late onset after congenital rubella. *N Engl J Med* 1975; **292**: 990–3.

83. Desmond MM, Fisher ES, Vorderman AL, *et al.* The longitudinal course of congenital rubella encephalitis in nonretarded children. *J Pediatr* 1978; **93**: 584–91.

84. McIntosh ED, Menser MA. A fifty-year follow-up of congenital rubella. *Lancet* 1992; **340**: 414–5.

85. Noticeboard. Congenital rubella: 50 years on. *Lancet* 1991; **337**: 668.

86. Chess S, Fernandez P, Korn S. Behavioral consequences of congenital rubella. *J Pediatr* 1978; **93**: 699–703.

87. Brown AS, Cohen P, Greenwald S, *et al.* Nonaffective psychosis after prenatal exposure to rubella. *Am J Psychiatry* 2000; **157**: 438–43.

88. Tanemura M, Suzumori K, Yagami Y, *et al.* Diagnosis of fetal rubella infection with reverse transcription and nested polymerase chain reaction: a study of 34 cases diagnosed in fetuses. *Am J Obstet Gynecol* 1996; **174**: 578–82.

89. Bart KJ, Orenstein WA, Preblud SR, *et al.* Elimination of rubella and congenital rubella from the United States. *Pediatr Infect Dis* 1985; **4**: 14–21.

90. Reef SE, Cochi SL. The evidence for the elimination of rubella and congenital

rubella syndrome in the United States: a public health achievement. *Clin Infect Dis* 2006; **43**: S123–5.

91. Badilla X, Morice A, Avila-Aguero ML, *et al*. Fetal risk associated with rubella vaccination during pregnancy. *Pediatr Infect Dis J* 2007; **26**: 830–5.

92. Minussi L, Mohrdieck R, Bercini M, *et al*. Prospective evaluation of pregnant women vaccinated against rubella in southern Brazil. *Reprod Toxicol* 2008; **25**: 120–3.

93. Klass PE, Brown ER, Pelton SI. The incidence of prenatal syphilis at the Boston City Hospital: a comparison across four decades. *Pediatrics* 1994; **94**: 24–8.

94. Reyes MP, Hunt N, Ostrea EM, Jr., *et al*. Maternal/congenital syphilis in a large tertiary-care urban hospital. *Clin Infect Dis* 1993; **17**: 1041–6.

95. Sison CG, Ostrea EM, Reyes MP, *et al*. The resurgence of congenital syphilis: a cocaine-related problem. *J Pediatr* 1997; **130**: 289–92.

96. Wharton M, Chorba TL, Vogt RL, *et al*. Case definitions for public health surveillance. *MMWR Recomm Rep* 1990; **39**: 1–43.

97. Centers for Disease Control and Prevention. 1993 sexually transmitted diseases treatment guidelines. *MMWR Recomm Rep* 1993; **42**: 1–102.

98. Centers for Disease Control and Prevention. Congenital syphilis: United States, 1998. *MMWR Morb Mortal Wkly Rep* 1999; **48**: 757–61.

99. Centers for Disease Control and Prevention. Congenital syphilis: United States, 2000. *MMWR Morb Mortal Wkly Rep* 2001; **50**: 573–7.

100. Centers for Disease Control and Prevention. Congenital syphilis: United States, 2002. *MMWR Morb Mortal Wkly Rep* 2004; **53**: 716–19.

101. Ingall D, Sanchez P, Baker C. Syphilis. In Remington JS, Klein JO, eds., *Infectious Diseases of the Fetus and Newborn Infant*, 6th edn. Philadelphia, PA: Elsevier Saunders, 2006: 545–80.

102. Sung L, MacDonald NE. Syphilis: a pediatric perspective. *Pediatr Rev* 1998; **19**: 17–22.

103. Stoll BJ. Congenital syphilis: evaluation and management of neonates born to mothers with reactive serologic tests for syphilis. *Pediatr Infect Dis J* 1994; **13**: 845–53.

104. Sanchez PJ, Wendel GD, Grimprel E, *et al*. Evaluation of molecular

methodologies and rabbit infectivity testing for the diagnosis of congenital syphilis and neonatal central nervous system invasion by *Treponema pallidum*. *J Infect Dis* 1993; **167**: 148–57.

105. Sanchez PJ. Laboratory tests for congenital syphilis. *Pediatr Infect Dis J* 1998; **17**: 70–1.

106. Srinivasan G, Ramamurthy RS, Bharathi A, *et al*. Congenital syphilis: a diagnostic and therapeutic dilemma. *Pediatr Infect Dis* 1983; **2**: 436–41.

107. Risser WL, Hwang LY. Problems in the current case definitions of congenital syphilis. *J Pediatr* 1996; **129**: 499–505.

108. Michelow IC, Wendel GD, Jr., Norgard MV, *et al*. Central nervous system infection in congenital syphilis. *N Engl J Med* 2002; **346**: 1792–8.

109. American Academy of Pediatrics. Syphilis. In Pickering LK, Baker CJ, Long SS, *et al*., eds., *Red Book: 2006 Report of the Committee on Infectious Diseases*, 27th edn. Elk Grove Village, IL: American Academy of Pediatrics, 2006: 631–44.

110. Workowski KA, Berman SM. Sexually transmitted diseases treatment guidelines, 2006. *MMWR Recomm Rep* 2006; **55**: 1–94.

111. Glaser JH. Centers for Disease Control and Prevention guidelines for congenital syphilis. *J Pediatr* 1996; **129**: 488–90.

112. Platou R. Treatment of congenital syphilis with penicillin. *Adv Pediatr* 1949; **4**: 35.

113. Ahmed A, Hickey SM, Ehrett S, *et al*. Cerebrospinal fluid values in the term neonate. *Pediatr Infect Dis J* 1996; **15**: 298–303.

114. Sarff LD, Platt LH, McCracken GH. Cerebrospinal fluid evaluation in neonates: comparison of high-risk infants with and without meningitis. *J Pediatr* 1976; **88**: 473–7.

115. Beeram MR, Chopde N, Dawood Y, *et al*. Lumbar puncture in the evaluation of possible asymptomatic congenital syphilis in neonates. *J Pediatr* 1996; **128**: 125–9.

116. Lapunzina PD, Altcheh JM, Flichman JC, *et al*. Neurosyphilis in an eight-year-old child: usefulness of the SPECT study. *Pediatr Neurol* 1998; **18**: 81–4.

117. Fiumara NJ, Lessell S. Manifestations of late congenital syphilis: an analysis of 271 patients. *Arch Dermatol* 1970; **102**: 78–83.

118. Zenker PN, Berman SM. Congenital syphilis: trends and recommendations for evaluation and management. *Pediatr Infect Dis J* 1991; **10**: 516–22.

119. Dorfman DH, Glaser JH. Congenital syphilis presenting in infants after the newborn period. *N Engl J Med* 1990; **323**: 1299–302.

120. Ikeda MK, Jenson HB. Evaluation and treatment of congenital syphilis. *J Pediatr* 1990; **117**: 843–52.

121. Paryani SG, Vaughn AJ, Crosby M, *et al*. Treatment of asymptomatic congenital syphilis: benzathine versus procaine penicillin G therapy. *J Pediatr* 1994; **125**: 471–5.

122. Gershon AA. Chickenpox, measles and mumps. In Remington JS, Klein JO, eds., *Infectious Diseases of the Fetus and Newborn Infant*, 6th edn. Philadelphia, PA: Elsevier Saunders, 2006: 693–737.

123. Pastuszak AL, Levy M, Schick B, *et al*. Outcome after maternal varicella infection in the first 20 weeks of pregnancy. *N Engl J Med* 1994; **330**: 901–5.

124. Dufour P, de Bievre P, Vinatier D, *et al*. Varicella and pregnancy. *Eur J Obstet Gynecol Reprod Biol* 1996; **66**: 119–23.

125. Harger JH, Ernest JM, Thurnau GR, *et al*. Frequency of congenital varicella syndrome in a prospective cohort of 347 pregnant women. *Obstet Gynecol* 2002; **100**: 260–5.

126. Laforet L. Multiple congenital defects following maternal varicella. *N Engl J Med* 1947; **236**: 534–7.

127. Paryani SG, Arvin AM. Intrauterine infection with varicella-zoster virus after maternal varicella. *N Engl J Med* 1986; **314**: 1542–6.

128. Kent A, Paes B. Congenital varicella syndrome: a rare case of central nervous system involvement without dermatological features. *Am J Perinatol* 2000; **17**: 253–6.

129. Jones KL, Johnson KA, Chambers CD. Offspring of women infected with varicella during pregnancy: a prospective study. *Teratology* 1994; **49**: 29–32.

130. Enders G, Miller E, Cradock-Watson J, *et al*. Consequences of varicella and herpes zoster in pregnancy: prospective study of 1739 cases. *Lancet* 1994; **343**: 1548–51.

131. Da Silva O, Hammerberg O, Chance GW. Fetal varicella syndrome. *Pediatr Infect Dis J* 1990; **9**: 854–5.

132. Alkalay AL, Pomerance JJ, Rimoin DL. Fetal varicella syndrome. *J Pediatr* 1987; **111**: 320–3.

133. Higa K, Dan K, Manabe H. Varicella-zoster virus infections during pregnancy: hypothesis concerning the mechanisms of congenital malformations. *Obstet Gynecol* 1987; **69**: 214–22.

134. Ong CL, Daniel ML. Antenatal diagnosis of a porencephalic cyst in congenital varicella-zoster virus infection. *Pediatr Radiol* 1998; **28**: 94.

135. Bassett DC. Varicella infection in pregnancy. *N Engl J Med* 1994; **331**: 482.

136. Scharf A, Scherr O, Enders G, *et al.* Virus detection in the fetal tissue of a premature delivery with a congenital varicella syndrome: a case report. *J Perinat Med* 1990; **18**: 317–22.

137. Mouly F, Mirlesse V, Meritet JF, *et al.* Prenatal diagnosis of fetal varicella-zoster virus infection with polymerase chain reaction of amniotic fluid in 107 cases. *Am J Obstet Gynecol* 1997; **177**: 894–8.

138. Salzman MB, Sharrar RG, Steinberg S, *et al.* Transmission of varicella-vaccine virus from a healthy 12-month-old child to his pregnant mother. *J Pediatr* 1997; **131**: 151–4.

139. Myers J. Congenital varicella in term infants: risk reconsidered. *J Infect Dis* 1974; **128**: 215–19.

140. Gershon AA, Raker R, Steinberg S, *et al.* Antibody to varicella-zoster virus in parturient women and their offspring during the first year of life. *Pediatrics* 1976; **58**: 692–6.

141. Gustafson TL, Shehab Z, Brunell PA. Outbreak of varicella in a newborn intensive care nursery. *Am J Dis Child* 1984; **138**: 548–50.

142. Varicella vaccine. *Med Lett Drugs Ther* 1995; **37**: 55–7.

143. Centers for Disease Control and Prevention. Prevention of varicella: recommendations of the Advisory Committee on Immunization Practices (ACIP). *MMWR Recomm Rep* 1996; **45**: 1–36.

144. Centers for Disease Control and Prevention. Establishment of VARIVAX pregnancy registry. *MMWR Morb Mortal Wkly Rep* 1996; **45**: 239.

145. Wilson E, Goss MA, Marin M, *et al.* Varicella vaccine exposure during pregnancy: data from 10 years of the pregnancy registry. *J Infect Dis* 2008; **197** (Suppl 2): S178–84.

146. American Academy of Pediatrics. Committee on Infectious Diseases. Prevention of varicella: recommendations for use of varicella vaccines in children, including recommendations for a routine 2-dose varicella immunization schedule. *Pediatrics* 2007; **120**: 221–31.

147. American Academy of Pediatrics. Varicella-zoster infections. In Pickering LK, Baker CJ, Long SS, *et al.*, eds., *Red Book: 2006 Report of the Committee on Infectious Diseases*, 27th edn. Elk Grove Village, IL: American Academy of Pediatrics, 2006: 711–25.

148. Miller E, Cradock-Watson JE, Ridehalgh MK. Outcome in newborn babies given anti-varicella-zoster immunoglobulin after perinatal maternal infection with varicella-zoster virus. *Lancet* 1989; **2**: 371–3.

149. Meyberg-Solomayer GC, Fehm T, Muller-Hansen I, *et al.* Prenatal ultrasound diagnosis, follow-up, and outcome of congenital varicella syndrome. *Fetal Diagn Ther* 2006; **21**: 296–301.

150. Arvin AM, Whitley RJ, Gutierrez KM. Herpes simplex virus infections. In Remington JS, Klein JO, eds., *Infectious Diseases of the Fetus and Newborn Infant*, 6th edn. Philadelphia, PA: Elsevier Saunders, 2006: 845–65.

151. American Academy of Pediatrics. Herpes simplex. In Pickering LK, Baker CJ, Long SS, *et al.*, eds., *Red Book: 2006 Report of the Committee on Infectious Diseases*, 27th edn. Elk Grove Village, IL: American Academy of Pediatrics, 2006: 361–71.

152. Whitley RJ, Corey L, Arvin A, *et al.* Changing presentation of herpes simplex virus infection in neonates. *J Infect Dis* 1988; **158**: 109–16.

153. Whitley RJ, Nahmias AJ, Visintine AM, *et al.* The natural history of herpes simplex virus infection of mother and newborn. *Pediatrics* 1980; **66**: 489–94.

154. Brown ZA, Benedetti J, Ashley R, *et al.* Neonatal herpes simplex virus infection in relation to asymptomatic maternal infection at the time of labor. *N Engl J Med* 1991; **324**: 1247–52.

155. Hutto C, Arvin A, Jacobs R, *et al.* Intrauterine herpes simplex virus infections. *J Pediatr* 1987; **110**: 97–101.

156. Vasileiadis GT, Roukema HW, Romano W, *et al.* Intrauterine herpes simplex infection. *Am J Perinatol* 2003; **20**: 55–8.

157. Whitley R, Arvin A, Prober C, *et al.* A controlled trial comparing vidarabine with acyclovir in neonatal herpes simplex virus infection. Infectious Diseases Collaborative Antiviral Study Group. *N Engl J Med* 1991; **324**: 444–9.

158. Whitley R, Arvin A, Prober C, *et al.* Predictors of morbidity and mortality in neonates with herpes simplex virus infections. The National Institute of Allergy and Infectious Diseases Collaborative Antiviral Study Group. *N Engl J Med* 1991; **324**: 450–4.

159. Kimberlin DW, Lakeman FD, Arvin AM, *et al.* Application of the polymerase chain reaction to the diagnosis and management of neonatal herpes simplex virus disease. National Institute of Allergy and Infectious Diseases Collaborative Antiviral Study Group. *J Infect Dis* 1996; **174**: 1162–7.

160. ACOG Practice Bulletin No. 82. Management of herpes in pregnancy. *Obstet Gynecol* 2007; **109**: 1489–98.

161. Brown ZA, Wald A, Morrow RA, *et al.* Effect of serologic status and cesarean delivery on transmission rates of herpes simplex virus from mother to infant. *JAMA* 2003; **289**: 203–9.

162. Prober CG, Hensleigh PA, Boucher FD, *et al.* Use of routine viral cultures at delivery to identify neonates exposed to herpes simplex virus. *N Engl J Med* 1988; **318**: 887–91.

163. Arvin AM, Hensleigh PA, Prober CG, *et al.* Failure of antepartum maternal cultures to predict the infant's risk of exposure to herpes simplex virus at delivery. *N Engl J Med* 1986; **315**: 796–800.

164. Brown ZA, Vontver LA, Benedetti J, *et al.* Effects on infants of a first episode of genital herpes during pregnancy. *N Engl J Med* 1987; **317**: 1246–51.

165. Coleman RM, Pereira L, Bailey PD, *et al.* Determination of herpes simplex virus type-specific antibodies by enzyme-linked immunosorbent assay. *J Clin Microbiol* 1983; **18**: 287–91.

166. Jacobs RF. Neonatal herpes simplex virus infections. *Semin Perinatol* 1998; **22**: 64–71.

167. Kimberlin DW, Lin CY, Jacobs RF, *et al.* Safety and efficacy of high-dose intravenous acyclovir in the management of neonatal herpes simplex virus infections. *Pediatrics* 2001; **108**: 230–8.

168. Kimberlin DW. Herpes simplex virus infections of the newborn. *Semin Perinatol* 2007; **31**: 19–25.

Chapter 33

Perinatal human immunodeficiency virus infection

Avinash K. Shetty and Yvonne A. Maldonado

Introduction

Since the initial description of acquired immune deficiency syndrome (AIDS) cases in infants and children more than 25 years ago [1], the epidemiology of the pediatric human immunodeficiency virus type 1 (HIV-1) epidemic has changed significantly [2–4]. Most pediatric HIV infections occur through perinatal transmission [5]. Dramatic declines in the number of perinatally HIV infected children have been reported in the USA and Europe due to prompt implementation of strategies to prevent mother-to-child transmission of HIV (PMTCT) [3,4]. Further, availability of highly active antiretroviral therapy (HAART) has led to improved survival of HIV-infected children into adolescence and adulthood, changing most HIV infections into a chronic rather than an acute disease [6]. In contrast, prevention of mother-to-child HIV transmission is a major public health challenge in many resource-limited countries [2]. Although several effective, simple, and less expensive prophylactic antiretroviral regimens are available to prevent perinatal HIV transmission, these interventions have not been widely implemented in the developing world [2].

Pediatricians and obstetricians play a crucial role in the prevention of perinatal HIV transmission, including identification of HIV-infected women during pregnancy, treatment of the pregnant women with appropriate antiretroviral therapy, ensuring evaluation for HIV infection in early infancy, and subsequent provision of ongoing care for children and families affected by HIV [7]. The purpose of this chapter is to review advances in the prevention of perinatal HIV transmission and highlight certain unique features of HIV infection in infants with a focus on early diagnosis, clinical manifestations, treatment, and prognosis.

Epidemiology

Cases of AIDS in children have accounted for 1% of all reported cases in the USA [8]. Since the beginning of the epidemic, 9441 cases of AIDS in children under 13 years of age have been reported in the USA. Perinatal transmission is the most common source of pediatric HIV infection, accounting for

91% of cases, whereas 4% acquired infection through receipt of blood or blood products, and another 2% acquired HIV from transfusion due to hemophilia. Fewer than 3% of cases have been reported to have no identifiable risk factor [9].

The racial, ethnic and geographic distribution of AIDS cases in children parallels that of women with AIDS. Perinatally acquired HIV infection has occurred more frequently among black non-Hispanic (61%) and Hispanic (23%) children than among white non-Hispanic children, whereas infection related to blood or blood-product transfusion is more proportional to the racial and ethnic distribution of the general population [9]. Most children with vertically acquired AIDS are diagnosed before 5 years of age (83%) compared with children with hemophilia or transfusion-acquired AIDS, who often are diagnosed at 5 years of age or older (95% and 73% respectively) [9].

The number of infants born with HIV has dropped from a high of 2000 per year in the early 1990s to fewer than 200 [10]. At the same time, new pediatric AIDS cases and AIDS deaths also have dramatically declined, primarily due to availability of HAART. In 1992, 858 AIDS cases were reported in children under 13 years of age, compared to only 41 cases in 2004 [11]. New York and Florida reported the highest number of cases. Adolescents now represent a growing population of HIV-1 infection, with at least 5000 young people 13–19 years of age living with HIV [12]. Blacks and Hispanics are disproportionately affected. A significant number of HIV-infected adolescents acquired their infection perinatally.

Globally, the perinatal HIV-1 epidemic continues to advance at an alarming rate; approximately 2.1 million HIV-infected children are currently living with HIV/AIDS [13]. More than 90% of HIV-infected children reside in sub-Saharan Africa, where approximately 1500 infants are newly infected daily [13]. Over 50% of HIV-infected children in sub-Saharan Africa die by their second birthday [14].

Perinatal transmission: rates, timing, mechanisms and risk factors

Mother-to-child transmission of HIV can take place in utero via transplacental infection, intrapartum by exposure to maternal blood at the time of labor and delivery, and postnatally through breastfeeding [3–5,15–17]. Perinatal HIV transmission rates in the absence of specific interventions vary

Fetal and Neonatal Brain Injury, 4th edition, ed. David K. Stevenson, William E. Benitz, Philip Sunshine, Susan R. Hintz, and Maurice L. Druzin. Published by Cambridge University Press. © Cambridge University Press 2009.

from about 15–30% among non-breastfeeding HIV-infected women in the USA and Europe to 25–45% among breastfeeding populations in sub-Saharan Africa [5,18–21]. Variability in estimated rates likely reflects differences in breastfeeding patterns, maternal and obstetric risk factors, and viral factors, as well as methodological differences among studies.

Knowledge about the precise timing of transmission is crucial for the design of potential preventive strategies [15]. In the non-breastfed infant, about one-third of transmissions occur during gestation and the remaining two-thirds during delivery [18]. The absolute risk for intrauterine transmission is approximately 5%, and for intrapartum transmission it is approximately 13–18%. In the breastfed infant, one-third to one-half of overall transmission may occur after delivery during lactation [16,17]. In 1992, Bryson *et al.* proposed a working definition of timing of vertical transmission in non-breastfeeding infants: infants with a positive HIV culture or DNA PCR test in the first 48 hours of life are usually considered to have had in utero infection, while those with a negative virologic test in the first week of life who subsequently become positive before 90 days of life are probably infected during the intrapartum period [22].

In utero transmission may occur through HIV infection in the placenta or fetal exposure to HIV in the amniotic fluid, and has been documented by isolation of HIV from the tissue of aborted or miscarried fetuses as early as 8 weeks of gestation [23–25]. Intrapartum transmission may occur in a variety of ways, including direct exposure of the fetus/infant to infected maternal secretions during birth, ascending infection after rupture of membranes, or maternal–fetal microtransfusions during uterine contractions [26]. Intrapartum transmission is supported by studies failing to detect HIV in infants born to HIV-infected women in the first month of life but subsequently detecting virus after 1–3 months of life [27–30]. Retrospective studies of twins born to HIV-infected women found a higher HIV transmission rate among those born by vaginal delivery compared with those born by cesarean delivery, and among first-born compared with second-born twins. These data support exposure to maternal virus during delivery as a likely route of transmission [31–33]. The role of cesarean delivery in reducing the risk of perinatal transmission may be beneficial in certain situations, such as for women who are not receiving antiretroviral therapy or for those who have high levels of HIV-1 in their blood at the time of labor and delivery [32,33].

Although numerous maternal, obstetric, infant, and viral-related factors may modify perinatal HIV transmission risk [34], the strongest predictor of both intrauterine and intrapartum transmission is the maternal serum HIV RNA level [35–42]. However, transmission can occur rarely among pregnant women with low or undetectable serum levels of HIV around the time of labor and delivery [43]. Other maternal risk factors associated with higher rates of perinatal HIV infection include women with progressive symptoms of AIDS, acute HIV infection during pregnancy, and low CD4 counts [44–48]. HIV viral burden in cervicovaginal secretions is an independent risk factor for perinatal HIV transmission [49]. Obstetric risk factors associated with increased risk of transmission include vaginal delivery, rupture of membranes for more than 4 hours, chorioamnionitis, and invasive obstetric procedures [48,50,51]. Premature infants born to HIV-infected women have a higher rate of perinatal HIV infection than full-term infants [21,37,48,52,53]. Studies evaluating the relative risk of HIV transmission associated with vaginal (versus cesarean) delivery have demonstrated decreased transmission with cesarean delivery [32,33]. Increased transmission of HIV strains that are fetotropic is reported; isolation of HIV strains with highly conserved gene sequences from HIV-infected infants has been demonstrated, despite the large number of genetically diverse strains isolated from their mothers [54]. Maternal–fetal HLA concordance increases the risk of perinatal transmission [55], whereas CCR5 haplotype may be permissive or protective, depending on the specific mutation [56].

In resource-poor settings, where breastfeeding is the cultural norm, postnatal transmission of HIV through breast milk remains a serious problem and carries an estimated risk of about 15% when breastfeeding is prolonged and continued into the second year of life [16,17,57,58]. HIV has been isolated from cellular and cell-free fractions of human breast milk from HIV-infected women [59,60]. Available data among breastfeeding African populations suggest that 33–50% of transmission may occur through breastfeeding [16,61–64]. A meta-analysis estimated the overall additional risk of breast-milk transmission as 14% (95% CI 7–22%) for established maternal infection and 29% (95% CI 16–42%) for primary infection [61]. Most breast-milk HIV-1 transmission occurs during the first few months of life, with a lower but continued risk thereafter [64,65]. In a randomized controlled trial of breastfeeding versus formula feeding on HIV-1 transmission in Kenya, investigators found that formula feeding reduced transmission by 44% at age 2 years and that 75% of infections were acquired during the first 6 months of life [64]. In a prospective breastfed cohort study in Malawi, Miotti *et al.* reported cumulative transmission rates of 3.5%, 7.0%, 8.9%, and 10.3% after 5 months, 11 months, 17 months, and 23 months of breastfeeding, respectively [65]. Several studies have evaluated the risks of late postnatal breast-milk transmission [58,66–69]. In a international multicenter pooled meta-analysis of over 900 mother–infant pairs, the risk of late postnatal transmission (after age 4 months) was 3.2 cases (95% CI 3.1–3.8) per year per 100 breastfed infants [68]. A more recent meta-analysis estimated the risk of postnatal HIV transmission to be 8.9 transmissions per 100 child-years of breastfeeding or 0.9% per month after the first month of life [58].

Risk factors for breast-milk HIV transmission include women seroconverting during lactation, high HIV DNA or RNA level in plasma and breast-milk, longer duration of breastfeeding, mixed infant feeding, bleeding or cracked nipples, subclinical and clinical mastitis, and breast abscesses [16,17,57,69–71].

Early diagnosis

Routine HIV antibody testing cannot be used for the diagnosis of infant HIV infection because of passively transferred maternal HIV-1 antibodies, which may be present in children up to 18 months of age [2]. HIV DNA or RNA PCR assays represent the gold standard for early diagnosis of HIV infection in children younger than 18 months [72–76]. HIV RNA PCR may be more sensitive than the HIV DNA PCR test for detection of non-B-subtype virus [77]. The sensitivity of HIV RNA PCR is not affected by the presence of maternal/infant zidovudine prophylaxis [77]. HIV DNA or RNA PCR testing is recommended within the first 2 weeks of life, at 1–2 months of age, and at 2–4 months of age [7]. Cord blood specimens should not be used because of possible contamination with maternal blood. Two separate positive HIV DNA or RNA PCR test results are needed for diagnosis of HIV infection. HIV-1 infection can be definitively excluded in non-breastfed HIV-exposed infants if two HIV DNA or RNA PCR assays obtained at > 1 month of age, and a third test obtained at > 4 months of age, are reported as negative if the maternal virus is subtype B [72]. Many physicians confirm the absence of HIV infection by documenting a negative HIV antibody test at 12–18 months of age. Detection of HIV antibody in a child > 18 months of age is diagnostic of HIV infection [7,72].

For any positive HIV DNA PCR result, the infant should be re-tested immediately for confirmatory PCR testing. If infection is confirmed, a pediatric infectious disease consultation should be requested, because of the rapidly evolving and complex nature of the disease. Plasma HIV RNA levels are characteristically very high in HIV-infected newborns and infants and are likely to reflect the immaturity of the immune system for bringing viral replication under control [78]. Early recognition of infant HIV infection is critical to allow early initiation of aggressive antiretroviral therapy and prophylaxis for *Pneumocystis jirovecii* (formerly *carini*) pneumonia with the potential to prevent the rapid disease progression observed in some perinatally HIV-infected infants [79].

Clinical manifestations of HIV-infected infants

The clinical manifestations of HIV infection in infants are highly variable and often non-specific [80]. Infants with perinatally acquired HIV infection are often asymptomatic, and physical examination is usually normal in the neonatal period. Although a distinctive craniofacial dysmorphism characterized by prominent boxlike forehead, hypertelorism, flattened nasal bridge, triangular philtrum, and patulous lips were suggested as a possible congenital HIV syndrome [81], these findings have not been confirmed in subsequent reports [82]. In a prospective cohort study of 200 children with perinatally acquired HIV-1 infection, the median age of onset of any HIV-related symptom or sign was 5.2 months; the probability of remaining asymptomatic was 19% at 1 year and 6.1% at 5 years [83]. In another large prospective cohort study, AIDS-defining conditions developed in approximately 23%

and 40% of perinatally infected infants by 1 and 4 years respectively [84,85].

Growth delay can be an early sign of untreated perinatal HIV infection, and the linear growth is most severely affected in infants with high HIV RNA levels [86]. Other features of infection in early infancy could include lymphadenopathy, often associated with hepatosplenomegaly. Also commonly encountered are oral candidiasis, developmental delay, and dermatitis [87].

The current AIDS case definitions devised by the Centers for Disease Control and Prevention (CDC) for surveillance and reporting purposes are similar, with some important exceptions [88]. Lymphoid interstitial pneumonia (LIP) and multiple or recurrent serious bacterial infections are AIDS-defining illness only for children. Also, certain herpes virus infections (cytomegalovirus, herpes simplex virus) and toxoplasmosis of the CNS are AIDS-defining conditions only for adults and children older than 1 month of age. In 1994, the CDC published a revised pediatric classification system for HIV infection in children less than 13 years of age according to parameters: (1) HIV infection status, (2) clinical disease, and (3) immunologic status [89].

Clinical categories range from N, indicating no signs or symptoms, through A, B, and C, for mild, moderate, and severe (AIDS-defining) symptoms and signs. PCP pneumonia is the leading AIDS-defining illness diagnosed during the first year of life and is associated with a high mortality rate [90]. Other common AIDS-defining conditions in US children with vertically acquired infection include lymphoid interstitial pneumonitis, multiple or recurrent serious bacterial infections, HIV encephalopathy, wasting syndrome, candida esophagitis, cytomegalovirus disease, and *Mycobacterium avium-intracellulare* complex infection [85].

The immunologic categories place emphasis on the CD4 T-cell lymphocyte count and percentages for age, and include stage 1, no evidence of immunosuppression; Stage 2, moderate immunosuppression; and Stage 3, indicating severe immunosuppression [89]. Once classified, a child cannot be reclassified into a less severe category, even if the child's clinical status or immune function improves in response to antiretroviral treatment or resolution of clinical events. HIV-exposed infants whose HIV infection status is indeterminate (unconfirmed) are classified by placing a prefix E (for perinatally exposed) before the appropriate classification code (e.g., EN2) [89].

Neurologic manifestations in the infant

Central nervous system (CNS) manifestations in patients with HIV infection may be due to direct effects of HIV viral infection or to secondary effects of opportunistic diseases of the central nervous system that may occur in advanced stages of HIV/AIDS [91]. The impact and neurologic manifestations of HIV infection occurring early in development are different from neurologic sequelae in adults infected at the time of central nervous system maturity (Table 33.1). This likely reflects the vulnerability of the immature infant brain to HIV infection [91,92].

Table 33.1. Neurologic manifestations of HIV in children and adults

Features	Children	Adults
Syndrome	HIV-associated encephalopathy	AIDS-dementia complex
Target cells	Macrophages, microglia, astrocytes (minor role)	Macrophages, microglia astrocytes (central role)
Latent period	Short	Long
	Encephalopathy often the first AIDS-defining illness	
Clinical features	Motor, cognitive and language functions impaired	Motor and cognitive functions deteriorate
Opportunistic CNS infections	Rare	Common
Cerebrovascular disease	Rare	Common

Neurologic disease in children with rapid progression of HIV infection has been commonly recognized as HIV encephalopathy, which can affect 8–20% of HIV-infected children [93–95]. In the current era of highly active antiretroviral therapy (HAART) for perinatal HIV infection, the incidence of overt and rapidly progressive HIV encephalopathy seems to have decreased, but it may be associated with more subtle and insidious central nervous system manifestations [96].

The neuropathogenesis of HIV encephalopathy is poorly understood [91,96]. Studies have shown that HIV enters the CNS soon after primary infection and may persist in this compartment during the course of HIV infection [91]. CNS targets of HIV infection may be different in children and adults. In contrast to terminally differentiated cells of the mature nervous system of adults, the immature nervous system of children has mitotically active cells. Blood-derived macrophages, microglial cells, and their derivatives harbor HIV in the CNS [91,96]. The neuropathogenesis of HIV encephalopathy appears to involve a cascade of viral proteins, various cytokines (i.e., TNF-α) and chemokines, and neurotransmitters which promote ongoing inflammation, excitation, and overstimulation of the N-methyl-D-aspartate type receptor (NMDAR) system [96,97]. This subsequently leads to neuronal injury and death secondary to apoptosis or necrosis, astrocytosis, as well as dendritic and synaptic damage [98]. Neural progenitor cells may also be involved in the neuropathogenesis of HIV encephalopathy [99].

Neuropathologic evidence of pediatric HIV-related CNS disease includes decreased brain weight, cortical atrophy, symmetric intracerebral calcifications, white-matter changes, reactive astrocytosis, and subcortical gray-matter abnormalities of the basal ganglia, thalamus, claustrum, caudate, putamen, globus pallidus, and hippocampus [100–102]. HIV has been isolated from the brain of aborted fetuses from HIV-infected women, and from the brain and cerebrospinal fluid of HIV-infected children and adults [100,101]. HIV RNA and DNA have been detected in CNS tissue [103]. Although virus

has been recovered from cerebrospinal fluid of patients at all stages of HIV disease, including asymptomatic individuals, the highest rate of viral recovery is from those with symptomatic HIV infection or neurologic complaints [104].

Children with HIV infection can suffer from progressive encephalopathy, static encephalopathy, neuropsychiatric disorders, motor impairment, and cognitive decline [104–110]. In the pre-HAART era, more than 50% of children with AIDS had progressive encephalopathy [108,109]. Hypertonicity of the extremities was the hallmark of early-onset severe encephalopathy [96]. These affected children typically had severe immunosuppression at the time of presentation, but neurologic signs can occur before immune suppression [111]. Other risk factors for developing HIV encephalopathy include intrauterine infection, and high HIV RNA in plasma and CSF [96]. More recently, because of the ability to identify asymptomatic and mildly symptomatic HIV-infected children, the prevalence of progressive encephalopathy has dropped significantly, accounting for about 15% of all pediatric AIDS-defining conditions reported to the CDC [112].

Criteria for the definitive diagnosis of HIV encephalopathy are listed in Table 33.2. The syndrome is characterized by a classic triad of developmental delay, secondary or acquired microcephaly, and pyramidal tract neuromotor deficits [108,109]. Computed tomographic findings characteristic of HIV encephalopathy include cerebral atrophy (85% of cases) and bilateral symmetric calcification of the basal ganglia (15% of cases) [109,113]. The cerebrospinal fluid profile is often normal; however, mild pleocytosis and elevated protein concentrations may be present [102,104]. Encephalopathy in children with HIV is associated with a 28-fold increase in death, a 22-fold increase in wasting, and a 16-fold increase in cardiomyopathy [93]. Thus the diagnosis of the most severe, rapidly progressive form of encephalopathy in an HIV-infected child is a marker of poor prognosis.

Children infected with HIV display a range of neuropsychological problems, including learning and attention disorders, emotional and behavioral problems, depression, autistic behavior, and social withdrawal [106,110,114,115]. Using various age-appropriate neuropsychological tests (Bayley Scales of Infant Development, McCarthy Scales of Children's Abilities, and the Wechsler Intelligence Scale for Children – Revised), researchers have demonstrated that the overall level

Table 33.2. Manifestations of HIV encephalopathy in infants

Clinical manifestations	Neuroimaging findings
Acquired microcephaly	Cerebral atrophy
Developmental delay or regression	Symmetric calcifications in basal ganglia
Spasticity	
Pathologic reflexes	
Dystonia	
Gait abnormalities	
Expressive language impairment	

of neuropsychological functioning in HIV patients is below normal. HIV-infected children have mean full-scale intelligence quotients (FIQ) of 85.9, compared with FIQs of 100 in non-infected controls [114]. Neuropsychological abnormalities are not observed in HIV-exposed but uninfected infants [115,116]. A recent study examined the effects of perinatal HIV infection, in combination with other health and social factors, on cognitive development. The investigators found that an early AIDS-defining illness increased the risk of chronic static encephalopathy during the preschool and early school-age years [117].

Neurologic consequences of HIV infection vary with the state of infection. For example, asymptomatic patients have infrequent or no neurologic deficits while children with advanced AIDS often have profound and persistent neurologic abnormalities [105,107,109,114,115]. It is important to recognize the difficulty in evaluating the impact of the direct effects of HIV infection on neurodevelopment. Multiple confounding variables impacting neurodevelopment are often present in HIV-infected children. These variables include prematurity, low birthweight, in utero drug exposure, antiviral drug toxicities, nutritional deficits, endocrine abnormalities, and the social impacts of disease [105,116]. Furthermore, secondary CNS complications of infection may be present. Thus it is often not possible to isolate HIV's direct impact on neurodevelopment from the effects of these other variables.

Secondary CNS complications of HIV infection include opportunistic infections, neoplasms, and strokes. Opportunistic infections of the CNS are less common in children than in adults with HIV infection [118]. When these infections do occur in children, they are often diagnosed in those over 6 years of age with CD4 counts below 200. Central nervous system opportunistic agents include *Cryptococcus*, toxoplasmosis, cytomegalovirus, herpes simplex virus, *Candida* spp., JC virus, and syphilis [118]. Primary CNS lymphomas, non-Hodgkin lymphoma with CNS metastasis, and strokes are rare in children.

The rate of progression and severity of HIV encephalopathy are variable. HAART in children may prevent, reduce, or improve neurologic manifestations of HIV infection [91,95,96,119]. The optimal HAART regimen to treat HIV encephalopathy has not been established [120]. In early studies, zidovudine (ZDV) continuous therapy improved cognitive performance and reduced brain atrophy in a small study of symptomatic HIV-infected children [121,122]. Combination therapy with ZDV and didanosine was more effective than monotherapy with either agent in improving age-appropriate neurocognitive scores in young children with symptomatic HIV [110,122–124]. Central nervous system penetration differs substantially among current antiretroviral drugs [122]. Of the available agents, zidovudine has the best penetration into the CSF, followed by stavudine and high-dose abacavir [120]. Thus physicians are challenged to find adequate drug combinations to prevent and treat both CNS and systemic manifestations of HIV infection.

Early treatment

HAART is the standard of care for pediatric HIV infection in the USA. HAART has evolved from simple nucleoside reverse transcriptase inhibitor (NRTI) regimens of the 1980s and early 1990s to current complex regimens of NRTI in combination with protease inhibitors (PIs) and/or non-nucleoside reverse transcriptase inhibitors (NNRTIs). The introduction of such combination antiretroviral therapy has resulted in dramatic reductions in mortality and morbidity in both adults and children [6,125,126].

However, there are currently no randomized clinical trials addressing the question of when to begin combination antiretroviral therapy in asymptomatic HIV-1-infected infants who are diagnosed early in life. Current US pediatric guidelines recommend immediate initiation of HAART in all vertically HIV-infected infants under 12 months of age who have symptoms or immune suppression, and recommend consideration of therapy for asymptomatic infected infants under 12 months of age who have normal immune function [127]. The European guidelines recommend initiation of HAART in young infants only if there is evidence of clinical AIDS, CD4 T cells less than 20%, or HIV RNA viral load consistently greater than 10^6 copies per milliliter [128].

The consideration of treatment initiation for asymptomatic infants is based on the rationale that infants are at highest risk of rapid disease progression to AIDS or death, even when immune degradation and virus replication are moderately well contained, and that there are no reliable clinical or laboratory markers to distinguish those infants who will progress from those who will not [129–132]. Studies have shown that the initiation of combination antiretroviral therapy within the first 3 months of life can result in complete cessation of viral replication and the preservation of normal immune function [133–135]. Several regimens of antiretroviral therapy are safe, effective, and well tolerated for long periods of time when started in early infancy [133,136].

Preferred drug regimens include combination antiretroviral therapy – generally two NRTIs plus a PI or an NNRTI [127]. Infants in whom HIV infection is detected while on ZDV prophylaxis should receive combination antiretroviral therapy [127]. Because of adverse effects and drug interactions, not all agents can be paired in the regimens [127]. Resistance testing should be considered before starting antiretroviral therapy in newly diagnosed infants under the age of 12 months, especially if the mother has known or suspected infection with drug-resistant virus [127].

Treatment of infected infants with combination antiretroviral therapy is complex, and high rates of virologic failure have been noted [137,138]. Other challenges include issues of medication compliance to complex and demanding regimens, difficulties in developing pediatric formulations, immature drug metabolism, and the lack of age-specific pharmacokinetic data to guide pediatric dosing [139]. In addition, toxicity and development of drug resistance are other serious concerns [140]. Fortunately, several promising second-generation agents as well as new classes of antiretroviral agents are currently being evaluated in pediatric clinical trials [141].

Other aspects of HIV management include TB screening, assessment of organ system involvement, maintaining indicated immunizations, PCP and MAI prophylaxis, development and psychosocial assessments and intervention [8,85]. A family-centered approach involving a multidisciplinary team to integrate medical, social, and psychosocial support is critical.

Prognosis

Considerable progress has been made in understanding the natural history of HIV infection in children. Infants with perinatally acquired HIV-1 infection have widely variable clinical courses and durations of survival. Early reports suggest a bimodal disease expression, with 20–25% of untreated HIV-1-infected infants rapidly progressing to AIDS or death over the first year of life, while others have a better prognosis, some now surviving into young adulthood [80,142–144]. The presence of high viral load ($> 300\,000$ copies/mL), and the development of AIDS-defining conditions such as PCP pneumonia, HIV encephalopathy, and severe wasting are associated with a poor prognosis [8,80,142], whereas slow loss of CD4 T-lymphocyte count, late onset of clinical symptoms, and occurrence of LIP are associated with improved survival. Advanced maternal HIV-1 disease during pregnancy and high maternal viral load late in pregnancy or shortly after delivery are independently associated with disease progression in HIV-1-infected infants [145,146]. In the infant, early clinical symptoms and depressed maternal and infant CD4 T-cell count are determinants of disease progression by 6 months of age; in contrast, progression by 18 months of age is associated with presence of moderate clinical symptoms and elevated infant viral load [147]. Since the introduction of combination antiretroviral therapy, prognosis and survival of perinatally HIV-infected children has improved significantly [6,125,126].

The natural course of HIV infection in children differs from infected adults in a variety of ways. Firstly, the disease often progresses more rapidly in children; secondly, children have higher viral loads than adults; thirdly, children have recurrent bacterial infections more often and LIP is seen almost exclusively in children; fourthly, opportunistic infections often present as primary diseases with a more aggressive course due to lack of prior immunity; and finally certain infections like toxoplasmosis, cryptococcal infection, and cancer, especially Kaposi's sarcoma, are less frequent in the HIV-infected children [148].

Prevention

Preventing MTCT became a reality in 1994 when the Pediatric AIDS Clinical Trials Group protocol showed that a long course of ZDV prophylaxis given to an HIV-1-infected mother at 14 weeks of gestation and labor and to her newborn infant reduced MTCT by nearly 70% in a non-breastfeeding population [149]. Since then, MTCT rates have decreased to $< 2\%$ due to widespread implementation of routine antenatal HIV testing (opt-out approach), use of antiretroviral prophylaxis and HAART, elective cesarean delivery, and avoidance of breastfeeding [2–10,32,33,150].

Use of HAART among pregnant women is an integral component of PMTCT strategies in the USA and Europe. HAART is recommended for all HIV-infected pregnant women if maternal viral load is > 1000 copies/mL, along with consideration of elective cesarean delivery. Because of the proven benefit of antiretroviral prophylaxis in preventing MTCT, including those with viral load < 1000 copies/mL [38], all HIV-1-infected women should receive ZDV prophylaxis alone or HAART [151]. ZDV monotherapy administered to HIV-infected women with viral load < 1000 copies/mL has been shown to reduce perinatal HIV transmission to 1% [152]. In addition, no long-term effects on women's health have been noted among US women enrolled in the PACTG 076 trial in terms of disease progression, mortality, viral load, or ZDV resistance between randomized treatment and placebo arms [153].

When the woman has not received any therapy during pregnancy, several efficacious intrapartum/postpartum regimens are available. When the woman has not received any therapy during pregnancy, or during labor, ZDV should be prescribed to the neonate for 6 weeks [151,154]. In such instances, other antiretroviral agents could be added to the postnatal ZDV regimen [5].

Challenges to perinatal HIV-1 prevention

Despite significant advances in PMTCT, around 150 HIV-1-infected babies are born annually in the USA, primarily due to missed prevention opportunities, including inadequate prenatal care or lack of antenatal HIV testing [10,155]. Recently, the Mother–Infant Rapid Intervention at Delivery (MIRIAD) study demonstrated the feasibility of rapid HIV-1 testing of women with unknown HIV status during labor [156]. The MIRIAD study results have important implications for populations in developed countries, but may have a greater impact in sub-Saharan Africa, where approximately 29% of women do not receive prenatal care [156,157]. Knowledge of a women's HIV status during labor is crucial for providing ZDV prophylaxis for those who test positive and their babies, to prevent perinatal transmission [156]. Other challenges include preventing new HIV infections in women of childbearing age, especially adolescent girls of minority race or ethnicity, and preventing unplanned pregnancy in adolescent women [155,158].

There are major barriers to the implementation of perinatal HIV prevention programs in resource-poor countries [2,155, 157,159]. Major challenges include limited prenatal care services and HIV counseling and testing centers, and transmission of HIV through breastfeeding [5,16,17]. Limited resources, social and cultural issues, and divergent political agendas further compound the dilemma [155]. There is a clear need to bridge the gap in PMTCT programs between resource-rich and resource-limited countries [5]. Future efforts must focus on rapid scale-up and sustaining effective, simpler, and low-cost PMTCT programs worldwide, and develop innovative strategies to prevent transmission of HIV via breastfeeding [17,155].

Developing a safe and effective preventive infant HIV vaccine would be an optimal strategy to reduce transmission of HIV via breastfeeding [155,160]. Finally, saving the lives of parents through access to HAART is critically important, in order to blunt the global orphan crisis in sub-Saharan Africa [161].

References

1. Centers for Disease Control. Unexplained immunodeficiency and opportunistic infections in infants: New York, New Jersey, California. *MMWR* 1982; **31**: 665–7.

2. Prendergast A, Tudor-Williams G, Jeena P, *et al.* International perspectives, progress, and future challenges of paediatric HIV infection. *Lancet* 2007; **370**: 68–80.

3. Thorne C, Newell ML. HIV. *Semin Fetal Neonatal Med* 2007; **12**: 174–81.

4. Shetty AK, Maldonado Y. Advances in the prevention of perinatal HIV-1 transmission. *NeoReviews* 2005; **6**: 12–25.

5. Mofenson LM. Advances in the prevention of vertical transmission of human immunodeficiency virus. *Semin Pediatr Infect Dis* 2003; **14**: 295–308.

6. Gortmaker SL, Hughes M, Cervia J, *et al.* Effect of combination therapy including protease inhibitors on mortality among children and adolescents infected with HIV-1. *N Engl J Med* 2001; **345**: 1522–8.

7. King SM. American Academy of Pediatrics Committee on Pediatric AIDS, American Academy of Pediatrics Infectious Diseases and Immunization Committee. Evaluation and treatment of the human immunodeficiency virus-1-exposed infant. *Pediatrics* 2004; **114**: 497–505.

8. American Academy of Pediatrics. Human immunodeficiency virus infection. In Pickering LK, Baker CJ, Long SS, eds., *Red Book: 2006 Report of the Committee on Infectious Diseases*, 27th edn. Elk Grove Village, IL, American Academy of Pediatrics, 2006: 378–401.

9. Lindegren ML, Steinberg S, Byers RH. Epidemiology of HIV/AIDS in children. *Pediatr Clin N Am* 2004; **47**: 1–20.

10. Centers for Disease Control and Prevention. Achievements in public health: reduction in perinatal transmission of HIV infection: United States, 1985–2005. *MMWR Morb Mortal Wkly Rep* 2006; **55**: 592–7.

11. McKenna MT, Hu X. Recent trends in the incidence and morbidity that are associated with perinatal human immunodeficiency virus infection in the United States. *Am J Obstet Gynecol* 2007; **197**: S10–16.

12. Brady MT. Pediatric human immunodeficiency virus-1 infection. *Adv Pediatr* 2005; **52**: 163–93.

13. UNAIDS/World Health Organization. *AIDS Epidemic Update, December, 2006.* Geneva: UNAIDS, 2006.

14. Newell ML, Coovadia H, Cortina-Borja M, *et al.* Ghent International AIDS Society (IAS) Working Group on HIV Infection in Women and Children. Mortality of infected and uninfected infants born to HIV-infected mothers in Africa: a pooled analysis. *Lancet* 2004; **364**: 1236–43.

15. Kourtis AP, Lee FK, Abrams EJ, *et al.* Mother-to-child transmission of HIV-1: timing and implications for prevention. *Lancet Infect Dis* 2006; **6**: 726–32.

16. Fowler MG, Newell ML. Breastfeeding and HIV-1 transmission in resource-limited settings. *J Acquir Immune Defic Syndr* 2002; **30**: 230–9.

17. Kourtis AP, Jamieson DJ, Vincenzi I, *et al.* Prevention of human immunodeficiency virus-1 transmission to the infant through breastfeeding: new developments. *Am J Obstet Gynecol* 2007; **197**: S113–22.

18. Thorne C, Newell ML. Prevention of mother-to-child transmission of HIV infection. *Curr Opin Infect Dis* 2004; **17**: 247–52.

19. Working Group on Mother-to-Child Transmission of HIV. Rates of mother-to-child transmission of HIV-1 in Africa, America and Europe: results from 13 perinatal studies. *J Acquir Immune Defic Syndr Hum Retrovirol* 1995; **8**: 506–10.

20. Blanche S, Rouzioux C, Moscato MLG, *et al.* A prospective study of infants born to women seropositive for human immunodeficiency virus type 1. *N Engl J Med* 1989; **320**: 1643–8.

21. European Collaborative Study. Children born to women with HIV-1 infection: natural history and risk of transmission. *Lancet* 1991; **337**: 253–60.

22. Bryson YJ, Luzuriaga K, Sullivan JL, *et al.* Proposed definitions for in utero versus intrapartum transmission of HIV-1. *N Engl J Med* 1992; **327**: 1246–7.

23. Lewis SH, Reynolds-Kohler C, Fox HE, *et al.* HIV-1 trophoblastic and villous Hofbauer cells, and haematological precursors in eight-week fetuses. *Lancet* 1990; **335**: 565–8.

24. Lyman WD, Kress Y, Kure K, *et al.* Detection of HIV in fetal central nervous system tissue. *AIDS* 1990; **4**: 917–20.

25. Mano H, Cherman JC. Fetal human immunodeficiency virus type 1 infection of different organs in the second trimester. *AIDS Res Hum Retroviruses* 1991; **7**: 83–8.

26. Newell ML. Mechanisms and timing of mother-to-child transmission of HIV-1. *AIDS* 1998; **12**: 831–7.

27. Rogers MF, Ou CY, Rayfield M, *et al.* Use of the polymerase chain reaction for early detection of the proviral sequences of human immunodeficiency virus in infants born to seropositive mothers. *N Engl J Med* 1989; **320**: 1649–54.

28. Weiblen BJ, Lee FK, Cooper ER, *et al.* Early diagnosis of HIV infection in infants by detection of IgA HIV antibodies. *Lancet* 1990; **335**: 988–90.

29. Quinn TC, Kline RL, Halsey N, *et al.* Early diagnosis of perinatal HIV infection by detection of viral-specific IgA antibodies. *JAMA* 1991; **266**: 3439–942.

30. Krivine A, Firtion G, Cao L, *et al.* HIV replication during the first weeks of life. *Lancet* 1992; **339**: 1187–9.

31. Goedert JJ, Duliege AM, Amos CI, *et al.* High risk of HIV-1 infection for firstborn twins. *Lancet* 1991; **338**: 1471–5.

32. The International Perinatal HIV Group. The mode of delivery and the risk of vertical transmission of human immunodeficiency virus type 11: a meta-analysis of 15 prospective studies. *N Engl J Med* 1999; **340**: 977–87.

33. The European Mode of Delivery Collaboration. Elective cesarean section versus vaginal delivery in prevention

of vertical HIV-1 transmission: a randomized clinical trial. *Lancet* 1999; **353**: 1035–9.

34. Havens PL, Waters D. Management of the infant born to a mother with HIV infection. *Pediatr Clin North Am* 2004; **51**: 909–37.

35. Garcia P, Kalish LA, Pitt J, *et al.* Maternal levels of plasma human immunodeficiency virus type-1 RNA and the risk of perinatal transmission. *N Engl J Med* 1999; **341**: 394–402.

36. Mofenson LM, Lambert JS, Stiehm ER, *et al.* Risk factors for perinatal transmission of human immunodeficiency virus type 1 in women treated with zidovudine. *N Engl J Med* 1999; **341**: 385–93.

37. Magder LS, Mofenson L, Paul ME, *et al.* Risk factors for in utero and intrapartum transmission of HIV. *J Acquir Immune Defic Syndr* 2005; **38**: 87–95.

38. Ioannidis JPA, Abrams EJ, Ammann A, *et al.* Perinatal transmission of human immunodeficiency virus type 1 by pregnant women with RNA virus loads < 1000 copies/ml. *J Infect Dis* 2001; **183**: 539–45.

39. O'Shea S, Newell ML, Dunn D, *et al.* Maternal viral load, CD4 cell count and vertical transmission of HIV-1. *J Med Virol* 1998; **54**: 113–17.

40. Mock P, Shaffer N, Bhadrakom C, *et al.* Maternal viral load and timing of mother-to-child HIV transmission, Bangkok, Thailand. *AIDS* 1999; **13**: 407–14.

41. St Louis ME, Kamenga M, Brown C, *et al.* Risk for perinatal HIV-1 transmission according to maternal immunologic, virologic, and placental factors. *JAMA* 1993; **269**: 2853–9.

42. Borkowsky W, Krasinski K, Cao Y, *et al.* Correlation of perinatal transmission of human immunodeficiency virus type 1 with maternal viremia and lymphocyte phenotypes. *J Pediatr* 1994; **125**: 345–51.

43. Sperling RS, Shapiro DE, Coombs RW, *et al.* Maternal viral load, zidovudine treatment, and the risk of transmission of human immunodeficiency virus type 1 from mother to infant. *N Engl J Med* 1996; **335**: 1621–9.

44. Newell ML, Peckham C. Risk factors for vertical transmission of HIV-1 and early markers of HIV-1 infection in children. *AIDS* 1993; **7**: S591–7.

45. Gabiano C, Tobo PA, de Martino M, *et al.* Mother-to-child transmission of

human immunodeficiency virus type 1: risk of infection and correlates of transmission. *Pediatrics* 1992; **90**: 369–74.

46. Thomas PA, Weedon J, Krasinski K, *et al.* Maternal predictors of perinatal human immunodeficiency virus transmission. *Pediatr Infect Dis J* 1994; **13**: 489–95.

47. Mayers MM, Davenny K, Schoenbaum EE, *et al.* A prospective study of infants of human immunodeficiency virus seropositive and seronegative women with a history of intravenous drug use or of intravenous drug-using sex partners, in the Bronx, New York City. *Pediatrics* 1991; **88**: 1248–56.

48. European Collaborative Study. Risk factors for mother-to-child transmission of HIV-1. *Lancet* 1992; **339**: 1007–12.

49. Chuachoowong R, Shaffer N, Siriwasin W, *et al.* Short-course antenatal zidovudine reduces both cervicovaginal human immunodeficiency virus type 1 RNA levels and risk of perinatal transmission. Bangkok Collaborative Perinatal HIV Transmission Study Group. *J Infect Dis* 2000; **181**: 99–106.

50. Landesman SH, Kalish LA, Burns D, *et al.* Obstetrical factors and the transmission of human immunodeficiency virus type 1 from mother to child. *N Engl J Med* 1996; **334**: 1617–23.

51. European Collaborative Study. Vertical transmission of HIV-1: maternal immune status and obstetric factors. *AIDS* 1996; **10**: 1675–81.

52. Goedert JJ, Mendez H, Drummond JE, *et al.* Mother-to-infant transmission of human immunodeficiency virus type 1: association with prematurity or low antigp120. *Lancet* 1989; **2**: 1351–4.

53. Tovo PA, de Martino M, Gabiano C, *et al.* Mode of delivery and gestational age influence perinatal HIV-1 transmission. *J Acquir Immune Defic Syndr Hum Retrovirol* 1996; **11**: 88–94.

54. Wolinsky SM, Wike CM, Korber BTM, *et al.* Selective transmission of human immunodeficiency virus type-1 variants from mothers to infants. *Science* 1992; **255**: 1134–7.

55. MacDonald KS, Embree J, Njenga S, *et al.* Mother–child class I HLA concordance increases perinatal human immunodeficiency virus type 1 transmission. *J Infect Dis* 1998; **177**: 551–6.

56. Kostrikis LG. Impact of natural chemokine receptor polymorphisms on perinatal transmission of human

immunodeficiency virus type 1. *Teratology* 2000; **61**: 387–90.

57. John-Stewart G, Mbori-Ngacha D, Ekpini R, *et al.* Breast-feeding and transmission of HIV-1. *J Acquir Immune Defic Syndr* 2004; **35**: 196–202.

58. Coutsoudis A, Dabis F, Fawzi W, *et al.* Late postnatal transmission of HIV-1 in breastfed children: an individual patient data meta-analysis. *J Infect Dis* 2004; **189**: 2154–66.

59. Lewis P, Nduati RW, Kreiss JK, *et al.* Cell-free HIV type 1 in breast milk. *J Infect Dis* 1998; **177**: 34–9.

60. Koulinska IN, Villamour E, Chaplin B, *et al.* Transmission of cell-free and cell-associated HIV-1 through breastfeeding. *J Acquir Immune Defic Syndr* 2006; **41**: 93–9.

61. Dunn DT, Newell ML, Ades AE, *et al.* Risk of human immunodeficiency virus type 1 transmission through breastfeeding. *Lancet* 1992; **340**: 585–8.

62. Tess BH, Rodrigues LC, Newell ML, *et al.* Breastfeeding, genetic, obstetric and other risk factors associated with mother-to-child transmission of HIV-1 in Sao Paulo State, Brazil. *AIDS* 1998; **12**: 513–20.

63. Bobat R, Moodley D, Coutsoudis A, *et al.* Breastfeeding by HIV-1 infected women and outcome in their infants: a cohort study from Durban, South Africa. *AIDS* 1997; **11**: 1627–33.

64. Nduati R, John G, Mbori-Ngacha D, *et al.* Effect of breastfeeding and formula feeding on transmission of HIV-1: a randomized controlled trial. *JAMA* 2000; **283**: 1167–74.

65. Miotti PG, Taha TET, Kumwenda NI, *et al.* HIV transmission through breastfeeding: a study in Malawi. *JAMA* 1999; **282**: 744–9.

66. Bertolli J, St Louis ME, Simonds RJ, *et al.* Estimating the timing of mother-to-child transmission of human immunodeficiency virus in a breast-feeding population in Kinshasa, Zaire. *J Infect Dis* 1996; **174**: 722–6.

67. Epkini ER, Wiktor SZ, Satten FA, *et al.* Late postnatal mother-to-child transmission of HIV-1 in Abidjan, Cote d'Ivoire. *Lancet* 1997; **349**: 1054–9.

68. Leroy V, Newell ML, Dabis F, *et al.* International multicentre pooled analysis of late postnatal mother-to-child transmission of HIV-1 infection. *Lancet* 1998; **352**: 597–600.

69. Taha TE, Hoover DR, Kumwenda NI, *et al.* Late postnatal transmission of

HIV-1 and associated risk factors. *J Infect Dis* 2007; **196**: 10–14.

70. Iliff PJ, Piwoz EG, Tacengwa NV, *et al.* Early exclusive breastfeeding reduces the risk of postnatal HIV-1 transmission and increases HIV-free survival. *AIDS* 2005; **19**: 699–708.

71. Coovadia HM, Rollins NC, Bland RM, *et al.* Mother-to-child transmission of HIV-1 infection during exclusive breastfeeding in the first 6 months of life: an intervention cohort study. *Lancet* 2007; **369**: 1107–16.

72. Read JS and the Committee on Pediatric AIDS, American Academy of Pediatrics. Diagnosis of HIV-1 infection in children younger than 18 months in the United States. *Pediatrics* 2007; **120**: 1547–62.

73. Owens DK, Holodniy M, McDonald TW, *et al.* A meta-analytic evaluation of the polymerase chain reaction for the diagnosis of HIV infection in infants. *JAMA* 1996; **275**: 1342–8.

74. Cunningham CK, Charbonneau TT, Song K, *et al.* Comparison of human immunodeficiency virus 1 DNA polymerase chain reaction and qualitative and quantitative RNA polymerase chain reaction in human immunodeficiency virus 1-exposed infants. *Pediatr Infect Dis J* 1999; **18**: 30–5.

75. Simonds RJ, Brown TM, Thea DM, *et al.* Sensitivity and specificity of a qualitative RNA detection assay to diagnose HIV infection in young infants. Perinatal AIDS Collaborative Transmission Study. *AIDS* 1998; **12**: 1545–9.

76. Rouet F, Montcho C, Rouzioux C, *et al.* Early diagnosis of paediatric HIV-1 infection among African breast-fed children using a quantitative plasma HIV RNA assay. *AIDS* 2001; **15**: 1849–56.

77. Young NL, Shaffer N, Chaowanachan T, *et al.* Early diagnosis of HIV-1-infected infants in Thailand using RNA and DNA PCR assays sensitive to non-B subtypes. *J Acquir Immune Defic Syndr* 2000; **24**: 401–7.

78. Luzuriaga K, Wu H, McManus M, *et al.* Dynamics of human immunodeficiency virus type 1 replication in vertically infected infants. *J Virol* 1999; **73**: 362–7.

79. Blanche S, Newell ML, Mayaux MJ, *et al.* Morbidity and mortality in European children vertically infected by HIV-1. The French Pediatric HIV Infection Study Group and European Collaborative Study. *J Acquir Immune Defic Syndr Hum Retrovirol* 1997; **14**: 442–50.

80. Scott GB, Hutto C, Makuch RW, *et al.* Survival in children with perinatally acquired human immunodeficiency virus type 1 infection. *N Engl J Med* 1989; **321**: 1791–6.

81. Marion RW, Wiznia AA, Hutcheon G, *et al.* Human T-cell lymphotropic virus type III (HTLV-III) embryopathy: a new dysmorphic syndrome associated with intrauterine HTLV-III infection. *Am J Dis Child* 1986; **140**: 638–40.

82. Qazi QH, Sheikh TM, Fikrig S, *et al.* Lack of evidence for craniofacial dysmorphism in perinatal human immunodeficiency virus infection. *J Pediatr* 1998; **112**: 7–11.

83. Galli L, deMartino M, Tovo PA, *et al.* Onset of clinical signs with HIV-1 perinatal infection. *AIDS* 1995; **9**: 455–61.

84. Newell ML, Peckham C, Dunn D, *et al.* Natural history of vertically-acquired human immunodeficiency virus-1 infection. The European Collaborative Study. *Pediatrics* 1994; **94**: 815–19.

85. Mofenson LM, Oleske J, Serchuck L, *et al.* Treating opportunistic infections among HIV-exposed and infected children: recommendations from CDC, the National Institutes of Health, and the Infectious Diseases Society of America. *MMWR Recomm Rep* 2004; **53**: 1–92.

86. Pollack H, Glasberg H, Lee E, *et al.* Impaired early growth of infants perinatally infected with human immunodeficiency virus: correlation with viral load. *J Pediatr* 1997; **130**: 915–22.

87. Kline MW. Vertically acquired human immunodeficiency virus infection. *Semin Pedatr Infect Dis* 1999; **10**: 147–53.

88. Centers for Disease Control. Revision of the CDC surveillance case definition for acquired immune deficiency syndrome. *MMWR* 1987; **36**: 1–15.

89. Centers for Disease Control and Prevention. 1994 revised classification system for human immunodeficiency virus infection in children less than 13 years of age. *MMWR* 1994; **43**: 1–11.

90. Simonds RJ, Oxtoby MJ, Caldwell MB, *et al. Pneumocystis carinii* pneumonia among US children with perinatally acquired HIV infection. *JAMA* 1993; **270**: 470–3.

91. Van Rie A, Harrington PR, Dow A, *et al.* Neurologic and neurodevelopmental manifestations of pediatric HIV/AIDS: a global perspective. *Eur J Paediatr Neurol* 2007; **11**: 1–9.

92. Gorry PR, Bristol G, Zack JA, *et al.* Macrophage tropism of human immunodeficiency virus type 1 isolates from brain and lymphoid tissues predict neurotropism independent of coreceptor specificity. *J Virol* 2001; **75**: 10073–89.

93. Cooper ER, Hanson C, Diaz C, *et al.* Encephalopathy and progression of human immunodeficiency virus disease in a cohort of children with perinatally acquired human immunodeficiency virus infection. *J Pediatr* 1998; **132**: 808–12.

94. Labato MN, Caldwell MB, Ng P, *et al.* Encephalopathy in children with perinatally acquired human immunodeficiency virus infection. *J Pediatr* 1995; **126**: 710–15.

95. Chiriboga CA, Fleishman S, Champion S, *et al.* Incidence and prevalence of HIV encephalopathy in children with HIV infection receiving highly active anti-retroviral therapy (HAART). *J Pediatr* 2005; **146**: 402–7.

96. Mitchell CD. HIV-1 encephalopathy among perinatally infected children: neuropathogenesis and response to highly active antiretroviral therapy. *Ment Retard Dev Disabil Res Rev* 2006; **12**: 216–22.

97. Kaul M, Zheng J, Okamoto S, *et al.* HIV-1 infection and AIDS: consequences for the CNS. *Cell Death Differ* 2005; **12**: 878–92.

98. Epstein LG, Gelbard HA. HIV-1-induced neuronal injury in the developing brain. *J Leukoc Biol* 1999; **65**: 453–7.

99. Schwartz L, Major EO. Neural progenitors and HIV-1-associated central nervous system disease in adults and children. *Curr HIV Res* 2006; **4**: 319–27.

100. Lyman YD, Kress Y, Kure K, *et al.* Detection of HIV in fetal central nervous tissue. *AIDS* 1990; **4**: 917–20.

101. Kozlowski PB, Brudkowska J, Kraszpulski M, *et al.* Microencephaly in children congenitally infected with human immunodeficiency virus: a gross-anatomical morphometric study. *Acta Neuropathol (Berl)* 1997; **93**: 136–45.

102. Levy JA, Shimabukuro J, Hollander H, *et al.* Isolation of AIDS-associated retroviruses from cerebrospinal fluid and brain of patients with neurological symptoms. *Lancet* 1985; **2**: 586–8.

103. Shaw GM, Harper ME, Hahn BH, *et al.* HTLV-III infection in brains of children and adults with AIDS encephalopathy. *Science* 1985; **227**: 177–82.

104. Hollander H, Levy JA. Neurologic abnormalities and recovery of human immunodeficiency virus from cerebrospinal fluid. *Ann Intern Med* 1987; **106**: 692–5.

105. Belman AL. Pediatric neuro-AIDS: update. *Neuroimaging Clin North Am* 1997; **7**: 593–613.

106. Brouwers P, De Carli C, Civitello L, *et al.* Correlation between computed tomographic brain scan abnormalities and neuropsychological function in children with symptomatic human immunodeficiency virus disease. *Arch Neurol* 1995; **52**: 39–44.

107. Cooper ER, Hanson C, Diaz C, *et al.* Encephalopathy and progression of human immunodeficiency virus disease in a cohort of children with perinatally acquired human immunodeficiency virus infection. Women and Infants Transmission Study Group. *J Pediatr* 1998; **132**: 808–12.

108. Belman AL, Ultmann MH, Horoupian D, *et al.* Neurologic complications in infants and children with acquired immune deficiency syndrome. *Ann Neurol* 1985; **18**: 560–6.

109. Epstein LG, Sharer LR, Oleske JM, *et al.* Neurologic manifestations of human immunodeficiency virus infection in children. *Pediatrics* 1986; **78**: 678–87.

110. Raskino C, Pearson DA, Baker CJ, *et al.* Neurologic, neurocognitive and brain growth outcomes in human immunodeficiency virus-infected children receiving different nucleoside antiretroviral regimens. *Pediatrics* 1999; **104**: e32.

111. Tardieu M, Le Chenadec J, Persoz A, *et al.* HIV-1 related encephalopathy in infants compared with children and adults. French Pediatric HIV Infection Study and the SEROCO Group. *Neurology* 2000; **54**: 1089–95.

112. Centers for Disease Control and Prevention. *HIV/AIDS Surveillance Report.* Atlanta, GA: CDC, 1993.

113. Johann-Liang R, Lin K, Cervia J, *et al.* Neuroimaging findings in children perinatally infected with the human immunodeficiency virus. *Pediatr Infect Dis J* 1998; **17**: 753–4.

114. Brouwers P, Tudor-Williams G, DeCarli C, *et al.* Relation between stage of disease and neurobehavioral measures in children with symptomatic HIV disease. *AIDS* 1995; **9**: 713–20.

115. Nozyce M, Hittelman J, Muenz L, *et al.* Effect of perinatally acquired human immunodeficiency virus infection on neurodevelopment in children during the first two years of life. *Pediatrics* 1994; **94**: 883–91.

116. Belman AL, Muenz LR, Marcus JC, *et al.* Neurologic status of human immunodeficiency virus 1-infected infants and their controls: a prospective study from birth to 2 years. Mothers and Infants Cohort Study. *Pediatrics* 1996; **98**: 1109–18.

117. Smith R, Malee K, Leighty R, *et al.* Women and Infants Transmission Study Group. Effects of perinatal HIV infection and associated risk factors on cognitive development among young children. *Pediatrics* 2006; **117**: 851–62.

118. Mintz M. Clinical features and treatment interventions for human immunodeficiency virus-associated neurologic disease in children. *Semin Neurol* 1999; **19**: 165–76.

119. Sanchez-Ramon S, Resino S, Bellon Cano JM, *et al.* Neuroprotective effects of early antiretrovirals in vertical HIV infection. *Pediatr Neurol* 2003; **29**: 218–21.

120. Saavedra-Lozano J, Ramos JT, Sanz F, *et al.* Salvage therapy with abacavir and other reverse transcriptase inhibitors for human immunodeficiency-associated encephalopathy. *Pediatr Infect Dis J* 2006; **25**: 1142–52.

121. DeCarli C, Fugate L, Falloon J, *et al.* Brain growth and cognitive improvement in children with human immunodeficiency virus-induced encephalopathy after 6 months of continuous infusion zidovudine therapy. *J Acquir Immune Defic Syndr* 1991; **4**: 585–92.

122. Pizzo PA, Eddy J, Falloon J, *et al.* Effect of continuous intravenous infusion of zidovudine (AZT) in children with symptomatic HIV infection. *N Engl J Med* 1988; **319**: 889–96.

123. Portegies P. HIV-1, the brain, and combination therapy. *Lancet* 1995; **346**: 1244–5.

124. McCoig C, Castrejon MM, Castano E, *et al.* Effects of combination antiretroviral therapy on cerebrospinal fluid HIV RNA, HIV resistance, and clinical manifestations of encephalopathy. *J Pediatr* 2002; **141**: 36–44.

125. Berk DR, Falkovitz-Halpern MS, Hill DW. Temporal trends in early clinical manifestations of perinatal HIV infection in a population-based cohort. *JAMA* 2005; **293**: 2221–31.

126. De Martino M, Tovo PA, Balducci M, *et al.* Reduction in mortality with availability of antiretroviral therapy for children with perinatal HIV-1 infection. Italian Register for HIV infection in children and the Italian national AIDS registry. *JAMA* 2000; **284**: 190–7.

127. Working Group on Antiretroviral Therapy and Medical Management of HIV-infected Children. *Guidelines for the Use of Antiretroviral Agents in Pediatric HIV Infection.* Rockville, MD: AIDSInfo, 2005. aidsinfo.nih.gov. Accessed March, 2008.

128. Sharland N, di Zub GC, Ramos JT, *et al.* PENTA guidelines for the use of antiretroviral therapy in paediatric HIV infection. *HIV Med* 2002; **3**: 215–26.

129. Abrams EJ, Kuhn L. Should treatment be started among all HIV-infected children and then stopped? *Lancet* 2003; **362**: 1595–6.

130. Gray L, Newell ML, Thorne C, *et al.* Fluctuations in symptoms in human immunodeficiency virus-infected children: the first 10 years of life. *Pediatrics* 2001; **108**: 116–22.

131. Diaz C, Hanson C, Cooper ER, *et al.* Disease progression in a cohort of infants with vertically acquired HIV infection observed from birth: the Women and Infants Transmission Study (WITS). *J Acquir Immune Defic Syndr Hum Retrovirol* 1998; **18**: 221–8.

132. Anabwani GM, Woldetsadik EA, Kline MW. Treatment of human immunodeficiency virus (HIV) in children using antiretroviral drugs. *Semin Pediatr Infect Dis* 2005; **16**: 116–24.

133. Luzuriaga K, McManus M, Mofenson LM, *et al.* A trial of three antiretroviral regimens in HIV-1 infected children. *N Engl J Med* 2004; **350**: 2471–80.

134. Luzuriaga K, Bryson Y, Krogstad P, *et al.* Combination treatment with zidovudine, didanosine, and nevirapine in infants with human immunodeficiency virus type 1 infection. *N Engl J Med* 1997; **336**: 1343–9.

135. Luzuriaga K, McManus M, Catalina M, *et al.* Early therapy of vertical human immunodeficiency virus type 1 (HIV-1) infection: control of viral replication and absence of persistent HIV-1 specific immune responses. *J Virol* 2000; **74**: 6984–91.

136. Hainaut M, Peltier CA, Gerard M, *et al.* Effectiveness of antiretroviral therapy initiated before the age of 2 months in

infants vertically infected with human immunodeficiency virus type 1. *Eur J Pediatr* 2000; **159**: 778–82.

137. Faye A, Bertone C, Teglas JP, *et al.* Early multitherapy including a protease inhibitor for human immunodeficiency virus type 1 infected infants. *Pediatr Infect Dis J* 2002; **21**: 518–25.

138. Paediatric European Network for Treatment of AIDS (PENTA). Highly active antiretroviral therapy started in infants under 3 months of age: 72 week follow-up for CD4 cell count, viral load and drug resistance outcome. *AIDS* 2004; **18**: 237–45.

139. Litalien C, Faye A, Compagnucci A, *et al.* Pharmacokinetics of nelfinavir and its active metabolite, hydroxyl-tert-butylamide, in infants less than 1 year old perinatally infected with HIV-1. *Pediatr Infect Dis J* 2003; **22**: 48–56.

140. Hoody DW, Fletcher CV. Pharmacology considerations for antiretroviral therapy in human immunodeficiency virus (HIV)-infected children. *Semin Pediatr Infect Dis* 2003; **14**: 286–94.

141. McKinney RE, Cunningham CK. Newer treatment for HIV in children. *Curr Opin Pediatr* 2004; **16**: 76–9.

142. Blanche S, Tardieu M, Duliege AA, *et al.* Longitudinal study of 94 symptomatic infants with perinatally acquired human immunodeficiency virus infection. *Am J Dis Child* 1990; **144**: 1210–14.

143. Blanche S, Newell ML, Mayaux MJ, *et al.* Morbidity and mortality in European children vertically infected by HIV-1. The French Pediatric HIV Infection Study Group and European Collaborative Study. *J Acquir Immune Defic Syndr Hum Retrovirol* 1997; **14**: 442–50.

144. Thorne C, Newell ML, Botet FA, *et al.* Older children and adolescents surviving with vertically acquired infection. *J AIDS* 2002; **29**: 396–401.

145. Lambert G, Thea DM, Pliner V, *et al.* Effect of maternal CD4+ cell count, acquired immune deficiency syndrome, and viral load on disease progression in infants with perinatally acquired human immunodeficiency virus type 1 infection. *J Pediatr* 1997; **130**: 830–7.

146. Abrams EJ, Wiener J, Carter R, *et al.* Maternal health factors and early pediatric antiretroviral therapy influence the rate of perinatal HIV-1 disease progression in children. *AIDS* 2003; **17**: 867–77.

147. Rich KC, Fowler MG, Mofenson LM, *et al.* Maternal and infant factors predicting disease progression in human immunodeficiency virus type 1-infected infants. *Pediatrics* 2000; **105**: e8.

148. Maldonado Y. Acquired immunodeficiency syndrome in the infant. In Remington JS, Klein JO, Wilson C, *et al.* eds., *Infectious Diseases of the Fetus and Newborn Infant*, 6th edn. Philadelphia, PA: Saunders, 2006: 667–92.

149. Connor EM, Sperling RS, Gelber R, *et al.* Reduction of maternal–infant transmission of human immunodeficiency virus type 1 with zidovudine treatment. *N Engl J Med* 1994; **331**: 1173–80.

150. Cooper E, Charurat M, Mofenson L, *et al.* Combination antiretroviral strategies for the treatment of pregnant HIV-1 infected women and prevention of perinatal HIV-1 transmission. *J Acquir Immune Defic Syndr* 2002; **29**; 484–94.

151. Centers for Disease Control and Prevention. U.S. Public Health Service Task Force recommendations for use of antiretroviral drugs in pregnant women for maternal health and interventions to reduce perinatal HIV-1 transmission in the United States. *MMWR Recomm Rep* 2002; **51**: 1–40.

152. Shaffer N, Chuachoowong R, Mock PA, *et al.* Short-course zidovudine for perinatal HIV-1 transmission in

Bangkok, Thailand: a randomized controlled trial. *Lancet* 1999; **353**: 773–80.

153. Bardeguez AD, Shapiro DE, Mofenson LM, *et al.* Effect of cessation of zidovudine prophylaxis to reduce vertical transmission on maternal HIV disease progression and survival. *J Acquir Immune Defic Syndr* 2003; **32**: 170–81.

154. Wade NA, Birkhead GS, Warren BL, *et al.* Abbreviated regimens of zidovudine prophylaxis and perinatal transmission of the human immunodeficiency virus. *N Engl J Med* 1998; **339**: 1409–14.

155. Fowler MG, Lamper MA, Jamieson DJ, *et al.* Reducing the risk of mother-to-child human immunodeficiency virus transmission: past successes, current progress and challenges, and future directions. *Am J Obstet Gynecol* 2007; **197**: S3–9.

156. Bulterys M, Jamieson DJ, O'Sullivan MJ, *et al.* Rapid HIV-1 testing during labor: a multicenter study. *JAMA* 2004; **292**: 219–23.

157. Wilfert CM, Stringer JS. Prevention of pediatric human immunodeficiency virus. *Semin Pediatr Infect Dis* 2004; **15**: 190–8.

158. Mofenson LM. Successes and challenges in the perinatal HIV-1 epidemic in the United States as illustrated by the HIV-1 serosurvey of childbearing women. *Arch Pediatr Adolesc Med* 2004; **158**: 422–5.

159. Shetty AK, Maldonado M. Preventing mother-to-child transmission of human immunodeficiency virus type 1 in resource-poor countries. *Pediatr Infect Dis J* 2003; **22**: 553–5.

160. Gallo RC. The end or the beginning of the drive to an HIV-preventive vaccine: a view from over 20 years. *Lancet* 2005; **366**: 1894–8.

161. Drew RS, Makufa C, Foster G. Strategies for providing care and support to children orphaned by AIDS. *AIDS Care* 1998; **10**: S9–15.

Chapter 34

Inborn errors of metabolism with features of hypoxic–ischemic encephalopathy

Gregory M. Enns

Introduction

Inborn errors of metabolism that present in the neonatal period can have clinical, biochemical, and neuroradiologic features similar to those of hypoxic–ischemic encephalopathy (HIE). Both metabolic disorders and HIE are associated with severe neurologic distress, metabolic acidosis, and multiorgan system involvement. Perinatal asphyxia affects 2–4/1000 neonates, with encephalopathy occurring in 25% and death in an additional 30% [1]. In general, the patterns of brain injury are different when HIE and inborn errors of metabolism are compared. However, some metabolic disorders may have neuroradiologic findings similar to those seen in HIE. Inborn errors are rare individually, but as a group they affect approximately 1/1000 neonates [2]. It is crucial to consider these disorders in the differential diagnosis of patients who present with non-specific features suggestive of sepsis or asphyxia. Prompt diagnosis not only may prevent mortality or significant morbidity, but also allows the clinician to provide the family with accurate genetic counseling. Although expanded newborn screening using tandem mass spectrometry (MS/MS) will detect a number of metabolic disorders, this testing will miss many inborn errors of metabolism that present with HIE-like features. In such cases, specialized testing is required in order to establish a diagnosis. In this chapter, patterns of brain injury and systemic complications that occur in HIE and metabolic disorders are reviewed. Specific inborn errors of metabolism with clinical presentations that may be seen in patients with HIE are discussed further.

Patterns of brain injury in HIE and inborn errors of metabolism

Neonatal hypoxic–ischemic brain injury may be caused by localized infarction or a diffuse ischemic insult. Focal ischemic infarction in the neonate typically presents with lethargy, hypotonia, or seizures. Most infarcts occur in full-term infants and are localized to the distribution of an artery, especially the middle cerebral artery and its branches. Reported causes of focal infarction include cardiac disorders, emboli, infection, coagulation abnormalities, or birth asphyxia, although in

many cases an etiology is never found [3]. Metabolic causes of focal ischemia are listed in Table 34.1, but will not be reviewed in this chapter.

Diffuse hypoxic–ischemic injury affects different brain regions, depending on the duration and severity of the insult, the gestational age of the infant, and the presence or absence of systemic stress [4]. Mild to moderate cerebral hypotension, with impaired brain vascular autoregulation, results in the shunting of blood from the anterior to posterior circulation, in order to maintain blood flow to the basal ganglia, brainstem, and cerebellum. Brain damage is thus restricted to the cerebral hemisphere intervascular boundary zones ("watershed regions") [3,5,6]. Because the location of the watershed regions changes with brain maturation, different patterns of cerebral damage are encountered in premature and term infants. Mild to moderate cerebral hypotension in premature infants results in periventricular white-matter injury, with sparing of the cerebral cortex and subcortical white matter. By the 34th–36th week of gestation, the watershed areas have shifted peripherally to include the subcortical white matter and cerebral cortex. Therefore, term infants who sustain brain injury as a result of mild to moderate hypotension have damage primarily in the cortex and underlying subcortical and periventricular white matter [6].

Severe cerebral hypotension, with complete or near-complete interruption of the cerebral blood supply, results in deep gray-matter (especially thalami and basal ganglia) and brainstem damage [7]. In this case, the shunting of blood is not sufficient to prevent deep gray-matter damage. Damage to white matter and the cerebral cortex are later sequelae to profound hypotension. Profound cerebral hypotension also causes different patterns of brain injury depending on brain maturity [5,6]. In the early third trimester, the thalami and brainstem have the highest metabolic activity and relative blood flow. The thalami, brainstem, basal ganglia, and perirolandic region have the highest metabolic activity from the middle of the third trimester through 40 weeks of gestation. By the end of the first postnatal month, the visual cortex has an increased metabolic activity and is susceptible to damage. The basal ganglia remain highly vulnerable to injury from HIE or other environmental stress factors until approximately age 3 years [8].

The pattern of brain involvement is also dependent on the duration of injury. In mild to moderate hypoperfusion, the

Fetal and Neonatal Brain Injury, 4th edition, ed. David K. Stevenson, William E. Benitz, Philip Sunshine, Susan R. Hintz, and Maurice L. Druzin. Published by Cambridge University Press. © Cambridge University Press 2009.

Table 34.1. Inborn errors of metabolism associated with stroke in childhood

Organic acidurias

  Propionic acidemia

  Methylmalonic acidemia

  Isovaleric acidemia

  Glutaric aciduria type I

  Multiple acyl-coenzyme A (CoA) dehydrogenase deficiency (glutaric aciduria type II)

  3-Methylcrotonyl CoA carboxylase deficiency

  3-Hydroxy-3-methylglutaryl CoA lyase deficiency

Aminoacidemias

  Homocystinuria

  Methylene tetrahydrofolate reductase (MTHFR) deficiency

  Sulfite oxidase deficiency

  Molybdenum cofactor deficiency

Urea cycle disorders

  Ornithine transcarbamylase deficiency

  Carbamyl phosphate synthetase deficiency

Mitochondrial disorders

  MELAS (mitochondrial encephalomyopathy, lactic acidosis, and stroke-like episodes)

  Leigh syndrome

  Cytochrome oxidase (complex IV) deficiency

Lysosomal storage disorders

  Fabry disease

  Cystinosis

Other

  Congenital disorders of glycosylation[a]

  Phosphoglycerate kinase deficiency

  Hyperlipoproteinemia

  Menkes disease

  Purine nucleoside phosphorylase deficiency

Note:
[a]Formerly carbohydrate-deficient glycoprotein syndrome.
Source: Adapted from Barkovich AJ. *Pediatric Neuroimaging*, 3rd edn. Philadelphia, PA: Lippincott Williams & Wilkins, 2000.

areas affected by ischemia are limited to the watershed regions and periventricular white matter. Progression of damage beyond watershed regions does not occur unless the hypoperfusion becomes more severe. In severe hypoperfusion, no damage is present if the duration of circulatory arrest is less than approximately 10 minutes. Damage to the ventrolateral thalami, globus pallidus, posterior putamen, perirolandic cortex, and hippocampi may be seen in arrest lasting 10–15 minutes. The superior vermis, optic radiation, and calcarine cortex become involved with increasing duration of arrest. By 25–30 minutes of arrest, injury is present in nearly all the gray matter [9].

In contrast to the patterns of brain injury encountered in classic HIE, metabolic disorders typically affect different areas of the brain [8,9]. Whereas head magnetic resonance imaging

(MRI) evaluation in HIE often shows hyperintense signal in the putamen (with relative sparing of the anterior putamen) and thalamus, metabolic disorders affect other structures. Metabolic conditions with differential involvement of white and gray matter are listed in Tables 34.2–34.4. Disorders of mitochondrial energy metabolism may present with a wide spectrum of lesions, but abnormal hyperintense signal in the globus pallidus and periatrial white matter of the centrum semiovale are often present [8]. Pyruvate dehydrogenase deficiency, organic acidemias, carbon monoxide or cyanide poisoning, and hypothermic circulatory arrest during cardiac surgery have been associated with similar abnormal signals in the globus pallidus [8,9]. Mitochondrial disorders may also present with isolated white-matter disease, Leigh syndrome, or even normal MRI findings [9]. Different patterns of abnormality may suggest other underlying inborn errors of metabolism. For example, basal ganglia "metabolic strokes" have been associated with methylmalonic and propionic acidemias [10]. It is important to emphasize that normal head imaging does not exclude the presence of an inborn error of metabolism [8].

The mechanisms underlying the differential effects of HIE and metabolic disorders on the brain have been the subject of much study [1,11–18]. The position of deep gray-matter nuclei within the basal ganglia motor loop circuitry may be particularly important in determining the location of brain injury [1,16]. HIE following severe asphyxia results in electroencephalographic and positron emission tomographic patterns suggestive of activity in corticothalamic, thalamocortical, and corticoputaminal excitatory projections with strong glutamate innervations [16]. Such hyperexcitability in these circuits

Table 34.2. Inborn errors of metabolism involving gray matter only

Cortical gray matter

  Neuronal ceroid lipofuscinosis

  Sialidosis

Deep gray matter

  Prolonged striatal T2 signal

    Mitochondrial disorders: MELAS,[a] Leigh syndrome

    Hypoglycemia[b]

    Juvenile Huntington disease

  Shortened pallidum T2 signal

    Neurodegeneration with brain iron accumulation type 1 (NBIA1)[c]

  Prolonged pallidum T2 signal

    Methylmalonic acidemia

    Carbon monoxide poisoning

    Kernicterus

Notes:
[a]MELAS, mitochondrial encephalomyopathy, lactic acidosis, and stroke-like episodes.
[b]In older infants, adolescents, and adults.
[c]Formerly Hallervorden–Spatz disease.
Source: Adapted from Barkovich AJ. *Pediatric Neuroimaging*, 3rd edn. Philadelphia, PA: Lippincott Williams & Wilkins, 2000.

Table 34.3. Inborn errors of metabolism involving white matter only

Subcortical white matter early

  Macrocephaly

    Alexander disease

  Normal head circumference

    4-Hydroxybutyric aciduria[a]

  Galactosemia

Deep white matter early

  Pons/medulla corticospinal tract involvement

    Peroxisomal disorders

  No specific brainstem tracts involved

    Phenylketonuria

    Maple syrup urine disease[b]

    -5,10-Methylene tetrahydrofolate reductase (MTHFR) deficiency

    Disorders of cobalamin metabolism

    Metachromatic leukodystrophy

Lack of myelination

  Pelizaeus–Merzbacher disease

  Trichothiodystrophy

Non-specific white-matter pattern

  Glycine encephalopathy (non-ketotic hyperglycinemia)

  3-Hydroxy-3-methylglutaryl coenzyme A lyase deficiency

  Urea cycle disorders

Notes:
[a]Cerebellar atrophy may also be present.
[b]Cerebellar and cerebral peduncle involvement may also be present.
Source: Adapted from Barkovich AJ. *Pediatric Neuroimaging*, 3rd edn.
Philadelphia, PA: Lippincott Williams & Wilkins, 2000.

Table 34.4. Inborn errors of metabolism involving both gray and white matter

Cortical gray matter only

  Cortical dysplasia

    Muscle–eye–brain disease

    Walker–Warburg syndrome

    Fukuyama muscular dystrophy

    Other congenital muscular dystrophies

  Absent cortical dysplasia

    Alpers disease

    Menkes disease

  Abnormal bones

    Mucopolysaccharidoses

  Lipid storage disorders

  Peroxisomal disorders

Deep gray-matter-involvement

  Primary thalamic involvement

    GM1 gangliosidosis

    GM2 gangliosidosis

    Krabbe disease

  Primary globus pallidus involvement

    Canavan disease

    Methylmalonic acidemia

    L-2-Hydroxyglutaric aciduria

    Maple syrup urine disease

    Mitochondrial disorders: Kearns–Sayre syndrome

  Primary striatal involvement

    Organic acidemias: propionic acidemia, biotinidase deficiency, multiple carboxylase deficiency, glutaric aciduria type I, β-ketothiolase deficiency, 3-methylglutaconic aciduria, ethylmalonic acidemia

    Tricarboxylic acid cycle disorders: malonic acidemia, α-ketoglutaric aciduria

    Molybdenum cofactor deficiency

    Mitochondrial disorders: MELAS,[a] Leigh syndrome

  Wilson disease

Note:
[a]MELAS, mitochondrial encephalomyopathy, lactic acidosis, and stroke-like episodes.
Source: Adapted from Barkovich AJ. *Pediatric Neuroimaging*, 3rd edn.
Philadelphia, PA: Lippincott Williams & Wilkins, 2000.

may cause the characteristic thalamus and putamen lesions seen in HIE via glutamate-mediated toxicity [13]. Areas of the brain with a high concentration of glutamate innervations may be particularly vulnerable to injury during asphyxia, because of damage sustained to nerve terminal glutamate reuptake pumps and subsequent high levels of synaptic glutamate. Glutamate has the potential to bind to postsynaptic N-methyl-D-aspartate (NMDA) receptors, causing membrane-bound calcium channels to open and subsequent influx of Ca^{2+} and cell death, mediated in part by mitochondrial damage and augmentation of nitric oxide and carbon monoxide production [1,14,17]. Released nitric oxide combines with superoxide to form peroxynitrite, which, in turn, leads to DNA damage, depletion of cellular energy, and cell death [14]. While the cortex, putamen, and thalamus are activated by such a glutamate excitatory stimulus, the globus pallidus is inhibited, resulting in relative sparing of this structure from damage [16]. This neuronal circuitry hypothesis may explain the selective pattern of involvement of deep gray structures in HIE, despite the close proximity and similar vascular supply of these structures. Nitric oxide produced by nitric oxide synthase following NMDA receptor activation also inhibits mitochondrial respiratory chain complex IV (cytochrome oxidase), which elicits further production of superoxide and

peroxynitrate. Mitochondrial release of proapoptotic proteins follows, resulting in caspase- and apoptosis-inducing factor-dependent cell death [18].

In contrast, toxic and metabolic disorders that affect mitochondrial energy metabolism (e.g., kernicterus, pyruvate dehydrogenase complex deficiency, respiratory chain disorders) cause neuronal injury through different mechanisms, although glutamate release may also play a role. Disorders that cause mitochondrial dysfunction may lead to neuronal injury by diminishing the ability of mitochondria to maintain membrane potentials. Neuronal subacute membrane depolarization could result in subsequent opening of postsynaptic voltage-dependent NMDA and sodium channels with resultant cellular injury [12,16]. The globus pallidus appears to be particularly vulnerable in metabolic disorders, because of the relatively high basal firing rate of pallidal neurons [16]. This predisposition to oxidative stress could also be related to the relatively high concentration of brain NMDA receptors in neonates when compared to adults [11,15]. In addition, mitochondrial damage may lead to decreased expression of hypoxia-inducible factor 1 (HIF-1), a transcription factor that induces genes coding for erythropoietin, vascular endothelial growth factor, glycolytic enzymes, and glucose transporters. HIF-1 appears to be important in an adaptive response to hypoxia, because of its role in stimulating cellular glucose uptake, increasing glycolytic capacity, and enhancing tissue O_2 delivery [19].

Clinical features of HIE and inborn errors of metabolism

Neonates progress through distinctive stages of neurologic impairment following asphyxia severe enough to cause HIE [4]. Seizures occur in 50–70% of acutely asphyxiated neonates and tend to start between 30 minutes and 24 hours after birth, with an earlier occurrence signifying a more severe asphyxial insult [4]. In addition to central nervous system (CNS) complications seen in perinatal asphyxia, systemic involvement of multiple organs, including heart, liver, and kidneys, may also occur (Table 34.5). Such damage to other organs may contribute to the severity of brain injury. Asphyxia in the immediate perinatal period is associated with low Apgar scores (typically 3 or less at 1 minute and 6 or less at 5 minutes); bradycardia, pallor, cyanosis, decreased or absent respirations, and diminished or absent reflex activity may be present. A combined metabolic and respiratory acidosis is characteristic. Other metabolic findings include hypoglycemia, hypocalcemia, hyponatremia (secondary to the syndrome of inappropriate antidiuretic hormone secretion, SIADH), and multiple electrolyte abnormalities from renal dysfunction. Hyperammonemia may occur if hepatic dysfunction is severe [4,20].

Table 34.5. Systemic complications of hypoxic–ischemic encephalopathy

Cardiomyopathy
Hepatic necrosis
Acute tubular necrosis
Adrenal insufficiency
Necrotizing enterocolitis
Meconium aspiration syndrome
Persistent fetal circulation
Thrombocytopenia
Hypoglycemia
Hypocalcemia
Hyperammonemia
SIADH (syndrome of inappropriate antidiuretic hormone secretion)

Table 34.6. Laboratory investigations in neonates with a suspected inborn error of metabolism

Routine investigations
Complete blood count + differential
Urinalysis
Electrolytes, blood urea nitrogen, creatinine, calcium, phosphorus, magnesium
Liver enzymes
Creatine kinase
Blood gases
CSF glucose, protein, erythrocytes, and leukocytes
Cultures of blood, urine, and CSF
Basic metabolic investigations
Ammonia
Lactate, pyruvate
Quantitative serum amino acids
Quantitative urine organic acids
Carnitine levels (total, free, and esterified carnitine)
Acylcarnitine profile
Further metabolic investigations[a]
Blood ketone bodies
CSF lactate, glycine, serine, 4-aminobutyric acid levels[b]
Very-long-chain fatty acid analysis
Plasma and urine guanidinoacetate and creatine levels
Urine S-sulfocysteine
Urine homocitrulline
Urine purines and pyrimidines
Cultured fibroblasts for specific enzymology[c]
Muscle biopsy for histochemistry, mitochondrial respiratory chain activities
DNA analysis[d]

Notes:
CSF, cerebrospinal fluid.
[a]These investigations are performed on an individual basis depending on the presentation.
[b]Simultaneous serum glycine should be obtained for the investigation of glycine encephalopathy (non-ketotic hyperglycinemia). Other CSF studies, e.g., HPLC analysis for the characteristic compound seen in folinic-acid-responsive seizures or succinylpurine analysis, may be needed in some cases (see text).
[c]Fibroblast analysis is often used for assay of fatty acid oxidation disorders, some mitochondrial disorders, and disorders of pyruvate metabolism. Other tissues (e.g., liver, muscle) may also be useful for enzyme analysis.
[d]DNA analysis may be routinely available for certain metabolic disorders, including some mitochondrial disorders, but often is only available on a research basis.

Inborn errors of metabolism may also present with severe neurologic illness and the involvement of multiple organ systems. A high index of suspicion and specific laboratory investigations are necessary to diagnose a metabolic disorder presenting with symptoms and signs suggestive of HIE (Table 34.6). The onset of symptoms of metabolic disease is typically postnatal, appearing after an interval period of apparent good health, and following a normal pregnancy. This interval may be as short as a few hours, or last several days or even longer. Because an asphyxial insult may occur at any time in the prenatal period, the absence of a significant obstetric event does not exclude HIE as a cause of neonatal distress, but may raise the suspicion of an underlying metabolic condition. In general, if the degree of neonatal metabolic distress seems out of proportion to known obstetric or environmental factors, there is a higher likelihood that an inborn error of metabolism is present. The persistence, or increasing levels, of markers of metabolic disease (e.g., lactic acid and ammonia) despite vigorous therapy may also point to an underlying metabolic problem. Because most inborn errors of metabolism are characterized by autosomal recessive or maternal inheritance, obtaining a detailed family history is crucial. Parental consanguinity, or a history of a previously affected child, also increases the probability that neonatal distress is secondary to an underlying inborn error of metabolism.

Other indicators of metabolic imbalance include an anion gap acidosis, lactic acidosis, hyperammonemia, and hypoglycemia, but these markers are not invariably present (Table 34.7). It is apparent that the clinician may have difficulty distinguishing HIE from a metabolic disorder, because similar signs and symptoms occur in both conditions. Furthermore, these conditions are not mutually exclusive. An asphyxial insult may constitute the initial environmental stress that unmasks an underlying inborn error of metabolism, or a debilitating metabolism disorder may predispose an infant to a difficult delivery. The following sections summarize specific metabolic diseases according to their typical presentations in the neonatal period. These clinical classifications are general guidelines only, because metabolic disorders may present in atypical ways.

Isolated seizures

Up to 9% of infants admitted to neonatal intensive care units have seizures [21]. The most common causes of neonatal seizures are asphyxia, hypoglycemia, electrolyte abnormalities, infection, CNS malformations, drug exposure and withdrawal, and inborn errors of metabolism [22]. Metabolic disorders that may present with isolated neonatal seizures, without other obvious routine laboratory or clinical markers of an underlying inborn error of metabolism, are relatively rare and include glycine encephalopathy (non-ketotic hyperglycinemia), sulfite oxidase deficiency (either isolated or as part of molybdenum cofactor deficiency), α-amino adipic semialdehyde dehydrogenase deficiency (pyridoxine-dependent epilepsy), pyridox(am)ine 5'-phosphate oxidase deficiency (pyridoxal-dependent seizures), folinic-acid-responsive seizures, 4-aminobutyrate aminotransferase (GABA transaminase) deficiency, 3-phosphoglycerate dehydrogenase deficiency, dihydropyrimidine dehydrogenase deficiency, guanidinoacetate methyltransferase (GAMT) deficiency, glucose transporter (GLUT-1) deficiency, and mitochondrial glutamate transporter deficiency [22–33]. Peroxisomal disorders, mitochondrial disorders, congenital disorders of glycosylation, organic acidemias, and urea cycle defects may also have seizures as part of a neonatal presentation, but other organ-system involvement or characteristic routine laboratory

Table 34.7. Inborn errors of metabolism with features of hypoxic–ischemic encephalopathy

Isolated seizures
  Glycine encephalopathy (non-ketotic hyperglycinemia)
  Sulfite oxidase (molybdenum cofactor) deficiency
  Pyridoxine-dependent seizures
  Pyridoxal-dependent seizures
  Folinic-acid-responsive seizures
  4-Aminobutyrate aminotransferase (GABA transaminase) deficiency
  3-Phosphoglycerate dehydrogenase (3-PGD) deficiency[a]
  Dihydropyrimidine dehydrogenase (DPD) deficiency
  Guanidinoacetate methyltransferase (GAMT) deficiency
  Glucose transporter defect (GLUT-1 deficiency syndrome)
  Mitochondrial glutamate transporter deficiency
  Peroxisomal disorders[a]
  Mitochondrial disorders[a]
  Organic acidemias[a,b]

Lactic acidosis, hypotonia, and systemic involvement
  Pyruvate dehydrogenase deficiency[b]
  Pyruvate carboxylase deficiency[b]
  Fatty acid oxidation defects[b,c]
  Mitochondrial disorders
  3-Methylglutaconic aciduria
  α-Ketoglutarate dehydrogenase deficiency
  Fumaric aciduria[d]

Severe ketoacidosis
  Propionic acidemia
  Methylmalonic acidemia
  Isovaleric acidemia
  Multiple acyl coenzyme A dehydrogenase deficiency (MADD, glutaric aciduria type II)[d]
  Holocarboxylase synthetase deficiency (multiple carboxylase deficiency, MCD)
  3-Hydroxyisobutyric aciduria[d]

Lethargy without metabolic acidosis
  Maple syrup urine disease[e]
  Mevalonic aciduria[d]

Lethargy with hyperammonemia
  Urea cycle defects
  HHH (hyperammonemia, hyperornithinemia, homocitrullinuria) syndrome
  Lysinuric protein intolerance

Other disorders
  Glycogen storage disorders types I, II, III, VIII[f,g]
  Fructose 1,6-diphosphatase deficiency[f,g]
  Congenital disorders of glycosylation

Notes:
[a]These conditions commonly have other systemic manifestations (see text).
[b]Hyperammonemia may also be present.
[c]Lactic acidosis is usually not prominent, except in long-chain 3-hydroxyacyl coenzyme A dehydrogenase deficiency and trifunctional protein deficiency, or if there is systemic hypoperfusion.
[d]Dysmorphic features and head magnetic resonance imaging abnormalities are commonly present.
[e]Metabolic acidosis may occur later in the course of disease.
[f]Lactic acidosis may be severe.
[g]Hypoglycemia with hepatomegaly are commonly present. An enlarged heart is present in glycogen storage disorder type II and may be present in glycogen storage disorder type VIII.

abnormalities (e.g., hyperammonemia, lactic acidemia, or metabolic acidosis) should guide the clinician to the underlying diagnosis [34–37]. Disorders with an isolated seizure presentation, in contrast, may not have concomitant acidosis, hypoglycemia, or electrolyte abnormalities. Routine metabolic studies are also normal; specific investigations on blood, cerebrospinal fluid (CSF), or urine are required to make a diagnosis [29,38].

Glycine encephalopathy (non-ketotic hyperglycinemia)

Glycine encephalopathy is an autosomal recessive condition characterized by the accumulation of large amounts of glycine in body fluids because of defective glycine cleavage system function. Symptoms include lethargy, apnea, profound hypotonia, feeding difficulty, hiccups, and seizures. Approximately two-thirds of patients will have symptoms appear within 48 hours of delivery, but symptoms may occur as early as 6 hours of life. Routine laboratory evaluations and organic acid analysis are normal. The only consistent abnormality is an elevated glycine concentration in urine, plasma, and CSF. A CSF-to-plasma glycine ratio greater than 0.08 is diagnostic of glycine encephalopathy. CSF and blood samples for glycine analysis should be obtained as near to simultaneously as possible to allow for an accurate calculation of the glycine ratio. Elevated CSF glycine has also been reported in HIE, but a normal CSF-to-plasma glycine ratio would be expected in this case [39]. Definitive diagnosis requires enzymatic analysis of liver glycine cleavage system activity or mutation analysis. The electroencephalogram (EEG) is characterized by a burst–suppression pattern in the first 2 weeks of life. Head computed tomography (CT) evaluation may show cerebral and cerebellar volume loss with hypoattenuation of the periventricular white matter. Head MRI studies show delayed myelination early. Progressive cerebral atrophy, agenesis of the corpus callosum, and atrophic basal ganglia may also occur [40–42]. Treatment with sodium benzoate and dextromethorphan (a non-competitive NMDA receptor antagonist) may improve symptoms, but is not curative. Survivors often display minimal cognitive development and may have seizures recalcitrant to therapy.

Sulfite oxidase deficiency

Sulfite oxidase deficiency may occur in isolation or combined with xanthine oxidase deficiency (molybdenum cofactor deficiency). Inheritance is autosomal recessive. Patients typically present with drug-resistant seizures in the first few days of life. Routine laboratory evaluations and urine organic acid analysis are normal, although a low uric acid level may be noted in molybdenum cofactor deficiency. Elevated S-sulfocysteine in plasma or urine is diagnostic. (Note that S-sulfocysteine content is not routinely reported on serum or urine amino acid analyses; a specific assay must be performed.) EEG shows a burst–suppression pattern. In the neonatal period, head MRI shows T2 prolongation of the white matter and caudate nuclei,

consistent with edema. In the subacute phase, the basal ganglia may have abnormalities similar to those seen in acute asphyxia [43]. Encephalomalacia with cystic changes, especially in subcortical regions, may also mimic HIE [44]. There is no current therapy for sulfite oxidase deficiency, and most cases result in profound mental retardation or early fatality.

Pyridoxine-dependent seizures

Pyridoxine-dependent seizures are caused primarily by α-amino adipic semialdehyde dehydrogenase (antiquin) deficiency, a defect in the cerebral lysine degradation pathway [33]. Genetic heterogeneity exists, but the overall birth incidence is approximately 1/160 000 [27,33]. Patients may present on the first day of life with flaccidity, abnormal eye movements, and irritability. Shock, hypothermia, hepatomegaly, and abdominal distension suggestive of intestinal obstruction also occur [25]. EEG shows intermittent or continuous generalized slow-wave activity, with or without focal or multifocal spike or spike and wave activity. Patients may have structural brain abnormalities, including cerebellar hypoplasia, generalized brain atrophy, and a thin corpus callosum. Approximately 10% of neonatal cases have features suggestive of HIE [45]. Initial diagnosis is clinical, with documented response of seizures to intravenous pyridoxine (vitamin B$_6$). Markedly elevated pipecolic acid and α-amino adipic semialdehyde are present in urine, plasma, and CSF, but detection requires specialized laboratory methods. Antiquitin (ALDH7A1) mutation analysis provides final confirmation of the diagnosis [33].

Pyridoxal-dependent seizures

Pyridoxal phosphate is a cofactor for aromatic L-amino acid decarboxylase (AADC), threonine dehydratase, and the glycine cleavage enzyme. Some infants with intractable neonatal seizures have increased concentrations of threonine, glycine, and AADC metabolites in the CSF, suggesting a cellular deficiency of pyridoxal phosphate. Signs of fetal distress may be noted. These infants respond to pyridoxal phosphate, but not pyridoxine, supplementation (30 mg/kg/day) [32]. Mutations in the gene coding for pyridox(am)ine 5'-phosphate oxidase (PNPO) are associated with pyridoxal-dependent seizures [30]. Prompt treatment with pyridoxal phosphate results in amelioration of seizures and normal development or moderate psychomotor delay. Severe mental retardation with or without early demise occurs in children with late or no treatment [32].

Folinic-acid-responsive seizures

This is an entity of unknown etiology in which seizures may occur as early as 2 hours after birth [22,24]. Routine laboratory studies and metabolic tests are normal. EEG shows a diffuse discontinuous pattern with excessive spikes. Head imaging in two patients between 1 and 2 months of age showed dilated ventricles, cerebellar atrophy, and abnormal signal in frontal and parietal lobe white matter. High-pressure liquid chromatography analysis of CSF detects the presence of a characteristic compound, whose chemical structure has not yet been elucidated. Patients respond to folinic acid supplementation (5–20 mg/day in divided doses) [22].

GABA transaminase deficiency

GABA transaminase catalyzes the first step in the conversion of GABA (γ-aminobutyric acid), a CNS-inhibitory neurotransmitter, to succinic acid. Clinical features of GABA transaminase deficiency include neonatal seizures, lethargy, hypotonia, hyperreflexia, and a high-pitched cry. MRI findings include agenesis of the corpus callosum and cerebellar hypoplasia. Only a few patients with GABA transaminase deficiency have been reported, but diagnosis will be missed unless GABA is measured in plasma or CSF [28].

3-Phosphoglycerate dehydrogenase (3-PGD) deficiency

In addition to intractable seizures, 3-PGD deficiency is characterized by congential microcephaly, severe psychomotor retardation, hyperexcitability, and spastic tetraparesis. Brain MRI shows hypomyelination and cortical and subcortical atrophy. Decreased serine in fasting plasma and CSF is a biochemical marker for this disorder [46].

Dihydropyrimidine dehydrogenase (DPD) deficiency

DPD deficiency is a disorder of pyrimidine metabolism that is associated with a variety of neurologic findings, including isolated neonatal seizures and head imaging abnormalities, such as delayed myelination and brainstem white-matter abnormalities [47,48]. Disorders of purine metabolism (e.g., adenylosuccinate lyase deficiency) can also present with infantile seizures and developmental delay. A urine screen for purine and pyrimidine metabolites is helpful in detecting these conditions, although some cases of adenylosuccinate lyase deficiency may be detected only after measuring succinylpurines in the CSF.

Guanidinoacetate methyltransferase (GAMT) deficiency

GAMT deficiency is a disorder of creatine metabolism characterized by low plasma creatine levels and elevated guanidinoacetate. Patients typically present in infancy with seizures, developmental delay, unusual behavior, and extrapyramidal signs, but this condition has also been diagnosed in neonates. Guanidinoacetate may be assayed in plasma by tandem-mass spectrometry. Treatment with creatine monohydrate may be effective [26].

GLUT-1 deficiency syndrome

GLUT-1 protein is the major glucose transporter in the blood–brain barrier. Mutations in the *GLUT1* gene result in haploinsufficiency of this hexose carrier and severe clinical symptoms, including seizures, acquired microcephaly, and developmental delay. Patients have presented as early as the third week of life, but relatively few cases have been reported in the literature. The GLUT-1 deficiency syndrome is an autosomal dominant condition. Characteristic diagnostic findings are a reduced CSF glucose concentration (hypoglycorrhachia) and reduced erythrocyte glucose transporter activity. Peripheral blood glucose and other routine metabolic evaluations are normal. Seizures may stop and children may show a dramatic recovery with the institution of a ketogenic diet [23,49].

Peroxisomal disorders

Peroxisomal disorders that may present with neonatal seizures include neonatal adrenoleukodystrophy, Zellweger syndrome, and infantile Refsum disease [34]. Most are inherited as autosomal recessive traits, although X-linked adrenoleukodystrophy (which presents in childhood) and rhizomelic chondrodysplasia punctata are X-linked. Clinical features in the neonatal period include severe hypotonia and seizures refractory to therapy. Seizures may be grand mal or myoclonic, and EEG typically shows multifocal spike discharges [34]. Head imaging in Zellweger syndrome may show subependymal cysts reminiscent of those found in HIE, as well as profound hypomyelination, and cerebral cortex malformations [9,50]. Anterior frontal and temporal lobe microgyri or perisylvian and perirolandic cortex pachygyria may be present. A spectrum of similar brain abnormalities may occur in other peroxisomal disorders, although head imaging may also appear normal in these conditions [9]. Patients with peroxisomal disorders may also have prominent ophthalmologic and systemic findings, including large fontanel, cataracts, retinitis pigmentosa, dysmorphic features, hepatomegaly, hepatic fibrosis, and renal cysts. Despite the occasional presence of subependymal cysts, the presence of other characteristic features should make distinguishing these conditions from HIE relatively straightforward. Plasma elevation of very-long-chain fatty acids, bile acid intermediates, and phytanic acid, and decreased erythrocyte plasmalogens, are biochemical markers for these conditions. No effective therapy is currently available.

Mitochondrial disorders

These conditions may rarely present with neonatal seizures, but more commonly feature hypotonia and lactic acidosis. Multiple organ-system involvement is also typical of mitochondrial disease [35,36,51–56]. However, severe neonatal epilepsy with a burst–suppression pattern may occur in an autosomal recessive condition caused by impaired mitochondrial glutamate transport secondary to mutations in *SLC25A22*, the gene coding for a mitochondrial glutamate/H^+ symporter [31]. Mitochondrial respiratory chain disorders are discussed further below.

Organic acidemias and urea cycle disorders

Seizures may occur in neonates with classic organic acidemias and urea cycle defects, but are usually not the major manifestation of these disorders. Overwhelming ketoacidosis, hyperammonemic coma, and characteristic serum amino acids and urine organic acids are usually present. Combined D-2- and L-2-hydroxyglutaric aciduria is a condition that presents with neonatal-onset encephalopathy and intractable seizures [57]. Mevalonic aciduria may present with severe neurologic involvement and seizures, without a metabolic acidosis. However, other findings, including dysmorphic features, hepatosplenomegaly, recurrent fevers, and anemia are more typical [58]. Interestingly, an unusual pattern of organic acid excretion may occur in neonates with severe tissue hypoxia in the absence of an underlying genetic defect [59].

Lactic acidosis, hypotonia, and systemic involvement

Disorders of pyruvate metabolism, tricarboxylic acid cycle disorders, fatty acid oxidation defects, and mitochondrial disease may present in the neonatal period with neuromuscular abnormalities, lactic acidosis, and other systemic manifestations, including cardiomyopathy, liver disease, and renal tubular defects. Anomalies may be present on head imaging, including thinning or agenesis of the corpus callosum and basal ganglia lesions, but the classic findings of HIE are typically absent [9,16].

Disorders of pyruvate metabolism

Pyruvate dehydrogenase complex (PDHC) deficiency is the most common defect in oxidative metabolism that features persistent lactic acidosis [60,61]. Most often a defect in the $E_{1\alpha}$ component of the multimeric PDHC is the underlying cause of this disorder. $E_{1\alpha}$ deficiency is X-linked. Defects in the E_2, protein X, E_3, and PDH phosphatase components of the PDHC are rare autosomal recessive conditions. Although PDHC deficiency often presents later in infancy, a neonatal form exists that is characterized by lactic acidosis and severe neurologic compromise with hypotonia. Subtle dysmorphic features may be present. In contrast to the acidosis associated with tissue hypoxia, ketosis is often present in primary lactic acidemias. Hyperammonemia has also been reported in some patients [60,61]. Head MRI shows findings typical of Leigh syndrome in about 50% of patients. Cerebral and cerebellar atrophy, delayed myelination, and agenesis of the corpus callosum can be seen [9]. Patients may respond to a diet low in carbohydrate and high in fat. Dichloroacetate reduces lactate in most patients, but is not standard therapy. Some variants have also shown a response to high-dose thiamine administration.

The complex form of pyruvate carboxylase deficiency presents with severe neonatal lactic acidosis, hyperammonemia, citrullinemia, and hyperlysinemia. This disorder has been described in patients of European, Egyptian, and Saudi Arabian descent. Most patients with the severe form die by age 3 months. A simple (American Indian) form presents with developmental delay or lactic acidosis in infancy. Both forms are autosomal recessive. No effective treatment is available [61].

Tricarboxylic acid cycle defects

Alpha-ketoglutarate dehydrogenase deficiency may present with lactic acidemia, hypotonia, hepatomegaly, and elevated creatine kinase immediately after birth. Patients have elevated α-ketoglutarate in the urine and a low-normal plasma β-hydroxybutyrate-to-acetoacetate ratio [62]. A combined deficiency of α-ketoglutarate dehydrogenase and pyruvate dehydrogenase has also been described in neonates with lactic acidosis, hypoglycemia, and neurologic abnormalities, including seizures. The combined defects may be caused by lipoamide dehydrogenase deficiency, because this enzyme is integral to both α-ketoglutarate dehydrogenase and PDHC [63]. Patients with fumaric aciduria may have lactic acidosis, dysmorphic features, and congenital brain malformations, including polymicrogyria, decreased white-matter volume, ventriculomegaly, open operculum, angulation of the frontal horns, and brainstem hypoplasia [64]. Treatment of these conditions is supportive.

Fatty acid oxidation defects

Although the most common defect of fatty acid β-oxidation, medium-chain acyl-CoA dehydrogenase (MCAD) deficiency, typically presents later in infancy or childhood with a Reye-syndrome-like illness, significant neonatal disease may occur [65]. Other fatty acid oxidation disorders may present in the neonatal or early infantile periods with greater frequency. Short-chain 3-hydroxyacyl-CoA dehydrogenase (SCHAD) deficiency, long-chain 3-hydroxyacyl-CoA dehydrogenase (LCHAD) deficiency, trifunctional protein (TFP) deficiency, very-long-chain acyl-CoA dehydrogenase (VLCAD) deficiency, carnitine palmitoyl transferase II (CPT II) deficiency, and carnitine-acylcarnitine translocase (CAT) deficiency have been described in neonates [66–69]. Systemic manifestations include cardiomyopathy, hepatopathy, Reye-syndrome-like illness, and muscle weakness and hypotonia. The creatine kinase level may be very elevated, and prominent myoglobinuria may lead to renal tubular dysfunction and renal failure. A "salt-and-pepper" retinopathy has been reported in LCHAD deficiency, but usually appears in later childhood. A history of acute fatty liver of pregnancy and hemolysis, elevated liver enzymes, low platelets (HELLP) syndrome may be elicited from a heterozygous mother carrying a fetus with LCHAD deficiency [70]. Lactic acidosis is more commonly encountered in long-chain fatty acid oxidation disorders, but may not be a prominent feature unless present as part of terminal illness. Patients typically have hypoketotic or non-ketotic hypoglycemia, although increased production of ketone bodies may be seen in SCHAD deficiency. Marked hyperammonemia is atypical, but may occur (e.g., CAT and VLCAD deficiency) [67]. Urine organic acid analysis typically shows elevated dicarboxylic acids of characteristic chain length depending on the underlying disorder. Plasma total carnitine levels are typically low, with an elevation in the esterified carnitine fraction and esterified-to-free carnitine ratio. An acylcarnitine profile may detect pathognomonic compounds characteristic of specific fatty acid oxidation disorders. However, fibroblast enzymology or intracellular acylcarnitine profile analysis with or without DNA mutation analysis may be needed to establish the diagnosis with certainty. Treatment includes avoidance of fasting, low-fat diet, and carnitine supplementation in patients who survive the neonatal period. Medium-chain triglycerides may be useful in long-chain defects [66].

Mitochondrial disease

The mitochondrial electron transport chain is coded for by the coordinated action of both nuclear and mitochondrial genomes. These conditions, therefore, may exhibit either Mendelian (autosomal recessive, autosomal dominant, X-linked) or maternal (mitochondrial) inheritance [53]. Dysfunction of any organ system, either alone or in combination, may occur when mitochondrial function is abnormal. However, neuromuscular signs and symptoms occur most commonly. Children who have mitochondrial disorders, caused by either nuclear or mitochondrial DNA defects, may first come to medical attention as neonates [35,36,51,52,54–56,71–75]. Hypotonia, lethargy, deafness, dystonia, or seizures are common features. Cataracts and retinal pigmentary abnormalities may also be present. Systemic involvement includes cardiomyopathy, bone marrow suppression, hepatic disease, and renal dysfunction. Antenatal findings include polyhydramnios, oligohydramnios, hydrops fetalis, intrauterine growth retardation, arthrogryposis, decreased movement, and cardiomyopathy [35,36].

Although some patients with mitochondrial disease may only have non-specific white-matter abnormalities or delayed myelination, gray-matter involvement is relatively common, especially affecting the dorsal midbrain, thalami, and globi pallidi [16]. Leigh syndrome (subacute necrotizing encephalomyopathy) is another manifestation of mitochondrial dysfunction, although affected children tend to present after the neonatal period. The clinician must maintain a high index of suspicion, because these disorders are often difficult to diagnose. For example, a patient initially diagnosed with HIE after presenting with fetal distress, metabolic acidosis, and seizures at 4 hours of age was later documented to have complex IV (cytochrome oxidase) deficiency [56]. Elevated lactate-to-pyruvate ratio (> 25), β-hydroxybutyrate-to-acetoacetate ratio (> 1.0), and urine organic acids with tricarboxylic acid cycle intermediates or other compounds suggestive of mitochondrial dysfunction offer clues to diagnosis. Although a muscle biopsy may show changes suggestive of mitochondrial disease, ragged-red fibers are rarely encountered in children and histopathology may appear normal or have non-specific findings. Definitive diagnosis is made by mitochondrial respiratory chain analysis in muscle or other tissue or the detection of a pathogenic mutation in mitochondrial or nuclear DNA. Various vitamin "cocktails" have been attempted, but there is no proven effective therapy for these conditions.

Severe ketoacidosis

Classic organic acidemias often present in the neonatal period or infancy with overwhelming illness and ketoacidosis with an elevated anion gap. Prominent lactic acidosis is uncommon, but mild to moderate elevations may occur, especially if there is superimposed tissue hypoperfusion. Diagnosis of these disorders is relatively straightforward and is based on detection of characteristic metabolites in serum amino acids and urine organic acids.

Organic acidemias

Methylmalonic acidemia (MMA), propionic acidemia (PA), isovaleric acidemia (IVA), glutaric aciduria type II (multiple acyl CoA dehydrogenase deficiency, MADD), and holocarboxylase synthetase deficiency (multiple carboxylase deficiency, MCD) are autosomal recessive conditions that may present in neonates with lethargy, vomiting, and severe ketoacidosis. Neonatal seizures have also been reported, but are not common. Renal cysts and dysmorphic features frequently occur in MADD with neonatal presentation. An odor of "sweaty feet" may also be noted in patients with MADD or IVA. Routine labs often show neutropenia, hypoglycemia, and a metabolic acidosis. Lactic acidosis is usually not a prominent feature, except in MCD. Head MRI may show abnormal T2 prolongation in the periventricular white matter and lesions in the basal ganglia, especially the globus pallidus (MMA) or putamen and caudate nucleus (PA) [9]. Characteristic organic acids in urine make diagnosis of these conditions relatively straightforward.

Affected individuals with 3-hydroxyisobutyric aciduria may also present in the neonatal period with overwhelming ketoacidosis. In addition, patients may have lactic acidosis, dysmorphic features, and congenital brain malformations, including intracerebral calcifications, lissencephaly, pachygyria, polymicrogyria, agenesis of the corpus callosum, and an indistinct gray- and white-matter interface [76]. Glutaric aciduria type I may also feature severe brain anomalies, including frontotemporal atrophy, delayed myelination, and basal ganglia changes, but this disorder tends to present later in infancy [9].

Therapy of organic acidemias consists of dietary restriction of specific amino acids in some conditions, and the prompt treatment of acute episodes of ketoacidosis. Supplementation with carnitine and specific cofactors (e.g., vitamin B_{12} in some forms of MMA or biotin in MCD) are important therapeutic interventions.

Lethargy without metabolic acidosis or hyperammonemia
Maple syrup urine disease

Children with maple syrup urine disease (MSUD) typically present in the first few days to weeks of life, after appearing normal at birth. Feeding difficulty and vomiting may be the initial symptoms. By the end of the first week, lethargy and progressive neurologic deterioration occur unless appropriate treatment is started. A markedly hypertonic infant with opisthotonus is typical. The characteristic odor is present by the time neurologic symptoms develop, but not all patients have a "maple syrup" smell. Metabolic acidosis is uncommon until later in the course of disease. Neuroimaging is normal in the first few days of life. Characteristic head MRI findings develop with time, including profound localized edema in the deep cerebellar white matter, dorsal brainstem, cerebral peduncles, posterior limb of the internal capsule, perirolandic white matter, and globi pallidi. Generalized cerebral hemisphere edema may also be present. Delayed, or abnormal, myelination is common [9]. Emergency management includes measures to decrease the levels of branched-chain amino acids (BCAA) rapidly (e.g., hemodialysis, BCAA-free parenteral nutrition, and the prevention of catabolism). Restricting intake of branched-chain amino acids, while providing adequate nutrition, and prompt treatment of intercurrent illnesses are the cornerstones of chronic management. Thiamine supplementation may help in some cases of MSUD.

Mevalonic aciduria

Mevalonic aciduria is an autosomal recessive disorder of cholesterol biosynthesis that may present in the neonatal period with lethargy, hypotonia, or other signs of neurologic dysfunction, without a metabolic acidosis. Patients may have dysmorphic features, cataracts, hepatosplenomegaly, recurrent fevers without identifiable infectious agents, and anemia [58,77].

Lethargy with hyperammonemia

Neonatal hyperammonemia is the predominant laboratory finding in urea cycle disorders, although other inborn errors of metabolism cause hyperammonemia by a secondary inhibition of urea cycle function. Pyruvate carboxylase deficiency, organic acidemias, carnitine-acylcarnitine translocase deficiency, lysinuric protein intolerance, and the HHH (hyperammonemia, hyperornithinemia, homocitrullinuria) syndrome may be associated with neonatal hyperammonemia. Prominent hyperammonemia ($> 10 \times$ elevation) has also been reported in patients with perinatal asphyxia, likely secondary to hepatic dysfunction. Other common associations with perinatal asphyxia, such as severe fetal bradycardia, low Apgar scores, and the need for prolonged resuscitation following delivery typically are present in such instances [20]. In contrast, patients with inborn errors of metabolism, including urea cycle disorders, typically appear normal at birth, without perinatal distress, following an uneventful pregnancy.

Urea cycle disorders

Patients with urea cycle disorders (N-acetylglutamate synthetase deficiency, carbamyl phosphate synthetase deficiency, ornithine transcarbamylase deficiency, argininosuccinic acid synthetase deficiency (citrullinemia), and argininosuccinic acid lyase deficiency) typically present with lethargy, poor feeding, and hyperpnea with a respiratory alkalosis in the first few days of life. Sepsis is often initially suspected, and, unless an ammonia level is checked, these infants may die of unknown cause early in the neonatal period. Aside from ornithine transcarbamylase deficiency, which is X-linked, these are autosomal recessive conditions. Progression to deep coma supervenes, necessitating intubation and mechanical ventilation. Head imaging is non-specific in these disorders, but may show cerebral edema. Head MRI in the subacute phase (day of life 3–7) may resemble HIE, with edema in both gray and white matter and gray-matter T1 shortening. Damage to the cortex and underlying white matter, similar to ischemic injury, may be present in the chronic phase [9]. Diagnosis is based on characteristic serum amino acid patterns and urine orotic acid concentration. Enzymology on fibroblasts or hepatocytes may be needed to confirm the diagnosis. DNA analysis has limited availability. Initial emergency treatment consists of hemodialysis, protein restriction, provision of adequate fluids and calories to prevent catabolism, intravenous ammonia-scavenging medications (sodium benzoate and sodium phenylacetate), and intravenous arginine hydrochloride. Chronic therapy includes protein restriction, oral sodium phenylbutyrate and/or sodium benzoate, and arginine or citrulline supplementation.

HHH syndrome

This autosomal recessive condition is caused by defective transport of ornithine into mitochondria, resulting in a secondary inhibition of the urea cycle. Most patients present in infancy with lethargy, intermittent hyperammonemia, failure to thrive, developmental delay, and ataxia. Diagnosis is made by detecting characteristic metabolites in blood and urine. Treatment includes protein restriction.

Lysinuric protein intolerance

Defective transport of basic amino acids across the basolateral membrane of epithelial cells is the fundamental defect in lysinuric protein intolerance. Patients typically present in infancy with hyperammonemia, vomiting, diarrhea, and failure to thrive. Inheritance is autosomal recessive. Serum concentrations of ornithine, lysine, and arginine are low, while citrulline, glutamine, and alanine tend to be elevated. There is increased urinary excretion of lysine, ornithine, and arginine. Moderate protein restriction and citrulline supplementation are the primary therapies.

Other disorders

Glycogen storage disorders (GSD) and disorders of gluconeogenesis may cause hypoglycemia and lactic acidosis in neonates. However, differentiation from HIE and other inborn errors of metabolism should be straightforward.

Glycogen storage disorders

GSD type I patients may have hepatomegaly at birth and symptomatic hypoglycemia, but most patients become symptomatic in infancy. GSD type III (debrancher enzyme deficiency) tends to be a more mild condition, but may present in neonates. GSD type 0 (glycogen synthetase deficiency) may present with ketotic hypoglycemia and lactic acidosis, without prominent hepatomegaly. GSD type VIII (phosphorylase kinase deficiency) may be inherited as an autosomal recessive or X-linked condition. Clinical features include hepatomegaly, myopathy, and a fatal infantile variant with cardiomyopathy. Pompe disease (GSD type II, α-glucosidase deficiency) may also present with neonatal cardiomyopathy and marked hypotonia secondary to a skeletal myopathy [78].

Disorders of gluconeogenesis

Fructose 1,6-bisphosphatase deficiency may present with severe neonatal metabolic acidosis. Routine labs show hypoglycemia and lactic acidosis. Patients typically respond well to intravenous fluids containing dextrose and bicarbonate. Avoidance of fasting is the mainstay of therapy for gluconeogenesis disorders [78].

Congenital disorders of glycosylation (CDG)

These disorders are caused by abnormalities in enzymes responsible for the glycosylation of proteins and lipids. CDG-Ia, the most common subtype, is characterized by mild dysmorphic features, abnormal fat distribution, inverted nipples, strabismus, and hypotonia. Protein-losing enteropathy, nephrotic syndrome, cardiomyopathy, and pericardial effusion are other common features. The head MRI shows cerebellar hypoplasia, but this may not be obvious in neonates [37]. These conditions should be considered, in addition to mitochondrial disorders, in neonates who have multisystem involvement.

Other neonatal myopathies and encephalomyopathies

Patients with inherited myopathies (e.g., centronuclear myopathy) may also present with neonatal distress, hypotonia, and signs suggestive of HIE [78]. Boys with Rett syndrome have been described with a non-specific neonatal encephalopathy and periventricular leukomalacia [79]. Molecular testing for Rett syndrome should be considered in patients with unexplained encephalopathy and normal metabolic investigations.

Summary

Inborn errors of metabolism may present in neonates with features of HIE. In contrast to children with HIE, neonates with metabolic disorders often have an unremarkable delivery and an apparent normal period lasting hours to days. On the other hand, a traumatic delivery or prematurity may constitute environmental stress factors that unmask an underlying inborn error of metabolism; the absence of a normal period, therefore, does not exclude these disorders from consideration. Although patients with metabolic disorders and HIE, in general, have different obstetric histories and head-imaging findings, in practice it may be difficult to distinguish these conditions, because they also share many clinical and laboratory features. There is a tendency to evaluate neonates for a possible underlying metabolic disorder only after more common conditions have been excluded. It is crucial for the clinician to consider metabolic disorders in all neonates with non-specific features suggestive of sepsis or asphyxia upon initial presentation. Rapid diagnosis and management may prevent death or significant morbidity. By obtaining appropriate laboratory investigations, the clinician can provide the family with the best chance of arriving at a diagnosis for their child during an extremely stressful time. Establishing a diagnosis permits not only optimal management of the child, but also accurate genetic counseling. Tandem-mass spectrometry (MS/MS) testing for a wide variety of aminoacidemias, organic acidemias, and fatty acid oxidation defects is currently being integrated into newborn screening programs throughout the world. Such technology provides new hope for the early diagnosis and treatment of inborn errors of metabolism, which collectively account for significant neonatal morbidity and mortality. However, MS/MS newborn screening will not detect many metabolic disorders that may masquerade as HIE, so neonatologists must continue to have a high index of suspicion in order to arrive at a definitive diagnosis.

References

1. Biagas K. Hypoxic–ischemic brain injury: advancements in the understanding of mechanisms and potential avenues for therapy. *Curr Opin Pediatr* 1999; **11**: 223–8.

2. Greene CL, Goodman SI. Catastrophic metabolic encephalopathies in the newborn period: evaluation and management. *Clin Perinatol* 1997; **24**: 773–86.

3. Khong PL, Lam BC, Tung HK, *et al.* MRI of neonatal encephalopathy. *Clin Radiol* 2003; **58**: 833–44.

4. Vannucci RC. Hypoxic–ischemic encephalopathy. *Am J Perinatol* 2000; **17**: 113–20.

5. Barkovich AJ, Sargent SK. Profound asphyxia in the premature infant: imaging findings. *AJNR Am J Neuroradiol* 1995; **16**: 1837–46.

6. Barkovich AJ, Westmark K, Partridge C, *et al.* Perinatal asphyxia: MR findings in the first 10 days. *AJNR Am J Neuroradiol* 1995; **16**: 427–38.

7. Roland EH, Poskitt K, Rodriguez E, *et al.* Perinatal hypoxic–ischemic thalamic injury: clinical features and neuroimaging. *Ann Neurol* 1998; **44**: 161–6.

8. Hoon AH, Reinhardt EM, Kelley RI, *et al.* Brain magnetic resonance imaging in suspected extrapyramidal cerebral palsy: observations in distinguishing genetic–metabolic from acquired causes. *J Pediatr* 1997; **131**: 240–5.

9. Barkovich AJ. *Pediatric Neuroimaging*, 3rd edn. Philadelphia, PA: Lippincott Williams & Wilkins, 2000.

10. Haas RH, Marsden DL, Capistrano-Estrada S, *et al.* Acute basal ganglia infarction in propionic acidemia. *J Child Neurol* 1995; **10**: 18–22.

11. Greenamyre T, Penney JB, Young AB, *et al.* Evidence for transient perinatal glutamatergic innervation of globus pallidus. *J Neurosci* 1987; **7**: 1022–30.

12. Penn AA, Enzmann DR, Hahn JS, *et al.* Kernicterus in a full term infant. *Pediatrics* 1994; **93**: 1003–6.

13. Ankarcrona M, Dypbukt JM, Bonfoco E, et al. Glutamate-induced neuronal death: a succession of necrosis or apoptosis depending on mitochondrial function. Neuron 1995; 15: 961–73.

14. Eliasson MJ, Sampei K, Mandir AS, et al. Poly(ADP-ribose) polymerase gene disruption renders mice resistant to cerebral ischemia. Nat Med 1997; 3: 1089–95.

15. Johnston MV. Hypoxic and ischemic disorders of infants and children. Lecture for 38th meeting of Japanese Society of Child Neurology, Tokyo, Japan, July 1996. Brain Dev 1997; 19: 235–9.

16. Johnston MV, Hoon AH. Possible mechanisms in infants for selective basal ganglia damage from asphyxia, kernicterus, or mitochondrial encephalopathies. J Child Neurol 2000; 15: 588–91.

17. Shi Y, Pan F, Li H, et al. Role of carbon monoxide and nitric oxide in newborn infants with postasphyxial hypoxic–ischemic encephalopathy. Pediatrics 2000; 106: 1447–51.

18. Blomgren K, Hagberg H. Free radicals, mitochondria, and hypoxia–ischemia in the developing brain. Free Radic Biol Med 2006; 40: 388–97.

19. Agani FH, Pichiule P, Chavez JC, et al. The role of mitochondria in the regulation of hypoxia-inducible factor 1 expression during hypoxia. J Biol Chem 2000; 275: 35863–7.

20. Goldberg RN, Cabal LA, Sinatra FR, et al. Hyperammonemia associated with perinatal asphyxia. Pediatrics 1979; 64: 336–41.

21. Sheth RD, Hobbs GR, Mullett M. Neonatal seizures: incidence, onset, and etiology by gestational age. J Perinatol 1999; 19: 40–3.

22. Torres OA, Miller VS, Buist NM, et al. Folinic acid-responsive neonatal seizures. J Child Neurol 1999; 14: 529–32.

23. De Vivo DC, Trifiletti RR, Jacobson RI, et al. Defective glucose transport across the blood–brain barrier as a cause of persistent hypoglycorrhachia, seizures, and developmental delay. N Engl J Med 1991; 325: 703–9.

24. Hyland K, Buist NR, Powell BR, et al. Folinic acid responsive seizures: a new syndrome? J Inherit Metab Dis 1995; 18: 177–81.

25. Baxter P, Griffiths P, Kelly T, et al. Pyridoxine-dependent seizures: demographic, clinical, MRI and psychometric features, and effect of dose on intelligence quotient. Dev Med Child Neurol 1996; 38: 998–1006.

26. Stockler S, Isbrandt D, Hanefeld F, et al. Guanidinoacetate methyltransferase deficiency: the first inborn error of creatine metabolism in man. Am J Hum Genet 1996; 58: 914–22.

27. Baxter P. Epidemiology of pyridoxine dependent and pyridoxine responsive seizures in the UK. Arch Dis Child 1999; 81: 431–3.

28. Medina-Kauwe LK, Tobin AJ, De Meirleir L, et al. 4-Aminobutyrate aminotransferase (GABA-transaminase) deficiency. J Inherit Metab Dis 1999; 22: 414–27.

29. Hyland K, Arnold LA. Value of lumbar puncture in the diagnosis of infantile epilepsy and folinic acid-responsive seizures. J Child Neurol 2002; 17: 3S48–56.

30. Mills PB, Surtees RA, Champion MP, et al. Neonatal epileptic encephalopathy caused by mutations in the PNPO gene encoding pyridox(am)ine 5'-phosphate oxidase. Hum Mol Genet 2005; 14: 1077–86.

31. Molinari F, Raas-Rothschild A, Rio M, et al. Impaired mitochondrial glutamate transport in autosomal recessive neonatal myoclonic epilepsy. Am J Hum Genet 2005; 76: 334–9.

32. Hoffmann GF, Schmitt B, Windfuhr M, et al. Pyridoxal 5'-phosphate may be curative in early-onset epileptic encephalopathy. J Inherit Metab Dis 2007; 30: 96–9.

33. Plecko B, Paul K, Paschke E, et al. Biochemical and molecular characterization of 18 patients with pyridoxine-dependent epilepsy and mutations of the antiquitin (ALDH7A1) gene. Hum Mutat 2007; 28: 19–26.

34. Takahashi Y, Suzuki Y, Kumazaki K, et al. Epilepsy in peroxisomal diseases. Epilepsia 1997; 38: 182–8.

35. Gire C, Girard N, Nicaise C, et al. Clinical features and neuroradiological findings of mitochondrial pathology in six neonates. Childs Nerv Syst 2002; 18: 621–8.

36. von Kleist-Retzow JC, Cormier-Daire V, Viot G, et al. Antenatal manifestations of mitochondrial respiratory chain deficiency. J Pediatr 2003; 143: 208–12.

37. Enns GM, Steiner RD, Buist N, et al. Clinical and molecular features of congenital disorder of glycosylation in patients with type 1 sialotransferrin pattern and diverse ethnic origins. J Pediatr 2002; 141: 695–700.

38. Hoffmann GF, Surtees RA, Wevers RA. Cerebrospinal fluid investigations for neurometabolic disorders. Neuropediatrics 1998; 29: 59–71.

39. Roldan A, Figueras-Aloy J, Deulofeu R, et al. Glycine and other neurotransmitter amino acids in cerebrospinal fluid in perinatal asphyxia and neonatal hypoxic–ischaemic encephalopathy. Acta Paediatr 1999; 88: 1137–41.

40. Bekiesiniska-Figatowska M, Rokicki D, Walecki J. MRI in nonketotic hyperglycinaemia: case report. Neuroradiology 2001; 43: 792–3.

41. del Toro M, Arranz JA, Macaya A, et al. Progressive vacuolating glycine leukoencephalopathy with pulmonary hypertension. Ann Neurol 2006; 60: 148–52.

42. Mourmans J, Majoie CB, Barth PG, et al. Sequential MR imaging changes in nonketotic hyperglycinemia. AJNR Am J Neuroradiol 2006; 27: 208–11.

43. Eyaid WM, Al-Nouri DM, Rashed MS, et al. An inborn error of metabolism presenting as hypoxic–ischemic insult. Pediatr Neurol 2005; 32: 134–6.

44. Topcu M, Coskun T, Haliloglu G, et al. Molybdenum cofactor deficiency: report of three cases presenting as hypoxic–ischemic encephalopathy. J Child Neurol 2001; 16: 264–70.

45. Haenggeli CA, Girardin E, Paunier L. Pyridoxine-dependent seizures, clinical and therapeutic aspects. Eur J Pediatr 1991; 150: 452–5.

46. Jaeken J. Genetic disorders of gamma-aminobutyric acid, glycine, and serine as causes of epilepsy. J Child Neurol 2002; 17: 3S84–8.

47. Au KM, Lai CK, Yuen YP, et al. Diagnosis of dihydropyrimidine dehydrogenase deficiency in a neonate with thymine-uraciluria. Hong Kong Med J 2003; 9: 130–2.

48. Enns GM, Barkovich AJ, van Kuilenburg AB, et al. Head imaging abnormalities in dihydropyrimidine dehydrogenase deficiency. J Inherit Metab Dis 2004; 27: 513–22.

49. De Vivo DC, Leary L, Wang D. Glucose transporter 1 deficiency syndrome and other glycolytic defects. J Child Neurol 2002; 17: 3S15–25.

50. Norman MG, McGillivray BC, Kalousek DK, et al. Perinatal hemorrhagic and

hypoxic–ischemic lesions. In Norman MG, ed., *Congenital Malformations of the Brain: Pathological and Genetic Aspects.* Oxford: Oxford University Press, 1995: 419–23.

51. Birch-Machin MA, Shepherd IM, Watmough NJ, *et al.* Fatal lactic acidosis in infancy with a defect of complex III of the respiratory chain. *Pediatr Res* 1989; **25**: 553–9.

52. von Dobeln U, Wibom R, Ahlman H, *et al.* Fatal neonatal lactic acidosis with respiratory insufficiency due to complex I and IV deficiency. *Acta Paediatr* 1993; **82**: 1079–81.

53. Zeviani M, Bertagnolio B, Uziel G. Neurological presentations of mitochondrial diseases. *J Inherit Metab Dis* 1996; **19**: 504–20.

54. Muraki K, Goto Y, Nishino I, *et al.* Severe lactic acidosis and neonatal death in Pearson syndrome. *J Inherit Metab Dis* 1997; **20**: 43–8.

55. Procaccio V, Mousson B, Beugnot R, *et al.* Nuclear DNA origin of mitochondrial complex I deficiency in fatal infantile lactic acidosis evidenced by transnuclear complementation of cultured fibroblasts. *J Clin Invest* 1999; **104**: 83–92.

56. Willis TA, Davidson J, Gray RG, *et al.* Cytochrome oxidase deficiency presenting as birth asphyxia. *Dev Med Child Neurol* 2000; **42**: 414–17.

57. Muntau AC, Roschinger W, Merkenschlager A, *et al.* Combined D-2- and L-2-hydroxyglutaric aciduria with neonatal onset encephalopathy: a third biochemical variant of 2-hydroxyglutaric aciduria? *Neuropediatrics* 2000; **31**: 137–40.

58. Hoffmann GF, Charpentier C, Mayatepek E, *et al.* Clinical and biochemical phenotype in 11 patients with mevalonic aciduria. *Pediatrics* 1993; **91**: 915–21.

59. Bakkeren JA, Sengers RC, Trijbels JM, *et al.* Organic aciduria in hypoxic premature newborns simulating an inborn error of metabolism. *Eur J Pediatr* 1977; **127**: 41–7.

60. Byrd DJ, Krohn HP, Winkler L, *et al.* Neonatal pyruvate dehydrogenase deficiency with lipoate responsive lactic acidaemia and hyperammonaemia. *Eur J Pediatr* 1989; **148**: 543–7.

61. Robinson BH, MacKay N, Chun K, *et al.* Disorders of pyruvate carboxylase and the pyruvate dehydrogenase complex. *J Inherit Metab Dis* 1996; **19**: 452–62.

62. Bonnefont JP, Chretien D, Rustin P, *et al.* Alpha-ketoglutarate dehydrogenase deficiency presenting as congenital lactic acidosis. *J Pediatr* 1992; **121**: 255–8.

63. Haworth JC, Perry TL, Blass JP, *et al.* Lactic acidosis in three sibs due to defects in both pyruvate dehydrogenase and alpha-ketoglutarate dehydrogenase complexes. *Pediatrics* 1976; **58**: 564–72.

64. Kerrigan JF, Aleck KA, Tarby TJ, *et al.* Fumaric aciduria: clinical and imaging features. *Ann Neurol* 2000; **47**: 583–8.

65. Wilcken B, Haas M, Joy P, *et al.* Outcome of neonatal screening for medium-chain acyl-CoA dehydrogenase deficiency in Australia: a cohort study. *Lancet* 2007; **369**: 37–42.

66. Duran M, Wanders RJ, de Jager JP, *et al.* 3-Hydroxydicarboxylic aciduria due to long-chain 3-hydroxyacyl-coenzyme A dehydrogenase deficiency associated with sudden neonatal death: protective effect of medium-chain triglyceride treatment. *Eur J Pediatr* 1991; **150**: 190–5.

67. Stanley CA, Hale DE, Berry GT, *et al.* Brief report: a deficiency of carnitine-acylcarnitine translocase in the inner mitochondrial membrane. *N Engl J Med* 1992; **327**: 19–23.

68. Bertrand C, Largilliere C, Zabot MT, *et al.* Very long chain acyl-CoA dehydrogenase deficiency: identification of a new inborn error of mitochondrial fatty acid oxidation in fibroblasts. *Biochim Biophys Acta* 1993; **1180**: 327–9.

69. Hintz SR, Matern D, Strauss A, *et al.* Early neonatal diagnosis of long-chain 3-hydroxyacyl coenzyme A dehydrogenase and mitochondrial trifunctional protein deficiencies. *Mol Genet Metab* 2002; **75**: 120–7.

70. Ibdah JA, Bennett MJ, Rinaldo P, *et al.* A fetal fatty-acid oxidation disorder as a cause of liver disease in pregnant women. *N Engl J Med* 1999; **340**: 1723–31.

71. Agsteribbe E, Huckriede A, Veenhuis M, *et al.* A fatal, systemic mitochondrial disease with decreased mitochondrial enzyme activities, abnormal ultrastructure of the mitochondria and deficiency of heat shock protein 60. *Biochem Biophys Res Commun* 1993; **193**: 146–54.

72. Briones P, Vilaseca MA, Ribes A, *et al.* A new case of multiple mitochondrial enzyme deficiencies with decreased amount of heat shock protein 60. *J Inherit Metab Dis* 1997; **20**: 569–77.

73. Poggi GM, Lamantea E, Ciani F, *et al.* Fatal neonatal outcome in a case of muscular mitochondrial DNA depletion. *J Inherit Metab Dis* 2000; **23**: 755–7.

74. Valnot I, Osmond S, Gigarel N, *et al.* Mutations of the SCO1 gene in mitochondrial cytochrome c oxidase deficiency with neonatal-onset hepatic failure and encephalopathy. *Am J Hum Genet* 2000; **67**: 1104–9.

75. Seyda A, Newbold RF, Hudson TJ, *et al.* A novel syndrome affecting multiple mitochondrial functions, located by microcell-mediated transfer to chromosome 2p14–2p13. *Am J Hum Genet* 2001; **68**: 386–96.

76. Chitayat D, Meagher-Villemure K, Mamer OA, *et al.* Brain dysgenesis and congenital intracerebral calcification associated with 3-hydroxyisobutyric aciduria. *J Pediatr* 1992; **121**: 86–9.

77. Burlina AB, Bonafe L, Zacchello F. Clinical and biochemical approach to the neonate with a suspected inborn error of amino acid and organic acid metabolism. *Semin Perinatol* 1999; **23**: 162–73.

78. Tein I. Neonatal metabolic myopathies. *Semin Perinatol* 1999; **23**: 125–51.

79. Schanen NC, Kurczynski TW, Brunelle D, *et al.* Neonatal encephalopathy in two boys in families with recurrent Rett syndrome. *J Child Neurol* 1998; **13**: 229–31.

Chapter 35

Acidosis and alkalosis

Ronald S. Cohen

Introduction

As part of normal homeostasis, the pH of arterial blood is fairly tightly controlled by normal physiologic processes. Healthy adults maintain a reasonably stable pH, ranging from 7.35 to 7.45, and the initial pH after birth can range from 7.11 to 7.36. Acidosis (low pH) and alkalosis (high pH) occur commonly when there are disturbances of the body's normal physiology. This can result from either a pathologic process or medical interventions. When they are due to, or associated with, a pathologic process, the abnormal pH may be blamed for any long-term consequences of that event. Similarly, when a medication or treatment results in an abnormal pH, any long-term consequences may be assigned to that intervention. In both situations, it is not clear whether the underlying physiologic disturbance is responsible for the adverse long-term outcome, or whether the abnormal pH played a role, and if so, how important that role may have been.

Acidosis

Acidosis is known to accompany ischemia, and has been used as a marker for tissue hypoxia and damage. However, it is unclear whether or not acidosis per se is a cause of injury. To examine this issue, we need to separate the two clinical subtypes of acidosis – respiratory and metabolic.

Respiratory acidosis

Respiratory acidosis occurs when carbon dioxide (CO_2), produced by metabolism, builds up in the body and dissolves in the bloodstream. The reaction of CO_2 with water (H_2O) results in the production of hydrogen ions (H^+) and bicarbonate (HCO_3^-). Since pH is defined as the inverse log of the concentration of hydrogen ions, as more CO_2 builds up in the bloodstream, the more H^+ is produced, and the lower the pH becomes. In extrauterine life, the CO_2 that is produced by the body's metabolism is excreted through the lungs. Of course, in utero, CO_2 produced by fetal metabolism must cross the placenta and be excreted through the mother's lungs. Thus, after birth, respiratory acidosis usually indicates an inability of the lungs to meet the demands of the body's metabolism. Fetal

respiratory acidosis usually reflects failure of the placenta to meet the demands of fetal metabolism rather than failure of maternal lung function. If either lung or placental function is inadequate to meet the metabolic needs of the patient, hypoxemia can co-exist commonly with respiratory acidosis. In such a situation, apportioning the causality for any injury to either the hypoxemia or the acidosis is difficult, if not impossible. However, situations exist where there is predominantly respiratory acidosis, and these allow us to determine the effect of this alone.

Allowing a higher arterial partial pressure of CO_2 ($PaCO_2$), or "permissive hypercapnia," has been suggested as a safer method of mechanical ventilation [1–4]. Theoretically, permitting a moderate degree of respiratory acidosis to occur while on mechanical ventilation, by using less pressure or smaller tidal volumes, would be potentially less traumatic to the lungs than using more aggressive mechanical ventilation to achieve a lower "normal" $PaCO_2$. Since oxygenation target levels are not changed with this strategy, these patients generally are not any more hypoxemic than control patients ventilated utilizing standard $PaCO_2$ target levels. Thus the impact of respiratory acidosis per se might be discernible.

Increasing $PaCO_2$ results in lower pH, causing increased cerebral blood flow due to vasodilation. This has been demonstrated in animals and in human neonates [5–11]. The data suggest that newborn animals are less responsive than adults. Nevertheless, the possibility that hypercapnia could cause cerebral vasodilation in the neonate raises a concern for possible intraventricular hemorrhage (IVH), and there are some data to support this.

Early on, hypercapnic acidosis was identified as a risk factor for IVH [12, 13]. More recently, a retrospective review found that maximum $PaCO_2$ was a dose-dependent predictor of severe IVH [14]. The babies with IVH were smaller and more premature, and the retrospective nature of this study limits its strength, but the results are interesting. The patients with no IVH had a mean maximum $PaCO_2$ of about 61 mmHg, while the median maximum $PaCO_2$ for patients with grade 3 and 4 IVH was about 74 mmHg ($p < 0.0001$), somewhat higher than the usual target range even with "permissive hypercapnia." This was also higher than their target range, pointing out the risk of overshooting the upper limit in the clinical "real world." In a study that is not a randomized clinical trial (RCT), it is impossible to know whether the

Fetal and Neonatal Brain Injury, 4th edition, ed. David K. Stevenson, William E. Benitz, Philip Sunshine, Susan R. Hintz, and Maurice L. Druzin. Published by Cambridge University Press. © Cambridge University Press 2009.

$PaCO_2$ is causal or just a proxy for worse lung disease. Furthermore, severe IVH per se might result in an increased $PaCO_2$. In particular, these authors have pointed out the risk of developing acute hypercarbia, and thus increased cerebral blood flow, during surfactant administration [15]. They used an intra-arterial, continuous $PaCO_2$ monitoring device, which demonstrated marked acute swings that otherwise would not have been detected using standard, intermittent blood-gas sampling. They suggest that the incidence of undetected extreme hypercapnia could be much higher than suspected clinically.

Acute changes in $PaCO_2$ may be just as important, if not more so, as prolonged exposure to specific levels, for which there may be acclimatization by the cerebral vasculature. In newborn lambs, the cerebral blood flow returns to baseline after 6 hours of hyperventilation [16]. However, acute normalization of the $PaCO_2$ resulted in an abrupt increase (up to 140%) in cerebral blood flow. Theoretically, this abrupt overperfusion could result in hemorrhage. A recent large ($n = 849$) single-center retrospective analysis showed that the time-weighted average of $PaCO_2$ was less predictive of severe IVH than high, low, and changes in $PaCO_2$ levels [17]. This study, being retrospective, was not able to look at acute changes in $PaCO_2$. Nevertheless, the association of severe IVH with extremes of $PaCO_2$ and changes in $PaCO_2$, more than the time-weighted average, suggests that fluctuations may be significant. Furthermore, since the association was with severe (i.e., grade 3 and 4) IVH, and not with smaller bleeds, the authors speculate that the fluctuations may result in the extension of existing small hemorrhages.

Additional data supporting the theory that moderate hypoventilatory acidosis may be benign for both the lung and the brain are available from animal studies. Using the rat model with unilateral carotid ligation, Vannucci and coworkers studied the impact of hypoxia versus hypercarbia [18]. They exposed rats after ligation to hypoxic gas (8% O_2) mixed with varying levels of CO_2 (0, 3, 6, or 9%). All groups had similar PaO_2 levels, about 34.7 mmHg, with average $PaCO_2$ levels of 26, 42, 54, and 71 mmHg, respectively. Animals were exposed to the different gas mixtures for 2.5 hours, and then sacrificed at 30 days. Brain pathology was scored on a 0–5 scale. Exposure to hypocarbic conditions resulted in worse scores than normocarbia. Increasing CO_2 exposure to 6% further decreased brain pathology, with 9% doing about as well as 3%. They concluded that "hypocapnia aggravates perinatal hypoxic–ischemic brain damage while mild hypercapnia is neuroprotective, at least in the immature rat." Further studies by the same group suggest that higher levels of hypercarbia (greater than 80 mmHg) are associated with lower cerebral blood flow and worse brain damage [19]. Recent studies in rabbits on the effect of hypercarbia on the circulation also show improved cardiac output and tissue perfusion until $PaCO_2$ levels greater than 100 mmHg [20]. Studies on neurons in vitro show that acidosis resulted in decreased apoptosis [21]. Thus, the $PaCO_2$ levels associated with well-controlled permissive hypercarbia, if carefully maintained without rapid

swings, may be neuroprotective on the cellular level, whereas CO_2 levels that are either very high or swing dramatically may alter cardiovascular function in ways that may be deleterious.

Further animal studies demonstrate many theoretic benefits of moderate hypercapnia. Looking specifically at lung injury, studies have not only shown less lung injury with permissive hypercapnia, but have shown a protective effect of inhaled CO_2, without lowered ventilator settings [22]. Thus, CO_2 itself, not the altered ventilator strategy, may be lung-protective. These same authors found that buffering the pH while breathing CO_2 actually attenuated this protective effect [23]. The impact of hypercapnia on other organ systems has also been investigated. Hypercapnic acidosis appears to be protective of the myocardium in post-ischemic animal models [24].

Clinical trials of permissive hypercapnia have thus far been somewhat reassuring, though perhaps not definitive. Though most studies have been positive, including two RCTs [2,25], one study was stopped early when there was a trend towards worse outcome in the hypercapnic "minimal ventilation" group [26]. This small study did have target ranges for $PaCO_2$ of 55–65 mmHg, higher than most other studies. Combining these data with the results discussed above regarding higher levels of $PaCO_2$ and IVH does raise a concern about an upper limit to "how high can you go" with permissive hypercapnia [14]. Nevertheless, the authors of the stopped trial have continued to support studies of permissive hypercapnia, and consider it "a safe and effective management strategy to decrease morbidity from bronchopulmonary dysplasia" [27].

Metabolic acidosis

Metabolic acidosis in neonates usually is secondary to other pathologic processes such as significant hypoxemia, hypovolemia, shock, or an underlying genetic disorder. The presence of a significant metabolic acidosis is one of the generally accepted hallmarks of a perinatal hypoxic–ischemic event [28]. When a hypoxic–ischemic event results in metabolic acidosis, this generally is due to an increase in the serum lactate level induced by anaerobic metabolism [29]. Thus a metabolic acidosis frequently accompanies a hypoxic–ischemic event which results in neurological injury. Other chapters will address the implications of metabolic acidosis as a marker for perinatal hypoxia–ischemia. The question to address here is, can metabolic acidosis itself cause neurological injury? To sort this out, we need to look for evidence that lactic acidosis per se induces neurologic injury, and that treating metabolic acidosis has an impact on neurologic outcome.

The data linking metabolic acidosis itself to neurologic injury are remarkably slim. There are metabolic disorders (e.g., microvillus inclusion disease [30]) that are known to cause recurrent or prolonged episodes of acidosis without resultant central nervous system (CNS) injury. In a large cohort of patients with mitochondrial disorders known to cause lactic acidosis, poor outcome was associated with early onset of symptoms, but was not correlated with plasma lactate levels or metabolic status [31]. Patients with MELAS (mitochondrial encephalopathy, lactic acidosis, stroke) syndrome have qualified for cardiac transplantation [32].

Is there laboratory evidence for lactic acid toxicity? Interestingly, the data suggest that lactic acid may actually be neuroprotective. First, substantial evidence suggests that lactate is a metabolic substrate for the brain [33,34]. Additionally, recent studies on rat brain cells in culture have shown that exposure to very low pH, 6.6 or less, is toxic to brain cells [35]. However, incubation with very high concentrations of lactate, up to 100 mM, did not induce cell death. When lactate was perfused into the brains of unanesthetized rats, there was slowing and suppression of pyramidal cell firing that was completely reversible [36]. This appeared to be due to lactate suppression of glucose metabolism, but only occurred at supraphysiologically high concentrations (10 mM). With lactate alone at physiologic levels (1 mM), nerve cell ATP levels were reduced; with lactate (1 mM) and glucose present at physiologic levels, ATP levels increased. Thus it may be that lactate metabolism can keep brain cells alive when glucose cannot be metabolized, in part by reducing their metabolic activity.

Germane to this discussion is the question of the role of sodium bicarbonate therapy in the neonatal intensive care unit (NICU), since this is probably the most common treatment for metabolic acidosis. If metabolic acidosis is harmful, then treating it should be helpful. Indeed, despite minimal data to support its use, sodium bicarbonate is widely used in neonatology for varying indications [37]. It is commonly given during resuscitation to correct acidosis either documented or suspected. Nevertheless, its efficacy for this remains unclear. There are understandably few RCTs looking at this issue. One, from India, studied the impact of sodium bicarbonate 1.8 mEq/kg versus dextrose 5% given to "asphyxiated" neonates requiring positive-pressure ventilation. The cord pH of the two groups was low (7.01 base, 7.05 dextrose), but in follow-up at 1, 6, 12, and 24 hours, there were no differences in blood gases between the groups [38]. There was also no significant difference in long- or short-term outcomes [39]. If anything, the non-significant trend was worse for the bicarbonate-treated group for outcomes such as cerebral edema (52% vs. 30%), encephalopathy (74% vs. 63%), and need for inotropes (44% vs. 28.6%). Thus the most recent Cochrane analysis states, "There is insufficient evidence from randomized controlled trials to determine whether the infusion of sodium bicarbonate reduces mortality and morbidity in infants receiving resuscitation in the delivery room at birth" [40].

Alkalosis

Alkalosis, like acidosis, can either be respiratory or metabolic. Both are most commonly iatrogenic in the newborn period, though rare metabolic disorders can result in either. The neurologic implications of alkalosis, when accompanied by an underlying genetic disorder, are necessarily complicated by the inherent ramifications of the specific metabolic disorder, many of which can cause brain injury through other mechanisms. Thus, analogous to situations in which hypoxemia accompanies acidosis, it is sometimes difficult to ascribe outcome to alkalosis per se or the underlying genetic cause.

Respiratory alkalosis

Respiratory alkalosis occurs when $PaCO_2$ levels are decreased, a situation known as hypocapnia. This reverses the reaction described above under *respiratory acidosis*, decreasing the concentration of H^+ in the blood, thus raising the pH. In neonates, this usually occurs during mechanical ventilation, though less commonly CNS, cardiac, pulmonary, infectious, or metabolic disorders may cause an infant to hyperventilate while breathing spontaneously, resulting in respiratory alkalosis [41]. Hypocapnia, like its inverse hypercapnia, has effects on the circulation of several organ systems.

Both pH and $PaCO_2$ have long been known to affect pulmonary vasculature tone in newborn animals, with alkalosis causing decreased pulmonary vascular resistance [42,43]. Thus, Peckham and Fox advocated intentional hyperventilatory alkalosis (the opposite of permissive hypercapnia) as a treatment for persistent pulmonary hypertension of the newborn (PPHN) [44], which became a common treatment for this high-mortality condition for the next several years [45,46]. Initial follow-up studies reported good neurological outcomes [47–49]. However, concerns were soon raised about an association between respiratory alkalosis and hearing loss [46,50,51]. It is not completely clear that the hearing loss and other neurologic sequelae of PPHN were due to the treatment, or whether they were related to the perinatal factors associated with the disease itself, such as asphyxia, hypoxemia, meconium staining, and infection. However, the duration of hyperventilatory alkalosis appeared to correlate with poor neurologic outcome [52], suggesting that the alkalosis per se, and not other factors, may be the cause. Also, follow-up of babies with PPHN from the pre-hyperventilatory alkalosis era did not find this association with hearing loss, suggesting that it may be related to the treatment and not the disease or its causes [53]. More recent studies of long-term outcome for patients with PPHN treated with newer modalities, such as iNO and ECMO, show variable results for hearing outcomes, but it is unclear how many patients were hyperventilated, and for how long, before meeting criteria for the new treatment. At least one study correlated post-ECMO hearing loss with profound hypocarbia prior to initiating ECMO, further strengthening this association [54]. Interestingly, even though some animal and human data suggest that alkalosis induced by bicarbonate infusion would decrease pulmonary artery pressure as well as hyperventilation does [55–57], there are recent animal data to question the efficacy of bicarbonate buffering to reverse hypoxic pulmonary vasoconstriction [58]. Clinical data have not supported the efficacy of this treatment for neonatal PPHN. In fact, at least one study suggests that metabolic alkalosis treatment (e.g., sodium bicarbonate IV) may be associated with a worse outcome for PPHN [59].

The connection between hyperventilatory alkalosis and hearing loss may have a plausible biological explanation. Cerebral blood flow is pH-dependent, as discussed above, and may be reduced by alkalosis in animal and human neonates [16,60–63]. This relationship may be more important in term infants who get PPHN than in sick premature ones, whose cerebral circulation may lose the ability to respond to pH and become "pressure-passive" [64]. Animal data suggest that auditory centers may be particularly vulnerable in the newborn period because of a very high metabolic rate compared to other brain regions [65,66]. Thus it is reasonable to theorize that the high metabolic demand of auditory centers may not be met when cerebral blood flow is decreased by hypocapnic alkalosis. Again, there are animal data to support this theory, as decreased levels of brain energy stores have been reported in piglets exposed to normoxemic but hypocapnic ventilation [67,68]. The otherwise healthy normal human neonate might tolerate this. But if you add hypoxemia and hypotension, two situations that commonly co-exist with PPHN, then you may have a scenario where the high metabolic demands may not be met. Furthermore, experimental data mentioned above indicate that hypocarbia may potentiate hypoxemic brain injury in rats [18]. Given the current availability of both iNO and ECMO treatment, it would seem prudent today to minimize the duration of exposure of neonates with PPHN to hyperventilatory alkalosis. Alkalinization with sodium bicarbonate appears to offer little value, and may add risk, and thus should be limited, too [59]. Until more is known, all patients with PPHN need close neurodevelopmental follow-up and monitoring for sensorineural hearing loss. This hearing loss may be progressive, and may not show up for some years [69,70], and thus early screening alone is not adequate.

An association between hypocapnia and periventricular leukomalacia (PVL) has been noted in many studies over many years and with different modes of ventilation [71–74]. A study of high-frequency oscillatory ventilation (HFOV) found increased intracranial hemorrhages and hypocapnia with HFOV, but did not specifically look for a statistical association between hypocapnia and PVL [75]. One study with high-frequency jet ventilation (HFJV) could not link PVL statistically to hypocarbia, only to HFJV [76], though the same group had just reported an association of PVL to hypocarbia with HFJV and previously with conventional ventilation [72,73]. A larger, multicenter trial of HFJV did show an association between ventilator strategy, hypocapnia, and PVL [77]. However, they found a decreased risk of PVL with HFJV when used with a strategy that avoided hyperventilation.

There is also further evidence of hypocapnia being a risk for perinatal brain injury in the setting of hypoxic–ischemic injury. In a large Canadian cohort study of term infants meeting the rigorous definition of hypoxic–ischemic encephalopathy (HIE) [78], outcomes were analyzed for exposure to either high PaO_2 (> 200 mmHg) or low $PaCO_2$ (< 20 mmHg) during the first 2 hours of life. Multivariate analysis controlling for degree of illness showed a significant association of severe hypocapnia with adverse outcome (OR 2.34, 95% CI 1.02–5.37). The strongest association with bad outcome was with both severe hyperoxemia and severe hypocapnia (OR 4.56, 95% CI 1.4–14.9). Lower levels of hyperoxemia or hypocapnia were not significant. Interestingly, in this study, first available base deficit was not significant. Again, these authors postulate that an additive effect of hypocapnic alkalosis induced decreased cerebral blood flow upon underlying hypoxic–ischemic injury. Higher PaO_2 levels, which occur not infrequently during resuscitation, may have contributed to oxidative injury [79].

Metabolic alkalosis

Metabolic alkalosis occurs less commonly than respiratory alkalosis, and often is related to treatment with an alkalinizing agent, such as sodium bicarbonate. It may be associated with chloride depletion due to hyperemesis; the use of diuretics, primarily furosemide, and especially if there is inadequate replacement of potassium; severe dehydration resulting in a state of "contraction alkalosis"; and, more rarely, a number of uncommon renal, endocrine, and gastrointestinal disorders [80]. Interestingly, though some of the hereditary renal causes of persistent metabolic alkalosis are associated with developmental delay and sensorineural deafness, not all are, and the mechanism of the CNS abnormality may be part of the overall genetic syndrome [81,82]. Congenital chloride diarrhea can result in metabolic alkalosis, but when treated, even with a mean age of diagnosis over 2 months, neurologic outcome is good [83,84]. These observations suggest that the neonatal brain can tolerate metabolic alkalosis fairly well, especially considering that these diagnoses also commonly add hypovolemia and other electrolyte abnormalities, but generally not hypoxemia.

Since hyperventilatory alkalosis has been recommended for treatment of pulmonary hypertension (see above), metabolic alkalinization has also been proposed. Indeed, as recently as 1997 it was listed as part of the "basic therapy" in a European review [85]. However, a review of data from US multicenter trials actually showed that bicarbonate use resulted in a worse outcome, with an odds ratio for ECMO of 5.03 versus hyperventilatory alkalosis [59].

Given the current data on the use of sodium bicarbonate, there appear to be few if any indications, some significant concerns about risk, and virtually no documented benefits. Though it continues to be used to treat acidosis due to the lack of any readily available alternative, this does not necessarily mean it is better than no treatment. Thus, if used, it must be used minimally and cautiously, and not using it clearly should not be considered a breach of standard of care.

Conclusions

We have reviewed the literature on the impact of alkalosis and acidosis on the brain of the neonate. Though it is clear that much remains to be learned, it appears that the neonatal CNS has remarkable resilience. Respiratory alkalosis does seem to be associated with injury when prolonged or associated with pronounced swings in pH. Careful monitoring to avoid this is warranted. Furthermore, the benefits of sodium bicarbonate treatment remain at best unproven, with reasons to be concerned about complications thereof. However, it appears that the newborn brain can tolerate acidosis, both respiratory and metabolic, better than one might have imagined.

References

1. Hickling KG, Henderson SJ, Jackson R. Low mortality associated with low volume pressure limited ventilation with permissive hypercapnia in severe adult respiratory distress syndrome. *Intensive Care Med* 1990; **16**: 372–7.

2. Mariani G, Cifuentes J, Carlo WA. Randomized trial of permissive hypercapnia in preterm infants. *Pediatrics* 1999; **104**: 1082–8.

3. Ni Chonghaile M, Higgins B, Laffey JG. Permissive hypercapnia: role in protective lung ventilatory strategies. *Curr Opin Crit Care* 2005; **11**: 56–62.

4. Carlo WA. Permissive hypercapnia and permissive hypoxemia in neonates. *J Perinatol* 2007; **27**: S64–70.

5. Hernandez MJ, Brennan RW, Vannucci RC, *et al*. Cerebral blood flow and oxygen consumption in the newborn dog. *Am J Physiol* 1978; **234**: R209–15.

6. Reivich M, Brann AW, Shapiro H. Reactivity of cerebral vessels to CO_2 in the newborn rhesus monkey. *Eur Neurol* 1971; **6**: 132–6.

7. Rosenberg AA, Jones MD, Traystman RJ, *et al*. Response of cerebral blood flow to changes in pCO_2 in fetal, newborn, and adult sheep. *Am J Physiol* 1982; **242**: H862–6.

8. Griesen G. Cerebral blood flow and energy metabolism in the newborn. *Clin Perinatol* 1997; **24**: 531–46.

9. Dietz V, Wolf M, Keel M, *et al*. CO_2 reactivity of the cerebral hemoglobin concentration in healthy term newborns measured by near infrared spectrophotometry. *Biol Neonate* 1999; **75**: 85–90.

10. Jayasinghe D, Gill AB, Levene MI. CBF reactivity in hypotensive and normotensive preterm infants. *Pediatr Res* 2003; **54**: 848–53.

11. Kaiser JR, Gauss CH, Williams DK. The effects of hypercapnia on cerebral autoregulation in ventilated very low birth weight infants. *Pediatr Res* 2005; **58**: 931–5.

12. Kenny JD, Garcia-Prats JA, Hilliard JL, *et al*. Hypercarbia at birth: a possible role in the pathogenesis of intraventricular hemorrhage. *Pediatrics* 1978; **62**: 465–7.

13. Levene MI, Fawer, CL, Lamont RF. Risk factors in the development of intraventricular haemorrhage in the preterm neonate. *Arch Dis Child* 1982; **57**: 410–17.

14. Kaiser JR, Gauss CH, Pont MJ, *et al*. Hypercapnia during the first 3 days of life is associated with severe intraventricular hemorrhage in very low birth weight infants. *J Perinatol* 2006; **26**: 279–85.

15. Kaiser JR, Gauss CH, Williams DK. Surfactant administration acutely affects cerebral and systemic hemodynamics and gas exchange in very low birth weight infants. *J Pediatr* 2004; **144**: 809–14.

16. Gleason CA, Short BL, Jones Jr MD. Cerebral blood flow and metabolism during and after prolonged hypocapnia in newborn lambs. *J Pediatr* 1989; **115**: 309–14.

17. Fabres J, Carlo WA, Phillips V, *et al*. Both extremes of arterial carbon dioxide pressure and the magnitude of fluctuations in arterial carbon dioxide pressure are associated with severe intraventricular hemorrhage in preterm infants. *J Pediatr* 2007; **119**: 299–305.

18. Vannucci RC, Towfighi J, Heitjan DF, *et al*. Carbon dioxide protects the perinatal rat brain from hypoxic–ischemic damage. *Pediatrics* 1995; **95**: 868–74.

19. Vannucci RC, Towfighi J, Brucklacher RM, *et al*. Effect of extreme hypercapnia on hypoxic–ischemic brain damage in the immature rat. *Pediatr Res* 2001; **49**: 799–803.

20. Komori M, Takada K, Tomizawa Y, *et al*. Permissive range of hypercapnia for improved peripheral microcirculation and cardiac output in rabbits. *Crit Care Med* 2007; **35**: 2171–5.

21. Xu L, Glassford AJM, Giaccia AJ, *et al*. Acidosis reduces neuronal apoptosis. *NeuroReport* 1998; **9**: 875–9.

22. Laffey JG, Tanaka M, Engelberts D, *et al*. Therapeutic hypercapnia reduces pulmonary and systemic injury following *in vivo* lung reperfusion. *Am J Respir Crit Care Med* 2000; **162**: 2287–94.

23. Laffey JG, Engelberts D, Kavanagh BP. Buffering hypercapnic acidosis worsens acute lung injury. *Am J Respir Crit Care Med* 2000; **161**: 141–6.

24. Fujita M, Asanuma H, Hirata A, *et al*. Prolonged transient acidosis during early reperfusion contributes to the cardioprotective effects of postconditioning. *Am J Physiol Heart Circ Physiol* 2007; **292**: H2004–8.

25. Carlo WA, Stark AR, Wright LL, *et al*. Minimal ventilation to prevent bronchopulmonary dysplasia in extremely-low-birth-weight infants. *J Pediatr* 2002; **141**: 370–5.

26. Thome UH, Carroll W, Wu T-J, *et al*. Outcome of extremely preterm infants randomized at birth to different $PaCO_2$ targets during the first seven days of life. *Biol Neonate* 2006; **90**: 218–25.

27. Miller JD, Carlo WA. Safety and effectiveness of permissive hypercapnia in the preterm infant. *Curr Opin Pediatr* 2007; **19**: 142–4.

28. American College of Obstetricians and Gynecologists. Committee on Obstetric Practice. Umbilical cord blood gas and acid–base analysis. *Obstet Gynecol* 2006; **108**: 1319–22.

29. Evans OB. Lactic acidosis in childhood: Part I. *Pediatr Neurol* 1985; **1**: 325–8.

30. Bar A, Riskin A, Iancu T, *et al*. A newborn infant with protracted diarrhea and metabolic acidosis. *J Pediatr* 2007; **150**: 198–201.

31. Debray FG, Lamber M, Chevalier I, *et al*. Long-term outcome and clinical spectrum of 73 pediatric patients with mitochondrial diseases. *Pediatrics* 2007; **119**: 722–33.

32. Bhati RS, Sheridan BC, Mill MR, *et al*. Heart transplantation for progressive cardiomyopathy as a manifestation of MELAS syndrome. *J Heart Lung Transplant* 2005; **24**: 2286–9.

33. Schurr A. Lactate: the ultimate cerebral oxidative energy substrate? *J Cerebral Blood Flow Metabol* 2006; **26**: 142–52.

34. Bergersen LH. Is lactate food for neurons? Comparison of monocarboxylate transporter subtypes in brain and muscle. *Neuroscience* 2007; **145**: 11–19.

35. Pirchl M, Marksteiner J, Humpel C. Effects of acidosis on brain capillary endothelial cells and cholinergic neurons: relevance to vascular dementia and Alzheimer's disease. *Neurol Res* 2006; **28**: 657–64.

36. Gilbert E, Tang JM, Ludvig N, *et al*. Elevated lactate suppresses neuronal

firing *in vivo* and inhibits glucose metabolism in hippocampal slice cultures. *Brain Res* 2006; **1117**: 213–23.

37. Ammari AN, Schulze KF. Uses and abuses of sodium bicarbonate in the neonatal intensive care unit. *Curr Opin Pediatr* 2002; **14**: 151–6.

38. Murki S, Kumar P, Lingappa L, *et al.* Effect of a single dose of sodium bicarbonate given during neonatal resuscitation at birth on the acid–base status on first day of life. *J Perinatol* 2004; **24**: 696–9.

39. Lokesh L, Kumar P, Murki S, *et al.* A randomized controlled trial of sodium bicarbonate in neonatal resuscitation: effect on immediate outcome. *Resuscitation* 2000; **60**: 219–23.

40. Beveridge CJE, Wilkinson AR. Sodium bicarbonate infusion during resuscitation of infants at birth. *Cochrane Database Syst Rev* 2006; (1): CD004864.

41. Laffey JG, Kavanagh BP. Hypocapnia. *N Engl J Med* 2002; **347**: 43–53.

42. Cassin S, Dawes GS, Mott JC, *et al.* The vascular resistance of the foetal and newly ventilated lung of the lamb. *J Physiol* 1964; **171**: 61–79.

43. Rudolph AM, Yuan S. Response of the pulmonary vasculature to hypoxia and H^+ ion concentration changes. *J Clin Invest* 1966; **45**: 399–411.

44. Peckham GJ, Fox WW. Physiologic factors affecting pulmonary artery pressure in infants with persistent pulmonary hypertension. *J Pediatr* 1978; **93**: 1005–10.

45. Fox WW, Duara S. Persistent pulmonary hypertension in the neonate: diagnosis and management. *J Pediatr* 1983; **103**: 505–14.

46. Marron MJ, Crisafi MA, Driscoll JM, *et al.* Hearing and neurodevelopmental outcome in survivors of persistent pulmonary hypertension of the newborn. *Pediatrics* 1992; **90**: 392–6.

47. Brett C, Dekle M, Leonard CH, *et al.* Developmental follow-up of hyperventilated neonates: preliminary observations. *Pediatrics* 1981; **68**: 588–91.

48. Ferrara B, Johnson DE, Chang PN, *et al.* Efficacy and neurologic outcome of profound hypocapneic alkalosis for the treatment of persistent pulmonary hypertension in infancy. *J Pediatr* 1984; **105**: 457–61.

49. Bernbaum JC, Russell P, Sheridan PH, *et al.* Long-term follow-up of newborns with persistent pulmonary hypertension. *Crit Care Med* 1984; **12**: 579–83.

50. Ballard RA, Leonard CH. Developmental follow-up of infants with persistent pulmonary hypertension of the newborn. *Clin Perinatol* 1984; **11**: 737–44.

51. Leavitt AM, Watchko JF, Bennett FC, *et al.* Neurodevelopmental outcome following persistent pulmonary hypertension of the neonate. *J Perinatol* 1987; **7**: 288–91.

52. Bifano EM, Pfannenstiel A. Duration of hyperventilation and outcome in infants with persistent pulmonary hypertension. *Pediatrics* 1988; **81**: 657–61.

53. Cohen RS, Stevenson D, Malachowski N, *et al.* Late morbidity among survivors on respiratory failure treated with tolazoline. *J Pediatr* 1980; **97**: 644–7.

54. Graziani LJ, Baumgart S, Desai S, *et al.* Clinical antecedents of neurologic and audiologic abnormalities in survivors of extracorporeal membrane oxygenation. *J Child Neurol* 1997; **12**: 415–22.

55. Lyrene Rk, Welch KA, Godoy G, *et al.* Alkalosis attenuates hypoxic pulmonary vasoconstriction in neonatal lambs. *Pediatr Res* 1985; **19**: 1268–71.

56. Schreiber MD, Heymann MA, Soifer SJ. Increased arterial pH, not decreased PaCO2, attenuates hypoxia-induced pulmonary vasoconstriction in newborn lambs. *Pediatr Res* 1986; **20**: 113–17.

57. Chang AC, Zucker HA, Hickey PR, *et al.* Pulmonary vascular resistance in infants after cardiac surgery: role of carbon dioxide and hydrogen ion. *Crit Care Med* 1995; **23**: 568–74.

58. Lee KJ, Hernandez G, Gordon JB. Hypercapnic acidosis and compensated hypercapnia in control and pulmonary hypertensive piglets. *Pediatr Pulmonol* 2003; **36**: 94–101.

59. Walsh-Sukys MC, Tyson JE, Wright LL, *et al.* Persistent pulmonary hypertension of the newborn in the era before nitric oxide: practice variation and outcomes. *Pediatrics* 2000; **105**: 14–20.

60. Hansen NB, Nowicki PT, Miller RR, *et al.* Alterations in cerebral blood flow and oxygen consumption during prolonged hypocarbia. *Pediatr Res* 1986; **20**: 147–50.

61. Kusada S, Shisida N, Miyagi N, *et al.* Cerebral blood flow during treatment for pulmonary hypertension. *Arch Dis Child Fetal Neonatal Ed* 1999; **80**: F30–3.

62. Menke J, Michel E, Rabe H, *et al.* Simultaneous influence of blood pressure, PCO2, and PO2 on cerebral blood flow velocity in preterm infants of

less than 33 weeks' gestation. *Pediatr Res* 1993; **24**: 173–7.

63. Kaiser JR, Gauss CH, Williams DK. The effects of hypercapnia on cerebral autoregulation in ventilated very low birth weight infants. *Pediatr Res* 2005; **58**: 931–5.

64. Soul JS, Hammer PE, Tsuji P, *et al.* Fluctuating pressure-passivity is common in the cerebral circulation of sick premature infants. *Pediatr Res* 2007; **61**: 467–73.

65. Kennedy C, Sakurada O, Shinohara M, *et al.* Local cerebral glucose utilization in the newborn macaque monkey. *Ann Neurol* 1982; **12**: 333–40.

66. Vannucci RC, Vannucci SJ. Perinatal brain metabolism. In Polin RA, Fox WW, Abman SH, eds., *Fetal and Neonatal Physiology*, 3rd edn. Philadelphia, PA: Saunders, 2004: 1713–25.

67. Graham EM, Apostolou M, Mishra OP, *et al.* Modification of the *N*-methyl-D-aspartate (NMDA) receptor in the brain of newborn piglets following hyperventilation induced ischemia. *Neurosci Lett* 1996; **218**: 29–32.

68. Fritz KI, Zubrow AB, Ashraf QM, *et al.* The effect of moderate hypocapnic ventilation on nuclear Ca^{2+}-ATPase activity, nuclear Ca^{2+} flux, and Ca^{2+}/calmodulin kinase IV activity in the cerebral cortex of newborn piglets. *Neurochem Res* 2004; **29**: 791–6.

69. Naulty CM, Weiss IP, Herer GR. Progressive sensorineural hearing loss in survivors of persistent fetal circulation. *Ear Hear* 1986; **7**: 74–7.

70. Hendricks-Munoz KD, Walton JP. Hearing loss in infants with persistent fetal circulation. *Pediatrics* 1988; **81**: 650–6.

71. Calvert SA, Hoskins EM, Fong KW, *et al.* Etiological factors associated with the development of periventricular leukomalacia. *Acta Paediatr Scand* 1987; **76**: 254–9.

72. Graziani LJ, Spitzer AR, Mitchell DG, *et al.* Mechanical ventilation in preterm infants: neurosonographic and developmental studies. *Pediatrics* 1992; **90**: 515–22.

73. Wiswell TE, Graziani LJ, Kornhauser MS, *et al.* Effects of hypocarbia on the development of cystic periventricular leukomalacia in premature infants treated with high-frequency jet ventilation. *Pediatrics* 1996; **98**: 918–24.

74. Shankaran S, Langer JC, Kazzi SN, *et al.* Cumulative index of exposure to

hypocarbia and hyperoxia as risk factors for periventricular leukomalacia in low birth weight infants. *Pediatrics* 2006; **118**: 1654–9.

75. HiFO Study Group. Randomized study of high-frequency oscillatory ventilation in infants with severe respiratory distress syndrome. *J Pediatr* 1993; **122**: 609–19.

76. Wiswell TE, Graziani LJ, Kornhauser MS, *et al*. High-frequency jet ventilation in the early management of respiratory distress syndrome is associated with a greater risk for adverse outcomes. *Pediatrics* 1996; **98**: 1035–43.

77. Keszler M, Modanlou HD, Brudno DS, *et al*. Multicenter controlled clinical trial of high-frequency jet ventilation in preterm infants with uncomplicated respiratory distress syndrome. *Pediatrics* 1997; **100**: 593–9.

78. Klinger G, Beyene J, Shah P, *et al*. Do hyperoxaemia and hypocapnia add to the risk of brain injury after intrapartum asphyxia? *Arch Dis Child Fetal Neonatal Ed* 2005; **90**: F49–52.

79. Vento M, Asensi M, Sastre J, *et al*. Oxidative stress in asphyxiated term infants resuscitated with 100% oxygen. *J Pediatr* 2003; **142**: 240–6.

80. Laski ME, Sabatini S. Metabolic alkalosis, bedside and bench. *Semin Nephrol* 2006; **26**: 404–21.

81. Shaer AJ. Inherited primary renal tubular hypokalemic alkalosis: a review of Gitelman and Bartter syndromes. *Am J Med Sci* 2001; **322**: 316–32.

82. Naesens M, Steels P, Verberckmoes R, *et al*. Bartter's and Gitelman's syndromes: from gene to clinic. *Nephron Physiol* 2004; **96**: 65–78.

83. Kagalwalla AF. Congenital chloride diarrhea: a study in Arab children. *J Clin Gastroenterol* 1994; **19**: 36–40.

84. Hihnala S, Höglund P, Lammi L, *et al*. Long-term clinical outcome in patients with congenital chloride diarrhea. *J Pediatr Gastroenterol Nutr* 2006; **42**: 369–75.

85. Sasse S, Kribs A, Vierzig A, *et al*. A staged protocol for the treatment of persistent pulmonary hypertension of the newborn. *Klin Padiatr* 1997; **209**: 301–7.

Chapter 36

Meconium staining and the meconium aspiration syndrome

Thomas E. Wiswell

Introduction

Meconium-stained amniotic fluid (MSAF) occurs in approximately 10–15% of all pregnancies [1]. The presence of MSAF has been recognized as being associated with adverse fetal and neonatal outcomes for centuries [2]. Aristotle gave the substance the name *meconium-arion*, meaning "opium-like." This may have been because the philosopher believed it induced fetal sleep, recognizing fetal deaths and neonatal depression as being associated with meconium. Conversely, the name may have arisen because processed opium is a black, tarry substance resembling meconium. Obstetricians and pediatricians have long recognized the relationship of MSAF with stillborn infants, abnormal fetal heart-rate (FHR) tracings, neonatal encephalopathy, respiratory distress, and an abnormal neurologic outcome in some survivors. Nevertheless, the vast majority of infants born through MSAF do not have apparent antenatal, intrapartum, or postnatal problems. Thus we have somewhat limited ability to predict and prognosticate from the presence of MSAF. Healthcare providers should be appropriately concerned about both MSAF and meconium-stained neonates who subsequently develop respiratory distress, the meconium aspiration syndrome (MAS). Despite the frequent occurrence of MSAF and MAS, there remains a distinct paucity of literature describing the neurological development of either children born through MSAF or those with MAS.

Historical aspects

More than 80 years ago, Schulze reviewed several controversies concerning MSAF, including whether its presence reflected fetal asphyxia versus a physiologic process, as well as whether MSAF represented a grave prognostic omen [3]. She referred to publications from the 1600s in which MSAF was considered a sign of death or impending death of the fetus, and quoted several publications from the 1800s in which MSAF portended an endangered condition of the fetus. She referred to Jesse's 1888 report, in which MSAF was found in 9.5% of pregnancies. In this latter report, of 314 pregnancies in which MSAF was found, 74 of the infants were stillborn, while 74 were described as "asphyxiated." Grant referred to the work

of Kennedy in 1833 in which MSAF was described as a harbinger of stillbirth or fetal distress [4]. In 1918 Reed proposed that in utero anoxia would relax the anal sphincter and result in meconium passage, and was the first individual to describe in utero aspiration of meconium [5]. Clifford reported a 6% mortality rate and a 60% morbidity rate among infants born through MSAF [6]. He specifically commented on the frequent need for resuscitation of such infants. Brews subsequently hypothesized that meconium passage was a result of increased intestinal peristalsis as a response to asphyxia [7]. The degree of hypoxia needed for meconium passage was first described by Walker [8], who found that meconium passage was associated with umbilical venous oxygen saturations < 30%.

Some data concerning MSAF and MAS were reported from the National Institute of Neurological and Communicative Disorders and Stroke Collaborative Perinatal Project (CPP) of the late 1950s and 1960s. In this study, more than 42 000 children were followed from birth for the development of cerebral palsy (CP), mental retardation (MR), and other neurologic disorders [9,10]. Fujikura and Klionsky reported that 10.3% of all live-born infants in the CPP had meconium staining [9], and found the stained group to have a neonatal mortality death rate of 3.3% compared to 1.7% among non-meconium-stained babies. Fully 18.1% of the babies that died in the CPP were born through MSAF. Naeye found MAS to occur in 8.7% of the infants in the CPP who were born through MSAF [10]. Of those babies with such respiratory distress, 63% died. In the 1950s, Desmond and colleagues reported meconium-stained babies to be more likely to have abnormal neurologic findings [11].

During the 1970s several articles appeared supporting the benefits of aggressive airway management in meconium-stained neonates. These were summarized in a review article in 2000 [12]. Although they represented anecdotal experience and not randomized controlled trials (RCTs), these works led to virtually universal practices of obstetrical oro- and nasopharyngeal suctioning, as well as postpartum intratracheal suctioning, of meconium-stained infants in the delivery room. However, in a large RCT [12] we established that intratracheal intubation and suctioning did not improve the respiratory outcomes of apparently vigorous meconium-stained neonates. Additionally, other interventions aimed at preventing MAS have recently been evaluated in another large random RCT [13]. Vain and colleagues assessed the value of intrapartum

Fetal and Neonatal Brain Injury, 4th edition, ed. David K. Stevenson, William E. Benitz, Philip Sunshine, Susan R. Hintz, and Maurice L. Druzin. Published by Cambridge University Press. © Cambridge University Press 2009.

oro- and nasopharyngeal suctioning prior to delivery of the baby's shoulders [13]. They found no decrease in MAS with this maneuver. Amnioinfusion has been widely practiced since the late 1980s. Normal saline or lactated Ringer's solution is infused into the uteri of women with thick-consistency MSAF. The hope is that the fluid would dilute the meconium and make it less toxic, as well as alleviate umbilical cord compression. Fraser *et al.* performed an RCT enrolling approximately 2000 women with thick-consistency MSAF and found amnioinfusion to be of no benefit in preventing MAS [14].

Meconium-stained amniotic fluid and fetal distress

What is the evidence supporting the association of MSAF with fetal distress? Unquestionably, babies born through MSAF and those who subsequently develop MAS have a higher frequency of abnormal fetal heart-rate tracings [15,16]. The classic work of Walker [8] revealed the markedly low fetal oxygen saturations related to meconium passage. Meconium-stained infants are more likely to have lower scalp pHs or low umbilical cord artery pHs [16–18]. Additionally, meconium-stained infants have lower 1- and 5-minute Apgar scores [1,19]. When we previously reviewed the literature [1], we found approximately one-third of all reported babies (10 studies) were "depressed" at birth. Additionally, it is likely that in some cases the lower Apgar scores in meconium-stained babies are due to the intubation procedure itself [12].

Can there be abnormal outcomes in babies born through MSAF who have normal antenatal testing or normal FHR tracings? Various authors have found from 29% to 60% of infants with meconium-associated respiratory distress had normal FHR tracings [12,15]. Smith and colleagues reviewed a series of fetal deaths which followed antepartum heart-rate testing [20]. They found 16 of 53 stillborn infants had passed meconium. Thirteen of these 16 had had normal, reactive non-stress tests (NSTs). Fleischer's group reported that even with the presence of normal intrapartum FHR tracings and normal 5-minute Apgar scores, infants with MSAF had an incidence of respiratory complications many times greater than those born through clear amniotic fluid [21]. I conclude that the finding of MSAF is associated with many markers of fetal distress. The evidence definitely supports that one should not be at ease in cases of MSAF with normal FHR tracings, as adverse outcomes may still occur.

Non-neurologic adverse outcomes

Fleischer and colleagues found meconium-stained, term-gestation infants to be 100 times more likely to develop respiratory distress than their counterparts born through clear amniotic fluid [21]. The MAS is the most frequently noted adverse outcome found among infants subsequent to being born through MSAF. The term "meconium aspiration syndrome" refers to infants born through MSAF who have respiratory distress and whose symptoms cannot be otherwise explained. In two large reviews of the disorder [2,22], we have

found approximately 5% of infants born through MSAF will subsequently develop MAS, one-third to one-half of those with MAS will require mechanical ventilation, one-quarter will develop pneumothoraxes, and one in 20 will die. The death rate has varied over time, from as many as 63% of those in the CPP to as low as 0% in more recent, smaller populations. The death rate has declined over time [1], a finding which likely has been influenced by aggressive airway management in the delivery room, better ventilatory techniques, and improvements in supportive care (thermoregulation, parenteral nutrition, etc.). Two-thirds of neonates with persistent pulmonary hypertension have MAS as an associated disorder [16]. The proportion of babies admitted to newborn intensive care units (NICUs) is increased among those born through MSAF compared to those born through clear MSAF. Nathan *et al.* found 24% of meconium-stained babies were admitted to their NICU compared to 7% of those born through clear fluid [16]. Among premature infants born through MSAF, Wagner and associates found lower 1- and 5-minute Apgar scores, as well as a fourfold higher mortality rate [24]. Thus, among babies born through MSAF, there is considerable morbidity not related to neurologic outcome.

Adverse neurologic outcomes

There are no prospective investigations that have specifically followed a group of meconium-stained infants, or even the sicker group of children with MAS, for a minimum of at least 2–6 years to adequately assess how such children develop. Nonetheless, there exists abundant literature, which links some adverse neurologic findings with meconium.

Grafe described brain injury in 83 stillborn and 13 infants dying within 1 hour after birth [25]. She found neurological damage to be more common if there had been meconium staining of the placenta. The major change was white-matter gliosis/necrosis. Redline found meconium-associated vascular necrosis of the placenta to be a major factor associated with neurologic impairment in infants [26].

Desmond and colleagues found infants born through MSAF to be more likely to have hypotonia, lethargy, and seizures [11]. Several investigators have examined data from the CPP. Naeye reported that if infants were born through MSAF [10] they had a significantly increased risk for neurologic abnormalities at 7 years of age, including quadriplegic CP, chronic seizures, and severe MR. These children were also more likely to have hyperactivity at this age. Nelson and Broman assessed a group of 50 children from the CPP who had marked neurological abnormalities [27], characterized by moderate or severe motor disability and severe MR, and compared them to a large control population. Those with severe handicaps were more than twice as likely to have been born through MSAF (40.8% vs. 19.1%). Nelson found the rate of CP among the children with birthweight > 2500 g in the project to be approximately 3/1000 if there was no history of obstetrical complications [28]. When there was a history of MSAF and no other complications, 4/1000 survivors developed CP. However, when there was a history of MSAF and a 5-minute Apgar score ≤ 3, the rate of CP increased to 94/1000. Among CPP infants of birthweight ≤ 2500 g born through MSAF, Nelson and Ellenberg reported the frequency of CP to be 15/1000 [29]. Additionally, 12/1000 of the low-birthweight meconium-stained babies had no CP, but developed seizures.

Shields and Schifrin examined a group of 75 babies with cerebral palsy who had been born between 1976 and 1983 [30]. They found that 41% had been born through MSAF, and that overall 21% of the 75 babies with CP had been affected with MAS. Gaffney and colleagues in England similarly examined a group of infants with CP ($n = 141$) [31]. They found MSAF to be significantly more common in those with CP versus control (non-CP) infants (24.2% vs. 9.9%). Spinillo et al. reported an increased risk for CP and periventricular leukomalacia (PVL) among meconium-stained premature infants [32,33].

Seizures during the neonatal period are an important predictor of subsequent neurological handicap. Neonatal seizures occur in approximately 0.4–0.8% of all live-born infants. Berkus et al. found a sevenfold increased risk for neonatal seizures, as well as a fivefold increased risk for hypotonia, among infants born through moderately thick or thick MSAF [15]. Similarly, Nathan et al. described a fivefold increased risk for seizures during the first 24 hours of life if infants had been born through MSAF (2.0% vs. 0.4%) [16]. Lien et al. reviewed a group of term-gestation infants that had neonatal seizures [34]. Of 40 such infants, 40% had been born through MSAF, while 12.5% had a history of MAS. Sato and colleagues described three infants born through MSAF without signs of hypoxic–ischemic encephalopathy (HIE) that developed seizures and were found to have perisagittal cerebral infarcts [35]. Blackwell et al. described a group of 48 infants with severe MAS (needing mechanical ventilation for > 48 hours) [36]. Of these, 29 had umbilical cord artery pH levels ≥ 7.20, while 19 had levels < 7.20. Approximately 21% of the infants in both groups subsequently developed seizures. The latter authors speculated that pre-existing neurological injury prior to birth occurs in many meconium-stained babies, rather than intrapartum injury. They also conjectured that non-hypoxic–ischemic mechanisms may cause neuronal injury in this population. Finer's group reviewed 95 infants of ≥ 37 weeks gestation that had evidence of HIE [37]. Almost half of these children (48.4%) had a history of MAS, while 28% of those with MAS subsequently developed moderate to severe neurologic handicaps. In a recent review from Australia, Walstab et al. similarly reported increased risk for subsequent CP in infants with MAS [38]. Beligere's group recently described a 3-year follow-up of 29 infants with MAS requiring mechanical ventilation [39]. None of these neonates was treated with extracorporeal membrane oxygenation (ECMO), high-frequency ventilation, or inhaled nitric oxide (iNO). These authors described normal outcomes in 38% of the population, while 7% developed CP, 14% had global developmental delays, and 41% had mild developmental delays.

Matsuishi and colleagues prospectively evaluated the incidence of autistic disorder among 5271 survivors of a NICU [40]. The children were assessed sequentially for neurodevelopmental disorders for a 5-year period following discharge. Autistic disorder was identified in 18 of the infants, while 57 had CP. The authors found that a history of MAS was significantly higher in children with autistic disorder (22%) or CP (8.8%) compared to the control population of NICU graduates without MAS.

The data I have discussed in this section indicate a relationship between certain adverse neurodevelopmental outcomes and MSAF/MAS. Presumably, most infants born through MSAF will ultimately be neurologically intact. As a group, babies born through MSAF or who develop MAS are generally not followed to assess long-term morbidity. Unfortunately, because there are no prospective epidemiologic studies of various adverse neurodevelopmental outcomes and MSAF, one cannot generally prognosticate about infants either born through MSAF or those who develop MAS.

Pathophysiology of meconium passage

Meconium is a viscous green liquid consisting of gastrointestinal secretions, bile, bile acids, mucus, pancreatic juice, cellular debris, amniotic fluid, and swallowed vernix caseosa, lanugo, and blood [2]. Between the 10th and 16th weeks of gestation, the substance may first be noted in the fetal gastrointestinal tract. Typically, 60–200 g of the substance is found in a term infant's intestine. Because of the lack of strong peristalsis, as well as the presence of good anal sphincter tone and a terminal cap of particularly viscous meconium, in utero passage of the substance is uncommon.

In utero passage of meconium has been thought to reflect ante- or intrapartum asphyxia. Reed suggested that hypoxia would relax anal sphincter tone [5], while Brews hypothesized that hypoxia would increase intestinal peristalsis [7]. In addition, it has been speculated that compression of the fetal head or umbilical cord (often seen in the post-term infant with oligohydramnios) could cause a vagal response and result in meconium passage [41]. Walker documented hypoxia causing meconium passage [8]. The finding of fetal acidosis among many infants with MSAF is consistent with a hypoxic environment [17]. Nevertheless, for most infants, passage of meconium is likely a physiologic maturational event. Meconium passage is rare before 37 weeks' gestation, but may occur in 35% or more of pregnancies lasting longer than 42 weeks [16]. In addition, motilin is a hormone responsible for bowel peristalsis and defecation. Motilin levels are higher in term and post-dates infants than in premature infants [42], additionally supporting the maturity concept of the physiologic passage of meconium.

A seldom-recognized mechanism causing fetal defecation is that of intrauterine infection. Naeye reported that 64% of cases of MSAF were associated with acute chorioamnionitis [10]. Wen and colleagues found a significantly higher rate of clinical intra-amniotic infection in women with MSAF compared to those with clear amniotic fluid [43]. Romero's group found the prevalence of positive amniotic fluid cultures to be significantly higher among women with MSAF than in those with clear fluid [44]. Piper and colleagues reported MSAF to be associated with higher rates of clinical maternal infection both pre- (chorioamnionitis) and post- (endometritis) delivery [45]. As inflammation plays an important role in the course of neonates with meconium-associated respiratory distress, the infectious mechanism of meconium passage needs to be explored further.

Unfortunately, for any given fetus, neither obstetricians nor pediatricians may be able to ascertain prenatally the specific mechanism of passage, nor is the rationale readily apparent postnatally. Indeed, conceivably a combination of mechanisms could affect any given fetus. Whatever the reason for fetal defecation, it will occur in 10–15% of all deliveries.

Potential mechanisms of neurologic injury

What are the potential mechanisms of injury in these children? Because of the dearth of prospective data on a large group of infants born through MSAF or who develop MAS, one may only speculate. The infants at highest risk appear to be those who have prolonged depression in the post-delivery stage. Data from the CPP indicate that the combination of MSAF and a 5-minute Apgar score ≤ 3 resulted in a 9.4% incidence of CP among surviving infants > 2500 g birthweight [46]. Very real culprits which one must consider include the events potentiating meconium passage. Meconium staining among infants in the CPP was strongly associated with disorders that could affect the fetus: chorioamnionitis, premature rupture of membranes, abruptio placentae, and large placental infarcts [10]. One must recognize the concept of in utero recovery. Some fetuses suffer acute or chronic episodes which are severe enough to cause neurological injury, but not severe enough to result in death. The stress may disappear and the fetus resumes its normal status. Such an infant may not demonstrate postpartum depression with low umbilical cord pHs or low Apgar scores, and may appear neurologically intact for months after birth, only to end up with major neurodevelopmental disabilities.

The post-dates fetus is at high risk for oligohydramnios, uteroplacental insufficiency, and meconium passage [47]. These fetuses may suffer from chronic insults insufficient to cause death or even signs of fetal distress, but sufficient to cause neurologic damage. The pathophysiologic mechanisms that cause CP remain elusive and usually cannot be ascribed to birth injury or hypoxic–ischemic insults during delivery [48]. Recurrent neonatal seizures predict CP better than other perinatal characteristics [27,48]. However, although such seizures are significantly more likely in infants born through MSAF, they are likely the consequence, rather than the cause, of the processes leading to CP. Similarly, an abnormal fetal heart rate tracing or persistently low Apgar scores may be reflective of an insult that occurred long before birth (hours to days to even weeks or months), rather than of more immediate intrapartum difficulties.

Are there substances in the meconium itself that make it harmful? Altshuler and colleagues have investigated a mechanism of fetal ischemia caused by vasoconstriction of placental or umbilical vessels [49,50]. Conceivably, vasoactive substances could cross into the circulation of the fetus and cause ischemia of cerebral vessels or make pulmonary vessels more reactive, hence persistent pulmonary hypertension of the newborn (PPHN). The latter investigators initially performed an in vitro experiment in which they exposed excised umbilical venous tissue to solutions of meconium and found substantial vasocontraction. Although no specific constituent in the substance was identified as the vasoactive substance, they found the agent to be heat-labile. They hypothesized that MSAF could cause in vivo placental and umbilical cord vasoconstriction. Additionally, the vasoconstricting agents could cross into the fetal circulation and lead to cerebral or other organ hypoperfusion. Additionally, this group described meconium-induced necrosis of placental and umbilical cord vessels. Holcberg and colleagues more recently confirmed the vasoconstrictive effects of meconium on the fetal–placental vasculature [51]. Altshuler has described that with the presence of meconium in the fetal sac, it takes a minimum of 4–12 hours for the meconium to diffuse to and into the lumens of placental and umbilical cord vessels and become a pathogenetic means of inducing placental and umbilical vasocontraction [50].

Burgess and Hutchins have presented further evidence implicating meconium's role in producing injury [52]. In a series of 123 autopsied cases in which there was meconium passage, these investigators described substantial placental and fetal lung inflammation due to the meconium, as well as abundant umbilical cord pathology. Kaspar and colleagues assessed the relationship between the immediate neonatal outcome and the presence of placental lesions in 96 pregnancies complicated by MSAF [53]. They found an increased prevalence of severe placental lesions (vascular thromboses, placental infarcts, etc.) and adverse immediate neonatal outcomes (lower 5-minute Apgar scores, lower umbilical artery pHs, and more NICU admissions) associated with the duration of exposure to meconium.

Kojima and colleagues have described meconium-induced oxidant injury to the lungs caused by activation of alveolar macrophages [54], while Jones et al. found increased production of proinflammatory cytokines in MAS (including tumor necrosis factor and interleukin 8) [55]. Moreover, both human infants and piglets with MAS may have increased levels of eicosanoids such as leukotriene B4 and thromboxane B2, substances that may cause pulmonary vasoconstriction [56,57]. Both oxidant- and cytokine-induced injury could also damage the brain, while eicosanoids could result in ischemia of the brain. We know little about the potentially deleterious effects on neural tissue by the increased levels of oxidants, cytokines, and eicosanoids found with MAS.

Naeye suggested that meconium-induced brain damage may be a subacute rather than an acute process [10]. He reported that only three of 31 non-Perinatal Project children with meconium-associated spastic quadriplegia whose cases he had reviewed had more than brief occurrences of neonatal renal or myocardial failure.

Benirschke has commented on the important toxic vasoconstrictive properties of meconium, suggesting this as an etiology of fetal hypoperfusion and PPHN, as well as brain injury [58]. He wrote that meconium's damage to the umbilical cord vessels occurs after the "noxious agent" seeps through Wharton's jelly. He has also suggested that umbilical venous and placental vessel vasocontraction may reduce the venous return of oxygenated blood from the placenta to the child, and has commented that we know virtually nothing about the long-term function of meconium-injured vessels, nor of meconium's diffusion or transportation through the umbilical cord and placental membranes [59]. He also reminds us about the effect of cytokines and other infection-related factors, which may additionally affect vascular injury in the presence of MSAF.

The increased incidence of chorioamnionitis in the presence of MSAF, as well as the frequent finding of inflammatory changes in the placenta, umbilical cord, fetal membranes, and lungs, suggests that inflammation may play an important role in brain injury in this population. The precise mechanism(s), however, remain unclear. Theoretically, vasoconstriction or cytokine-mediated injury likely play a role. Sienko and Altshuler assessed four cases of meconium-induced umbilical vascular necrosis [60]. These were in three fetal demises and one live-born, growth-retarded infant. Bilirubin was found in macrophages between umbilical vascular myocytes and in the Wharton's jelly. Additionally, immunocytochemical staining revealed the presence of interleukin 1β in these same macrophages. These authors speculated that cytokines and other meconium-associated factors may contribute to the pathogenesis of fetal death or neonatal morbidity (such as PVL) (see Chapter 20).

Neonates with severe MAS, particularly those with concomitant PPHN, may be severely hypoxic and acidotic due to the lung disorder itself, factors which of themselves may contribute to neurologic injury [61]. Some authors have reported a high incidence of seizures, cerebral infarction, and intracranial hemorrhage among infants with PPHN [61,62]. Additionally, therapies used for the management of MAS could potentially injure a child's brain. Hyperventilation is often used to treat MAS, particularly if PPHN is evident [61]. The aim of this therapy is to achieve respiratory alkalosis, often with arterial pH above 7.55 and/or hypocapnia to $PaCO_2$ levels of 25 torr or less. Hyperventilation to these extremes has been shown to decrease cerebral blood flow and oxygen consumption in animal models and adult humans [63–66]. Follow-up data from children managed with hyperventilation have shown impairment in neurological outcomes (e.g., CP) and sensorineural hearing loss. However, it is unclear whether or not the changes can be attributed to the hyperventilation or to pre-existing damage due to the effects of the child's illness or the degree of acidosis, hypoxemia, and hypocapnia often present (see Chapter 37).

Table 36.1. Adverse neurological findings in neonates requiring ECMO. Those with MAS are compared to those with all other disorders (included are all infants in the ELSO registry through mid-2001)

	MAS	Other disorders	Significance
Total number of infants	5754	10649	
Seizures (%)	642 (11.2%)	1308 (12.3%)	$p = 0.034$
Cerebral infarct (%)	374 (6.5%)	1262 (11.9%)	$p < 0.0001$
Cerebral hemorrhage (%)	125 (2.2%)	666 (6.3%)	$p < 0.0001$
Brain death (%)	48 (0.8%)	126 (1.2%)	$p = 0.015$

Notes:
Data courtesy of Robert E. Schumacher, M.D. and the ECMO Registry of the Extracorporeal Life Support Organization (ELSO), Ann Arbor, Michigan, July 2001.

The therapy of last resort for PPHN is extracorporeal membrane oxygenation (ECMO) [60], a form of long-term cardiopulmonary bypass used when children failing conventional therapy have a projected high rate of mortality. Many children requiring this therapy have been profoundly acidotic, hypoxemic, and hypotensive. The most common way of performing ECMO over the past three decades involves permanent ligation of the right carotid artery and jugular vein. There are relatively scant data concerning survivors of ECMO, particularly concerning neurodevelopmental outcome beyond 1–2 years of age. At least 60% of survivors are intact, approximately 25% have substantial neurodevelopmental impairment, and 15% have findings which are potentially indicative of neurologic damage [68]. Children with MAS make up the largest proportion of newborn infants who are treated with this therapy (approximately 35%). The occurrence of adverse short-term neurological findings among infants treated with ECMO is significantly lower in babies with MAS compared to those with other disorders (Table 36.1) [68]. Unfortunately, there are no long-term data comparing neurological outcomes (such as the occurrence of CP) or developmental testing in a large population of infants who were managed with ECMO (see Chapter 37).

Timing of meconium passage

Can one make estimates of the amount of time that has passed from fetal defecation to delivery? There are some elements which may, perhaps, assist estimation of this interval: the color of the MSAF, the consistency of the MSAF, staining of the neonate, and placental/membrane alterations due to the meconium. Freshly passed meconium in a healthy newborn is a thick, viscous shimmering black-green colored substance. When passed by a fetus, the early color of MSAF is also black-green. However, the dilutional effect of the amount of amniotic fluid plays a role in the visually appreciated color of the MSAF [69]. As time progresses, the color of MSAF will progress to a brown and then to tan or yellow. Classically, yellow-brown MSAF has been considered to reflect "old" meconium [6,9,11]. Some believe the tan/yellow color change is due to the concomitant presence of vernix caseosa, the white cheesy substance whose presence may "lighten up" the darker meconium (K. Bernischke, personal communication). Altshuler comments that the color of placental staining reflects duration since fetal defecation: "acute" staining is slimy and has a dark-green appearance, "chronic" staining is muddy-brown in appearance, while "very remotely passed" meconium is light tan [70]. Sienko and Altshuler have correlated the degree of meconium-associated placental and umbilical cord damage, as well as the color of the meconium staining, with the duration of time the fetus was exposed to the meconium [60]. The "fresh" meconium staining was green-brown in color and was not associated with substantial changes. Long-term placental staining (> 6 hours of exposure) progressively manifested in color as greenish tan, muddy brown, and then light tan. The latter-colored membranes and fetal surfaces were more likely to be associated with adverse placental, membrane, and umbilical cord findings.

We performed a prospective in vitro study to assess the effect of time and other factors on the color changes of meconium [69]. We sought to evaluate factors that might influence the color changes of MSAF. We obtained uncontaminated amniotic fluid from women at the time of elective cesarean sections and mixed it with human meconium to produce concentrations of 10% and 40% by volume. To 5 mL aliquots of these solutions we added either: (1) nothing (control); (2) 2 g of human vernix; (3) antibiotics (ampicillin and gentamicin); (4) 1 mEq $NaHCO_3$; or (5) 1 mL of 12-N hydrochloric acid. Specimens were placed in an incubator at 37 °C and serially examined for color changes at 0, 6, 12, 24, 48, 72, 96, 168, and 336 hours. Photographs were taken at each time point. We used a nine-point color gradation scale (from black-green to yellow-tan) to score the specimens. Seven individuals blinded to solution content and time of photograph assigned color scores for the specimens. The 10% specimens were lighter in color than the 40% solutions at all periods. Regardless of meconium concentration, the specimens containing vernix were lighter throughout the study. All specimens became progressively lighter over time, most notably between 24 and 72 hours. Neither the presence of antibiotics nor pH changes independently affected the color changes of the solutions. A factor we could not assess was the influence of natural, in vivo uptake and degradation of meconium by living tissue. Nonetheless, the color changes of MSAF are independently affected by meconium concentration, the presence of vernix, and the duration of time since initial passage.

When meconium is passed and diluted by a normal volume of amniotic fluid, it will be of thin consistency. If there is oligohydramnios, often seen with post-maturity or chronic uteroplacental insufficiency, the MSAF will be thicker in consistency [47]. This will often result in the tenacious, "pea-soup" consistency seen in these children. In addition, in the presence of a normal or near-normal amount of amniotic fluid, when greater quantities of meconium are passed the fluid becomes thicker in consistency. Meconium passed in utero will be absorbed after several days [50,71]; this may

be reflected in decreased fluid consistency and a thinner, more watery appearance. There may be repeated defecations by a fetus under stress. This could progressively increase the thickness of the MSAF. A clinician may not be able to appreciate that there were repeated defecations. Thus, the thickness of the MSAF is a relatively unreliable marker of the interval since passage.

Staining of the external fetus is a better indicator of the amount of time since the child passed the substance. Desmond et al. immersed the feet of normal babies in rubber gloves containing meconium-stained solutions [72]. They found that it took at least 4–6 hours for the toenails to manifest yellow staining. They further assessed the amount of time it took for vernix placed into MSAF to become stained, and found that it took at least 12–14 hours for vernix to achieve definite yellow staining. In an in vitro experiment, Miller et al. obtained umbilical cords from normal term newborn infants [73]. They also obtained meconium samples from normal term infants less than 18 hours of age and froze these specimens at 4 °C for later evaluation. The authors subsequently exposed transverse sections of the umbilical cords to various concentrations of meconium (5%, 10%, and 20%). They found minimal staining after 1 hour and maximal staining of all specimens at 3 hours. We do not know if cold storage of the meconium or exposure of the fluid to diverse antibiotics could have affected the uptake of the pigment causing the cords to become colored.

Examination of the placenta and membranes may assist in timing meconium's passage. One should recognize, however, that if a placenta sits unrefrigerated with meconium covering the membranes, postpartum transport in macrophages may proceed for some time. Nurses often report MSAF in a particular woman may have different color and consistency over time. The in vitro study of Miller, Coen and Benirschke is a frequently cited work delineating changes due to meconium over time in the placenta and membranes [73]. They exposed placentas and membranes to various meconium solutions. Within 1 hour, meconium pigment-laden macrophages could be found in the amnion. After 3 hours, pigmented macrophages could be found in all of the chorions. In addition, Miller and colleagues found a time correlation with amniotic epithelial degeneration: pseudostratification was exhibited in the epithelium after 1–3 hours. Epithelial disorganization was present after 3 hours of exposure. These investigators found the depth of penetration and uptake by macrophages to be related to length of exposure and to be independent of meconium concentration. Finally, these authors stated that meconium may be cleared from the amniotic fluid by both fetal swallowing and macrophage uptake. In such an instance, although the amniotic fluid would be seemingly clear, they felt that one could detect meconium placental macrophages for at least a week after initial meconium passage. Altshuler opines that the temporal development of meconium-induced tissue changes may be influenced by co-existing conditions such as chorioamnionitis [50]. Almost 25 years before the Miller report, Bourne performed a similar experiment [74].

He exposed amniotic membranes to varying concentrations of meconium. Bourne found gross staining of the amnion to occur in 2–6 hours. Furthermore, although 10% formalin apparently removed or dissolved the gross pigment, the pigment could still be found within the vacuoles of the macrophages of the amnion. Bourne conjectured that meconium from different fetuses may be phagocytized at different rates in such an artificial situation, and cautioned readers concerning any conclusions from an in vitro experiment.

We examined the issue in our in vivo fetal rabbit model [75]. Initial meconium staining could be seen at 3 hours in the amnion. However, it took from 6 to 12 hours for macrophages in both the chorion and amnion to exhibit meconium staining, with no differences in rate of uptake between the two concentrations (10% and 40%) of meconium-stained fluid. The amnion initially became reactive and edematous and would disappear, probably due to the toxicity of the meconium. We first found epithelial degeneration at 3 hours, with some vacuolization within 3 hours. We found squamous regeneration of the epithelium at 24 hours. The chorion responded to the meconium by becoming edematous at 1–3 hours and accumulating macrophages with vacuoles.

Altshuler opines that in the presence of MSAF, acute amniotic epithelial necrosis is the light-microscopic counterpart of grossly observed acute (< 4 hours since passage) meconium staining [50]. He states that chronic meconium staining is manifested by amniotic epithelial vacuolization and balloon degeneration, as well as by the presence of balls of squamous epithelium across the placental surface and meconium-laden macrophages within the extraplacental membranes, placenta, and umbilical cord. He states that in the absence of chorioamnionitis, meconium-laden macrophages deep within the umbilical cord indicate meconium has been in the fetal sac for at least 2 days. Benirschke is not as definite, stating that there is less certainty as to the chronology of umbilical cord staining and the temporal evolution of meconium-induced vascular injury [58,59]. The timing of meconium passage is complex. We must keep in mind that the majority of babies who subsequently are noted to have CP, as well as those who are stillborn, are not born through meconium-stained amniotic fluid. Clearly, severe enough stress to result in brain injury or even death may not always result in meconium passage. Furthermore, the vast majority of babies born through MSAF apparently do not suffer any neurologic morbidity. Again, there are no specific longitudinal follow-up studies concerning the neurodevelopmental outcome of this latter group of infants. Perhaps there could be more subtle neurologic changes that would only manifest later in life, such as learning disorders, behavior problems, or attention-deficit disorders. Conceivably, with in utero recovery, a fetus could suffer a substantial insult, pass meconium, suffer brain injury, recover over a period of days, have some or all of the meconium resorbed, be born through either MSAF or apparently clear amniotic fluid, appear completely normal neurologically in the neonatal period, and subsequently manifest long-term neurodevelopmental abnormalities.

Thick- versus thin-consistency meconium

What does the thickness of meconium represent? There are several factors that come into play, most importantly the total quantity of defecated material and the amount of amniotic fluid present. However, one should consider that the meconium at the most distal end of the intestinal tract is more viscous and likely to result in a thicker-consistency MSAF. Additionally, if meconium is present for a period of time, it will gradually be resorbed by surrounding tissue, or swallowed by the fetus. Is "thick" meconium clinically worse than "thin" or watery meconium? Clearly, infants born through "thick" MSAF are more likely to develop MAS [12,76,77]. Presumably, the thicker substance is more likely to cause obstructive airway problems. Greenwood et al. have found those born through thick-consistency MSAF to be more likely to have seizures, low 1-minute Apgar scores, and require NICU admission [77]. Nonetheless, as many as 44% of those who develop MAS were born through "thin-consistency" MSAF [1]. Infants born through thin-consistency meconium may still develop substantial respiratory distress, need ECMO, or die [78].

Estimating the consistency of MSAF is a very subjective matter. Reasonable definitions are: (1) *thin* (synonymous with "watery" or "light"): only discoloration of the fluid – one could read through this liquid; (2) *moderate* (synonymous with "moderately thick"): particulate suspension present – the solution would be opaque and you could not read through it; and (3) *thick* (synonymous with "heavy"): tenacious fluid of pea-soup viscosity and appearance. Although babies born through thicker-consistency meconium are more likely to have lower Apgar scores and umbilical cord artery pHs [15,76], there are no data comparing the long-term neurodevelopmental outcome on the basis of MSAF consistency. Until such investigations are performed, I believe clinicians have to be wary with all infants born through MSAF of any consistency.

Summary

Meconium staining of the amniotic fluid is an everyday occurrence for healthcare providers. The last several decades have resulted in an increased understanding of meconium passage, the pathophysiology of MAS, and mechanisms of brain injury associated with MSAF and MAS. We are learning more about how the substance itself may be both directly and indirectly toxic to tissue. Unfortunately, our knowledge remains scant. Most studies that review the outcomes of infants with MAS are subsets of those focusing on ECMO, surfactant, or iNO. I am of the opinion that we need a new project on the scale of the CPP in order to assess factors involved in the development of CP, mental retardation, and other abnormal neurodevelopmental outcomes. This is not just because of meconium-related issues. The current rate of CP is virtually the same among term-gestation neonates as it was 40–50 years ago when babies were enrolled in the CPP. Perhaps babies who would have died during the time of the CPP will now survive and manifest CP, while those who were found to have CP in the late 1950s and early 1960s will have had improved prenatal care, nutrition, and intra- and postpartum care and not develop CP. Thus, while the overall percentage of babies who have CP would remain the same, the characteristics of the children could be different.

We continue to make technological advances in how we support and manage critically ill infants. Our resuscitative skills have improved since the early 1960s, while our methods of managing neonatal pulmonary disease have also considerably improved. We have made advances in our ability to image the brain of term and preterm gestation neonates, as well as in interpreting other techniques of assessing brain injury (near-infrared spectroscopy, electroencephalography, etc.). I believe our understanding of brain injury and development of methods to prevent such injury could only be enhanced by a future study enrolling at least as many infants as the CPP.

Despite our best efforts, a finite number of infants will be harmed by the effects of meconium. We may not be able to predict or prevent the stresses that lead to meconium passage. Moreover, babies who suffer in utero aspiration or those who develop remodeling of the pulmonary vasculature may not be responsive to current therapies. There is no evidence that current obstetrical management of women who exhibit meconium-stained amniotic fluid has resulted in improved neurodevelopmental outcomes of their progeny. Moreover, although we have decreased the death rate due to MAS, there is no evidence that improved delivery room or newborn intensive care unit management has led to improved neurologic outcomes in infants born through MSAF. As MSAF and MAS are such common entities, further research efforts need to be made to increase our knowledge and, hopefully, to develop therapies to prevent or mitigate the consequences of meconium. I continue to reflect on how much we do not understand about MSAF and MAS. One fact remains a certainty: the greatest importance of MSAF is to alert us to the potential for problems.

References

1. Wiswell TE, Tuggle JM, Turner BS. Meconium aspiration syndrome: have we made a difference? *Pediatrics* 1990; **85**: 715–21.

2. Wiswell TE, Bent RC. Meconium staining and the meconium aspiration syndrome: unresolved issues. *Pediatr Clin N Am* 1993; **50**: 955–81.

3. Schulze M. The significance of the passage of meconium during labor. *Am J Obstet Gynecol* 1925; **10**: 83–8.

4. Grant A. Monitoring the fetus during labor. In Chalmers I, Enking M, Keirse MJNC, eds., *Effective Care in Pregnancy and Childbirth*. Oxford: Oxford University Press, 1989: 846–82.

5. Reed CB. Fetal death during labor. *Surg Gynecol Obstet* 1918; **26**: 545–51.

6. Clifford SH. Clinical significance of yellow staining of the vernix caseosa, skin, nails, and umbilical cord of the newborn. *Am J Dis Child* 1945; **69**: 327–8.

7. Brews A. Fetal asphyxia. In *Eden & Hollands Manual of Obstetrics*, 9th edn. London: Churchill, 1948: 609–12.

8. Walker J. Foetal anoxia. *J Obstet Gynecol Br Empire* 1954; **61**: 162–80.

9. Fujikura T, Klionsky B. The significance of meconium staining. *Am J Obstet Gynecol* 1975; **121**: 45–50.

10. Naeye RL. *Disorders of the Placenta, Fetus, and Neonate: Diagnosis and Clinical Significance*. St. Louis, MO: Mosby Year Book, 1992: 257–68, 330–52.

11. Desmond MM, Moore J, Lindley JE, *et al.* Meconium staining of the amniotic fluid: a marker of fetal hypoxia. *Obstet Gynecol* 1957; **9**: 91–103.

12. Wiswell TE, Gannon CM, Jacob JJ, *et al.* Delivery room management of the apparently vigorous meconium-stained neonate: results of the multicenter, international collaborative trial. *Pediatrics* 2000; **105**: 1–7.

13. Vain NE, Szyld EG, Prudent LM, *et al.* Oropharyngeal and nasopharyngeal suctioning of meconium-stained neonates before delivery of their shoulders: multicentre, randomized controlled trial. *Lancet* 2004; **364**: 597–602.

14. Fraser WD, Hofmeyer J, Lede R, *et al.* Amnioinfusion for the prevention of the meconium aspiration syndrome. *N Engl J Med* 2004; **353**: 909–17.

15. Berkus MD, Langer O, Samueloff A, *et al.* Meconium-stained amniotic fluid: increased risk for adverse neonatal outcome. *Obstet Gynecol* 1994; **84**: 115–20.

16. Nathan L, Leveno KJ, Carmody TJ, *et al.* Meconium: a 1990s perspective on an old obstetric hazard. *Obstet Gynecol* 1994; **83**: 329–32.

17. Ramin K, Leveno K, Kelly M, *et al.* Observations concerning the pathophysiology of meconium aspiration syndrome. *Am J Obstet Gynecol* 1994; **170**: 312 (#124).

18. Starks GD. Correlation of meconium-stained amniotic fluid, early intrapartum fetal pH, and Apgar scores as predictors of perinatal outcome. *Obstet Gynecol* 1980; **56**: 604–9.

19. Steer PJ, Eigbe F, Lissauer TJ, *et al.* Interrelationships among abnormal cardiotocograms in labor, meconium staining of the amniotic fluid, arterial cord blood pH, and Apgar scores. *Obstet Gynecol* 1989; **74**: 715–21.

20. Smith CV, Nguyen HN, Kovacs B, *et al.* Fetal death following antepartum fetal heart rate testing: a review of 65 cases. *Obstet Gynecol* 1987; **70**: 18–20.

21. Fleischer A, Anyaegbunam A, Guidetti E, *et al.* A persistent clinical problem: profile of the term infant with significant respiratory complications. *Obstet Gynecol* 1992; **79**: 185–90.

22. Cleary GM, Wiswell TE. Meconium-stained amniotic fluid and the meconium aspiration syndrome: an update. *Pediatr Clin N Am* 1998; **45**: 511–29.

23. Abu-Osa YK. Treatment of persistent pulmonary hypertension of the newborn: update. *Arch Dis Child* 1991; **66**; 74–7.

24. Wagner W, Druzin M, Rond A, *et al.* Meconium-stained amniotic fluid (MSAF) ≤ 32 weeks predicts poor perinatal outcome. *Am J Obstet Gynecol* 1991; **164**: 357 (#409).

25. Grafe MR. The correlation of prenatal brain damage with placental pathology. *J Neuropathol Exp Neurol* 1994; **53**: 407–15.

26. Redline RW. Severe fetal placental vascular lesions in term infants with neurologic impairment. *Am J Obstet Gynecol* 2005; **192**: 452–7.

27. Nelson KB, Broman SH. Perinatal risk factors in children with serious motor and mental handicaps. *Ann Neurol* 1977; **2**: 371–7.

28. Nelson KB. Perspective on the role of perinatal asphyxia in neurologic outcome: its role in developmental deficits in children. *CMAJ* 1989; **141**: 3–10.

29. Nelson KB, Ellenberg JH. Obstetric complications as risk factors for cerebral palsy or seizure disorders. *JAMA* 1984; **251**: 1843–8.

30. Shields JR, Schifrin BS. Perinatal antecedents of cerebral palsy. *Obstet Gynecol* 1988; **71**: 899–905.

31. Gaffney G, Sellers S, Flavell V, *et al.* Case–control study of intrapartum care, cerebral palsy, and perinatal death. *BMJ* 1994; **308**: 743–50.

32. Spinillo A, Fazzi E, Capuzzo E, *et al.* Meconium-stained amniotic fluid and risk for cerebral palsy in preterm infants. *Obstet Gynecol* 1997; **90**: 519–23.

33. Spinillo A, Capuzzo E, Stronati M, *et al.* Obstetric risk factors for periventricular leukomalacia among preterm infants. *Br J Obstet Gynaecol* 1998; **105**: 865–71.

34. Lien JM, Towers CV, Quilligan EJ, *et al.* Term early-onset neonatal seizures: obstetric characteristics, etiologic classifications, and perinatal care. *Obstet Gynecol* 1995; **85**: 163–9.

35. Sato S, Okumura A, Kato T, *et al.* Hypoxic ischemic encephalopathy associated with neonatal seizures without other neurological abnormalities. *Brain Dev* 2003; **25**: 215–19.

36. Blackwell SC, Moldenhauer J, Hassan SS, *et al.* Meconium aspiration syndrome in term neonates with normal acid-base status at delivery: is it different? *Am J Obstet Gynecol* 2001; **184**: 1422–6.

37. Finer NN, Robertson CM, Richards RT, *et al.* Hypoxic ischemic encephalopathy in term neonates: perinatal factors and outcome. *J Pediatr* 1981; **98**: 112–17.

38. Walstab JE, Bell RJ, Reddihough DS, *et al.* Factors identified during the neonatal period associated with risk of cerebral palsy. *Aust NZ J Obstet Gynaecol* 2004; **44**: 342–6.

39. Beligere N, Rao R. Neurodevelopmental outcome of infants with meconium aspiration syndrome (MAS). *Pediatr Res* 2002; **51**: 293A.

40. Matsuishi T, Yamashita Y, Ohtani Y, *et al.* Brief report: incidence of and risk factors for autistic disorder in neonatal intensive care unit survivors. *J Autism Dev Disorders* 1999; **29**: 161–6.

41. Miller FC, Read JA. Intrapartum assessment of the postdate fetus. *Am J Obstet Gynecol* 1981; **141**: 516–20.

42. Lucas A, Adrian TE, Christofides N, *et al.* Plasma motilin, gastrin, and enteroglucagon and feeding in the human newborn. *Arch Dis Child* 1980; **55**: 673–7.

43. Wen TW, Eriksen NL, Blanco JD, *et al.* Association of clinical intra-amniotic infection and meconium. *Am J Perinatol* 1993; **10**: 438–40.

44. Romero R, Hanaoka S, Mazo M, *et al.* Meconium-stained amniotic fluid: a risk factor for microbial invasion of the amniotic cavity. *Am J Obstet Gynecol* 1991; **164**: 859–62.

45. Piper JM, Newton ER, Berkus MD, *et al.* Meconium: a marker for peripartum infection. *Obstet Gynecol* 1998; **91**: 741–5.

46. Nelson KB. Relationship of intrapartum and delivery room events to long-term neurologic outcome. *Clin Perinatol* 1989; **16**: 995–1007.

47. Crowley P. Post-term pregnancy: induction or surveillance? In Chalmers I, Enking M, Keirse MJNC., eds., *Effective Care in Pregnancy and Childbirth*. Oxford: Oxford University Press, 1989: 776–91.

48. Kuban KCK, Leviton A. Cerebral palsy. *N Engl J Med* 1994; **330**: 188–95.

49. Altshuler G, Hyde S. Meconium-induced vasocontraction: a potential cause of cerebral and other fetal hypoperfusion and of poor pregnancy outcome. *J Child Neurol* 1989; **4**: 137–42.

50. Altshuler G. Placental insights into neurodevelopmental and other childhood diseases. *Semin Pediatr Neurol* 1995; **2**: 90–9.

51. Holcberg G, Huleihel M, Katz M, *et al.* Vasoconstrictive activity of meconium stained amniotic fluid in the human placental vasculature. *Eur J Obstet Gynecol Reprod Biol* 1999; **87**: 147–50.

52. Burgess AM, Hutchins GM. Inflammation of the lungs, umbilical cord, and placenta associated with meconium passage *in utero*: review of 123 autopsied cases. *Pathol Res Prac* 1996; **192**: 1121–8.

53. Kaspar HG, Abu-Musa A, Hannoun A, *et al.* The placenta in meconium staining: lesions and early neonatal outcome. *Clin Exp Obstet Gynecol* 2000; **27**: 63–6.

54. Kojima T, Hattori K, Fujiwara T, *et al.* Meconium-induced lung injury mediated by activation of alveolar macrophages. *Life Sci* 1994; **54**: 1559–62.

55. Jones CA, Cayabyab RG, Hamdan H, *et al.* Early production of proinflammatory cytokines in the pathogenesis of neonatal adult respiratory distress syndrome (ARDS) associated with meconium aspiration. *Pediatr Res* 1994; **35**: 339A (#2019).

56. Bui KC, Martin G, Kammerman LA, *et al.* Plasma thromboxane and pulmonary artery pressure in neonates treated with extracorporeal membrane oxygenation. *J Thoracic Cardiovasc Surg* 1992; **104**: 124–9.

57. Wu JM, Yeh TF, Lin YJ, *et al.* Increases of leukotriene B4 (LTB4) and D4 (LTD4) and cardio-hemodynamic changes in newborn piglets with meconium aspiration (MAS). *Pediatr Res* 1995; **37**: 357A (#2122).

58. Benirschke K. Placenta pathology questions to the perinatologist. *J Perinatol* 1994; **14**: 371–5.

59. Benirschke K. Fetal consequences of amniotic fluid meconium. *Contemp Obstet Gynecol* 2001; **46**: 76–83.

60. Sienko A, Altshuler G. Meconium-induced umbilical vascular necrosis in abortuses and fetuses: a histopathologic study for cytokines. *Obstet Gynecol* 1999; **94**: 415–20.

61. Walsh-Sukys MC. Persistent pulmonary hypertension of the newborn: the black box revisited. *Clin Perinatol* 1993; **20**: 127–43.

62. Klesh KW, Murphy TF, Scher MS, *et al.* Cerebral infarction in persistent pulmonary hypertension of the newborn. *Am J Dis Child* 1987; **141**: 852–7.

63. Hansen NB, Nowicki PT, Miller RR, *et al.* Alterations in cerebral blood flow and oxygen consumption during prolonged hypocarbia. *Pediatr Res* 1986; **20**: 147–50.

64. Reuter JH, Disney TA. Regional blood flow and cerebral metabolic rate of oxygen during hyperventilation in the newborn dog. *Pediatr Res* 1986; **29**: 1102–6.

65. Bifano EM, Pfannenstiel A. Duration of hyperventilation and outcome in infants with persistent pulmonary hypertension. *Pediatrics* 1988; **81**: 657–61.

66. Marron MJ, Crisafi MA, Driscoll JM, *et al.* Hearing and neurodevelopmental outcome in survivors of persistent pulmonary hypertension of the newborn. *Pediatrics* 1992; **90**: 392–6.

67. Page J, Frisk V, Whyte H. Developmental outcome of infants treated with extracorporeal membrane oxygenation (ECMO) in the neonatal period: is the evidence all in? *Paediatr Perinat Epidemiol* 1994: **8**; 123–39.

68. Extracorporeal Life Support Organization (ELSO). *ECMO Registry* Ann Arbor, MI: ELSO, July 2001.

69. Wiswell TE, Tencer HL. What causes the color changes of meconium-stained amniotic fluid? *Pediatr Res* 1994; **35**: 261A (#1551).

70. Altshuler G. Placenta within the medicolegal imperative. *Arch Pathol Lab Med* 1991; **115**: 688–95.

71. Naeye RL. Functionally important disorders of the placenta, umbilical cord, and fetal membranes. *Hum Pathol* 1987; **18**: 680–91.

72. Desmond MM, Lindley JE, Moore J, *et al.* Meconium staining of newborn infants. *J Pediatr* 1956; **49**: 540–9.

73. Miller PW, Coen RW, Benirschke K. Dating the time interval from meconium passage to birth. *Obstet Gynecol* 1985; **66**: 459–62.

74. Bourne G. Meconium transport. In *The Human Amnion and Chorion*. Chicago, IL: Year Book, 1962: 143–54.

75. Wiswell TE, Popek E, Barfield WD, *et al.* The effect of intra-amniotic meconium on histologic findings over time in a fetal rabbit model. *Pediatr Res* 1994; **35**: 261A (#1550).

76. Rossi EM, Philipson EH, Williams TG, *et al.* Meconium aspiration syndrome: Intrapartum and neonatal attributes. *Am J Obstet Gynecol* 1989; **161**: 1106–10.

77. Greenwood C, Lalchandani S, MacQuillan K, *et al.* Meconium passed in labor: how reassuring is clear amniotic fluid. *Obstet Gynecol* 2003; **102**: 89–93.

78. Wiswell TE, Henley MA. Intratracheal suctioning, systemic infection, and the meconium aspiration syndrome. *Pediatrics* 1992; **89**: 203–6.

Chapter 37

Persistent pulmonary hypertension of the newborn

Alexis S. Davis, William D. Rhine, and Krisa P. Van Meurs

Introduction

Persistent pulmonary hypertension of the newborn (PPHN) is characterized by markedly elevated pulmonary vascular resistance and pulmonary arterial pressure, along with striking pulmonary vasoreactivity, which produces right-to-left shunting through the ductus arteriosus and foramen ovale [1,2]. With severe PPHN, this extrapulmonary shunting results in severe hypoxemia, which typically is poorly responsive to treatment with high concentrations of inspired oxygen, assisted ventilation, and pharmacologic manipulation of the circulation.

Elevated pulmonary vascular resistance with right-to-left extrapulmonary shunting also often occurs in association with severe pulmonary parenchymal disease, including meconium aspiration syndrome (MAS), bacterial pneumonia, lung hypoplasia, or hyaline membrane disease, and may be compounded by co-existent impairment of systemic cardiac output and/or systemic arterial pressures due to impaired myocardial function, hypovolemia, or systemic vasodilation [3]. In addition, pulmonary hypertension is often very difficult to distinguish from total anomalous pulmonary venous return, and may complicate a variety of other congenital cardiac malformations. These associated conditions may occur with or without intrinsic structural and functional abnormalities of the pulmonary vascular bed, and treatment needs not only to be specific for the underlying or associated conditions, but also must account for the behavior of the pulmonary blood vessels. As a consequence, infants with PPHN present one of the most difficult diagnostic and therapeutic challenges in neonatal intensive care. The complexity of these relationships has also led to a complicated and inconsistent nosology in the medical literature [4]. Some clinicians apply the label of PPHN to nearly all neonates with hypoxemia unresponsive to administration of 100% oxygen, excluding only those with cyanotic congenital heart disease, some use this term for all infants with elevated pulmonary artery pressures and right-to-left shunting, and others reserve this terminology for only those with excessive pulmonary arterial reactivity associated with pathognomonic excessive muscularization of the pulmonary

arteries, with or without associated parenchymal disease (e.g., meconium aspiration) or other congenital malformations (e.g., pulmonary hypoplasia, congenital diaphragmatic hernia (CDH), or cardiac disease). The following discussion addresses the latter, more narrowly defined, syndrome of PPHN, for which some authors have reserved the label of "persistent fetal circulation." Because the fetal circulation includes the placenta, however, this is somewhat of a misnomer for a description of abnormal physiology in the infant after birth.

Differential diagnosis of persistent pulmonary hypertension of the newborn

The diagnosis of PPHN must be considered in any infant who remains hypoxemic, with a PaO_2 less than 100 mmHg, while breathing 100% oxygen [3]. This clinical observation provides strong evidence for right-to-left shunting, but provides no information regarding the location or cause of such shunting. The prerequisites for right-to-left shunting include pressures on the right (pulmonary) side of the circulation exceeding those on the left (systemic) side, along with a communication between the right and left sides through which shunting can occur. In addition to the fetal channels (ductus arteriosus and foramen ovale), which are present and patent in almost every infant, shunting may occur at atrial or ventricular septal defects, aortopulmonary windows, or at other sites where cardiac malformations permit admixture of venous and arterial blood (e.g., atrioventricular canal, truncus arteriosus). Since right-to-left shunting may result from reduced systemic pressures even if pulmonary arterial pressures are normal, pulmonary hypertension should not be considered until it has been established that systemic cardiac output is adequate. Because the right ventricle can sustain systemic pressures, it is essential that normal systemic arterial pressures should not be taken as proof of adequacy of left ventricular output.

Presently, color Doppler echocardiography provides the most direct approach to assessment of systemic blood flow, allowing diagnosis of structural obstructions (covering the entire spectrum of hypoplastic left heart syndromes) as well as intrinsic (hypoglycemia, hypocalcemia, asphyxial or toxic cardiomyopathy) and extrinsic (tamponade, hypovolemia) left ventricular dysfunction. If these conditions have been excluded, and there is echocardiographic evidence of elevated pulmonary arterial pressures, the cause of the elevation in

Fetal and Neonatal Brain Injury, 4th edition, ed. David K. Stevenson, William E. Benitz, Philip Sunshine, Susan R. Hintz, and Maurice L. Druzin. Published by Cambridge University Press. © Cambridge University Press 2009.

pulmonary artery pressures must be ascertained. Since high pressures may result from increased flow as well as from increased resistance, conditions which may produce an obligatory increase in pulmonary blood flow, such as intracardiac left-to-right shunts or large arteriovenous malformations, must be identified or excluded. Hyperviscosity, most commonly due to a hematocrit greater than 65%, has a larger effect on pulmonary than on systemic vascular resistance and pressures, and may produce intractable right-to-left shunting until corrected by partial exchange transfusion. Constriction of otherwise normal pulmonary arteries may occur with any significant pulmonary parenchymal process, mediated by reflex vasoconstriction of blood vessels in poorly ventilated and hypoxic regions of the lungs. Specific diagnosis is important, since adequate treatment of the primary process will ameliorate secondary pulmonary vasoconstriction, increase systemic cardiac output, and reduce or eliminate right-to-left shunting. These conditions do not require interventions primarily intended to alter pulmonary vascular tone.

Intrinsic disease of the pulmonary arteries may be recognized by its association with other congenital malformations, especially pulmonary hypoplasia (e.g., CDH, thoracic dystrophies, chronic intrauterine pleural effusions) [5,6], or by the infant's characteristic response to induction of systemic alkalosis, typically by acute hyperventilation [7]. Infants with mild to moderately severe pulmonary arterial disease respond to this stimulus with at least a transient pulmonary vasodilation, reflecting the dynamic component of their pulmonary vascular obstruction, which is clinically evident as a reduction in pulmonary pressures to below systemic levels, reversal of right-to-left shunting, and a marked increase in PaO_2. Typically, these infants exhibit a pH threshold below which they have right-to-left shunting and are hypoxemic and above which they have a well-saturated arterial blood; this threshold may be relatively low early in the course of mild disease, but may be much higher later in the course or in infants with

severe disease. Infants with severe pulmonary vascular disease, however, may fail to respond perceptibly to alkalosis, either because structural remodeling of the pulmonary vessels is so advanced that vasodilation is impossible or insufficient, or because early intrauterine growth failure has produced not only pulmonary hypoplasia but also a deficient number of arteries and arterioles beyond the third or fourth branching generation [6], so that the maximal cross-sectional area of the pulmonary arterial tree is severely compromised, even with maximal dilation of these vessels. In summary, clinical diagnosis of PPHN involves exclusion of other causes of right-to-left shunting, confirmation of elevated pulmonary artery pressures usually by echocardiography, and demonstration of a threshold response to elevation of the systemic pH.

Pathogenesis of persistent pulmonary hypertension of the newborn

PPHN, defined narrowly as above, is characterized by striking intrinsic structural and functional abnormalities of the pulmonary arteries [8]. During normal pulmonary development, the muscular investment of the pulmonary arteries extends from proximal to distal vessels, and the thickness of the medial smooth-muscle layer increases in the already muscular proximal vessels. In normal infants at term, the arteries and arterioles found within the respiratory acinus (distal to terminal bronchioles) are all non-muscular, and a muscular arterial media is present only in the more proximal, extra-acinar arteries. Infants with PPHN exhibit precocious development of the muscular layer of the pulmonary arteries, with extension of the smooth muscular investment into smaller and more peripheral intra-acinar arteries, as far peripherally as the pleura, and the thickness of the muscular media in more proximal vessels is markedly increased, as shown in Figure 37.1 [9]. In addition, there is marked thickening of the adventitial connective tissue surrounding the pulmonary

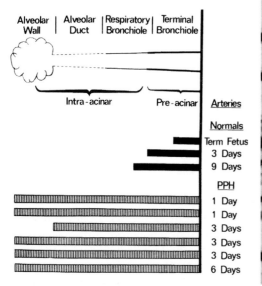

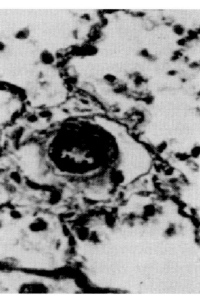

Fig. 37.1. Vascular maldevelopment is a hallmark of PPHN. The pulmonary vessels show thickened walls with smooth-muscle hyperplasia. Further, the smooth muscle extends to the level of the intra-acinar arteries, which does not normally occur until much later in the postnatal period.

arteries, with increased deposition of adventitial collagen and elastin. These changes are associated with abnormal pulmonary vascular sensitivity to a variety of stimuli, ranging from hypercarbia, acidosis, and hypoxia to stimulation from tracheal suctioning, handling, or a noisy environment. Excessive vasoconstrictive responses appear to be mediated by excessive production of endothelin and possibly other vasoconstrictive substances, and by deficient local production of nitric oxide (NO), presumably due to loss of NO synthase activity in these pulmonary vessels [10]. Normal activity of these vasoregulatory mechanisms appears to recover a few days after birth, accounting for the clinical observation that pulmonary vasoconstriction becomes much less problematic at about 4 days of age in infants with PPHN who can be supported through that period [11]. On the other hand, the structural abnormalities in the pulmonary arteries of these infants probably resolve much more slowly, and normal pulmonary arterial structure may be achieved only after months or years, when lung development catches up with the precocious arteries.

The antecedents of accelerated arterial development and abnormal vasoregulatory function remain uncertain [8]. Clinical observations suggest that antenatal hypoxia or increased intrauterine pulmonary blood flow may be important predisposing factors. The archetypal infant with PPHN is a meconium-stained post-term baby with wasted subcutaneous fat and epidermal peeling, suggesting chronic placental insufficiency. Infants with intrauterine closure or constriction of the ductus arteriosus (resulting from exposure to non-steroidal anti-inflammatory agents) or with cardiac malformations that impose increased pulmonary blood flow and elevated pulmonary arterial pressures in utero have been associated with both pulmonary arterial remodeling and clinical pulmonary hypertension in the immediate postnatal period. Increased sensitivity of the ductus to the constrictor effects of prostaglandin synthetase inhibitors and the more advanced development of the pulmonary arteries with increasing gestation, particularly near term, may both contribute to the lower risk of PPHN in preterm infants and the predilection for this disorder to occur in post-term infants. In many cases, however, no predisposing intrauterine condition can be identified.

In sheep, fetal hypoxia resulting from maternal hypotension [12], placental embolization [13], or umbilical cord compression produces pulmonary arterial remodeling [14], elevated pulmonary vascular resistance and pressures, and accentuated and more prolonged vasoconstrictor responses to asphyxial stimuli, but pulmonary arterial pressures remain substantially below systemic levels during normoxic ventilation in these models. Ligation of the ductus arteriosus several days before delivery in fetal lamb, or partial occlusion of the ductus using an inflatable occluder for 9–14 days in fetal lambs [15–18], with consequent diversion of right ventricular output into the lungs, causes an acute increase in pulmonary artery flow and pressure. Although the elevated pressure is sustained, the increment in flow is reversed as the pulmonary vascular resistance increases, and these animals exhibit elevation of pulmonary artery pressures to equal or exceed those in

the aorta, along with the right-to-left extrapulmonary shunting and refractory hypoxemia that is characteristic of infants with PPHN. These animals also have increased muscularity of the pulmonary arteries, analogous to that observed in infants who die with PPHN. Notably, these structural and functional changes in the pulmonary arteries occur only 5–8 days or more after induction of the hypoxic or pulmonary hypertensive condition, and there is no evidence that even repeated or severe acute asphyxial episodes can rapidly elicit the intractable pulmonary vasoconstriction that epitomizes this condition. These observations have several implications for infants with PPHN who subsequently manifest neurodevelopmental impairments. It is clear that these infants have been subject to a significantly disturbed intrauterine environment for a period of at least several days. Reduced arterial oxygen content, due to impaired placental function or increased arteriovenous admixture at the atrial level with premature constriction of the ductus, may impair cerebral oxygen delivery, placing these infants at increased risk for intrauterine hypoxic–ischemic cerebral insults. Redistribution of cardiac output in a fetus who is hypoxic or has reduced flow from the ductus into the descending aorta may impair renal perfusion, causing oligohydramnios, increasing the risk of cord compression events prior to and during labor and delivery. The primary events may also reduce the capacity for the fetus to tolerate the stress of labor and delivery, either directly or by blunting the metabolic and endocrine responses to this stress, enhancing the potential for intrapartum insults. Abnormal developmental outcomes in these infants therefore often have several antecedents, most of which are not amenable to diagnosis or treatment, and attribution of a poor outcome exclusively to intrapartum or obstetrical events is not easily justified.

Treatment of persistent pulmonary hypertension of the newborn

Review articles demonstrate the wide variety of practice patterns in the treatment of PPHN [10,19–22]. As there is no singular cause of PPHN, or a singular pathophysiologic effect on the body, there is clearly no defined strategy to treat it. Whenever PPHN is secondary, such as in severe respiratory distress syndrome (RDS) or sepsis, therapeutic intervention must include addressing the underlying disease. Similarly, when there are secondary effects from PPHN (e.g., pulmonary hemorrhage), treatment must also correct those perturbations.

Non-specific physiologic interventions to ameliorate PPHN

The initial approach to treat PPHN includes normalization of physiologic perturbations that can exacerbate PPHN, including normalization of serum glucose, calcium, and partial exchange transfusion for polycythemia. Optimization of cardiac function may require colloid volume infusion or inotropic pressor support (e.g., dopamine or epinephrine infusions). Intravenous vasodilators (e.g., nitroprusside) are usually non-selective and affect both systemic and pulmonary vascular resistance, so are often not successful in reversing right-to-left shunting associated with PPHN. Tolazoline, usually given intravenously to achieve pulmonary vasodilation, was never proven to reduce mortality rates in PPHN, and is no longer available in the United States [23]. Oxygen-carrying capacity should be optimized by red blood cell transfusion; it should be appreciated that increasing the hematocrit from 30% to 40% will be associated with an approximately 33% increase in oxygen delivery, an increase that is difficult to attain with changes in ventilator strategies. Sedation is often used to decrease agitation and resistance to mechanical ventilation.

Ventilator management

Although neonates with clinically significant PPHN are almost always on mechanical respiratory support, ventilator management remains a controversial arena for the treatment of PPHN. Alkalosis, induced by hyperventilation and hypocapnia, has been shown to reduce pulmonary vascular resistance in PPHN [7,24], and for many physicians this historically represented the cornerstone of the treatment of severe PPHN [19]. However, the excessive barotrauma and/or volutrauma that may be necessary to achieve hyperventilation may delay lung repair or even cause further injury. Furthermore, extreme hypocarbia has been shown to reduce cerebral blood flow in human adults and neonatal animal models [25,26]. In neonatal humans, this response might not be fully present or it may be transient, with subsequent adjustment of cerebral blood flow at a reduced $PaCO_2$. If there is a reduction in cerebral blood flow, any improvement in oxygen content in the blood achieved by hyperventilation may be more than counterbalanced, leading to a net overall reduction in cerebral oxygen delivery and consumption. Regional cerebral blood flow reduction and accompanying oxygen deficits may account for specific neurologic injury in PPHN such as sensorineural hearing loss (SNHL). Measurement of the relative effects of hyperventilation and other strategies upon cerebral metabolism and integrity may be achieved by portable bedside monitoring techniques such as near-infrared optical spectroscopy. An alternative to extreme hyperventilation is more modest hypocapnia ($PaCO_2$ 30–40 mmHg or 3.3–4.7 kPa) combined with more aggressive alkali (bicarbonate or tromethamine) administration. In a review by Walsh-Sukys et al., achieving alkalosis by alkali administration was associated with a fivefold increase in the use of extracorporeal membrane oxygenation (ECMO), while hyperventilation seemed to reduce the risk of ECMO without increasing the use of oxygen at 28 days of age [22]. Peak inspiratory pressures may be reduced with the implementation of high-frequency ventilation or synchronous ventilator techniques.

An alternative approach to ventilator management advocated by Wung and others is "gentle ventilation," with more modest blood gas goals such as PaO_2 50–70 mmHg (6.7–9.3 kPa) and $PaCO_2$ 40–60 mmHg (5.3–8.0 kPa), along with avoidance of paralysis [27,28]. This strategy, which seeks to minimize ventilator-induced injury, has been shown in several uncontrolled reports to reduce the need for ECMO in neonates with severe PPHN, and was associated with favorable neurologic outcomes, including intact sensorineural hearing [29]. The absence of any controlled trials comparing hyperventilation to "gentle ventilation" or any other specific ventilator strategy makes it difficult to state definitely which approach is superior. However, there have several reviews of experience with treatment strategies for PPHN associated with CDH showing marked improvements in outcome when there is more tolerance of hypercarbia and lower oxygen saturation [30,31]. Animal studies have shown the ability to achieve oxygenation and ventilation through the use of novel perfluorocarbons (e.g., perflubron), with less lung injury than would be induced by the use of conventional ventilators [32,33]. However, there has been little reported experience with the use of liquid ventilation in human neonates with respiratory failure and PPHN [34]; it appears that this approach will not be available for many years.

High-frequency ventilation

The use of high-frequency ventilation (HFV), be it by flow-interruption, oscillation, or jet ventilation, has been advocated for neonatal respiratory disease [35–38]. HFV maintains lung expansion and achieves ventilation with rapid (5–15 Hz) delivery of breaths at tidal volumes that may be smaller than the nominal physiological dead space. The maximal distension during HFV is less than in conventional tidal volume ventilation, thereby decreasing barotrauma. In patients nearing or meeting ECMO criteria, HFV strategies seem to reduce the need for bypass in 10–50% of patients, depending upon the underlying lung disease [39–41]. HFV may also improve alveolar expansion and therefore the availability and distribution of exogenously administered inhaled nitric oxide (iNO). This may account for the improvement in the physiologic response to iNO when HFV is used to deliver iNO in the treatment of neonatal PPHN [42,43].

Pharmacologic approaches to treat neonatal PPHN

Exogenous surfactant

Patients with severe PPHN have several reasons for inadequate surfactant activity. Meconium, infection-related inflammation, and pulmonary hemorrhage may decrease surfactant effectiveness. In patients with CDH or severe RDS, there may be insufficient surfactant present [44,45]. Improving alveolar expansion via surfactant administration may be important in optimizing the effect of iNO [46]. Lotze et al. have shown that surfactant replacement improves pulmonary mechanics and reduces duration of ECMO bypass in patients with respiratory failure [47]. Given the relatively rare, limited, and transient adverse side effects seen with surfactant administration, some advocate a test dose (1 mL/kg) in patients with severe PPHN approaching ECMO criteria. A large multicenter randomized trial has shown that administration of surfactant led to a 30% reduction in the need for ECMO in a high-risk population of neonates, most of whom had PPHN [48]. Meta-analysis of four clinical trials supports the use of surfactant for infants with MAS, based on the decreased need for ECMO [49].

Inhaled nitric oxide

The intracellular mediator of vascular smooth-muscle dilation released by the neighboring endothelial cell appears to be NO [50]. Within the smooth muscle, NO activates guanylate cyclase to form cyclic guanosine monophosphate, which causes muscle relaxation. Administration of exogenous NO by inhalation reduces pulmonary vascular resistance [51,52]. In neonates with severe PPHN, reduced pulmonary vascular resistance should decrease right-to-left shunting at the foramen ovale or patent ductus arteriosus and thereby improve oxygenation. Besides reducing extrapulmonary right-to-left shunting, iNO may also improve intrapulmonary ventilation perfusion matching. iNO is rapidly metabolized by conversion of hemoglobin to methemoglobin, and has little or no effect on systemic vascular resistance and cardiac output.

Initial clinical trials of iNO in neonates with respiratory failure and PPHN showed dramatic improvements in oxygenation, and an apparent decrease in the subsequent need for ECMO [21,53,54]. Two multicenter randomized controlled trials (RCTs) demonstrated that iNO decreased the incidence of ECMO or death in term and near-term newborns with PPHN [55,56], which led to Food and Drug Administration (FDA) approval in December 1999. While the most recent Cochrane review supports the use of iNO in term and near-term infants with severe respiratory failure, a meta-analysis of recent trials of iNO in premature infants with respiratory failure (which also may be accompanied by PPHN) concluded that there is not enough evidence to support the use of iNO for this population [57,58]. Most clinicians use iNO to treat severe respiratory failure with some component of PPHN based on some physiologic measurement of respiratory failure, such as an oxygenation index (OI) ≥ 25 (OI = ((mean airway pressure × FiO$_2$)/ PaO$_2$) × 100). Treatment is usually initiated at a dose between 5 and 20 ppm, although the commercially available delivery system allows for dosing as high as 80 ppm. Most centers have protocols in place to promote weaning of iNO leading to its eventual discontinuation, typically within 3–7 days.

iNO is not without potential risks that could possibly affect prognosis and neurologic outcome. Methemoglobinemia and hypoxia can result from excess NO administration or in the rare patient with decreased methemoglobin reductase. NO and its metabolites, including nitrogen dioxide and peroxynitrites, may directly cause lung injury. iNO increases bleeding time in normal adult humans, presumably through platelet-mediated effects [59]. However, in patients with acute respiratory distress syndrome, NO affected platelet aggregation tests without changing the bleeding time [60]. The effects of NO on coagulation could theoretically place neonatal iNO recipients at higher hemorrhagic risk, although this has not been seen to be a significant side effect in the clinical trials to date. Given these potential risks, it is understandable that the clinical trials of iNO in neonates with severe PPHN have

examined secondary outcomes, including neurodevelopment. In a follow-up to one of the pivotal studies used for FDA approval, iNO was not associated with an increase in neurodevelopmental, behavioral, or medical abnormalities at 2 years of age [61].

Phosphodiesterase inhibitors

In the pulmonary smooth muscle, NO, be it endogenous or exogenously administered via inhalation, increases formation of cyclic guanosine monophosphate, which is vasodilatory until it is degraded by phosphodiesterase (PDE). There are several types of PDE, of which type V dominates in the pulmonary vascular bed. Inhibitors of PDE such as dypyramidole have been used to potentiate the effects of iNO, although their use has been associated with deleterious side effects, including severe hypotension [62]. Other type V selective PDE inhibitors, such as zaprinast, have been used in animal models to affect pulmonary vasodilation, often to potentiate the effects of iNO [63–65], but have yet to be used clinically in humans in any prospective randomized trials.

Sildenafil, an FDA-approved drug whose primary mechanism is inhibition of PDE, has recently been studied as a treatment in animal models of PPHN [66,67]. There have been some case reports of neonates with PPHN who apparently responded well to enteral administration of sildenafil, but there are only a few recent randomized studies of its use to treat PPHN [68,69]. In a study by Baquero et al., babies were dosed at 1 mg/kg every 6 hours, with allowance for doubling the dose if oxygenation did not improve. This intensive care unit did not have iNO, HFV, or ECMO available [69]. A statistically significant improvement in oxygenation in sildenafil-treated babies versus controls, as well as a trend to reduced mortality, was seen. Another small randomized trial showed that 2 mg/kg of sildenafil given via orogastric tube every 6 hours for a total of 72 hours lowered the OI more than placebo control [70]. Intravenous sildenafil has also been shown to augment the pulmonary vasodilator effects of iNO in infants early after cardiac surgery, although sildenafil administration was also associated with significant hypotension [71]. A lower dose (0.4 mg/kg) of sildenafil has been shown to reduce the rebound pulmonary hypertension associated with the withdrawal of iNO in older infants and children treated with iNO [72]. This approach has yet to be studied in neonates with PPHN. Two other recent reports retrospectively reviewed the experience of using sildenafil for neonates with chronic pulmonary hypertension, such as that seen in CDH [73,74]. Clinical trials are under way to study the pharmacology of intravenous sildenafil and its clinical efficacy in the treatment of neonatal PPHN.

Milrinone, a PDE III inhibitor that is a cardiopressor with known vasodilatory effects, also recently has been used to treat neonatal PPHN. In one small series, nine babies with poor initial response to iNO were treated with a milrinone drip for approximately 72 hours, and they demonstrated improved oxygenation, especially in the first 24 hours of milrinone treatment, without systemic hypotension [75]. In another case report, four neonates with PPHN not responding to iNO had improved oxygenation and survived after treatment with milrinone drip for 3–7 days, although two of four suffered severe intraventricular hemorrhage [76]. Randomized trials will be needed to establish the safety and efficacy of milrinone in the treatment of neonatal PPHN.

Magnesium sulfate

Magnesium sulfate is a potent vasodilator, and its mechanism of action is only partially understood. It may help due to its sedative, muscle-relaxant, and bronchodilator effects. Improvements in oxygenation have been seen in four observational studies. A 2007 Cochrane review concluded that there was no evidence from RCTs to support the use of magnesium for PPHN [77]. However, a more recent article describes a retrospective experience of 58 neonates in six Italian intensive care units, where 27 of 28 babies with PPHN were treated with magnesium sulfate with improvement in OI, compared to 100% response in matched controls treated with iNO. However, the response to iNO was more rapid. No significant differences in immediate and long-term consequences, including neurological evaluation at 18 months of age, were reported [78].

Other drugs targeted to reduce pulmonary vasoconstriction

Administration of tolazoline and nitroprusside via the endotracheal tube has been used to target these vasodilator therapies more selectively to the pulmonary vascular bed [79–82]. However, no prospective randomized studies have investigated their effects on major outcomes, such as the need for ECMO. Adenosine infusion has been shown to dilate the pulmonary vessels of fetal and newborn lambs [83], and has also been associated with improved oxygenation in a small series of newborns with PPHN [84]. Because adenosine presumably acts upon adenylate cyclase, its action may be additive to that of iNO, as suggested by the data of Aranda *et al.* in an experimental model of PPHN [85].

Prostacyclin (prostaglandin I2) is a potent vasodilator that upon binding to a specific receptor stimulates adenylate cyclase to form cyclic adenosine monophosphate, thereby activating protein kinase A, which induces vasodilation. There has been limited experience using either inhaled or intravenous prostacyclin or its analogue, iloprost, in neonates, sometimes as an adjunct to the use of iNO; however, intravenous use has been associated with significant side effects including hypotension [86]. Prostacyclin administration seems to be more effective in neonates with pulmonary hypertension secondary to chronic conditions, such as bronchopulmonary dysplasia (BPD) or CDH, rather than PPHN from acute respiratory failure. There is a case report of inhaled prostacyclin in neonates with PPHN not responding to iNO, with one of four such infants surviving [87]. There remains inadequate experience to recommend its use in neonates with PPHN at this time.

Hyperoxia frequently occurs in neonates being treated for PPHN and may cause oxidative injury that can inactivate NO and exacerbate pulmonary vasoconstriction. In a recent study

of PPHN in a lamb model, recombinant human superoxide dismutase (rhSOD) was administered intratracheally, leading to sustained improvement in oxygenation similar to that seen when animals were given iNO [88]. Combined treatment with rhSOD and iNO resulted in a more rapid and sustained increase in oxygenation and reduced ventilator settings when compared to iNO alone. rhSOD treatment in PPHN may be efficacious by scavenging superoxide, prolonging the biologic half-life of endogenous and exogenous iNO, and preventing peroxynitrite formation. It is a therapeutic strategy on the horizon for the term and near-term infant with hypoxic respiratory failure and PPHN to be used in conjunction with iNO. Clinical trials performed in premature infants have not identified any safety concerns [89,90].

Extracorporeal membrane oxygenation

ECMO is a form of heart–lung bypass providing cardio-respiratory support for days to weeks, which is available at approximately 120 US centers and another 60 outside the USA [91]. Venoarterial (VA) ECMO bypass, using right jugular venous drainage and right carotid arterial return, can provide respiratory and cardiac support; the latter is often needed in patients with PPHN associated with sepsis or cardiac disease. Venovenous (VV) ECMO, usually performed via a double-lumen catheter placed in the right jugular vein with the tip in the right atrium, returns oxygenated blood preferentially towards the right ventricle, thereafter relying on the patient's cardiac function to achieve adequate systemic oxygen delivery. Once on bypass, ventilator settings are weaned, thereby avoiding or minimizing further oxygen toxicity and barotrauma, and permitting pulmonary recovery and reversal of PPHN.

Both VA and VV ECMO require systemic heparinization titrated based on bedside coagulation studies to prevent circuit clotting. This places ECMO patients at increased risk for hemorrhagic complications, including risk for intracranial hemorrhage, which occurs in approximately 7% of patients, but varies depending on gestational age, diagnosis, and coagulation status [91–93]. Strategies to decrease the incidence of intracranial hemorrhage of ECMO include administration of aminocaproic acid, a fibrinolysis inhibitor [94], as well as the use of cephalad venous drainage catheters [95]. Besides pre-ECMO and hemorrhagic risks for neurologic sequelae, ECMO patients have additional risks, including nosocomial and transfusion-related infection, thromboembolism, and potential effects of neck vessel ligation. Jugular venous ligation may impair cerebral venous drainage and lead to superior vena cava syndrome. Carotid artery ligation leads to collateral flow to the right side of the brain. VV ECMO obviates the need for carotid artery ligation. Some centers advocate post-ECMO carotid artery repair, but there may be subsequent stenosis, and there are no data to date demonstrating improved neurobehavioral outcomes with such repair.

Given the relatively invasive nature of ECMO therapy and its attendant risks, ECMO is reserved for neonates with severe PPHN or other forms of cardiorespiratory disease only after failure of presumably less risky medical management. Criteria predicting high mortality rates between 60% and 80% have been developed, based on arterial blood gases and ventilator settings. It is also important that there must be adequate time to transport such critically ill patients to an ECMO center and to place them on bypass before cardiac arrest or hypoxic brain injury occurs. While ECMO was used for over 1500 neonates with respiratory failure in 1991, since then its utilization rate has been reduced nearly in half, which is likely due to the increased use of HFV, surfactant, and iNO, as well as improved obstetrical practices including Group B *Streptococcus* prophylaxis, and avoiding post-dates deliveries. Current ECMO patients have more severe and complex illnesses, such as CDH; this explains why survival rates for neonatal ECMO have fallen from 86% to 64% over the past 20 years [91].

Outcome of persistent pulmonary hypertension of the newborn

Infants with PPHN are among the most critically ill patients cared for in the neonatal intensive care unit. These infants often have a wide variety of pre-existing perinatal conditions such as low Apgar scores or fetal distress that place them at high risk for abnormal outcomes. The treatment of PPHN involves the use of therapies, including high-frequency ventilation, ECMO, and iNO, which may also adversely affect outcome.

Outcome for PPHN survivors treated with medical therapy

Outcome for PPHN survivors treated with conventional medical therapy

Conventional medical therapy (CMT) for PPHN often includes periods of mechanical ventilation with high pressure and high oxygen concentrations that increase the risk for chronic lung disease (CLD), historically defined in term infants as a persistent oxygen requirement beyond 28 days of life. CLD has been shown to be associated with worse cognitive outcome [96,97]. Hyperventilation with production of a respiratory alkalosis has been used to treat PPHN and has been shown to decrease pulmonary artery pressures and increase arterial PaO_2 [7]. Although hyperventilation has been shown to attenuate pulmonary vasoconstriction, the resulting hypocarbia can produce cerebrovascular vasoconstriction with a subsequent reduction in cerebral blood flow [98]. Whether hyperventilation is specifically responsible for the neurodevelopmental sequelae seen in PPHN survivors is difficult to determine, because of the multitude of potential causes of neurologic injury present in this population.

The literature describing the neurodevelopmental outcome of infants treated with CMT is summarized in Table 37.1. Cohen *et al.* reported on the outcomes of 29 survivors of PPHN treated with tolazoline, 50% of whom had abnormal EEGs or seizures in the newborn period [23]. Overall, 28% of the children had evidence of significant neurologic impairment

at age 3. When examining the infants with perinatal hypoxia and an Apgar score less than 6, there was a similar incidence of significant handicaps, leading the authors to conclude that the morbidity from PPHN was related to the degree of perinatal hypoxia.

Brett *et al.* reported on the neurologic and developmental assessment of nine infants with PPHN treated with hyperventilation [99]. The infants in this cohort were exposed to a $PaCO_2 < 20$ for 51.8 hours and a pH > 7.5 for 64.4 hours; exposure to a $PaCO_2 < 15$ and a pH > 7.6 was also present, but for shorter time periods. All had normal neurologic examinations at follow-up, and seven of the eight had normal developmental quotient (DQ) on standardized testing. The authors concluded that the outcome following hyperventilation was reassuring.

Bernbaum *et al.* evaluated 11 survivors of PPHN managed with hyperventilation strategies [100]. The authors attempted to correlate neurologic and developmental outcome with physiologic parameters such as pH, $PaCO_2$, PaO_2, and blood pressure. Of the three patients with an abnormal neurologic outcome, there were significant differences in the duration of mean arterial pressure < 50 and $PaCO_2 < 25$ compared to the infants with a normal outcome. The authors speculated that hypocarbia may potentiate hypoxic–ischemic encephalopathy by further compromising cerebral blood flow.

In a review of the developmental follow-up of PPHN survivors at their institution, Ballard and Leonard reported on the outcome of 11 infants treated with hyperventilation [101]. Subjects were assessed at 4–6 years of age, and all had a normal neurologic exam. Assessment of cognitive development using the McCarthy scales revealed a mean General Cognitive Index (GCI) of 95, with scores ranging from 79 to 120. The authors concluded there was no evidence for a negative effect of hyperventilation, and the presence of a specific motor or mental deficit in patients with PPHN was attributed to perinatal asphyxia.

Ferrara *et al.* studied the outcome of 16 infants treated with hypocapneic alkalosis for PPHN [102]. All infants studied (n = 11) had EEG abnormalities during hyperventilation, nine demonstrated transient hypotonia, and there was a statistically significant discrepancy between Bayley Mental Developmental Index (MDI) and Psychomotor Developmental Index (PDI) scores. The authors urged further long-term studies to investigate potential detrimental effects of hyperventilation.

Sell *et al.* examined the neurodevelopmental status of 40 patients between the ages of 1 and 4 years who received hyperventilation as treatment for PPHN [103]. Cerebral palsy (CP) was reported in 15%, profound impairment in 7.5%, and mild motor delay in 2%. Of the 37 functional children, mean Bayley and McCarthy scores were within the normal range.

Bifano and Pfannenstiel examined 21 PPHN survivors treated with hyperventilation at 1 year of age [96]. Using a stepwise regression analysis, an association was observed between the duration of hyperventilation and abnormal neurodevelopmental outcome. Although the mean Bayley MDI

Table 37.1. Outcome following conventional medical therapy

Study	Description	Age	n	Neurologic outcome	n	Cognitive outcome	
						Stanford–Binet IQ	
Cohen *et al.* 1980 [23]	PPHN Tolazoline	1–3 years	29	Seizures: 3.5% CP: 10% Microcephaly: 34%	12	97.7 (range 66–132)	
						Developmental Quotient	
Brett *et al.* 1981 [99]	PPHN Hyperventilation	1–3 years	9	Normal: 100%	8	107.6 (range 89–130)	
						Developmental Quotient	
Bernbaum *et al.* 1984 [100]	PPHN Hyperventilation	6 months – 4 years	11	Normal: 73% Abnormal: 27% (1 hemiparesis, 2 increased tone/reflexes)	11	92 (range 70–110)	
						McCarthy GCI	
Ballard & Leonard 1984 [101]	PPHN Hyperventilation	4–6 years	11	Normal: 100%	9	95 (range 76–120)	
						Bayley MDI	*Bayley PDI*
Ferrara *et al.* 1984 [102]	PPHN Hyperventilation	1 year	16	Normal: 88% Abnormal: 12% (1 hemiparesis, 1 gross motor delay)	11	106	93
						Bayley MDI	*Bayley PDI*
Sell *et al.* 1985 [103]	PPHN Hyperventilation	1–4 years	40	Normal: 40% CP: 15% Severely impaired: 7.5%	37	116 (1 year) 102 (2 year) *McCarthy GCI* 110 (3 year) 103 (4 year)	102 (1 year) 91 (2 year)
						Bayley MDI	*Bayley PDI*
Bifano & Pfannenstiel 1988 [96]	PPHN Hyperventilation	1 year	21	Normal: 52% Suspect: 29% Abnormal: 19% (4 CP)	21	106	91
						Bayley MDI	
Hageman *et al.* 1988 [104]	PPHN Hyperventilation	1 year	10	Not reported	10	98 for AaDO$_2$ > 600 93 for AaDO$_2$ < 599	
						Stanford–Binet IQ	
Marron *et al.* 1992 [29]	PPHN Gentle ventilation	2–6 years	27	Normal: 63% Mild abnormality: 22% Severe abnormality: 15%	13	96 for children with normal or mildly abnormal neurologic examination	

Notes:
Unless otherwise noted, all scores are mean values. PPHN, persistent pulmonary hypertension of the newborn; CP, cerebral palsy; MDI, Mental Developmental Index; PDI, Psychomotor Developmental Index; GCI, General Cognitive Index. "Suspect" neurologic outcome defined as Bayley MDI or PDI 70–85.

and PDI scores were within the normal range, the infants with abnormal neurologic examinations or below-average Bayley scores were more likely to have had a PaCO$_2$ < 25, leading the authors to conclude that prolonged hypocarbia was associated with poor neurodevelopmental outcome.

Hageman *et al.* studied the relationship between the alveolar–arterial oxygen difference (AaDO$_2$) and outcome and found that AaDO$_2$ values were significantly higher in non-survivors [104]. Bayley assessment of survivors failed to demonstrate a correlation between AaDO$_2$ values and neurodevelopmental outcome at age 1.

Marron *et al.* reported the neurologic and cognitive outcomes for a cohort of PPHN survivors treated with conservative ventilation strategies [29]. Sixty-three percent of infants had a normal neurologic examination, while 22% and 15% had mild and severe abnormalities, respectively. A significant

relationship between low Apgar scores and poor neurologic outcome was observed, and three of the four children with severe impairment had biochemical evidence of asphyxia at birth. Stanford–Binet IQ testing in the 13 children tested was normal.

Outcome for PPHN survivors treated with inhaled nitric oxide

iNO is now the standard treatment for term and near-term infants with hypoxemic respiratory failure and PPHN. The outcome data for iNO trials are summarized in Table 37.2.

Rosenberg *et al.* first documented the medical and neurodevelopmental outcome of PPHN patients treated with iNO [105]. They reported a 12.1% incidence of severe neurologic disability at 2 years, defined as MDI or PDI < 68, abnormal neurologic exam, or both. Of note, children tested serially at

Table 37.2. Outcome following inhaled nitric oxide therapy

Study	Description	Age	n	Neurologic outcome	n	Cognitive outcome	
						Bayley MDI	*Bayley PDI*
Rosenberg *et al.* 1997 [105]	iNO	2 years	33	Mild disability: 9.1% Severe disability: 12.1%	33	107	109
						Bayley MDI	*Bayley PDI*
NINOS 2000 [61]	iNO	18–24 months	85	Normal: 77.6% CP: 11.8%	79	85	85.7
	Controls		87	Normal: 79.3% CP: 10.3%	75	87	93.6
						Developmental Quotient	
Ellington *et al.* 2001 [106]	iNO	1–4 years	35	Disability: 9%	33	102	
	Controls		25	Disability: 20%		99	
						Bayley MDI	*Bayley PDI*
Lipkin *et al.* 2002 [107]	iNO	1 year	92	Normal: 82% Mild disability: 4% Major disability: 14% CP: 8%	87	≥ 85: 69% < 85: 31%	≥ 85: 76% < 85: 24%
	Controls		35	Normal: 80% Mild disability: 9% Major disability: 11% CP: 6%	33	≥ 85: 71% < 85: 29%	≥ 85: 82% < 85: 18%
						Bayley MDI	*Bayley PDI*
CINRGI 2003 [108]	iNO	1 year	74	Normal: 81% Mild hypotonia: 6.7% CP: 4%	81	95	92
	Controls		71	Normal: 86% Mild hypotonia: 2.8% CP: 1.4%		95	85
						Kyoto Scale of Psychological Development	
Ichiba *et al.* 2003 [109]	iNO	3 years	15	Mild disability: 6.7% Severe disability: 6.7%	14	98.4	
						Bayley MDI	*Bayley PDI*
Konduri *et al.* 2006 [110]	iNO	18–24 months	121	NDI: 27.9% CP: 8.2%	121	83.3	89
	Controls		113	NDI: 24.6% CP: 6.3%	113	86.1	98

Notes:
Unless otherwise noted, all scores are mean values. CP, cerebral palsy; MDI, Mental Developmental Index; PDI, Psychomotor Developmental Index; GCI, General Cognitive Index; NDI, Neurodevelopmental impairment, defined as moderate or severe CP, Bayley MDI or PDI < 70, blindness, or permanent hearing impairment requiring amplification.

1 and 2 years demonstrated significant improvement in MDI and PDI scores.

The Neonatal Inhaled Nitric Oxide Study (NINOS) Group reported on the outcome of infants enrolled in an RCT of iNO for hypoxemic respiratory failure [61]. Comprehensive neurodevelopmental assessment of survivors was performed at 18–24 months of age, and the rates of neurologic abnormality, CP, and low Bayley scores were not significantly different. Infants treated with iNO had lower Bayley PDI scores, but this difference was not statistically significant. The rate of disability was not affected by the need for ECMO, and the authors concluded that the timing of injury was most likely before ECMO.

Ellington *et al.* reported on the neurodevelopmental outcome of 60 of 83 survivors enrolled in a single center RCT of iNO for PPHN [106]. All results reported in this study were obtained by telephone interview, and disability was defined by the presence of a seizure disorder, cerebral palsy, or DQ < 70. Although a 20% rate of disability was found in the control group compared to 9% in the iNO group, this difference was not statistically significant, given the sample size.

Lipkin *et al.* reported the 1-year outcome of 133 survivors enrolled in the I-NO/PPHN Study [107]. This multicenter RCT sought to recruit 320 patients but was halted after 155 patients due to decreasing enrollment rate. The overall rate of impairment, including neurologic abnormalities, CP, and motor and cognitive outcomes assessed using the Bayley scales, was similar between control and treatment groups.

Clark et al. reported outcomes of 145 survivors enrolled in the Clinical Inhaled Nitric Oxide Research Group (CINRGI) [108]. The rate of a normal neurologic outcome was similar to previously published trials and there was no difference between the iNO and control groups (iNO 19% vs. control 14%). Notably, the rates of CP were lower than the average 11% previously cited by studies using CMT and reported for the NINOS trial (iNO 4% vs. control 1.4%, NS). The authors did not report any significant neurologic impairment at 1 year in this cohort. Assessment in 81 infants using the Bayley scales did not demonstrate a significant difference between groups. Although the authors concluded that treatment with iNO was not associated with an increase in adverse neurologic injury, they were cautious to note this study was not adequately powered to discern small but meaningful differences in neurologic outcome, and follow-up at 1 year of age is inadequate to assess future school performance.

Ichiba et al. presented 3-year outcome data on 15 infants treated with iNO and correlated clinical data with long-term outcome [109]. Hyperventilation was not used in this cohort. Infants were categorized by response to iNO into early, late, and poor responders based on the OI following initiation of therapy. The frequency of survival with a normal neurodevelopmental outcome was significantly higher in the early responders. The severity of PPHN as measured by OI was not associated with outcome. The authors suggested that a worse outcome in late or poor responders was related to prolonged exposure to hypoxia.

Konduri et al. reported on the 18- to 24-month outcomes of infants enrolled in the Early iNO Trial [110]. This multi-center RCT differed from previous trials by randomizing and initiating iNO at an OI of 15, whereas prior studies utilized an OI of 25 as the primary criterion for enrollment. Although earlier initiation of iNO did not reduce the combined incidence of ECMO/mortality, it did limit the progression of respiratory failure to an OI > 25. However, this did not translate into improved neurodevelopmental outcomes. Neurodevelopmental impairment (NDI), defined as the presence of moderate or severe CP, Bayley MDI or PDI < 70, blindness, or permanent hearing impairment requiring amplification, was similar in the two treatment groups. As seen previously in the NINOS trial, the investigators noted a non-significant decrease in the Bayley PDI in the iNO-treated group when compared to controls. This difference persisted even when infants with moderate to severe CP were excluded. The authors concluded that a possible adverse effect of iNO exposure could not be excluded.

Outcome for PPHN survivors treated with ECMO

More than 22 000 newborns have been treated with ECMO for respiratory failure, with a cumulative overall survival to discharge of 76% [91]. Therapies such as iNO, surfactant, and HFV have led to a decrease in the utilization of ECMO treatment, and those infants who currently receive treatment

have longer, more complicated ECMO runs [111]. Although life-saving, ECMO is an invasive therapy with many potential complications.

Risks associated with ECMO

Due to the patient's critical status, dependence on heart–lung bypass, and the inherent complexity of the ECMO equipment, patients are at risk for equipment failure, user error, and other ECMO-related complications, which can result in significant morbidity and mortality. The overall incidence of mechanical complications for neonates on ECMO reported to the Extracorporeal Life Support Organization (ELSO) is 82% [91].

Numerous studies have attempted to correlate findings on head ultrasound, head computed tomography (CT), and brain magnetic resonance imaging (MRI) with later neurodevelopmental outcome [112–115]. Some authors have suggested that a strong correlation exists between the severity of abnormality on neuroimaging and neurodevelopmental outcome. Although individual outcomes cannot be predicted, neuroimaging can be useful in assigning ECMO survivors to different risk categories. The presence of abnormalities is associated with an increased risk of developmental delay, but the sensitivity and specificity values for normal neuroimaging in predicting normal neurodevelopmental outcome are relatively low [112]. Cerebrovascular injury in the ECMO population is likely to be multifactorial. Prematurity, hypoxemia, asphyxia, and mechanical ventilation have all been associated with intracranial hemorrhage and infarction in critically ill newborns. Thus, even before ECMO, these infants are at high risk for cerebrovascular injury.

Ligation of both the right carotid artery and jugular vein was required for all patients receiving ECMO prior to the development of the double-lumen VV catheter in 1990. Ligation of the right common carotid artery (RCCA) has been shown to result in decreased right and left hemispheric flow [116]. Following RCCA ligation, the vertebrobasilar and the contralateral internal carotid systems are the main sources of flow for the right hemisphere via the circle of Willis. The circle of Willis provides a unique anatomic arrangement: it is able to redistribute and balance flow and thereby theoretically can avoid any deficit in cerebral perfusion due to unilateral carotid ligation. Numerous studies have attempted to determine if hemispheric brain injury occurs as a result of RCCA ligation [113,117–121]. Schumacher et al. reported on eight children with evidence of right hemispheric brain injury on either neurologic examination or neuroimaging study [117]. In a larger study, Taylor et al. found intracranial abnormalities in 95 of 207 infants; 21 were right-sided, 16 were left-sided, and 58 were bilateral [114]. The authors concluded that there was no increased injury in the distribution of the middle cerebral artery. Campbell et al. documented an increased risk of left-sided focal seizures following ECMO [119]. However, a follow-up study in the same children failed to find a significant difference in lateralization of motor findings [122]. In a study of ECMO survivors with unilateral brain injury, Bulas and Glass noted an increased rate of right-hand dominance

(94% ECMO vs. 85% control) and a suggestion of poorer performance by the left hand on psychometric testing [123]. However, this right-hand dominance persisted irrespective of the side of injury.

Electroencephalographic studies of ECMO infants have had conflicting findings. Streletz *et al.* found no consistently lateralized electroencephalographic abnormalities during or after ECMO when compared to tracings obtained before cannulation of the RCCA [124]. Hahn *et al.* found more repetitive or periodic discharges arising from the right hemisphere in ECMO patients compared to conventionally treated infants [125]. Pappas *et al.* evaluated the amplitude-integrated EEG (aEEG) characteristics of infants undergoing ECMO [126]. No acute changes were seen in aEEG amplitude during cannulation, and there was no difference seen between hemispheres. All infants studied demonstrated an improvement in aEEG background patterns at discharge compared to those obtained during the ECMO course.

Near-infrared spectroscopy (NIRS) has been applied to the ECMO population to investigate the effects of right carotid cannulation on cerebral oxygenation. Van Heijst *et al.* documented a transient decrease in cerebral oxygenation during cannulation for VA ECMO in both hemispheres in 10 infants using NIRS [127]. One hour following cannulation, an increase in cerebral oxygenation was observed, with no differences between the right and left hemispheres. Three infants in this cohort demonstrated asymmetric lesions on neuroimaging, but the authors were unable to associate cerebral oxygenation measurements with these abnormalities. Ejike *et al.* reported on cerebral oxygenation characteristics of 11 patients undergoing VA ECMO [128]. A transient decrease in cerebral oxygenation on the right was noted, followed by recovery toward baseline, and ultimately an increase in cerebral oxygenation was noted in both hemispheres. There was no association between ECMO flow rates and cerebral oxygenation in this cohort. Further studies are needed to determine the significance of cerebral oximetry and aEEG measurements during right carotid cannulation for VA ECMO.

ECMO follow-up studies

ECMO survivors have been identified as being at high risk for neurodevelopmental sequelae, but it remains unclear whether the neurologic sequelae seen in ECMO survivors are more indicative of the primary disease process, pre-ECMO therapy, or as a result of ECMO. The following studies are summarized in Table 37.3.

Krummel *et al.* published the first study of six ECMO survivors [129]. Five of the six were functioning normally with normal neurologic, neurodevelopmental, and neuroimaging examinations. One infant experienced an air embolus and had significant delay and bilateral cortical atrophy. The authors concluded that the early results with ECMO were encouraging considering the degree of illness.

Towne *et al.* reported the outcome of ECMO survivors among the first cohort of patients treated by Dr. Robert Bartlett between 1973 and 1980 [130]. Ten of the 16 had

normal neurologic outcomes, three had minor mental or motor problems, and five had moderate to severe handicap. Mean McCarthy GCI scores were in the normal range for the nine children tested. Two children were found to have a discrepancy between verbal and perceptual scores, and this was thought to reflect differences in the function of the two hemispheres.

Andrews *et al.* reported on the outcome of 14 survivors of ECMO evaluated using the Bayley scales [131]. Ten children (71%) had a normal MDI and nine (64%) had a normal PDI. The remaining children had scores less than 60. They concluded that the majority of these critically ill infants treated with ECMO have normal or near-normal outcomes.

Glass *et al.* examined 42 infants at 1 year of age [132]. Fifty-nine percent were found to be functioning in the normal range, with 20% suspect and 20% delayed. Sepsis, CLD, and neuroimaging abnormalities were associated with a poor outcome. No lateralizing signs consistent with a right hemispheric injury were found on neurologic or neuroimaging studies.

Adolph *et al.* evaluated ECMO survivors between the ages of 6 and 48 months [133]. Neurologic examination was normal in all but one child. Twenty-four children were evaluated with the Bayley scales, and 71% were classified as normal, 21% as suspect, and 8% as delayed. Twelve patients were evaluated using the McCarthy scales, with 75% obtaining normal scores. An abnormal outcome was found to be associated with the presence of CLD.

A large study of 80 ECMO survivors between the ages of 1 and 7 years by Schumacher *et al.* found 20% to be handicapped [134]. "Handicapped" was defined as having moderate to severe neurologic abnormality or SNHL requiring amplification. The oldest group of ECMO survivors had the highest incidence of handicap (45%), and this was felt to be due to a learning-curve effect. Improvements in patient selection criteria and ECMO management were felt to result in a subsequent lower rate of handicap. Speech and language abnormalities were identified in 15% of the ECMO survivors, with SNHL in 4%. The authors concluded that the outcome post-ECMO was similar to that reported in PPHN survivors treated with CMT.

Campbell *et al.* compared the 1- to 2-year neurologic and neurodevelopmental outcome of ECMO survivors with and without seizures in the neonatal period [122]. Twelve of the 41 ECMO survivors (29%) had neonatal seizures. The neurologic examination was abnormal in 50% of the children who had seizures. There was no predominance of left motor abnormalities and no association between the side of neonatal seizures and the lateralization of disability. The Cattell DQ scales were significantly lower for ECMO survivors with seizures than for those ECMO survivors without seizures. The authors concluded that carotid artery ligation was not responsible for lateralizing findings in ECMO survivors, but that seizures were associated with a higher risk for CP and developmental delay.

Hofkosh *et al.* reported on the neurodevelopmental outcome of 67 ECMO survivors between the ages of 6 months

Table 37.3. Outcome following ECMO therapy

Study	Description	Age	n	Neurologic outcome	n	Cognitive outcome	
						Bayley MDI and PDI	
Krummel *et al.* 1984 [129]	ECMO	15–21 months	6	Normal: 83% Abnormal: 17%	5	Range: 98–100	
						McCarthy GCI	
Towne *et al.* 1985 [130]	ECMO	4–11 years	16	Normal: 63% Abnormal: 37%	9	99 (range 78–122)	
						Bayley MDI	*Bayley PDI*
Andrews *et al.* 1986 [131]	ECMO	1–3 years	14	CP: 21% Microcephaly: 29% Seizures: 7%	14	≥ 85: 71% < 85: 29%	≥ 85: 64% < 85: 36%
						Bayley MDI and PDI	
Glass *et al.* 1989 [132]	ECMO	1 year	42	Normal: 75% Minor abnormality: 19% Definite abnormality: 5%	42	MDI and PDI > 90: 59% MDI or PDI < 90: 20% MDI and PDI < 90: 11% MDI and PDI < 70: 10%	
						Bayley MDI	*Bayley PDI*
Adolph *et al.* 1990 [133]	ECMO	6–48 months	57	Normal: 98% Abnormal: 2%	36	105 *McCarthy GCI* 95	99
						Bayley MDI	*Bayley PDI*
Schumacher *et al.* 1991 [134]	ECMO	1–7 years	80	Seizures: 3.7% Hearing loss: 3.7% Microcephaly: 6%	80	109 103 *McCarthy GCI* 96 (3 year) 115 (4 year) 93 (≥ 5 yr)	99 (1 year) 102 (2 years)
						Cattell DQ	
Campbell *et al.* 1991 [122]	ECMO Seizures	1–2 years	12	Seizures: 50% normal 50% abnormal	12	89	
			15	No seizures: 100% normal	15	105	
						Bayley MDI	*Bayley PDI*
Hofkosh *et al.* 1991 [135]	ECMO	6 months – 10 years	67	Normal: 81% Abnormal: 19%	67	101 *Pre-school IQ* 91	98 *School-age IQ* 109
						Bayley MDI	*Bayley PDI*
Flusser *et al.* 1993 [136]	ECMO	1 year	30	Normal: 63% Suspect: 13% Abnormal: 13%	30	> 85: 83% 70–85: 7% < 70: 10%	> 85: 80% 70–85: 7% < 70: 13%
Van Meurs *et al.* 1994 [121]	ECMO VV VA	4–24 months	40	Normal: 100% Normal: 100%	40	*Bayley MDI* 111 112	*Bayley PDI* 111 102
						Bayley MDI	*Bayley PDI*
Wildin *et al.* 1994 [137]	ECMO	6–24 months	22	Normal: 77% Abnormal: 23%	22	108 (6 mo) 106 (1 yr) 100 (2 yr)	110 (6 mo) 106 (1 yr) 100 (2 yr)
	Controls		29	Not reported	29	126 (6 mo) 112 (1 yr) 115 (2 yr)	122 (6 mo) 106 (1 yr) 112 (2 yr)
						WIPPSI-R Full Scale IQ	
Glass *et al.* 1995 [138]	ECMO	5 years	102	Seizures: 2% Hearing loss: 3% CP: 6% Visual problem: 2%	102	96	
	Controls		37		37	115	

Table 37.3. (cont.)

Study	Description	Age	n	Neurologic outcome	n	Cognitive outcome	
						Bayley MDI	*Bayley PDI*
Kornhauser et al. 1998 [139]	ECMO – BPD	2 years	17	Normal: 18% Mild: 34% Severe: 16%	17	76	74
	No BPD		47	Normal: 62% Mild: 34% Severe: 4%	47	103	97
						WIPPSI-R Full Scale IQ	
Desai et al. 2000 [140]	ECMO – RCA ligation	5 years	28	CP: 0%	28	95	
	No RCA ligation		35	CP: 14%	35	96	
						Stanford-BinetIQ	
Parish et al. 2004 [141]	ECMO + seizures	7–9 years	16	CP: 31%	16	85	
	ECMO no seizures		16	CP: 0%	16	95	
						SGS-II DQ	
Khambekar et al. 2006 [142]	ECMO VV VA	1 year	93	Not reported	93	105 100	
Taylor et al. 2007 [143]	ECMO	14 months–26 years	35	Normal: 69% Mild disability: 17% Moderate disability: 11% Severe disability: 3%		Not reported	

Notes:
Unless otherwise noted, all scores are mean values. CP, cerebral palsy; MDI, Mental Developmental Index; PDI, Psychomotor Developmental Index; GCI, General Cognitive Index; BPD, bronchopulmonary dysplasia; RCA, right carotid artery; WIPPSI-R, Weschler Preschool and Primary Scale of Intelligence-Revised; VV, venovenous; VA, venoarterial; SGS-II, Schedule for Growing Skills-II. "Suspect" neurologic outcome is defined as MDI or PDI 70–85.

and 10 years [135]. Using the Bayley scales and Stanford–Binet, mean scores were within the normal range for all ages, with 64% normal, 25% suspect, and 11% delayed. The 10 school-age ECMO survivors were compared with normal controls and no statistically significant differences were noted. Two children in the ECMO group were found to have behavioral concerns noted by classroom teachers, consisting of immaturity in one and impulsivity, distractibility, and hyperactivity in the second. The authors noted that an abnormal outcome was significantly associated with CLD, seizures, and cerebral infarction, but not with other perinatal variables.

In a study by Flusser et al., 30 children treated with ECMO underwent follow-up evaluation at 1 year of age [136]. Neurologic examination was normal in 63% of the population. Bayley MDI and PDI were normal in 83% and 80%, respectively. No relationship was found between neurodevelopmental outcome and perinatal factors such as Apgar scores, diagnosis, length of time on ECMO, neuroimaging abnormalities, seizures, or electroencephalographic findings. Ten infants in their study had congenital anomalies, including pulmonary defects such as CDH, cystic malformation of the lung, and pulmonary atresia. They found that adverse outcomes were associated with the presence of congenital anomalies.

Van Meurs et al. reported on the neurodevelopmental and neuroimaging findings in 24 VV ECMO survivors and 24 VA

ECMO survivors matched by diagnosis, gestational age, sex, and Apgar scores [121]. Comparison of the Bayley scores and neuroimaging results for VA and VV survivors found no statistically significant differences. The authors concluded that no differences attributable to carotid artery ligation were identified with either short-term neurodevelopmental evaluation or neuroimaging.

A study by Wildin et al. reported on 22 ECMO survivors and 29 healthy control infants matched by race, sex, maternal age, maternal education, and socioeconomic status [137]. Bayley scales were performed at 6, 12, and 24 months. Healthy term infants scored significantly better than ECMO infants at 6 and 24 months, though mean Bayley scores for the ECMO cohort were within the normal range. The authors concluded that the overall rate of developmental delay found in this study (23%) was comparable to that reported in prior studies.

A large and comprehensive study by Glass et al. of the neuropsychological outcome and educational adjustment of 102 ECMO survivors at age 5 compared with 37 age-matched controls found lower full-scale IQ scores and a higher incidence of neuropsychological deficits and behavioral problems in ECMO survivors [138]. Although the mean full-scale IQ for the ECMO survivors was average, 77% were found to have one or more deficits in the following areas: language, fine motor efficiency/planning, visual/motor integration, lateralization, academic achievement, verbal memory, or attention/impulse control. Major handicapping conditions were identified in 17%. The authors concluded that, although the IQ scores were average and the incidence of major disability is similar to that in other high-risk populations, there exists an increased rate of behavioral problems and neuropsychological deficits which place ECMO survivors at increased risk for school failure.

Kornhauser et al. examined the impact of bronchopulmonary dysplasia (BPD) on the outcome of ECMO survivors [139]. Complete follow-up data were available for 64 of 145 ECMO-treated patients; BPD was present in 17 (27%). The diagnosis of respiratory distress syndrome was significantly more common in the BPD group (53% vs. 13%). In addition, the mean age of initiation of ECMO was later and the length of ECMO treatment longer for the BPD group. Developmental testing at ages 2 and 4 years revealed significantly lower scores for the BPD group, and a significantly higher rate of disability (72% vs. 38%).

A study by Desai et al. sought to determine if reconstruction of the RCCA following ECMO therapy resulted in improved neurodevelopmental outcome [140]. Thirty-four children who underwent RCCA construction were compared to 35 children who had permanent ligation of the RCCA. RCCA reconstruction was successful in 76% of cases, with success defined as less than 50% stenosis. Both neuroimaging abnormalities and CP were seen less frequently in the children who received RCCA reconstruction. No differences in neurodevelopmental scores performed at ages 30 months and 5–6 years were noted. The authors suggest that RCCA reconstruction may result in improved cerebral circulation, but the long-term risks and benefits of this procedure remain undetermined.

Parish et al. expanded the short-term results published by Campbell regarding the outcome of ECMO survivors with seizures by following 32 children until the ages of 7–9 years [141]. Although mean full-scale IQ scores using Stanford–Binet testing were not significantly different between ECMO survivors with and without neonatal seizures, 50% of the children who had experienced seizures had IQ scores ≤ 84. CP was present in five of 16 infants (31%) with a history of seizures, compared to none in the seizure-free group.

Khambekar et al. described the outcome of 93 ECMO survivors in the era following the UK ECMO trial [142]. Infants underwent developmental assessment at 11–19 months of age using the Schedule for Growing Skills-II. Eighty-two infants (88%) were classified as normal, seven as "impairment," and four as "severe disability." One of the infants with severe disability had Trisomy 21. The developmental quotient did not differ between VA and VV ECMO survivors.

Taylor et al. reported the outcome of 95 neonates treated with ECMO [143]. Outcome was assessed through a standardized telephone interview, and the distinction between "favorable" and "unfavorable" outcome was based on the ability to function independently; infants with mild or moderate disability were considered to have a "favorable" outcome. Ninety-seven percent of survivors had a favorable outcome; only one child (3%) was considered severely disabled.

However, the survival rate in this cohort was 37%, much lower than in previously published reports. The authors cited a high rate of elective discontinuation of therapy as contributing to the higher than normal incidence of favorable outcomes.

Outcome studies comparing conventional medical therapy and ECMO

Several studies have directly compared the outcomes of CMT and ECMO. The six studies are discussed below and summarized in Table 37.4.

A comparison of the morbidity, mortality, and outcome of survivors treated with conventional medical management and ECMO between 1987 and 1989 was performed by Walsh-Sukys et al. [144]. Survival in the conventionally treated group was 69%, compared to a survival of 90% in the ECMO group. Reasons for not initiating ECMO therapy in survivors of the conventionally treated group included improvement with additional treatment (89%) and suspected neurologic injury (11%). CLD occurred in 35% of the conventionally treated patients and in 16% of the ECMO-treated patients. No differences were seen in neurologic outcomes or cognitive testing of survivors. Lower PDI scores were seen in the conventionally treated children, but this was not statistically significant. The authors concluded that infants treated with and without ECMO have similar neurodevelopmental outcomes, but there is a worse pulmonary outcome in conventionally treated patients, despite the ECMO patients having higher $AaDO_2$ values and being assessed to be more critically ill.

A small study by Gratny et al. compared the neurodevelopmental outcome and incidence of significant morbidity in 10 ECMO and 10 CMT survivors at 18 months of age [145]. No statistically significant differences in the incidence of intracranial hemorrhage, motor impairment, SNHL, or developmental delay were identified.

Robertson et al. examined the outcome of 38 ECMO-treated and 26 CMT survivors [146]. The CMT group was described as near-miss ECMO patients who had a lower severity of illness as measured by OI. The underlying diagnoses were similar, except for a higher percentage with a diagnosis of respiratory distress syndrome in the conventionally treated group. The reported neurologic outcomes were not statistically different. The mean MDI and PDI scores were lower in the ECMO-treated group, but the difference was not statistically significant. Further analysis of the results suggested that an underlying diagnosis of sepsis identified the infants most likely to have lower Bayley scores. The distance transported and socioeconomic status were not found to be good predictors of neurodevelopmental outcome.

A large study by Vaucher et al. compared the outcome of ECMO survivors to a group of ECMO-eligible infants who did not receive ECMO due to improvement with conventional medical management [147]. Children were seen between 12 and 30 months of age for neurologic and developmental evaluation. The follow-up rate for the CMT group was lower (39% vs. 69%). CP occurred in 6% of ECMO survivors versus

Table 37.4. Outcome following ECMO when compared to conventional medical therapy

Study	Description	Age	n	Neurologic outcome	n	Cognitive outcome	
						Bayley MDI	*Bayley PDI*
Walsh-Sukys *et al.* 1994 [144]	CMT	20 months	17	Normal: 88% Abnormal: 12%	12	95	83
	ECMO		38	Normal: 82% Abnormal: 18%	32	96	98
						Bayley MDI	*Bayley PDI*
Gratny *et al.* 1992 [145]	CMT	18 months	10	Normal: 90% Abnormal: 10%	7	97	101
	ECMO		10	Normal: 80% Abnormal: 20%	10	104	94
						Bayley MDI	*Bayley PDI*
Robertson *et al.* 1995 [146]	CMT	2 years	26	Disabled: 4% CP: 4%	26	100.5	96.4
	ECMO		38	Disabled: 16% CP: 5%	38	91.8	87.2
						Bayley MDI	*Bayley PDI*
Vaucher *et al.* 1996 [147]	CMT	12–30 months	20	Normal: 68% Major disability: 25%		92	92
	ECMO		95	Normal: 74% Major disability: 11%		100	99
						Stanford-Binet IQ	
Parish *et al.* 2004 [141]	CMT	4–6 years	12	CP: 0%	12	100	
	ECMO		39	CP: 5.1%	39	96	
	ECMO + seizure		25	CP: 36%	25	83	
						Griffiths Mental Development Scale	
UK ECMO 1998 [148]	CMT	1 year	37	Normal: 73%		Overall ≥ 85: 92% Motor ≥ 85: 92%	
	ECMO		62	Normal: 73%		Overall ≥ 85: 92% Motor ≥ 85: 84%	
						British Ability Scales II-GCAS	
UK ECMO 2001 [149]	CMT	4 years	35	Normal: 37%		92	
	ECMO		60	Normal: 50%		93	
UK ECMO 2006 [150]	CMT	7 years	34	Normal: 50%		96	
	ECMO		56	Normal: 55%		95	

Notes:
Unless otherwise noted, all scores are mean values. CMT, conventional medical therapy; CP, cerebral palsy; MDI, Mental Developmental Index; PDI, Psychomotor Developmental Index; GCI, General Cognitive Index; GCAS, General Conceptual Ability Score.

22% of CMT survivors ($p = 0.06$). CLD was seen more frequently in the CMT group, and it independently increased the risk of neurodevelopmental delay after adjusting for other perinatal and neonatal variables. Moderate to severe neuroimaging abnormalities also identified infants with abnormal neurodevelopmental outcome. The authors found that the assumption that ECMO-treated infants had higher rates of disability was incorrect; in this study, ECMO survivors had lower rates of major disability and higher Bayley scores.

Parish *et al.* examined the neurologic and neurodevelopmental outcomes of infants treated with VA ECMO, with and without seizures, in comparison to a cohort of infants referred for ECMO but treated with CMT [141]. Similar rates of CP,

language impairment, and performance on Stanford–Binet were found in the CMT and ECMO survivors. ECMO-treated infants who had the additional complication of seizures in the neonatal period had a significantly higher rate of CP and lower performance on developmental testing. The authors concluded that seizures associated with neonatal ECMO were a primary risk factor for later neurologic and neurodevelopmental sequelae.

The UK Collaborative Randomized Trial of ECMO included neurodevelopmental assessments at ages 1, 4, and 7 years. There was a higher rate of death before age 1 in the conventionally treated group (59%) compared to the ECMO-treated group (32%) [148]. Survivors demonstrated similar rates of impairment or disability at the 1-year follow-up. Children receiving anticonvulsant therapy, tube feeding, or supplemental oxygen were included in the disabled group. At the 4-year follow-up, there was a higher proportion of survivors without disability in the ECMO-treated group (50%) compared to the CMT group (37%) [149]. At the 7-year follow-up, the rate of survival without disability was similar (55% ECMO vs. 50% CMT) [150]. Cognitive functioning using British Ability Scales-II General Conceptual Ability Score was similar between the groups at age 4 and age 7. The authors concluded that ECMO therapy improves survival in neonates with severe respiratory failure without an increase in disability up to 7 years of age, and that the underlying disease process, rather than the treatment, is the major influence on neurodevelopmental outcome.

Comparing the outcome of ECMO patients with CDH to other diagnoses

Infants with CDH treated with ECMO have significantly lower survival rates than infants with other diagnoses (CDH 51% vs. MAS 94%) [91]. Several authors have sought to compare the outcome of CDH infants with those of other diagnoses. These studies are reviewed and the results presented in Table 37.5.

Van Meurs et al. found that the 18 CDH survivors had a longer time on ECMO, time to extubation, and length of hospitalization when compared to other ECMO survivors [151]. In addition, a higher percentage were discharged home on oxygen. In this study, the neurodevelopmental outcome was not different from that in other ECMO-treated survivors.

Stolar et al. reported on the neurocognitive outcome of 25 CDH infants who were treated with ECMO and compared them to 26 ECMO-treated infants with other diagnoses [152]. The age at follow-up ranged from 2 months to 7 years. The neurologic outcomes did not differ significantly, but the cognitive outcome was noted to be poorer in the CDH children. Male sex and limited maternal education were found to be additional risk factors for poor outcome. In this CDH cohort, none was discharged home on oxygen or had SNHL, but gastroesophageal reflux (GER) and nutritional problems were common.

A study by Bernbaum et al. also found a longer ECMO duration and more complicated hospital course for CDH infants when compared to infants with meconium aspiration syndrome [153]. At hospital discharge, there was a higher rate of CLD, GER, and hypotonia. At 1 year, 79% of CDH infants remained hypotonic compared with 8% of the comparison

Table 37.5. Comparison of outcome following ECMO therapy for CDH versus for other diagnoses

Study	Description	Age	n	Neurologic outcome			n	Cognitive outcome		
								Bayley or Stanford-Binet		
Van Meurs et al. 1993 [151]	CDH	1–4 years	18	Not reported			15	MDI and PDI > 90: 47% MDI or PDI < 90: 40% MDI and PDI < 90: 13% MDI and PDI < 70: 0%		
	Other diagnoses	1 year					42	MDI and PDI > 90: 59% MDI or PDI < 90: 19% MDI and PDI < 90: 12% MDI and PDI < 70: 10%		
				Normal	*Suspect*	*Abnormal*		*Normal*	*Suspect*	*Abnormal*
Stolar et al. 1995 [152]	CDH	2 months –	25	56%	24%	20%	25	60%	16%	24%
	Other diagnoses	7 years	26	50%	35%	15%	26	88%	4%	8%
								Bayley MDI	*Bayley PDI*	
Bernbaum et al. 1995 [153]	CDH	1 year	14	Hypotonia: 79%			14	87	75	
	MAS		12	Hypotonia: 8%			12	98	99	
Jaillard et al. 2000 [154]	CDH	2 years	11	CP: 18%				Not reported		
	Other diagnoses		25	CP: 12% Developmental delay: 4%						
								Peabody test score		
Nield et al. 2000 [155]	CDH	3.5 years	17	Not different			17	96		
	MAS		67				67	89		
	Sepsis		29				29	93		

Notes:
Unless otherwise noted, all scores are mean values. CDH, congenital diaphragmatic hernia; MDI, Mental Developmental Index; PDI, Psychomotor Developmental Index; MAS, meconium aspiration syndrome; CP, cerebral palsy.

group. On Bayley scales at 1 year, CDH infants had lower MDI and significantly lower PDI.

Jaillard et al. compared the 2-year outcome for 23 infants with CDH compared to 34 non-CDH infants who required ECMO for severe respiratory failure [154]. Infants with CDH had a higher incidence of death prior to 2 years (47% CDH vs. 17% non-CDH). Although a higher rate of CP in survivors was seen in the CDH group (18%) compared to the non-CDH group (12%), this was not statistically significant. The authors concluded that ECMO therapy resulted in increased survival and decreased morbidity in non-CDH infants compared to those with CDH.

Nield et al. analyzed the neurodevelopmental outcome at 3.5 years of age for 130 ECMO survivors with six different diagnoses [155]. No significant differences were found between diagnostic groups in functional status or neurologic sequelae. Length of hospitalization was the only variable to have an influence on neurodevelopmental testing, functional status, and major neurologic sequelae. The authors noted that the neurodevelopmental test results in the CDH population done between 1 and 2 years were more worrisome than later testing, possibly due to the early medical conditions associated with this group.

Comorbidities associated with PPHN

Hearing loss

NICU graduates are known to be at increased risk for hearing loss. Several studies have specifically addressed the hearing outcome of PPHN survivors. Sell et al. were the first to note an increase in the incidence of hearing abnormalities (20%) in the PPHN population compared to other high-risk infants without PPHN [103]. Naulty et al. found three of 11 infants with progressive SNHL [156]. A subsequent study by Hendricks-Munoz and Walton reported a 52.5% incidence of hearing impairment in a study of 40 infants treated for PPHN [157]. In this study, a longer duration of hyperventilation and ventilation were highly associated with hearing loss. Leavitt et al. corroborated the high incidence of SNHL (25%) in PPHN survivors treated with hyperventilation [158]. Cheung et al. reported that 62% of their CDH population had SNHL on long-term follow-up, with similar rates between the ECMO-treated group (65%) and the conventionally treated group (59%) [159]. An unexpected finding in this study was that survivors with SNHL had a higher cumulative exposure to pancuronium bromide. The cohort published by Marron et al., which used conservative ventilatory management, resulted in no SNHL [29]. The authors speculated that hyperventilation or alkalosis might be the causative factor for the high incidence of SNHL in other studies of PPHN survivors. Animal studies have shown that one of the highest areas of blood flow is the auditory nucleus [160]; decreased cerebral blood flow with hyperventilation may cause injury to this area. Alkalosis could also potentially induce hearing abnormalities by affecting the sodium–potassium pump in the cochlea or the chemical composition of the endolymph [161].

Because a high rate of SNHL was noted in the survivors of PPHN treated with CMT, several outcome studies for the iNO trials have reported audiologic outcomes. Using interview techniques, Ellington et al. found an overall incidence of hearing loss or speech difficulties of 18.3%, with no difference between iNO and control groups [106]. The CINRGI trial reported an overall rate of hearing loss of 2% at 1 year of age, though the methods of interview technique and relatively early follow-up may have resulted in under-reporting [108]. Formal audiologic testing was performed at 1 year in the I-NO/PPHN Study and found 19% of infants with hearing loss, with no differences between treatment and control groups [107]. The NINOS trial followed infants to 18–24 months and reported an overall incidence of abnormal hearing of 30%, with rates up to 59% in the subgroup of infants with CDH [162]. Only 8.9% of infants required the use of hearing aids. Robertson et al. reported on the Canadian cohort enrolled in the NINOS trial and performed audiologic testing at 4 years of age [163]. Forty-three of the 81 infants tested (53%) demonstrated hearing loss, despite only three infants failing the audiologic screen prior to discharge from the NICU. The authors examined the age of onset of hearing loss and found that 13 (30%) infants were diagnosed with hearing loss after age 2. A subsequent retrospective analysis of this cohort was performed to further elucidate clinical factors that may contribute to hearing loss, including neuromuscular blockers and ototoxic medications [164]. Multivariate analysis revealed that prolonged use of loop diuretics (> 14 days) and neuromuscular blockers were significantly associated with the development of hearing loss. The authors speculated that inhibition of the protective acoustic stapedius reflex through prolonged neuromuscular blockade in the setting of a noisy NICU environment could explain this correlation. None of the 15 infants reported by Ichiba et al. using iNO and gentle ventilation had hearing loss when evaluated at 18 months [109]. The overall incidence of hearing loss in the Early iNO trial was 24%, with no difference between treatment groups [110].

Bilateral SNHL has been reported in 3–21% (average 7.5%) of infants treated with neonatal ECMO [134,135,138,165]. Robertson et al. reported on the audiologic status of infants with CDH treated with ECMO and medical therapy [166]. A similar but very high rate of SNHL was detected in both groups (60% ECMO vs. 59% CMT). All infants diagnosed with SNHL who had been tested in the neonatal period passed initial audiologic screening tests. Fligor et al. reported on 111 survivors of ECMO who underwent audiologic testing at follow-up evaluation [167]. Twenty-six percent of children tested had SNHL, with the median age of onset at 19 months (range 4 months to 8 years). In this study, factors significantly associated with the development of SNHL included a primary diagnosis of CDH, length of ECMO therapy, and the number of days children received aminoglycoside antibiotics.

These studies highlight the increased risk of hearing loss in infants with PPHN, regardless of therapy utilized. An important aspect of the hearing loss seen in PPHN survivors is the delayed onset and progressive nature of the problem, making diagnosis problematic. Hearing loss in PPHN survivors often occurs in children who had normal hearing documented in the newborn period [168,169]. Although the most recent position statement from the Joint Committee on Infant Hearing does not recognize PPHN as a specific risk indicator for delayed SNHL, all infants who received assisted ventilation or ECMO therapy are recommended to undergo early and more frequent audiologic testing, because of the risk of delayed-onset hearing loss [170].

Respiratory morbidities

Survivors of PPHN are at increased risk of long-term respiratory difficulties including CLD, asthma, and susceptibility to respiratory tract infections. Sell *et al.* cited a 30% rate of CLD in PPHN survivors treated with a hyperventilation strategy [103]. Bernbaum *et al.* also utilized hyperventilation, and reported 18% of survivors had wheezing and required daily bronchodilators [100]. In contrast, the gentle ventilation techniques employed by Marron *et al.* resulted in a CLD rate of 7% [29]. Ichiba *et al.* also used a gentle ventilation strategy in their iNO cohort; five infants (33%) had reactive airways disease at the 18-month follow-up, and two continued to report wheezing at the 3-year follow-up [109]. The authors noted that the risk of wheezing was correlated with the duration of mechanical ventilation.

A protective effect of ECMO treatment compared to CMT on respiratory outcomes could be hypothesized, owing to the nature of cardiopulmonary bypass permitting a period of lung rest during an acute respiratory insult. Walsh-Sukys *et al.* reported a CLD incidence of 35% in infants treated with CMT, compared to 16% in infants treated with ECMO [144]. Vaucher *et al.* reported an overall incidence of CLD of 15% in their cohort; ECMO-treated infants were less likely to have CLD than infants treated with CMT (12% ECMO vs. 25% CMT) [147]. The UK ECMO Collaborative Trial followed the respiratory outcomes of its survivors. At the 4-year follow-up, 77% of CMT infants were noted to wheeze, compared to 42% of infants treated with ECMO [149]. Wheezing improved at the 7-year follow-up but continued to be more prevalent in the CMT group (32% CMT vs. 11% ECMO) [150].

Majaesic *et al.* examined the 8-year respiratory outcome of 54 survivors of neonatal respiratory failure of various etiologies, including MAS, sepsis, CDH, RDS, and other diagnoses [171]. Fifty-seven percent of this cohort had required ECMO therapy. Using spirometry measurements, the authors found that ECMO-treated infants had significantly worse pulmonary outcomes than non-ECMO infants, but there was no difference in the requirement for supplemental oxygen.

Rehospitalization is common in survivors of PPHN. In a study of PPHN survivors treated with CMT, Bernbaum *et al.* reported that 36% of their cohort had required rehospitalization for pulmonary illness [100]. Ellington *et al.* reported an overall rehospitalization rate of 27% for the infants enrolled in their RCT of iNO [106]. Twenty-two percent of infants in the I-NO/PPHN study required rehospitalization; of these,

67% were hospitalized for respiratory indications [107]. In the NINOS and Early iNO trials, 36% of infants required rehospitalization [110,162].

Infants with CDH are at particular risk for respiratory difficulties outside the newborn period. In reports of infants with CDH who required ECMO therapy, D'Agostino *et al.* found that 54% of survivors had CLD at 1-year follow-up [172], and Jaillard *et al.* reported a CLD rate of 22% in their CDH subgroup [154]. Bernbaum *et al.* reported a higher percentage of CDH infants had CLD compared to infants treated with ECMO for other reasons (50% vs. 17%) [153]. In a small series, Kamata *et al.* reported recurrent pneumonia as the most prevalent morbidity among CDH survivors [173]. Because infants with CDH are at increased risk for bronchiolitis, prophylaxis against respiratory syncytial virus may be warranted [174].

Growth and nutritional difficulties

Growth and feeding difficulties are commonly reported in follow-up studies of survivors of PPHN, and outcomes are often linked to the degree of residual pulmonary disease. In the cohort reported by Walsh-Sukys *et al.*, 36% of the PPHN survivors treated with CMT had weight percentiles less than 2 SD below the mean at the 8-month follow-up, compared to 17% of infants treated with ECMO [144]. By the 20-month follow-up, however, the majority of the CMT group had demonstrated catch-up growth (only 6% less than 5th percentile), whereas the ECMO-treated group had failed to demonstrate the same degree of growth (16% less than 5th percentile). Vaucher *et al.* noted similar growth rates between ECMO- and CMT-treated infants, but infants with CLD had consistently lower weight percentiles through 18 months [147]. Survivors of PPHN may also require gavage feeding to maintain adequate nutrition. At the 18- to 24-month follow-up of infants enrolled in the NINOS trial, 8.7% continued to require gavage feedings [162], and 6% of the infants in the Early iNO trial required gavage feedings at the 2-year follow-up [110].

Infants with CDH are at particular risk for growth failure, and GER is a major comorbidity of CDH. The precise correlation between GER and CDH is unproven, though speculation exists that anatomical derangements caused by CDH during fetal life predispose these infants to GER [175]. Van Meurs *et al.* noted an extremely high rate of GER and failure to thrive (FTT) in CDH infants treated with ECMO. At both 1 and 2 years, 50% were less than the 5th percentile weight-to-length ratio. Eighty-nine percent had clinical evidence of GER, and 44% were discharged home on nasogastric feedings. The authors suggested that more aggressive nutritional intervention was needed for CDH survivors [151]. D'Agostino *et al.* reported that 81% of CDH survivors had symptoms of GER following repair, and 50% remained symptomatic at 1 year of age [172]. All 11 infants with CDH reported by Jaillard *et al.* demonstrated GER, compared to none of the 25 infants treated with ECMO for other diagnoses; 90% of the CDH infants demonstrated growth retardation at the 2-year follow-up [154]. Muratore *et al.* reported that 56% of CDH survivors were below the 25th percentile for weight at 1 year of age, and 24% demonstrated severe oral aversion [176]. Infants treated with ECMO or those requiring oxygen at discharge were more likely to demonstrate growth difficulties. Furthermore, CDH requiring a patch repair was highly associated with a diagnosis of FTT, the need for a gastrostomy tube (GT), and the need for a Nissen fundoplication. Cortes *et al.* reported growth failure rates (weight < 2 SD below mean) in CDH survivors of 69% and 29% at the 1- and 2-year follow-up, respectively [177]. Chiu *et al.* examined the impact of ventilation technique in 143 CDH survivors [178]. Although gentle ventilation resulted in improved survival (51% CMT vs. 80% gentle ventilation), infants treated with gentle ventilation were more likely to require GT placement at the 3-year follow-up.

Conclusions

In the era prior to the use of ECMO, HFV, and iNO, the mortality rate for infants with PPHN was as high as 50%, but it is currently less than 20% [55,56,179]. A wide variety of pre-existing perinatal conditions, such as low Apgar scores or fetal distress, place these infants at increased risk for abnormal neurodevelopmental outcomes. Furthermore, treatment of PPHN may include use of aggressive therapies that also have the potential to affect outcome adversely, either directly or because of iatrogenic complications. Because PPHN occurs in as many as 1/1000 live births, infants with this condition have the potential to contribute substantially to the prevalence of neurodevelopmental disorders. Recent improvements in treatment have resulted in significant reduction in mortality rates, but there is concern that this may have been achieved at the expense of increasing the number of survivors with neurodevelopmental impairment.

Analysis of the outcome studies performed in PPHN survivors treated with CMT, iNO, and ECMO yield grossly equivalent morbidities and outcomes. These findings suggest that the neurodevelopmental outcome is more closely related to the severity of the underlying illness than to the therapeutic intervention utilized. Overall, the majority of PPHN survivors have good outcomes, but approximately one-third of survivors have some neurodevelopmental impairment. Significant comorbidities which place survivors at higher risk for developmental delay include CLD, hearing loss, or a primary diagnosis of CDH.

Limitations imposed by some follow-up studies are the types of neurodevelopmental examinations performed, small sample sizes, the absence of an appropriate control population, and the length of follow-up. The most frequently performed neurodevelopmental assessment was the Bayley Scales of Infant Development, which is known not to be predictive of long-term outcome [180]. In addition, many studies have been small, with no control populations, and limited conclusions can be drawn from these cohorts. Some of the more recent randomized controlled studies have had large sample sizes with appropriate control groups and have significantly improved our information. The continuation of these outcome studies into school age is critical, yet few of the outcome studies have included the school-age child. Infants with PPHN due to CDH represent a population at particular risk for adverse outcomes. Further research is needed to understand the full impact of the varying therapies for PPHN so that developmental and educational services can be developed to serve the needs of PPHN survivors.

References

1. Levin DL, Heymann MA, Kitterman JA, *et al.* Persistent pulmonary hypertension of the newborn infant. *J Pediatr* 1976; **89**: 626–30.

2. Drummond WH, Peckham GJ, Fox WW. The clinical profile of the newborn with persistent pulmonary hypertension: observations in 19 affected neonates. *Clin Pediatr* 1977; **16**: 335–41.

3. Benitz WE, Stevenson DK. Refractory neonatal hypoxemia: diagnostic evaluation and pharmacologic management. *Resuscitation* 1988; **16**: 49–64.

4. Gersony W. Neonatal pulmonary hypertension: pathophysiology, classification, and etiology. *Clin Perinatol* 1984; **11**: 517–24.

5. Long WA. Structural cardiovascular abnormalities presenting as persistent pulmonary hypertension of the newborn. *Clin Perinatol* 1984; **11**: 601–26.

6. Geggel R, Reid L. The structural basis of PPHN. *Clin Perinatol* 1981; **11**: 525–49.

7. Peckham GJ, Fox WW. Physiologic factors affecting pulmonary artery pressure in infants with persistent pulmonary hypertension. *J Pediatr* 1978; **93**: 1005–10.

8. Morin FC, Stenmark KR. Persistent pulmonary hypertension of the newborn. *Am J Respir Crit Care Med* 1995; **151**: 2010–32.

9. Murphy JD, Rabinovitch M, Goldstein JD, *et al.* The structural basis of persistent pulmonary hypertension of the newborn infant. *J Pediatr* 1981; **98**: 962–67.

10. Kinsella JP, Abman SH. Recent developments in the pathophysiology and treatment of persistent pulmonary hypertension of the newborn. *J Pediatr* 1995; **126**: 853–64.

11. Fox WW, Duara S. Persistent pulmonary hypertension in the neonate: diagnosis and management. *J Pediatr* 1983; **103**: 505–14.

12. Gersony WM, Morishima HO, Daniel SS, *et al.* The hemodynamic effects of intrauterine hypoxia: an experimental model in newborn lambs. *J Pediatr* 1976; **89**: 631–5.

13. Drummond WH, Bissonnette JM. Persistent pulmonary hypertension in the neonate: development of an animal model. *Am J Obstet Gynecol* 1978; **131**: 761–3.

14. Soifer SJ, Kaslow D, Roman C, *et al.* Umbilical cord compression produces pulmonary hypertension in newborn lambs: a model to study the pathophysiology of persistent pulmonary hypertension in the newborn. *J Dev Physiol* 1987; **9**: 239–52.

15. Morin FC. Ligating the ductus arteriosus before birth causes persistent pulmonary hypertension in the newborn lamb. *Pediatr Res* 1989; **25**: 245–50.

16. Wild LM, Nickerson PA, Morin FC. Ligating the ductus arteriosus before birth remodels the pulmonary vasculature of the lamb. *Pediatr Res* 1989; **25**: 245–50.

17. Morin FC, Egan EA. The effect of closing the ductus arteriosus on the pulmonary circulation of the fetal sheep. *J Dev Physiol* 1989; **11**: 283–7.

18. Abman SH, Shanley PF, Accurso FJ. Failure of postnatal adaptation of the pulmonary circulation after chronic intrauterine pulmonary hypertension in fetal lambs. *J Clin Invest* 1989; **83**: 1849–58.

19. Walsh-Sukys MC, Cornell DJ, Houston LN, *et al.* Treatment of persistent pulmonary hypertension of the newborn without hyperventilation: an assessment of diffusion of innovation. *Pediatrics* 1994; **94**: 303–6.

20. Walsh-Sukys MC. Persistent pulmonary hypertension of the newborn: the black box revisited. *Clin Perinatol* 1993; **20**: 127–43.

21. Roberts JD, Shaul PW. Advances in the treatment of persistent pulmonary hypertension of the newborn. *Pediatr Clin North Am* 1993; **40**: 983–1004.

22. Walsh-Sukys MC, Tyson JE, Wright LL, *et al.* Persistent pulmonary hypertension of the newborn in the era before nitric oxide: practice variation and outcomes. *Pediatrics* 2000; **105**: 14–20.

23. Cohen RS, Stevenson DK, Malachowski N, *et al.* Late morbidity among survivors of respiratory failure treated with tolazoline. *J Pediatr* 1980; **97**: 644–7.

24. Fineman JR, Wong J, Soifer SJ. Hyperoxia and alkalosis produce pulmonary vasodilation independent of endothelium-derived nitric oxide in newborn lambs. *Pediatr Res* 1993; **33**: 341–6.

25. Lou HC, Skov H and Pedersen H. Low cerebral blood flow: a risk factor in the neonate. *J Pediatr* 1979; **95**: 606–9.

26. Kusuda S, Shishida N, Miyagi N, *et al.* Cerebral blood flow during treatment for pulmonary hypertension. *Arch Dis Child Fetal Neonatal Ed* 1999; **80**: F30–3.

27. Wung JT, James LS, Kilchevsky E, *et al.* Management of infants with severe respiratory failure and persistence of the fetal circulation, without hyperventilation. *Pediatrics* 1985; **76**: 488–94.

28. Dworetz AR, Moya FR, Sabo B, *et al.* Survival of infants with persistent pulmonary hypertension without extracorporeal membrane oxygenation. *Pediatrics* 1989; **84**: 1–6.

29. Marron MJ, Crisafi MA, Driscoll JM, *et al.* Hearing and neurodevelopmental outcome in survivors of persistent pulmonary hypertension of the newborn. *Pediatrics* 1992; **90**: 392–6.

30. Ng GY, Derry C, Marston L, *et al.* Reduction in ventilator-induced lung injury improves outcome in congenital diaphragmatic hernia? *Pediatr Surg Int* 2008; **24**: 145–50.

31. Migliazza L, Bellan C, Alberti D, *et al.* Retrospective study of 111 cases of congenital diaphragmatic hernia treated with early high-frequency oscillatory ventilation and presurgical stabilization. *J Pediatr Surg* 2007; **42**: 1526–32.

32. Greenough A. High frequency oscillation and liquid ventilation. *Paediatr Respir Rev* 2006; **7**: S186–88.

33. Wolfson MR, Shaffer TH. Pulmonary applications of perfluorochemical liquids: ventilation and beyond. *Paediatr Respir Rev* 2005; **6**: 117–27.

34. Hirschl RB. Current experience with liquid ventilation. *Paediatr Respir Rev* 2004; **5**: S339–45.

35. Martin LD. New approaches to ventilation in infants and children. *Curr Opin Pediatr* 1995; **7**: 250–61.

36. Ring JC, Stidham GL. Novel therapies for acute respiratory failure. *Pediatr Clin North Am* 1994; **41**: 1325–63.

37. Clark RH. High-frequency ventilation. *J Pediatr* 1994; **124**: 661–70.

38. Frantz ID. High-frequency ventilation. *Crit Care Med* 1993; **21**: S370.

39. deLemos R, Yoder B, McCurnin D, *et al.* The use of high-frequency oscillatory ventilation (HFOV) and extracorporeal membrane oxygenation (ECMO) in the management of the term/near term infant with respiratory failure. *Early Hum Dev* 1992; **29**: 299–303.

40. Ito Y, Kawano T, Miyasaka K, *et al.* Alternative treatment may lower the need for use of extracorporeal membrane oxygenation. *Acta Paediatr Jpn* 1994; **36**: 673–7.

41. Varnholt V, Lasch P, Suske G, *et al.* High frequency oscillatory ventilation and extracorporeal membrane oxygenation in severe persistent pulmonary hypertension of the newborn. *Eur J Pediatr* 1992; **151**: 769–74.

42. Waffarn F, Turbo R, Yang L, *et al.* Treatment of PPHN: a randomized trial comparing intermittent mandatory ventilation and HFOV for delivering NO. *Pediatr Res* 1995; **37**: 243A.

43. Lampland AL, Mammel MC. The role of high-frequency ventilation in neonates: evidence-based recommendations. *Clin Perinatol* 2007; **34**: 129–44, viii.

44. Lotze A, Stroud CY, Soldin SJ. Serial lecithin/sphingomyelin ratios and surfactant/albumin ratios in tracheal aspirates from term infants with respiratory failure receiving extracorporeal membrane oxygenation. *Clin Chem* 1995; **41**: 1182–8.

45. Lotze A, Knight GR, Anderson KD, *et al.* Surfactant (beractant) therapy for infants with congenital diaphragmatic hernia on ECMO: evidence of persistent surfactant deficiency. *J Pediatr Surg* 1994; **29**: 407–12.

46. Karamanoukian HL, Glick PL, Wilcox DT, *et al.* Pathophysiology of congenital diaphragmatic hernia. VIII: Inhaled nitric oxide requires exogenous surfactant therapy in the lamb model of congenital diaphragmatic hernia. *J Pediatr Surg* 1995; **30**: 1–4.

47. Lotze A, Knight GR, Martin GR, *et al.* Improved pulmonary outcome after exogenous surfactant therapy for respiratory failure in term infants requiring extracorporeal membrane oxygenation. *J Pediatr* 1993; **122**: 261–8.

48. Lotze A, Mitchell BR, Bulas DI, *et al.* Multicenter study of surfactant (beractant) use in the treatment of term infants with severe respiratory failure. Survanta in Term Infants Study Group. *J Pediatr* 1998; **132**: 40–7.

49. El Shahed AI, Dargaville P, Ohlsson A, *et al.* Surfactant for meconium aspiration syndrome in full term/near term infants. *Cochrane Database Syst Rev* 2007; (3): CD002054.

50. Johns RA. EDRF/nitric oxide: the endogenous nitrovasodilator and a new cellular messenger. *Anesthesiology* 1991; **75**: 927–31.

51. Fratacci MD, Frostell CG, Chen TY, *et al.* Inhaled nitric oxide: a selective pulmonary vasodilator of heparin-protamine vasoconstriction in sheep. *Anesthesiology* 1991; **75**: 990–9.

52. Pepke-Zaba J, Higenbottam T, Dinh-Xuan A, *et al.* Inhaled nitric oxide as a cause of selective pulmonary vasodilatation in pulmonary hypertension. *Lancet* 1991; **338**: 1173–4.

53. Kinsella JP, Abman SH. Efficacy of inhalational nitric oxide therapy in the

clinical management of persistent pulmonary hypertension of the newborn. *Chest* 1994; **105**: 92S–94S.

54. Finer NN, Etches PC, Kamstra B, *et al.* Inhaled nitric oxide in infants referred for extracorporeal membrane oxygenation: dose response. *J Pediatr* 1994; **124**: 302–8.

55. The Neonatal Inhaled Nitric Oxide Study Group (NINOS). Inhaled nitric oxide in term and nearly full-term infants with hypoxic respiratory failure. *N Engl J Med* 1997; **336**: 597–604.

56. Clark RH, Kueser TJ, Walker MW, *et al.* Low-dose nitric oxide therapy for persistent pulmonary hypertension of the newborn. Clinical Inhaled Nitric Oxide Research Group. *N Engl J Med* 2000; **342**: 469–74.

57. Finer NN, Barrington KJ. Nitric oxide for respiratory failure in infants born at or near term. *Cochrane Database Syst Rev* 2006; (4): CD000399.

58. Barrington KJ, Finer NN. Inhaled nitric oxide for respiratory failure in preterm infants. *Cochrane Database Syst Rev* 2007; (3): CD000509.

59. Högman M, Frostell C, Arnberg H, *et al.* Bleeding time prolongation and NO inhalation. *Lancet* 1993; **341**: 1664–5.

60. Samama CM, Diaby M, Fellahi JL, *et al.* Inhibition of platelet aggregation by inhaled nitric oxide in patients with acute respiratory distress syndrome. *Anesthesiology* 1995; **83**: 56–65.

61. The Neonatal Inhaled Nitric Oxide Study Group (NINOS). Inhaled nitric oxide in term and near-term infants: neurodevelopmental follow-up of the neonatal inhaled nitric oxide study group (NINOS). *J Pediatr* 2000; **136**: 611–17.

62. Thébaud B, Saizou C, Farnoux C, *et al.* Dipyridamole, a cGMP phosphodiesterase inhibitor, transiently improves the response to inhaled nitric oxide in two newborns with congenital diaphragmatic hernia. *Intensive Care Med* 1999; **25**: 300–3.

63. Dukarm RC, Russell JA, Morin FC, *et al.* The cGMP-specific phosphodiesterase inhibitor E4021 dilates the pulmonary circulation. *Am J Respir Crit Care Med* 1999; **160**: 858–65.

64. Nagamine J, Hill LL, Pearl RG. Combined therapy with zaprinast and inhaled nitric oxide abolishes hypoxic pulmonary hypertension. *Crit Care Med* 2000; **28**: 2420–4.

65. Steinhorn RH, Gordon JB, Todd ML. Site-specific effect of guanosine 3',5-cyclic monophosphate phosphodiesterase inhibition in isolated lamb lungs. *Crit Care Med* 2000; **28**: 490–5.

66. Ryhammer PK, Shekerdemian LS, Penny DJ, *et al.* Effect of intravenous sildenafil on pulmonary hemodynamics and gas exchange in the presence and absence of acute lung injury in piglets. *Pediatr Res* 2006; **59**: 762–6.

67. Binns-Lovemann KM, Kaplowitz MR, Fike CD. Sildenafil and an early stage of chronic hypoxia-induced pulmonary hypertension in newborn piglets. *Pediatr Pulmonol* 2005; **40**: 72–80.

68. Shah PS, Ohlsson A. Sildenafil for pulmonary hypertension in neonates. *Cochrane Database Syst Rev* 2007; (3): CD005494.

69. Baquero H, Soliz A, Neira F, *et al.* Oral sildenafil in infants with persistent pulmonary hypertension of the newborn: a pilot randomized blinded study. *Pediatrics* 2006; **117**: 1077–83.

70. Herrea J, Castillo R, Conch E, *et al.* Oral sildenafil treatment as an alternative to inhaled NO therapy for persistent pulmonary hypertension of the newborn. *E-PAS* 2006; **59**: 3724.3.

71. Stocker C, Penny DJ, Brizard CP, *et al.* Intravenous sildenafil and inhaled nitric oxide: a randomised trial in infants after cardiac surgery. *Intensive Care Med* 2003; **29**: 1996–2003.

72. Namachivayam P, Theilen U, Butt WW, *et al.* Sildenafil prevents rebound pulmonary hypertension after withdrawal of nitric oxide in children. *Am J Respir Crit Care Med* 2006; **174**: 1042–7.

73. Noori S, Friedlich P, Wong P, *et al.* Cardiovascular effects of sildenafil in neonates and infants with congenital diaphragmatic hernia and pulmonary hypertension. *Neonatology* 2007; **91**: 92–100.

74. Keller RL, Moore P, Teitel D, *et al.* Abnormal vascular tone in infants and children with lung hypoplasia: findings from cardiac catheterization and the response to chronic therapy. *Pediatr Crit Care Med* 2006; **7**: 589–94.

75. McNamara PJ, Laique F, Muang-In S, *et al.* Milrinone improves oxygenation in neonates with severe persistent pulmonary hypertension of the newborn. *J Crit Care* 2006; **21**: 217–22.

76. Bassler D, Choong K, McNamara P, *et al.* Neonatal persistent pulmonary hypertension treated with milrinone: four case reports. *Biol Neonate* 2006; **89**: 1–5.

77. Ho JJ, Rasa G. Magnesium sulfate for persistent pulmonary hypertension of the newborn. *Cochrane Database Syst Rev* 2007; (3): CD005588.

78. Raimondi F, Migliaro F, Capasso L, *et al.* Intravenous magnesium sulphate vs. inhaled nitric oxide for moderate, persistent pulmonary hypertension of the newborn: a multicentre, retrospective study. *J Trop Pediatr* 2008; **54**: 196–9.

79. Curtis J, O'Neill JT, Pettett G. Endotracheal administration of tolazoline in hypoxia-induced pulmonary hypertension. *Pediatrics* 1993; **92**: 403–8.

80. Welch JC, Bridson JM, Gibbs JL. Endotracheal tolazoline for severe persistent pulmonary hypertension of the newborn. *Br Heart J* 1995; **73**: 99–100.

81. Parida SK, Baker S, Kuhn R, *et al.* Endotracheal tolazoline administration in neonates with persistent pulmonary hypertension. *J Perinatol* 1997; **17**: 461–4.

82. Palhares DB, Figueiredo CS, Moura AJ. Endotracheal inhalatory sodium nitroprusside in severely hypoxic newborns. *J Perinat Med* 1998; **26**: 219–24.

83. Crowley MR. Oxygen-induced pulmonary vasodilation is mediated by adenosine triphosphate in newborn lambs. *J Cardiovasc Pharmacol* 1997; **30**: 102–9.

84. Patole S, Lee J, Buettner P, *et al.* Improved oxygenation following adenosine infusion in persistent pulmonary hypertension of the newborn. *Biol Neonate* 1998; **74**: 345–50.

85. Aranda M, Bradford KK, Pearl RG. Combined therapy with inhaled nitric oxide and intravenous vasodilators during acute and chronic experimental pulmonary hypertension. *Anesth Analg* 1999; **89**: 152–8.

86. Gessler T, Seeger W, Schmehl T. Inhaled prostanoids in the therapy of pulmonary hypertension. *J Aerosol Med* 2008; **21**: 1–12.

87. Kelly LK, Porta NF, Goodman DM, *et al.* Inhaled prostacyclin for term infants with persistent pulmonary hypertension refractory to inhaled nitric oxide. *J Pediatr* 2002; **141**: 830–2.

88. Lakshminrusimha S, Russell JA, Wedgwood S, *et al.* Superoxide dismutase improves oxygenation and reduces oxidation in neonatal pulmonary hypertension. *Am J Respir Crit Care Med* 2006; **174**: 1370–7.

89. Davis JM, Rosenfeld WN, Richter SE, *et al.* Safety and pharmacokinetics of multiple doses of recombinant human CuZn superoxide dismutase administered intratracheally to premature neonates with respiratory distress syndrome. *Pediatrics* 1997; **100**: 24–30.

90. Davis JM, Richter SE, Biswas S, *et al.* Long-term follow-up of premature infants treated with prophylactic, intratracheal recombinant human CuZn superoxide dismutase. *J Perinatol* 2000; **20**: 213–16.

91. Extracorporeal Life Support Organization (ELSO). *Neonatal ECMO Registry*. Ann Arbor, MI: ELSO, 2008.

92. Radack DM, Baumgart S, Gross GW. Subependymal (grade 1) intracranial hemorrhage in neonates on extracorporeal membrane oxygenation: frequency and patterns. *Clin Pediatr* 1994; **33**: 583–7.

93. Upp JR, Bush PE, Zwischenberger JB. Complications of neonatal extracorporeal membrane oxygenation. *Perfusion* 1994; **9**: 241–56.

94. Wilson JM, Bower LK, Fackler JC, *et al.* Aminocaproic acid decreases the incidence of intracranial hemorrhage and other hemorrhagic complications of ECMO. *J Pediatr Surg* 1993; **28**: 536–41.

95. O'Connor TA, Haney BM, Grist GE, *et al.* Decreased incidence of intracranial hemorrhage using cephalic jugular venous drainage during neonatal extracorporeal membrane oxygenation. *J Pediatr Surg* 1993; **28**: 1332–5.

96. Bifano EM, Pfannenstiel A. Duration of hyperventilation and outcome in infants with persistent pulmonary hypertension. *Pediatrics* 1988; **81**: 657–61.

97. Landry SH, Chapieski L, Fletcher JM, *et al.* Three year outcomes for low birthweight infants: differential effects of early medical complications. *J Pediatr Psychol* 1988; **13**: 317–27.

98. Gleason CA, Short BL, Jones MD. Cerebral blood flow and metabolism during and after prolonged hypocapnia in newborn lambs. *J Pediatr* 1989; **115**: 309–14.

99. Brett C, Dekle M, Leonard CH, *et al.* Developmental follow-up of hyperventilated neonates: preliminary observations. *Pediatrics* 1981; **68**: 588–91.

100. Bernbaum JC, Russell P, Sheridan PH, *et al.* Long-term follow-up of newborns with persistent pulmonary hypertension. *Crit Care Med* 1984; **12**: 579–83.

101. Ballard RA, Leonard CH. Developmental follow-up of infants with persistent pulmonary hypertension of the newborn. *Clin Perinatol* 1984; **11**: 737–44.

102. Ferrara B, Johnson D, Chang PN, *et al.* Efficacy and neurologic outcome of profound hypocapneic alkalosis for the treatment of persistent pulmonary hypertension in infancy. *J Pediatr* 1984; **105**: 457–61.

103. Sell EJ, Gaines JA, Gluckman C, *et al.* Persistent fetal circulation: neurodevelopmental outcome. *Am J Dis Child* 1985; **139**: 25–8.

104. Hageman JR, Dusik J, Keuler H, *et al.* Outcome of persistent pulmonary hypertension in relation to severity of presentation. *Am J Dis Child* 1988; **142**: 293–6.

105. Rosenberg AA, Hennaugh JM, Moreland SG, *et al.* Longitudinal follow-up of a cohort of newborn infants treated with inhaled nitric oxide for persistent pulmonary hypertension. *J Pediatr* 1997; **131**: 70–5.

106. Ellington MJ, O'Reilly D, Allred E, *et al.* Child health status, neurodevelopmental outcome, and parental satisfaction in a randomized, controlled trial of nitric oxide for persistent pulmonary hypertension of the newborn. *Pediatrics* 2001; **107**: 1351–6.

107. Lipkin PH, Davidson D, Spivak L, *et al.* Neurodevelopmental and medical outcomes of persistent pulmonary hypertension in term newborns treated with nitric oxide. *J Pediatr* 2002; **140**: 306–10.

108. Clark RH, Huckaby JL, Kueser TJ, *et al.* Low-dose inhaled nitric-oxide therapy for persistent pulmonary hypertension: 1-year follow-up. *J Perinatol* 2003; **23**: 300–3.

109. Ichiba H, Matsunami S, Itoh F, *et al.* Three-year follow up of term and near-term infants treated with inhaled nitric oxide. *Pediatr Int* 2003; **45**: 290–3.

110. Konduri GG, Vohr B, Robertson C, *et al.* Early inhaled nitric oxide therapy for term and near-term newborn infants with hypoxic respiratory failure: neurodevelopmental follow-up. *J Pediatr* 2007; **150**: 235–40.

111. Hintz SR, Suttner DM, Sheehan AM, *et al.* Decreased use of neonatal extracorporeal membrane oxygenation (ECMO): how new treatment modalities have affected ECMO utilization. *Pediatrics* 2000; **106**: 1339–43.

112. Taylor GA, Glass P, Fitz CR, *et al.* Neurologic status in infants treated with extracorporeal membrane oxygenation: correlation of imaging findings with developmental outcome. *Radiology* 1987; **165**: 679–82.

113. Taylor GA, Fitz CR, Glass P, *et al.* CT of cerebrovascular injury after neonatal extracorporeal membrane oxygenation: implications for neurodevelopmental outcome. *AJR Am J Roentgenol* 1989; **153**: 121–6.

114. Taylor GA, Short BL, Fitz CR. Imaging of cerebrovascular injury in infants treated with extracorporeal membrane oxygenation. *J Pediatr* 1989; **114**: 635–9.

115. Wiznitzer M, Masaryk TJ, Lewin J, *et al.* Parenchymal and vascular magnetic resonance imaging of the brain after extracorporeal membrane oxygenation. *Am J Dis Child* 1990; **144**: 1323–6.

116. Raju TN, Kim SY, Meller JL, *et al.* Circle of Willis blood velocity and flow direction after common carotid artery ligation for neonatal extracorporeal membrane oxygenation. *Pediatrics* 1989; **83**: 343–7.

117. Schumacher RE, Barks JD, Johnston MV, *et al.* Right-sided brain lesions in infants following extracorporeal membrane oxygenation. *Pediatrics* 1988; **82**: 155–61.

118. Schumacher RE, Spak C, Kileny PR. Asymmetric brain stem auditory evoked responses in infants treated with extracorporeal membrane oxygenation. *Ear Hear* 1990; **11**: 359–62.

119. Campbell L, Bunyapen C, Holmes GL, *et al.* Right common carotid artery ligation in extracorporeal membrane oxygenation. *J Pediatr* 1988; **113**: 110–13.

120. Mendoza JC, Shearer LL, Cook LN. Lateralization of brain lesions following extracorporeal membrane oxygenation. *Pediatrics* 1991; **88**: 1004–9.

121. Van Meurs KP, Nguyen HT, Rhine WD, *et al.* Intracranial abnormalities

and neurodevelopmental status after venovenous extracorporeal membrane oxygenation. *J Pediatr* 1994; **125**: 304–7.

122. Campbell LR, Bunyapen C, Gangarosa ME, *et al.* Significance of seizures associated with extracorporeal membrane oxygenation. *Pediatrics* 1991; **119**: 789–92.

123. Bulas D, Glass P. Neonatal ECMO: neuroimaging and neurodevelopmental outcome. *Semin Perinatol* 2005; **29**: 58–65.

124. Streletz LJ, Bej MD, Graziani LJ, *et al.* Utility of serial EEGs in neonates during extracorporeal membrane oxygenation. *Pediatr Neurol* 1992; **8**: 190–6.

125. Hahn JS, Vaucher Y, Bejar R, *et al.* Electroencephalographic and neuroimaging findings in neonates undergoing extracorporeal membrane oxygenation. *Neuropediatrics* 1993; **24**: 19–24.

126. Pappas A, Shankaran S, Stockmann PT, *et al.* Amplitude-integrated electroencephalography in neonates treated with extracorporeal membrane oxygenation: a pilot study. *J Pediatr* 2006; **148**: 125–7.

127. van Heijst A, Liem D, Hopman J, *et al.* Oxygenation and hemodynamics in left and right cerebral hemispheres during induction of veno-arterial extracorporeal membrane oxygenation. *J Pediatr* 2004; **144**: 223–8.

128. Ejike JC, Schenkman KA, Seidel K, *et al.* Cerebral oxygenation in neonatal and pediatrics patients during veno-arterial extracorporeal life support. *Pediatr Crit Care Med* 2006; **7**: 154–8.

129. Krummel TM, Greenfield LJ, Kirkpatrick BV, *et al.* The early evaluation of survivors after extracorporeal membrane oxygenation for neonatal pulmonary failure. *J Pediatr Surg* 1984; **19**: 585–90.

130. Towne BH, Lott IT, Hicks DA, *et al.* Long-term follow-up of infants and children treated with extracorporeal membrane oxygenation (ECMO): a preliminary report. *J Pediatr Surg* 1985; **20**: 410–14.

131. Andrews AF, Nixon CA, Cilley RE, *et al.* One- to three-year outcome for 14 survivors of extracorporeal membrane oxygenation. *Pediatrics* 1986; **78**: 692–8.

132. Glass P, Miller M, Short B. Morbidity for survivors of extracorporeal

membrane oxygenation: neurodevelopmental outcome at 1 year of age. *Pediatrics* 1989; **83**: 72–8.

133. Adolph V, Ekelund C, Smith C, *et al.* Developmental outcome of neonates treated with extracorporeal membrane oxygenation. *J Pediatr Surg* 1990; **25**: 43–6.

134. Schumacher RE, Palmer TW, LaClaire PA, *et al.* Follow-up of infants treated with extracorporeal membrane oxygenation for newborn respiratory failure. *Pediatrics* 1991; **87**: 451–7.

135. Hofkosh D, Thompson AE, Nozza RJ, *et al.* Ten years of extracorporeal membrane oxygenation: neurodevelopmental outcome. *Pediatrics* 1991; **87**: 549–55.

136. Flusser H, Dodge NN, Engle WE, *et al.* Neurodevelopmental outcome and respiratory morbidity for extracorporeal membrane oxygenation survivors at 1 year of age. *J Perinatol* 1993; **13**: 266–71.

137. Wildin SR, Landry SH, Zwischenberger JB. Prospective, controlled study of developmental outcome in survivors of extracorporeal membrane oxygenation: the first 24 months. *Pediatrics* 1994; **93**: 404–8.

138. Glass P, Wagner AE, Papero PH, *et al.* Neurodevelopmental status at age five years of neonates treated with extracorporeal membrane oxygenation. *J Pediatr* 1995; **127**: 447–57.

139. Kornhauser MS, Baumgart S, Desai SA, *et al.* Adverse neurodevelopmental outcome after extracorporeal membrane oxygenation among neonates with bronchopulmonary dysplasia. *J Pediatr* 1998; **132**: 307–11.

140. Desai SA, Stanley C, Gringlas M, *et al.* Five-year follow-up of neonates with reconstructed right common carotid arteries after extracorporeal membrane oxygenation. *J Pediatr* 1999; **134**: 428–33.

141. Parish AP, Bunyapen C, Cohen MJ, *et al.* Seizures as a predictor on long-term neurodevelopmental outcome in survivors of neonatal extracorporeal membrane oxygenations (ECMO). *J Child Neurol* 2004; **19**: 930–4.

142. Khambekar K, Nichani S, Luyt DK, *et al.* Developmental outcome in newborn infants treated for acute respiratory failure with extracorporeal membrane oxygenation: present experience. *Arch Dis Child Fetal Neonatal Ed* 2006; **91**: F21–5.

143. Taylor AK, Cousins R and Butt WW. The long-term outcome of children managed with extracorporeal life support: an institutional experience. *Crit Care Resusc* 2007; **9**: 172–7.

144. Walsh-Sukys M, Bauer RE, Cornell DJ, *et al.* Severe respiratory failure in neonates: mortality and morbidity rates and neurodevelopmental outcomes. *J Pediatr* 1994; **125**: 104–10.

145. Gratny L, Haney B, Hustead V, *et al.* Morbidity and developmental outcome of ECMO survivors compared to concurrent control group. *Soc Pediatr Res* 1992; **31**: 248A.

146. Robertson C, Finer N, Suave R, *et al.* Neurodevelopmental outcome after neonatal extracorporeal membrane oxygenation. *CMAJ* 1995; **152**: 1981–8.

147. Vaucher YE, Dudell GG, Bejar R, *et al.* Predictors of early childhood outcome in candidates for extracorporeal membrane oxygenation. *J Pediatr* 1996; **128**: 109–17.

148. UK Collaborative ECMO Group. The Collaborative UK ECMO Trial: follow-up to 1 year of age. *Pediatrics* 1998; **101**: e1.

149. Bennett CC, Johnson A, Field DJ, *et al.* UK collaborative randomized trial of neonatal extracorporeal membrane oxygenation: follow-up to age 4 years. *Lancet* 2001; **357**: 1094–6.

150. McNally H, Bennett CC, Elbourne D, *et al.* United Kingdom collaborative randomized trial of neonatal extracorporeal membrane oxygenation: follow-up to age 7 years. *Pediatrics* 2006; **117**: e845–54.

151. Van Meurs KP, Robbins ST, Reed VL, *et al.* Congenital diaphragmatic hernia: long-term outcome in neonates treated with extracorporeal membrane oxygenation. *J Pediatr* 1993; **122**: 893–9.

152. Stolar CJ, Crisafi MA, Driscoll YT. Neurocognitive outcome for neonates treated with extracorporeal membrane oxygenation: are infants with congenital diaphragmatic hernia different? *J Pediatr Surg* 1995; **30**: 355–71.

153. Bernbaum J, Schwartz I, Gerdes M, *et al.* Survivors of extracorporeal membrane oxygenation at 1 year of age: the relationship of primary diagnosis with health and neurodevelopmental sequelae. *Pediatrics* 1995; **96**: 907–13.

154. Jaillard S, Pierrat V, Truffert P, *et al.* Two years' follow-up of newborn infants after extracorporeal membrane oxygenation (ECMO). *Eur J Cardiothorac Surg* 2000; **18**: 328–33.

155. Nield TA, Langenbacher D, Pulsen MK, *et al.* Neurodevelopmental outcome at 3.5 years of age in children treated with extracorporeal life support: relationship to primary diagnosis. *J Pediatr* 2000; **136**: 338–44.

156. Naulty CM, Weiss IP, Herer GR. Progressive sensorineural hearing loss in survivors of persistent fetal circulation. *Ear Hear* 1986; **7**: 74–7.

157. Hendricks-Munoz KD, Walton JP. Hearing loss in infants with persistent fetal circulation. *Pediatrics* 1988; **81**: 650–6.

158. Leavitt AM, Watchko JF, Bennett FC, *et al.* Neurodevelopmental outcome following persistent pulmonary hypertension of the neonate. *J Perinatol* 1987; **7**: 288–91.

159. Cheung P, Tyebkhan J, Peliowski A, *et al.* Prolonged use of pancuronium bromide and sensorineural hearing loss in childhood survivors of congenital diaphragmatic hernia. *J Pediatr* 1999; **135**: 233–9.

160. Kennedy C, Sakurada O, Shinohara M, *et al.* Local cerebral glucose utilization in the newborn macaque monkey. *Ann Neurol* 1982; **12**: 333–40.

161. Pickles J. *An Introduction to the Physiology of Hearing.* New York, NY: Academic Press, 1982.

162. The Neonatal Inhaled Nitric Oxide Study Group. Inhaled nitric oxide in term and near-term infants: neurodevelopmental follow-up of the Neonatal Inhaled Nitric Oxide Study Group (NINOS). *J Pediatr* 2002; **136**: 611–17.

163. Robertson C, Tyebkhan J, Hagler M, *et al.* Late-onset, progressive sensorineural hearing loss after severe neonatal respiratory failure. *Otol Neurotol* 2002; **23**: 353–6.

164. Robertson C, Tyebhkan J, Peliowski A, *et al.* Ototoxic drugs and sensorineural hearing loss following severe neonatal respiratory failure. *Acta Paediatr* 2006; **95**: 214–33.

165. Cheung PY, Robertson CMT. Sensorineural hearing loss in survivors of neonatal extracorporeal membrane oxygenation. *Pediatr Rehabil* 1997; **1**: 127–30.

166. Robertson CMT, Cheung PY, Haluschak MM, *et al.* High prevalence of sensorineural hearing loss among survivors of neonatal congenital diaphragmatic hernia. Western Canadian ECMO Follow-up Group. *Am J Otol* 1998; **19**: 730–6.

167. Fligor BJ, Neault MW, Mullen CH, *et al.* Factors associated with sensorineural hearing loss among survivors of extracorporeal membrane oxygenation therapy. *Pediatrics* 2005; **115**: 1519–28.

168. Desai S, Kollros PR, Graziani LJ, *et al.* Sensitivity and specificity of the neonatal brain-stem auditory evoked potential for hearing and language deficits in survivors of extracorporeal membrane oxygenation. *J Pediatr* 1997; **131**: 233–9.

169. Hutchin ME, Gilmer C, Yarbrough WG. Delayed-onset sensorineural hearing loss in a 3-year-old survivor of persistent pulmonary hypertension of the newborn. *Arch Otolaryngol Head Neck Surg* 2000; **126**: 1014–17.

170. Joint Committee on Infant Hearing. Year 2007 position statement: principles and guidelines for early hearing detection and intervention programs. *Pediatrics* 2007; **120**: 898–921.

171. Majaesic CM, Jones R, Dinu IA, *et al.* Clinical correlations and pulmonary function at 8 years of age after severe neonatal respiratory failure. *Pediatr Pulmonol* 2007; **42**: 829–37.

172. D'Agostino JA, Bernbaum JC, Gerdes M, *et al.* Outcome for infants with congenital diaphragmatic hernia requiring extracorporeal membrane oxygenation: the first year. *J Pediatr Surg* 1995; **30**: 10–15.

173. Kamata S, Usui N, Kamiyama M, *et al.* Long-term follow-up of patients with high-risk congenital diaphragmatic hernia. *J Pediatr Surg* 2005; **40**: 1833–8.

174. Muratore CS, Kharash V, Lund DP, *et al.* Pulmonary morbidity in 100 survivors of congenital diaphragmatic hernia monitored in a multidisciplinary clinic. *J Pediatr Surg* 2001; **36**: 133–40.

175. Bagolan P, Morini F. Long-term follow up of infants with congenital diaphragmatic hernia. *Semin Pediatr Surg* 2007; **16**: 134–44.

176. Muratore C, Utter S, Jaksic T, *et al.* Nutritional morbidity in survivors of congenital diaphragmatic hernia. *J Pediatr Surg* 2001; **36**: 1171–6.

177. Cortes RA, Keller RL, Townsend T, *et al.* Survival of severe congenital diaphragmatic hernia has morbid consequences. *J Pediatr Surg* 2005; **40**: 36–46.

178. Chiu PL, Sauer C, Mihailovic A, *et al.* The price of success in the management of congenital diaphragmatic hernia: is improved survival accompanied by an increase in long-term morbidity? *J Pediatr Surg* 2006; **41**: 888–92.

179. Hageman JR, Adams MA, Gardner TH. Persistent pulmonary hypertension of the newborn: trends in incidence, diagnosis, and management. *Am J Dis Child* 1984; **138**: 592–5.

180. Hack M, Taylor HG, Drotar D, *et al.* Poor predictive validity of the Bayley Scales of Infant Development for cognitive function of extremely low birth weight children at school age. *Pediatrics* 2005; **116**: 333–41.

Chapter 38

Pediatric cardiac surgery: relevance to fetal and neonatal brain injury

Giles J. Peek and Susan R. Hintz

Introduction

In this chapter the impact of congenital heart disease and its surgical treatment on the neonatal brain will be discussed. Babies may have congenital cardiac disease as an isolated malformation or may have a heart defect as part of a larger spectrum of abnormalities, which may in turn be associated with a syndrome. In addition, these babies are often profoundly ill, presenting to medical attention on the verge of cardiac arrest with severe hypoxia, hypotension, or both. The treatment of the condition usually involves a trip to the catheterization laboratory or operating room (or both). We therefore have great potential for neurological morbidity, with a combination of possible underlying abnormality of the brain, preoperative, perioperative, and postoperative insults all conspiring to injure the cardiac surgery patient's brain. Despite these problems, the majority of babies do extremely well following heart surgery in the newborn period, although it is important to recognize that many of them will have a subtle neurological deficit if they are compared to the normal population. These are evidenced as cognitive and intellectual impairment, behavioral difficulties, speech delays, etc. [1,2,3]. The incidence of major neurological insult postoperatively as manifest by seizures, stroke, coma, or choreo-athetoid movements has fallen to around 2–11% in the current era [4,5].

Congenital heart disease and common genetic associations

Fortunately, congenital heart disease (CHD) is rare, affecting 2.8/1000 live births [6]. It does not have a clear solely genetic causation, as the risk of ostium secundum atrial septal defect (ASD) in sisters of patients with secundum ASD is 1/3, and the chances of a mother of a child with secundum ASD having the same defect is only 22.5% [7]. The incidence of CHD in dizygotic twins is only 13.6%, but in one series they all had the same type of defect, pointing to a shared environmental risk during pregnancy [8]. Nevertheless there are clearly familial clusters of congenital heart defects [9], especially in consanguineous families, so there are definite genetic components

involved [10]. Approximately one-third of children with CHD have an associated non-cardiac abnormality [11]. There are also certain genetic syndromes which are associated with specific cardiac defects.

DiGeorge syndrome/velocardiofacial syndrome (VCFS)

This is caused by microdeletion of chromosome 22q11. It occurs in 1/4000 live births. This entity is now more appropriately referred to as 22q11.2 deletion, as the presentation encompasses a broad phenotypic spectrum including thymic aplasia, hypocalcemia, facial dysmorphism, velopharyngeal dysfunction, impairment in neurodevelopmental outcome, and cono-truncal abnormalities such as interrupted aortic arch and truncus arteriosus. The deletion can be inherited in an autosomal dominant fashion, but the majority are thought to be new deletions. It has been estimated that 77% of these babies have a deficit of cell-mediated immunity [12]. All blood for transfusion to these patients must be irradiated blood to prevent graft versus host disease from live leucocytes in the transfused blood, although this procedure is standard practice in many institutions. Although clinical variability is marked, 40–50% of patients with 22q11.2 deletion have cognitive or learning difficulties. The neurodevelopmental prognosis for children with 22q11.2 deletion and CHD requiring surgery in the neonatal period appears to be even more guarded (see *Neurodevelopmental outcomes*, below). These children also have been reported to be at significantly higher risk for schizophrenia and other behavioral disorders than the general population [13].

Down syndrome

Caused by trisomy 21, this well-known syndrome is the most common chromosomal anomaly, affecting approximately 1/700 to 1/1000 live births. It is associated with congenital heart disease in 40% of cases, nearly half of which are atrioventricular septal defects (AVSD) [14]. Indeed, 40–60% of children with AVSD have a chromosomal abnormality, usually Down syndrome [15]. It is unusual for a newborn with Down and AVSD to require surgery, most patients being operated on electively at around the age of 6 months. If there is severe left AV valve regurgitation and heart failure in the newborn period requiring surgery the prognosis is usually guarded.

Fetal and Neonatal Brain Injury, 4th edition, ed. David K. Stevenson, William E. Benitz, Philip Sunshine, Susan R. Hintz, and Maurice L. Druzin. Published by Cambridge University Press. © Cambridge University Press 2009.

Other syndromes

Polymorphism for apolipoprotein E, which is involved in neuronal repair, can cause susceptibility to neurological injury following heart surgery [16]. Williams syndrome, a micro-deletion of chromosome 7q11.23 (elastin gene) affecting 1/20 000 live births, is associated with valvar and supra-valvar aortic stenosis, pulmonary artery stenosis, developmental impairments, and elfin facies. There is also a clear association between congenital heart disease and congenital malformation of the brain [3].

Presurgical neurological injury

We have seen in the last section how some babies have congenital anomalies which can contribute to their ultimate neurological outcome. However, even children who have anatomically normal brains can suffer injury from hypoxia and ischemia as a result of their cardiac malformation, and this can occur in 15–30% of patients preoperatively [17,18]. Congenital heart disease often presents in the first few days of life when the ductus arteriosus closes. Patients can then be largely divided into cyanotic lesions, where the duct had been supplying the pulmonary blood flow (i.e., pulmonary atresia with intact ventricular septum, PAIVS), and obstructive lesions, where the duct had been supplying the systemic blood flow (i.e., coarctation of the aorta). Babies with transposition of the great arteries (TGA) do not fit neatly into this categorization, because their duct acts to increase mixing of oxygenated blood between the pulmonary and systemic circulations, neither do children with obstructed total anomalous pulmonary venous connections (TAPVC), but since both may present with cyanosis and collapse in the first few days of life this is largely an academic issue. Patients may present with profound desaturation, collapse, cardiogenic shock, or cardiac failure. Obviously any condition that reduces oxygen delivery to the brain by reducing the oxygen content of the blood and the cardiac output can cause neurological injury. Thus, as in preterm infants, the white matter of term infants with CHD is exquisitely vulnerable to injury [19]. Hypoxic–ischemic insults as well as proinflammatory mediators may injure the developing oligodendrocytes in the term infant with CHD, causing periventricular leukomalacia (PVL), which is detectable by MRI in as many as 50% of neonates following cardiac surgery [20,21]. Yet it is important to recognize that many studies do not include MRI *prior* to cardiac surgery. Therefore, although peri- and postoperative hypotension or hypoxemia may play a role, PVL or white-matter injury detected after surgery may actually have been present in some cases before. Oligodendrocytes may also be damaged by inflammatory cytokines and therefore can be injured by cardiopulmonary bypass (CPB) itself, as well as by other inflammatory states such as meningitis [22].

Recognition of the possibility of duct-dependent congenital heart disease in a collapsed newborn and early resuscitation with prostaglandin infusion to re-open the duct restores oxygenation of the tissues and limits brain injury in most cases. The exception to this is obstructed TAPVC: these babies have severe consolidation of the lungs and may present in the first few hours of life with apparent respiratory failure which may be refractory to ventilation and nitric oxide. Prostaglandin infusion does not help, and may be detrimental, and many of these babies are referred for ECMO as cases of persistent fetal circulation. Sometimes the correct diagnosis is not made until after they have been cannulated for ECMO. Since ECMO is a good way to restore oxygenation this is not actually a bad thing, and allows resuscitation before surgery.

Aside from presurgical brain injury, there is likely a high rate of unrecognized structural brain abnormality in children with CHD. For example, in a postmortem series of 41 babies with hypoplastic left heart syndrome (HLHS), 29% had a major structural brain abnormality, including absent corpus callosum, holoprosencephaly, and immature cortical mantle [23]. Fetal brain growth may also be impaired in CHD, potentially due to inappropriate fetal cerebral oxygen delivery, particularly in those with single ventricle physiology and TGA [23,24]. Carefully performed cranial ultrasound (CUS) may be sufficient to reveal significant preoperative structural abnormalities. In a retrospective series, te Pas *et al.* reported that 42% of term and near-term infants with CHD had preoperative brain abnormalities detected by CUS [25]. These included ventriculomegaly, wide subarachnoid spaces, lenticulostriate vasculopathy, and acute ischemic changes, and were most likely to occur in those with HLHS. More recently, MRI and diffusion tensor imaging (DTI) have been employed to delineate both macro- and microstructural preoperative brain abnormalities among term infants with HLHS and TGA compared with control infants without CHD [26]. On preoperative imaging, 41% of those with TGA and 17% of those with HLHS had brain injury; none of the control infants had white-matter injury on MRI. Using more advanced microstructural interrogation with DTI, white-matter fractional anisotropy (a measure of directionality of water movement, which should increase with maturation) was significantly lower among those with CHD compared with controls. Average diffusivity (a measure of overall diffusion of water, which should decrease with maturation) was significantly higher among infants with CHD. These concerning findings indicate that the pattern of brain microstructural development in term infants with HLHS and TGA is similar to that of premature infants. Furthermore, because observations were made soon after birth, the DTI results suggest impaired fetal brain development is likely to be associated with these congenital cardiac anomalies. In light of these important findings, advanced neuroimaging prior to surgical intervention may become increasingly important to clinical management and decision making. Substantial opportunities for further investigation into preoperative neuroprotective strategies exist.

In some cases, the standard treatment for TGA is balloon atrial septostomy (BAS) as a resuscitative measure to improve mixing across the atrial septum and then a switch operation at some point a week or more later. There has recently been demonstration of neurological morbidity associated with the septostomy itself [27]. In a series of 29 patients with TGA studied with brain MRI prior to definitive switch repair, 12 of the 19 patients who required BAS as a resuscitative measure had focal or multifocal stroke; none of the patients without BAS had such injury. In a larger series of patients with a range of congenital cardiac defects, 39% had preoperative brain injury by MRI, most commonly stroke, and this was independently associated with BAS [28]. On the basis of this evidence, some centers appear to be moving towards immediate surgery in more TGA cases, as septostomy itself appears to be a risk factor for neurological injury.

Preoperative injury: timing of surgery

All babies who have had a significant hypoxic or ischemic neurological insult should undergo neuroimaging after resuscitation. If intracranial hemorrhage (ICH) is detected surgery should be deferred for as long as practicable to reduce the risk of extension of the ICH when the patient undergoes cardiopulmonary bypass. It can take several weeks for an ICH to organize sufficiently to make CPB "safe," but a delay of as little as 1 week can reduce the risk of ICH substantially.

Limitation of perioperative neurological injury

Unfortunately the process of surgical correction of congenital heart defects causes neurological injury, when surgical patients are compared to the general population [29]. This is inherent in the technology that is available and the diseases being treated. Fortunately, however, modern surgical and anesthetic techniques have evolved so that this damage is limited. It requires a neurophysiologist armed with sophisticated psychomotor tests and an MRI scanner to detect. The majority of children who undergo cardiac surgery will probably function within the normal range during childhood and beyond. It is likely that if these children had been born without a heart defect they would have had higher IQs and better psychomotor function. However, comparing these children with the ideal situation is futile; in the majority of cases, these infants with CHD would not survive, or at the very least would have a far more guarded neurologic prognosis, without surgical intervention. Thus we must focus on optimizing operative and perioperative management and techniques to ensure the best possible outcomes.

Anesthesia

In a baby with duct-dependent congenital heart disease the usual anesthetic technique of pre-oxygenation prior to intubation causes pulmonary vasodilation resulting in steal from the systemic circulation. This can paradoxically cause a massive reduction in tissue oxygen delivery with systemic hypotension. Ventilation is therefore tailored to avoid this. Animal studies have shown neuroprotective effects of various different anesthetic agents including the volatiles, which have calcium channel-blocking effects, and the barbiturates [11,30,31], but these have not been borne out in clinical practice and so the anesthesiologist's focus is to maintain cardiovascular stability and tissue oxygen delivery by use of a variety of techniques. Barbiturates may have a protective effect against air embolism in the warm brain, and are sometimes used following catastrophic air embolism [32]. Surface cooling in the anesthetic room is a useful adjunct to cooling on CPB.

Cardiopulmonary bypass

CPB is what makes surgery possible, but it is an abnormal non-pulsatile circulation and requires full anticoagulation with heparin to the extent that the blood will not clot at all. This is achieved with a heparin dose of 3 mg/kg, and is necessary to prevent the patient's blood clotting in the extracorporeal circuit. CPB causes dilution and consumption of clotting proteins and activation and consumption of platelets, resulting in a typical coagulopathy [33]. There is also a pan-endothelial injury caused by activation of inflammatory cytokines such as complement factors, interleukins, and tumor necrosis factor (TNF), although there is no clear correlation between the degree of inflammation and the clinical outcome [34]. Blood shed into the surgical field is aspirated back to the CPB machine and re-infused into the patient. This blood can contain particulate debris such as pieces of bone, bone wax, small clots, fat, and also microbubbles. The addition of arterial line filters and avoidance of embolism has reduced the neurological injury that was attendant on the re-infusion of these particles into the aorta [35,36]. Children with cyanotic heart disease often have many collateral vessels between the systemic and pulmonary circulations; these may be anatomical structures such as major aortopulmonary collateral arteries (MAPCAs) or smaller vessels which open up as a result of the chronic hypoxia. When CPB is established these vessels can result in a huge amount of blood returning to the heart despite the diversion of all the vena-caval blood to the machine. This open-heart return can obscure the surgical field and make repair impossible. The use of systemic hypothermia reduces the metabolic rate by a factor of approximately 2.5 for every 10 °C and thus allows lower CPB flows, which reduces the collateral return and makes surgery possible [37]. Hypothermia in turn causes increased viscosity in the blood, and historically it was routine to hemodilute patients to offset this, as it was thought that a lower viscosity would result in higher tissue oxygen delivery. In addition, this reduced blood transfusion requirements [38]. Modern practice has moved away from this concept, as it has been shown that a relatively normal hematocrit of 30% is preferable on bypass to optimize tissue oxygen delivery and improve neurological outcome [39,40,41]. During open-heart surgery air enters the heart and great vessels, but this must not enter the cerebral circulation and must be removed at the end of the procedure as it is a potent cause of neurological injury; even if a blood vessel is not blocked the mere passage of an air bubble can cause injury [22]. In addition to these factors, the newborn brain appears more susceptible to neurological injury following CPB, in that MRI evidence of PVL can be seen in 50% of newborns following CPB while in older babies only 5% are affected [19]. The clinician has little influence over most of these factors, as they are inherent in the use of the technology [22], but there are some aspects that the clinician can influence to affect the outcome and limit neurological injury. These factors are discussed below.

Cooling strategy

Cooling is the main neuroprotective tool used during CPB. It is important to ensure that the brain cools evenly. To this end cooling (and warming) should be relatively slow, to allow thorough equilibration of temperature throughout the tissues. It is agreed that cooling prior to deep hypothermic circulatory arrest (DHCA) should take at least 20 minutes [22]. Also barbiturates (if used) should not be given until the desired temperature is reached, because they can cause cerebral vasoconstriction and prevent even cooling. The blood gas management during cooling is also important. CPB was run using an alpha-stat profile for many years, as this was felt to provide the best perfusion conditions as well as being easy to manage. During alpha-stat management the blood gas machine is not adjusted for temperature; in other words the pH is measured at 37 °C, even though the patient may be at 25 °C. The upshot of this is that the patient becomes more alkalotic during cooling, and this in turn leads to cerebral vasoconstriction, reduced oxygen delivery to boundary areas, and uneven cooling. The alternative method is pH-stat, when the blood gas machine is adjusted for temperature, and CO_2 is added to the bypass oxygenator sweep gas to offset the alkalosis. The relative acidosis keeps the brain vasodilated and maintains cerebral blood flow, especially once cerebral autoregulation is abolished as the patient becomes poikilothermic during cooling [11,42]. There is substantial evidence that neurological outcomes are better when pH-stat is used during cooling, and some to support the use of alpha-stat during rewarming [43–46]. A typical protocol employs pH-stat during cooling, switching to alpha-stat prior to circulatory arrest and using alpha-stat during warming. Most units also employ some form of topical brain cooling.

DHCA versus low-flow CPB versus head perfusion

When the brain temperature is sufficiently low (around 15 °C), the circulation can be stopped for a period of time and restarted with few sequelae, this is termed deep hypothermic circulatory arrest (DHCA). There is much discussion about how long that period of time is, but less than 25 minutes is indistinguishable from low-flow CPB and therefore relatively safe [47,48]. All children in the Boston DHCA study whose arrest time exceeded 35 minutes had postoperative seizure activity [49], and there was an incremental decrease in intellectual ability which correlated closely with duration of DHCA beyond the very short "safe period" [48,50]. In addition, the children in the Boston study whose DHCA time exceeded 41 minutes had worse late neurodevelopmental outcome than the children in the low-flow continuous bypass group. DHCA is useful because it allows the bypass cannulae to be removed and provides excellent operative conditions with a bloodless field

[51]. It is therefore helpful for some operations in very small patients, and for some parts of operations around the arch of the aorta (e.g., Damus–Kaye–Stansell procedure). Some surgeons use DHCA routinely, but most prefer to limit its use [47]. There is currently much controversy regarding this issue, as surgeons have realized that they can perform most of the operation on CPB and that long periods of DHCA are no longer mandatory [47]. The use of low-flow CPB at around 50 mL/kg/min, with a cerebral perfusion pressure of 13 mmHg [11] and isolated anterograde head perfusion at flows of 20–30 mL/kg/min, has meant that periods of circulatory arrest can often be reduced to just a few minutes [52]. In addition, periods of reperfusion during DHCA may also reduce the neurological insult [11]. Most surgeons adopt a combination of techniques which they adapt to the individual patient's condition.

NIRS intraoperative monitoring of cerebral oxygen delivery

Near-infrared spectroscopy (NIRS) is now commercially available as transcutaneous devices which can continually monitor cerebral oxygen delivery (Somanetics, Hamamatsu). It has been shown in a retrospective study that their use during heart surgery improves the general condition of the patient as well as the neurological outcome, reducing length of stay [53]. This is likely to be due to the ability of this device to identify periods of occult cerebral hypoxia. These can occur when the cerebral perfusion pressure decreases below 13 mmHg without being noticed [11], which in turn can occur when a child has bi-caval venous cannulation with a transiently obstructed superior vena-caval cannula, causing intracranial venous hypertension [54]. It can also occur when the perfusion pressure decreases because of vasodilation, run-off via aortopulmonary collaterals or a shunt, or when CPB flow is reduced to allow improved visualization of the surgical field. By immediately identifying cerebral hypoxia and correcting it, brain injury is limited and neurological outcome may be improved. Most CPB circuits have a continuous display of the venous line oxygen saturation, using devices like the CDI500 (Terumo). Maintaining the $SvO_2 > 65\%$ ensures global tissue oxygen delivery, but does not identify regional tissue hypoxia. Since the brain has the fastest metabolic rate of any organ it will be the first to suffer from a global decrease in oxygen delivery during CPB, and using NIRS in addition to SvO_2 monitoring acts to prevent cerebral hypoxia.

CO_2 flooding

Open-heart surgery inevitably allows air to enter the heart, and this must be removed at the end of the procedure before the heart is allowed to beat. This is an imperfect process and can result in air embolus to the brain, with disastrous consequences. By flooding the surgical field with CO_2 any gas left in the heart at the end of the procedure will be soluble and theoretically less dangerous if not completely removed [55].

Corticosteroids

Intravenous steroids are used routinely in a number of centers preoperatively (dexamethasone 1 mg/kg or methyl-prednisolone 30 mg/kg) to reduce the inflammatory activation associated with CPB, but there is little consensus on dosing protocols [56,57]. There is good evidence that this is effective in limiting postoperative inflammatory markers and that this translates into improved pulmonary, renal, and general clinical outcome, but specific neurological outcome was not studied [56].

MUF

Modified ultra-filtration (MUF) can also act to remove inflammatory mediators, and can result in improved myocardial function. MUF may reduce brain injury associated with DHCA [22,58]. However, use of arteriovenous MUF can result in hypotension, and this may contribute to reduced cerebral oxygen delivery [59].

Postoperative management

Once patients have undergone successful surgery they are taken to the pediatric intensive care unit (PICU), where their organ functions are further optimized as they recover from the operation. Hypotension and hypoxia are both predictive of PVL postoperatively [20]. A full discussion of PICU management is beyond the scope of this chapter, but three specific treatments which could help to improve neurological outcome are discussed.

NOMO-VAD

In some cases the cardiac output is marginal following a successful corrective operation. Some of these patients will deteriorate and die, and some will survive. It has been suggested that early or even elective mechanical support of the cardiac output can improve survival as well as improving the neurological outcome in these borderline cases [60]. NOMO-VAD uses an ECMO circuit without an oxygenator (hence NOMO) to provide ventricular assist (VAD) via venoarterial cannulation to children with arteriopulmonary shunts. The flow in the circuit is set at around 200 mL/kg/min, approximately double that used for VA ECMO. Pulmonary blood flow comes from the shunt flow, augmented by the flow from the circuit. Children with biventricular circulations and normal pulmonary blood flow anatomy can be supported with VA ECMO in the event of low cardiac output postoperatively [61]. Larger children can be supported with ventricular assist devices such as the Berlin Heart [62].

Cooling

Cooling has been used as a neuroprotective treatment in many different arenas following cardiac arrest in adults and children, birth asphyxia, and head trauma [63,64]. There are two potential mechanisms by which cooling could help improve neurological outcome following cardiac surgery. Firstly, by reducing the metabolic rate of the brain the balance between oxygen supply and usage can be restored in the presence of a limited cardiac output, and further improvement of this equation occurs because of a reduction in excitotoxic neurotransmitters in the cooled brain [65]. Secondly, many children suffer tachycardia after heart surgery, which can impair the cardiac output, and many of these tachycardias (e.g., junctional ectopic tachycardia, JET) respond well to cooling, which thus boosts the cardiac output and improves cerebral oxygen delivery.

Tight glycemic control

There is evidence that tight glycemic control with prevention of hyperglycemia can improve outcome after head injury in children [66,67]. Whether this is also true following cardiac surgery in children is currently the subject of a national multi-center randomized controlled trial in the UK (CHIP: Control of Hyperglycaemia In Paediatric intensive care, ISRCTN61735247). It is also important to avoid hypoglycemia, as this is associated with seizures [68].

Neurodevelopmental outcomes

With substantial advances in intraoperative and perioperative management, and remarkable improvements in surgical technique and approach allowing for better short-term outcomes, the focus of attention both for families and for further research turns to long-term neurodevelopmental outcomes [69]. Studies reporting neurodevelopmental follow-up assessments in children after complex congenital heart surgery have been challenging to interpret for several reasons. Given the rapidly changing and improving strategies for operative and perioperative management, the outcomes of infants born years ago may not be generalizable to the present. The morbidities associated with approaches used in the past may be related to adverse neurocognitive outcomes reported now; similarly, the potential modifying effects of newer techniques may not be fully understood for several years. Specific CHD lesions and numerous other intrinsic and extrinsic patient variables may be associated with differing outcomes. Thus, if a small but very diverse cohort of CHD survivors is examined, such predictors may be difficult to assess. In addition, most of these studies do not include contemporaneous control groups.

Intrinsic genetic variables

As discussed previously, several genetic syndromes known to be associated with CHD are also known to be associated with increased risk for developmental impairment [69,70]. These include trisomy 21, Williams syndrome, and CHARGE association. More subtle genetic variables have also been recognized as potentially important determinant factors for adverse outcomes after complex congenital heart surgery.

Polymorphisms of the apolipoprotein E (*APOE*) gene are associated with impaired recovery after brain ischemic injury, and with neurologic decline after surgery for CHD [16]. In a recent neurodevelopmental follow-up study by Gaynor *et al.*, 188 patients who had undergone two-ventricle repair for a range of CHD lesions were assessed at 1 year of age using the Bayley Scales of Infant Development II (BSID) Mental

Developmental Index (MDI) and Psychomotor Developmental Index (PDI) (population normed mean = 100, standard deviation = 15), as well as neurologic exam [71]. For the entire cohort, mean scores were within or slight lower than those expected for the general population (MDI 90.6 ± 14.9, PDI 81.6 ± 17.2). Although numerous potentially important pre-, intra-, and postoperative variables were evaluated, only preoperative factors were independently associated with worse MDI scores on multivariate analyses. These intrinsic factors included low birthweight, presence of a genetic syndrome, and presence of the *APOE ε2* polymorphism.

The outcomes of children with CHD affected by 22q11.2 deletion spectrum have also recently been evaluated. The Western Canadian Complex Pediatric Therapies Project Follow-up Group reported on the 18-month outcomes of a regional cohort of 85 patients who had undergone a range of interventions including arterial switch, Norwood, TAPVC repair, as well as other procedures [72]. For the entire cohort, BSID scores were lower than would be expected for the population (MDI 84 ± 17, PDI 80 ± 22). However, for the subgroup with genetic abnormalities, the majority of whom had 22q11.2 deletion, mean BSID scores were substantially lower (mean MDI and PDI scores < 70). Another study from this group compared 2-year outcomes of a small group of CHD patients with 22q11.2 deletion to patients without deletion [73], matched on cardiac lesion, socioeconomic status, and hospital and year of operation. There were significant differences between the groups. Of the group with 22q11.2 deletion, 61.5% had MDI < 70, 84.6% had PDI < 70, and 69% were in a developmental intervention program. Of the group without deletion, only 13.8% had MDI < 70, 6.7% had PDI < 70, and 20% were in developmental intervention. Forbess *et al.* reported on the 5-year outcomes of children who had had definitive repair or palliative surgery for a range of CHD lesions in the neonatal period [74]. In this analysis, the presence of 22q11.2 deletion was significantly associated with lower full-scale IQ, performance IQ, and verbal IQ, independent of numerous other variables. Taken together, these data suggest the critical importance of making the diagnosis of 22q11.2 deletion as soon as possible – preferably in the prenatal period – to allow appropriate and better-informed counseling as to long-term outcomes. The diagnosis is now easy to make with the use of fluorescent in-situ hybridization (FISH).

Socioeconomic factors

The association of socioeconomic status (SES) with cognitive and developmental outcomes has been demonstrated in numerous neurodevelopmental follow-up studies of high-risk neonatal groups, including extremely low-birthweight and extremely preterm infants [75,76]. This association is also true for children followed after congenital cardiac surgery [69]. Forbess and colleagues reported that lower SES was independently correlated with lower full-scale IQ and verbal IQ at 5 years of age in a cohort with a range of CHD lesions [74]. After Fontan operation specifically, Wernovsky *et al.* found that SES was also significantly independently associated with cognitive outcome [77].

Congenital heart lesion type

Robust assessment of neurodevelopmental outcomes by CHD lesion has been challenging, given the limitation of patient numbers of any single diagnostic category in any single institution. However, special interest has been given to HLHS, because of improved survival, the severity of the lesion and the complexity of the intervention needed, early reports of extremely poor neurodevelopmental outcomes, and recognition that cerebral blood flow is impaired among infants with HLHS [3,69,70,78,79]. More recent investigations of early development and school-age outcomes of patients with HLHS after either staged palliation or transplant have reported low to low-normal IQ [3,78,80,81]. In young children who had undergone transplantation for HLHS, Ilke *et al.* found mean full-scale IQ to be 88.5, verbal IQ 89.9, and performance IQ 90.5 [80]. Mahle and colleagues compared school-age outcomes of patients who had undergone transplant (*n* = 21) to those who had undergone Norwood (*n* = 26) for HLHS [78]. They found no significant differences between the groups in IQ, expressive or receptive language, motor function, or behavior. For the overall cohort, mean full-scale IQ was 86, mean expressive and receptive language scores, and mean math, reading, and spelling achievement scores were all approximately one standard deviation below the population-expected mean. In multivariate analyses, only prolonged length of stay was associated with lower full-scale IQ.

The Western Canadian Complex Pediatric Therapies Project Follow-up Group reported that, among patients who had undergone Norwood procedures (*n* = 16), 18-month mean BSID MDI was 84, and mean PDI was 68; 25% had MDI < 70 and 56% had PDI < 70 [72]. However, very early childhood BSID scores may not be predictive of later outcome [82,83]. This group also reported on early childhood outcomes after TAPVC repair in the neonatal period [84]. Mean BSID scores were also in the low-normal range, with mean MDI 87 and mean PDI 89. Comparing developmental outcomes as a function of single-ventricle or biventricular repairs, Forbess and colleagues found significant differences between the patients at 5 years of age [74]. Mean full-scale IQ was 89.9 and performance IQ was 88.4 in the single-ventricle group, compared with 98.2 and 97.8 in the biventricular repair group. Results of visual-motor tests were significantly worse for single-ventricle patients, although mean scores were still within the low-normal range.

Intraoperative factors

One of the most comprehensive trials of intraoperative interventions is the Boston Circulatory Arrest Study (BCAS), in which infants with d-TGA were randomized to DHCA or continuous low-flow CPB and received neurodevelopmental follow-up at several points during childhood [1,29,51]. At 4 years of age, there were no differences between the DHCA and CPB groups in terms of IQ, although the DHCA group were more likely to have gross and fine motor impairment and speech and language delay. The mean full-scale IQ (92.6) and performance (91.6) scores for the cohort as a whole were in the low-normal range. Assessment at 8 years of age revealed impaired outcomes for the overall cohort in areas including cognitive and executive function, fine motor skills, and speech and language. Although there were no differences between the DHCA and CPB groups in full-scale, verbal, or performance IQ, the length of time under DHCA was significantly correlated with lower full-scale and performance IQ. Of note, at 1-year follow-up, significantly lower BSID PDI scores and a trend toward lower MDI scores were observed in the DHCA group; this disparity between 1-year and 8-year findings underscores the poor predictive validity of very early neurodevelopmental testing, and the importance of long-term follow-up [82,83]. Forbess *et al.* also found an independent correlation of length of time under DHCA with lower performance IQ scores at 5 years of age, and this correlation approached significance in other IQ domains [73].

Hematocrit strategy during CPB has also been investigated [39,85]. Combined results at 1 year of age from two trials ($n = 271$) suggest that hematocrit at the initiation of CPB is linearly associated with increasing BSID PDI score to a threshold hematocrit level of 23.5%; beyond this point, the effect plateaus and no apparent improvement is achieved. There was no significant association between pre-CPB hematocrit level and BSID MDI scores at 1 year. These are very early childhood results; extended follow-up to school age will be valuable.

Length of hospital stay

In the BCAS, in which infants with TGA were randomized to DHCA or continuous low-flow CPB, follow-up at 8 years of age revealed impaired outcomes for the overall study group in areas including executive function, fine motor skills, and speech and language [1,29,51]. Although treatment group and other variables were associated with some outcomes, longer postoperative stay in the intensive care unit was an independent risk factor for lower IQ [86]. Others have also found significant or nearly significant independent correlations of length of stay with lower IQ in middle childhood [74,78].

This finding suggests that unmeasurable or unmeasured variables may influence hospital course and are associated with adverse long-term outcomes. Events and findings that traditionally keep a child in the hospital longer, such as infection and significant feeding issues, may portend larger and more complex issues. Data on variables such as these should be collected and reported meticulously in future studies. A continued search to define significant modifiable clinical factors will be critical for the development of protective strategies.

Conclusions

Congenital heart disease may be associated with intrinsic brain malformations, especially when part of a dysgenetic syndrome. Hypoxia and hypotension can then cause preoperative brain injury which can be minimized by appropriate resuscitation. Definitive or palliative repair is then performed, usually with the aid of cardiopulmonary bypass using hypothermia as neuroprotection and avoiding DHCA except where absolutely necessary or minimizing the length of exposure to this maneuver. A range of neurodevelopmental outcomes have been reported for patients after surgery for CHD. Patients with CHD requiring surgery in the neonatal period are at risk for cognitive, academic, and neurologic impairment compared to the general population. Meticulous attention to preoperative and intraoperative management strategies that protect the patient from ischemic or hemorrhagic injury is critical. However, intrinsic factors such as socioeconomic status also influence developmental progress. Genetic variables, such as presence of 22q11.2 deletion, are extremely significant predictors of adverse neurocognitive outcomes. Congenital heart disease is more manageable and its treatment much safer today than at any time in history, but there is still much more to be learned and understood to improve the ultimate outcome for these high-risk infants. Continued vigorous research of the short- and long-term neurologic progress of patients with CHD, and identification of factors linked with improved outcomes, will allow us to better care for these vulnerable patients and their families.

References

1. Bellinger DC, Wypij D, Kuban KC, *et al.* Developmental and neurological status of children at 4 years of age after heart surgery with hypothermic circulatory arrest or low-flow cardiopulmonary bypass. *Circulation* 1999; **100**: 526–32.

2. Majnemer A, Limperopoulos C. Developmental progress of children with congenital heart defects requiring open heart surgery. *Semin Pediatr Neurol* 1999; **6**: 12–19.

3. Mahle WT, Wernovsky G. Neurodevelopmental outcomes in hypoplastic left heart syndrome. *Semin*

Thorac Cardiovasc Surg Pediatr Card Surg Annu 2004; **7**: 39–47.

4. Trittenwein G, Nardi A, Pansi H, *et al.* Early postoperative prediction of cerebral damage after pediatric cardiac surgery. *Ann Thorac Surg* 2003; **76**: 576–80.

5. Menache CC, du Plessis AJ, Wessel DL, *et al.* Current incidence of acute neurologic complications after open heart operations in children. *Ann Thorac Surg* 2002; **73**: 1752–8.

6. Pradat P. Epidemiology of major congenital heart defects in Sweden, 1981–1986. *J Epidemiol Community Health* 1992; **46**: 211–15.

7. Caputo S, Capozzi G, Russo MG, *et al.* Familial recurrence of congenital heart disease in patients with ostium secundum atrial septal defect. *Eur Heart J* 2005; **26**: 2179–84.

8. Caputo S, Russo MG, Capozzi G, *et al.* Congenital heart disease in a population of dizygotic twins: an echocardiographic study. *Int J Cardiol* 2005; **102**: 293–6.

9. Cymbron T, Anjos R, Cabral R, *et al.* Epidemiological characterization of congenital heart disease in Sao Miguel Island, Azores, Portugal. *Community Genet* 2006; **9**: 107–12.

10. Stollenberg C, Magnus P, Skrondal A, *et al.* Consanguinity and recurrence risk

of birth defects: a population-based study. *Am J Med Genet* 1999; **82**: 423–8.

11. Williams GD, Ramamoorthy C. Brain monitoring and protection during pediatric cardiac surgery. *Semin Cardiothorac Vasc Anesth* 2007; **11**: 23.

12. Sullivan KE, Jawad KF, Randall P, *et al.* Lack of correlation between impaired T cell production, immunodeficiency, and other phenotypic features in chromosome 22q11.2 deletion syndromes. *Clin Immunol Immunopathol* 1998; **86**: 141–6.

13. Gothelf D. Velocardiofacial syndrome. *Child Adolesc Psychiatr Clin N Am* 2007; **16**: 677–693.

14. Mokhtar MM, Abdel-Fattah M. Major birth defects amongst infants with Down syndrome in Alexandria, Egypt (1995–2000): trends and risk factors. *East Mediterr Health J* 2001; **7**: 441–51.

15. Ashok M, Thangavel G, Indrani S, *et al.* Atrioventricular septal defect: associated anomalies and aneuploidy in prenatal life. *Indian Pediatr* 2003; **40**: 659–64.

16. Gaynor JW, Gerdes M, Zackai EH, *et al.* Apolipoprotein E genotype and neurodevelopment sequelae on infant cardiac surgery. *J Thorac Cardiovasc Surg* 2003; **126**: 1736–45.

17. Mahle WT, Tavani F, Zimmerman RA, *et al.* An MRI study of neurological injury before and after congenital heart surgery. *Circulation* 2002; **106**: I109–14.

18. Limperopoulos C, Majnemer A, Shevell MI, *et al.* Predictors of developmental disabilities after open heart surgery in young children with congenital heart defects. *J Pediatr* 2002; **141**: 51–8.

19. Miller SP, McQuillen PS. Neurology of congenital heart disease: insight from brain imaging. *Arch Dis Child Fetal Neonatal Ed* 2007; **92**: F435–7.

20. Gaynor JW. Periventricular leukomalacia following neonatal and infant cardiac surgery. *Semin Thorac Cardiovasc Surg Pediatr Card Surg Annu* 2004; **7**: 133–40.

21. Galli KK, Zimmerman RA, Jarvik GP, *et al.* Periventricular leukomalacia is common after neonatal cardiac surgery. *J Thorac Cardiovasc Surg* 2004; **127**: 692–704.

22. Hsia TY, Gruber PJ. Factors influencing neurological outcome after neonatal cardiopulmonary bypass: what we can and cannot control. *Ann Thorac Surg* 2006; **81**: S2381–8.

23. Glauser TA, Rorke LB, Weinberg PM, *et al.* Congenital brain anomalies associated with the hypoplastic left heart syndrome. *Pediatrics* 1990; **85**: 984–90.

24. Rosenthal GL. Patterns of prenatal growth among infants with cardiovascular malformations: possible fetal hemodynamic effects. *Am J Epidemiol* 1996; **143**: 505–13.

25. Te Pas AB, van Wezel-Meijler G, Bokenkamp-Gramann R, *et al.* Preoperative cranial ultrasound findings in infants with major congenital heart disease. *Acta Paediatr* 2005; **94**: 1597–603.

26. Miller SP, McQuillen PS, Hamrick S, *et al.* Abnormal brain development in newborns with congenital heart disease. *N Engl J Med* 2007; **357**: 1928–38.

27. McQuillen PS, Hamrick SEG, Perez MJ, *et al.* Balloon atrial septostomy is associated with preoperative stroke in neonates with transposition of the great arteries. *Circulation* 2006; **113**: 280–5.

28. McQuillen PS, Barkovic AJ, Hamrick SEG, *et al.* Temporal and anatomic risk profile of brain injury with neonatal repair of congenital heart defects. *Stroke* 2007; **38**: 736–41.

29. Bellinger DC, Wypij D, duPlessis AJ, *et al.* Neurodevelopmental status at eight years in children with Dextro-transposition of the great arteries: the Boston Circulatory Arrest Trial. *J Thorac Cardiovasc Surg* 2003; **126**: 1385–96.

30. Kurth CD, Priestley M, Watzman HM, *et al.* Desflurane confers neurologic protection for deep hypothermic circulatory arrest in newborn pigs. *Anesthesiology* 2001; **95**: 959–64.

31. Kawaguchi M, Furuya H, Patel PM. Neuroprotective effects of anesthetic agents. *J Anesth* 2005; **19**: 150–6.

32. Reid RW, Warner DS. Pro: arguments for use of barbiturates in infants and children undergoing deep hypothermic circulatory arrest. *J Cardiovasc Anesth* 1998; **12**: 591–4.

33. Peek GJ, Firmin RK. The inflammatory and coagulative response to prolonged extracorporeal membrane oxygenation, a review. *ASAIO J* 1999; **45**: 250–63.

34. Westaby S, Saatvedt K, White S, *et al.* Is there a relationship between cognitive dysfunction and systemic inflammatory response after cardiopulmonary bypass? *Ann Thorac Surg* 2001; **71**: 667–72.

35. Stump DA. Embolic factors associated with cardiac surgery. *Semin Cardiothorac Vasc Anesth* 2005; **9**: 151–2.

36. Prasongsukarn K, Borger MA. Reducing cerebral emboli during cardiopulmonary bypass. *Semin Cardiothorac Vasc Anesth* 2005; **9**: 153–8.

37. Ehrlich MP, McCullough JN, Zhang N, *et al.* Effect of hypothermia on cerebral blood flow and metabolism in the pig. *Ann Thorac Surg* 2002; **73**: 191–7.

38. Neptune WB, Bougas JA, Panico FG. Open-heart surgery without the need for donor-blood priming in the pump oxygenator. *N Engl J Med* 1960; **263**: 111–15.

39. Jonas RA, Wypij D, Roth SJ, *et al.* The influence of hemodilution on outcome after hypothermic cardiopulmonary bypass: results of a randomized trial in infants. *J Thorac Cardiovasc Surg* 2003; **126**: 1765–74.

40. Jaggers JJ, Ungerleider RM. Cardiopulmonary bypass in infants and children. In Mavroudis C, Backer CL, eds., *Pediatric Cardiac Surgery*. Philadelphia, PA: Mosby, 2003: 171–93.

41. del Nido PJ, McGowan FX. Surgical approaches, cardiopulmonary bypass in pediatric cardiac surgery. In Sellke FW, Swanson SCJ, del Nido P, eds., *Surgery of the Chest*. Philadelphia, PA: Elsevier Saunders, 2005: 1821–58.

42. du Plessis AJ, Jonas RA, Wypij D, *et al.* Perioperative effects of alpha-stat versus pH-stat strategies for deep hypothermic cardiopulmonary bypass in infants. *J Thorac Cardiovasc Surg* 1997; **114**: 991–1001.

43. Hiramatsu T, Miura T, Forbess JM, *et al.* pH strategies and cerebral energetics before and after circulatory arrest. *J Thorac Cardiovasc Surg* 1995; **109**: 948–57.

44. Jonas RA. Optimal pH strategy for CPB in neonates, infants and children. *Perfusion* 1998; **13**: 377–87.

45. Scallan MJH. Cerebral injury during pediatric heart surgery: perfusion issues. *Perfusion* 2004; **19**: 221–8.

46. Gravlee GP, Davis RF, Kurusz M, *et al. Cardiopulmonary Bypass: Principles and Practice*, 2nd edn. Philadelphia, PA: Lippincott Williams & Wilkins, 2000: Chapter 30.

47. Hanley FL. Religion, politics . . . deep hypothermic circulatory arrest. *J Thorac Cardiovasc Surg* 2005; **130**: 1236.

48. Gaynor JW, Nicholson SC, Jarvik GP, *et al.* Increasing duration of deep hypothermic circulatory arrest is associated with an increased incidence of postoperative electroencephalographic

seizures. *J Thorac Cardiovasc Surg* 2005; **130**: 1278–86.

49. Newburger JW, Jonas RA, Wernozsky G, *et al.* A comparison of the perioperative neurologic effects of hypothermic circulatory arrest versus low-flow cardiopulmonary bypass in infant heart surgery. *N Engl J Med* 1993; **329**: 1057–64.

50. Ungerleider RM, Gaynor JW. The Boston Circulatory Arrest Study: an analysis. *J Thorac Cardiovasc Surg* 2004; **127**: 1256–61.

51. Wypij D, Newburger JW, Rappaport LA, *et al.* The effect of duration of deep hypothermic circulatory arrest in infant heart surgery on late neurodevelopment: the Boston Circulatory Arrest Trial. *J Thorac Cardiovasc Surg* 2003; **126**: 1397–403.

52. Amir G, Ramamoorthy C, Riemer RK, *et al.* Neonatal brain protection and deep hypothermic circulatory arrest: pathophysiology of ischemic neuronal injury and protective strategies. *Ann Thorac Surg* 2005; **80**: 1955–64.

53. Austin EH, Edmonds HL, Auden SM, *et al.* Benefit of neurophysiologic monitoring for pediatric cardiac surgery. *J Thorac Cardiovasc Surg* 1997; **114**: 707–16.

54. Sakamoto T, Duebener LF, Laussen PC, *et al.* Cerebral ischemia caused by obstructed superior vena cava cannula is detected by near-infrared spectroscopy. *J Cardiothorac Vasc Anesth* 2004; **18**: 293–303.

55. Svenarud P, Persson M, van der Linden J. Effect of CO_2 insufflation on the number and behaviour of air microemboli in open-heart surgery: a randomized clinical trial. *Circulation* 2004; **109**: 1127–32.

56. Bronicki RA, Backer CL, Baden HP, *et al.* Dexamethasone reduces the inflammatory response to cardiopulmonary bypass in children. *Ann Thorac Surg* 2000; **69**: 1490–5.

57. Checchia PA, Bronicki RA, Costello JM, *et al.* Steroid use before pediatric cardiac operations using cardiopulmonary bypass: an international survey of 36 centers. *Pediatr Crit Care Med* 2005; **6**: 441–4.

58. Elliott M. Modified ultrafiltration and open heart surgery in children. *Pediatr Anaesth* 1999; **9**: 1–5.

59. Rodriguez RA, Ruel M, Broecker L, *et al.* High flow rates during modified ultrafiltration decrease cerebral blood flow velocity and venous oxygen saturation in infants. *Ann Thorac Surg* 2005; **80**: 22–8.

60. Ungerleider RM, Shen I, Yeh T, *et al.* Routine mechanical ventricular assist following the Norwood procedure improved neurologic outcome and excellent hospital survival. *Ann Thorac Surg* 2004; **77**: 18–22.

61. Peek GJ, Firmin RK. Extracorporeal membrane oxygenation for pediatric cardiac support. *Coron Artery Dis* 1997; **8**: 371–89.

62. Hetzer R, Loebe M, Potapov EV, *et al.* Circulatory support with pneumatic paracorporeal ventricular assist device in infants and children. *Ann Thorac Surg* 1998; **66**: 1498–506.

63. Edwards AD, Azzopardi D. Hypothermic neural rescue treatment: from laboratory to cotside? *Arch Dis Child Fetal Neonatal Ed* 1998; **78**: F88–91.

64. Liu WG, Qiu WS, Zhang Y, *et al.* Effects of selective brain cooling in patients with severe traumatic brain injury: a preliminary study. *J Int Med Res* 2006; **34**: 58–64.

65. Gunn AJ, Gunn TR, de Haan HH, *et al.* Dramatic neuronal rescue with prolonged selective head cooling after ischemia in fetal lambs. *J Clin Invest* 1997; **99**: 248–56.

66. Paret G, Tirosh R, Lotan D, *et al.* Early prediction of neurological outcome after falls in children: metabolic and clinical markers. *J Accid Emerg Med* 1999; **16**: 186–8.

67. Chiaretti A, De Benedictis R, Langer A, *et al.* Prognostic implications of hyperglycaemia in paediatric head injury. *Childs Nerv Syst* 1998; **14**: 455–9.

68. Steward DJ, DaSilva CA, Flegel T. Elevated blood glucose levels may increase the danger of neurological deficit following profound hypothermic cardiac arrest. *Anesthesiology* 1998; **68**: 653.

69. Ballweg JA, Wernovsky G, Gaynor JW. Neurodevelopmental outcomes following congenital heart surgery. *Pediatr Cardiol* 2007; **28**: 126–33.

70. Mahle WT. Neurologic and cognitive outcomes in children with congenital heart disease. *Curr Opinion Pediatr* 2001; **13**: 482–6.

71. Gaynor JW, Wernovsky G, Jarvik GP, *et al.* Patient characteristics are important determinants of neurodevelopmental outcome at one year of age after neonatal and infant cardiac surgery. *J Thorac Cardiovasc Surg* 2007; **133**: 1344–53.

72. Robertson CMT, Joffe AR, Sauve RS, *et al.* Outcomes from an interprovincial program of newborn open heart surgery. *J Pediatr* 2004; **144**: 86–92.

73. Atallah J, Joffe AR, Robertson CMT, *et al.* Two-year general and neurodevelopmental outcomes after neonatal complex cardiac surgery in patients with deletion 22q11.2: a comparative study. *J Thorac Cardiovasc Surg* 2007; **134**: 772–9.

74. Forbess JM, Visconti KJ, Hancock-Friesen C, *et al.* Neurodevelopmental outcome after congenital heart surgery: results from an institutional registry. *Circulation* 2002; **106**: I95–102.

75. Hack M, Wilson-Costello D, Friedman H, *et al.* Neurodevelopment and predictors of outcomes of children with birth weights of less than 1000 g: 1992–1995. *Arch Pediatr Adolesc Med* 2000; **154**: 725–31.

76. Hintz SR, Kendrick DE, Vohr BR, *et al.* Changes in neurodevelopmental outcomes at 18–22 months corrected age among infants born at less than 25 weeks gestation 1993–1999. *Pediatrics* 2005; **115**: 1645–51.

77. Wernovsky G, Stiles KM, Gauvreau K, *et al.* Cognitive development after Fontan operation. *Circulation* 2000; **102**: 883–9.

78. Mahle WT, Viconti KJ, Freier C, *et al.* Relationship of surgical approach to neurodevelopmental outcomes in hypoplastic left heart syndrome. *Pediatrics* 2006; **117**: e90–7.

79. Licht DJ, Wang J, Silvestre DW, *et al.* Preoperative cerebral blood flow is diminished in neonates with severe congenital heart defects. *J Thorac Cardiovasc Surg* 2004; **128**: 841–9.

80. Ilke L, Hale K, Fashaw L, *et al.* Developmental outcome of patients with hypoplastic left heart syndrome treated with heart transplantation. *J Pediatr* 2003; **142**: 20–5.

81. Mahle WT, Clancy RR, Moss EM, *et al.* Neurodevelopmental outcome and lifestyle assessment in school-aged and adolescent children with hypoplastic left heart syndrome. *Pediatrics* 2000; **105**: 1082–9.

82. Hack M, Taylor HG, Drotar D, *et al.* Poor predictive validity of the Bayley Scales of Infant Development for

cognitive function of extremely low birth weight children at school age. *Pediatrics* 2005; **116**: 333–41.

83. McGrath E, Wypij D, Rappaport LA, *et al.* Prediction of IQ and achievement at age 8 years from neurodevelopmental status at age 1 year in children with D-transposition of the great arteries. *Pediatrics* 2004; **114**: e572–6.

84. Alton GY, Robertson CMT, Sauve R, *et al.* Early childhood health, growth, and neurodevelopmental outcomes after complete repair of total anomalous pulmonary venous connection at 6 weeks or younger. *J Thorac Cardiovasc Surg* 2007; **133**: 905–11.

85. Wypij D, Jonas RA, Bellinger DC, *et al.* The effect of hematocrit during hypothermic cardiopulmonary bypass in infant heart surgery: results from the combined Boston hematocrit trials. *J Thorac Cardiovasc Surg* 2008; **135**: 355–60.

86. Newburger JW, Wypij D, Bellinger DC, *et al.* Length of stay after infant heart surgery is related to cognitive outcome at age 8 years. *J Pediatr* 2003; **143**: 67–73.

Management of the depressed or neurologically dysfunctional neonate
Neonatal resuscitation: immediate management

Louis P. Halamek and Julie M. R. Arafeh

Introduction

Despite the fact that recent studies suggest that postpartum events account for only a fraction of untoward outcomes such as cerebral palsy, mental retardation, and chronic seizure disorders, management of the newborn during the immediate postpartum period is often subject to rigorous scrutiny by malpractice attorneys and their medical consultants. Because the potential for cerebral injury during the intrapartum period is real, it is critical that evidence-based principles of neonatal resuscitation as described in the Neonatal Resuscitation Program (NRP) of the American Academy of Pediatrics (AAP) be applied in an effort to attenuate or even reverse pathologic processes originating in utero.

Adequate maternal cardiac output and arterial oxygen content, in addition to a functioning placenta, serve to support the metabolic needs of the fetus. Disruption of oxygen supply to the fetus may have consequences after birth depending on the severity and duration of decreased oxygen delivery. Anything that impacts the health of the pregnant woman may also have adverse effects on the fetus. Fetal oxygen delivery may be impaired by poor maternal cardiopulmonary function such as that seen in cystic fibrosis and cardiomyopathy; altered uterine blood flow as in maternal hemorrhage; chronically or acutely diminished placental perfusion due to pregnancy-induced hypertension and uterine hyperstimulation; or umbilical cord dysfunction as in umbilical cord prolapse. Detection of fetal stress during the intrapartum period relies mainly on monitoring of the fetal heart rate. When a non-reassuring fetal heart rate is present, maneuvers to restore adequate oxygen delivery to the fetus are indicated. These attempts at intrauterine resuscitation include maternal repositioning, intravenous fluid administration, and delivery of oxygen to the mother. While these maneuvers are standard of care for fetal resuscitation during labor and delivery, there is little scientific evidence to support their use. One randomized prospective trial did find an increase in fetal oxygen saturation during labor in term infants with a reassuring fetal heart tracing following placement of the mother in the lateral recumbent position, administration of a 1000 mL fluid bolus, and application of

oxygen with a tight fitting non-rebreather face mask at 10 liters/minute [1]. In cases where persistent severe variable decelerations (attributed to umbilical cord compression) are noted, infusion of fluid into the uterine cavity in a procedure known as amnioinfusion should be considered, according to the American College of Obstetricians and Gynecologists [2]. Replacement of the cushioning effect of amniotic fluid on areas of the umbilical cord vulnerable to compression has been shown to be successful in resolving variable decelerations [3].

When maternal conditions exist that have the potential to negatively affect the fetus, or in fact fetal stress has been detected, communication of this information to the neonatal resuscitation team is mandatory. Of particular importance is the transfer of information concerning events that clearly impact the fetus, such as the presence of severe blood loss at the time of delivery; because the source of the blood loss often cannot be prospectively determined to be maternal or fetal in origin, the team caring for the neonate must be prepared to replace large amounts of volume rapidly in order to successfully resuscitate the potentially hypovolemic newborn. Lack of clear communication and coordination of efforts between obstetric and neonatal healthcare professionals places the stressed newborn in a dangerous situation. In July of 2004, the United States Joint Commission on Accreditation of Healthcare Organizations (JCAHO) issued a Sentinel Event Alert detailing 47 cases of neonatal mortality or severe neonatal morbidity reported since 1996 [4]. This alert was updated at the end of 2005 to include a total of 109 cases. Root cause analyses performed in these cases revealed that inadequate communication played a significant role in the outcome of more than 70% of the cases. In response to these findings JCAHO recommended that healthcare facilities where newborns are delivered conduct team training and debriefings such as those pioneered at the Center for Advanced Pediatric and Perinatal Education (CAPE, http://www.cape.lpch.org).

Cardiopulmonary resuscitation of the newborn
Anticipation and planning

The majority of newborns will not require resuscitation in the delivery room. Prenatal findings that are consistent with a smooth transition to extrauterine life include full-term gestation, no history or evidence of fetal infection, clear amniotic

Fetal and Neonatal Brain Injury, 4th edition, ed. David K. Stevenson, William E. Benitz, Philip Sunshine, Susan R. Hintz, and Maurice L. Druzin. Published by Cambridge University Press. © Cambridge University Press 2009.

fluid, and no evidence of fetal stress on fetal heart-rate monitoring. In circumstances where these conditions are present, the newborn should be dried and stimulated, airway cleared if necessary, heart rate and respiratory effort assessed, and placed on the mother's chest to maintain euthermia if her condition allows [5]. Because it is impossible to predict with absolute certainty which fetuses will present as neonates in distress, those responsible for caring for the newborn in the delivery room must always be prepared to deliver whatever level of care is required. Approximately 10% of newborns will require support of breathing efforts in the delivery room, and 1% will require more extensive resuscitation [6]. Anticipation of the infant who will require resuscitation will be facilitated by clear communication with the obstetric team. Essential information that needs to be obtained prior to or immediately upon entry into the delivery room by the neonatal resuscitation team includes the gestational age of the fetus, whether meconium is present in the amniotic fluid, and the number of fetuses being delivered. This information allows the neonatal team to begin preparations for resuscitation. Other information specific to the condition of the mother or fetus(es), including chronic conditions such as intrauterine growth restriction and acute emergencies like uterine rupture, will also prove helpful to the neonatal team.

Appropriately trained personnel

Professionals trained in neonatal resuscitation must be readily available 24 hours a day in any hospital that offers obstetrical services [7]. According to the NRP Provider Manual:

> At every delivery, there should be at least 1 person who can be immediately available to the baby as his or her only responsibility and who is capable of initiating resuscitation. Either this person or someone else who is immediately available should have the skills required to perform a complete resuscitation, including endotracheal intubation and administration of medications. It is not sufficient to have someone "on-call" (either at home or in a remote area of the hospital) for newborn resuscitation in the delivery room.
>
> [6, p. 1–16]

When delivery of a stressed infant is anticipated, responsibility for various aspects of the resuscitation should be delegated to each team member prior to delivery. These tasks depend on the problems anticipated. One team member should attend to the airway and assist breathing, if necessary. Another member should palpate the umbilical cord or ausculate the chest to assess the heart rate, provide this information to the team, and initiate chest compressions if required. A third professional should assume responsibility for other procedures such as umbilical venous cannulation or thoracentesis. If necessary, other team members should prepare and administer drugs and record the progress of the resuscitation. Ideally the team member directing the resuscitation should not be responsible for any of these tasks in order that he or she can focus full attention on the overall condition of the neonate and the performance of the entire team. Also, in an ideal situation, documentation of the

techniques used, timing of interventions, the use and dosage of medications, and the response of the newborn to these procedures should be delegated to an individual who is not directly involved in the resuscitation. Documentation of the events of a resuscitation in a post-hoc manner via recall is suboptimal at best and creates a situation that is ripe for misrepresentation and misunderstanding, potentially leading to serious legal consequences.

Equipment

In any situation where resuscitation may be needed, appropriate equipment must be readily available (Table 39.1). A clearly identified clean and warm environment in close proximity to the location of birth where all potentially necessary resuscitation equipment is easily located must be available. This equipment must be checked periodically to insure that all items are readily accessible and are in working order. If the newborn nursery is not adjacent to the delivery room, additional equipment may need to be located in the delivery room to allow more thorough stabilization of the newborn prior to transfer to the nursery. Ready access to equipment allowing blood gas, hematocrit, and glucose determinations is also important. Other equipment, supplies, and items may also be required. For example, blood products (preferably cross-matched against maternal blood) should be available for infants with severe isoimmune hemolytic disease or blood loss due to placenta abnormalities such as vasa previa; large-bore intravenous catheters should be available to drain large pleural or pericardial effusions; and other items may be mandated by unique clinical situations. Finally, universal precautions should be observed by all professionals in the delivery room. Every team member should wear gloves and other protective devices as necessary.

Rapid cardiopulmonary assessment in the delivery room

Immediate assessment of the stressed infant by experienced professionals is critically important. This should begin with immediate assessment of the neonate's heart rate, respiratory effort, color, tone, and response to stimulation in the first 10–20 seconds after birth. Re-evaluation of heart rate, respirations, and color every 30 seconds during the resuscitation provides an assessment of the efficacy of the resuscitative measures and the need for continued or more aggressive interventions. Apgar scores should be assigned and recorded at 1 minute and every 5 minutes thereafter until a score of seven or more is attained.

The algorithm for neonatal resuscitation described in the NRP Provider Manual has been developed to guide healthcare professionals in caring for the newborn regardless of the setting or cause of stress (Figure 39.1) [6]. After the initial rapid cardiopulmonary assessment is complete, during which time drying, wiping, and placing the infant on pre-warmed dry linens in a warm environment is taking place, the ABCD (Airway, Breathing, Circulation, Drugs) approach to resuscitation

Table 39.1. Equipment for neonatal resuscitation

Suction equipment	Bulb syringe
	Wall/mechanical suction and tubing
	Catheters: 5–6F, 8F, 10F, 12–14F
	Feeding tube 8F, syringe (20 mL)
	Meconium aspirator
Bag/mask equipment	Self-inflating or flow-inflating bag or T-piece resuscitator
	Face masks: cushioned or soft rims
	Oxygen wall regulator or tank
	Oxygen tubing
Intubation equipment	Laryngoscope handle, batteries
	Laryngoscope blades (#0, #1), bulbs
	Endotracheal tubes: 2.5, 3.0, 3.5, 4.0
	Scissors
	Device to secure endotracheal tube or tape
	Alcohol wipes
	CO_2 detector
Medications	Epinephrine 1:10 000 (1.0 mg/mL)
	100–250 mL isotonic crystalloid
	Sodium bicarb 4.2% (5 mEq/10 mL)
	Naloxone HCl (0.4 mg/mL)
	Dextrose 10%, 250 mL
	Normal saline flushes
	Umbilical vessel catheterization kit
	Syringes: 1, 3, 5, 10, 20, 50 mL
	Needles: needleless or 25, 21, 18 g
Miscellaneous	Personal protection gear
	Radiant warmer or heat source
	Resuscitation area: firm, padded
	Apgar timer or timer with second hand
	Warm blankets or towels
	Stethescope (neonatal)
	Tape
	Oropharyngeal airways: 0, 00, 000
Optional equipment	Stylet
	Laryngeal mask airway
	Cardiac monitor and pulse oximetry (optional in delivery room)
	Compressed air
	Oxygen blender
	Plastic wrap or gallon-size plastic bag
	Warming pad (chemical activated)
	Transport incubator

Note:
From Kattwinkel, *Neonatal Resuscitation Textbook*, 5th edn. [6].

should be carried out. During this time the newborn should be protected from heat loss in order to decrease oxygen consumption [8]. Hypothermia and hyperthermia should be avoided and, in the immediate minutes after birth, it is recommended that the neonate be maintained in a neutral thermal environment.

Airway

Several techniques may be utilized to clear the upper airway. Secretions near the surface can be wiped away with a towel or gauze pad. A bulb syringe can be used to clear the mouth and nose after delivery. Suction catheters may be used to reach deeper into the airway, but team members must be aware that vigorous and aggressive suctioning of the pharyngeal region can cause laryngeal spasm and vagally mediated bradycardia [9]. The approach to the newborn delivered through meconium-stained amniotic fluid is discussed later in this chapter.

Breathing (ventilation)

Newborns should be placed supine with the head and neck in a "sniffing" position to open the airway. Effective stimulation may be all that is required to elicit an appropriate response in an infant who is cyanotic and/or bradycardic. For those requiring additional support, positive-pressure ventilation (PPV) with a face mask may be used. The face mask should have a cushioned rim and provide a seal around the mouth and nose to prevent leakage of air. Creating and maintaining a good seal on the newborn's face is a critical component of ventilation with a face mask, and acquisition and maintenance of this technical skill requires practice. A small dead space of 5 mL or less is desired. The pressure required to establish effective ventilation varies with each patient, but the peak inspiratory pressure (PIP) and duration of inspiration (inspiratory time) should be sufficient to achieve chest excursion, audible breath sounds, and improvement in heart rate. PIPs up to 40 cm of H_2O and inspiratory times of 1 second may be required during the first few breaths in order to establish a normal functional residual capacity (FRC), and respiratory rates of 40–60 breaths per minute should be used. As the patient begins to generate effective spontaneous respirations, PIP and rate should be decreased. Gastric distension is one of the side effects of PPV, but it can be treated by insertion of either a 5- or an 8-French orogastric tube to achieve decompression.

The types of resuscitation devices used to provide PPV with a face mask include the self-inflating bag, the flow-inflating bag, and the T-piece resuscitator. Bennett *et al.* compared these three devices and found that while the T-piece increased the PIP over a longer period of time, the maximum pressure delivered decreased with each ventilation. The T-piece and the flow-inflating bag were better able to maintain a more sustained inflation pressure than the self-inflating bag. The technical skill necessary to use the flow-inflating bag effectively requires more practice than either the self-inflating bag or the T-piece resuscitator [10].

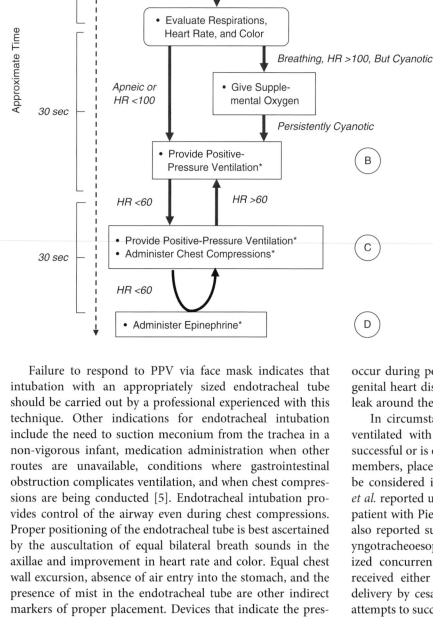

BIRTH

Fig. 39.1. Algorithm for neonatal resuscitation. From Kattwinkel, *Neonatal Resuscitation Textbook*, 5th edn. [6].

Failure to respond to PPV via face mask indicates that intubation with an appropriately sized endotracheal tube should be carried out by a professional experienced with this technique. Other indications for endotracheal intubation include the need to suction meconium from the trachea in a non-vigorous infant, medication administration when other routes are unavailable, conditions where gastrointestinal obstruction complicates ventilation, and when chest compressions are being conducted [5]. Endotracheal intubation provides control of the airway even during chest compressions. Proper positioning of the endotracheal tube is best ascertained by the auscultation of equal bilateral breath sounds in the axillae and improvement in heart rate and color. Equal chest wall excursion, absence of air entry into the stomach, and the presence of mist in the endotracheal tube are other indirect markers of proper placement. Devices that indicate the presence of CO_2 in exhaled breaths by a change in color can also be used to confirm proper endotracheal tube placement. However, caution must be exercised, as false-negative readings may

occur during poor pulmonary perfusion, cardiac arrest, congenital heart disease, incomplete exhalation, and excessive air leak around the tube [11,12].

In circumstances where the infant cannot be adequately ventilated with a face mask and intubation has not been successful or is outside of the skill set of the resuscitation team members, placement of a laryngeal mask airway (LMA) may be considered in order to provide a temporary airway. Yao *et al.* reported using an LMA successfully for several days in a patient with Pierre-Robin syndrome [13]. Johr and colleagues also reported successful management of a patient with a laryngotracheoesophageal cleft using an LMA [14]. In a randomized concurrent control study of 40 term newborns who received either endotracheal intubation or LMA following delivery by cesarean, Esmail *et al.* compared insertion time, attempts to successful insertion, duration of PPV and continuous positive airway pressure (CPAP), hemoglobin oxygen saturation, Apgar scores, and trauma related to insertion, and concluded that the LMA is an easy and effective means of managing a neonatal airway [15]. In a review of the literature on LMA use, Udaeta and Weiner reported a lack of studies comparing use of LMAs to the more traditional methods of ventilation such as bag-mask and endotracheal intubation [16]. They found a single study suggesting that LMA insertion is comparable to endotracheal intubation during neonatal resuscitation. Evidence supporting LMA use with anatomically difficult airways is stronger, but limited to case studies.

Continuous positive airway pressure (CPAP) has been proposed as a way to support ventilation in newborns who are spontaneously breathing but who continue to display increased work of breathing or suboptimal oxygenation, as in preterm infants with respiratory distress syndrome (RDS). CPAP delivers oxygen to the lungs under sustained pressure and has been found to be effective at establishing FRC, reducing work of breathing, and facilitating exchange of oxygen and carbon dioxide. Maintaining patency of the upper airway and establishing FRC can be problematic for preterm infants due to surfactant deficiency and inadequate inspiratory pressure [17–20]. CPAP effectively expands the lung, establishes FRC, and improves gas exchange [21–24]. Excessive CPAP, however, can increase pressure in the chest, reducing cardiac output and increasing the work of breathing for the newborn; it has also been associated with pneumothorax. Despite the literature supporting the beneficial effects of CPAP in newborns with RDS, data are currently insufficient to definitively support or refute its use during neonatal resuscitation, and many questions remain to be answered regarding the optimal methods and pressures to be used [25]. Thus an individualized approach is recommended. Currently, CPAP has not been adequately studied in the human neonate compared to PPV, and therefore its use cannot be routinely recommended.

Management of the infant with meconium staining of the amniotic fluid

The presence of meconium in the amniotic fluid places the newborn at risk for meconium aspiration. Meconium aspiration is a potentially life-threatening pulmonary disease and is discussed at length in Chapter 36. Obstetric and neonatal management of the infant with meconium-stained fluid at delivery has changed dramatically in the past decade as more evidence regarding the efficacy of traditional therapies has been generated. A large prospective multicenter randomized controlled international trial did not show a reduction in meconium aspiration syndrome with perineal suctioning; thus suctioning of the naso- and oropharynx while the fetal head is on the perineum is no longer routinely recommended [26]. Another large prospective multicenter randomized controlled international trial revealed that infants with meconium-stained fluid who are *vigorous* at birth (i.e., demonstrating adequate respirations, heart rate above 100 beats per minute, and good muscle tone) do not benefit from endotracheal intubation and suctioning immediately after birth, and this once routine practice is no longer indicated [27,28]. If,

however, the newborn is depressed (bradycardic, bradypneic, hypotonic) direct laryngoscopy and suctioning with an appropriate-sized endotracheal tube and meconium aspirator should be performed without delay. After suction is applied and the endotracheal tube and meconium aspirator are removed from the airway, PPV is indicated. Repeated attempts at intubation and suctioning in an effort to remove all of the particulate matter in the trachea are not indicated in newborns with persistent low heart rate and poor respiratory effort.

Use of oxygen

Oxygen is a drug, and like all drugs it possesses potentially toxic as well as therapeutic actions. Inappropriate use of oxygen has been associated with the development of acute lung injury (acute respiratory distress syndrome or ARDS), chronic lung injury (bronchopulmonary dysplasia or BPD), and retinopathy of prematurity (ROP). While historically most centers in the USA have utilized 100% oxygen in neonatal resuscitation, recent studies have indicated that the use of concentrations as low as room air (21%) are equally as or more effective than 100% oxygen [29–32]. Saugstad et al. conducted a prospective, multicenter, international (both developed and developing countries) controlled trial of 21% versus 100% oxygen in 609 newborns weighing more than 999 g at birth. The study involved 288 neonates in the 21% oxygen group and 321 in the 100% oxygen group. The incidence of grade II/III hypoxic–ischemic encephalopathy (HIE) did not differ between the groups, but the newborns resuscitated with 21% oxygen recovered more quickly than those resuscitated with 100% oxygen. Neurologic follow-up of 213 infants at 18 and 24 months of age revealed no significant differences in the incidence of neurodevelopmental handicap or rate of growth between the two groups [30,32]. Vento et al. confirmed these results in another study involving fewer patients and also showed that oxidative stress (as measured by the ratio of reduced to oxidized glutathione) was significantly higher in those patients resuscitated with 100% oxygen [33]. In a follow-up study, the same authors confirmed their earlier findings of increased oxidative stress in 106 full-term asphyxiated infants randomized to resuscitation with either 21% or 100% oxygen [34].

The NRP Update, available online at the NRP website (www.aap.org/nrp/nrpmain.html), states the following:

> Current evidence is insufficient to resolve all questions regarding supplemental oxygen use during neonatal resuscitation. For babies born at term, the Guidelines recommend use of 100% supplemental oxygen when a baby is cyanotic or when positive-pressure ventilation is required during neonatal resuscitation. However, research suggests that resuscitation with something less than 100% may be just as successful. If resuscitation is started with less than 100% oxygen, supplemental oxygen up to 100% should be administered if there is no appreciable improvement within 90 seconds following birth. If supplemental oxygen is unavailable, use room air to deliver positive-pressure ventilation. To reduce

excessive tissue oxygenation if a very preterm baby (less than approximately 32 weeks) is being electively delivered at your facility:

- Use an oxygen blender and pulse oximeter during resuscitation.
- Begin PPV with oxygen concentration between room air and 100% oxygen. No studies justify starting at any particular concentration.
- Adjust oxygen concentration up or down to achieve an oxyhemoglobin concentration that gradually increases toward 90%. Decrease the oxygen concentration as saturations rise over 95%.
- If the heart rate does not respond by increasing rapidly to > 100 beats per minute, correct any ventilation problem and use 100% oxygen. If your facility does not have use of an oxygen blender and pulse oximeter in the delivery room, and there is insufficient time to transfer the mother to another facility, the resources and oxygen management described for a term baby are appropriate. There is no convincing evidence that a brief period of 100% oxygen during resuscitation will be detrimental to the preterm infant. [35]

Determination of optimal oxygen concentration during resuscitation is an intense area of interest and research today. As new data become available in the next few years the guidelines are sure to evolve and become more definitive in their recommendations.

Cardiac output

If the heart rate remains less than 60 beats per minute despite adequate PPV with 100% oxygen for at least 30 seconds, cardiac compressions should be initiated [6]. Chest compressions may be performed via two methods: two fingers placed on the lower third of the sternum, or hands encircling the thorax with the thumbs placed on the lower third of the sternum. The compression depth varies depending upon the size of the infant, but should be one-third to one-half of the anterior–posterior diameter of the chest. Compressions and breaths should be coordinated in a compression : breath ratio of 3 : 1 with 90 compressions and 30 breaths occurring each minute. Heart rate should be reassessed every 30–60 seconds and compressions continued until a heart rate greater than 60 beats per minute is achieved.

In most situations ventilation and chest compressions will be sufficient to stimulate an improvement in heart rate and restore adequate cardiac output. Should the heart rate remain less than 60 beats per minute even with chest compressions, the use of inotropic and chronotropic medications and volume is indicated. The endotracheal tube may serve as an initial route of delivery for drugs, including epinephrine and atropine, and delivery via this route typically requires a higher dose than if given intravascularly. Endotracheal administration of medication should not delay securing intravascular access via the umbilical vein. Vascular access is usually achievable within minutes by cannulation of the umbilical vein, and only the presence of an omphalocele, gastroschisis, or other major anomaly in the abdominal area precludes access via this route [36]. Under emergency conditions the catheter is inserted to a depth of 2–4 cm below the skin surface until blood can be withdrawn freely; once in this position medications and volume can be given just as through a central venous

line. The catheter should not be advanced beyond this point, as in the absence of radiologic conformation of its position it could cause injury to the liver, intestine, or heart. Any umbilical venous catheter placed emergently should be removed once the patient has been resuscitated, and a new catheter placed under sterile conditions and confirmed by x-ray to be in good position if central venous access continues to be required. The umbilical artery is less than an ideal site for the administration of vasoactive medications, due to risk of vasospasm, and cannulation of the artery typically requires more time than cannulation of the vein; thus the umbilical vein is the recommended route for delivery of medications to the newborn in distress in the delivery room. An umbilical venous catheter also provides a portal for sampling of blood gases; this is a useful adjunct to physical examination during extended resuscitations.

When intravascular access is warranted but the healthcare professionals in attendance in the delivery room lack sufficient skill in umbilical venous catheter placement, the team should consider placement of an intraosseous catheter. These catheters should be readily available on IV access and code carts, and can be quickly placed into the marrow space of the tibia when emergent conditions dictate. Any medication or fluid that can be delivered into a central venous catheter can be delivered into the marrow. Physicians in hospital emergency departments should be very familiar with the placement and use of these devices, and should be called upon to assist with or perform the procedure if needed [37–39]. This technique is not recommended in small preterm neonates, who have fragile bones and relatively small intraosseus spaces. Medications should never be given directly into the heart, as the risk of coronary artery laceration, myocardial infarction, and pneumo- or hemopericardium with resultant cardiac tamponade is too great.

Epinephrine

Epinephrine has both α-adrenergic and β-adrenergic effects and is the medication used during resuscitation when the heart rate remains below 60 beats per minute despite adequate PPV and chest compressions. It should be delivered intravenously but can also be given via an endotracheal tube while intravenous access is being secured. The intravenous dose is 0.1–0.3 mL/kg of the 1/10 000 solution, and this dose may be repeated every 3–5 minutes until the heart rate improves to above 60 beats per minute. When delivered by the endotracheal tube a higher dose (0.3–1.0 mL/kg) is required [40]. The efficacy of epinephrine is reduced when the systemic pH is less than 7.1. Side effects include tachycardia, vasospasm, and tissue necrosis should extravasation occur.

Volume resuscitation

Because the cardiac ventricles of the neonate are less compliant than those of an adult, increased cardiac output does not result from expansion of an already adequate vascular volume [41]. Nonetheless, inadequate end-diastolic pressure due to decreased intravascular volume is one of the most common correctable causes of decreased cardiac output in the neonate, and hypovolemia should always be suspected in a newborn who appears to be poorly perfused in spite of an adequate heart rate and PPV. This condition should be expected in several clinical conditions such as abruptio placentae, vasa previa, and hydrops fetalis. Hypovolemia may manifest as respiratory distress in the absence of readily apparent pulmonary disease or refractory hypoxemia in a newborn who is easily ventilated. If hypovolemia is suspected, the best diagnostic procedure is also therapeutic: administration of 10 mL/kg of isotonic saline, repeated as necessary. In a delivery-room resuscitation situation, clinical indicators of efficacy include improved perfusion, better color, and correction of tachycardia. When possible, invasive measurement of central venous pressure is a useful guide to assess the adequacy of intravascular volume and any need for replacement.

Crystalloid and colloid solutions

Isotonic saline and lactated Ringer's solutions should always be readily available, as they have the advantages of being both inexpensive and in general well tolerated when used empirically. Isotonic crystalloid is effective in the treatment of hypotension, as demonstrated in several randomized controlled trials [42–44]. Colloid, in the form of cytomegalovirus-seronegative, type-specific or type O, Rh-negative blood crossmatched against the mother's blood, should be made available when acute blood loss or anemia is anticipated. Uncrossmatched type O, Rh-negative blood can also be used in emergencies, although transfusion reactions may occur. The hematocrit level should be measured approximately 4 hours after administration of the blood to determine whether additional transfusions are required.

Stabilization after cardiopulmonary resuscitation

Glucose

The cessation of glucose delivery via the placenta at the time of birth predisposes the neonate to hypoglycemia, yet under normal circumstances the term neonate is able to initiate gluconeogenesis and mobilize hepatic glycogen to maintain blood glucose levels in the normal range (40–60 mg/dL). Blood glucose levels do fall after birth, often to less than 30 mg/dL, typically achieving a nadir at about 1 hour of age; this decrease in glucose level acts as a stimulus to glycogen breakdown and gluconeogenesis, resulting in normal glucose levels by 2 hours of age in healthy term newborns even without feeding or other intervention [45]. Neonates who are small for gestational age or premature are at much higher risk of hypoglycemia secondary to diminished glycogen stores and impaired gluconeogenesis. Infants of diabetic mothers are another at-risk group, as they have increased glucose utilization, impaired gluconeogenesis, and a relative inability to mobilize hepatic glycogen stores. Fetal exposure to β-mimetic drugs (such as tocolytics) results in increased insulin secretion and exhaustion of hepatic glycogen. Hypoxia, hypothermia, hyperthermia, and infection also predispose the newborn

to hypoglycemia. When hypoglycemia is suspected during resuscitation appropriate therapy should be initiated even in the absence of a documented low blood glucose level from the laboratory. Intravenous administration of glucose (100–200 mg/kg or 1–2 mL/kg of 10% dextrose solution in water) should be followed by a continuous infusion of glucose at 6–8 mg/kg per minute. Management of hypoglycemia in the neonate is discussed in more detail in Chapter 26.

Sodium bicarbonate

Oxidative metabolism is dependent on maintaining a balance between oxygen delivery and oxygen consumption. As the delivery-to-consumption ratio approaches 2 : 1, tissues begin to shift to anaerobic metabolism and generate lactic acid. Metabolic acidosis caused by the accumulation of lactic acid after a short period of either decreased oxygen delivery or increased oxygen consumption usually corrects spontaneously once oxidative metabolism is re-established and the lactate is converted to pyruvate. When the oxygen delivery-to-consumption ratio remains unbalanced for a sustained period of time because of inadequate oxygen content in the blood (anemia, hypoxia), low oxygen delivery (bradycardia, hypotension), or increased oxygen consumption (sepsis, hyperthermia), sodium bicarbonate may be administered to ameliorate alterations in pH that may impair cellular functions. Correction of acidemia can result in improved cardiac output, tissue perfusion, and substrate utilization by reversing diminished myocardial function, increased systemic and pulmonary vascular resistance, impaired response to catecholamines, and inhibition of oxidative glucose metabolism. During cardiac arrest, or following severe asphyxia, sodium bicarbonate may be given empirically at a dose of 1 mEq/kg of a 4.2% solution; additional doses are ideally guided by blood gas analysis. It is important to remember that:

- Sodium bicarbonate is eventually converted to CO_2, which must be exhaled from the lungs before it, too, adds to the acid load in the body; therefore adequate ventilation must be established prior to administering sodium bicarbonate [46]. In fact, the blood pH does not increase and the cerebrospinal fluid pH decreases after bicarbonate administration unless adequate alveolar ventilation insures excretion of the carbon dioxide generated by the buffer reaction [47].
- Overcorrection of the pH early in resuscitation may be detrimental, because significant metabolic alkalosis impairs the dissociation of oxygen from hemoglobin and may actually impede oxygen delivery.
- Rapid infusion of sodium bicarbonate should be avoided, as hypertonic solutions have been associated with altered blood flow and subsequent organ injury [48,49]. The drug should be infused slowly over 5–10 minutes, and the concentration should not exceed 0.5 mEq/ml.
- Sodium bicarbonate administration only "buys time" in providing a temporary correction in pH, and ultimately the underlying cause of the acidosis must be treated for the patient to survive.

Naloxone

Naloxone is a pure opiate antagonist that is useful for the reversal of respiratory depression resulting from narcotic administration. Two conditions must be present in order to justify administration of naloxone to a newborn: (1) the newborn must continue to have apnea or poor respiratory effort after PPV has produced normal heart rate and color (there is no apparent cardiopulmonary etiology for the respiratory depression), and (2) the mother must have been given a narcotic in the past 4 hours but have no prior history of narcotic exposure (use or abuse) outside of labor. Administration of naloxone to a neonate whose mother is a narcotic abuser or who is enrolled in a methadone maintenance program may precipitate seizures. Because the half-life of naloxone is shorter than that of all narcotics except for fentanyl and its derivatives, any neonate receiving naloxone should be monitored continuously by skilled personnel for a minimum of 24 and preferably 48 hours to ensure that the respiratory depression due to the narcotic does not recur once the naloxone is metabolized. Naloxone is given in a dose of 0.1 mg/kg of a 1.0 mg/mL solution via either the intravenous or intramuscular route. In general naloxone should *not* be given in the delivery room. The most appropriate management of the neonate with respiratory depression suspected to be secondary to maternal narcotic administration usually is to support the patient's respirations as needed and transfer him or her to the nursery, where the patient can be monitored continuously and more information can be obtained from the obstetrical team and from ongoing examination of the newborn. Naloxone is no longer included in the NRP as a delivery-room medication. Naloxone has not been shown in human neonates to affect respiratory depression due to asphyxia, and is not recommended for use in that circumstance [50].

Cerebral resuscitation

While the focus during neonatal resuscitation has historically been on restoring cardiac and pulmonary function, protecting the brain is now receiving increasing attention as a burgeoning body of evidence suggests that it is possible to ameliorate if not reverse the cerebral dysfunction and injury caused by inadequate oxygen delivery. An evolving therapy that specifically addresses cerebral injury is the use of hypothermia. In randomized controlled trials, cooling of the head or the entire body was accomplished in term infants with indicators of hypoxic–ischemic injury including a need for resuscitation beyond 10 minutes of age, an Apgar score of < 5 at 10 minutes, pH < 7.0 or base deficit > 16 mmol/L on initial blood gas, seizures, or laboratory tests consistent with a diagnosis of hypoxic–ischemic encephalopathy (HIE). While the early results of these trials are promising, the long-term effects of this treatment remain unknown and it has not been evaluated in preterm or small-for-gestational-age neonates. A registry has been established for HIE to continue to collect data on this emerging therapy [51]. A more thorough discussion of hypothermia for HIE is found in Chapter 42 of this text.

Evidence-based resuscitation medicine

Over the past several decades a concerted effort has been made to improve the care for the new born infant by basing all treatment guidelines on the best evidence available in the medical literature. Spearheading this effort is the International Liaison Committee on Resuscitation (ILCOR). ILCOR is composed of representatives from the American Heart Association (AHA), the European Resuscitation Council, the Heart and Stroke Foundation of Canada, the Resuscitation Council of Southern Africa, the Australia and New Zealand Council on Resuscitation, and the InterAmerican Heart Foundation, with observers hailing from the Japan Resuscitation Council and the Ministry of Health in China. The mission of ILCOR is to provide a regular international forum for review and discussion of resuscitation practices and the evidence (or lack thereof) supporting them. Task forces composed of ILCOR members are assigned to review the scientific literature on specific issues in resuscitation, and to prepare both written and verbal reports on their findings. The task forces meet with other scientists and clinicians over a period of 5 years; their work culminates in a meeting of the ILCOR group at large, where consensus is reached as to the quality of the science behind current clinical practices. This review of the science is published as a document called the International Consensus on Cardiopulmonary Resuscitation and Emergency Cardiovascular Care Science and Treatment Recommendations (CoSTR) [52,53]. Once the review of the science is available, each national or regional resuscitation council then uses this review to determine its own treatment recommendations.

Delivery-room decision making

The delivery room is the scene of many emotionally laden and ethically challenging situations that potentially carry lifelong consequences for the newborn and parents alike. However, it should not be a place where difficult and irrevocable decisions are made without the availability of important objective data and the knowledge of parental desires. Deciding whether to initiate, forgo, or terminate resuscitation is often both intellectually challenging and emotionally draining, and in situations where the presumed gestational age is at the borderline of viability, or where the presence of malformations or other conditions clouds potential long-term outcome, or where the wishes of the parents are unknown, discordant, or at odds with those of the healthcare professionals charged with caring for the newborn, it becomes even more so [54,55]. An editorial by Saigal on the limits of viability points out the fact that predicting survival based on outcomes of groups of patients is intrinsically inaccurate when applied to an individual patient [56]. Furthermore, the likelihood of impairment in individual patients is even less predictable [57–61]. The same critical issues apply to all infants who have birth injuries and uncertain prognoses. In all of these instances parental input becomes of paramount importance [62–64].

Stevenson and Goldworth point out that the emotionally exhausting decision to withhold or withdraw life support in the early transitional period after birth is common but should never be routine [65]. The potential for development of functional status in the fetus or newborn is the single most important factor affecting immediate intervention and long-term outcome. The dilemma is that, although there is a threshold of maturity or extent of brain injury beyond which survival, or survival without devastating sequelae, is not possible, the exact threshold for a particular individual is typically not known prior to the attempt to assist the person to survive. Although the proportion of individuals who must face an ultimate threshold increases dramatically below 25 weeks' gestation, there is considerable variation in performance by neonates provided with appropriate technical assistance. Thus it is usually impossible at the onset of resuscitative efforts to know whether such efforts, if successful, will result in intact survival, survival with devastating neurologic injury, or prolonged dying with gradually worsening organ failure.

So what recommendations can be made to assist those faced with this tremendous responsibility? While there are no simple answers, the most important component of this process is to establish and maintain effective communication. Communication from the obstetrical team to the neonatal team of the best available information regarding gestational age, fetal condition, and other important factors is critical; without this, the neonatal team will not be able to deliver optimal care in the delivery room or in the NICU after delivery. Communication among neonatal members is necessary so that the plan of care, regardless of degree of intervention, can be carried out in a coordinated and professional manner. Finally, all of the obstetric and neonatal healthcare professionals involved in the care of the pregnant woman and her newborn must establish open lines of communication with the mother and any significant other who is involved in the decision-making process. Clear communication of medical facts, likely clinical outcomes (ideally based on objective, relevant, valid, institution-specific data), and medically acceptable options for care is an integral component of any counseling process and mandatory for establishing an atmosphere of trust and mutual respect between family members and the healthcare team.

Many times in caring for sick full-term neonates who, despite their current illness, have a high likelihood of recovery and good outcome there is a clear consensus as to the medical choices to be made on behalf of the patient. A similar circumstance exists at the other end of the spectrum of care when death is determined to be inevitable and relief of pain and discomfort coupled with emotional support of the patient and family is of paramount importance. There are clinical situations where the medically acceptable choices include options ranging from comfort care to initiation/continuation of aggressive intensive care – this is where the decision making is most complex and the consequences of the decisions made arguably carry the most potential for serious long-term physical, emotional, psychological, and financial harm. It is in these situations that the physician bears the greatest responsibility in clearly spelling out the various options for care and

the potential or likely consequences of each of these; it is also at these times that physicians must bear in mind that they share the privilege of caring for the patient for what amounts to a relatively brief period of time, and it is the parents who bear the long-term responsibility, and potentially the burden, of caring for their child. It is not the physician but the parents who are the appropriate surrogates for the child, provided that they are educated as to what is possible or not possible and what is likely or not likely, and are informed of the societal perspective represented by court precedents as pertinent to their situation. Thus, while a reasonable legal argument might be that, when there is any doubt as to outcome, initiation of resuscitative measures should always be undertaken, the moral imperative would be to defer to the parents when the outcome is in question and the medical choices are unclear.

Summary

Management of difficult deliveries and the subsequent resuscitation of the newborn are among the most intensely scrutinized and frequently criticized medical activities in medicolegal litigation (Table 39.2). Those professionals charged with caring for newborns immediately after birth are both obligated and well advised to ensure that resuscitation of the neonate is consistently performed skillfully and expeditiously according to the guidelines issued by the NRP. Optimal resuscitation

Table 39.2. A partial listing of aspects of neonatal resuscitation creating medicolegal risk

Failure to recognize a newborn in need of resuscitation
Failure to anticipate the need for extended resuscitation
Failure to assemble appropriately trained personnel in a timely fashion
Failure to follow hospital policies regarding treatment of the newborn
Ineffective communication between obstetric team and neonatal team
Ineffective communication among neonatal team members
Poorly performed cardiopulmonary resuscitation
Failure to recognize and treat an incorrectly placed endotracheal tube
Failure to achieve timely umbilical venous access for medication or volume delivery
Incorrectly placed umbilical venous catheter
Over- or under-dosage of medication
Failure to recognize a pneumothorax, pneumomediastinum, or pneumopericardium in a patient receiving positive-pressure ventilation
Failure to suction a depressed neonate with meconium
Failure to recognize the hypovolemic/anemic newborn
Delivery of peak inspiratory pressures that are too low or too high
Delivery of positive-pressure ventilations at too slow or too fast a rate
Delivery of medications through the endotracheal tube that should be administered only via the intravascular route
Failure to effectively communicate with parents
Initiating/continuing/discontinuing resuscitation against parental wishes
Lack of accurate and comprehensive documentation
Conflicting or incorrect documentation

requires anticipation and preparation, and demands intense collaboration and effective communication between the obstetric and neonatal team members. Resuscitation should begin as soon as needed after delivery, and should follow the evidence-based algorithm for assessment and intervention. Conducting an effective resuscitation requires cognitive (knowledge), technical (hands-on), and behavioral (working effectively as a team under pressure) skills, and these skills must be regularly practiced in order to maintain a high level of performance. Skillful resuscitation is capable of preventing postnatal organ injury and may also act to ameliorate the severity of any prenatal injury. This will continue to be an area of active research for the foreseeable future.

Acknowledgment

The authors wish to acknowledge the contributions of William E. Benitz, David K. Stevenson, Susan R. Hintz, and Philip Sunshine to the previous version of this chapter, large portions of which appear in this edition.

References

1. Simpson KR, James DC. Efficacy of intrauterine resuscitation techniques in improving fetal oxygen status during labor. *Obstet Gynecol* 2005; **105**: 1362–8.

2. American College of Obstetricians and Gynecologists. ACOG Practice Bulletin, Number 70, December 2005. Intrapartum fetal heart rate monitoring. *Obstet Gynecol* 2005; **106**: 1453–60.

3. Rinehart BK, Terrone DA, Barrow JH, *et al.* Randomized trial of intermittent or continuous amnioinfusion for variable decelerations. *Obstet Gynecol* 2000; **96**: 571–4.

4. The Joint Commission. *Sentinel Event Alert* 30, July 21, 2004. http://www.jointcommission.org/sentinelevents/sentineleventalert/sea_30.htm. Accessed February, 2008.

5. American Heart Association. Part 13: neonatal resuscitation guidelines. *Circulation* 2005; **112**: IV-188–95.

6. Kattwinkel J. *Neonatal Resuscitation Textbook*, 5th edn. Elk Grove Village, IL: American Academy of Pediatrics, American Heart Association, 2006.

7. Lockwood CJ, Lemons JA, eds. *Guidelines for Perinatal Care*, 6th edn. Elk Grove Village, IL: American Academy of Pediatrics, American College of Obstetricians and Gynecologists, 2007.

8. Gandy GM, Adamson SK, Cunningham N, *et al.* Thermal environment and acid base homeostasis in human infants during the first few hours of life. *J Clin Invest* 1964; **43**: 751–8.

9. Halbower AC, Jones MD. Physiologic reflexes and their impact on resuscitation of the newborn. *Clin Perinatol* 1999; **26**: 621–7.

10. Bennett S, Finer NN, Rich W, *et al.* A comparison of three neonatal resuscitation devices. *Resuscitation* 2005; **67**: 113–18.

11. Aziz HF, Martin JB, Moore JJ. The pediatric disposable end-tidal carbon dioxide detector role in endotracheal intubation in newborns. *J Perinatol* 1999; **19**: 110–13.

12. Repetto JE, Donohue PCP, Baker SF, *et al.* Use of capnography in the delivery room for assessment of endotracheal tube placement. *J Perinatol* 2001; **21**: 284–7.

13. Yao C, Wang J, Tai Y, *et al.* Successful management of a neonate with Pierre-Robin syndrome and severe upper airway obstruction by long term placement of a laryngeal mask airway. *Resuscitation* 2004; **61**: 97–9.

14. Johr M, Berger TM, Ruppen W, *et al.* Congenital laryngotracheo-oesophageal cleft: successful ventilation with the Laryngeal Mask Airway™. *Paediatr Anaesth* 2003; **13**: 68–71.

15. Esmail N, Saleh M, Ali A. Laryngeal mask airway versus endotracheal intubation for Apgar score improvement in neonatal resuscitation. *Eg J Anesth* 2002; **18**: 115–21.

16. Udaeta ME, Weiner GM. Alternative ventilation strategies: laryngeal masks. *Clin Perinatol* 2006; **33**: 99–110.

17. Milner AD, Saunders RA. Pressure and volume changes during the first breath of human neonates. *Arch Dis Child* 1977; **52**: 918–24.

18. Avery ME, Mead J. Surface properties in relation to atelectasis and hyaline membrane disease. *AMA J Dis Child* 1959; **97**: 517–23.

19. Gerhardt T, Bancalari E. Chest wall compliance in full term and preterm infants. *Acta Paediatr Scand* 1980; **69**: 359–64.

20. Heldt G, McIlroy MB. Dynamics of chest wall in preterm infants. *J Appl Physiol* 1987; **62**: 170–4.

21. Morley CJ. Continuous distending pressure. *Arch Dis Child Fetal Neonatal Ed* 1999; **81**: F152–6.

22. Saunders RA, Milner AD, Hopkin IE. The effects of continuous positive airway pressure on lung mechanics and lung volumes in the neonate. *Biol Neonate* 1976; **29**: 178–86.

23. Richardson CP, Jung AL. Effects of continuous positive airway pressure on pulmonary function and blood gases of infants with respiratory distress syndrome. *Pediatr Res* 1978; **12**: 771–4.

24. Cotton RB, Lindstom DP, Kanarek KS, *et al.* Effect of positive-end-expiratory-pressure on right ventricular output in lambs with hyaline membrane disease. *Acta Paediatr Scand* 1980; **69**: 603–6.

25. Halamek LP, Morley C. Continuous positive airway pressure during neonatal resuscitation. *Clin Perinatol* 2006; **33**: 83–98.

26. Vain NE, Szyld EG, Prudent LM, *et al.* Oropharyngeal and nasopharyngeal suctioning of meconium-stained neonates before delivery of their shoulders: multicentre, randomized controlled trial. *Lancet* 2004; **364**: 597–602.

27. Wiswell TE, Gannon CM, Jacob J, *et al.* Delivery room management of the apparently vigorous meconium-stained neonate: results of the multicenter, international collaborative trial. *Pediatrics* 2000; **106**: 1–7.

28. Halliday HL. Endotracheal intubation at birth for preventing morbidity and mortality in vigorous, meconium-stained infants born at term. *Cochrane Database Syst Rev* 2001; (1): CD000500.

29. Ramji S, Ahuja S, Thirupuram S, *et al.* Resuscitation of asphyxic newborn infants with room air or 100% oxygen. *Pediatr Res* 1993; **34**: 809–12.

30. Saugstad OD, Rootwelt T, Aalen O. Resuscitation of asphyxiated newborn infants with room air or oxygen: an international controlled trial. The Resair 2 study. *Pediatrics* 1998; **102**: e1.

31. Ramji S, Rasaily R, Mishra PK, *et al.* Resuscitation of asphyxiated newborns

with room air or 100% oxygen at birth: a multicentric trial. *Indian Pediatr* 2003; **40**: 510–17.

32. Saugstad OD, Ramji S, Irani SF, *et al.* Resuscitation of newborn infants with 21% or 100% oxygen: follow-up at 18 to 24 months. *Pediatrics* 2003; **112**: 296–300.

33. Vento M, Asensi M, Sastre J, *et al.* Resuscitation with room air instead of 100% oxygen prevents oxidative stress in moderately asphyxiated term neonates. *Pediatrics* 2001; **107**: 642–7.

34. Vento M, Asensi M, Sastre J, *et al.* Oxidative stress in asphyxiated term infants resuscitated with 100% oxygen. *J Pediatr* 2003; **142**: 240–6.

35. Neonatal Resuscitation Program. Update. www.aap.org/nrp/nrpmain. html. Accessed March 30, 2008.

36. Kitterman JA, Phibbs RH, Tooley WH. Catheterization of umbilical vessels in newborn infants. *Pediatr Clin North Am* 1970; **17**: 895–912.

37. Heinild S, Søndergaard T, Tudvad F. Bone marrow infusion in childhood: experiences from a thousand infusions. *J Pediatr* 1947; **30**: 400–12.

38. Glaeser PW, Losek JD, Nelson DB, *et al.* Pediatric intraosseous infusions: impact on vascular access time. *Am J Emerg Med* 1988; **6**: 330–2.

39. Ellemunter H, Burkhart S, Trawoger R, *et al.* Intraosseous lines in preterm and full term neonates. *Arch Dis Child Fetal Neonatal Ed* 1999; **80**: F74–5.

40. International Liaison Committee on Resuscitation. The International Liaison Committee on Resuscitation (ILCOR) consensus on science with treatment recommendations for pediatric and neonatal patients: neonatal resuscitation. *Pediatrics* 2006; **117**: e978–88.

41. Romero T, Friedman WF. Limited left ventricular response to volume overload in the neonatal period: a comparative study with the adult animal. *Pediatr Res* 1979; **13**: 910–15.

42. So KW, Fok TF, Ng PC, *et al.* Randomized controlled trial of colloid or crystalloid in hypotensive preterm infants. *Arch Dis Child Fetal Neonatal Ed* 1997; **76**: F43–6.

43. Oca MJ, Nelson M, Donn SM. Randomized trial of normal saline versus 5% albumin for the treatment of neonatal hypotension. *J Perinatol* 2003; **23**: 473–6.

44. Emery EF, Greenough A, Gamsu HR. Randomised controlled trial of colloid infusions in hypotensive preterm infants. *Arch Dis Child* 1992; **67**: 1185–8.

45. Srinivasan G, Pildes RS, Caughey M, *et al.* Plasma glucose values in normal neonates: a new look. *J Pediatr* 1986; **109**: 114–17.

46. Bishop RL, Weisfeldt ML. Sodium bicarbonate administration during cardiac arrest: effect on arterial pH, PCO_2 and osmolality. *JAMA* 1976; **235**: 506–9.

47. Berenyi KJ, Wolk M, Killip T. Cerebrospinal fluid acidosis complicating therapy of experimental cardiopulmonary arrest. *Circulation* 1975; **52**: 319–24.

48. Simmons MA, Adcock EW, Bard H, *et al.* Hypernatremia and intracranial hemorrhages in neonates. *N Engl J Med* 1974; **291**: 6–10.

49. Papile L, Burnstein J, Burnstein R, *et al.* Relationship of intravenous sodium bicarbonate infusions and cerebral intraventricular hemorrhage. *J Pediatr* 1978; **93**: 834–6.

50. Chernick V, Manfreda J, De Booy V, *et al.* Clinical trial of naloxone in birth asphyxia. *J Pediatr* 1988; **113**: 519–25.

51. Higgins RD, Raju TN, Perlman J, *et al.* Hypothermia and perinatal asphyxia: executive summary of the NICHD workshop. *J Pediatr* 2006; **148**: 170–5.

52. American Heart Association. 2005 International Consensus on CPR and ECC science with treatment recommendations. www.americanheart. org/presentor.jhtml?identifier=3022512. Accessed Nov 27, 2007.

53. American Heart Association. Part 1: introduction. *Circulation* 2005; **112**: IV-1–5.

54. Halamek, LP. The advantages of prenatal consultation by a neonatologist. *J Perinatol* 2001; **21**: 116–20.

55. Halamek LP. Prenatal consultation at the limits of viability. *NeoReviews* 2003; **4**: e153–6.

56. Saigal S. The limits of viability. *Pediatr Res* 2001; **49**: 451.

57. Wood NS, Marlow N, Costeloe K, *et al.* Neurologic and developmental disability after extremely preterm birth. EPICure Study Group. *N Engl J Med* 2000; **343**: 378–84.

58. Costeloe K, Hennessy E, Gibson AT, *et al.* The EPICure Study: outcomes to discharge from hospital for infants born at the threshold of viability. *Pediatrics* 2000; **106**: 659–71.

59. deLeeuw R, Cuttini M, Nadai M, *et al.* Treatment choices for extremely preterm infants: an international perspective. *J Pediatr* 2000; **137**: 608–15.

60. Vohr BR, Wright LL, Dusick AM, *et al.* Neurodevelopment and functional outcomes of extremely low birth weight infants in the National Institute of Child Health and Human Development Neonatal Research Network, 1993–1994. *Pediatrics* 2000; **105**: 1216–26.

61. El-Metwally D, Vohr B, Tucker R. Survival and neonatal morbidity at the limits of viability in the mid 1900s: 22 to 25 weeks. *J Pediatr* 2000; **137**: 616–22.

62. Watts J, Saigal S. Replies to malcontent: fumes from the spleen. *Pediatr Perinat Epidemiol* 1995; **9**: 375–9.

63. Saigal S, Stoskopf BL, Feeny D, *et al.* Differences in preferences for neonatal outcomes among health care professionals, parents and adolescents. *JAMA* 1999; **281**: 1991–7.

64. Lorenz JM, Paneth N. Treatment decisions for the extremely premature infant. *J Pediatr* 2000; **137**: 593–5.

65. Stevenson DK, Goldworth A. Ethical dilemmas in the delivery room. *Semin Perinatol* 1998; **22**: 198–206.

Improving performance, reducing error, and minimizing risk in the delivery room

Louis P. Halamek

Introduction

In 1999 the Institute of Medicine (IOM) published *To Err is Human: Building a Safer Health System*, a report on human error and patient safety in the USA [1]. In this report the authors estimate that between 44 000 and 98 000 Americans die each year as a result of medical errors. Although this figure has been highly debated, it is based on extrapolation of the data contained in published studies out of Colorado, Utah, and New York [2–4]. The 1999 report was followed in 2001 by another from the IOM, *Crossing the Quality Chasm: A New Health System for the 21st Century*, where the type of interventions, including training methodologies, necessary to improve patient safety were discussed [5]. Subsequently in 2004 the Joint Commission for the Accreditation of Healthcare Organizations (JCAHO) published a *Sentinel Event Alert* describing ineffective communication as a major cause in almost three-quarters of the cases of neonatal mortality or severe neonatal morbidity (lifelong serious neurological compromise) reported to that agency [6]. JCAHO recommended that hospitals that deliver newborns establish a system of training that incorporates behavioral skills such as teamwork and effective communication, and that they conduct regular clinical drills in delivery-room emergencies with these drills followed by constructive debriefings. Despite the recommendations by the IOM and JCAHO, healthcare has yet to fully examine the complex relationship among training, human performance, and medical error, and development and implementation of such training programs remains challenging.

While many factors influence the incidence of medical error in the USA today, this chapter will focus on training and education. Similarly, while medical errors occur across every medical specialty and affect all patients, this chapter will center on the newborn in the first minutes of life in the delivery room. First, the history of medical training will be reviewed. Next, new methodologies designed to improve the performance of professionals working in dynamic environments will be highlighted. Finally, the impediments to future enhancements of medical training and potential solutions to these will be discussed.

Fetal and Neonatal Brain Injury, 4th edition, ed. David K. Stevenson, William E. Benitz, Philip Sunshine, Susan R. Hintz, and Maurice L. Druzin. Published by Cambridge University Press. © Cambridge University Press 2009.

Historical perspective

Traditional medical training is essentially a two-step process. First, trainees read about the many different aspects of medical practice. This begins in the first two years of medical school, when much time is spent either studying and working from textbooks or listening to lectures describing the basic science underlying modern medical practice. Second, trainees then begin to care for real human patients. Caring for patients typically begins with trainees observing senior colleagues in the practice of medicine, followed by trainees' efforts to mimic the performance of their colleagues while under varying degrees of supervision. This has historically been described as "see one, do one, teach one;" while that phrase is an unfair criticism of medical training in many respects, certain elements continue to ring true [7].

Several assumptions underlie the traditional two-step model of medical training. First, this model assumes that current methodologies in medical education are optimal for all adult learners. Second, there exists an assumption that the close of a training period implies that the trainee is competent to practice all aspects of medicine in his or her specialty. Yet the limitations to these assumptions are obvious. Adults learn best via active participation; passive training exercises such as reading or observing others tend to be less effective than active immersion on the part of the trainee. Adults also have different strengths and weaknesses. Training models that more or less offer the same content in the same fashion to all adult learners in essence demand that these learners accommodate the training model. This failure to recognize the inherent differences in trainees impairs their ability to succeed and suppresses unique contributions from trainees with different life experiences.

In a similar fashion, acquisition of skills occurs at different rates for different trainees, and retention of skills is not uniform across trainees. Training programs that assume that exposure of the trainee to a particular environment for a defined period of time is adequate preparation for the practice of medicine fail to recognize that all training programs are by definition limited in time and depth. As an example, the Residency Review Committee for Residency Training Programs in General Pediatrics in the USA revised the requirements for residency training in 2001 by reducing the amount of time that residents spend in intensive care environments [8]. Yet there are few objective data in the medical literature regarding the time required for skill acquisition and retention in intensive care domains. Therefore it is not currently known whether the decrease in time spent in intensive care units by pediatric residents as directed by the Residency Review Committee goes too far or not far enough. In addition, there appear to be no objective measures in place for monitoring the effects of this change over time.

Other limitations to the traditional model include the relative lack of a systematic approach to clinical training due to the very random nature of patient care experiences. This model of training, based upon whatever patients are admitted to the hospital or seen in the clinic, is accurately termed "education by random opportunity" [9] (T. M. Krummel, personal communication). Because common things are common, such a model usually provides adequate training in the management of common clinical situations. However, this model is sorely deficient in preparing trainees to handle those rare but potentially devastating events that eventually occur during a professional career. Another weakness of the traditional training model is its focus on the individual trainee as the one solely responsible for patient care. In reality many medical domains are characterized by a need for communication among and coordination of multidisciplinary teams of professionals. Individuals trained in different specialties, typically in isolation from one another, are often forced in emergencies to attempt to function as an integrated team despite a lack of any real experience in doing so. Unfortunately, teams of experts do not necessarily make an expert team [10]. Because health care as a profession lacks a universally accepted theoretical model of effective team performance it has proven difficult to develop appropriate training programs and assessment tools [11]. The limitations listed previously indicate that a re-examination of the very foundations of education and training in health care is necessary in order to optimize its impact on human performance and patient safety.

First of all it must be recognized that there is a difference between *teaching* and *learning* [12]. Teaching is something that is done (passively) *to* trainees while learning is something that is done (actively) *by* trainees. Thus not everything that is *taught* is necessarily *learned*. Second, it is important to consider what can be learned. Delivering safe and effective care to patients requires mastery of three types of expertise or skill: cognitive skills or content knowledge (what we know in our brains), technical skills (what we do with our hands), and behavioral skills (what we use to employ the first two skill sets while caring for patients while working under realistic time pressure). Knowledge of the normal and abnormal physiologies manifested in the delivery room and how to treat them, together with proficiency in the technical aspects of that treatment, are prerequisites to delivering care to the pregnant woman in labor and her newborn. Nevertheless, cognitive and technical skills alone are insufficient for the modern practice of medicine. Both the evidence currently available in the literature (albeit limited) and rational conjecture indicate that behavioral skills such as teamwork and effective communication are also critically important to successful outcomes for patients undergoing cardiopulmonary resuscitation [13]. Unfortunately behavioral skills have rarely been addressed in conventional training programs for healthcare professionals in the USA or elsewhere.

New methodologies

How can the limitations of the traditional medical training model be overcome? In looking for answers to this question it is useful to examine other dynamic domains where the risk to human life is high and where similar limitations have been successfully surmounted. Dynamic medical domains like the delivery room are similar to other domains such as commercial aviation and aerospace in that they are all characterized by an inherent risk to human life, short-time constant action/feedback loops, and intense time pressure. There is a direct relationship between actions and outcomes. Communication in these domains is primarily verbal and immediate, involves multiple personnel, and is characterized by changes in pitch, intensity, and word compression as well as non-verbal cues including eye movement and body language. Effective human interface with technology is critical both in flying air- and spacecraft and in resuscitating neonates in the delivery room. The tradition of the pilot as commander-in-chief is similar to that of the physician bearing ultimate responsibility for the care of the newborn. Thus medicine shares many characteristics with aerospace and aviation, and stands to benefit from adopting similar training methodologies.

Flying large aircraft has been described as "hours and hours of boredom interspersed by moments of terror" (this is also a reasonable description of working in a busy delivery room!). The downing of a commercial aircraft is devastating, in terms of both loss of human life and destruction of expensive technology. Because of this, the commercial aviation industry long ago recognized the need to develop a better understanding of why planes crash, in an effort to reduce the incidence of such events. One of the first steps in this effort was to equip the cockpits of commercial aircraft with devices that record the communications of the crew and the readings of the plane's instruments. These devices provide an objective, time-coded record of the events as they occur during flight. Analysis of the data from these "black boxes" indicated that approximately two-thirds of airline accidents occurred not because of major mechanical failures or lack of technical knowledge on the part of the crew but rather because of suboptimal communication and teamwork by those responsible for flying the plane [9]. This information was surprising in that the pilots, copilots, and flight engineers flying these large commercial aircraft were some of the most experienced in the industry, having logged thousands of hours of flight time in a variety of aircraft under a wide array of conditions, yet were unable to utilize and integrate their collective skills during in-flight crises.

In response to these findings the aerospace industry developed a training program known as Crew (or Cockpit)

Resource Management (CRM) [14]. In CRM crews are taught the appropriate technical responses to in-flight crises. In addition, heavy emphasis is placed upon the necessary behavioral responses (effective teamwork and communication) vital to optimal crew performance. The key to effective CRM training is creating a "suspension of disbelief" in those participating in the exercise; this is greatly enhanced by creating a training environment that simulates a cockpit with high fidelity. Flight simulators are designed to be identical to the physical layout of a real cockpit and provide realistic visual, auditory, tactile, and kinesthetic cues to those training within the simulator. The simulator contains working controls, alarms, and other devices; these must be operated as in real life or the desired responses by the simulated aircraft will not occur. It is not possible simply to talk one's way out of a problem, nor pick the correct solution from a list of multiple-choice options, in a flight simulator. If the crew does not exhibit the correct technical and behavioral responses to the events in the simulator exactly as would be necessary in the real cockpit during actual flight, the scenario cannot be successfully completed and the simulator "crashes."

The aerospace industry has succeeded in overcoming many of the barriers to effective error detection, analysis, and prevention. Error detection is enhanced by a system that encourages crews to report near-miss and adverse events to a national agency, the Federal Aviation Administration (FAA), without risk of liability. The FAA database serves as a valuable resource to flight crews and the industry in general, and allows for early recognition of systematic problems. The industry's experience with error analysis is unsurpassed; this experience includes recognition of good decisions on the part of crews in addition to detailed analysis of suboptimal aspects of performance. The FAA and other agencies, such as the National Aeronautics and Space Administration (NASA), provide ongoing support for human performance research, including efforts to study optimal modes of communication, effects of sleep deprivation, and other human factors. Ultimately, the goal of these efforts is to prevent errors and improve the safety of passengers and crew. Evaluation of the effects of simulation-based flight training indicates that the experience gained in realistic simulators improves crew performance; although confounded by concomitant advances in technology, passenger safety has improved since the initiation of mandatory annual CRM training by all flight crews of major commercial airlines.

Given the similarities between these high-risk domains, what has been done in medicine to mimic the successes in training (as in CRM) experienced by commercial aviation? Videotape has been used to record the actions and words of physicians and nurses in emergency rooms and trauma centers [15–18]. This video record of events augments the written record and memories of team members and is used in debriefing the teams after major events. Anesthesiologists have combined videotape with human patient simulators in creating the medical equivalent of a flight simulator. Their course, anesthesia crisis resource management (ACRM),

was one of the first simulation-based medical training programs [19].

The delivery room possesses many similarities to the operating room. It is characterized by high risk, intense time pressure, and reliance upon technical skills and verbal communication. Unlike the operating room, there are at least two (and occasionally three or more) patients present, demanding coordinated team action between groups of physicians and nurses who in many institutions spend most of their time working in isolation from one another on separate adult and pediatric units. The use of videotape to record the actions of delivery-room resuscitation teams as a quality assurance instrument has been reported [20]. This study found that the videotape record provides a useful quality assurance tool for monitoring the conduct of newborn resuscitation and providing constructive feedback.

These innovations in the real delivery room have been augmented by highly realistic training experiences carried out in a simulated delivery room where everything is real except for the patients. NeoSim™ is a simulation-based training program based upon the CRM program in commercial aviation and focused on the individuals responsible for resuscitation of the neonate [21]. It is one of a number of programs developed and conducted at the Center for Advanced Pediatric and Perinatal Education at Packard Children's Hospital at Stanford, or CAPE (www.cape.lpch.org). The objectives of NeoSim are to: recognize the collective responsibility of delivery-room personnel for the health of mothers and babies; identify the cognitive, technical, and behavioral skills necessary for optimal human performance; and practice these skills in a realistic and safe environment. Each program begins with a general introduction to the principles of simulation-based training, followed by review of videotapes depicting simulation-based training in aviation/ aerospace and medicine. Review of these videotapes is meant to stimulate the trainees to think about the technical and behavioral skills (or lack thereof) exhibited by those captured on these "trigger" videos. Trainees are then oriented to the equipment, supplies (including medications and fluids), patients, and colleagues in the simulated delivery room. Once this familiarization is complete, trainees are immersed in multiple realistic, challenging clinical scenarios involving problems with patients, devices, colleagues, and multisystem failures. The details of these scenarios are captured on time-coded videotape used during debriefings facilitated by the simulator faculty that are conducted immediately after each scenario. Typically a thorough debriefing requires at least twice the length of time required for the conduct of the scenario itself.

OBSim™ is similar to NeoSim, but it addresses the needs of the obstetric team in handling difficult deliveries and managing maternal cardiorespiratory decompensation and arrest. Sim DR™ is another training program developed at CAPE that is directed at *all* of the individuals caring for both the mother (obstetrician/perinatologist, anesthesiologist/obstetric anesthesiologist, scrub nurse, circulating nurse) and the newborn (pediatrician/neonatologist, neonatal nurse practitioner, nursery nurse) in the delivery room. Even though these two groups of professionals must work together on a regular basis in the same physical space, joint training programs such as Sim DR are a novel concept. The success of these programs demonstrates that it is possible to overcome the difficulties inherent in simultaneous training and debriefing of multiple groups of medical professionals.

There are many aspects of simulation-based training that intuitively appear to be significant advantages over traditional training methodologies:

- The ability to create specific scenarios eliminates the dependence on "education by random opportunity" described earlier.

- The capacity for numerous scenarios during the conduct of a single training program provides for a very intense experience in a relatively short period of time, maximizing time, money, and other resources.

- Scenarios can be scaled to challenge both the novice and the experienced clinician.

- Use of videotape provides an unbiased, objective, detailed, time-coded record of the actions of the trainees, reducing dependence on more subjective records such as human memory, as occurs in reviewing the events during a real medical emergency.

- Debriefings conducted immediately after each scenario provide detailed constructive feedback unparalleled in quantity and quality.

- Finally, simulation-based medical training presents no risk to patients and very minimal risk to trainees (a small risk of injury to users is present whenever real working medical equipment is used, as in the simulator).

Thus the use of simulation-based methodologies represents a significant advance in healthcare training and has the potential to revolutionize efforts to improve human performance and patient safety.

The Neonatal Resuscitation Program (NRP) of the American Academy of Pediatrics (AAP) sets the standard for neonatal resuscitation in the USA and serves as the basis for similar programs elsewhere in the world. Development of a career-long learning program in neonatal resuscitation that is relevant to professionals from multiple disciplines at all levels of experience, and that is embedded with robust learning opportunities and valid performance metrics, is the focus of the NRP [22]. Similar to what is happening in other healthcare domains, a major shift in learning methodology is occurring within the NRP. The NRP Instructor Development Task Force began meeting in early 2007 to plan how to prepare NRP instructors to shift from the role of an instructor in control of the learning process for trainees to someone who facilitates acquisition of knowledge and skills by trainees charged with responsibility for their own education. The NRP is poised to transition from a single learning opportunity experienced once every 2 years to a career-long learning model where trainees are required to regularly review different aspects of neonatal resuscitation

using an assortment of learning methodologies that are best suited to their individual learning styles. This transition will result in new learning materials accessible online from anywhere in the world, and will allow rapid updating of content to reflect new evidence as it becomes available.

The body of evidence in support of the impact of simulation-based training on patient safety is growing. One of the most intriguing is a retrospective multicenter cohort observational study of 19 460 infants by Draycott et al., who looked at the effect of a training program on the management of difficult deliveries on neonatal outcome [23]. The training program consisted of review of interpretation of fetal heart-rate tracings and hands-on drills in the management of shoulder dystocia, postpartum hemorrhage, eclampsia, twin delivery, breech presentation, and maternal and neonatal resuscitation. After completion of the program the incidence of newborns with 5-minute Apgar scores ≤ 6 decreased from 86.6 to 44.6/10 000 births ($p < 0.001$); in addition the incidence of hypoxic–ischemic encephalopathy decreased from 27.3 to 13.6/10 000 births ($p = 0.032$).

Virtual-reality-based learning opportunities represent another technologic and methodologic innovation that puts the learner in control of his or her learning opportunities. Virtual reality refers to depictions of reality that exist only in a computer. Learning programs such as VIDERO (VIrtual DElivery ROom) and Virtual Worlds place the user in a virtual clinical scenario and require interaction with patients and other healthcare professionals in the context of a multidisciplinary team [24–28]. Online interactive virtual environments will continue to evolve in utility and complexity, and are certain to become important learning tools in the future.

The future

What is a safe delivery room from the perspective of training? A safe delivery room is one that is staffed by professionals who not only have mastered the appropriate body of content knowledge specific to their domain and are highly trained in the necessary technical skills but also have practiced and demonstrated behavioral skills such as teamwork and effective communication with their colleagues on a regular basis in the context of multidisciplinary teams. These professionals are supported by clinical information systems that use artificial intelligence to assimilate, analyze, and display patient data in a format that can be easily visualized and interpreted, in real time, in the real environment. The delivery room itself is highly sophisticated: patient monitors, infusion pumps and other "smart" devices are not only servo-regulated but their data streams are archived in a central repository from which they can be recovered at any time. All of the activities that occur in the delivery room are recorded on time-coded video, also stored on secure servers. When it becomes necessary to examine the recorded video and data streams they can be played back in a simulator, allowing a high-fidelity re-creation of those events of interest for detailed analysis by teams of healthcare professionals, human-factors experts, industrial psychologists, risk managers, and hospital administrators. How close are we to a truly safe delivery room?

While some technical barriers persist, all of the technologies described previously exist already in some form. Perhaps the area in greatest need of innovation is the simulation of birth. Human birth is a complex process, characterized by numerous continuous changes in the physiology, anatomy, and spatial relationships among various physical structures in both mother and baby. While these technical barriers to high-fidelity simulation of birth may seem daunting at first glance, it is important to understand that highly effective simulation can be achieved with far less than 100% fidelity to actual biologic processes. Close collaboration among physicians, computer scientists, biomedical engineers, medical artists, and others will allow the remaining technical challenges to be overcome in a timely and cost-efficient manner. Work also needs to continue in the area of methodology, as useful metrics to assess human technical and behavioral performance in the delivery room need to be developed and validated.

Medicine is currently faced with tremendous financial pressures to improve efficiency and lower cost, ostensibly to deliver more care to more people. This means that it will not be adequate simply to develop and implement new training methodologies and technologies. Validation of new training programs and devices will be necessary to insure that the skills learned in medical simulators can be effectively transferred to the real medical domain and result in improved human performance, reduced medical error rates, and better patient outcomes. This will require appropriate evaluation of these new methodologies. Any improvements over historically accepted training models should be weighed against the costs of these newer methodologies averaged over time. Financial resources to conduct this research and development must be made available, and the funds to conduct training must be secured, either by finding "new" money (always a difficult undertaking) or by re-allocating funds already dedicated to training.

Most importantly, the culture of health care must change, from one of silence about (and blame and punishment for) mistakes to one where mistakes are acknowledged and preventive actions are widely disseminated. There is much about the legal climate within the USA that discourages recognition of, detailed open discussion about, and widespread dissemination of information regarding medical errors. The threat of loss of reputation, current income, and long-term financial security thwarts any substantive effort to examine systematically the issue of patient safety. There is no method by which medical errors are logged and this database made universally accessible to practicing physicians, nurses, and allied healthcare personnel. In the absence of this shared knowledge, the same errors, many of which are preventable, continue to occur repeatedly in the hospitals, clinics, and other healthcare delivery sites throughout this country. Whenever an adverse event occurs, the question typically asked is "Who is responsible?" in order to assign blame to an individual rather than closely examine the system for the inherent flaws that set up these individuals for failure. The burden of error prevention must shift from the shoulders of individual practitioners to the healthcare system as a whole. Strict patient confidentiality must be insured, and healthcare professionals must be protected from any type of accusation or retribution if they are to be willing participants in such a process as has been described. Until a system that encourages responsible, blameless reporting of "medical near-misses" and adverse patient outcomes exists, medicine will never begin to approach the safety record of high-risk industries such as commercial aviation. Only then will the promise of new training methodologies and technologies designed to enhance the safety of patients be fulfilled.

Conclusions

Improvement in the safety of newborns and their mothers will require a new paradigm of education and training. Faster microprocessors, advanced algorithms, and sophisticated haptic interfaces will lead to the development of sophisticated fetal, neonatal, and maternal patient simulators based on realistic physiologic models. Regional centers that utilize the tremendous potential of these simulation- and virtual-reality-based technologies in their curricula will be established to serve as resources for the physicians and nurses seeking training and accreditation. The traditional two-step model of medical education will evolve. This new model will consist of four steps, and will be more in line with the successful training models found in aerospace and other industries like nuclear power where the risk to human life is high:

(1) Read about health and disease in textbooks and journals.
(2) Interact with virtual patients (computer-generated renderings).
(3) Practice on simulated patients (sophisticated physical manikins).
(4) Care for real patients.

Rather than asking "Can we afford to do this?" the proper question to be asked is "Can we afford not to do this?" The Institute of Medicine, in its 1999 report, states: "The status quo is not acceptable and cannot be tolerated any longer. Despite the cost pressures, liability constraints, resistance to change and other seemingly insurmountable barriers, it is simply not acceptable for patients to be harmed by the same health care system that is supposed to offer healing and comfort . . . A comprehensive approach to improving patient safety is needed" [1]. Adopting a new paradigm of training and education in delivery-room medicine, one that incorporates the use of simulation- and virtual-reality-based technologies, should be a major component of this comprehensive approach to improving the care and safety of newborns and their mothers.

References

1. Kohn LT, Corrigan JM, Donaldson MS, eds. *To Err is Human: Building a Safer Health System*. Washington, DC: National Academy Press, 1999.

2. Thomas EJ, Studdert DM, Burstin HR, *et al.* Incidence and types of adverse events and negligent care in Utah and Colorado. *Med Care* 2000; **38**: 261–71.

3. Brennan TA, Leape LL, Laird NM, *et al.* Incidence of adverse events and negligence in hospitalized patients: results of the Harvard Medical Practice Study I. *N Engl J Med* 1991; **324**: 370–6.

4. Leape LL, Brennan TA, Laird NM, *et al.* The nature of adverse events in hospitalized patients: results of the Harvard Medical Practice Study II. *N Engl J Med* 1991; **324**: 377–84.

5. Committee on Quality of Health Care in America. *Crossing the Quality Chasm: a New Health System for the 21st Century*. Washington, DC: National Academy Press, 2001.

6. The Joint Commission. Preventing infant death and injury during delivery. *Sentinel Event Alert* 30, July 21, 2004. www.jointcommission.org/sentinelevents/sentineleventalert/sea_30.htm. Accessed February, 2008.

7. Hall JG. See one, do one, teach one. *Pediatrics* 1991; **103**: 155–6.

8. Accreditation Council for Graduate Medical Education. Program Requirements for Residency Education in Pediatrics. www.acgme.org/acWebsite/RRC_320/320_prIndex.asp. Accessed February, 2008.

9. Billings CE, Reynard WD. Human factors in aircraft incidents: results of a 7-year study. *Aviat Space Environ Med* 1984; **55**: 960–5.

10. Burke CS, Salas E, Wilson-Donnelly K, *et al.* How to turn a team of experts into an expert medical team: guidance from the aviation and military communities. *Qual Saf Health Care* 2004; **13**: i96–104.

11. Baker DP, Gustafson S, Beaubien J, *et al. Medical Teamwork and Patient Safety: The Evidence-based Relation. Literature Review.* AHRQ Publication No. 05-0053, April 2005. Rockville, MD: Agency for Healthcare Research and Quality. www.ahrq.gov/qual/medteam. Accessed February, 2008.

12. Halamek LP. Teaching vs. learning and the role of simulation-based training in pediatrics. *J Pediatr* 2007; **151**: 329–30.

13. Weinstock P, Halamek LP. Teamwork during resuscitation. *Pediatr Clin North Am* 2008; **55**: 1011–24, xi–xii.

14. Weiner EL, Kanki BG, Helmreich RL, eds. *Cockpit Resource Management*. San Diego, CA: Academic Press, 1993.

15. Ellis DG, Lerner EB, Jehle D, *et al.* A multi-state survey of videotaping practices for major trauma resuscitations. *J Emerg Med* 1999; **17**: 597–604.

16. Ritchie PT, Cameron PA. An evaluation of trauma team leader performance by video recording. *Aust NZ J Surg* 1999; **69**: 183–6.

17. Mann CJ, Heyworth J. Comparison of cardiopulmonary resuscitation techniques using video camera recordings. *J Accid Emerg Med* 1996; **13**: 198–9.

18. Weston C, Richmond P, McCabe MJ, *et al.* Video recording of cardiac arrest management: an aid to training and audit. *Resuscitation* 1992; **24**: 13–15.

19. Howard SK, Gaba DM, Fish KJ, *et al.* Anesthesia crisis resource management training: teaching anesthesiologists to handle critical incidents. *Aviat Space Environ Med* 1992; **63**: 763–70.

20. Carbine DN, Finer NN, Knodel E, *et al.* Video recording as a means of evaluating neonatal resuscitation performance. *Pediatrics* 2000; **106**: 654–8.

21. Halamek LP, Kaegi DM, Gaba DM, *et al.* Time for a new paradigm in pediatric medical education: teaching neonatal resuscitation in a simulated delivery room environment. *Pediatrics* 2000; **106**: e45.

22. Halamek LP. Educational perspectives: the genesis, adaptation and evolution of the Neonatal Resuscitation Program. *Neo Reviews* 2008; **9**: e142–9.

23. Draycott T, Sibanda T, Owen L, *et al.* Does training in obstetric emergencies improve neonatal outcome? *BJOG* 2006; **113**: 177–82.

24. Koročsec D, Holobar A, Divjak M, *et al.* Building interactive virtual environments for simulated training in medicine using VRML and Java/JavaScript. *Comput Methods Programs Biomed* 2005; **80**: S61–70.

25. System Software Laboratory. *VIDERO: Virtual Delivery Room*. storm.uni-mb.si/videro. Accessed February, 2008.

26. Stockholm Challenge. Virtual delivery room (VIDERO). www.stockholmchallenge.se/data/virtual_delivery_room_vid. Accessed February, 2008.

27. Dev P, Youngblood P, Heinrichs WL, *et al.* Virtual worlds and team training. *Anesthesiol Clin* 2007; **25**: 321–36.

28. Dev P, Montgomery K, Senger S, *et al.* Simulated medical learning environments on the Internet. *J Am Med Inform Assoc* 2002; **9**: 437–4.

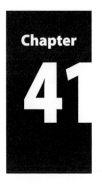

Chapter 41

Extended management following resuscitation

William E. Benitz, Susan R. Hintz, David K. Stevenson, Ronald J. Wong, and Philip Sunshine

Introduction

After the initial resuscitation of an encephalopathic infant, the extended management of the patient becomes critical in order to prevent as much secondary damage as possible. There are many different management protocols that are acceptable, and it is not the intent of this chapter to review all of them used for the various conditions encountered in neonatal intensive care. Rather, we focus on the early transitional period following birth and resuscitation, during which the condition of the depressed infant can be substantially improved by expert care.

As noted in Chapters 2 and 42, the encephalopathic period involves a continuum of biologic events associated with secondary energy failure lasting up to 48–72 hours after the initial insult. These include the reperfusion period with the elaboration of oxygen free radicals and various cytokines as well as necrosis and apoptosis that then ensue. It is imperative that the extended management of these infants be carried out in an optimal fashion at a center that can provide hypothermia or other novel neuroprotective interventions that may be developed.

Unfortunately, the windows of opportunity may be short and variable depending upon the nature of the intervention, and could change as further research informs practice. Thus there is an obligation for the practitioner to be well informed about progress in the standard of care and to stay current with respect to neuroprotective strategies. Various neuroprotective mechanisms after hypoxic–ischemic injury are discussed in detail in Chapter 42.

The condition of the infant during this period may have been determined by circumstances that occurred prior to or during the delivery and initial resuscitation, many of which are beyond the control of the obstetrician and neonatologist. It is also important to recognize that significant neurologic or physiologic compromise is not always evident during the early evaluation; and an infant with good initial Apgar scores may present with significant problems later after an apparently successful resuscitation. Nonetheless, it is possible to identify many infants who require continued intensive care, including all those who require vigorous resuscitation and those who

remain depressed or dependent on cardiopulmonary support. The roles of pharmacologic therapy in extended intensive care and in the management of refractory neonatal hypoxemia have been reviewed in detail [1]. In this chapter, we provide an overview of the aspects of extended intensive care, which addresses the maintenance of cerebral integrity in appropriate facilities that can provide specialized therapy, and provides recommendations for the implementation of these interventions by the primary care practitioner [2]. These interventions consist of sustaining ventilation, supporting cardiac output, correcting anemia, and evaluating and initiating therapy for hypoxemia.

Fluid management

Although there is little evidence to guide fluid administration in infants with hypoxic–ischemic injury and encephalopathy, the risk for exacerbating cerebral edema is real. Hyponatremia may exist if excessive free water is administered or in the context of the syndrome of inappropriate secretion of antidiuretic hormone (SIADH). In addition, capillary leak syndrome associated with asphyxia may lead to intravascular volume depletion; with appropriate secretion of ADH and any relative water load, this can set the stage for hyponatremia. Thus, intravascular volume depletion should be treated with crystalloid or colloid, while continuous intravenous (IV) fluid administration should be restricted, limiting free water in the context of low glomerular filtration rate (GFR) or oliguric renal failure. On the other hand, it is paramount to avoid dehydration and possible hypotension and to maintain good cardiac output and perfusion. Enteral feeding is usually avoided in the first several days of life in consideration of damage to or impaired perfusion of the gastrointestinal tract, particularly in the setting of continued need for inotropic support. This is discussed in Chapter 44.

Supporting ventilation

Assisted ventilation should be provided for any infant who is not able to maintain acceptable arterial blood gas levels without such assistance, or who does so only with extreme effort. The range of desired arterial oxygen tensions depends on the clinical circumstances, as indicated in Chapter 39. In the premature infant, a PaO_2 of 50–60 mmHg (6.7–8.0 kPa) is usually adequate, but a PaO_2 slightly higher than 100 mmHg (13.3 kPa) may be more desirable in an infant with persistent

Fetal and Neonatal Brain Injury, 4th edition, ed. David K. Stevenson, William E. Benitz, Philip Sunshine, Susan R. Hintz, and Maurice L. Druzin. Published by Cambridge University Press. © Cambridge University Press 2009.

pulmonary hypertension of the newborn (PPHN). In some situations, extreme vigorous support (with a concomitant risk of adverse effects, such as pneumothorax, adult respiratory distress syndrome [ARDS], or bronchopulmonary dysplasia [BPD]) may be required to achieve optimal blood gas parameters. In such high-risk clinical scenarios, one may decide to accept lower oxygen tensions (35–50 mmHg or 4.7–6.7 kPa) if this allows less vigorous utilization of positive-pressure ventilation or greatly reduced inspired oxygen concentrations, as long as both the oxygen-carrying capacity of the blood and the cardiac output are maintained.

Similarly, higher than normal $PaCO_2$ target ranges are often accepted as long as the arterial pH level is not excessively depressed, because these values may be achieved with less aggressive mandatory ventilation. Hyperventilation to achieve elevated pH values has been utilized in the treatment of PPHN [3,4]. However, extreme hyperventilation results in hypocapnia and alkalosis, and shifts the hemoglobin–oxygen dissociation curve to the left, which is unfavorable to tissues. The effects of hyperventilation on cerebral metabolism are not fully understood, but cerebral blood flow may be compromised by this maneuver [5]. Cerebral vascular autoregulation may also be impaired in critically ill neonates and blood flow patterns may change after hypocapnia [6–8]. Retrospective clinical studies have also suggested an association of hyperventilation, as part of a therapeutic approach to PPHN, with later sensorineural hearing loss and poorer neurodevelopmental outcome [9–11]. Moreover, significant risks of pulmonary injury, including pneumothorax and pulmonary interstitial emphysema (PIE), may be incurred with excessively vigorous mechanical ventilation. Cognizant of the potential short- and long-term complications associated with hyperventilation, and with the assistance of improved adjuvant therapies (see below), tertiary care centers now employ more conservative ventilation strategies in the management of PPHN [12,13]. However, support for any specific ventilatory regimen is limited by the paucity of randomized controlled trials.

Recent evidence has suggested that changes in lung volume rather than changes in applied proximal airway pressures may be most important in the development of chronic lung disease (CLD) in ventilated infants. This has led to the adoption of high-frequency ventilation (HFV), including high-frequency oscillatory ventilation (HFOV), high-frequency jet ventilation (HFJV), high-frequency flow interruption (HFFI), and high-frequency positive-pressure ventilation (HFPPV), as strategies for supporting gas exchange while minimizing pulmonary injury [14]. In general, the strategy for use of these devices is to maintain the lung volume above functional residual capacity using a constant distending pressure and delivering small tidal volumes at 2–20 Hz. HFV appears to be at least as effective as conventional positive-pressure ventilation for management of premature infants with respiratory distress syndrome (RDS), and may be the preferred mode of ventilation in infants with PIE or other air-leak syndromes. Both HFOV and HFJV have been studied as methods for rescue

of infants with severe respiratory failure who qualify for extracorporeal membrane oxygenation (ECMO) while on conventional ventilation [14–16]. Such HFV rescue has been shown to be most likely to succeed in infants with severe RDS, and less so for those with meconium aspiration or congenital diaphragmatic hernia (CDH). However, there are very few randomized controlled trials in this area [17], making establishment of clear recommendations difficult. Plans for further trials of ventilatory strategies alone will be complicated by use of other adjuvant interventions, as well as by dissimilar diagnoses and responses among infants with pulmonary failure. Increasing utilization of HFV in combination with other therapies is likely responsible for a dramatic decrease in the need for ECMO in neonates with PPHN [18].

To facilitate safe and effective ventilatory management, it is occasionally necessary to provide pharmacologic neuromuscular blockade. The administration of pancuronium bromide or vecuronium iodide allows for neuromuscular relaxation, produces significant improvement in gas exchange, and reduces the risk of barotrauma [19,20]. Vecuronium has weak atropine-like and histamine-releasing effects, which may cause hypotension, tachycardia, and an apparent increase in skin perfusion. In contrast, pancuronium has been shown to decrease blood histamine levels and is less likely to cause hypotension because of direct effects on heart function. It is also possible that these drugs may increase the risk of intracranial hemorrhage. Provision of analgesia with morphine sulfate or fentanyl and sedation with midazolam is recommended during neuromuscular blockade.

A major advance in the management of respiratory insufficiency in preterm infants occurred with the introduction of surfactant replacement therapy. Investigational use of surfactants became widespread by 1989, and commercial products were introduced in 1990 (Exosurf, an entirely synthetic surfactant) and 1991 (Survanta, a bovine surfactant-based product). Other exogenous surfactant preparations such as Infasurf and Curosurf have since been marketed in the USA and Europe. Use of exogenous surfactant in preterm infants with RDS has been associated with reduced mortality, fewer pneumothoraces, and lower oxygen requirements and ventilatory settings in these patients [21–23]. Weight-specific mortality has been substantially reduced, especially in infants of less than 28 weeks' gestation. This single therapeutic innovation reduced the total neonatal mortality rate in the USA by 10% in the year it was introduced. Unfortunately, the prevalence of BPD appears not to have changed significantly. This is most likely explained by improved survival among the sickest premature infants since the implementation of surfactant therapy, and a concomitant change in the pathophysiology of BPD [24]. However, a recent meta-analysis of randomized controlled trials of synthetic surfactant treatment in preterm infants does suggest a decrease in the risk of BPD as well as neonatal mortality [23].

Term infants with severe respiratory failure have also been shown to benefit from surfactant therapy. Meconium, blood, and infection may inactivate or wash out endogenously produced surfactant; thus replacement with exogenous surfactant has been added to the armamentarium of treatments for severe respiratory failure in newborns [25]. A multicenter, randomized, double-blind, placebo-controlled trial demonstrated that a four-dose regimen of beractant (Survanta) decreases the need for ECMO without increasing complications in critically ill term and near-term infants with meconium aspiration, sepsis, or PPHN, especially if the treatment was administered early in the course [26]. In term infants, surfactant treatment is most often utilized in combination with other advanced ventilatory and therapeutic modalities. Administration of surfactant occasionally results in desaturation episodes, which could prove life-threatening for the patient with severe pulmonary hypertension. Therefore, prudence and safety dictate that surfactant treatment of critically ill and unstable neonates be initiated in a facility where other therapies such as inhaled nitric oxide (iNO) and ECMO may be offered.

Surfactant use has not been associated with significant adverse effects. Neither the incidence of intraventricular hemorrhage (IVH) nor that of patency of the ductus arteriosus has been consistently increased in clinical trials. Some trials have suggested an increased frequency of pulmonary hemorrhage, but this appears to result from increased recognition rather than a true increase in the incidence of this complication. The major hazards of surfactant use relate to hypoxic episodes if the agent is given too rapidly and air-leak complications if ventilatory support is not reduced appropriately as lung mechanics improve after surfactant administration. Finally, although the course of illness is much less severe in treated infants, the time to recovery is not greatly reduced, and infants with significant RDS can still be expected to require assisted ventilation and careful monitoring. For these reasons, it is important that all infants who are treated with exogenous surfactant receive their care in nurseries that are appropriately equipped and staffed to provide this ongoing care.

iNO has dramatically impacted the way in which term and near-term infants with respiratory failure are managed. The Neonatal Inhaled Nitric Oxide Study (NINOS) Group demonstrated that iNO significantly reduced the need for ECMO in term infants with hypoxic respiratory failure other than CDH, but did not reduce mortality [27,28]. Food and Drug Administration approval of iNO for specific use in term and near-term newborns with hypoxic respiratory failure was obtained in 1999. Investigations of applications of iNO therapy for other indications, such as severe respiratory failure in premature infants, are ongoing. A multicenter randomized controlled trial of early administration of iNO in term and near-term infants with respiratory failure demonstrated that iNO can decrease the need for ECMO, but had no apparent effect on mortality [27]. Nonetheless, neurodevelopmental impairment or hearing loss was not increased at follow-up. Many centers have also now made iNO available for transport, allowing stabilization of extremely critical neonates who may otherwise not survive transfer to a higher level of care. Complacency as to the reliable effectiveness of iNO therapy in avoiding ECMO may be developing, however, and a temptation to use iNO routinely at non-ECMO centers has followed. The potential danger in this scenario should not be underestimated. The appropriate and safe use of iNO requires an integrated team comprised of respiratory therapists, nurses, and physicians, and is best carried out at a center where ECMO is readily available.

Sustaining cardiac output

If the cardiac output remains impaired after correction of bradycardia (by assisted ventilation or the administration of epinephrine, isoproterenol, or atropine), hypovolemia, and metabolic disorders (acidemia, hypoglycemia, and hypocalcemia), as described in Chapter 39, inotropic or vasodilator drug therapy may be required.

Inotropic drugs

Infants may be at risk for myocardial injury and dysfunction because of sepsis or severe asphyxia. Less commonly, myocardial edema, as with hydrops, may compromise myocardial contractility. Administration of β-mimetic catecholamines may increase the stroke volume and cardiac output under such conditions with a structurally normal heart. Infants of poorly controlled diabetic mothers may have a temporary congenital defect characterized by hypertrophic cardiomyopathy. These infants respond with a reduced cardiac output when treated with such drugs because of narrowing of the right ventricular infundibulum [29]; the use of such drugs would be relatively contraindicated in such a scenario. Finally, benefit with inotropes is unlikely if the heart rate or diastolic ventricular volume is inadequate, the pH is below 7.1, or they are inactivated by admixture with alkaline solutions for infusion. In general, peripheral IV administration of the drug should be avoided due to the potential for severe local ischemia following extravasation, but it can be tolerated for short periods in larger term or near-term infants. Intra-arterial infusions or catecholamines are contraindicated.

Dopamine

Dopamine is the cardiotonic drug most frequently used in the level III nursery. Its effects are dose-dependent and similar to those seen in adult patients. Measurable beneficial effects may occur at doses as low as 0.8 µg/kg per minute. Typically, however, the initial dose is 2 µg/kg per minute. At this rate of administration the effect is predominantly dopaminergic receptor-mediated dilation of renal and splanchnic vessels, causing an increase in the GFR, urine output, and urinary sodium excretion. β-Adrenergic effects result in improved cardiac contractility, a moderate increase in the heart rate, and mild peripheral vasodilation, all contributing to an increased cardiac output [30,31]. Such effects can be observed with doses over 5 µg/kg per minute, but α-adrenergic effects dominate at doses over 15 µg/kg per minute. These effects may result in increased systemic vascular resistance and arterial blood pressures, with a reduction in cardiac output and renal perfusion. The effects on the pulmonary vascular resistance and pulmonary artery pressure may be less pronounced under some conditions, and the α-adrenergic effects of dopamine may be useful in establishing a favorable ratio of systemic to pulmonary vascular resistance, leading to decreased right-to-left shunting in infants with hypoxemia refractory to mechanical ventilation. This differential systemic vasoconstriction may be observed at doses between 10 and 25 µg/kg per minute, particularly when combined with vasodilator infusion.

Despite its frequent use in newborn intensive care, dopamine is not a harmless medicine. It should only be used for appropriate indications, and its use requires continued monitoring. Even when used properly, it can increase myocardial oxygen demands and sometimes causes tachyarrhythmias. In unusual infants, it can also cause intensive vasoconstriction and hypertension at doses that would be considered dopaminergic. This phenomenon is most common with excessive doses.

Dobutamine

This selective β-adrenergic drug can increase cardiac contractility and cardiac output but has minimal effects on heart rate and vascular tone [30]. It has been used primarily for cardiac shock refractory to dopamine infusion and is often used in conjunction with dopamine. It is administered at a dose between 2.5 and 15 µg/kg per minute, titrated to achieve the desired improvement in cardiac performance. It may be the drug of choice in the initial management of the hypotensive neonate with myocardial dysfunction who does not have evidence of significant peripheral vasodilation [30].

Epinephrine (adrenaline)

For cardiogenic shock unresponsive to other catecholamines, epinephrine infusion (50–250 ng/kg per minute) may have to be used [30]. However, the benefits of increased contractility are often balanced against the adverse effects of increased vascular resistance.

Afterload reduction

Another strategy for the management of severely compromised myocardial function is to decrease the systemic vascular resistance (afterload). This should be attempted only after aggressive management of the heart rate, preload, and inotropic therapy has been optimized to improve the cardiac output. Administration of a vasodilator may improve the Frank–Starling relationship between cardiac output and end-diastolic ventricular volumes, moving the curve upward and to the left [32], without affecting myocardial function itself. Dilation of arterioles and precapillary sphincters may reduce the systemic vascular resistance, resulting in increased cardiac output. However, cardiac output may decrease because of reduced preload, which is due to increased venous capacitance, or it may be unchanged if these effects are balanced. Therefore, use of these drugs requires meticulous monitoring and management. This treatment is seldom used in neonatal intensive care, and agents that have been used include nitroprusside and milrinone. The use of bipyridine phosphodiesterase inhibitors such as milrinone may provide an alternative to nitroprusside for treating low cardiac output in neonates without adversely affecting endogenous catecholamine levels.

Management of anemia

The oxygen-carrying capacity of the blood is especially important for the newborn infant. Hemoglobin F interacts less well with 2,3-diphosphoglycerate, thus limiting any compensatory response to hypoxia by a shift in the hemoglobin–oxygen dissociation curve [33]. Practically, an oxygen-carrying capacity of at least 16 ml of oxygen per deciliter may provide a margin of safety for oxygenation in the asphyxiated infant with a normal cardiac output. This translates to a hemoglobin concentration of 12 mg/dL, because 1 g of hemoglobin can bind 1.34 ml of oxygen. The minimal desirable hematocrit level of approximately 40% for a distressed neonate is thus derived. In infants for whom optimal oxygen tensions can not be achieved, the increased oxygen-carrying capacity imparted by elevation of the hematocrit level to 50% may ensure adequate tissue oxygen delivery, allowing marginal oxygen tensions to be better tolerated.

Evaluation and management or refractory hypoxemia

The infant who remains hypoxemic in spite of ventilation with 100% oxygen is at risk for cerebral injury, depending on the severity and duration of the hypoxemic episode. Although the metabolic hallmark of severe hypoxemia is metabolic acidosis, it is better to suspect hypoxemia and initiate a thorough evaluation and appropriate therapy than to identify its late consequences. The practitioner should recognize that hypoxemia might be present despite a normal arterial oxygen tension (PaO_2 level > 50 mmHg or 6.7 kPa) or hemoglobin saturation ($> 90\%$). In particular, severe anemia (or normotonic hypoxemic infants) is a common and easily correctable problem, which may have consequences as serious as those created by a low oxygen tension. In fact, infants with severe anemia may present with respiratory distress despite having normal arterial oxygen tensions and oxygen saturations. A normal PaO_2 value with an arterial blood gas sample may be falsely reassuring in the presence of pallor caused by anemia or acidosis. Thus, one should remember that cyanosis might not always be observed with clinically significant hypoxemia. Conversely, a PaO_2 level as low as 40 mmHg (5.3 kPa) may be associated with an oxygen saturation exceeding 90% and adequate oxygen delivery to tissues, especially if hemoglobin F is the predominant hemoglobin and the oxygen-carrying capacity (red cell mass) is normal. Conditions in normotonic hypoxemic infants (methemoglobinemia, hemoglobinopathies) are uncommon causes of hypoxemia in the newborn. From a practical perspective most infants with reduced arterial oxygen contents have arterial oxygen tensions below 50 mmHg (6.7 kPa) and present with respiratory difficulties. The physiologic processes contributing to this syndrome include alveolar hypoventilation, impaired diffusion of oxygen from alveoli into blood, ventilation–perfusion

Table 41.1. Evaluation of the neonate with hypotonic hypoxemia

Test	Result	Probable diagnosis	Potential causes of error	Additional studies
Hyperoxia	$PaO_2 > 150$ mmHg (20 kPa)	Pulmonary parenchymal disease	Reactive pulmonary hypertension	Consider pre- and postductal PaO_2 or echocardiography
	PaO_2 100–150 mmHg (13–20 kPa)		All diagnoses possible	
	$PaO_2 < 100$ mmHg (13 kPa)	Right-to-left shunting	Severe pulmonary parenchymal disease	Compare pre- and postductal PaO_2; consider trial of continuous positive airway pressure
Preductal and postductal PaO_2	Preductal < postductal	Transposition of great arteries	Venous preductal sample	Echocardiogram
	Preductal = postductal	Intracardiac or intrapulmonary right-to-left shunting	May result from cardiac disease, severe parenchymal disease, or severe pulmonary hypertension	Echocardiogram, electrocardiogram
	Preductal > postductal	Ductal right-to-left shunting	Must distinguish pulmonary hypertension from reduced left ventricular output	Assess systemic blood pressure and cardiac output

Source: From Stevenson and Benitz [2].

mismatching, and right-to-left shunting. Studies useful in evaluation of the neonate with hypotonic hypoxemia (PaO_2 < 50 mmHg or 6.7 kPa), listed in Table 41.1, are discussed below. In addition, the medical record should include a careful history and physical examination, which may contribute to the diagnosis suggested by those studies. Metabolic disorders (acidosis, hypoglycemia, hypocalcemia) and rheologic abnormalities (hyperviscosity) should always be ruled out before this evaluation is initiated.

It should be noted that many of the procedures that have been used in the past to differentiate primary pulmonary disease from cardiac abnormalities have been replaced by the use of echocardiography. We continue to describe these evaluations in case an echocardiogram is not available.

Hyperoxia test

By definition, infants with refractory hypoxemia have already been subjected to the hyperoxia test, which consists simply of determining the PaO_2 level during the administration of 100% oxygen. Most infants who have low arterial oxygen tensions under these conditions have right-to-left shunting as a result of congenital heart disease or pulmonary vascular disease. However, some infants with severe pulmonary parenchymal disease may have persistently low PaO_2 levels owing to diffusion block or ventilation–perfusion mismatching. Those with the latter conditions often respond well to administration of continuous positive airway pressure at 5–6 cm of water (0.5–0.6 kPa), with a significant increment in the PaO_2 value. Contrarily, infants with pulmonary hypertension or congenital heart disease usually do less well during such administration and require additional evaluation.

Detection of ductal shunting

Simultaneous measurements of preductal (temporal or right radial artery) and postductal (umbilical, dorsalis pedis, or posterior tibial artery) oxygen tensions can be performed at the crib side while the infant is breathing 100% oxygen. If the postductal PaO_2 level exceeds the preductal value, transposition of the great arteries can be suspected clinically. Right-to-left ductal shunting is present if the preductal PaO_2 level exceeds the postductal value by more than 15–20 mmHg (2.0–2.7 kPa). If both the preductal and postductal PaO_2 values are low, the absence of such a difference does not exclude ductal shunting. Shunting at other levels (foramen ovale, intrapulmonary) cannot be either excluded or detected by this test. Measurement of the systemic blood pressure and assessment of the systemic cardiac output are essential in interpreting this observation, because right-to-left shunting may result from a decrease in the systemic arterial pressure or cardiac output, as well as increased pulmonary arterial pressures. These hemodynamic abnormalities must be corrected before evaluation of the cause of refractory hypoxemia can be completed, using the studies described below.

In current practice, measurement of pre- and postductal arterial oxygen tensions to detect right-to-left ductal shunting is complemented by color Doppler echocardiography. This technology permits detection of cardiac structural abnormalities, as well as shunt flows at the foramen ovale or ductus arteriosus, and should be readily available in all high-level or regional intensive care nurseries.

Information obtained from these diagnostic maneuvers must be combined with that obtained from other studies, including chest radiography and echocardiography. These data often do not correspond precisely to a description of a typical infant with any of the conditions listed in Table 41.2, and may appear to be contradictory or confusing. Thoughtful synthesis of all available information, including that from the history, physical examination, and laboratory studies, is required. All diagnostic information must be re-evaluated frequently if it becomes apparent that the infant's condition

Table 41.2. Pathophysiologic categories of refractory hypoxemia

Category	Characteristics
Reduced systemic pressure	Ductal or intracardiac right-to-left shunting
	Usually no improvement in PaO_2 during hyperventilation
	Reduced systemic blood pressure or cardiac output
Pulmonary hypertension	Ductal or intracardiac right-to-left shunting
	Hyperventilation produces $PaO_2 > 100$ mmHg (13 kPa) in those conditions associated with partially reversible pulmonary arterial constriction
	If the cause of pulmonary hypertension is not associated with reversible arterial constriction of the pulmonary vasculature, the diagnosis depends upon recognition of prolonged right ventricular systolic time intervals and exclusion of intrapulmonary right-to-left shunting, cardiac malformations, and systemic hypotension
Congenital heart disease	Ductal or intracardiac right-to-left shunting
	No improvement in PaO_2 during hyperventilation
	Echocardiogram usually diagnostic
Intrapulmonary shunting	No demonstrable ductal shunt
	Modest or no improvement in PaO_2 during hyperventilation
	Usually no evidence for pulmonary hypertension

Source: From Stevenson and Benitz [2].

Table 41.3. Priorities in the management of neonatal hypoxemia

Promote oxygenation by administering appropriate oxygen and assisted ventilation
Correct hypotension and/or anemia by correcting bradycardia and administering plasma and/or blood
Correct metabolic acidosis
Correct hypoglycemia
Correct hypocalcemia
Maintain acid–base homeostasis
Avoid hyperthermia, hypoxia, hyperoxia, severe hypocarbia, and severe hypercarbia
Correct polycythemia, if present
Obtain cultures and treat potential infection with antibiotics

Note:
Although these interventions are listed sequentially, it is imperative that they are carried out as expeditiously as possible; it is not appropriate to delay subsequent items while observing the response to initial measures.
Source: Adapted from Stevenson and Benitz [2].

has changed or that the initial diagnostic impression was incorrect or incomplete.

The physician should have a clear understanding of the priorities in the management of neonatal hypoxemia. These priorities are summarized in Table 41.3. The management of any infant with the syndrome of refractory hypoxemia should be discussed with the neonatologist at the regional high-level intensive care nursery while transport is being arranged. The details of this management depend on the diagnosis, the facilities available, and the input of the consulting neonatologist. A comprehensive discussion of the management of conditions that cause refractory hypoxemia is beyond the scope of this work; a brief review of three common categories of disease is given in the following sections.

Severe pulmonary parenchymal disease

Pulmonary parenchymal disease, such as bacterial pneumonia or severe hyaline membrane disease, that is refractory to surfactant therapy, administration of 100% oxygen, and assisted ventilation at low to moderate pressures and rates is most commonly treated by increasingly aggressive mechanical ventilation. This can be achieved in a variety of ways, most of which result in increasing mean airway pressure. These maneuvers must be used with caution because of the risk of air leaks. In addition, excessive distending pressures may

compromise pulmonary perfusion, resulting in increased extrapulmonary right-to-left shunting and exacerbation of hypoxemia. Sedation or neuromuscular blockade may be useful.

Diuretic therapy may help improve pulmonary gas exchange, if there is significant pulmonary edema. Diuretics are most effective in patients with hypervolemia or pulmonary overperfusion, but should be used with great caution in infants with pulmonary edema due to increased capillary permeability (e.g., in postasphyxial or septic infants), in whom intravascular volumes may already be diminished. The effects of diuretics result primarily from the decrease in vascular volume achieved by diuresis, but furosemide also increases venous capacitance, allowing translocation of pulmonary interstitial fluid into the venous system. Prolonged use of furosemide may lead to hypokalemia, hyponatremia, hypochloremia, and metabolic alkalosis. Moreover, long-term furosemide use may be associated with renal calculi, related to hypercalciuria [34]. Thus the use of other diuretics, such as chlorothiazide, may be considered.

Persistent patency of the ductus arteriosus beyond the first 48 hours of life may be associated with the shunting of blood from the aorta into the pulmonary artery, causing pulmonary congestion, increased interstitial lung fluid, and congestive heart failure. This can exacerbate pulmonary disease in premature infants, leading to a requirement for increased mechanical ventilatory support and consequent complications. There is no uniform agreement regarding the optimal overall approach to ductal closure (medical vs. surgical) or the protocol for medical management. In most centers active intervention is reserved for selected infants with demonstrable cardiovascular effects and respiratory compromise due to left-to-right shunting. Initial management often consists of fluid restriction and diuretic therapy, and may be successful.

If symptomatic ductal patency persists, attempted closure of the ductus with indomethacin is appropriate, if there are no contraindications to administration of the drug. Indomethacin is most effective if given in the first few days of life. Closure is achieved most consistently in premature infants with birthweight greater than 1000 g. A multicenter randomized trial demonstrated that ibuprofen may be as effective as indomethacin in the pharmacological treatment of patent ductus arteriosus in preterm infants [35]. Surgical ligation may be required for infants who do not improve after treatment with indomethacin. The effect of prophylactic treatment with indomethacin on short-term outcome in preterm infants has also been studied by a number of groups, and is routinely used in some institutions. Dosage regimens have varied enormously. A meta-analysis of randomized controlled trials concluded that prophylactic treatment with IV indomethacin results in significant reductions in symptomatic patent ductus arteriosus and severe IVH [36]. Available long-term follow-up studies suggest that such therapy is not associated with adverse neurodevelopmental outcome at 36 or 54 months' corrected age [37]. In a follow-up evaluation by Ment *et al.* it was found that males who received prophylactic indomethacin had significantly less intraventricular and parenchymal hemorrhage and improved verbal scores at 3 and 8 years of age [38]. This improvement was not noted in the girls who were given prophylactic indomethacin. The incidence of clinically significant ductus arteriosus, in fact, varies greatly among institutions, also reflecting differences in fluid management and ventilator management.

Glomerular filtration, urinary sodium excretion, and urine output can be affected adversely after treatment with indomethacin, especially in infants who already have compromised renal function because of large ductus arteriosus [39]. Indomethacin should not be given to an infant with impaired renal function as evidenced by a creatinine level greater than 1.8 mg/dl or oliguria (urine output < 0.5 mL/kg per hour in the preceding 8 hours). Because platelet function may also be compromised, indomethacin should not be used in infants with a bleeding diathesis or a platelet count less than 60 000 per microliter. Because necrotizing enterocolitis and focal gastrointestinal perforation have been associated with oral indomethacin use, the drug should not be used in infants with clinical or radiographic evidence of gastrointestinal dysfunction. Intracranial hemorrhage may also be a relative contraindication to treatment with indomethacin.

Refractory hypoxemia secondary to severe RDS has become much less common since the widespread introduction of surfactant replacement therapy. This treatment significantly reduces the incidence of RDS and markedly reduces its severity in infants who develop RDS in spite of surfactant therapy. Numerous studies of differing design evaluating the potential benefit of elective or rescue HFV in the management of RDS have arrived at different conclusions. Reviews and meta-analyses of available studies were unable to recommend conclusively any particular ventilatory strategy [40,41]. A recent multicenter, randomized, double-blinded controlled clinical trial of iNO for preterm infants with severe respiratory failure sponsored by the National Institute of Child Health and Human Development (NICHD) Neonatal Research Network

suggested in a post hoc analysis that the rates of death and BPD are reduced for infants with birthweights over 1000 g and up to 1500 g, in contrast to those 1000 g or less, who had more severe IVH and death [42]. These data suggest the need for further study.

Pulmonary arterial disease

Intrinsic disease of the pulmonary arteries is encountered most frequently in cases of PPHN. Pulmonary vascular disease is also a common correlate of disorders which produce an imbalance between pulmonary blood flow and the ability of the pulmonary vascular bed to accommodate flow in utero, such as may occur with pulmonary hypoplasia (e.g., with CDH), premature (intrauterine) closure of the ductus arteriosus, and cardiac malformations associated with increased pulmonary blood flow or pulmonary venous obstruction. Infants with these disorders have both structural and functional abnormalities of the pulmonary arteries, typified by excessive muscularity and hyperreactivity to a variety of stimuli, including hypoxia and acidemia. These conditions are characterized by increased pulmonary arterial and right heart pressures, and right-to-left shunting via the ductus arteriosus and foramen ovale. The diagnosis and management of these disorders are addressed in greater detail in Chapter 37.

Cyanotic congenital heart disease

Maintaining patency of the ductus arteriosus may be life-saving in a variety of congenital cardiac malformations, including those in which pulmonary blood flow must be derived from the aorta via the ductus arteriosus (because of obstruction of the right heart), those in which systemic perfusion is dependent on blood flow from the pulmonary artery to the aorta via the ductus arteriosus (due to left-sided heart obstruction), and those in which admixture of blood from the systemic and pulmonary circulations is essential for maintaining a reasonable systemic arterial oxygen content (Table 41.4). This can be accomplished with the infusion of 50–100 ng/kg per minute of prostaglandin E (PGE), gradually decreasing to 10–30 ng/kg per minute in many cases once patency is established [43]. Higher doses of PGE can be associated with diarrhea, fever, tachyarrhythmias, and systemic hypertension. Apnea can also be associated with use of PGE.

Management of cerebral edema

The management of cerebral edema in infants with hypoxic–ischemic encephalopathy (HIE) remains a controversial issue. Although data in human adults and in intrauterinely asphyxiated fetal monkeys demonstrated that cerebral edema is a major complication of HIE and begins soon after the asphyxial episode, extrapolation of these observations to the human infant is speculative at best [44–46]. Studies in neonatal rats and dogs suggest that the immature brain is relatively resistant to the development and severity of the edema that is seen in

Table 41.4. Patent ductus arteriosus-dependent cardiac malformations

Right-sided heart obstruction
Tricuspid atresia
Pulmonary atresia or severe stenosis
Truncus arteriosus with ductus-dependent pulmonary arteries
Tetralogy of Fallot
Left-sided heart obstruction
Coarctation of the aorta (preductal or juxtaductal)
Interruption of the aortic arch
Severe aortic stenosis
Mitral atresia/aortic atresia (HLHS Spectrum)
Mixing-dependent lesions
Transposition of the great arteries

Source: Modified from Benitz *et al.* [1].

Table 41.5. Methods of treatment for increased intracranial pressure

Fluid restriction
Hyperventilation
Corticosteroids
Mannitol

the mature animal [47,48]. Based upon studies by Myers and Brann & Myers in fetal monkeys [44–46], it has been postulated that intrauterine asphyxia leads to intracellular edema, followed by generalized cerebral edema and increased intracranial pressure (ICP). This in turn leads to decreased cerebral blood flow and necrosis of brain tissue. Excellent reviews by Volpe, Lupton and coworkers, and Hill suggest an alternative theory [49–51]. That is, following the asphyxial episode there is loss of vascular autoregulation of cerebral blood flow. This, coupled with systemic hypotension, leads to brain injury and brain necrosis, which are then followed by the development of cerebral edema.

Not only is there controversy regarding the mechanisms by which cerebral edema occurs, but the incidence and severity of the brain swelling following HIE have not been clearly elucidated. Lupton and coworkers evaluated 32 asphyxiated term infants during their first week of life with serial ICP measurements, using the Ladd ICP monitor; and 26 of the 32 infants had correlative CT scans performed as well [50]. They found that 22% of the infants had increased ICP, and that the pressure reached maximum levels between 36 and 72 hours rather than within the first few hours of life. Levene and Evans, using catheters placed in the subarachnoid space to measure ICP, found that 70% of severely asphyxiated newborns had a sustained increase in ICP of greater than 10 mmHg, for at least 60 minutes [52]. In 23 severely asphyxiated infants, nine infants did not have increased ICP at any time, nine had marked and sustained ICP that was resistant to medical therapy consisting of hyperventilation and infusions of mannitol, and five infants had sustained but mild elevations of ICP, which did not respond to infusions of mannitol. Of these five infants, three died, but two infants survived and were subsequently found to be normal. In this series, intracranial monitoring of the 23 infants was of benefit to two infants who responded to mannitol and survived (see further discussion of mannitol, below). In later reviews, Levene noted that "there is no evidence that routine monitoring of ICP and appropriate management of the elevation of ICP makes

any improvement in outcome" in the severely asphyxiated newborn [53,54].

Methods of decreasing cerebral edema

Since many infants with HIE have IADH, fluid restriction and the avoidance of fluid overload are of primary concern. Careful monitoring of fluid intake and output as well as serum electrolytes is indicated in the asphyxiated infant. Other methods of decreasing cerebral edema are listed in Table 41.5.

Hyperventilation

Infants have variable respiratory responses to HIE. Some will hyperventilate, some will have normal respiratory rates, and some will hypoventilate and be unresponsive to hypercarbia. By hyperventilating to hypocarbic ranges, cerebral blood flow can be reduced significantly. By decreasing the $PaCO_2$ by 1 mmHg, the cerebral blood flow will be decreased by 3% over the physiological $PaCO_2$ range [6,55]. The response is lessened when the $PaCO_2$ is decreased to 20 mmHg or less [6]. Follow-up of infants with PPHN demonstrated that infants with abnormal neurological findings in early childhood had both longer periods of hypotension and of hypocarbia ($PaCO_2 < 25$ mmHg) than did infants without neurological sequelae [56].

Bifano and Pfannenstiel also demonstrated that the surviving infants with PPHN who had adverse neurological sequelae had longer periods of hypocarbia than did survivors without neurological impairment [9]. Similar to the data of Bernbaum *et al.* [56], the infants who were treated with prolonged hyperventilation were most likely those infants who were most severely affected with PPHN.

Gleason and coworkers, studying paralyzed and sedated newborn lambs, evaluated the effects of 6 hours of hypocarbia with $PaCO_2$ levels down to 15 ± 2 mmHg on cerebral blood flow. Although the cerebral blood flow was decreased by 35% initially, it returned to baseline levels by 6 hours. Abrupt termination of the hyperventilation resulted in a marked increase in cerebral blood flow within 30 minutes [6]. These authors cautioned that if hypocarbia occurs after hyperventilation is stopped, it could possibly increase the incidence of intracranial hemorrhage. Such situations occur clinically in neonates who fail to respond to hyperventilation and then require treatment with iNO or with ECMO.

Wiswell and coworkers studied a group of prematurely born infants of 33 weeks' gestation or less who were treated with HFJV during the first 72 hours of life [57]. They found that the incidence of cystic periventricular leukomalacia (cPVL) was much greater in infants with greater cumulative periods of hypocarbia during the first 24 hours of life. Other factors, such as degree of hypertension, acidosis, or hypoxemia, did not increase the incidence of cPVL.

A study of 790 infants of 28 weeks' gestation or less who had hypocarbia during their first day of life also reported an increased risk for echo lucency on univariate analysis, although the association was diminished in a multivariate analysis [58]. Nevertheless, it is apparent that hypocarbia should be avoided in the infant if at all possible.

Studies by Vannucci et al., using an asphyxiated neonatal model, demonstrated a protective effect of mild to moderate hypercarbia in animals with asphyxia [59]. Severe hypocarbia did not offer this protective effect [60].

To date, there have been no reported clinical studies evaluating hyperventilation and subsequent hypocarbia as an adjunct in the therapy of infants with HIE. Recommendations that hyperventilation be used to prevent or treat cerebral edema must be viewed with caution. It is currently recommended that normocarbic levels be maintained in these infants, and that hyper- or hypocarbia be avoided.

Corticosteroids

Corticosteroids have been used effectively in reducing vasogenic cerebral edema, but they have had little, if any, effect in edema secondary to HIE, meningitis, or edema following trauma to the cranium [61,62]. Controlled studies in comatose adults secondary to trauma failed to alleviate the increased ICP or to mitigate neurological sequelae [61]. Similar results have been reported using corticosteroids following strokes in mature laboratory animals [63]. Svenningsen et al., in their evaluation of the protective effect of phenobarbital in the treatment of severe neurological asphyxia, used betamethasone and furosemide as adjuncts to their therapy, but did not specifically study the effects of either of these two agents [64]. Levene and Evans found no improvement of cerebral perfusion pressure when using dexamethasone in the treatment of infants with HIE [65].

Interestingly, Barks et al. and Tuor et al. have shown that when neonatal rats were pretreated 24 hours or more with dexamethasone, even at low doses, they were protected from subsequent episodes of cerebral damage due to asphyxia [66,67]. Treatment with dexamethasone, even in large amounts, had no protective effects if given less than 24 hours prior to or within 24 hours of the asphyxial event. These data are interesting in light of the fact that preterm infants of mothers who had been pretreated with betamethasone and dexamethasone had a decreased incidence and severity of IVH in the neonatal period [68]. Since there are numerous side effects of steroids, including hypertension, hyperglycemia, and electrolyte aberrations, the use of these agents in an already fragile patient is not recommended.

Mannitol

Mannitol and other hyperosmolar agents have been used to reduce the amount of cerebral edema following brain injury [69]. Mujsce et al., studying brain injury due to HIE in immature rats, infused mannitol immediately after the event and every 12 hours thereafter for a total of four infusions [47].

Although mannitol reduced the amount of edema and brain water, it did not alter the severity of the brain damage when compared to control animals.

Adhikari and coworkers treated 12 severely asphyxiated infants with a single infusion of 1 g/kg of mannitol and compared them with 13 similarly affected infants who were not given mannitol [69]. No differences were found in the mortality rate, the severity of cerebral edema as measured ultrasonographically, or in short-term outcome.

In an uncontrolled study, Marchal and coworkers treated over 200 asphyxiated infants with IV mannitol either before or after 2 hours of age [70]. There were fewer deaths and better neurological outcome in those infants who were treated early than in those treated after 2 hours. Unfortunately the types of infants treated and the variability in the severity of disease processes make the interpretation of these data difficult.

Although some investigators report that IV mannitol reduces ICP in asphyxiated newborns with cerebral edema, brain injury may not be altered, and most authorities currently do not recommend its use as an adjunct in the treatment of infants with HIE [49,60].

Other potential strategies as adjuncts in the management of infants with hypoxic–ischemic encephalopathy (Table 41.6)
Barbiturates

While barbiturates are readily used to control seizures that often accompany severe HIE (see Chapter 43), their use to prevent further brain damage after an asphyxial episode has also been recommended. Since the early 1970s, investigators have demonstrated that barbiturates decrease the rates of cerebral metabolism, decrease ICP, and reduce cellular injury due to the elaboration of free radicals.

Svenningsen et al. evaluated 35 term infants with neonatal asphyxia in two separate time periods. During the first 3 years of the study, 1973–76, affected infants received what was considered conservative management. During the second 3-year period, infants were ventilated early and effectively, had aggressive plasma and blood transfusions, and were given 10 mg/kg of phenobarbital within 60 minutes after birth and then daily thereafter [64]. Betamethasone and furosemide were also added to this regime. Both the mortality rates and the incidence of neurodevelopmental handicaps were reduced significantly during this latter aggressive period.

Goldberg et al. studied 32 consecutively admitted term neonates with severe asphyxia, all of whom required supportive ventilation [71]. Half of the group was given thiopental infusions beginning 1 and 3 hours after birth. Sustained elevation of ICP was encountered infrequently in all patients, and the outcome was the same in the two groups. Those infants receiving thiopental required pressor support more frequently than did the control group (14/16 vs. 7/15). These authors could not recommend thiopental for term asphyxiated

Table 41.6. Potential strategies that have been used as adjuncts in the management of infants with hypoxic–ischemic encephalopathy

Barbiturates
Excitatory amino acid receptor inhibitors
Oxygen free radical inhibitors
Monosialgangliosides
Lazaroids
Growth factors, including erythropoietin
Hypothermia

neonates. Similar data were obtained in adult patients who received thiopental following cardiac arrest [72].

Hall et al. studied the effects of phenobarbital given to term infants with severe asphyxia in a randomized controlled prospective trial [73]. After the infant's blood pressure, ventilation, and acid–base status were stabilized, the infants were given 40 mg/kg of the drug. Seizures occurred in nine of 15 study infants and 14 of 16 infants in the control group. A follow-up evaluation 3 years later revealed that 11 of 15 infants in the treatment group had a normal outcome, but only three of 16 in the control group were normal [73]. There were a few drawbacks to the study, in that a placebo was not used, after the babies were randomized the caretakers were not blinded to the type of treatment, and five infants were lost to follow-up, two in the treatment group and three in the control group. Nevertheless, this was an important study in that no adverse effects were encountered with a drug that is often used in an intensive care nursery, and that it appeared to result in a significant decrease in neurological damage. As the authors note, more comprehensive studies using continuous electroencephalographic monitoring, magnetic resonance spectroscopy (MRS), and monitoring of cerebral blood flow would enhance the study of a much larger group of patients in a randomized, blinded, and prospectively carried-out trial. A systematic review of anticonvulsant treatment of infants with perinatal asphyxia has concluded that such therapy should be reserved for treatment of clinical seizures. Prophylactic therapy with barbiturates has not been shown to be effective, but aggressive treatment of seizures should be initiated [74].

Excitatory amino acid (EAA) receptor inhibitors

EAAs, especially glutamate and aspartate, are the major neurotransmitters found in mammalian brain. The EAAs also have a trophic effect on differentiating neurons and are involved in the regulation of neuroendocrine function as well [75]. When hypoxic–ischemic insults occur, there is increased release of these EAAs up to 100-fold in the brains of adult animals, and to a much lesser extent in fetal and neonatal brain tissues [75]. EAAs activate postsynaptic receptors which, in turn, are coupled to channels that regulate the flow of sodium and calcium ions into the cell. There are two major types of receptors, metabotropic and ionotropic, the latter of which has been extensively studied. The major subtypes of the ionotropic receptors are N-methyl-D-aspartate (NMDA)

and α-amino-3-hydroxy-5-methyl-4-isoxazole propionic acid (AMPA). This latter receptor also mediates the effects of kainic acid and is referred to as the AMPA/kainic acid (KA) receptor [76].

Antagonists to these receptors have been studied and utilized, and have also been divided into the subtypes competitive and non-competitive antagonists. The competitive antagonists block the glutamate site directly, but because they are polar substances they do not cross the blood–brain barrier readily. The non-competitive antagonists to NMDA are utilized more frequently as they do cross the blood–brain barrier readily. These compounds include ketamine, phencyclidine (PCP or "angel dust"), dizocilpine (MK-801), aptiganel hydrochloride (CNS 112, Cerestat), and dextrorotary opioid derivatives, such as dextrorphan and dextromethorphan [76,77].

MK-801, which has the highest affinity for the ion-channel site, has demonstrated significant neuroprotective effects in both adult and newborn animals. This agent is effective when given prior to or following the asphyxial event in decreasing, but not abolishing, the neuronal damage. However, the toxicity of the agent is profound, even when used in low dosage, and neurobehavioral changes in the surviving animals have been noted as well [77].

Dextromethorphan is another non-competitive NMDA antagonist and has demonstrated neuroprotective effects in a rabbit model of transient ischemia [78]. The use of this agent as an adjunct to prophylactic therapy in patients undergoing neurosurgical procedures has also demonstrated beneficial effects with modest and reversible side effects [76]. Whether this agent will prove to have neuroprotective effects remains to be seen.

A competitive NMDA receptor antagonist, selfotel, which binds directly to the NMDA site of the glutamate receptor, had been shown to limit neuronal damage in several animal stroke studies. Unfortunately, in humans it was shown to be ineffective after acute ischemic stroke, and even exhibited neurotoxic effects in brain ischemia patients [79].

The magnesium ion also acts as a non-competitive NMDA antagonist [80], and has improved survival following myocardial infarctions and has been associated with decreased neurological damage following traumatic brain injury and strokes in adults [81]. Magnesium sulfate ($MgSO_4$) has been used as a tocolytic agent, as an antihypertensive agent, and as protection against the development of seizures in women with pre-eclampsia [82].

$MgSO_4$ has reduced the severity of asphyxial brain damage in immature rats and mice, but when studied in near-term fetal lambs and piglets, it did not reduce injury to the cerebral cortex [83–86].

Levene et al. evaluated two different doses of $MgSO_4$ in a group of infants when 10-minute Apgar scores were less than 6, or a 5-minute Apgar score was less than 6 with other clinical and laboratory evidence of fetal distress [87]. The infants received either 250 or 400 mg/kg IV. All of the infants receiving 400 mg/kg had cessation of respiratory function for 3–6 hours, but since the infants had already been intubated and ventilated, no harm was encountered. The electroencephalogram did not change, but muscle tone and activity were diminished. The infants also had significant lowering of blood pressure. The lower dose did not cause hypotension but did cause some respiratory depression. These authors have advised against using the higher dose of $MgSO_4$, and also cautioned that respiratory failure can occur even with the lower dose. A multicenter randomized controlled trial was designed to evaluate whether $MgSO_4$ is neuroprotective after birth asphyxia has been suspended [88]. In a recent review by Marret et al. the results of four major randomized controlled trials of antenatal $MgSO_4$ therapy in fetuses of less than 34 weeks' gestation were collated and analyzed [89]. Overall, there were no significant differences in mortality or the development of CP at follow-up. One of the studies did demonstrate that significant motor dysfunction was found in fewer of the $MgSO_4$-treated infants when they were studied at 2 years of age [90]. The Maternal-Fetal Medicine Unit Network of the NICHD is currently conducting the BEAM (Beneficial Effects of Antenatal Magnesium Sulfate) trial, which is investigating the use of $MgSO_4$ in preventing cerebral palsy.

Calcium-channel blockers

Because of the toxicity of increased intracellular calcium accumulation that occurs when a cell is damaged, various drugs have been developed to prevent the influx of the ion into neurons. Investigators from New Zealand demonstrated a neuroprotective effect of one of these blockers, flunarizine, in immature rats [91], as well as in fetal sheep [92]. However, when Levene et al. used nicardipine, another calcium-channel blocker, in four severely asphyxiated neonates, they had severe complications [93]. The mean arterial blood pressure decreased in three infants and two developed sudden and dramatic hypotension. They strongly cautioned against the use of this drug in infants with HIE.

Oxygen free radical inhibitors

The mechanisms by which oxygen free radicals initiate and perpetuate cellular damage are clearly elucidated in Chapter 3. Although the body produces naturally occurring antioxidants such as catalase, superoxide dismutase, endoperoxidases, glutathione, and cholesterol, as well as using vitamins C and E in such situations, the elaboration of the oxygen free radicals following an asphyxial event may exceed the infant's ability to generate adequate protection [94]. Drugs such as superoxide dismutase, glutathione peroxidase, and catalase have been used primarily in laboratory animals, but they have limitations such as a prolonged period to traverse the blood–brain barrier and a narrow therapeutic dosage range. They also have to be given hours before the insult.

Vitamins C and E have also been proven ineffective in these infants. Allopurinol, a xanthine oxidase inhibitor that is converted to oxypurinol, has been shown by Palmer et al. to be of benefit in rats during the reperfusion period [95]. Several investigators have evaluated allopurinol in postasphyxial infants. Van Bel et al. studied 22 infants of 35 weeks' or more gestation who had severe HIE [96], of whom 11 were given

40 mg/kg IV allopurinol and 11 served as controls. In their report, as well as in a follow-up abstract, a beneficial neurological outcome was observed. However, in a more recent study from the same center, infants with severe encephalopathy treated with allopurinol showed no differences in mortality or short-term morbidity as compared to control infants [97].

Lastly, Gunes et al. evaluated 60 infants with mild, moderate, and severe encephalopathy. Half were treated with 40 mg/kg of IV allopurinol daily for 3 days, while the other half were given saline [98]. Those with mild encephalopathy did well in both groups, but those with moderate or severe encephalopathy who were treated with allopurinol had decreased nitric oxide concentrations on their sera and cerebral spinal fluid compared to controls, and also had better neurological and neurodevelopmental outcome at 12 months of age.

Obviously, there is still much to be learned regarding the use of allopurinol, especially in the timing of the initiation of therapy, the dosage, and the length of treatment required.

Monosialogangliosides

These glycosphingolipids, found throughout the body, are found in high concentrations in the nervous system and are important components of cell membranes. Monosialoganglioside (GMI) crosses the placenta and blood–brain barriers and can be incorporated into neural cell membranes. Tan et al., in elegant studies using a fetal sheep model, showed that GMI given prior to and following repeated episodes of asphyxial damage protected the animals from neurological sequelae that would ordinarily have taken place [99]. They demonstrated that "systemic treatment with GMI reduced morphologic, biochemical, neurophysiological and behavioral manifestation of hypoxic–ischemic brain damage" [99]. The agent did not cause hypotension or metabolic disturbances in the animals. To date, this form of therapy has not been reported in human neonates.

Lazaroids (21-aminosteroids)

Methylprednisone has been used for many years to diminish the severity of sequelae following brain and spinal cord injury [100]. When given in high doses, some beneficial effect was noted in a few patients. Subsequent studies demonstrated that the therapeutic effect was not related to the glucocorticoid or mineralocorticoid actions of the drug, but to its effect of limiting lipid peroxidation [101]. Thus 21-aminosteroids were developed as inhibitors of lipid peroxidation. These agents have neither glucocorticoid nor mineralocorticoid activity and are essentially non-toxic. The 21-aminosteroid that has been selected for the acute treatment of brain and spinal injury, ischemic stroke, and subarachnoid hemorrhage is tirilazad mesylate, which is a potent inhibitor of oxygen-radical-induced, ion-catalyzed lipid peroxidation. It appears to exert its effect by a radical scavenging activity and by stabilization of the cellular membrane. This agent also prevents the post-traumatic permeability of the blood–brain barrier, reduces the extent of cerebral edema, and maintains and preserves endogenous vitamin E levels in tissue [102].

The vast majority of studies with the lazaroids have been accomplished in laboratory animals, including subhuman primates, and phase I trials in humans showed that tirilazad mesylate did not affect cardiovascular parameters, nor did it have any adverse interaction with the calcium-channel blocker nimodipine. In phase II studies of 245 patients with aneurysmal subarachnoid hemorrhage, symptomatic vasospasm was reduced and the Glasgow outcome score was improved in the lazaroid-treated patients compared to controls [102]. Kavanagh and Kam have reviewed studies evaluating the efficacy of lazaroids in the treatment of trauma to the brain, ischemic and subarachnoid hemorrhage, and noted that the routine clinical use of these agents was not warranted [103]. Further studies utilizing this agent in acute head and spinal injury, aneurysmal subarachnoid hemorrhage, and ischemic stroke should be forthcoming; and if the drugs have beneficial effects in these patients, use in neonates with HIE may prove beneficial as well. To date, no reports of the use of lazaroids in human neonates have been published.

Growth factors

The use of various growth factors in the treatment of neonatal encephalopathy is described in Chapter 42. One of the additional neuroprotective agents is erythropoietin. This endogenously produced cytokine promotes red blood cell maturation. McPherson and Juul have reviewed the neuroprotective effects of the agent in the treatment of extremely premature infants and those with neonatal encephalopathy [104]. Most of the studies have been carried out in laboratory animals, and they have demonstrated a remarkable benefit of erythropoietin as a neuroprotective agent. However, higher doses of the agent were required as only a small fraction, less than 2%, crossed the blood–brain barrier. Thus, even 10 times the dose used to treat anemias has been required if neuroprotection is to be achieved. In newborn rat studies, erythropoietin has been shown to significantly protect brain tissues and improve functional recovery 2 weeks following stroke [105]. Certainly, more research is to be required if this agent is to be used in neonatal encephalopathy.

Hypothermia

The use of hypothermia has been evaluated intensively over the past 10 years and is described at length in Chapter 42. Because an encephalopathic infant has a decreased ability to regulate his/her temperature, it is at the mercy of the environment. Perinatal *hyperthermia*, due to maternal fever and/or increased temperature levels in the delivery room, has been shown to be associated with increased risks for developing neonatal encephalopathy and cerebral palsy [106–108].

Conclusions

Following the resuscitation and stabilization of the encephalopathic infant, it is imperative that the newborn continues to receive intensive observation and care in order to obtain optimal outcome. Knowledge of the factors involved in the encephalopathic process, and the provision of meticulous and intensive therapy are paramount if the infant is to survive with as few handicaps as possible. The avoidance of over- and under-ventilation, hypo- and hyperoxia, appropriate correction of chemical and metabolic abnormalities, judicious monitoring of blood pressure and adequacy of the circulation, and avoidance of hyperthermia are key in enhancing improved outcome. In addition, treatment of definite and suspected bacterial, viral, and fungal infections, after appropriate cultures have been obtained, is also extremely important in the management of the obtunded child. Immediate referrals to centers that can provide specialized therapy such as hypothermia within a small window of opportunity are critical as well. As newer therapies are developed for these infants, it is hoped that we can limit the severity of brain injury and thereby improve neurodevelopmental outcomes. This is an exciting time for our ability to provide these innovative therapies for affected infants, and newer techniques including the use of stem cell therapy are on the horizon. However, it is also important to recognize that many of the encephalopathic infants may have sustained injury days to weeks prior to delivery; in such unfortunate situations, all of the technology and therapeutic advantages that we currently have at our disposal will be ineffective in altering the ultimate outcome.

References

1. Benitz WE, Frankel LR, Stevenson DK. The pharmacology of neonatal resuscitation and cardiopulmonary intensive care. Part II: extended intensive care. *West J Med* 1986; **145**: 47–51.

2. Stevenson DK, Benitz WE. A practical approach to diagnosis and immediate care of the cyanotic neonate: stabilization and preparation for transfer to level III nursery. *Clin Pediatr* 1987; **26**: 325–31.

3. Bruce DA. Effects of hyperventilation on cerebral blood flow and metabolism. *Clin Perinatol* 1984; **11**: 673–80.

4. Walsh-Sukys MC, Tyson JE, Wright LL, *et al.* Persistent pulmonary hypertension of the newborn in the era before nitric oxide: practice variation and outcomes. *Pediatrics* 2000; **105**: 14–20.

5. Kusuda S, Shishida N, Miyagi N, *et al.* Cerebral blood flow during treatment for pulmonary hypertension. *Arch Dis Child Fetal Neonatal Ed* 1999; **80**: F30–3.

6. Gleason CA, Short BL, Jones MD. Cerebral blood flow and metabolism during and after prolonged hypocapnia in newborn lambs. *J Pediatr* 1989; **115**: 309–14.

7. Liem KD, Hopman JC, Oeseburg B, *et al.* Cerebral oxygenation and hemodynamics during induction of extracorporeal membrane oxygenation as investigated by near infrared spectrophotometry. *Pediatrics* 1995; **95**: 555–61.

8. Toft PB, Leth H, Lou HC, *et al.* Local vascular CO_2 reactivity in the infant brain assessed by functional MRI. *Pediatr Radiol* 1995; **25**: 420–4.

9. Bifano EM, Pfannenstiel A. Duration of hyperventilation and outcome in infants with persistent pulmonary hypertension. *Pediatrics* 1988; **81**: 657–61.

10. Hendricks-Munoz KD, Walton JP. Hearing loss in infants with persistent fetal circulation. *Pediatrics* 1988; **81**: 650–6.

11. Leavitt AM, Watchko JF, Bennett FC, *et al.* Neurodevelopmental outcome

following persistent pulmonary hypertension of the neonate. *J Perinatol* 1987; **7**: 288–91.

12. Walsh-Sukys MC, Cornell DJ, Houston LN, *et al.* Treatment of persistent pulmonary hypertension of the newborn without hyperventilation: an assessment of diffusion of innovation. *Pediatrics* 1994; **94**: 303–6.

13. Wung JT, James LS, Kilchevsky E, *et al.* Management of infants with severe respiratory failure and persistence of the fetal circulation, without hyperventilation. *Pediatrics* 1985; **76**: 488–94.

14. Clark RH, Yoder BA, Sell MS. Prospective, randomized comparison of high-frequency oscillation and conventional ventilation in candidates for extracorporeal membrane oxygenation. *J Pediatr* 1994; **124**: 447–54.

15. Baumgart S, Hirschl RB, Butler SZ, *et al.* Diagnosis-related criteria in the consideration of extracorporeal membrane oxygenation in neonates previously treated with high-frequency jet ventilation. *Pediatrics* 1992; **89**: 491–4.

16. deLemos R, Yoder B, McCurnin D, *et al.* The use of high-frequency oscillatory ventilation (HFOV) and extracorporeal membrane oxygenation (ECMO) in the management of the term/near term infant with respiratory failure. *Early Hum Dev* 1992; **29**: 299–303.

17. Bhuta T, Henderson-Smart DJ. Rescue high frequency oscillatory ventilation versus conventional ventilation for pulmonary dysfunction in preterm infants. *Cochrane Database Syst Rev* 2000; (2): CD000438.

18. Hintz SR, Suttner DM, Sheehan AM, *et al.* Decreased use of neonatal extracorporeal membrane oxygenation (ECMO): how new treatment modalities have affected ECMO utilization. *Pediatrics* 2000; **106**: 1339–43.

19. Crone RK, Favorito J. The effects of pancuronium bromide on infants with hyaline membrane disease. *J Pediatr* 1980; **97**: 991–3.

20. Goudsouzian NG, Liu LM, Savarese JJ. Metocurine in infants and children: neuromuscular and clinical effects. *Anesthesiology* 1978; **49**: 266–9.

21. Jobe AH. Pulmonary surfactant therapy. *N Engl J Med* 1993; **328**: 861–8.

22. Kendig JW, Ryan RM, Sinkin RA, *et al.* Comparison of two strategies for surfactant prophylaxis in very premature infants: a multicenter randomized trial. *Pediatrics* 1998; **101**: 1006–12.

23. Soll RF. Synthetic surfactant for respiratory distress syndrome in preterm infants. *Cochrane Database Syst Rev* 2000; (2): CD001149.

24. Bancalari E, del Moral T. Bronchopulmonary dysplasia and surfactant. *Biol Neonate* 2001; **80** Suppl 1: 7–13.

25. Greenough A. Expanded use of surfactant replacement therapy. *Eur J Pediatr* 2000; **159**: 635–40.

26. Lotze A, Mitchell BR, Bulas DI, *et al.* Multicenter study of surfactant (beractant) use in the treatment of term infants with severe respiratory failure. Survanta in Term Infants Study Group. *J Pediatr* 1998; **132**: 40–7.

27. The Neonatal Inhaled Nitric Oxide Study Group (NINOS). Inhaled nitric oxide in full-term and nearly full-term infants with hypoxic respiratory failure. *N Engl J Med* 1997; **336**: 597–604.

28. The Neonatal Inhaled Nitric Oxide Study Group (NINOS). Inhaled nitric oxide and hypoxic respiratory failure in infants with congenital diaphragmatic hernia. *Pediatrics* 1997; **99**: 838–45.

29. Breitweser JA, Meyer RA, Sperling MA, *et al.* Cardiac septal hypertrophy in hyperinsulinemic infants. *J Pediatr* 1980; **96**: 535–9.

30. Seri I. Systemic and pulmonary effects of vasopressors and inotropes in the neonate. *Biol Neonate* 2006; **89**: 340–2.

31. Zaritsky A, Chernow B. Use of catecholamines in pediatrics. *J Pediatr* 1984; **105**: 341–50.

32. Friedman WF, George BL. Treatment of congestive heart failure by altering loading conditions of the heart. *J Pediatr* 1985; **106**: 697–706.

33. Bard H. Hemoglobin synthesis and metabolism during the neonatal period. In Christensen RD, ed., *Hematologic Problems of the Neonate*. Philadelphia, PA: Saunders, 2000: 374–7.

34. Yeh TF, Shibli A, Leu ST, *et al.* Early furosemide therapy in premature infants (less than or equal to 2000 gm) with respiratory distress syndrome: a randomized controlled trial. *J Pediatr* 1984; **105**: 603–9.

35. Van Overmeire B, Smets K, Lecoutere D, *et al.* A comparison of ibuprofen and indomethacin for closure of patent ductus arteriosus. *N Engl J Med* 2000; **343**: 674–81.

36. Fowlie PW. Intravenous indomethacin for preventing mortality and morbidity in very low birth weight infants.

Cochrane Database Syst Rev 2000; (3): CD000174.

37. Ment LR, Vohr B, Allan W, *et al.* Outcome of children in the indomethacin intraventricular hemorrhage prevention trial. *Pediatrics* 2000; **105**: 485–91.

38. Ment LR, Vohr BR, Makuch RW, *et al.* Prevention of intraventricular hemorrhage by indomethacin in male preterm infants. *J Pediatr* 2004; **145**: 832–4.

39. Clyman RI. Recommendations for the postnatal use of indomethacin: an analysis of four separate strategies. *J Pediatr* 1996; **128**: 601–7.

40. Cools F, Offringa M. Meta-analysis of elective high frequency ventilation in preterm infants with respiratory distress syndrome. *Arch Dis Child Fetal Neonatal Ed* 1999; **80**: F15–20.

41. Henderson-Smart DJ, Bhuta T, Cools F, *et al.* Elective high frequency oscillatory ventilation versus conventional ventilation for acute pulmonary dysfunction in preterm infants. *Cochrane Database Syst Rev* 2000; (2): CD000104.

42. Van Meurs KP, Wright LL, Ehrenkranz RA, *et al.* Inhaled nitric oxide for premature infants with severe respiratory failure. *N Engl J Med* 2005; **353**: 13–22.

43. Heymann MA. Pharmacologic use of prostaglandin E$_1$ in infant with congenital heart disease. *Am Heart J* 1981; **101**: 837–43.

44. Brann AW, Myers RE. Central nervous system findings in the newborn monkey following severe in utero partial asphyxia. *Neurology* 1975; **25**: 327–38.

45. Myers RE. Two patterns of perinatal brain damage and their conditions of occurrence. *Am J Obstet Gynecol* 1972; **112**: 246–76.

46. Myers RE. Experimental models of perinatal brain damage: relevance to human pathology. In Gluck L, ed., *Intrauterine Asphyxia and the Developing Fetal Brain*. Chicago, IL: Year-Book, 1977: 37–97.

47. Mujsce DJ, Christensen MA, Vannucci RC. Cerebral blood flow and edema in perinatal hypoxic–ischemic brain damage. *Pediatr Res* 1990; **27**: 450–3.

48. Young RS, Yagel SK. Cerebral physiological and metabolic effects of hyperventilation in the neonatal dog. *Ann Neurol* 1984; **16**: 337–42.

49. Volpe JJ. Hypoxic–ischemic encephalopathy. In Volpe JJ, ed., *Neurology of the Newborn*. Philadelphia, PA: Saunders, 2001: 217–394.

50. Lupton BA, Hill A, Roland EH, *et al.* Brain swelling in the asphyxiated term newborn: pathogenesis and outcome. *Pediatrics* 1988; **82**: 139–46.

51. Hill A. Current concepts of hypoxic–ischemic cerebral injury in the term newborn. *Pediatr Neurol* 1991; **7**: 317–25.

52. Levene MI, Evans DH. Continuous measurement of subarachnoid pressure in the severely asphyxiated newborn. *Arch Dis Child* 1983; **58**: 1013–15.

53. Levene MI. Management and outcome of birth asphyxia. In Levene MI, Lilforde RJ, eds., *Fetal and Neonatal Neurology and Neurosurgery*. Edinburgh: Churchill Livingstone, 1995: 427–42.

54. Levene MI, Evans DH, Forde A, *et al.* Value of intracranial pressure monitoring of asphyxiated newborn infants. *Dev Med Child Neurol* 1987; **29**: 311–19.

55. Rosenberg AA, Jones MD, Traystman RJ, *et al.* Response of cerebral blood flow to changes in PCO_2 in fetal, newborn, and adult sheep. *Am J Physiol* 1982; **242**: H862–6.

56. Bernbaum JC, Russell P, Sheridan PH, *et al.* Long-term follow-up of newborns with persistent pulmonary hypertension. *Crit Care Med* 1984; **12**: 579–83.

57. Wiswell TE, Graziani LJ, Kornhauser MS, *et al.* Effects of hypocarbia on the development of cystic periventricular leukomalacia in premature infants treated with high-frequency jet ventilation. *Pediatrics* 1996; **98**: 918–24.

58. Dammann O, Allred EN, Kuban KC, *et al.* Hypocarbia during the first 24 postnatal hours and white matter echolucencies in newborns ≤ 28 weeks gestation. *Pediatr Res* 2001; **49**: 388–93.

59. Vannucci RC, Towfighi J, Heitjan DF, *et al.* Carbon dioxide protects the perinatal brain from hypoxic–ischemic damage: an experimental study in the immature rat. *Pediatrics* 1995; **95**: 868–74.

60. Vannucci RC, Towfighi J, Brucklacher RM, *et al.* Effect of extreme hypercapnia on hypoxic–ischemic brain damage in the immature rat. *Pediatr Res* 2001; **49**: 799–803.

61. Cooper PR, Moody S, Clark WK, *et al.* Dexamethasone and severe head injury: a prospective double-blind study. *J Neurosurg* 1979; **51**: 307–16.

62. Dearden NM, Gibson JS, McDowall DG, *et al.* Effect of high-dose dexamethasone on outcome from severe head injury. *J Neurosurg* 1986; **64**: 81–8.

63. Lee MC, Mastri AR, Waltz AG, *et al.* Ineffectiveness of dexamethasone for treatment of experimental cerebral infarction. *Stroke* 1974; **5**: 216–18.

64. Svenningsen NW, Blennow G, Lindroth M, *et al.* Brain-orientated intensive care treatment in severe neonatal asphyxia: effects of phenobarbitone protection. *Arch Dis Child* 1982; **57**: 176–83.

65. Levene MI, Evans DH. Medical management of raised intracranial pressure after severe birth asphyxia. *Arch Dis Child* 1985; **60**: 12–16.

66. Barks JD, Post M, Tuor UI. Dexamethasone prevents hypoxic–ischemic brain damage in the neonatal rat. *Pediatr Res* 1991; **29**: 558–63.

67. Tuor UI, Simone CS, Barks JD, *et al.* Dexamethasone prevents cerebral infarction without affecting cerebral blood flow in neonatal rats. *Stroke* 1993; **24**: 452–7.

68. National Institutes of Health Consensus Development Panel on the Effect of Corticosteroids for Fetal Maturation of Perinatal Outcomes. Effect of corticosteroids for fetal maturation on perinatal outcomes. *JAMA* 1994; **273**: 413–8.

69. Adhikari M, Moodley M, Desai PK. Mannitol in neonatal cerebral oedema. *Brain Dev* 1990; **12**: 349–51.

70. Marchal C, Costagliolu P, Leaveau P, *et al.* Treatment de la souffrance cérébrale néonatale d'orisivie anoxique par le mannitol. *Rev Pediatr* 1974; **9**: 581–9.

71. Goldberg RN, Moscoso P, Bauer CR, *et al.* Use of barbiturate therapy in severe perinatal asphyxia: a randomized controlled trial. *J Pediatr* 1986; **109**: 851–6.

72. Brain Resuscitation Clinical Trial I Study Group. Randomized clinical study of thiopental loading in comatose survivors of cardiac arrest. *N Engl J Med* 1986; **314**: 397–403.

73. Hall RT, Hall FK, Daily DK. High-dose phenobarbital therapy in term newborn infants with severe perinatal asphyxia: a randomized, prospective study with three-year follow-up. *J Pediatr* 1998; **132**: 345–8.

74. Evans DJ, Levene MI, Tsakmakis M. Anticonvulsants for preventing mortality and morbidity in full term newborns with perinatal asphyxia.

Cochrane Database Syst Rev 2007; (3): CD001240.

75. Giacoia GP. Asphyxial brain damage in the newborn: new insights into pathophysiology and possible pharmacologic interventions. *South Med J* 1993; **86**: 676–82.

76. Muir KW, Lees KR. Clinical experience with excitatory amino acid antagonist drugs. *Stroke* 1995; **26**: 503–13.

77. Levene M. Role of excitatory amino acid antagonists in the management of birth asphyxia. *Biol Neonate* 1992; **62**: 248–51.

78. Steinberg GK, Bell TE, Yenari MA. Dose escalation safety and tolerance study of the N-methyl-D-aspartate antagonist dextromethorphan in neurosurgery patients. *J Neurosurg* 1996; **84**: 860–6.

79. Davis SM, Lees KR, Albers GW, *et al.* Selfotel in acute ischemic stroke: possible neurotoxic effects of an NMDA antagonist. *Stroke* 2000; **31**: 347–54.

80. Parikka H, Toivonen L, Naukkarinen V, *et al.* Decreases by magnesium of QT dispersion and ventricular arrhythmias in patients with acute myocardial infarction. *Eur Heart J* 1999; **20**: 111–20.

81. Lampl Y, Gilad R, Geva D, *et al.* Intravenous administration of magnesium sulfate in acute stroke: a randomized double-blind study. *Clin Neuropharmacol* 2001; **24**: 11–15.

82. Lucas MJ, Leveno KJ, Cunningham FG. A comparison of magnesium sulfate with phenytoin for the prevention of eclampsia. *N Engl J Med* 1995; **333**: 201–5.

83. McDonald JW, Silverstein FS, Johnston MV. Magnesium reduces N-methyl-D-aspartate (NMDA)-mediated brain injury in perinatal rats. *Neurosci Lett* 1990; **109**: 234–8.

84. Marret S, Gressens P, Gadisseux JF, *et al.* Prevention by magnesium of excitotoxic neuronal death in the developing brain: an animal model for clinical intervention studies. *Dev Med Child Neurol* 1995; **37**: 473–84.

85. de Haan HH, Gunn AJ, Williams CE, *et al.* Magnesium sulfate therapy during asphyxia in near-term fetal lambs does not compromise the fetus but does not reduce cerebral injury. *Am J Obstet Gynecol* 1997; **176**: 18–27.

86. Penrice J, Amess PN, Punwani S, *et al.* Magnesium sulfate after transient hypoxia–ischemia fails to prevent delayed cerebral energy failure in the newborn piglet. *Pediatr Res* 1997; **41**: 443–7.

87. Levene M, Blennow M, Whitelaw A, *et al.* Acute effects of two different doses of magnesium sulphate in infants with birth asphyxia. *Arch Dis Child Fetal Neonatal Ed* 1995; **73**: F174–7.

88. Robertson NJ, Edwards AD. Recent advances in developing neuroprotective strategies for perinatal asphyxia. *Curr Opin Pediatr* 1998; **10**: 575–80.

89. Marret S, Doyle LW, Crowther CA, *et al.* Antenatal magnesium sulphate neuroprotection in the preterm infant. *Semin Fetal Neonatal Med* 2007; **12**: 311–17.

90. Crowther CA, Hiller JE, Doyle LW, *et al.* Effect of magnesium sulfate given for neuroprotection before preterm birth: a randomized controlled trial. *JAMA* 2003; **290**: 2669–76.

91. Gunn AJ, Mydlar T, Bennet L, *et al.* The neuroprotective actions of a calcium channel antagonist, flunarizine, in the infant rat. *Pediatr Res* 1989; **25**: 573–6.

92. Gunn AJ, Williams CE, Mallard EC, *et al.* Flunarizine, a calcium channel antagonist, is partially prophylactically neuroprotective in hypoxic–ischemic encephalopathy in the fetal sheep. *Pediatr Res* 1994; **35**: 657–63.

93. Levene MI, Gibson NA, Fenton AC, *et al.* The use of a calcium-channel blocker, nicardipine, for severely asphyxiated newborn infants. *Dev Med Child Neurol* 1990; **32**: 567–74.

94. Buonocore G, Groenendaal F. Anti-oxidant strategies. *Semin Fetal Neonatal Med* 2007; **12**: 287–95.

95. Palmer C, Towfighi J, Roberts RL, *et al.* Allopurinol administered after inducing hypoxia–ischemia reduces brain injury in 7-day-old rats. *Pediatr Res* 1993; **33**: 405–11.

96. Van Bel F, Shadid M, Moison RM, *et al.* Effect of allopurinol on postasphyxial free radical formation, cerebral hemodynamics, and electrical brain activity. *Pediatrics* 1998; **101**: 185–93.

97. Benders MJ, Bos AF, Rademaker CM, *et al.* Early postnatal allopurinol does not improve short term outcome after severe birth asphyxia. *Arch Dis Child Fetal Neonatal Ed* 2006; **91**: F163–5.

98. Gunes T, Ozturk MA, Koklu E, *et al.* Effect of allopurinol supplementation on nitric oxide levels in asphyxiated newborns. *Pediatr Neurol* 2007; **36**: 17–24.

99. Tan WK, Williams CE, Mallard CE, *et al.* Monosialoganglioside GM1 treatment after a hypoxic–ischemic episode reduces the vulnerability of the fetal sheep brain to subsequent injuries. *Am J Obstet Gynecol* 1994; **170**: 663–9.

100. Hall ED. The neuroprotective pharmacology of methylprednisolone. *J Neurosurg* 1992; **76**: 13–22.

101. Amar AP, Levy ML. Pathogenesis and pharmacological strategies for mitigating secondary damage in acute spinal cord injury. *Neurosurgery* 1999; **44**: 1027–3.

102. Hall ED, McCall JM, Means ED. Therapeutic potential of the lazaroids (21-aminosteroids) in acute central nervous system trauma, ischemia and subarachnoid hemorrhage. *Adv Pharmacol* 1994; **28**: 221–68.

103. Kavanagh RJ, Kam PC. Lazaroids: efficacy and mechanism of action of the 21-aminosteroids in neuroprotection. *Br J Anaesth* 2001; **86**: 110–19.

104. McPherson RJ, Juul SE. Recent trends in erythropoietin-mediated neuroprotection. *Int J Dev Neurosci* 2008; **26**: 103–11.

105. Gonzalez FF, McQuillen P, Mu D, *et al.* Erythropoietin enhances long-term neuroprotection and neurogenesis in neonatal stroke. *Dev Neurosci* 2007; **29**: 321–30.

106. Adamson SJ, Alessandri LM, Badawi N, *et al.* Predictors of neonatal encephalopathy in full-term infants. *BMJ* 1995; **311**: 598–602.

107. Badawi N, Kurinczuk JJ, Keogh JM, *et al.* Intrapartum risk factors for newborn encephalopathy: the Western Australian case–control study. *BMJ* 1998; **317**: 1554–8.

108. Shankaran S. The postnatal management of the asphyxiated term infant. *Clin Perinatol* 2002; **29**: 675–92.

42

Endogenous and exogenous neuroprotective mechanisms after hypoxic–ischemic injury

Alistair J. Gunn, Robert D. Barrett, and Laura Bennet

Introduction

Nearly all infants are exposed to periods of compromised gas exchange before and during labor (see Chapter 13), and yet only a remarkably small minority of newborns develop hypoxic–ischemic encephalopathy (HIE). Indeed, even severe metabolic acidosis at birth is associated with HIE in less than half of cases [1]. Similarly, experimental studies typically report that cerebral injury occurs only in a very narrow temporal window between survival with complete recovery and death [2,3]. Partly this is a reflection of the efficiency of the fetal adaptations that maintain perfusion to the essential organs. Partly, an acute event activates a cascade not only of damaging processes but also of protective endogenous processes that help limit neural injury, as illustrated in Figure 42.1. These processes may be modified, raising the possibility of treating acute encephalopathy.

Biphasic cell death after hypoxic–ischemic injury

The seminal observation, both from experimental studies in vivo and in vitro, and from clinical observations, is that HIE is not a single "event" but rather an evolving process. During actual hypoxia–ischemia (which may be termed the "primary" phase of the insult) high-energy metabolites are depleted, with progressive depolarization of cells, severe cytotoxic edema (cell swelling), and extracellular accumulation of excitatory amino acids (EAAs) due to failure of reuptake by astroglia and excessive depolarization-mediated release [4,5]. Although neurons may die during a sufficiently prolonged period of ischemia or asphyxia, many neurons initially recover at least partially from the insult in a so-called "latent" phase, only to die many hours or even days later (secondary or delayed cell death). Using magnetic resonance spectroscopy, it was shown that many infants with evidence of moderate to severe asphyxia show initial, transient recovery of cerebral oxidative metabolism after birth, followed by secondary deterioration with cerebral energy failure from 6 to 15 hours after birth [6,7]. It is this delay which offers the tantalizing possibility for therapeutic intervention. The severity of this secondary deterioration is closely correlated with neurodevelopmental outcome at 1 and 4 years of age [8], and infants

with encephalopathy who do not show initial recovery of cerebral oxidative metabolism have extremely poor outcomes [6]. An identical pattern of initial recovery of cerebral oxidative metabolism followed by delayed (secondary) energy failure is also seen after hypoxia–ischemia in the piglet, rat, and fetal sheep and is closely correlated to the severity of neuronal injury [9–12]. The timing of energy failure after hypoxia–ischemia is tightly coupled with histologic brain damage [13], implying that it is primarily a function of evolving cell death.

Because oxidative synthesis of ATP is mediated through the mitochondrial electron transport chain, loss of the terminal electron acceptor, cytochrome oxidase (CytOx) [14], is a close surrogate for loss of production of high-energy phosphates [15–17]. Continuous, non-invasive measurements with near-infrared spectroscopy (NIRS) demonstrate that severe asphyxia in fetal sheep leads to a consistent pattern of initial recovery of CytOx values after the end of the asphyxic insult, followed by a progressive fall, starting from approximately 3–4 hours, and continuing until approximately 48 hours after asphyxia (Fig. 42.1) [12]. Delayed loss of mitochondrial activity was associated with a marked *increase* in relative intracerebral oxygenation, consistent with an impaired ability to use oxygen [11,12].

Characteristic pathophysiological events may be distinguished during the early recovery (latent) phase compared with the secondary phase (Fig. 42.2). After restoration of circulation and oxygenation the initial hypoxia-induced impairments of cerebral oxidative metabolism, cytotoxic edema, and accumulation of EAAs resolve over approximately 30–60 minutes [4,5]. Despite normalization of oxidative cerebral energy metabolism and mitochondrial activity [12], mean electroencephalogram (EEG) activity remains depressed, while cerebral blood flow (CBF) initially recovers, followed by a transient secondary fall [4,12,18]. During the subsequent secondary deterioration, starting many hours later (approximately 6–15 hours after the insult) and continuing over many days, delayed seizures develop [4,12], accompanied by secondary cytotoxic edema (cell swelling) [4] and accumulation of excitotoxins as well as failure of cerebral mitochondrial activity and, ultimately, cell death [5,9,12,19]. There is no secondary energy failure after lesser insults that do not produce brain dysfunction [20].

The concepts that an acute, global insult can trigger evolving injury and that characteristic events are seen at different times

Fetal and Neonatal Brain Injury, 4th edition, ed. David K. Stevenson, William E. Benitz, Philip Sunshine, Susan R. Hintz, and Maurice L. Druzin. Published by Cambridge University Press. © Cambridge University Press 2009.

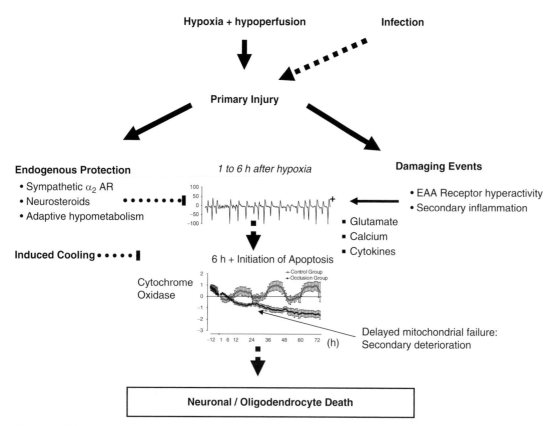

Fig. 42.1. Schematic representation of the hypothesized balance between protective and damaging events in the latent phase of recovery following asphyxia, leading to secondary loss of mitochondrial activity (cytochrome oxidase), and then cell death. Data derived in part from Bennet *et al.* [12,84].

after the insult, are central to understanding the causes and treatment of neonatal encephalopathy.

When is neuroprotection viable?

There is now overwhelming evidence that the "latent" phase in the early recovery period, before the start of the secondary deterioration, represents the effective window of opportunity for intervention therapies. The largest body of evidence comes from the lead therapeutic modality, induced hypothermia. As reviewed, the efficacy of hypothermia is highly dependent on a number of interdependent factors, including *the timing of initiation*, and the *duration* and *depth* of cooling [21–23].

The timing of initiation of hypothermia

For example, in the near-term fetal sheep, moderate hypothermia induced 90 minutes after reperfusion from a severe episode of cerebral ischemia, in the early latent phase, and continued until 72 hours after ischemia, prevented secondary cytotoxic edema, and improved electroencephalographic recovery [4]. There was a concomitant substantial reduction in cortical infarction and improvement in neuronal loss scores in all regions (Fig. 42.3). When the start of hypothermia was delayed until just before the onset of secondary seizures in this paradigm (5.5 hours after reperfusion) partial neuroprotection was seen [24]. With further delay after seizures were established (8.5 hours after reperfusion), there was no electrophysiological or overall histological protection with cooling [25].

Similar results have been reported in a wide range of species and paradigms. For example, in unanesthetized infant rats subjected to moderate hypoxia–ischemia mild hypothermia (2–3 °C decrease in brain temperature) for 72 hours from the end of hypoxia prevented cortical infarction, whereas cooling delayed until 6 hours after the insult had an intermediate, non-significant effect [26]. In anesthetized piglets exposed either to hypoxia with bilateral carotid ligation or to hypoxia with hypotension, either 12 hours of mild whole-body hypothermia (35 °C) or 24 hours of head cooling with mild systemic hypothermia started immediately after hypoxia prevented delayed energy failure [27], reduced neuronal loss, and suppressed post-hypoxic seizures [28,29].

Longer is better

Relatively extended periods of cooling, of between 12 and 72 hours, have been associated with the most consistent evidence of neuroprotection [26,27,30,31]. Critically for clinical practice, the more that initiation of hypothermia is delayed or the more severe the insult, the greater the duration of cooling required for protection [19]. For example, in the adult gerbil when the delay before initiating a 24-hour period of cooling was increased from 1 to 4 hours, neuroprotection in the CA1 region of the hippocampus after 6 months recovery fell from 70% to 12% [32]. Subsequent studies demonstrated that protection could be restored by extending the duration of moderate (32–34 °C) hypothermia to 48 hours or more, even when

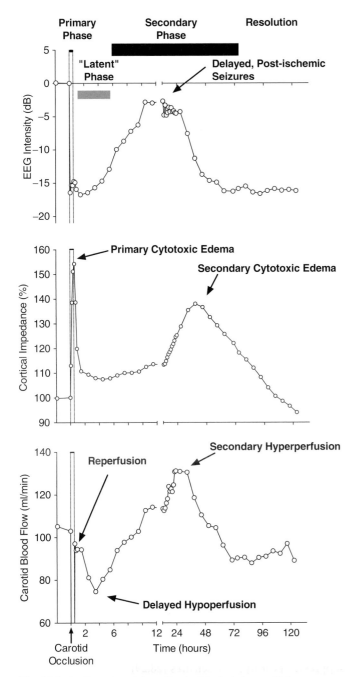

Fig. 42.2. An illustration of the pathophysiological phases of injury after 30 minutes of global cerebral ischemia in fetal sheep (*n* = 7). Data derived from Gunn *et al.* 1997 [4]. See text for details.

the start of cooling was delayed until 6 hours after reperfusion [33,34]. Similarly, in the near-term fetal sheep, cooling started after 5.5 hours and continued until 72 hours was still partially protective (Fig. 42.3) [24].

If some is good, is more better?

Similarly to the effect of duration, the critical depth of hypothermia required for protection seems to vary depending on the delay before initiation and the severity and nature of the

insult. For example, in the infant rat, mild cooling of just 1–2 °C was highly protective, provided it was started immediately after hypoxia [26]. In contrast, when cooling was delayed until 6 hours, in both adult rodents and the fetal sheep greater functional and histological neuroprotection was seen with a 5 °C reduction than with 3 °C [35].

Neuroprotection is maintained in the long term

There have been some reports that hypothermia only delayed, rather than prevented, neuronal degeneration after global ischemia in the adult rat [36–38], and severe hypoxia–ischemia in the 7-day-old rat [39]. However, subsequent studies suggest that the duration of hypothermia in those studies was inadequate. Seventy-two hours of very mild cooling in the infant rat after carotid occlusion and hypoxia was associated with long-term improvement, whereas 6 hours was not [26]. Subsequent studies, both in the 7-day rat and in adult animals of several species, have confirmed that prolonged cooling for 24–72 hours initiated within 6 hours of injury is associated with persistent behavioral and histological protection [31,33,35,40,41]. Nevertheless, it is important to accept that at least some attenuation of effect over time has been reported with virtually all therapies, such as early treatment with endogenous growth factors [42,43]. Indeed, it is strongly suggested that failure to consistently perform long-term evaluation is one of the major factors underlying the disappointing outcome of clinical trials of many putative cytoprotectants [44].

Clinical evidence

This compelling experimental evidence in multiple paradigms led to two major randomized controlled trials (RCTs) of hypothermia for neonatal HIE and many smaller trials. Systematic meta-analysis of data from all published RCTs available in 2007 (*n* = 5) of either selective head cooling or whole-body cooling initiated within 6 hours of birth in term neonates with acute HIE (a combined total of 552 randomized infants) reported a significant effect of therapeutic hypothermia on the primary composite outcome of death or disability at 18–22 months of age (RR 0.78, 95% CI 0.66–0.92; NNT 8, 95% CI 5–20). Further, subgroup analysis suggested significant effects on mortality (RR 0.75, 95% CI 0.59–0.96) and neurodevelopmental disability at 18–22 months (RR 0.72, 95% CI 0.53–0.98) [45]. Potentially, relatively greater improvements may be able to be obtained if we can target therapy more effectively, as suggested by the CoolCap trial [46]. The only minor side effects overall were sinus bradycardia not requiring treatment, mild thrombocytopenia, and a borderline increase in use of inotrope support [47]. The CoolCap trial reported scalp edema under the cap in many infants, which resolved rapidly after removal of the cap, and a transient increase in mean glucose levels during cooling [46]. Clearly there are many practical questions about how hypothermia should be optimally used in clinical practice [48], and the long-term effects, at school age and later, are not yet known.

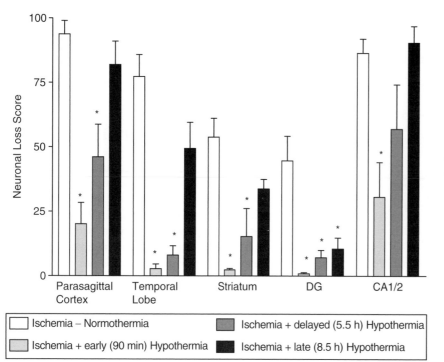

Fig. 42.3. The effect of cerebral cooling in the fetal sheep, started at different times after reperfusion and continued until 72 hours, on neuronal loss after 5 days' recovery from 30 minutes of cerebral ischemia [4,24,25]. Compared with sham cooling ($n = 13$), cooling started 90 minutes after reperfusion ($n = 7$) was dramatically protective. In contrast, cooling started just before the end of the latent phase (5.5 hours after reperfusion, $n = 11$) was partially protective, and cooling started shortly after the start of the secondary phase (8.5 hours after reperfusion, $n = 5$) was not. DG, dentate gyrus of the hippocampus; CA 1/2; cornu ammonis fields 1 and 2 of the hippocampus. *$p < 0.005$ compared with sham-cooled (control) fetuses; data are mean ± SEM.

Therapeutic targets for neuroprotection

These clinical and experimental data suggest that critical events occur within the latent phase after hypoxia–ischemia which materially contribute to further injury, and in turn that the delay between the initial insult and secondary energy failure reflects the time required for activation of cell death processes during the latent phase. Major initial triggers of the delayed death cascade during exposure to hypoxia–ischemia include exposure to oxygen free radical toxicity, excessive levels of EAAs ("excitotoxicity"), and intracellular calcium accumulation, both passively down the concentration gradient due to failure of energy-dependent pumps during hypoxia, and actively through channels linked to excitatory neurotransmitters [49]. However, these events rapidly resolve during reperfusion from the insult and thus cannot readily be related to the effects of post-insult interventions such as cooling. It is striking that even in vitro neuronal degeneration can be prevented by cooling initiated well after exposure to an insult [50]. Thus, the critical effect of hypothermia must be on secondary consequences, such as the intracellular progression of programmed cell death (apoptosis), the inflammatory reaction, and abnormal receptor activity.

Programmed cell death

There is good histological evidence that activation of pre-existing programmed cell death is a significant contributor to post-hypoxic cell death in the developing human brain. The morphological appearances include a mixture of necrosis and apoptosis. Necrosis is defined by loss of plasma membrane integrity associated with a random pattern of DNA degradation. Typically there is swelling of the cytoplasm and organelles, with little change initially to the nucleus. This pattern has been suggested to reflect biophysical damage to the cell (cell membrane instability, ion shifts, etc.), particularly lysis in the primary phase [51]. Apoptosis is defined morphologically by the development of "karyohexis". Karyohexis is the classic microscopic picture of condensation of chromatin (i.e., a dark shrunken nucleus) with loss of the reticular formation in the cytoplasm (leading to eosinophilia on light microscopy); ultimately, the shrunken cell breaks into small fragments [52]. By analogy with the active process of developmental loss of excess cells (including neurons), it was suggested that an apoptotic morphology reflected active or "programmed" cell death [53]. The intracytoplasmic stage of apoptosis involves alterations in the ratio of various intracellular factors such as the proto-oncogene *Bcl-2*, which inhibits apoptosis, and *Bax*, which promotes apoptosis, release of cytochrome c from mitochondria, and activation of cysteine proteases (caspases) [54,55]. The final, irreversible execution phase of apoptosis is intranuclear, involving endonuclease-mediated DNA fragmentation [56].

In practice, however, it has become clear that post-hypoxic cell death includes elements of both apoptotic and necrotic processes, with one or the other being most prominent depending on factors such as maturity and the severity of insult [57,58]. It is notable that apoptosis appears to be more prominent in the developing brain; for example, expression of caspase-3 after hypoxic–ischemic injury declines with maturation [59]. In the 7-day-old rat most neuronal loss in the first 24 hours after hypoxia–ischemia was associated with ultrastructural features of both apoptosis and necrosis [58]. Of critical importance, there was evidence of involvement of apoptotic pathways, including activation of caspase-3, even in neurons dying with a non-apoptotic morphology. Thus, despite the mixed mode of cell death, the concept remains an important one, since if neuronal and glia cell death includes a substantial element of active death (preprogrammed or triggered by secondary mechanisms such as cytotoxin exposure), then it should logically be possible to interrupt these events.

Consistent with the hypothesis that apoptotic processes are a key therapeutic target, post-insult hypothermia started after severe hypoxia–ischemia was reported to reduce apoptotic cell death, but not necrotic cell death, in the piglet [28]. Similarly, protection with post-hypoxic–ischemic hypothermia in fetal sheep has been closely linked with suppression of activated caspase-3 [60,61]. Further evidence comes from studies of endogenous antiapoptotic growth factors.

Other evidence for apoptosis: treatment with insulin-like growth factors (IGFs)

While a large array of growth factors are involved in regulating brain growth, IGF-1 is known to be a key mediator, with overexpression of the *IGF-1* gene leading to brain overgrowth and *IGF-1* knockouts or excess expression of IGF binding proteins leading to reduced growth [62–64]. IGF-1 is potently antiapoptotic, as well as promoting neural stem cell proliferation, differentiation, maturation, myelination, neurite outgrowth, and synaptogenesis [65]. There is marked upregulation of endogenous IGF-1 in injured areas of the brain after injury, which is suggested to contribute to cerebral repair and functional recovery [65]. However, it is unlikely that this response can be considered to be neuroprotective, because it occurs days after the insult, well after the latent phase, and is only beginning at a time when extensive cell death is already present. Indeed, in the neonatal rat there is a global *reduction*, not an increase, in all components of the IGF system during the early phase of recovery from hypoxia-ischemia [66].

Recent data have confirmed that post-ischemic administration of exogenous IGF-1 can attenuate the severe delayed, post-ischemic neuronal and oligodendrocyte cell loss and associated demyelination after cerebral ischemia or hypoxia-ischemia in the rat and in near-term fetal sheep (Fig. 42.4) [67–69]. For example, in term-equivalent fetal sheep IGF-1 given as a 1-hour infusion intracerebroventricularly (i.c.v.) was associated with dramatically reduced loss of oligodendrocytes after severe ischemia in the intragyral white matter, reduced demyelination, reduced tissue swelling, but upregulation of astrocytes and microglia [69]. IGF-1 treatment was associated with reduced caspase-3 activation and increased glial proliferation in a similar dose-dependent manner [70]. Caspase-3 was only expressed in oligodendrocytes that showed apoptotic morphology. Proliferating cell nuclear antigen co-localized with oligodendrocytes, astrocytes, and microglia. Thus, increased oligodendrocyte numbers after IGF-1 treatment are partly

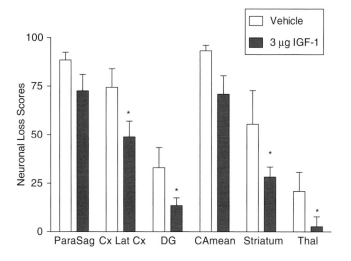

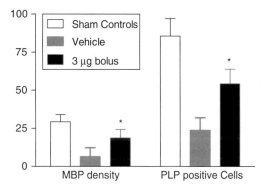

Fig. 42.4. Improvement in histological injury with IGF-1 therapy given intracerebroventricularly 2 hours after 30 minutes of cerebral ischemia in the fetal sheep, assessed after 96 hours' recovery. This insult leads to a watershed pattern of neuronal loss, greatest in the parasagittal cortex (ParaSag Cx). Note the significant improvement in the lateral (Lat Cx, i.e., temporal cortex) and subcortical structures, including the dentate gyrus of the dorsal hippocampus (DG), striatum and thalamus (Thal, top panel), and in myelin basic protein (MBP) and in numbers of proteolipid protein (PLP)-expressing mature oligodendrocytes (bottom panel). There was no significant improvement in the mean of the cornu ammonis regions of the hippocampus (CAmean). Data derived in part from [143]. *$p < 0.05$ vs. vehicle control.

due to suppression of apoptosis, and partly to increased proliferation. In contrast, the increase in reactive glia was related only to proliferation. These intriguing data raise the possibility that protective effects by reactive glia may partly mediate white-matter protection by IGF-1 [71], and thus, speculatively, that chronic treatment with this or other growth factors could help restore production of oligodendrocytes in premature infants.

Inflammatory second messengers

Brain injury leads to induction of the inflammatory cascade, with increased release of cytokines and interleukins (IL) [72]. These compounds are believed to exacerbate delayed injury, whether by direct neurotoxicity and induction of apoptosis or by promoting stimulation of leukocyte adhesion and infiltration into the ischemic brain. Experimentally, cooling can potently suppress this inflammatory reaction [19]. For example, in vitro, hypothermia inhibits proliferation, super-oxide and NO production by cultured microglia, and in adult rats hypothermia suppresses the post-traumatic release of interleukin-1β and accumulation of polymorphonuclear leukocytes. Similarly, neuroprotection with post-insult hypothermia was associated with suppression of microglial activation in fetal sheep [60,61].

Other receptor- and non-receptor-mediated toxic factors are likely to contribute to neural injury in the latent phase. For example, there is now some evidence from the preterm fetal sheep for delayed production of oxygen free radicals [73], which may be of particular importance for oligodendroglial survival. Further, post-hypoxic production of nitric oxide may contribute to further neuroinflammation, and a transient increase in neuronal nitric oxide synthase has been observed in the brain during the first few hours of recovery from hypoxia–ischemia in the rodent [74]. Against this, however, in preterm fetal sheep there was no change in the ratio of citrulline to arginine, an index of nitric oxide synthase activity, in the latent phase after exposure to severe cerebral ischemia that was associated with white-matter injury [75]. Further, although 2-iminobiotin, a selective inhibitor of neuronal and inducible nitric oxide synthase, reduced hypoxia–ischemia-induced brain damage in neonatal rats, this protection was selective to female rats only, and curiously was not associated with any change in indices of nitric oxide activity [76]. Thus 2-iminobiotin may have been acting through non-NO-related pathways.

Excitotoxicity after hypoxia–ischemia

Classically, cell death due to abnormal glutamate receptor activation (excitotoxicity) is related to pathologically elevated levels of extracellular glutamate, as occurs *during* hypoxia–ischemia. Following reperfusion, we and others have shown that glutamate levels rapidly return to control values [5,77], and thus naively we might predict that excitotoxicity should not be an important therapeutic target after reperfusion. More recent data, however, show that pathological hyperexcitability of glutamate receptors can continue for many hours following hypoxia–ischemia [78], and that it promotes intracellular neuronal calcium accumulation [79], which may help accelerate or increase programmed cell death.

In vitro, a large increase in the amplitude and duration of excitatory postsynaptic potentials was observed in hippocampal slice CA1 pyramidal neurons after exposure to 15–20 minutes of hypoxia in P10–11 rats (equivalent to term in humans) [78]. This hyperexcitability was greatest in the immature brain, and could be inhibited by NMDA receptor blockade [80]. In adult rat hippocampal slices, transient episodes of anoxia induced long-term potentiation of excitatory glutaminergic postsynaptic transmission in CA1 pyramidal neurons, the strength of which was related to the number of preceding anoxic episodes [81]. Similarly, CA1 pyramidal neurons in hippocampal slices from adult gerbils that were exposed to 5 minutes of ischemia demonstrated enhanced NMDA and non-NMDA receptor excitatory postsynaptic currents 1–12

hours after ischemia, accompanied by increased intracellular neuronal calcium accumulation [79]. Supporting these observations, following recovery from transient forebrain ischemia in the adult rat, evoked excitatory postsynaptic potentials of hippocampal CA1 pyramidal neurons in vivo were increased by up to 150% for 24 hours [82]. This activity occurred before the onset of histological signs of neuronal cell death and was reduced by treatment with dizocilpine, suggesting that enhanced synaptic NMDA receptor transmission was closely linked with the evolution of delayed neuronal death.

Evolving epileptiform transient events have also been demonstrated during the first few hours of recovery from severe asphyxia in preterm fetal sheep (Fig. 42.5), at a maturational stage equivalent to the 28–32-week human infant [83]. In this model, overall EEG activity was profoundly suppressed for many hours after hypoxia, regardless of whether injury subsequently developed or not [3]. In contrast, epileptiform EEG transient activity was only seen in the early recovery phase after a severe insult that was associated with severe injury. Other studies have shown that there is a strong, linear within-group correlation between the frequency of these events and the severity of neuronal loss [84,85]. Further, the maximal frequency of these events corresponded with a fall in cerebral oxygenation on near-infrared spectroscopy [12], and occurred well before secondary failure of mitochondrial oxidative activity on continuous near-infrared spectroscopic monitoring; in contrast, overt seizures did not occur until after the onset of the secondary fall [12]. There is considerable evidence suggesting that delayed failure of mitochondrial function is closely linked with the development of cell death [13], and thus these data strongly imply that the epileptiform transients precede the onset of cell death by a considerable margin.

Such epileptiform EEG transients are well described clinically, and in preterm infants their frequency is strongly associated overall with poor outcome [86–91]. However, there has been no detailed evaluation of their role or time course in perinatal brain injury, in part because typically clinical EEG recordings are not started until several days after birth, and in part because most bedside monitoring involves amplitude-integrated EEG (aEEG) cerebral function monitoring that does not permit assessment of such fast low-amplitude discrete events. Thus, their potential importance has not been systematically studied in the crucial first hours after birth.

Clearly EEG transients recorded from the surface of the brain could simply be a manifestation of injury rather than a cause. A possible causal relationship is supported by the observations that increased EEG transient activity during blockade of inhibitory α2-adrenergic receptor activity was associated with increased neuronal loss and, conversely, suppression of EEG transients with NMDA glutamate receptor blockade reduces cell loss in the striatum [85,92]. Further supporting a potential causal role, moderate, delayed cerebral hypothermia from 90 minutes to 70 hours after prolonged umbilical cord occlusion in fetal sheep markedly suppressed early-onset epileptiform EEG transients (Fig. 42.5), which correlated with reduced striatal damage. The effect of hypothermia

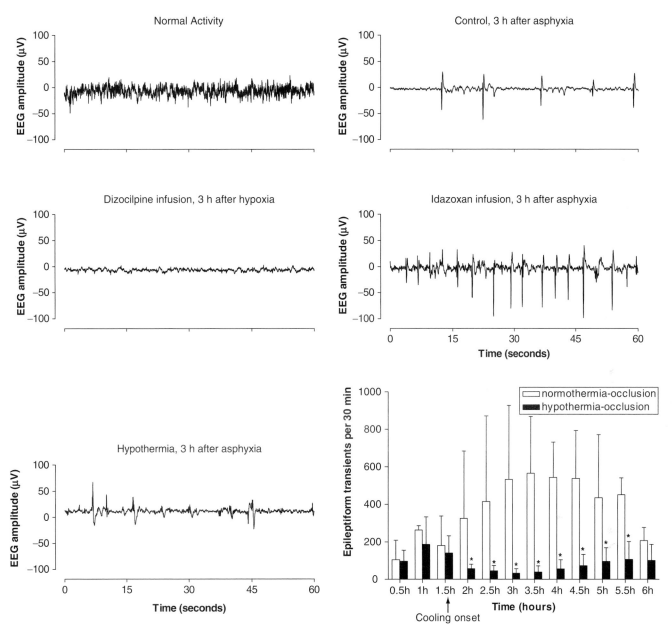

Fig. 42.5. Examples of raw EEG data from preterm fetal sheep showing normal discontinuous mixed frequency EEG activity, epileptiform transients superimposed on a suppressed EEG background 3 hours after an episode of reversible severe asphyxia. Postasphyxial infusion of an inhibitory α_2-adrenergic receptor antagonist, idazoxan, was associated with a marked increase in numbers of transients [85]. Conversely, these EEG transients were almost completely suppressed by N-methyl-D-aspartate blockade with dizocilpine [92], and were partially suppressed by cerebral hypothermia [84]. The time course of epileptiform transients during the latent phase, and the effect of cerebral hypothermia, are shown in the bottom-right panel [84]. *$p < 0.05$ hypothermia-occlusion vs. normothermia-occlusion.

on EEG transients is consistent with the well-established effect of hypothermia to reduce the slope of excitatory post-synaptic potentials in vitro and of glutamate release after depolarization and following reperfusion from severe hypoxia–ischemia in the piglet [93–95]. Focal cerebral cooling can reduce epileptiform activity in animals and in patients without changing the motor threshold for electrical stimulation [96,97]. Nevertheless, it is likely that neuroprotection with hypothermia was only partially related to suppression of N-methyl-D-aspartate receptor activity, as improvement in neuronal loss with hypothermia was markedly greater than

observed after an infusion of the highly selective antagonist dizocilpine in this model [92].

There is a fascinating contrast between the apparent importance of these brief, low-amplitude epileptiform transients, compared with the still unclear significance of the much larger sustained seizures seen later on in the secondary phase of recovery. NMDA receptor blockade delayed until the start of overt seizures in the near-term fetal sheep was associated only with modest protection, with no effect in the major parasagittal area of infarction [98]. Similarly, in the P7 rat, induced seizures did not increase damage after hypoxia–ischemia when secondary hyperthermia was prevented [99]. It is unknown whether these different outcomes reflect a true difference in underlying mechanisms, or whether it is simply that the setting of epileptiform events in a time of critical vulnerability, i.e., the latent phase, is more important than their magnitude.

Spreading depression

Alternatively, hypothermia may protect the brain from secondary extension of ischemic injury by inhibition of spreading depression [100]. Spreading depression is a rapid and nearly complete depolarization of a sizable population of brain cells with massive redistribution of ions between intracellular and extracellular compartments, which propagates in a wave [101]. Spreading depression-like events have been associated with epileptiform activity, and may further increase the excitability in human brain tissue [102]. There is increasing evidence that spreading depression-like events during ischemia increase the extent of neural injury by altering ion gradients or increasing glutamate release [103,104]. In contrast, the role of these events *after* hypoxia–ischemia is not well defined. However, there is in vitro evidence that the juvenile brain shows spontaneous spreading depression-like events during recovery from hypoxia, and is more likely to do so than the adult brain [105]. Further, whereas these events are not injurious to the normoxic adult brain [101], in juvenile normoxic hippocampal slice cultures repetitive spreading depression-like events led to deterioration of evoked fast field potentials and cell damage [106]. Mild hypothermia slowed the rate of propagation and frequency of spreading depression-like events in adult rats both after direct induction and during focal ischemia [100,107–109]. Consistent with this, during focal ischemia in adult rats mild hypothermia decreased the frequency of spreading depression-like events and associated transient reductions in apparent diffusion coefficient of water [108,109]. Thus, this is a plausible contributory mechanism of hypothermic neuroprotection.

Endogenous neuroprotection

While hypoxia can trigger many cytotoxic pathways within the brain, an important observation from experimental studies is that these damaging events are often associated with endogenous inhibitory neuroprotective responses that help to limit the degree of injury. For example, it is well established that the dramatic rise in extracellular glutamate during hypoxia-ischemia in gray matter is accompanied by accumulation of endogenous inhibitory neuromodulators such as γ-aminobutyric acid (GABA) and adenosine in near-term (0.8–0.9 of gestation) fetal sheep [5,110–112]. Indeed, the relative rise in GABA is reported to be greater than that of glutamate in the near-term fetus [5], and there is compelling evidence that intrahypoxic accumulation of adenosine mediates the initial rapid depression of EEG activity, and that this reduces hippocampal, striatal, and parasagittal neuronal loss after 72 hours recovery [112]. Conversely, in newborn adenosine A_{2A} receptor knockout mice, the degree of brain injury and behavioral

impairment after recovery from hypoxia–ischemia was significantly increased at 3 months compared to controls, without any differences in intra-insult cerebral blood flow [113]. This actively regulated suppression of metabolic rate during hypoxia or ischemia before energy stores are depleted has been termed *adaptive hypometabolism* [114].

After hypoxia, extracellular levels of GABA and adenosine quickly return to control values [5,110,115,116], suggesting their protective role is largely limited to the acute phase of insult. There is increasing evidence that other endogenous neuroinhibitory systems may be activated *after* the insult. These inhibitory systems may contribute, in part, to the marked suppression of EEG activity and cerebral hypoperfusion observed both clinically and experimentally during the initial few hours of recovery from severe asphyxia [3,117].

Evidence for post-insult adaptive hypometabolism

Experimentally, a classical feature of the latent (i.e., early recovery) phase after severe hypoxia in fetal, neonatal, and adult life is secondary cerebral and peripheral hypoperfusion despite normal or even elevated arterial blood pressure [4,12,18,118–120]. Corresponding with this transient fall in CBF, NIRS has confirmed that infants with HIE show a reduction in cerebral blood volume during the first 12 hours after birth [121]. The duration and speed of onset, and to a lesser extent the degree of the hypoperfusion, are reported to be broadly related to the severity of the insult, at least in the brain, where the phenomenon has mostly been assessed [122,123]. However, surprisingly, despite its near ubiquity, it has been rather controversial whether secondary hypoperfusion represents a period of true, deleterious secondary ischemia, leading to impaired cerebral oxygenation, or is merely a reflection of reduced cerebral metabolism [124,125].

For example, during this early recovery period after exposure to severe asphyxia, NIRS has shown a marked transient reduction in oxygenated hemoglobin despite normal blood pressure in fetal sheep and newborn infants [12,121,126]. However, a fall in HbO_2 could merely reflect the fall in total blood flow. However, the difference between oxygenated and deoxygenated hemoglobin, which is a reliable measure of changes in intracerebral oxygenation [127], showed only a minimal fall for a few hours [12], suggesting little change in tissue oxygenation. Supporting this conclusion, there was no significant change in arteriovenous oxygen content differences in either lambs or near-term fetal sheep after hypoxic-ischemic injury [4,128], and delayed post-hypoxic cerebral hypoperfusion after severe asphyxia in near-term fetal sheep was associated with suppression of cerebral metabolism and increased, not decreased, cortical tissue oxygenation [18]. Similarly, recent studies of infants with moderate to severe HIE have confirmed that there is an increase in intracerebral oxygenation and a fall in fractional oxygen extraction after 24 hours in the infants with an adverse outcome [129].

Thus, these data strongly suggest that post-asphyxial cerebral hypoperfusion occurs as part of an actively regulated response to reduced cerebral metabolism, with intact coupling of cerebral blood flow and metabolism. The mechanisms and the potential neuroprotective role for adaptive hypometabolism *after* hypoxia are discussed below.

Evidence for endogenous sympathoinhibition after hypoxia–ischemia

Extracellular noradrenalin levels increase dramatically during hypoxia, similarly to adenosine and GABA, and are believed to contribute to hypoxic-depression of synaptic activity through the inhibitory α_2-adrenergic receptor [130], as shown in vitro [131]. Although there is little information on levels after hypoxia, recent data in fetal sheep have shown that secondary central and peripheral hypoperfusion during the first few hours of recovery from severe asphyxia can be prevented by an infusion of an α_1/α_2-adrenergic receptor antagonist, phentolamine [132]. Further, the onset of post-asphyxial seizures was significantly earlier than in vehicle-treated animals, suggesting a loss of neural inhibition with phentolamine infusion [132]. A subsequent study demonstrated that a short infusion of the specific α_2-adrenergic receptor antagonist idazoxan in the early recovery phase, from 15 minutes until 4 hours after occlusion, significantly increased overall neuronal cell death, mainly in regions of the hippocampus, with a corresponding reduction in numbers of surviving neurons in the CA3 region [85]. This regional increase in neuronal loss was associated with an increase in numbers of cleaved caspase-3-positive cells and activated microglia. There was no effect of this infusion on cerebral blood flow. These data are consistent with sympathetic nervous system activation during the early recovery phase, and indicate that α_1-adrenergic activity mediates the hypoperfusion, while α_2-adrenergic activity in this critical phase helps mitigate evolving neuronal damage.

Sympathoinhibition and epileptiform activity

Intriguingly, in preterm fetal sheep blockade of the α_2-adrenergic receptor with idazoxan after asphyxia significantly increased epileptiform EEG transient activity in the early recovery phase from severe hypoxia (Fig. 42.5) [85], but did not significantly affect numbers of subsequent post-hypoxic seizures, consistent with the short duration of infusion. Moreover, there was a significant positive correlation between numbers of these events and severity of hippocampal neuronal loss, supporting a potentially causal role [85]. These data are consistent with postnatal data that implicate noradrenergic activity as an important modulator of the threshold for "classic" delayed stereotypic slow-wave seizures [133,134].

Other inhibitory neuromodulators

Other potential inhibitory neuromodulators are known to be elevated after severe hypoxia in the term fetus, including the $GABA_A$ receptor agonist allopregnanolone [135], which is neuroprotective in adult models [136,137]. This elevation is reported to resolve to pre-occlusion levels by 3–4 hours after asphyxia [135], consistent with the time course of secondary hypoperfusion. Thus it is likely that the full impact of endogenous protective responses after severe hypoxia represents the summation, or even a synergistic effect, of multiple systems.

Hypothesis

Based on these findings, we propose the *hypothesis* (Fig. 42.1) that during the *early* or *latent phase* of recovery from hypoxia, the long-term survival of vulnerable, injured neurons and white-matter cells in the immature brain is determined by a dynamic balance between damaging events (such as abnormal glutamate receptor activity and secondary inflammation) and active endogenous neural protection by neural systems (such as activation of the inhibitory component of the sympathetic nervous system). The limits and effectiveness of these systems are not known. However, for injury to occur, any endogenous neuroprotective system must only partly suppress damaging factors; i.e., there is an imbalance between protective and damaging processes. This concept, that the injured brain is not simply a passive target for toxic factors, but rather is actively defending itself, is an important insight into the resilience of newborn infants to hypoxic–ischemic injury [138].

Implications
Can we identify the "latent" phase after hypoxia?

The issues discussed reinforce the overwhelming importance of both targeting treatment to children who are at high risk of injury, and to a time when treatment is likely to be beneficial. At present, there is no easy way of identifying these patients in a timely manner. The studies discussed in this chapter strongly suggest that the *latent phase* may be able to be identified by the combination of post-hypoxic EEG transients with overall EEG suppression. To date, no such systemic early electrophysiological clinical monitoring data are available in newborn infants that would allow us to evaluate the utility of this EEG pattern. A major limitation of existing data is that, typically, formal EEG recordings are started several days after birth, so it is unknown whether these EEG transients are present in the early hours of recovery from hypoxia–ischemia. Further, the widely used method of aEEG cerebral function monitoring does not permit assessment of the real-time EEG, and so does not reveal or permit evaluation of these fast, discrete events. It is perhaps unwise to place too much hope on a single clinical parameter. Coupling early EEG monitoring with other non-invasive bedside monitoring techniques such as near-infrared spectroscopy, which has been used clinically in asphyxiated term newborns as early as 2 hours [121] to monitor changes in cerebral blood flow and oxygenation [121,126,139], and mitochondrial redox state, would likely be more effective than either alone [12].

Can we manipulate the window of opportunity for therapy?

A number of studies in adult and newborn animals have reported that short periods of active post-insult cerebral cooling can substantially delay the evolution of neuronal death even if there is no significant effect on long-term outcome [36,39,140]. This effect may be of some clinical utility in its own right. The timely selection and enrollment of patients for therapeutic trials of acute encephalopathy presents formidable logistic difficulties [48]. Recent studies have confirmed that such early but mild cooling can critically extend the window of opportunity for neuronal rescue with IGF-1 from 2 hours after hypoxia–ischemia, up to as long as 6 hours [141]. This approach may increase the number of patients who can be enrolled in therapeutic trials after hypoxia–ischemia [142].

Conclusions

Experimental studies of hypoxia–ischemia have shown that neural injury is an evolving process, characterized by an early "latent" phase, followed by the ultimate development of delayed neuronal death. The latent phase appears to be the foundation period during which the processes mediating delayed cell death are active and potentially reversible, and is thus the key period when treatment is most likely to be successful. There is now compelling evidence from two large well-conducted randomized controlled trials and a number of smaller studies that therapeutic hypothermia is protective [45]. It is the personal view of the authors that given the

remarkable safety profile under intensive care conditions, the strong foundation in basic science, and supporting evidence from related disease states such as encephalopathy after cardiac arrest, practicing clinicians may now cautiously use this first ever treatment for neonatal encephalopathy in consultation with the affected families, while they wait for the questions around its optimal use to be answered.

Because the trial sizes required to address the remaining questions will be very large, ideally all patients should be centrally registered with universal follow-up, and where possible treatment should be centralized to larger intensive care units, helping to increase local expertise in the use of hypothermia. These steps are critical to allow the first ever proven treatment for neonatal encephalopathy to be made safely available, while facilitating the ability of large consortia of neonatal units to examine incremental modifications to the treatment protocols such as the timing, mode, length, or degree of cooling, and the effects of additional therapies.

Acknowledgments

The authors' work reported in this review has been supported by the Health Research Council of New Zealand, the Lottery Health Board of New Zealand, the Auckland Medical Research Foundation, and the March of Dimes Birth Defects Foundation.

References

1. Low JA, Lindsay BG, Derrick EJ. Threshold of metabolic acidosis associated with newborn complications. *Am J Obstet Gynecol* 1997; **177**: 1391–4.

2. Gunn AJ, Parer JT, Mallard EC, *et al.* Cerebral histologic and electrocorticographic changes after asphyxia in fetal sheep. *Pediatr Res* 1992; **31**: 486–91.

3. George S, Gunn AJ, Westgate JA, *et al.* Fetal heart rate variability and brainstem injury after asphyxia in preterm fetal sheep. *Am J Physiol Regul Integr Comp Physiol* 2004; **287**: R925–33.

4. Gunn AJ, Gunn TR, de Haan HH, *et al.* Dramatic neuronal rescue with prolonged selective head cooling after ischemia in fetal lambs. *J Clin Invest* 1997; **99**: 248–56.

5. Tan WK, Williams CE, During MJ, *et al.* Accumulation of cytotoxins during the development of seizures and edema after hypoxic–ischemic injury in late gestation fetal sheep. *Pediatr Res* 1996; **39**: 791–7.

6. Azzopardi D, Wyatt JS, Cady EB, *et al.* Prognosis of newborn infants with hypoxic–ischemic brain injury assessed by phosphorus magnetic resonance spectroscopy. *Pediatr Res* 1989; **25**: 445–51.

7. Roth SC, Edwards AD, Cady EB, *et al.* Relation between cerebral oxidative metabolism following birth asphyxia, and neurodevelopmental outcome and brain growth at one year. *Dev Med Child Neurol* 1992; **34**: 285–95.

8. Roth SC, Baudin J, Cady E, *et al.* Relation of deranged neonatal cerebral oxidative metabolism with neurodevelopmental outcome and head circumference at 4 years. *Dev Med Child Neurol* 1997; **39**: 718–25.

9. Lorek A, Takei Y, Cady EB, *et al.* Delayed ("secondary") cerebral energy failure after acute hypoxia–ischemia in the newborn piglet: continuous 48-hour studies by phosphorus magnetic resonance spectroscopy. *Pediatr Res* 1994; **36**: 699–706.

10. Blumberg RM, Cady EB, Wigglesworth JS, *et al.* Relation between delayed impairment of cerebral energy metabolism and infarction following transient focal hypoxia–ischaemia in the developing brain. *Exp Brain Res* 1997; **113**: 130–7.

11. Marks KA, Mallard EC, Roberts I, *et al.* Delayed vasodilation and altered oxygenation after cerebral ischemia in fetal sheep. *Pediatr Res* 1996; **39**: 48–54.

12. Bennet L, Roelfsema V, Pathipati P, *et al.* Relationship between evolving epileptiform activity and delayed loss of mitochondrial activity after asphyxia measured by near-infrared spectroscopy in preterm fetal sheep. *J Physiol* 2006; **572**: 141–54.

13. Vannucci RC, Towfighi J, Vannucci SJ. Secondary energy failure after cerebral hypoxia–ischemia in the immature rat. *J Cereb Blood Flow Metab* 2004; **24**: 1090–7.

14. Cooper CE, Springett R. Measurement of cytochrome oxidase and mitochondrial energetics by near-infrared spectroscopy. *Philos Trans R Soc Lond B Biol Sci* 1997; **352**: 669–76.

15. Chang YS, Park WS, Lee M, *et al.* Near infrared spectroscopic monitoring of secondary cerebral energy failure after transient global hypoxia–ischemia in the newborn piglet. *Neurol Res* 1999; **21**: 216–24.

16. Peeters-Scholte C, van den Tweel E, Groenendaal F, *et al.* Redox state of near infrared spectroscopy-measured cytochrome aa(3) correlates with delayed cerebral energy failure following perinatal hypoxia–ischaemia in the newborn pig. *Exp Brain Res* 2004; **156**: 20–6.

17. Tsuji M, Naruse H, Volpe J, *et al.* Reduction of cytochrome aa3 measured by near-infrared spectroscopy predicts cerebral energy loss in hypoxic piglets. *Pediatr Res* 1995; **37**: 253–9.

18. Jensen EC, Bennet L, Hunter CJ, *et al.* Post-hypoxic hypoperfusion is

associated with suppression of cerebral metabolism and increased tissue oxygenation in near-term fetal sheep. *J Physiol* 2006; **572**: 131–9.

19. Gunn AJ, Thoresen M. Hypothermic neuroprotection. *NeuroRx* 2006; **3**: 154–69.

20. Williams CE, Gunn A, Gluckman PD. Time course of intracellular edema and epileptiform activity following prenatal cerebral ischemia in sheep. *Stroke* 1991; **22**: 516–21.

21. Floyer J. *An Enquiry into the Right Use and Abuses of the Hot, Cold, and Temperate Baths in England.* London, printed for R. Clavel at the Peacock, in St. Paul's-Church-yard, 1697.

22. Westin B, Nyberg R, Miller JA, *et al.* Hypothermia and transfusion with oxygenated blood in the treatment of asphyxia neonatorum. *Acta Paediatr* 1962; **51**: 1–80.

23. Miller JA, Miller FS, Westin B. Hypothermia in the treatment of asphyxia neonatorum. *Biol Neonat* 1964; **20**: 148–63.

24. Gunn AJ, Gunn TR, Gunning MI, *et al.* Neuroprotection with prolonged head cooling started before postischemic seizures in fetal sheep. *Pediatrics* 1998; **102**: 1098–106.

25. Gunn AJ, Bennet L, Gunning MI, *et al.* Cerebral hypothermia is not neuroprotective when started after postischemic seizures in fetal sheep. *Pediatr Res* 1999; **46**: 274–80.

26. Sirimanne ES, Blumberg RM, Bossano D, *et al.* The effect of prolonged modification of cerebral temperature on outcome after hypoxic–ischemic brain injury in the infant rat. *Pediatr Res* 1996; **39**: 591–7.

27. Thoresen M, Penrice J, Lorek A, *et al.* Mild hypothermia after severe transient hypoxia–ischemia ameliorates delayed cerebral energy failure in the newborn piglet. *Pediatr Res* 1995; **37**: 667–70.

28. Edwards AD, Yue X, Squier MV, *et al.* Specific inhibition of apoptosis after cerebral hypoxia–ischaemia by moderate post-insult hypothermia. *Biochem Biophys Res Commun* 1995; **217**: 1193–9.

29. Tooley JR, Satas S, Porter H, *et al.* Head cooling with mild systemic hypothermia in anesthetized piglets is neuroprotective. *Ann Neurol* 2003; **53**: 65–72.

30. Thoresen M, Bagenholm R, Loberg EM, *et al.* Posthypoxic cooling of neonatal rats provides protection against brain injury. *Arch Dis Child Fetal Neonatal Ed* 1996; **74**: F3–9.

31. Bona E, Hagberg H, Loberg EM, *et al.* Protective effects of moderate hypothermia after neonatal hypoxia–ischemia: short- and long-term outcome. *Pediatr Res* 1998; **43**: 738–45.

32. Colbourne F, Corbett D. Delayed postischemic hypothermia: a six month survival study using behavioral and histological assessments of neuroprotection. *J Neurosci* 1995; **15**: 7250–60.

33. Colbourne F, Li H, Buchan AM. Indefatigable CA1 sector neuroprotection with mild hypothermia induced 6 hours after severe forebrain ischemia in rats. *J Cereb Blood Flow Metab* 1999; **19**: 742–9.

34. Colbourne F, Corbett D, Zhao Z, *et al.* Prolonged but delayed postischemic hypothermia: a long-term outcome study in the rat middle cerebral artery occlusion model. *J Cereb Blood Flow Metab* 2000; **20**: 1702–8.

35. Colbourne F, Auer RN, Sutherland GR. Characterization of postischemic behavioral deficits in gerbils with and without hypothermic neuroprotection. *Brain Res* 1998; **803**: 69–78.

36. Dietrich WD, Busto R, Alonso O, *et al.* Intraischemic but not postischemic brain hypothermia protects chronically following global forebrain ischemia in rats. *J Cereb Blood Flow Metab* 1993; **13**: 541–9.

37. Nurse S, Corbett D. Neuroprotection after several days of mild, drug-induced hypothermia. *J Cereb Blood Flow Metab* 1996; **16**: 474–80.

38. Coimbra C, Drake M, Boris-Moller F, *et al.* Long-lasting neuroprotective effect of postischemic hypothermia and treatment with an anti-inflammatory/ antipyretic drug: evidence for chronic encephalopathic processes following ischemia. *Stroke* 1996; **27**: 1578–85.

39. Trescher WH, Ishiwa S, Johnston MV. Brief post-hypoxic–ischemic hypothermia markedly delays neonatal brain injury. *Brain Dev* 1997; **19**: 326–38.

40. Nedelcu J, Klein MA, Aguzzi A, *et al.* Resuscitative hypothermia protects the neonatal rat brain from hypoxic–ischemic injury. *Brain Pathol* 2000; **10**: 61–71.

41. Wagner BP, Nedelcu J, Martin E. Delayed postischemic hypothermia improves long-term behavioral outcome after cerebral hypoxia–ischemia in neonatal rats. *Pediatr Res* 2002; **51**: 354–60.

42. Guan J, Miller OT, Waugh KM, *et al.* TGFβ-1 and neurological function after hypoxia–ischemia in adult rats. *Neuroreport* 2004; **15**: 961–4.

43. Guan J, Miller OT, Waugh KM, *et al.* Insulin-like growth factor-1 improves somatosensory function and reduces the extent of cortical infarction and ongoing neuronal loss after hypoxia–ischemia in rats. *Neuroscience* 2001; **105**: 299–306.

44. DeBow SB, Clark DL, MacLellan CL, *et al.* Incomplete assessment of experimental cytoprotectants in rodent ischemia studies. *Can J Neurol Sci* 2003; **30**: 368–74.

45. Shah PS, Ohlsson A, Perlman M. Hypothermia to treat neonatal hypoxic ischemic encephalopathy: systematic review. *Arch Pediatr Adolesc Med* 2007; **161**: 951–8.

46. Gluckman PD, Wyatt JS, Azzopardi D, *et al.* Selective head cooling with mild systemic hypothermia to improve neurodevelopmental outcome following neonatal encephalopathy. *Lancet* 2005; **365**: 663–70.

47. Jacobs S, Hunt R, Tarnow-Mordi W, *et al.* Cooling for newborns with hypoxic ischaemic encephalopathy. *Cochrane Database Syst Rev* 2007; (4): CD003311.

48. Gunn AJ, Gluckman PD. Head cooling for neonatal encephalopathy: the state of the art. *Clin Obstet Gynecol* 2007; **50**: 636–51.

49. Johnston MV. Excitotoxicity in perinatal brain injury. *Brain Pathol* 2005; **15**: 234–40.

50. Bruno VM, Goldberg MP, Dugan LL, *et al.* Neuroprotective effect of hypothermia in cortical cultures exposed to oxygen-glucose deprivation or excitatory amino acids. *J Neurochem* 1994; **63**: 1398–406.

51. Scott RJ, Hegyi L. Cell death in perinatal hypoxic–ischaemic brain injury. *Neuropathol Appl Neurobiol* 1997; **23**: 307–14.

52. Raff MC, Barres BA, Burne JF, *et al.* Programmed cell death and the control of cell survival: lessons from the nervous system. *Science* 1993; **262**: 695–700.

53. Beilharz EJ, Williams CE, Dragunow M, *et al.* Mechanisms of delayed cell death following hypoxic–ischemic injury in the immature rat: evidence for apoptosis

during selective neuronal loss. *Mol Brain Res* 1995; **29**: 1–14.

54. Northington FJ, Ferriero DM, Flock DL, *et al.* Delayed neurodegeneration in neonatal rat thalamus after hypoxia–ischemia is apoptosis. *J Neurosci* 2001; **21**: 1931–8.

55. Northington FJ, Graham EM, Martin LJ. Apoptosis in perinatal hypoxic–ischemic brain injury: how important is it and should it be inhibited? *Brain Res Brain Res Rev* 2005; **50**: 244–57.

56. Samejima K, Tone S, Kottke TJ, *et al.* Transition from caspase-dependent to caspase-independent mechanisms at the onset of apoptotic execution. *J Cell Biol* 1998; **143**: 225–39.

57. Portera-Cailliau C, Price DL, Martin LJ. Non-NMDA and NMDA receptor-mediated excitotoxic neuronal deaths in adult brain are morphologically distinct: further evidence for an apoptosis–necrosis continuum. *J Comp Neurol* 1997; **378**: 88–104.

58. Northington FJ, Zelaya ME, O'Riordan DP, *et al.* Failure to complete apoptosis following neonatal hypoxia–ischemia manifests as "continuum" phenotype of cell death and occurs with multiple manifestations of mitochondrial dysfunction in rodent forebrain. *Neuroscience* 2007; **149**: 822–33.

59. Hu BR, Liu CL, Ouyang Y, *et al.* Involvement of caspase-3 in cell death after hypoxia–ischemia declines during brain maturation. *J Cereb Blood Flow Metab* 2000; **20**: 1294–300.

60. Roelfsema V, Bennet L, George S, *et al.* The window of opportunity for cerebral hypothermia and white matter injury after cerebral ischemia in near-term fetal sheep. *J Cereb Blood Flow Metab* 2004; **24**: 877–86.

61. Bennet L, Roelfsema V, George S, *et al.* The effect of cerebral hypothermia on white and grey matter injury induced by severe hypoxia in preterm fetal sheep. *J Physiol* 2007; **578**: 491–506.

62. Ye P, Li L, Richards RG, *et al.* Myelination is altered in insulin-like growth factor-I null mutant mice. *J Neurosci* 2002; **22**: 6041–51.

63. Ye P, Carson J, D'Ercole AJ. In vivo actions of insulin-like growth factor-I (IGF-I) on brain myelination: studies of IGF-I and IGF binding protein-1 (IGFBP-1) transgenic mice. *J Neurosci* 1995; **15**: 7344–56.

64. Gutierrez-Ospina G, Calikoglu AS, Ye P, *et al.* In vivo effects of insulin-like growth factor-I on the development of sensory pathways: analysis of the primary somatic sensory cortex (S1) of transgenic mice. *Endocrinology* 1996; **137**: 5484–92.

65. Guan J, Bennet L, Gluckman PD, *et al.* Insulin-like growth factor-1 and post-ischemic brain injury. *Prog Neurobiol* 2003; **70**: 443–62.

66. Clawson TF, Vannucci SJ, Wang GM, *et al.* Hypoxia–ischemia-induced apoptotic cell death correlates with IGF-I mRNA decrease in neonatal rat brain. *Biol Signals Recept* 1999; **8**: 281–93.

67. Guan J, Williams C, Gunning M, *et al.* The effects of IGF-1 treatment after hypoxic–ischemic brain injury in adult rats. *J Cereb Blood Flow Metab* 1993; **13**: 609–16.

68. Johnston BM, Mallard EC, Williams CE, *et al.* Insulin-like growth factor-1 is a potent neuronal rescue agent after hypoxic–ischemic injury in fetal lambs. *J Clin Invest* 1996; **97**: 300–8.

69. Guan J, Bennet L, George S, *et al.* Insulin-like growth factor-1 reduces postischemic white matter injury in fetal sheep. *J Cereb Blood Flow Metab* 2001; **21**: 493–502.

70. Cao Y, Gunn AJ, Bennet L, *et al.* Insulin-like growth factor (IGF)-1 suppresses oligodendrocyte caspase-3 activation and increases glial proliferation after ischemia in near-term fetal sheep. *J Cereb Blood Flow Metab* 2003; **23**: 739–47.

71. Corley SM, Ladiwala U, Besson A, *et al.* Astrocytes attenuate oligodendrocyte death in vitro through an α_6 integrin-laminin-dependent mechanism. *Glia* 2001; **36**: 281–94.

72. Hagberg H, Mallard C, Jacobsson B. Role of cytokines in preterm labour and brain injury. *BJOG* 2005; **112**: 16–18.

73. Welin AK, Sandberg M, Lindblom A, *et al.* White matter injury following prolonged free radical formation in the 0.65 gestation fetal sheep brain. *Pediatr Res* 2005; **58**: 100–5.

74. van den Tweel ER, Nijboer C, Kavelaars A, *et al.* Expression of nitric oxide synthase isoforms and nitrotyrosine formation after hypoxia–ischemia in the neonatal rat brain. *J Neuroimmunol* 2005; **167**: 64–71.

75. Fraser M, Bennet L, van Zijl PL, *et al.* Extracellular amino acids and peroxidation products in the periventricular white matter during and after cerebral ischemia in preterm fetal sheep. *J Neurochem* 2008, epub ahead of print.

76. Nijboer CH, Groenendaal F, Kavelaars A, *et al.* Gender-specific neuroprotection by 2-iminobiotin after hypoxia–ischemia in the neonatal rat via a nitric oxide independent pathway. *J Cereb Blood Flow Metab* 2007; **27**: 282–92.

77. Obrenovitch TP, Richards DA. Extracellular neurotransmitter changes in cerebral ischaemia. *Cerebrovasc Brain Metab Rev* 1995; **7**: 1–54.

78. Jensen FE, Wang C, Stafstrom CE, *et al.* Acute and chronic increases in excitability in rat hippocampal slices after perinatal hypoxia in vivo. *J Neurophysiol* 1998; **79**: 73–81.

79. Mitani A, Namba S, Ikemune K, *et al.* Postischemic enhancements of N-methyl-D-aspartic acid (NMDA) and non-NMDA receptor-mediated responses in hippocampal CA1 pyramidal neurons. *J Cereb Blood Flow Metab* 1998; **18**: 1088–98.

80. Wang C, Jensen FE. Age dependence of NMDA receptor involvement in epileptiform activity in rat hippocampal slices. *Epilepsy Res* 1996; **23**: 105–13.

81. Kalemenev SV, Savin AV, Levin SG, *et al.* Long-term potentiation of glutamatergic transmission and epileptiform activity induced by transient episodes of anoxia in slices of rats hippocampus field CA1. *Neurosci Behav Physiol* 2002; **32**: 431–4.

82. Gao TM, Pulsinelli WA, Xu ZC. Prolonged enhancement and depression of synaptic transmission in CA1 pyramidal neurons induced by transient forebrain ischemia in vivo. *Neuroscience* 1998; **87**: 371–83.

83. Barlow RM. The foetal sheep: morphogenesis of the nervous system and histochemical aspects of myelination. *J Comp Neurol* 1969; **135**: 249–62.

84. Bennet L, Dean JM, Wassink G, *et al.* Differential effects of hypothermia on early and late epileptiform events after severe hypoxia in preterm fetal sheep. *J Neurophysiol* 2007; **97**: 572–8.

85. Dean JM, Gunn AJ, Wassink G, *et al.* Endogenous α_2-adrenergic receptor-mediated neuroprotection after severe hypoxia in preterm fetal sheep. *Neuroscience* 2006; **142**: 615–28.

86. Hughes JR, Guerra R. The use of the EEG to predict outcome in premature infants with positive sharp waves. *Clin Electroencephalogr* 1994; **25**: 127–35.

87. Marret S, Parain D, Menard JF, *et al.* Prognostic value of neonatal electroencephalography in premature newborns less than 33 weeks of gestational age. *Electroencephalogr Clin Neurophysiol* 1997; **102**: 178–85.

88. Okumura A, Hayakawa F, Kato T, *et al.* Abnormal sharp transients on electroencephalograms in preterm infants with periventricular leukomalacia. *J Pediatr* 2003; **143**: 26–30.

89. Biagioni E, Bartalena L, Boldrini A, *et al.* Electroencephalography in infants with periventricular leukomalacia: prognostic features at preterm and term age. *J Child Neurol* 2000; **15**: 1–6.

90. Rowe JC, Holmes GL, Hafford J, *et al.* Prognostic value of the electroencephalogram in term and preterm infants following neonatal seizures. *Electroencephalogr Clin Neurophysiol* 1985; **60**: 183–96.

91. Vecchierini-Blineau MF, Nogues B, Louvet S, *et al.* Positive temporal sharp waves in electroencephalograms of the premature newborn. *Neurophysiol Clin* 1996; **26**: 350–62.

92. Dean JM, George SA, Wassink G, *et al.* Suppression of post hypoxic–ischemic EEG transients with dizocilpine is associated with partial striatal protection in the preterm fetal sheep. *Neuropharmacology* 2006; **50**: 491–503.

93. Aihara H, Okada Y, Tamaki N. The effects of cooling and rewarming on the neuronal activity of pyramidal neurons in guinea pig hippocampal slices. *Brain Res* 2001; **893**: 36–45.

94. Nakashima K, Todd MM. Effects of hypothermia on the rate of excitatory amino acid release after ischemic depolarization. *Stroke* 1996; **27**: 913–18.

95. Thoresen M, Satas S, Puka-Sundvall M, *et al.* Post-hypoxic hypothermia reduces cerebrocortical release of NO and excitotoxins. *Neuroreport* 1997; **8**: 3359–62.

96. Baldwin M, Frost LL. Effect of hypothermia on epileptiform activity in the primate temporal lobe. *Science* 1956; **124**: 931–2.

97. Karkar KM, Garcia PA, Bateman LM, *et al.* Focal cooling suppresses spontaneous epileptiform activity without changing the cortical motor threshold. *Epilepsia* 2002; **43**: 932–5.

98. Tan WK, Williams CE, Gunn AJ, *et al.* Suppression of postischemic epileptiform activity with MK-801 improves neural outcome in fetal sheep. *Ann Neurol* 1992; **32**: 677–82.

99. Yager JY, Armstrong EA, Jaharus C, *et al.* Preventing hyperthermia decreases brain damage following neonatal hypoxic–ischemic seizures. *Brain Res* 2004; **1011**: 48–57.

100. Ueda M, Watanabe N, Ushikubo Y, *et al.* The effect of hypothermia on CSD propagation in rats. *No Shinkei Geka* 1997; **25**: 523–8.

101. Somjen GG. Mechanisms of spreading depression and hypoxic spreading depression-like depolarization. *Physiol Rev* 2001; **81**: 1065–96.

102. Gorji A, Speckmann EJ. Spreading depression enhances the spontaneous epileptiform activity in human neocortical tissues. *Eur J Neurosci* 2004; **19**: 3371–4.

103. Hossmann KA. Periinfarct depolarizations. *Cerebrovasc Brain Metab Rev* 1996; **8**: 195–208.

104. Mies G, Iijima T, Hossmann KA. Correlation between peri-infarct DC shifts and ischaemic neuronal damage in rat. *Neuroreport* 1993; **4**: 709–11.

105. Luhmann HJ, Kral T. Hypoxia-induced dysfunction in developing rat neocortex. *J Neurophysiol* 1997; **78**: 1212–21.

106. Pomper JK, Haack S, Petzold GC, *et al.* Repetitive spreading depression-like events result in cell damage in juvenile hippocampal slice cultures maintained in normoxia. *J Neurophysiol* 2006; **95**: 355–68.

107. Takaoka S, Pearlstein RD, Warner DS. Hypothermia reduces the propensity of cortical tissue to propagate direct current depolarizations in the rat. *Neurosci Lett* 1996; **218**: 25–8.

108. Chen Q, Chopp M, Bodzin G, *et al.* Temperature modulation of cerebral depolarization during focal cerebral ischemia in rats: correlation with ischemic injury. *J Cereb Blood Flow Metab* 1993; **13**: 389–94.

109. Mancuso A, Derugin N, Hara K, *et al.* Mild hypothermia decreases the incidence of transient ADC reduction detected with diffusion MRI and expression of c-fos and hsp70 mRNA during acute focal ischemia in rats. *Brain Res* 2000; **887**: 34–45.

110. Blood AB, Hunter CJ, Power GG. Adenosine mediates decreased cerebral metabolic rate and increased cerebral blood flow during acute moderate hypoxia in the near-term fetal sheep. *J Physiol* 2003; **553**: 935–45.

111. Lotgering FK, Bishai JM, Struijk PC, *et al.* Ten-minute umbilical cord occlusion markedly reduces cerebral blood flow and heat production in fetal sheep. *Am J Obstet Gynecol* 2003; **189**: 233–8.

112. Hunter CJ, Bennet L, Power GG, *et al.* Key neuroprotective role for endogenous adenosine A1 receptor activation during asphyxia in the fetal sheep. *Stroke* 2003; **34**: 2240–5.

113. Aden U, Halldner L, Lagercrantz H, *et al.* Aggravated brain damage after hypoxic ischemia in immature adenosine A2A knockout mice. *Stroke* 2003; **34**: 739–44.

114. Mortola JP. Implications of hypoxic hypometabolism during mammalian ontogenesis. *Respir Physiol Neurobiol* 2004; **141**: 345–56.

115. Andine P, Sandberg M, Bagenholm R, *et al.* Intra- and extracellular changes of amino acids in the cerebral cortex of the neonatal rat during hypoxic-ischemia. *Dev Brain Res* 1991; **64**: 115–20.

116. Engidawork E, Loidl F, Chen Y, *et al.* Comparison between hypothermia and glutamate antagonism treatments on the immediate outcome of perinatal asphyxia. *Exp Brain Res* 2001; **138**: 375–83.

117. Sarnat HB, Sarnat MS. Neonatal encephalopathy following fetal distress: a clinical and electroencephalographic study. *Arch Neurol* 1976; **33**: 696–705.

118. Frerichs KU, Siren AL, Feuerstein GZ, *et al.* The onset of postischemic hypoperfusion in rats is precipitous and may be controlled by local neurons. *Stroke* 1992; **23**: 399–406.

119. Rosenberg AA, Murdaugh E, White CW. The role of oxygen free radicals in postasphyxia cerebral hypoperfusion in newborn lambs. *Pediatr Res* 1989; **26**: 215–19.

120. Hossmann KA. Reperfusion of the brain after global ischemia: hemodynamic disturbances. *Shock* 1997; **8**: 95–101.

121. van Bel F, Dorrepaal CA, Benders MJ, *et al.* Changes in cerebral hemodynamics and oxygenation in the first 24 hours after birth asphyxia. *Pediatrics* 1993; **92**: 365–72.

122. Huang J, Kim LJ, Poisik A, *et al.* Titration of postischemic cerebral hypoperfusion by variation of ischemic severity in a murine model of stroke. *Neurosurgery* 1999; **45**: 328–33.

123. Karlsson BR, Grogaard B, Gerdin B, *et al.* The severity of postischemic hypoperfusion increases with duration

of cerebral ischemia in rats. *Acta Anaesthesiol Scand* 1994; **38**: 248–53.

124. Michenfelder JD, Milde JH. Postischemic canine cerebral blood flow appears to be determined by cerebral metabolic needs. *J Cereb Blood Flow Metab* 1990; **10**: 71–6.

125. Gold L, Lauritzen M. Neuronal deactivation explains decreased cerebellar blood flow in response to focal cerebral ischemia or suppressed neocortical function. *Proc Natl Acad Sci USA* 2002; **99**: 7699–704.

126. Bennet L, Rossenrode S, Gunning MI, *et al.* The cardiovascular and cerebrovascular responses of the immature fetal sheep to acute umbilical cord occlusion. *J Physiol* 1999; **517**: 247–57.

127. Brun NC, Moen A, Borch K, *et al.* Near-infrared monitoring of cerebral tissue oxygen saturation and blood volume in newborn piglets. *Am J Physiol* 1997; **273**: H682–6.

128. Rosenberg AA. Regulation of cerebral blood flow after asphyxia in neonatal lambs. *Stroke* 1988; **19**: 239–44.

129. Toet MC, Lemmers PM, van Schelven LJ, *et al.* Cerebral oxygenation and electrical activity after birth asphyxia: their relation to outcome. *Pediatrics* 2006; **117**: 333–9.

130. Nakajima W, Ishida A, Takada G. Effect of anoxia on striatal monoamine metabolism in immature rat brain compared with that of hypoxia: an in vivo microdialysis study. *Brain Res* 1996; **740**: 316–22.

131. Pearson T, Frenguelli BG. Adrenoceptor subtype-specific acceleration of the hypoxic depression of excitatory synaptic transmission in area CA1 of the rat hippocampus. *Eur J Neurosci* 2004; **20**: 1555–65.

132. Quaedackers JS, Roelfsema V, Heineman E, *et al.* The role of the sympathetic nervous system in post-asphyxial intestinal hypoperfusion in the preterm sheep fetus. *J Physiol* 2004; **557**: 1033–44.

133. Weinshenker D, Szot P. The role of catecholamines in seizure susceptibility: new results using genetically engineered mice. *Pharmacol Ther* 2002; **94**: 213–33.

134. Mishra PK, Kahle EH, Bettendorf AF, *et al.* Anticonvulsant effects of intracerebroventricularly administered norepinephrine are potentiated in the presence of monoamine oxidase inhibition in severe seizure genetically epilepsy-prone rats (GEPR-9s). *Life Sci* 1993; **52**: 1435–41.

135. Nguyen P, Yan EB, Castillo-Melendez M, *et al.* Increased allopregnanolone levels in the fetal sheep brain following umbilical cord occlusion. *J Physiol* 2004; **560**: 593–602.

136. He J, Hoffman SW, Stein DG. Allopregnanolone, a progesterone metabolite, enhances behavioral recovery and decreases neuronal loss after traumatic brain injury. *Restor Neurol Neurosci* 2004; **22**: 19–31.

137. Lapchak PA. The neuroactive steroid 3-alpha-ol-5-beta-pregnan-20-one hemisuccinate, a selective NMDA receptor antagonist improves behavioral performance following spinal cord ischemia. *Brain Res* 2004; **997**: 152–8.

138. Gunn AJ, Quaedackers JS, Guan J, *et al.* The premature fetus: not as defenseless as we thought, but still paradoxically vulnerable? *Dev Neurosci* 2001; **23**: 175–9.

139. Tsuji M, Saul JP, du Plessis A, *et al.* Cerebral intravascular oxygenation correlates with mean arterial pressure in critically ill premature infants. *Pediatrics* 2000; **106**: 625–32.

140. Coimbra C, Boris-Moller F, Drake M, *et al.* Diminished neuronal damage in the rat brain by late treatment with the antipyretic drug dipyrone or cooling following cerebral ischemia. *Acta Neuropathol (Berl)* 1996; **92**: 447–53.

141. Guan J, Gunn AJ, Sirimanne ES, *et al.* The window of opportunity for neuronal rescue with insulin-like growth factor-1 after hypoxia–ischemia in rats is critically modulated by cerebral temperature during recovery. *J Cereb Blood Flow Metab* 2000; **20**: 513–19.

142. Schubert A. Side effects of mild hypothermia. *J Neurosurg Anesthesiol* 1995; **7**: 139–47.

143. Guan J, Bennet L, George S, *et al.* Selective neuroprotective effects with insulin-like growth factor-1 in phenotypic striatal neurons following ischemic brain injury in fetal sheep. *Neuroscience* 2000; **95**: 831–9.

Chapter 43

Neonatal seizures: an expression of fetal or neonatal brain disorders

Mark S. Scher

Introduction

Neonatal seizures are one of the few neonatal neurological conditions that require immediate medical attention. While prompt diagnostic and therapeutic plans are needed, multiple challenges impede the physician's evaluation of the newborn with suspected clinical and electroencephalographic (EEG) manifestations of neonatal seizures, which vary dramatically from those in older children. Recognition of the seizure state remains the foremost challenge to overcome. This dilemma is underscored by the brevity and subtlety of the clinical repertoire of the neonatal neurological examination.

Basic issues still remain regarding the recognition and treatment of neonatal seizures (Table 43.1). Which newborns with seizures to treat, and how to treat them, continues to occupy much discussion and controversy in written and oral presentations. While clinical seizures remain a common occurrence in neonatal intensive care settings, with an incidence as high as 2.6/1000 live births for term infants and 30–130/1000 live preterm births, increasing use of bedside EEG monitoring has resulted in the growing recognition that the incidence of seizures may be even higher. Yet the "who" question in the algorithm to diagnose and treat neonatal seizures includes a heterogeneous cohort of newborns who may present throughout the neonatal period (i.e., 30 days post-term). The manner of clinical presentation will reflect alternative diagnostic explanations for seizure recurrence based on timing, etiology, or brain region of injury [1]. Presentation may imply part of a longer-standing encephalopathic process prior to and/or during parturition in some newborns. Other infants present with isolated seizures or ictal events that herald the onset of new postnatal disease or an otherwise silent antepartum process.

The identification of seizure occurrence relies on both clinical sign recognition and coincident electrographic expression to define the exact onset and offset of seizure duration. This is also essential to more accurately define status epilepticus (SE). The issue of seizure recognition highlights the controversy regarding the assessment of treatment efficacy, linking to etiologic process, as well as location and timing of

injury. Unresolved questions also include the unknown duration of treatment for a neonate who experienced seizures after emergent treatment in the neonatal intensive care unit. Long-term treatment may be required for the child who is at an increased risk for childhood seizures and neurocognitive/neurobehavioral sequelae at an older age. Medications with antiepileptogenic properties rather than those used for anti-ictal purposes need to be tested.

Finally, there remains a controversy concerning whether electrical or clinical seizures are more detrimental to normal brain structure and function. Based on current epilepsy models in immature and older populations, epileptic-induced brain damage can occur either as a direct result of the metabolic consequences of the seizures themselves, and/or due to the underlying etiologies in which seizures are imbedded. Therefore the final section of this review will discuss the current innovations which augment our understanding of seizures in the immature brain. Current and proposed research may lead to novel therapeutic approaches that are relevant to the pathophysiologic mechanisms responsible for both seizures and non-epileptic paroxysmal movement disorders, in the context of the associated etiologies, location, and timing of injury in the immature brain.

Recognition of neonatal seizures

There remains a fundamental controversy regarding seizure recognition [2]. Many intensivists continue to rely primarily on clinical criteria for the diagnosis of neonatal seizures, while acknowledging that electrographic confirmation of seizures may also be necessary. This controversy has been fueled by the technological advances at the bedside using synchronized video EEG monitoring. Simultaneous documentation of suspicious clinical behaviors with electrographic seizures is considered the neurophysiologic gold standard. With this technology, new classifications of neonatal seizures can draw a clearer distinction between "epileptic" and "non-epileptic" events. Failure to document electrographic seizures by scalp recordings suggests the possibility that clinical events may be either non-epileptic paroxysmal behaviors or subcortical seizure events. While commonly diagnosed in older childhood and adult populations, such explanations for neonates are less frequently described. However, several authors argue that traditionally described "subtle seizures" have no coincidental electrographic seizure occurrence on

Fetal and Neonatal Brain Injury, 4th edition, ed. David K. Stevenson, William E. Benitz, Philip Sunshine, Susan R. Hintz, and Maurice L. Druzin. Published by Cambridge University Press. © Cambridge University Press 2009.

Table 43.1. Dilemmas regarding neonatal seizures

(1) Diagnostic choices – reliance on clinical vs. electroencephalographic criteria

(2) Etiologic explanations – multiple prenatal/neonatal conditions as a function of time.

(3) Treatment decisions – who, when, how, and for how long?

(4) Prognostic questions – consider mechanisms of injury based on etiologies vs. intrinsic vulnerability of the immature brain to prolonged seizures

Table 43.2. Caveats concerning recognition of neonatal seizures

(1) Specific stereotypic behaviors occur in association with normal neonatal sleep or waking states, medication effects, and gestational maturity

(2) Consider that any abnormal repetitive activity may be a clinical seizure if out of context for expected neonatal behavior

(3) Attempt to document coincident electrographic seizures with the suspected clinical event

(4) Abnormal behavioral phenomena may have inconsistent relationships with coincident electroencephalographic seizures, suggesting a subcortical seizure focus

(5) Non-epileptic pathologic movement disorders are events that are independent of the seizure state, and may also be expressed by neonates

scalp recordings, and this underscores the controversy. EEG recordings are therefore helpful to avoid treatment choices with traditional antiepileptic medications for paroxysmal non-epileptic events. Treatment protocols are needed after recognizing neonatal movement disorders that require alternative therapies.

The advocacy for electrographic confirmation may also require the preliminary use of automated screening devices in concert with traditional EEG studies. A prototype was designed in the late 1960s using a one-channel EEG. Current devices rely on either one or two channels, with a single computerized algorithm to detect a "pattern" for neonatal seizures. However, a limited number of channels and an arbitrary computer algorithm for automated detection will be suboptimal to document the electrographic expression of seizures that may originate distant from the electrode site or that are of such low intensity or duration as to avoid definitive conclusions regarding the presence or duration of seizures [3]. There is as yet no consensus regarding the comparison of screening recordings with conventional EEG studies with respect to the detection of seizures with acceptable false-negative and false-positive results. Two-tiered recording paradigms need to be incorporated in future studies, to combine the results from screening devices with more comprehensive neurophysiologic protocols.

Clinical seizure criteria

Neonatal seizures are presently listed separately from the traditional classification of seizures and epilepsy during childhood. The International League Against Epilepsy's classification, adopted by the World Health Organization (WHO), still considers neonatal seizures within an unclassified category [4]. A recent classification scheme now suggests a more strict distinction of clinical seizure (non-epileptic) events from electrographically confirmed (epileptic) seizures, with respect to possible treatment interventions [5]. Continued refinement of such novel classifications is needed to reconcile the variable agreement between clinical and EEG criteria for establishing a seizure diagnosis in the context of non-epileptic movement disorders caused by acquired diseases, malformations, and/or medications [6,7].

Several caveats (Table 43.2) may be useful in the identification of suspected neonatal seizures, and these raise questions regarding our diagnostic acumen using only clinical criteria.

The clinical criteria for neonatal seizure diagnosis were historically subdivided into five clinical categories: focal clonic, multifocal or migratory clonic, tonic, myoclonic, and subtle seizures [8]. A more recent classification expands the clinical subtypes, adopting a strict temporal occurrence of specific clinical events with coincident electrographic seizures, to distinguish neonatal clinical "non-epileptic" seizures from "epileptic" seizures (Tables 43.3 and 43.4) [5].

Subtle seizure activity

This is the most frequently observed category of neonatal seizures and includes repetitive buccolingual movements, orbital–ocular movements, unusual bicycling or pedaling, and autonomic findings (Fig. 43.1a). Subtle paroxysmal events which interrupt the expected behavioral repertoire of the neonatal state, and which appear stereotypic or repetitive, should heighten the clinician's level of suspicion for seizures. However, alterations in cardiorespiratory regularity, body movements, and other behaviors during active (REM) sleep, quiet (NREM) sleep, or waking segments also must be recognized before proceeding to a seizure evaluation [9,10]. Within the subtle category of neonatal seizures are stereotypic changes in heart rate, blood pressure, oxygenation, or other autonomic signs, particularly during pharmacological paralysis for ventilatory care. Other autonomic events include penile erections, skin changes, salivation, and tearing. Autonomic expressions may be intermixed with motoric findings. Isolated autonomic signs such as apnea, unless accompanied by other clinical findings, are rarely associated with coincident electrographic seizures (Fig. 43.1b). Since subtle seizures are both clinically difficult to detect and only variably coincident with EEG seizures [11,12], synchronized video/EEG/polygraphic recordings are recommended to document temporal relationships between clinical behaviors and coincident electrographic events [5,13–15]. Despite the "subtle" expression of this seizure category, these children may still have suffered significant brain injury.

Clonic seizures

Rhythmic movements of muscle groups in a focal distribution which consist of a rapid phase followed by a slow return movement are clonic seizures, to be distinguished from the

Table 43.3. Clinical characteristics, classification, and presumed pathophysiology of neonatal seizures

Classification	Characterization
Focal clonic	Repetitive, rhythmic contractions of muscle groups of the limbs, face, or trunk
	May be unifocal or multifocal
	May occur synchronously or asynchronously in muscle groups on one side of the body
	May occur simultaneously but asynchronously on both sides
	Cannot be suppressed by restraint
	Pathophysiology: epileptic
Focal tonic	Sustained posturing of single limbs
	Sustained asymmetrical posturing of the trunk
	Sustained eye deviation
	Cannot be provoked by stimulation or suppressed by restraint
	Pathophysiology: epileptic
Generalized tonic	Sustained symmetrical posturing of limbs, trunk, and neck
	May be flexor, extensor, or mixed extensor/flexor
	May be provoked by stimulation
	May be suppressed by restraint or repositioning
	Presumed pathophysiology: non-epileptic
Myoclonic	Random single rapid contractions of muscle groups of the limbs, face, or trunk
	Typically not repetitive, or may recur at a slow rate
	May be generalized, focal, or fragmentary
	May be provoked by stimulation
	Presumed pathophysiology: may be epileptic or non-epileptic

Classification	Characterization
Spasms	May be flexor, extensor, or mixed extensor/flexor
	May occur in clusters
	Cannot be provoked by stimulation or suppressed by restraint
	Pathophysiology: epileptic
Motor automatisms: ocular signs	Random and roving eye movements or nystagmus (distinct from tonic eye deviation)
	May be provoked or intensified by tactile stimulation
	Presumed pathophysiology: non-epileptic
Oral–buccal–lingual movements	Sucking, chewing, tongue protrusions
	May be provoked or intensified by stimulation
	Presumed pathophysiology: non-epileptic
Progression movements	Rowing or swimming movements
	Pedaling or bicycling movements of the legs
	May be provoked or intensified by stimulation
	May be suppressed by restraint or repositioning
	Presumed pathophysiology: non-epileptic
Complex purposeless movements	Sudden arousal with transient increased random activity of limbs
	May be provoked or intensified by stimulation
	Presumed pathophysiology: non-epileptic

Source: From Mizrahi EM, Kellaway P, *Diagnosis and Management of Neonatal Seizures*. Philadelphia, PA: Lippincott-Raven, 1998 [5].

Table 43.4. Classification of neonatal seizures based on electroclinical findings

Clinical seizures with a consistent electrocortical signature (pathophysiology: epileptic)
- *Focal clonic*
  - Unifocal
  - Multifocal
  - Hemiconvulsive
  - Axial
- *Focal tonic*
  - Asymmetrical truncal posturing
  - Limb posturing
  - Sustained eye deviation
- *Myoclonic*
  - Generalized
  - Focal
- *Spasms*
  - Flexor
  - Extensor
  - Mixed extensor/flexor

Clinical seizures without a consistent electrocortical signature (pathophysiology: presumed non-epileptic)
- *Myoclonic*
  - Generalized
  - Local
  - Fragmentary
- *Generalized tonic*
  - Flexor
  - Extensor
  - Mixed extensor/flexor
- *Motor automatisms*
  - Oral–buccal–lingual movements
  - Ocular signs
  - Progression movements
  - Complex purposeless movements
- *Electrical seizures without clinical seizure activity*

Source: From Mizrahi EM, Kellaway P, *Diagnosis and Management of Neonatal Seizures*. Philadelphia, PA: Lippincott-Raven, 1998 [5].

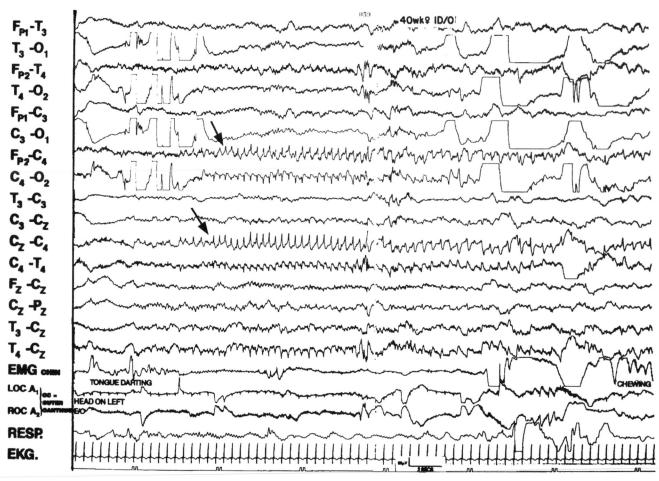

Fig. 43.1. (a) Electroencephalographic (EEG) segment of a 40-week-gestation, 1-day-old female following severe asphyxia resulting from rupture of velamentous insertion of the umbilical cord during delivery. An electrical seizure in the right central/midline region is recorded (arrows), coincident with buccolingual and eye movements (see comments and eye channels on record). From Scher MS, Painter MJ. Electrographic diagnosis of neonatal seizures: issues of diagnostic accuracy, clinical correlation and survival. In: Wasterlain CG, Vert P, eds., *Neonatal Seizures.* New York, NY: Raven Press. 1990: 17, with permission.

symmetric "to and fro" movements of tremulousness or jitteriness [1]. Gentle flexion of the affected body part easily suppresses the tremor, while clonic seizures persist. Clonic movements can involve any body part such as the face, arm, leg, and even diaphragmatic or pharyngeal muscles. Generalized clonic activities can occur in the newborn but rarely consist of a classical tonic followed by clonic phase, characteristic of the generalized motor seizure noted in older children and adults. Focal clonic and hemiclonic seizures have been described with localized brain injury, usually from cerebrovascular lesions (Fig. 43.2a), but can also be seen with generalized brain abnormalities [13,16–18]. As with older patients, focal seizures in the neonate may be followed by transient motor weakness, historically referred to as a transient Todd's paresis or paralysis [19], and are to be distinguished by a more persistent hemiparesis over multiple days to weeks. Electrographic seizures without clinical manifestations may also be seen (Fig. 43.2b). Clonic movements without EEG-confirmed seizures have been described in neonates with normal EEG backgrounds (Fig. 43.2c), and their neurodevelopment

outcome will more likely be normal [14]. The less experienced clinician may misclassify myoclonic as clonic movements. Recent computational studies suggest strategies to extract quantitative information from video recordings of neonatal seizures as a method by which clinicians can differentiate myoclonic from focal clonic seizures, as well as distinguish normal infant behaviors [20].

Multifocal (fragmentary) clonic seizures

Multifocal or migratory clonic activities spread over body parts either in a random or in an anatomically appropriate fashion. Such seizure movements may alternate from side to side and appear asynchronously between the two halves of the child's body. The word "fragmentary" was historically applied to distinguish this event from the more classical generalized tonic–clonic seizure seen in the older child. Multifocal clonic seizures may also resemble myoclonic seizures, which alternatively consist of brief shock-like muscle twitching of the midline and/or extremity musculature. Neonates with this

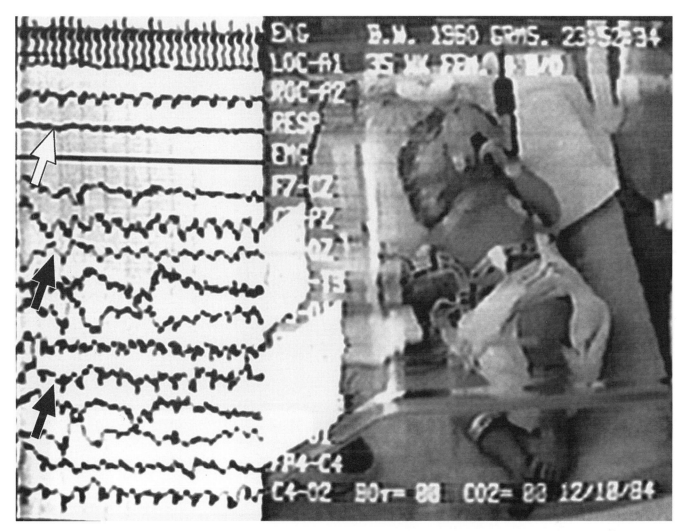

Fig. 43.1. (b) Synchronized video EEG record of a 35-week, 1-day-old female with *Escherichia coli* meningitis and cerebral abscesses. The open arrow notes apnea coincident with prominent right hemispheric and midline electrographic seizures (closed arrows). In addition to apnea, other motoric signs coincident to EEG seizures were noted at other times during the record. From Scher MS, Painter MJ. Controversies concerning neonatal seizures. *Pediatr Clin North Am* 1989; 36: 281–310, with permission.

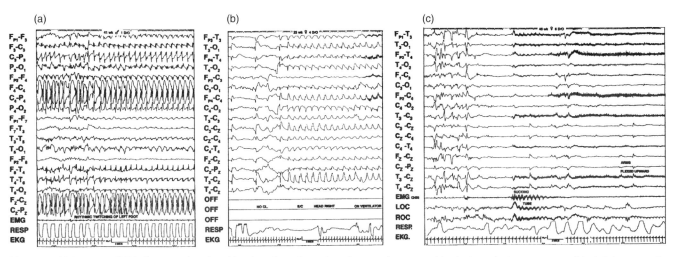

Fig. 43.2. (a) Segment of EEG of a 41-week, 1-day-old male with an electroclinical seizure characterized by rhythmic clonic movements of the left foot coincident with bihemispheric electrographic discharges of higher amplitude in the right hemisphere. This seizure was documented prior to antiepileptic medication. (b) Segment of EEG of a 25-week, 4-day-old female with an electrographic seizure without clinical accompaniment. (c) Segment of an EEG of a 40-week, 6-day-old infant with stereotypic flexion posturing in the absence of electrographic seizures (note muscle artifact). From Scher MS. Pediatric electroencephalography and evoked potentials. In: Swaiman KS, ed., *Pediatric Neurology: Principles and Practice*. St. Louis, MO: Mosby, with permission.

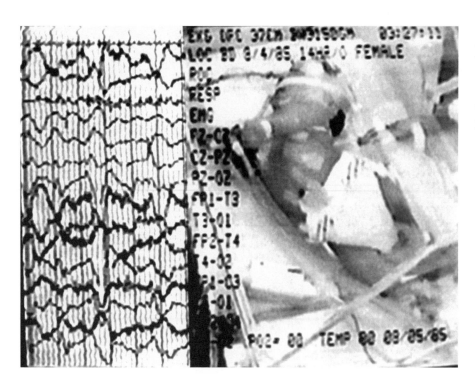

Fig. 43.3. (a) Segment of a synchronized video EEG recording of a 37-week, 1-day-old female who suffered asphyxia, demonstrating prominent opisthotonos with left arm extension in the absence of coincident electrographic seizure activity. From Scher MS, Painter MJ. Controversies concerning neonatal seizures. *Pediatr Clin North Am* 1989; **36**: 281–310, with permission.

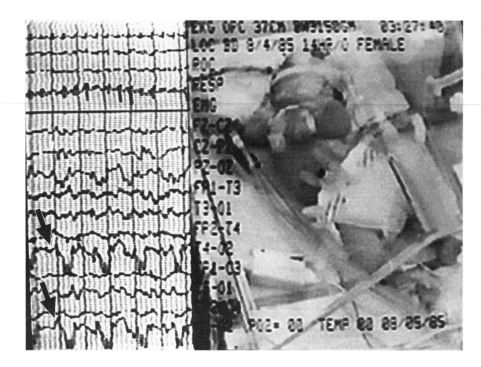

Fig. 43.3. (b) Synchronized video EEG recording of the same patient as in Fig. 43.3a, documenting electrographic seizure in the right posterior quadrant (arrows), following cessation of left arm tonic movements and persistent opisthotonos.

seizure description often suffer death or significant neurological morbidity [21].

Tonic seizures

Tonic seizures refer to a sustained flexion or extension of axial or appendicular muscle groups. Tonic movements of a limb or sustained head or eye turning may also be noted. Tonic activity with coincident EEG needs to be carefully documented, since 30% of such movements lack a temporal correlation with electrographic seizures [22] (Fig. 43.3a,b,c). "Brainstem release" resulting from functional decortications after severe neocortical dysfunction or damage is one physiologic explanation for this non-epileptic activity, to be discussed below. Extensive neocortical damage or dysfunction permits the emergence of uninhibited subcortical expressions of extensor movements [23] (Fig. 43.4). Tonic seizures may also be misidentified, when the non-epileptic movement disorder of dystonia is the more appropriate behavioral description (Figs. 43.2c, 43.3a).

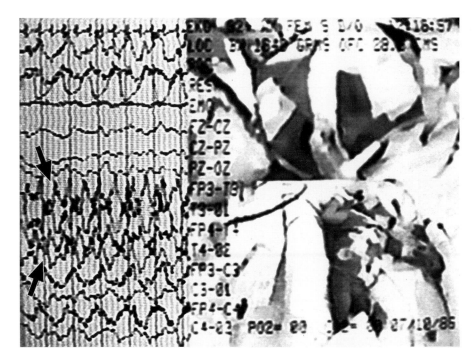

Fig. 43.3. (c) Segment of a video EEG recording documenting a fixed tonic neck reflex with coincident electrographic seizures in the temporal regions (arrows), described as a tonic seizure.

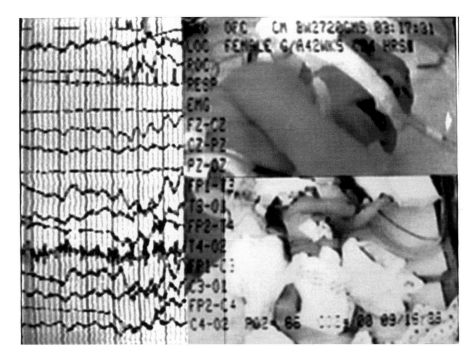

Fig. 43.4. Segment of a video EEG of a 42-week, < 24-hour-old growth-restricted female demonstrating stereotypic posturing and eye opening with no coincident electrographic seizure. The child presented with non-immune hydrops fetalis with significant neocortical injury from a fetal time period. The EEG background is markedly slow and suppressed, representing a severe interictal electrographic abnormality. From Scher MS. Seizures in the newborn infant: diagnosis, treatment, and outcome. *Clin Perinatol* 1997; **24**: 735–72, with permission.

Both tonic movements and dystonic posturing may also simultaneously occur.

Myoclonic seizures

Myoclonic movements are rapid, isolated jerks which can be generalized, multifocal, or focal in an axial or appendicular distribution. Myoclonus lacks the slow return phase of the clonic movement complex described above. Healthy preterm infants commonly exhibit myoclonic movements without seizures or a brain disorder. EEG, therefore, is recommended to confirm the coincident appearance of electrographic discharges with these movements (Fig. 43.5a). Pathologic myoclonus in the absence of EEG seizures also can occur in severely ill preterm or full-term infants after suffering severe brain dysfunction or damage [24]. As with older children and adults, myoclonus may reflect injury at multiple levels of the neuraxis from the spine, brainstem, or cortical regions. Stimulus-evoked myoclonus with either single coincident

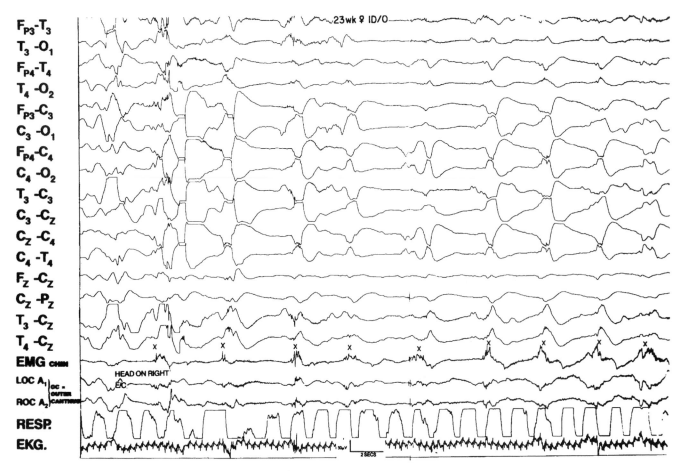

Fig. 43.5. (a) EEG segment of a 23-week, 1-day-old female with grade III intraventricular hemorrhage and progressive ventriculomegaly. An electroclinical seizure is noted coincident with mycolonic movements of the diaphragm (*x* marks). From Scher MS. Pathological myoclonus of the newborn: electrographic and clinical correlations. *Pediatr Neurol* 1985; **1**: 342–8, with permission.

spike discharges or sustained electrographic seizures has been reported [24] (Fig. 43.5a). An extensive evaluation must be initiated to exclude metabolic, structural, and genetic causes. Rarely, healthy sleeping neonates exhibit abundant myoclonus that subsides with arousal to the waking state [25,26], termed "benign sleep myoclonus of the newborn".

Non-epileptic behaviors of neonates

Specific non-epileptic neonatal movement repertoires continually challenge the physician's attempt to reach an accurate diagnosis of seizures and avoid the unnecessary use of anti-epileptic medications. Coincident synchronized video/EEG/polygraphic recordings are now the suggested diagnostic tool to confirm the temporal relationship between the suspicious clinical phenomena and electrographic expression of seizures [27]. The following three examples of pathologic non-epileptic movement disorders incorporate a new classification scheme [5], based on the absence of coincident EEG seizures. Clinicians should maintain an objective perspective regarding gestational age- and state-specific movements which reflect the healthy immature nervous system as well as the varied normal physiologic repertoire seen during sleep, awake, or transitional states.

Tremulousness or jitteriness with EEG correlates

Tremors are frequently misidentified as clonic activity. Unlike the unequal phases of clonic movements described above, the flexion and extension phases of tremor are equal in amplitude. Children are generally alert or hyperalert but may also appear somnolent. Passive flexion and repositioning of the affected tremulous body part diminishes or eliminates the movement. Such movements are usually spontaneous but can be provoked by tactile stimulation. Metabolic or toxin-induced encephalopathies including mild asphyxia, drug withdrawal, hypoglycemia–hypocalcemia, intracranial hemorrhage, hypothermia, and growth restriction are common clinical scenarios when such movements occur. Neonatal tremors generally decrease with age. For example, 38 full-term infants with excessive tremulousness resolved spontaneously over a 6-week period, with 92% neurologically normal at 3 years of age [28]. Medications are rarely considered to treat this particular movement disorder [29].

Neonatal myoclonus without EEG seizures

Myoclonic movements are bilateral and synchronous, or asymmetric and asynchronous in appearance. Clusters of

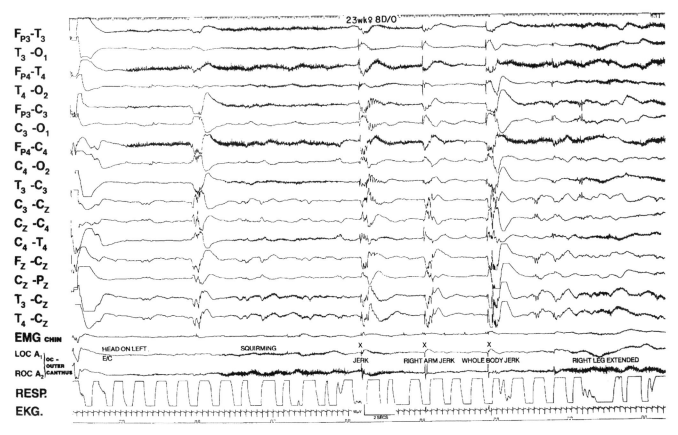

Fig. 43.5. (b) Segment of an EEG recording of an asymptomatic 23-week, 8-day-old female with spontaneous generalized focal myoclonus without electrographic discharges other than myogenic spike potentials.

myoclonic activity occur more predominantly during active (REM) sleep, and are more predominant in the preterm infant [9,30] (Fig. 43.5b), although they can occur in healthy full-term infants. Benign movements are not stimulus-sensitive, have no coincident electrographic seizure correlates, and are not associated with EEG background abnormalities. When these movements occur in the healthy full-term neonate, the activity is suppressed during wakefulness. The clinical description of benign neonatal sleep myoclonus must be a diagnosis of exclusion, after careful consideration of pathologic diagnoses [25].

Infants with severe central nervous system (CNS) dysfunction also may present with non-epileptic spontaneous or stimulus-evoked myoclonus. Different forms of metabolic encephalopathies (such as glycine encephalopathy), cerebrovascular lesions, brain infections, or congenital malformations may present with non-epileptic pathologic myoclonus (Figure 43.5c) [24]. Encephalopathic neonates may respond to tactile or painful stimulation by isolated focal, segmental, or generalized myoclonic movements. Rarely, cortically generated spike or sharp-wave discharges as well as seizures may be noted on the EEG recordings that are coincident with these myoclonic movements (Fig. 43.6a; the coronal section of the brain of this infant is depicted in Fig. 43.6b) [31]. Medication-induced myoclonus and other stereotypic movements have also been described [32], which resolve when the responsible drug is withdrawn.

A rare familial disorder has been described in the neonatal and early infancy periods, specifically termed hyperekplexia.

These movements usually are misinterpreted as a hyperactive startle reflex. Infants are stiff, with severe hypertonia which may lead to apnea and bradycardia. Forced flexion of the neck or hips sometimes alleviates these events. EEG background rhythms are generally age-appropriate. The postulated defect for these individuals involves regulation of brainstem centers which facilitate myoclonic movements [33]. Occasionally benzodiazepines or valproic acid lessen the startling, stiffening, or falling events [34]. Neurologic prognosis is reported to be variable.

Neonatal dystonia without EEG seizures

Dystonia is a third commonly misdiagnosed movement disorder that is often misrepresented as tonic seizures. It represents one of three pathologic hypertonic states present in the neonate besides spasticity and rigidity. Dystonia is classically defined as a distortion of a body part centered around one or multiple joints reflecting imbalance between agonist and antagonist muscle groups. It is not velocity-dependent, and is triggered many times by movement or stimulation. Dystonia can be associated with either acute or chronic disease states involving basal ganglia structures or the complex extrapyramidal pathways (i.e., striatal and cerebellar structures) which connect these regions with brainstem, cerebellum, and other cortical areas. Antepartum or intrapartum adverse events, such as commonly severe asphyxia (termed status mamoratus) or rarely specific inherited metabolic

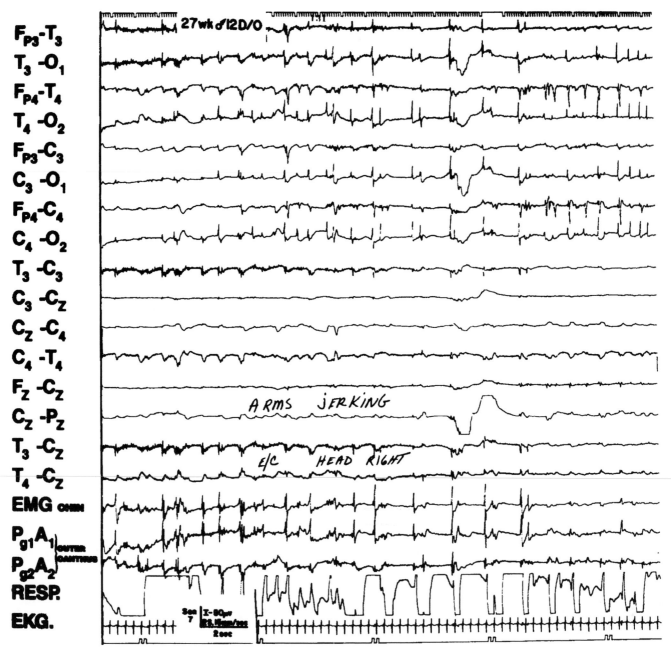

Fig. 43.5. (c) Segment of an EEG recording of an encephalopathic 27-week, 12-day-old male with herpes encephalitis who exhibits non-epileptic multifocal myoclonus (myogenic potentials as EEG artifacts).

diseases [35,36], result in injury to these structures. Alternatively, posturing may reflect subcortical motor pathways that are functionally unopposed because of a diseased or malformed neocortex [23] (Figs. 43.2c, 43.3a, 43.4). Documentation of EEG seizures with coincident video/EEG/polygraphic recordings helps avoid misdiagnosis as seizures and inappropriate treatment.

Electrographic seizure criteria

Over the last several decades, electrographic/polysomnographic studies have become invaluable tools for the assessment of suspected seizures [5,13,22,27,37–39]. Technical and interpretative skills of normal and abnormal neonatal EEG sleep patterns must be mastered before one can develop a confident visual-analysis style for seizure recognition [9,10,40–42].

Corroboration with the EEG technologist is always an essential part of the diagnostic process, since physiologic and non-physiologic artifacts can masquerade as EEG seizures. The physician must also anticipate expected behaviors for the child for a specific gestational maturity, medication use, and state of arousal, in the context of potential artifacts. Synchronized video EEG documentation permits careful offline analysis for more accurate documentation.

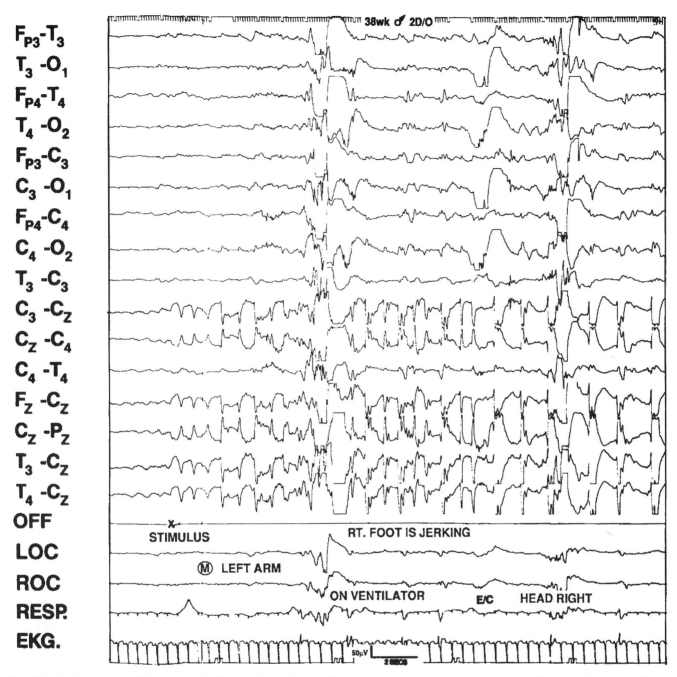

Fig. 43.6. (a) Segment of an EEG recording of a 38-week, 2-day-old male with glycine encephalopathy who has stimulus-sensitive generalized and multifocal myoclonus. Note the onset of a midline (C_z-onset) electrographic seizure with a painful stimulus, followed by right foot myoclonus. From Scher MS. *Pathological myoclonus of the newborn: electrographic and clinical correlations. Pediatr Neurol* 1985; 1: 342–8, with permission.

Hospital-based neurophysiological services must provide prompt interpretation of all bedside studies, depending on the diagnostic demand, as part of an integrated neurointensive program.

As with the epileptic older child and adult, it is generally accepted that the epileptic seizure is a clinical paroxysm of altered brain function with the simultaneous presence of an electrographic event on an EEG recording. Therefore, when assessing the suspected clinical event in the neonate, synchronized video/EEG/polygraphic monitoring is the preferred tool to distinguish an epileptic from a non-epileptic event. Some investigators advocate the use of single- or dual-channel computerized devices for continuous prolonged monitoring, given the multiple logistical challenges with the use of conventional multichannel recording devices at the cribside of a critically ill newborn [43]. This specific device may fail to detect focal or regional seizures if the single channel recording is not near the brain region involved with seizure expression, or if it is not sufficiently short in duration or low in amplitude [3]. For example, a recent study reported that suspected

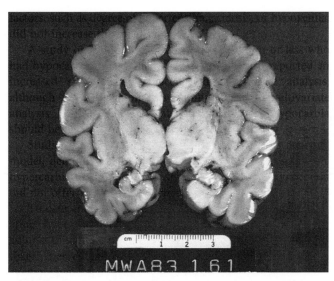

Fig. 43.6. (b) Coronal section of the brain for the patient shown in Figure 43.6a, with agenesis of the corpus callosum and bat-winged shape of lateral ventricles. Spongy myelinosis was noted on microscopic examination.

seizures on a single-channel device could be verified in fewer than three out of ten neonates by conventional EEG [44]. Others have suggested that modified four, five or nine channels of EEG can efficiently detect seizures when verified by continuous video EEG telemetry [3,45].

Epilepsy monitoring services for older children and adults readily utilize intracerebral or surface electrocorticography to detect seizures. Such recording strategies, however, are not ethically appropriate or technologically possible for the neonatal patient. Subcortical foci are consequently difficult to definitively eliminate from consideration, as will be discussed below.

Ictal EEG patterns: a more reliable marker for seizure onset, duration, and severity

Neonatal EEG seizure patterns commonly consist of a repetitive sequence of waveforms which evolve in frequency, amplitude, electrical field, and/or morphology. Four types of ictal patterns have been described: focal ictal patterns with normal background, focal patterns with abnormal background, multifocal ictal patterns, and focal monorhythmic periodic patterns of various frequencies. It is generally suggested that a minimal duration of 10 seconds for the evolution of discharges is required to distinguish electrographic seizures from repetitive but non-ictal epileptiform discharges [13,42,46,47] (Figs. 43.1a, 43.2a,b). Clinical neurophysiologists separately classify brief or prolonged repetitive discharges which lack an electrographic evolution as non-ictal abnormal epileptiform patterns but not confirmatory of seizures [48]. The unique features of neonatal electrographic seizure duration and topography are discussed below.

Seizure duration and topography

The duration and electrographic spread of paroxysmal discharges have been discussed with respect to "seizure burden" to assess antiepileptic drug (AED) efficacy, and consequently

will be needed to predict higher risk for neurologic sequelae. Continuous monitoring can increase the detection rate of neonatal seizures at least during the first 48 hours after birth [49,50]. Longer monitoring periods will depend on the onset and etiology of seizures for specific subsets of newborns.

Few studies have quantified minimal or maximal seizure durations in neonates [5,13,46]. Most notably, the definition of the most severe expression of seizures, status epilepticus (SE), which potentially promotes brain injury, can be problematic. For the older patient, SE is defined as at least 30 minutes of continuous seizures or two consecutive seizures with an interictal period during which the patient fails to return to full consciousness. This definition is not easily applied to the neonate, in whom the level of arousal may be difficult to assess, particularly if sedative medications are given. One study arbitrarily defined neonatal SE as continuous seizure activity for at least 30 minutes, or 50% of the recording time [46], and found that 33% (11/34) of full-term infants had SE, with a mean duration of 29.6 minutes prior to antiepileptic drug use, while 9% (3/34) of the preterm infants also had SE, with an average duration of 5.2 minutes per seizure (i.e., 50% of the recording time). The mean seizure duration was longer in the full-term infant (5 minutes) than in the preterm infant (2.7 minutes). Given that more than 20% of this study group fit the criteria for SE based on EEG documentation, concerns must be raised regarding underdiagnosis of the more severe form of seizures that potentially contributes to brain injury, if only clinical criteria are applied. Another study documented greater risk for neurologic sequelae in the neonatal cohort who exhibited SE [47].

Uncoupling of the clinical and electrographic expressions of neonatal seizures after antiepileptic medication administration also contributes to an underestimation of the true seizure duration, including SE (Fig. 43.7). One study estimated that 25% of neonates expressed persistent electrographic seizures despite resolution of their clinical seizure behaviors after receiving antiepileptic medications [51], termed electroclinical uncoupling. Other pathophysiological mechanisms besides medication effect also might explain uncoupling [7].

Most neonatal electrographic seizures arise focally from one brain region. Generalized synchronous and symmetrical repetitive discharges can also occur. In one study, 56% of seizures were seen in a single location at onset; specific sites included temporal–occipital (15%), temporal–central (15%), central (10%), frontotemporal–central (6%), frontotemporal (5%), and vertex (5%). Multiple locations at the onset of the electrographic seizures were noted in 44% [13]. Electrographic discharges may be expressed as specific EEG frequency ranges from fast to slow, including beta, alpha, theta, or delta activities. Multiple electrographic seizures can also be expressed independently in anatomically unrelated brain regions.

Subcortical seizures versus non-ictal functional decortication

Experimental animal models offer conflicting neuronal mechanisms to explain clinical events which do not have coincident

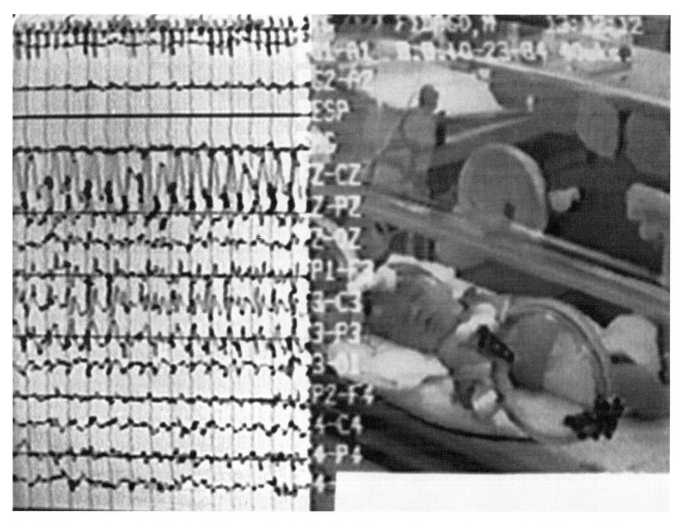

Fig. 43.7. Segment of a synchronized video EEG of a 40-week, 1-day-old male with electrographic status epilepticus noted in the left central/midline regions, after antiepileptic medication administration. Focal right shoulder clonic activity was only intermittently noted, while continuous electrographic seizures were documented mostly without clinical expression. This phenomenon of uncoupling of electrical and clinical seizure activities is associated with antiepileptic drug administration use (see text). From Scher MS, Painter MJ. Controversies concerning neonatal seizures. *Pediatr Clin North Am* 1989; **36**: 281–310, with permission.

EEG confirmation. There is experimental evidence with animal models supporting the existence of subcortical sites for seizure initiation [52,53], although most clinical neurophysiologists require documentation of an ictal pattern by surface EEG electrodes. However, subcortical seizures with only intermittent propagation to the surface may occur, as described for a neonatal cohort [6]. Alternatively, non-ictal "brainstem release" phenomena must be considered, particularly if EEG seizures are never expressed [22]. A more integrated electroclinical approach has been suggested to classify clinical events as seizures versus non-epileptic movement disorders, based on documentation by synchronized video EEG monitoring [5].

Brainstem release phenomena

Synchronized video EEG polygraphic monitoring provides the physician with documentation of a suspicious event with a concurrent electrographic pattern on surface recordings [15].

The temporal relationship between clinical and electrographic phenomena has been described, based on the synchronized video EEG polygraphic monitoring. Based on 415 clinical seizures in 71 babies, clonic seizure activity had the best correlation with coincident electrographic seizures. "Subtle" clinical events, on the other hand, had a more inconsistent relationship with coincident EEG seizure activity, suggesting a non-epileptic brainstem release phenomenon for at least a proportion of such events. Functional decortication resulting from neocortical damage without coincident EEG seizures has therefore been suggested, such as with tonic posturing, as illustrated in Figure 43.3a [22]. Newborns with non-seizure brainstem release activity may express a different functional pattern of metabolic dysfunction, detected as altered glucose uptake on single photon emission tomography (PET) studies, than neonates with seizures [54]. A recent suggestion to document increased prolactin levels with clinical seizures has also been reported [55], but such levels have not yet been correlated with electrographic seizures.

Electroclinical dissociation suggesting subcortical seizures

Experimental studies of immature animals also support the possibility that subcortical structures may initiate seizures, which subsequently, although intermittently, propagate to the cortical surface [56–58]. While EEG depth recordings in adults and adolescents help document subcortical seizures both with and without clinical expression, this technology is not applicable or appropriate to the neonate. Only one anecdotal report of a human infant documented seizures possibly emanating from deep gray-matter structures [59]. A recent symposium re-emphasized the contribution of subcortical networks to cortical excitability using animal models [60]. Documentation in the human neonate will remain problematic until technological advances permit us to monitor directly from subcortical locations, as with depth electrodes by epileptologists.

Electroclinical dissociation (ECD) is one proposed mechanism by which subcortical seizures may only intermittently appear on surface-recorded EEG studies [6]. ECD has been defined as a reproducible clinical event that occurs both with and without coincidental electrographic seizures. In one group of 51 infants with electroclinical seizures, 33 simultaneously expressed both electrical and clinical seizure phenomena. Extremity movements were more significantly associated with synchronized electroclinical seizures. However, a subset of 34% (18/51) also expressed ECD on EEG recordings. For neonates who expressed ECD, the clinical seizure component always preceded the electrographic seizure expression, suggesting that a subcortical focus may have initiated the seizure state. Some of these children also expressed synchronized electroclinical seizures, even on the same EEG record. It may be useful to classify clinical events without either simultaneous or disassociated electrographic patterns as non-epileptic movement disorders, requiring alternative treatment pathways.

Controversy remains whether subcortical seizures or non-ictal functional decortication best categorizes suspicious clinical behaviors without coincident EEG seizure documentation. This dilemma should encourage the clinician to use the EEG as a neurophysiologic yardstick by which more exact seizure start and end points can be assigned, before offering pharmacologic treatment with AEDs [27]. Neonates certainly exhibit electrographic seizures that go undetected unless EEG is utilized [61–66]. Two examples are neonates who are pharmacologically paralyzed for ventilatory assistance (Fig. 43.8a), and clinical seizures which are suppressed by the use of antiepileptic drugs (Fig. 43.8b) [13,51,61,64–66]. In one cohort of 92 infants, 60% of whom were pretreated with antiepileptic medications, 50% had electrographic seizures with no clinical accompaniment [51]. Both clinical and electrographic seizure criteria were noted for 45% of 62 preterm and 53% of 33 full-term infants. Seventeen infants

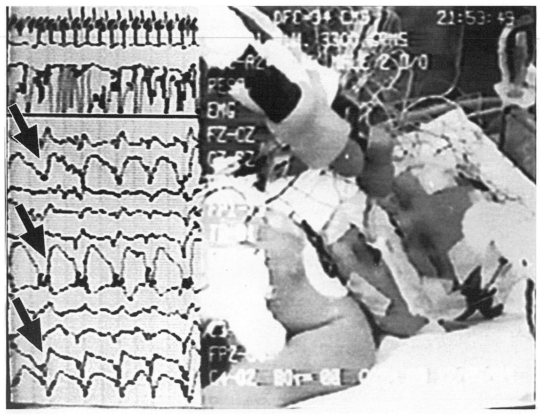

Fig. 43.8. (a) Segment of a synchronized video EEG record of a 36-week, 2-day-old male who is pharmacologically paralyzed for ventilatory care. A seizure is noted in the right posterior quadrant and midline (arrows). From Scher MS, Painter MJ. Controversies concerning neonatal seizures. *Pediatr Clin North Am* 1989; **36**: 281–310, with permission.

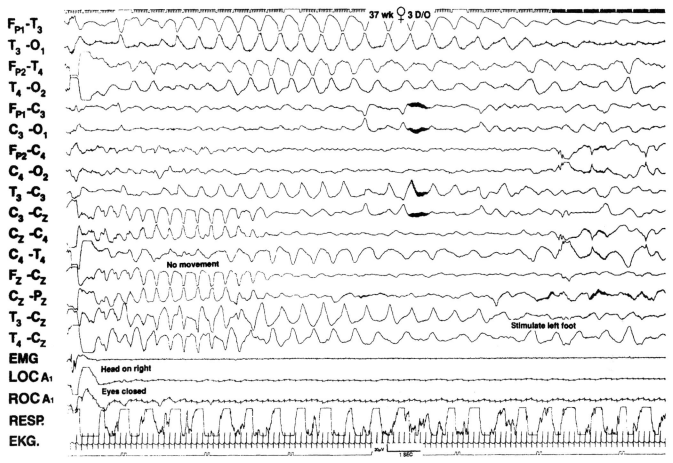

Fig. 43.8. (b) EEG segment for a 37-week, 3-day-old female after antiepileptic drug use with multifocal electrical seizures in the delta frequency range in the temporal and midline regions. Note the marked suppression of normal EEG background. From Scher MS. Neonatal seizures: seizures in special clinical settings. In: Wyllie E, ed., *The Treatment of Epilepsy: Principles and Practice*, 2nd edn. Baltimore, MD: Williams & Wilkins, 1997: 608, with permission.

were pharmacologically paralyzed when the EEG seizure was first documented. A later cohort of 60 infants, none of whom were pretreated with antiepileptic medications, included 7% of infants with only electrographic seizures prior to AED administration [51], and 25% who expressed electroclinical uncoupling after AED use.

The underestimation of seizures in the newborn period may also result from inadequate monitoring for specific neurologic signs. Autonomic changes in respirations, blood pressure, oxygenation, heart rate, pupillary size, skin color, and salivation are examples of subtle ictal signs (Fig. 43.9a,b). In one study, autonomic seizures accompanied electrographic seizures in 37% of 19 preterm neonates [61]. Newer classifications of neonatal seizures should emphasize documentation of autonomic findings on EEG recordings [5].

Variation in the incidence of neonatal seizures based on clinical versus EEG criteria

Over- and under-estimation of neonatal seizures are reported whether clinical or electrical criteria are used. Using clinical criteria, seizure incidences ranged from 0.5% in term infants to 22.2% in preterm neonates [67–70]. Discrepancies in incidence reflect not only varying post-conceptional ages of the

study populations chosen, but also poor interobserver reliability and the hospital setting in which the diagnosis was made [71]. Hospital-based studies which include high-risk deliveries generally report a higher seizure incidence [61]. Population studies which include less medically ill infants from general nurseries report lower percentages [72]. Incidence figures based only on clinical criteria without EEG confirmation include "false positives," consisting of the neonates with either normal or non-epileptic pathologic neonatal behaviors. Conversely, the absence of scalp-generated EEG seizures may include a subset of "false negatives" who express seizures only from subcortical brain regions without expression on the cortical surface. Closer consensus between clinical and EEG criteria is still needed.

Major etiologies for seizure: multiple overlapping conditions along a variable timeline

Neonatal seizures are not disease-specific, and can be associated with a variety of medical conditions which occur before or after parturition, as well as during the postnatal period (Table 43.5). Documentation of asphyxia is the most frequently diagnosed entity when seizures occur. Seizures can occur as part of an asphyxial injury before, during, and/or after labor

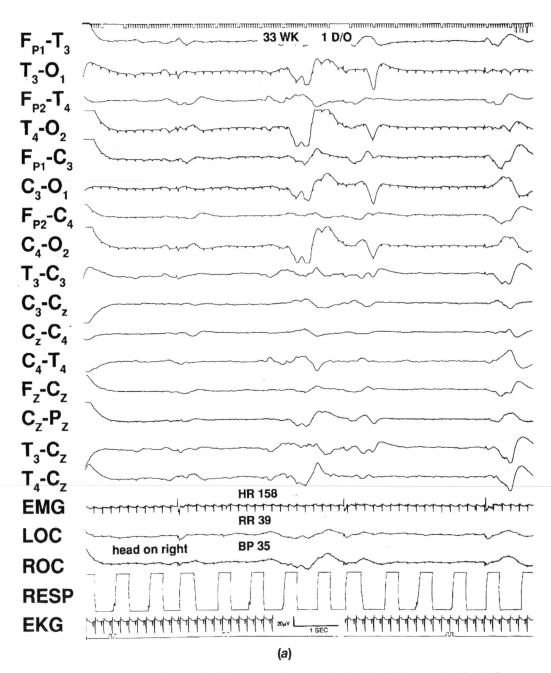

(a)

Fig. 43.9. (*a* and *b*) Electroencephalographic (EEG) segments of a 31-week, 1-day-old male documenting drops in heart rate and blood pressure measurements after the onset of an electrographic seizure.

and delivery, associated with a neonatal encephalopathy or brain disorder. Alternatively, other etiologies for neonatal encephalopathy besides asphyxia must be considered. Seizures may also be an isolated clinical sign without other neurological signs of a postnatal encephalopathy. A study using a logistic model to predict seizures emphasized the accumulation of both antepartum and intrapartum factors, which increases the likelihood of neonatal seizure occurrence [73]. While separately these same factors had low positive predictive values, a significant cumulative risk profile included factors

such as antepartum maternal anemia, bleeding, and asthma, meconium-stained amniotic fluid, abnormal fetal presentation, fetal distress, and shoulder dystocia.

Hypoxia–ischemia (i.e., asphyxia) is traditionally considered the most common cause associated with neonatal seizures [74]. However, children suffer asphyxia either before or during parturition; only 10% of asphyxia results from postnatal causes [8].

Intrauterine factors prior to labor can result in fetal asphyxia without later documentation of acidosis at birth. Both antepartum and intrapartum maternal and placental illnesses

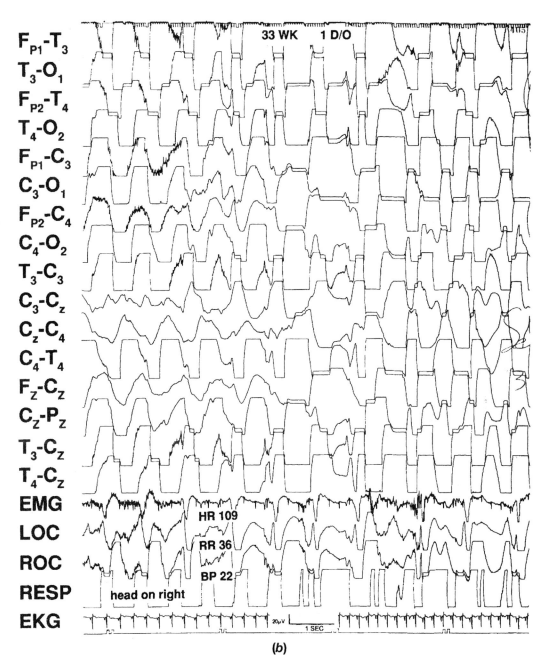

Fig. 43.9. (cont.)

associated with thrombophilia, pre-eclampsia, or specific utero-placental abnormalities such as abruptio placentae or cord compression may contribute to fetal asphyxial stress leading to metabolic acidosis. Antepartum maternal trauma and chorioamnionitis are additional conditions which also contribute to the intrauterine asphyxia secondary to uteroplacental insufficiency. Intravascular placental thromboses and infarctions of the placenta or umbilical cord documented after birth are markers for possible fetal asphyxia. Meconium passage into the amniotic fluid also promotes an inflammatory response within the placental membranes, potentially causing

vasoconstriction and resultant asphyxia. Neuroimaging, particularly using MRI, can define specific patterns of injury that result from asphyxia, either before or during labor and delivery, depending when the MRI was obtained and whether diffusion-weighted images are included [75].

Postnatal medical illnesses also cause or contribute to asphyxia-induced brain injury. Persistent pulmonary hypertension of the newborn, cyanotic congenital heart disease, sepsis, meningitis, encephalitis, and primary intracranial hemorrhage are leading diagnoses. A recent case–control study of term infants with clinical seizures reported a previously

Table 43.5. Selected differential diagnosis of neonatal seizures

Metabolic

  Hypoxia–ischemia (i.e., asphyxia)

    Hypoglycemia

    Hypocalcemia

    Hypomagnesemia

  Hypoglycemia

    Intrauterine growth retardation

    Infant of a diabetic mother

    Glycogen storage disease

    Galactosemia

    Idiopathic

  Hypocalcemia

    Hypomagnesemia

    Infant of a diabetic mother

    Neonatal hypoparathyroidism

    Maternal hyperparathyroidism

    High phosphate load

  Other electrolyte imbalances

    Hypernatremia

    Hyponatremia

Intracranial hemorrhage

  Subarachnoid hemorrhage

  Subdural/epidural hematoma

  Intraventricular hemorrhage

Cerebrovascular lesions (other than trauma)

  Cerebral infarction

    Thrombotic vs. embolic

    Ischemic vs. hemorrhagic

  Cortical vein thrombosis

  Circulatory disturbances from hypoperfusion

Trauma

Infections

  Bacterial meningitis

  Viral-induced encephalitis

  Congenital infections

    Herpes

    Cytomegalovirus

    Toxoplasmosis

    Syphilis

    Coxsackie meningoencephalitis

    Acquired immune deficiency syndrome (AIDS)

  Brain abscess

Brain anomalies (i.e., cerebral dysgenesis from either congenital or acquired causes)

Drug withdrawal or toxins

  Prenatal substance – methadone, heroin, barbiturate, cocaine, etc.

  Prescribed medications – propoxyphene, isoniazid

  Local anesthetics

Hypertensive encephalopathy

Amino acid metabolism

  Branched-chain amino acidopathies

  Urea-cycle abnormalities

  Nonketotic hyperglycinemia

  Ketotic hyperglycinemia

Familial seizures

  Neurocutaneous syndromes

    Tuberous sclerosis

    Incontinentia pigmenti

  Autosomal dominant neonatal seizures

Selected genetic syndromes

  Zellweger syndrome

  Neonatal adrenoleukodystrophy

  Smith–Lemli–Opitz syndrome

Note:
Etiology independent of timing from fetal to neonatal periods.
Source: Adapted from Scher [77].

unrecognized entity called fetal inflammatory response. A fourfold increase in the risk of unexplained early-onset seizures after intrapartum maternal fever was reported. In this study, all known causes of seizures were eliminated, including meningitis or sepsis. A cohort of 38 newborns, compared to 152 controls, experienced intrapartum fever as an independent risk factor on logistic regression which predicted seizures. The authors speculated on the role of circulating maternal cytokines which trigger "physiologic events" mimicking asphyxia and seizures [76].

A discussion of neonatal seizures should include prenatal contributions which contribute to neonatal encephalopathy with seizures in neonates who are at later risk for epilepsy and developmental delay during childhood [77]. A recently published consensus report by a multidisciplinary task force reviewed medical literature concerning the association of neonatal encephalopathy and cerebral palsy, emphasizing antepartum as well as intrapartum factors that need to be considered in the pathogenesis of neonatal brain disorders [78]. Children may experience brain injury from asphyxia during the antepartum period, sometimes associated with maternal or placental disease, worsened by genetic vulnerabilities such as from inherited thrombophilia. Vascular or parenchymal diseases on the maternal side of the placenta, for example, can lead to hypoperfusion-induced asphyxial injuries to the newborn brain, which initiate during the antepartum period, with or without continuation during parturition.

Clinicians should therefore consider a continuum of injury for some neonates presenting with encephalopathy, beginning in the antepartum and possibly extending into the intrapartum and neonatal periods. The epileptologist's description of "dual pathology" may have relevance for the fetal and neonatal patient. Dual pathology implies the existence of more than one cerebral lesion in addition to temporal lobe abnormalities, principally mesial temporal sclerosis. Historically, the concept of "dual pathology" referred to febrile SE during infancy in humans in association with cortical dysplasias that were acquired earlier during gestation. The concept of "dual pathology" was initially defined for populations of children and adults who had intractable seizures requiring evaluation for epilepsy surgery.

Cumulative risks for brain injury throughout the three trimesters of pregnancy, including parturition and the neonatal period, may include both malformations from genetic defects and lesions from acquired injuries. Multiple sites of brain injury in the fetus and the neonate underscore the importance of recognizing that brain lesions in different locations may occur at different time periods, cumulatively adding to the negative effects on developmental neural plasticity, initially expressed as neonatal encephalopathy with subsequent epilepsy and developmental delay at older ages [79,80]. Metabolic pathways for neurogenesis and epileptogenesis are shared; microdysgenesis found in surgical pathologic specimens at the time of epilepsy surgery in adults and children can be prenatal in origin from both genetic and acquired causes [81]. Different patterns of heterotopic neurons and abnormal cortical architecture may occur early or late during the first or second half of pregnancy from different disease states as well as from genetic defects. Epigenetic effects also may result when the fetus is exposed to harmful environmental conditions in utero. This may involve toxic, infectious, or metabolic (including asphyxial) stresses that alter genetic expression. For example, hippocampal sclerosis was uncommon in children who had fetal strokes before 28 weeks' gestation compared with children whose strokes occurred later in gestation [82]. This type of analysis provides evidence that the timing of prenatal insults has profound influences on subsequent brain pathology and clinical outcome. Neonatal encephalopathy with seizures underscores the importance of dual pathology as it relates to fetal and neonatal brain injuries acquired both before and during parturition and expressed after birth by encephalopathic signs [83]. Consideration of time, region, and etiologic-specific contributions to dual pathology will then alter the definition of intractable epilepsy later during childhood. These findings should lead to reconsideration of novel pharmacologic interventions and more aggressive surgical intervention strategies for epilepsy management for the fetus and neonate with dual pathology.

Historical data, clinical findings, and laboratory information must be placed along a timeline that considers prenatal time periods during which brain malformations or damage occur in the context of the child's genetic endowment. The pediatric neurologist who appreciates fully the child's risk for epilepsy and comorbidities involving cognition and behavior applies an ontogenetic approach to the neurologic evaluation beginning before birth to consider the epileptic condition from a fetal neurologic perspective. This fetal perspective consequently influences the type and timing of medical or surgical interventions, even as early as the neonatal period.

Placental findings can be associated with either antepartum or intrapartum conditions. Meconium staining through the chorionic and amnion layers suggests a longer-standing asphyxial stress of 12 hours or greater. Placental weights below the 10th or above the 90th percentile may suggest chronic hypoperfusion to the fetus if verified by histological examination. In a study of preterm and full-term neonates (23–42 weeks conceptional age) with electrically confirmed seizures, a significant association between seizures and chronic (with or without acute) placental lesions was noted [84]. Examples of chronic placental injuries included vasculopathies, stromal infarction, and villus maldevelopment when histologic specimens were examined.

Specific clinical examination findings in the neonate suggest the occurrence of antepartum injury even after signs of acute neurologic depression after delivery. Intrauterine growth restriction, hydrops fetalis, or joint contractures (including arthrogryposis) are specific findings that support an antepartum process that later was expressed as intrapartum fetal distress followed by neonatal depression. Spasticity, often with cortical thumbs, suggests longer-standing fetal neurological dysfunction, since neonates after intrapartum asphyxia are traditionally noted to be hypotonic. While antepartum brain injury can result from maternal, placental, or fetal conditions, intrapartum asphyxial injury can certainly add to brain injury in these children. Neonates may then exhibit signs of neonatal encephalopathy from both pre-existing antepartum brain injury and subsequent intrapartum events.

Seizures in the clinical context of maternal–fetal–placental diseases: following a diagnostic algorithm

Once seizures are confirmed by EEG, the neurologist must place these events into the context of clinical, historical and laboratory findings to determine the pathogenesis and timing of an encephalopathic process in the symptomatic neonate. Seizures associated with neonates after asphyxia support either acute intrapartum events and/or antepartum disease processes. Does the child with seizures also express clinical and laboratory signs of evolving cerebral edema? The presence of a bulging fontanel with neuroimaging evidence of increased intracranial-pressure cerebral edema (i.e., obliterated ventricular outline and abnormal diffusion-weighted MRI images) strongly suggests a more recent asphyxial disease process, in or around the intrapartum period. Hyponatremia and increased urine osmolality suggest the syndrome of inappropriate secretion of antidiuretic hormone accompanying acute or subacute cerebral edema.

Alternatively, failure to document evolving cerebral edema during the first 3 days after asphyxia, or documentation of encephalomalacia or cystic brain lesions on neuroimaging shortly after birth (i.e., even in the encephalopathic newborn), suggests a more chronic disease process and remote antepartum brain injury. Liquefaction necrosis requires longer than 2 weeks after the presumed in utero asphyxial event to produce a cystic cavity [85], which is then visible on neuroimaging.

Isolated seizures in an otherwise asymptomatic neonate also suggest a disease process that occurs during either the postnatal or antepartum periods. Neonates present with seizures as a result of postnatal illnesses from intracranial infection, cardiovascular lesions, drug toxicity, or inherited metabolic diseases. Children with antepartum injury may express isolated seizures after in utero cerebrovascular injury on the basis of thrombolytic and/or embolic disease of the mother, placenta, or fetus. Fetal injury alternatively may occur after ischemic hypoperfusion events from circulatory disturbances, such as maternal shock, chorioamnionitis, or placental fetal vasculopathy [86]. Other antepartum congenital or acquired factors may include familial epilepsy or pre-eclampsia.

Only a percentage of neonates with remote in utero cerebrovascular disease before labor and delivery present with neonatal seizures [87]. Many remain asymptomatic until later during infancy or childhood. Neonatal expression of seizures may reflect acute or subacute physiologic stress during or in proximity to parturition, which lowers the seizure threshold in vulnerable brain regions that have been previously damaged.

Following a careful review of the medical histories of the mother, fetus, and newborn, determination of serum glucose, electrolytes, ammonia, lactate, pyruvate, magnesium, calcium, and phosphorus levels may diagnose correctable metabolic conditions in newborns with seizures who will not require antiepileptic medications. Spinal fluid analyses include cell count, protein, glucose, lactate, pyruvate, amino acids, and culture studies to consider central nervous system infection, intracranial hemorrhage, and metabolic disease. Metabolic acidosis on serial arterial blood gas determinations may alternatively suggest an inherited metabolic disease, particularly if intrapartum asphyxia was not judged to be severe. Absence of multiorgan dysfunction may alert the clinician to other etiologies for seizures besides intrapartum asphyxia. Signs of chronic in utero stress such as growth restriction, early hypertonicity after neonatal depression, joint contractures, or elevated nucleated red blood cell values all suggest longer-standing antepartum stress to the fetus.

Careful review of placental and cord specimens can also be extremely useful [88]. Attention to the complete cord length, placental/fetal weight ratio, and specific anatomical lesions can help approximate the timing of the disease process when a brain disorder occurred, and the possible etiology [88].

Neuroimaging, preferably using MRI, can help localize, grade the severity of, and possibly time an insult [89]. The use of computerized programs using MRI illustrates how diffusion-weighted images help time the approximate window during which a brain disorder occurred [90].

Genetic or syndromic conditions can contribute to the expression of neonatal encephalopathies independent of asphyxial injury [91]. Ancillary genetic studies may also include long chain fatty acids, biotinidase glucose co-transporters, and chromosomal/DNA analyses, as deemed necessary by family and clinical histories. Finally, serum and urine organic acid and amino acid determinations may be needed to delineate a specific biochemical disorder for the child with a persistent metabolic acidosis. Lysosomal enzyme studies are also occasionally considered to diagnose specific enzymatic deficiencies in children with neonatal seizures.

Prognosis

Mortality of infants who present with clinical neonatal seizures has been reported to decline from 40% to 15% [92]. Studies of EEG-confirmed seizures documented 50% mortality in preterm and 40% in full-term infants during the 1980s [62,93]. During the 1990s, in the same institution, this mortality dropped below 20% [2]. Adverse neurologic sequelae, however, remain high for approximately two-thirds of survivors. Even if major neurodevelopmental sequelae such as motor deficits and mental retardation were avoided in survivors after neonatal seizures, subtle neurodevelopmental vulnerability may manifest in late teenage years as specific learning difficulties or poor social adjustment [94], underscoring more recent experimental findings of long-term deficits in animal populations [95].

Prediction of outcome should also consider the etiology for seizures, such as severe asphyxia, significant craniocerebral trauma, and brain infections. More accurate imaging procedures have heightened our awareness of destructive as well as congenital brain lesions, with a higher risk for compromised outcome.

Interictal EEG pattern abnormalities are extremely helpful in predicting neurologic outcome in the neonate with seizures [96,97]. Major background disturbances such as burst–suppression (Fig. 43.10) are highly predictive of poor outcome, particularly when persistently abnormal findings are still present on serial EEG studies into the second week of life. Ictal patterns alone may not be as accurate to predict outcome, unless quantified to high numbers, long durations, and multifocal distribution [98]. Normal findings on interictal EEG were associated with an 86% chance of normal development at 4 years of age in 137 neonates with seizures [21]; by contrast, neonates with marked abnormal EEG background disturbances had only a 7% chance for normal outcome. Another study reported outcome in term and preterm infants with seizures, concluding that the EEG background was more predictive of outcome than the presence of isolated sharp-wave discharges [98]. Even the interpretation of severe EEG abnormalities by single-channel spectral EEG recordings after asphyxia carries a higher risk for sequelae [99].

Neonates with seizures have a risk for epilepsy during childhood [100]. Based on clinical seizure criteria, 20–25% of neonates with seizures later develop epilepsy [101]. Excluding febrile seizures, the prevalence of epilepsy by 6–7 years of age is also estimated to be between 15% and 30%; based on EEG-confirmed seizures for an inborn hospital population,

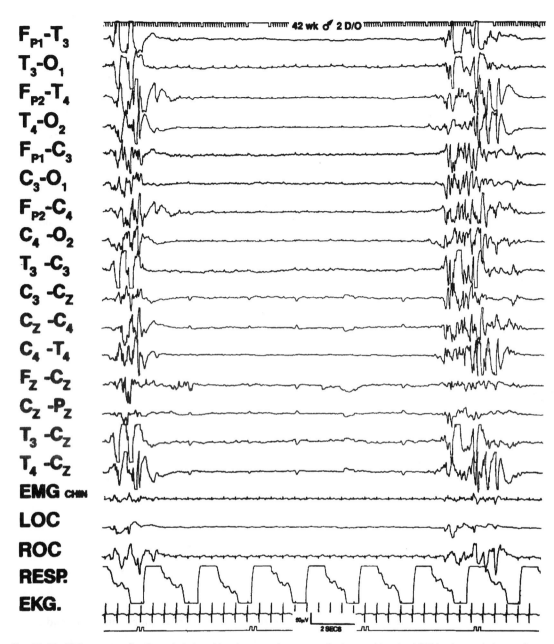

Fig. 43.10. EEG segment of a 42-week, 2-day-old male expressing a severely abnormal interictal EEG background abnormality, termed a burst–suppression or paroxysmal pattern.

two-thirds of this cohort were preterm neonates [102]. This is contrasted with an incidence of 56% with epilepsy for an exclusively outborn neonatal population of primarily full-term newborns with seizures [93]. Epilepsy risk therefore reflects selection bias of specific study groups, as well as referral patterns in different hospital settings.

Principles of therapy

The goal for treating neonatal seizures remains the prevention of long-term brain damage in the context of the medical management of the underlying etiology for a brain disorder. The two-tiered objective of medical management for neonatal seizures is the initial treatment of etiologic factors that may be responsible for seizure generation followed by the cessation of seizures of epileptic origin with either traditional anti-ictal medications or etiology-specific therapeutic agents. These goals may not be achievable since many etiologic factors are not determined for all neonates, and the potential causes for seizures are as yet unknown. As discussed in previous sections, certain clinical seizures with no electrographic expression on surface recordings may in fact be non-epileptic in physiologic origin and therefore may not respond to traditional antiepileptic medications. Alternative treatment choices that stop or lessen non-epileptic movement disorders may be required. Alternatively, antiepileptic medications may be ineffective in children with clinical and/or electrographic expression of presumed cortically propagated seizures, despite high doses of one or multiple antiepileptic medications. Finally, there is a "double-edged blade" to therapeutic interventions to prevent seizures. Antiepileptic medications used to control seizures may have short-term negative consequences by decreasing cerebral perfusion secondary to systemic hypotension, contributing to adverse consequences on brain growth and development.

There are three stages in the current acute management of neonates with seizures: (1) initial medical management, (2) etiology-specific therapy, and (3) antiepileptic medication treatment. These stages should be patient-specific for the clinical profile of the individual neonate. A hypothesized fourth level of treatment will be discussed which refers to the current level of understanding regarding seizure generation in the immature brain related to specific etiologies, brain region, and timing of injury.

General principles of medical management should always include maintaining the newborn's airway, providing adequate ventilation, and preserving cardiovascular circulation. In neonates with seizures, particularly those with recurrent or prolonged seizures, elevations in respiration, heart rate, and blood pressure may occur. Measures must therefore be taken to ensure adequate ventilatory support and circulatory perfusion of neonates with seizures during the initial stage of evaluation and therapy. This approach will potentially avoid the autonomic side effects that may occur as a result of recurrent seizures that can compromise multiorgan system function, leading to secondary brain damage.

If a specific reason for seizures has been identified as potentially treatable, specific etiology-specific therapy needs to be initiated. These treatable causes are critical to seizure management, and will not respond to traditional antiepileptic medications. Examples of common treatable metabolic etiologies include hypoglycemia, hypocalcemia, and hypomagnesemia. The neonatal intensivist must consider the associated brain disorders that may accompany such treatable metabolic derangements, such as asphyxia, intracranial infection, or craniocerebral trauma.

Although uncommon, there are other inherited metabolic conditions that may respond to specific nutritional supplementation. This form of treatment is exemplified by the therapy for pyridoxine deficiency, requiring 50–500 mg of pyridoxine with coincident EEG monitoring. This is a "potentially treatable" cause of medically refractory seizures. It is an exceedingly rare condition but should always be considered in an attempt to control seizures that do not respond to more conventional medical management. Other epileptic encephalopathies associated with metabolic disturbances include folinic acid deficiency and sulfite oxide/molybdenum deficiencies. Some of these metabolic disorders of metabolism can mimic traditional signs of postasphyxial encephalopathy [91].

Emergent antiepileptic drug treatment

It remains controversial which first-line antiepileptic drug agents should be used for neonatal seizure management. There have traditionally been three drug categories: barbiturates, phenytoin, and benzodiazepines. Adverse events must be anticipated with the administration of these antiepileptic medications, including alteration in levels of arousal, systemic hypotension, bradycardia, respiratory depression, and cardiac arrhythmias.

While the initial loading doses are approximated by the use of the neonate's body weight, certain researchers advocate the use of protein characteristics for antiepileptic medications in assigning the initial dosing. The unbound or free fraction of each of these drugs is pharmacologically active in the protein-binding characteristics of neonates, which vary to the extent that uniform dosing scheduled by weight does not provide the same efficacy and safety for the individual child. Preemptive binding profiles calculated for the individual neonate at risk for seizures may allow more accurate establishment of a customized loading dose of each drug for that child, thus avoiding toxicity for that individual neonate. This procedure is not universally available. However, these pharmacologic findings underscore the potential pharmacokinetic and pharmacodynamic variability among neonates regarding the utilizations of these drugs.

A "relative consensus" still exists regarding the choice of a specific antiepileptic medication as either a first- or second-line antiepileptic drug, while phenytoin remains the secondary choice [103]. Additional AEDs in the benzodiazepine family continue to be suggested. Controversy remains regarding these choices, given the evidence-based medicine which questions the efficacy to control seizures with specific AEDs [104].

If the decision to treat neonates with antiepileptic medications is reached, important questions must be addressed with respect to who should be treated, when to begin treatment, which drug to use, and for how long neonates should be treated. Some authors suggest that only neonates with clinical seizures should receive medications; brief electrographic seizures need not be treated. Others suggest more aggressive treatment of EEG seizures, since uncontrolled seizures potentially have an adverse effect on immature brain development. An alternative observation suggests that early administration of an AED, such as phenobarbital, may have adverse effects on outcome in term infants.

Phenobarbital and phenytoin, nonetheless, remain the most widely used antiepileptic medications; benzodiazepines, primidone, and valproic acid have been anecdotally reported. The half-life of phenobarbital ranges from 45 to 173 hours in the neonate [105–107]; the initial loading dose is recommended at 20 mg/kg, with a maintenance dose of 3–4 mg/kg per day. Therapeutic levels are generally suggested to be 16–40 µg/ml, but there is no consensus with respect to drug maintenance.

The preferred loading dose of phenytoin is 15–20 mg/kg [105,106]. Serum levels of phenytoin are difficult to maintain because this drug is rapidly redistributed to body tissues. Blood levels cannot be well maintained using an oral preparation.

Benzodiazepines may also be used to control neonatal seizures. The drug most widely used is diazepam. One study suggests a half-life of 54 hours in preterm infants to 18 hours in full-term infants [108]. Intravenous administration is recommended, since it is slowly absorbed after an intramuscular injection. Diazepam is highly protein bound; alteration of bilirubin binding is low. Recommended intravenous doses for acute management should begin at 0.5 mg/kg. Deposition into muscle precludes its use as a maintenance antiepileptic medication, since profound hypotonia and respiratory depression may result, particularly if barbiturates have also been administered. Lidocaine rather than diazepam infusion has more recently been suggested [109].

Efficacy of treatment

Conflicting studies report varying efficacy with phenobarbital or phenytoin. Most studies only apply a clinical endpoint to seizure cessation. One study found that only 36% of neonates with clinical seizures responded to phenobarbital [106], while another noted cessation of clinical seizures with phenobarbital in only 32% of neonates [105]. With doses as high as 40 mg/kg [110], seizure control was reported to be 85%. Another study reported that the earlier administration of high-dose phenobarbital in a group of asphyxiated infants was associated with a 27% reduction in clinical seizures and better outcome than a group who did not receive high dosages [111]. However, coincident EEG studies are now suggested to verify the resolution of electrographic seizures. A recent report suggests that 30% of neonates have persistent electrographic seizures after suppression of clinical seizure behaviors following drug administration [51]. With EEG as an endpoint to judge cessation of seizures, neither phenobarbital nor phenytoin was effective to control seizure activity [49].

The use of free or drug-bound fractions of AEDs has been suggested to better assess both efficacy and potential toxicity of antiepileptic drugs in pediatric populations [112]. Drug binding in neonates with seizures has only recently been reported, and can be altered in a sick neonate with organ dysfunction. Toxic side effects may result from elevated free fractions of a drug which adversely affect cardiovascular and respiratory function. To guard against untoward effects, evaluation of treatment and efficacy must take into account both total and free AED fractions, in the context of the newborn's progression or resolution of systemic illness.

Once an antiepileptic drug is chosen, the clinician must closely monitor that seizures are not worsened by the administration of such a drug choice. AED may cause worsening of seizures by either aggravating previous seizures or triggering new seizure types, as described in four neonates after midazolam was administered [113].

Discontinuation of drug use

The clinician's decision to maintain or discontinue antiepileptic drugs is also uncertain [92,114]. Discontinuation of drugs before discharge from the neonatal unit is generally recommended, since clinical assessments of arousal, tone, and behavior will not be hampered by medication effect. However,

newborns with congenital or destructive brain lesions on neuroimaging, or those with persistently abnormal neurologic examinations at the time of discharge, may suggest to the clinician that a slower taper off medication is required over several weeks or months. Most neonatal seizures rarely reoccur during the first 2 years of life, and prophylactic AED administration need not be maintained past 3 months of age, even in the child at risk. This is supported by a study suggesting a low risk of seizure recurrence after early withdrawal of AED therapy in the neonatal period [115]. Also, older infants who present with specific epileptic syndromes, such as infantile spasms, will not respond to the conventional antiepileptic drugs that were initially begun during the neonatal period. This honeymoon period without seizures commonly persists for many years in most children before isolated or recurrent seizures appear.

The potential damage of the developing central nervous system by antiepileptic drugs also emphasizes the need to consider early discontinuation of these agents in the newborn period. Adverse effects on the morphology and metabolism of neuronal cells have been extensively reported from collective research performed over the last several decades [116].

Novel antiepileptic drug approaches

Mechanisms of seizure generation, propagation, and termination are different during early brain development as compared with more mature ages. These age-related mechanisms have partially been elucidated [117]. Given that traditional antiepileptic medications have unacceptable efficacy to stop neonatal seizures for specific subsets of newborns, alternative medication options must be developed.

New antiepileptic alternatives to treat neonatal seizures are now being studied. One class of medications are the N-methyl-D-aspartate antagonists such as topiramate [118]. Experimental models of asphyxia-induced seizure activity in immature animal brains have indicated a certain degree of efficacy.

Such models provide data regarding pharmacological and physiological characteristics of neuronal responses after an asphyxial stress which cause excessive release of excitotoxic neurotransmitters [119], such as glutamate. Specific cell membrane receptors termed metabotropic glutamate receptors (MGluRs) are sensitive to extracellular glutamate release and may play a role in epileptogenesis and seizure-induced brain damage [120]. One class of membrane receptor, for example, has been studied in rat pups after hypoxia-induced seizures, suggesting that GluRs downregulation can be associated with epileptogenesis in the absence of cell loss [117]. Subclasses of MGluRs will lead to investigations of novel drugs which block these membrane receptors as the mode of treatment for neonatal seizures [121].

Another therapeutic approach is suggested by experimental studies that demonstrate enhanced seizure susceptibility in the developing brain because GABA exerts a depolarizing excitatory rather than repolarizing inhibitory action in immature subjects [122]. This paradoxical action of GABA early in development may be due in part to age-related differences in chloride homeostasis [123]. Chloride transport is a function of two membrane pumps with different time courses of expression. Early in development (i.e., in the rat, P3–P15 after birth), the Na^+-K^+-$2Cl^-$- co-transporter (NKCCl) imports large amounts of chloride into the neuron (along with sodium and potassium to maintain electroneutrality). This pump sets the chloride equilibrium potential positive to the resting potential, so that when the $GABA_A$ receptor is activated chloride flows out of the neuron, depolarizing it. Over time, NKCCl expression diminishes, and another chloride transporter, KCC2, is expressed. KCC2 has the opposite effect: it extrudes chloride out of the neuron, placing the equilibrium potential more negative than the resting potential so that $GABA_A$ receptor activation allows extracellular chloride to flow into the neuron, hyperpolarizing it and endowing GABA with inhibitory action.

Researchers have termed this the developmental "switch" in chloride homeostasis. This maturational aspect to the chloride ion may influence seizure susceptibility in the neonatal brain. The additional depolarization that is due to $GABA_A$ receptor activation augments excitation that may be initiated by the glutamate neurotransmission. As a result there is a shift in the excitation–inhibition balance towards excessive excitation, and thus towards seizure activity. These conclusions have been suggested by Dzhala *et al.* [124], who described the developmental profile of NKCCl in the human neonate. In the early postnatal period, NKCCl rises to a peak and then declines to adult levels. This rearrangement of membrane receptors occurs over the first several months of life. In the same time period, KCC2 expression gradually rises to adult levels. By blocking NKCCl function with a commonly used diuretic known as bumetanide there is a prevention of the accumulation of intercellular chloride which therefore counteracts the depolarizing action of $GABA_A$ receptor activation. Bumetanide reduces kainic-induced seizures in neonatal but not adult rats, and bursts firing in hippocampus slices. As further evidence, for genetically engineered mice who lack NKCCl, bumetanide is not effective in ameliorating seizures, supporting its role as a specific inhibitor of NKCCl. Therefore, bumetanide is now considered a promising antiepileptic drug with a developmental target, namely the immature chloride co-transporter NKCCl. Some claim that this particular diuretic can be safely used for the neonate, although its long-term safety profile needs to be better studied. It has also been recently suggested that pharmacologic agents that can diminish bursting behavior in neonatal neurons can add an additional level to the control of seizures. Dzhala *et al.* demonstrated that bumetanide rapidly suppresses synchronous bursts of network activity in P4–P8 hippocampus slices in the rat model [124]. This supports the use of this agent as a potential antiepileptic medication in this age group. Clinical trials need to demonstrate that bumetanide or other similar diuretics can inhibit seizure activity, with or without conventional medications such as phenobarbital [125]. One needs to

establish that these agents can reach the brain in appropriate concentrations, and that they lack short- as well as long-term adverse effects.

There are still crucial issues regarding the theory that GABA-mediated excitation may have an important role in human neonatal seizures, amenable to the treatment as discussed above. It is yet unknown why some GABAergic agents such as phenobarbital and benzodiazepine fail to have adequate efficacy for human neonatal seizure control for a substantial subset of patients. Though seizures can be halted in a percentage of newborns, additional understanding of epileptogenesis in the immature brain must consider the timing and etiology-specific aspects of GABA-mediated mechanisms of seizures as it relates to asphyxia, infection, or trauma. A specific etiology may alter seizure threshold by epigenetic modification, changing the specific genetic variability within individuals in a time-sensitive manner. Based on up- or down-regulation of genetic expression, individuals who suffer asphyxia, infection, or trauma may have variable vulnerability or resistance to GABA-mediated mechanisms for seizures. This generalization is further complicated not only by the timing of injury but also by the specific brain region of damage which may have occurred remotely either during the antepartum or during the intrapartum or neonatal periods. Seizures from selectively damaged deep gray matter, neocortical layers, or white-matter regions may respond differently to similar antiepileptic drug regimens. Therefore one must consider the question of whether neonatal seizures represent novel brain injury or are surrogates of injury resulting from etiologies either varied in brain location or during time periods beginning during fetal life [126]. The neurologist must place events leading to seizures in the context of clinical, historical, and laboratory findings to determine both the pathogenesis and the timing of an encephalopathic process in a neonate who is symptomatic with seizures. A new classification of neonatal seizures which integrates electrographic expression, brain region, etiology, and timing may then have more relevance to the choice of antiepileptic medication, both during the neonatal period and later in childhood [127].

Summary

Recognition and classification of seizures remain problematic. The clinician should rely on synchronized video/EEG/polygraphic recordings to correlate suspicious behaviors with electrographic seizures. This monitoring technique will limit misdiagnosis and overtreatment of non-epileptic abnormal behaviors, and define an exact endpoint for cortically propagated seizures. Pathologic non-epileptic behaviors can then be treated in a more appropriate manner. Diagnoses and treatment must be integrated with an appreciation of pathophysiologic mechanisms responsible for brain injury in a variety of anatomical sites during antepartum time periods from maternal–fetal–placental diseases as well as during the intrapartum and neonatal periods.

References

1. Scher MS. Seizures in the neonate: diagnostic and therapeutic considerations. In Spitzer AR, ed., *Intensive Care of the Fetus and Neonate*, 2nd edn. Philadelphia, PA: Saunders, 2004.

2. Scher MS. Neonatal seizures: an expression of fetal or neonatal brain disorders. In Stevenson DK, Benitz WE, Sunshine P, eds., *Fetal and Neonatal Brain Injury*, 3rd edn. Cambridge: Cambridge University Press, 2002: 735–84.

3. Clancy RR. Prolonged electroencephalogram monitoring for seizures and their treatment. *Clin Perinatol* 2006; **33**: 649–65.

4. Proposal for revised clinical and electroencephalographic classification of epileptic seizures. From the Commission on Classification and Terminology of the International League Against Epilepsy. *Epilepsia* 1981; **22**: 489–501.

5. Mizrahi EM, Kellaway P. *Diagnosis and Management of Neonatal Seizures*. Philadelphia, PA: Lippincott-Raven, 1998.

6. Weiner SP, Painter MJ, Geva D, *et al.* Neonatal seizures: electroclinical dissociation. *Pediatr Neurol* 1991; **7**: 363–8.

7. Biagioni E, Ferrari F, Boldrini A, *et al.* Electroclinical correlation in neonatal seizures. *Eur J Paediatr Neurol* 1998; **2**: 117–25.

8. Volpe JJ. Neonatal seizures. In *Neurology of the Newborn*, 4th edn. Philadelphia, PA: Saunders. 2001: 178–214.

9. Scher MS. Electroencephalography of the newborn: normal and abnormal features. In Niedermeyer E, Lopes da Silva F, eds., *Electroencephalography: Basic Principles, Clinical Applications, and Related Fields*, 5th edn. Philadelphia, PA: Lippincott Williams and Wilkins, 2005: 937–89.

10. Scher MS. Normal electrographic-polysomnographic patterns in preterm and fullterm infants. *Semin Pediatr Neurol* 1996; **3**: 2–12.

11. DaSilva O, Guzman GMC, Young GB. The value of standard electroencephalograms in the evaluation of the newborn with recurrent apneas. *J Perinatol* 1998; **18**: 377–80.

12. Fenichel GM, Olson BJ, Fitzpatrick JE. Heart rate changes in convulsive and nonconvulsive neonatal apnea. *Ann Neurol* 1980; **7**: 577–82.

13. Bye AM, Flanagan D. Spatial and temporal characteristics of neonatal seizures. *Epilepsia* 1995; **36**: 1009–16.

14. Boylan GB, Pressler RM, Rennie JM, *et al.* Outcome of electroclinical, electrographic, and clinical seizures in the newborn infant. *Dev Med Child Neurol* 1999; **41**: 819–25.

15. Mizrahi EM, Kellaway P. Characterization and classification of neonatal seizures. *Neurology* 1987; **37**: 1837–44.

16. Scher MS, Klesh KW, Murphy TF, *et al.* Seizures and infarction in neonates with persistent pulmonary hypertension. *Pediatr Neurol* 1986; **2**: 332–9.

17. Clancy R, Malin S, Laraque D, *et al.* Focal motor seizures heralding stroke in full-term neonates. *Am J Dis Child* 1985; **139**: 601–6.

18. Levy SR, Abroms IF, Marshall PC, *et al.* Seizures and cerebral infarction in the full-term newborn. *Ann Neurol* 1985; **17**: 366–70.

19. Holmes G. Diagnosis and management of seizures in childhood. In Markowitz M, ed., *Major Problems in Clinical Pediatrics*. Philadelphia, PA: Saunders, 1987: 237–61.

20. Karayiannis NB, Srinivasan S, Bhattacharya R, *et al.* Extraction of motion strength and motor activity signals from video recordings of neonatal seizures. *IEEE Trans Med Imaging* 2001; **20**: 965–80.

21. Rose AL, Lombroso CT. A study of clinical, pathological, and electroencephalographic features in 137 full-term babies with a long-term follow-up. *Pediatrics* 1970; **45**: 404–25.

22. Kellaway P, Hrachovy RA. Status epilepticus in newborns: a perspective on neonatal seizures. In Delgado-Escueta AV, Wasterlain CG, Treiman DM, *et al.*, eds., *Status Epilepticus: Mechanisms of Brain Damage and Treatment*. New York, NY: Raven Press, 1983: 93–9.

23. Sarnat HB. Anatomic and physiologic correlates of neurologic development in prematurity. In Sarnat HB, ed., *Topics in Neonatal Neurology*. Orlando, FL: Grune and Stratton, 1984: 1–25.

24. Scher MS. Pathologic myoclonus of the newborn: electrographic and clinical correlations. *Pediatr Neurol* 1985; **1**: 342–8.

25. Coulter DL, Allen RJ. Benign neonatal sleep myoclonus. *Arch Neurol* 1982; **39**: 191–2.

26. Resnick TJ, Moshe SL, Perotta L, *et al.* Benign neonatal sleep myoclonus: relationship to sleep states. *Arch Neurol* 1986; **43**: 266–8.

27. Clancy RR. The contribution of EEG to the understanding of neonatal seizures. *Epilepsia* 1996; **37**: S52–9.

28. Shuper A, Zalzberg J, Weitz R, *et al.* Jitteriness beyond the neonatal period: a benign pattern of movement in infancy. *J Child Neurol* 1991; **6**: 243–5.

29. Parker S, Zuckerman B, Bauchner H, *et al.* Jitteriness in full-term neonates: prevalence and correlates. *Pediatrics* 1990; **85**: 17–23.

30. Hakamada S, Watanabe K, Hara K, *et al.* Development of the motor behavior during sleep in newborn infants. *Brain Dev* 1981; **3**: 345–50.

31. Scher MS, Belfar H, Martin J, *et al.* Destructive brain lesions of presumed fetal onset: antepartum causes of cerebral palsy. *Pediatrics* 1991; **88**: 898–906.

32. Sexson WR, Thigpen J, Stajich GV. Stereotypic movements after lorazepam administration in premature neonates: a series and review of the literature. *J Perinatol* 1995; **15**: 146–51.

33. Brown P, Rothwell JC, Thompson PD, *et al.* The hyperekplexias and their relationship to the normal startle reflex. *Brain* 1991; **114**: 1903–28.

34. Andermann F, Andermann E. Startle disorders of man: hyperekplexia, jumping and startle epilepsy. *Brain Dev* 1988; **10**: 213–22.

35. Barth PJ. Inherited progressive disorders of the fetal brain: a field in need of recognition. In Fukuyama Y, Suzuki Y, Kamoshia S, *et al.*, eds., *Fetal and Perinatal Neurology*. New York, NY: Karger, 1992: 299–313.

36. Lyon G, Adams RD, Kolodny EH. Hypoglycemia. In *Neurology of Hereditary Metabolic Diseases of Children*, 2nd edn. New York, NY: McGraw-Hill, 1996: 6–44.

37. Scher MS. Seizures in the newborn infant: diagnosis, treatment, and outcome. *Clin Perinatol* 1997; **24**: 735–72.

38. Oliveira AJ, Nunes ML, da Costa JC. Polysomnography in neonatal seizures. *Clin Neurophysiol* 2000; **111**: S74–80.

39. Watanabe K, Kuroyanagi M, Hara K, *et al.* Neonatal seizures and subsequent epilepsy. *Brain Dev* 1982; **4**: 341–6.

40. Hrachovy R, Mizrahi E, Kellaway P. Electroencephalography of the newborn.

In Daly D, Pedley T, eds., *Current Practice of Clinical Electroencephalography*, 2nd edn. New York, NY: Raven Press, 1990: 201–42.

41. Stockard-Pope JE, Werner SS, Bickford RG. *Atlas of Neonatal Electroencephalography*, 2nd edn. New York, NY: Raven Press, 1992.

42. Lombroso CT. Neonatal polygraphy in full-term and premature infants: a review of normal and abnormal findings. *J Clin Neurophysiol* 1985; **2**: 105–55.

43. Hellstrom-Westas L. Comparison between tape-recorded and amplitude-integrated EEG monitoring in sick newborn infants. *Acta Paediatr* 1992; **81**: 812–9.

44. Klebermass K, Kuhle S, Kohlhauser-Vollmuth C, *et al.* Evaluation of the Cerebral Function Monitor as a tool for neurophysiological surveillance in neonatal intensive care patients. *Childs Nerv Syst* 2001; **17**: 544–50.

45. Alfonso I, Jayakar P, Yelin K, *et al.* Continuous-display four-channel electroencephalographic monitoring in the evaluation of neonates with paroxysmal motor events. *J Child Neurol* 2001; **16**: 625–8.

46. Scher MS, Hamid MY, Steppe DA, *et al.* Ictal and interictal electrographic seizure durations in preterm and term neonates. *Epilepsia* 1993; **34**: 284–8.

47. Clancy RR, Legido A. The exact ictal and interictal duration of electroencephalographic neonatal seizures. *Epilepsia* 1987; **28**: 537–41.

48. Sheth RD. Electroencephalogram confirmatory rate in neonatal seizures. *Pediatr Neurol* 1999; **20**: 27–30.

49. Painter MJ, Scher MS, Stein AD, *et al.* Phenobarbital compared with phenytoin for the treatment of neonatal seizures. *N Engl J Med* 1999; **341**: 485–9.

50. Scher MS, Steppe DA, Beggarly M. Timing of neonatal seizures and intrapartum obstetrical factors. *J Child Neurol* 2008; **23**: 640–3.

51. Scher MS, Alvin J, Gaus L, *et al.* Uncoupling of EEG-clinical neonatal seizures after antiepileptic drug use. *Pediatr Neurol* 2003; **28**: 277–80.

52. Veliskova J, Miller AM, Lunes, ML, *et al.* Regional neural activity within the substantia nigra during peri-ictal flurothyl generalized seizure stages. *Neurobiol Dis* 2005; **20**: 752–9.

53. Merrill MA, Clough RW, Dailey JW, *et al.* Localization of the serotonergic terminal fields modulating seizures in the genetically epilepsy-prone rat. *Epilepsy Res* 2007; **76**: 93–102.

54. Alfonso I, Papazian O, Litt R, *et al.* Single photon emission computed tomographic evaluation of brainstem release phenomenon and seizure in neonates. *J Child Neurol* 2000; **15**: 56–8.

55. Kilic S, Tarim O, Eralp O. Serum prolactin in neonatal seizures. *Pediatr Int* 1999; **41**: 61–4.

56. Browning RA. Role of the brain-stem reticular formation in tonic-clonic seizures: lesion and pharmacological studies. *Fed Proc* 1985; **44**: 2425–31.

57. Caveness WF, Kato M, Malamut BL, *et al.* Propagation of focal motor seizures in the pubescent monkey. *Ann Neurol* 1980; **7**: 213–21, 232–5.

58. Hosokawa S, Iguchi T, Caveness WF, *et al.* Effects of manipulation of the sensorimotor system on focal motor seizures in the monkey. *Ann Neurol* 1980; **7**: 222–9, 236–7.

59. Danner R, Shewmon DA, Sherman MP. Seizures in an atelencephalic infant: is the cortex essential for neonatal seizures? *Arch Neurol* 1985; **42**: 1014–16.

60. Subcortical Control of Cortical Excitability, Plenary Session. American Epilepsy Society Meeting, Philadelphia, PA, December, 2005.

61. Scher MS, Aso K, Beggarly ME, *et al.* Electrographic seizures in preterm and full-term neonates: clinical correlates, associated brain lesions, and risk for neurologic sequelae. *Pediatrics* 1993; **91**: 128–34.

62. Coen RW, McCutchen CB, Wermer D, *et al.* Continuous monitoring of the electroencephalogram following perinatal asphyxia. *J Pediatr* 1982; **100**: 628–30.

63. O'Meara MW, Bye AM, Flanagan D. Clinical features of neonatal seizures. *J Paediatr Child Health* 1995; **31**: 237–40.

64. Staudt F, Roth JG, Engel RC. The usefulness of electroencephalography in curarized newborns. *Electroencephalogr Clin Neurophysiol* 1981; **51**: 205–8.

65. Eyre JA, Oozeer RC, Wilkinson AR. Continuous electroencephalographic recording to detect seizures in paralyzed newborn babies. *Br Med J* 1983; **286**: 1017–18.

66. Goldberg RN, Goldman SL, Ramsay RE, *et al.* Detection of seizure activity in the paralyzed neonate using continuous monitoring. *Pediatrics* 1982; **69**: 583–6.

67. Ronen GM, Penney S, Andrews W. The epidemiology of clinical neonatal seizures in Newfoundland: a population-based study. *J Pediatr* 1999; **134**: 71–5.

68. Eriksson M, Zetterstrom R. Neonatal convulsions: incidence and causes in the Stockholm area. *Acta Paediatr Scand* 1979; **68**: 807–11.

69. Seay AR, Bray PF. Significance of seizures in infants weighing less than 2,500 grams. *Arch Neurol* 1977; **34**: 381–2.

70. Saliba RM, Annegers FJ, Waller DK, *et al.* Risk factors for neonatal seizures: a population-based study, Harris County, Texas, 1992–1994. *Am J Epidemiol* 2001; **154**: 14–20.

71. Lanska MJ, Lanska DJ, Baumann RJ, *et al.* Interobserver variability in the classification of neonatal seizures based on medical record data. *Pediatr Neurol* 1996; **15**: 120–3.

72. Lanska MJ, Lanska DJ, Baumann RJ, *et al.* A population-based study of neonatal seizures in Fayette County, Kentucky. *Neurology* 1995; **45**: 724–32.

73. Patterson CA, Graves WL, Bugg G, *et al.* Antenatal and intrapartum factors associated with the occurrence of seizures in the term infant. *Obstet Gynecol* 1989; **74**: 361–5.

74. Bergman I, Painter MJ, Hirsh RP, *et al.* Outcome in neonates with convulsions treated in an intensive care unit. *Ann Neurol* 1983; **14**: 642–7.

75. Evard P, Kadhim HJ, de Saint-George P, *et al.* Abnormal development and destructive processes of the human brain during the second half of gestation. In Evans P, Minkowski A, eds., *Developmental Neurobiology*. New York, NY: Raven Press, 1989: 21–39.

76. Lieberman E, Eichenwald E, Mathur G, *et al.* Intrapartum fever and unexplained seizures in term infants. *Pediatrics* 2000; **106**: 983–8.

77. Scher MS. Fetal neurologic consultations. *Pediatr Neurol* 2003; **29**: 193–202.

78. American College of Obstetricians and Gynecologists and American Academy of Pediatrics. *Neonatal Encephalopathy in Cerebral Palsy: Defining the Pathogenesis and Pathophysiology.* Washington, DC: ACOG, 2003.

79. Parent JM. The role of seizure-induced neurogenesis in epileptogenesis and brain repair. *Epilepsy Res* 2002; **50**: 179–89.

80. Swann JW. The effects of seizures on the connectivity and circuitry of the developing brain. *Ment*

Retard Dev Disabil Res Rev 2004;
10: 96–100.

81. Eriksson SH, Malmgren K, Nordborg C. Microdysgenesis in epilepsy. *Acta Neurol Scand* 2005; **111**: 279–90.

82. Squier M, Keeling JW. The incidence of prenatal brain injury. *Neuropathol Appl Neurobiol* 1991; **17**: 29–38.

83. Scher MS. Neonatal seizure classification: a fetal perspective concerning childhood epilepsy. *Epilepsy Res* 2006; **70**: S41–57.

84. Scher MS, Trucco J, Beggarly ME, *et al.* Neonates with electrically confirmed seizures and possible placental associations. *Pediatr Neurol* 1998; **19**: 37–41.

85. Friede RL. Porencephaly, hydranencephaly, multilocular cystic encephalopathy. In *Developmental Neuropathology*. New York, NY: Springer-Verlag, 1975: 102–13.

86. Miller V. Neonatal cerebral infarction. *Semin Pediatr Neurol* 2001; **7**: 278–88.

87. de Vries LS, Groenendaal F, Eken P, *et al.* Infarcts in the vascular distribution of the middle cerebral artery in preterm and fullterm infants. *Neuropediatrics* 1997; **28**: 88–96.

88. Baergen RN. The placenta as witness. *Clin Perinatol* 2007; **34**: 393–407.

89. Leth H, Toft PB, Herning M, *et al.* Neonatal seizures associated with cerebral lesions shown by magnetic resonance imaging. *Arch Dis Child Fetal Neonatal Ed* 1997; **77**: F105–10.

90. Rutherford M, Ward P, Allsop J, *et al.* Magnetic resonance imaging in neonatal encephalopathy. *Early Hum Dev* 2004; **81**: 13–25.

91. Enns GM. Inborn errors of metabolism masquerading as hypoxic–ischemic encephalopathy. *NeoReviews* 2005; **6**: e549–58.

92. Scher MS, Painter MJ. Controversies concerning neonatal seizures. *Pediatr Clin North Am* 1989; **36**: 281–310.

93. Clancy RR, Legido A. Postnatal epilepsy after EEG-confirmed neonatal seizures. *Epilepsia* 1991; **32**: 69–76.

94. Temple CM, Dennis J, Carney R, *et al.* Neonatal seizures: long-term outcome and cognitive development among "normal" survivors. *Dev Med Child Neurol* 1995; **37**: 109–18.

95. Holmes GL, Ben-Ari Y. The neurobiology and consequences of epilepsy in the developing brain. *Pediatr Res* 2001; **49**: 320–5.

96. Monod N, Pajot N, Guidasci S. The neonatal EEG: statistical studies and prognostic value in full-term and preterm babies. *Electroencephalogr Clin Neurophysiol* 1972; **32**: 529–44.

97. Tharp BR, Cukier F, Monod N. The prognostic value of the electroencephalogram in premature infants. *Electroencephalogr Clin Neurophysiol* 1981; **51**: 219.

98. McBride M, Laroia N, Guillet R. Electrographic seizures in neonates correlate with poor neurodevelopmental outcome. *Neurology* 2002; **55**: 506–13.

99. Hellström-Westas L. Comparison between tape-recorded and amplitude-integrated EEG monitoring in sick newborn infants. *Acta Paediatr* 1992; **81**: 812–19.

100. Watanabe K, Kuroyanagi M, Hara K, *et al.* Neonatal seizures and subsequent epilepsy. *Brain Dev* 1982; **4**: 341–6.

101. Holden KR, Mellits ED, Freeman JM. Neonatal seizures. I: Correlation of prenatal and perinatal events with outcomes. *Pediatrics* 1982; **70**: 165–76.

102. Scher MS, Aso K, Beggarley ME, *et al.* Electrographic seizures in preterm and full-term neonates: clinical correlates, associated brain lesions, and risk for neurological sequelae. *Pediatrics* 1993; **91**: 128–34.

103. Carmo KB, Barr P. Drug treatment of neonatal seizures by neonatologists and pediatric neurologists. *J Paediatr Child Health* 2005; **41**: 313–16.

104. Sankar R, Painter MJ. Neonatal seizures: after all these years we still love what doesn't work. *Neurology* 2005; **64**: 776–7.

105. Lockman LA, Kriel R, Zaske D, *et al.* Phenobarbital dosage for control of neonatal seizures. *Neurology* 1979; **29**: 1445–9.

106. Painter MJ, Pippenger C, MacDonald H, *et al.* Phenobarbital and diphenylhydantoin levels in neonates with seizures. *J Pediatr* 1978; **92**: 315–19.

107. Painter MJ, Pippenger C, Wasterlain C, *et al.* Phenobarbital and phenytoin in neonatal seizures: metabolism and tissue distribution. *Neurology* 1981; **31**: 1107–12.

108. Smith BT, Masotti RE. Intravenous diazepam in the treatment of prolonged seizure activity in neonates and infants. *Dev Med Child Neurol* 1971; **13**: 630–4.

109. Malingre MM, Van Rooij LG, Rademaker CM, *et al.* Development of an optimal lidocaine infusion strategy for neonatal seizures. *Eur J Pediatr* 2006; **165**: 598–604.

110. Gal P, Toback J, Boer HR, *et al.* Efficacy of phenobarbital monotherapy in treatment of neonatal seizures – relationship to blood levels. *Neurology* 1982; **32**: 1401–4.

111. Hall RT, Hall FK, Daily DK. High-dose phenobarbital therapy in term newborn infants with severe perinatal asphyxia: a randomized, prospective study with three-year follow-up. *J Pediatr* 1998; **132**: 345–8.

112. Painter MJ, Minnigh B, Mollica L, *et al.* Binding profiles of anticonvulsants in neonates with seizures. *Ann Neurol* 1987; **22**: 413.

113. Montenegro MA, Guerreiro MM, Caldas JP, *et al.* Epileptic manifestations induced by midazolam in the neonatal period. *Arq Neuropsiquiatr* 2001; **59**: 242–3.

114. Camfield PR, Camfield CS. Neonatal seizures: a commentary on selected aspects. *J Child Neurol* 1987; **2**: 244–51.

115. Hellstrom-Westas L, Blennow G, Lindroth M, *et al.* Low risk of seizure recurrence after early withdrawal of antiepileptic treatment in the neonatal period. *Arch Dis Child Fetal Neonatal Ed* 1995; **72**: F97–101.

116. Mizrahi EM. Acute and chronic effects of seizures in the developing brain: lessons from clinical experience. *Epilepsia* 1999; **40**: S42–50, S64–6.

117. Sanchez RM, Jensen FE. Maturational aspects of epilepsy mechanisms and consequences for the immature brain. *Epilepsia* 2001; **42**: 577–85.

118. Koh S, Jensen FE. Topiramate blocks perinatal hypoxia-induced seizures in rat pups. *Ann Neurol* 2001; **50**: 366–72.

119. Jensen FE, Wang C. Hypoxia-induced hyperexcitability in vivo and in vitro in the immature hippocampus. *Epilepsy Res* 1996; **26**: 131–40.

120. Aronica EM, Gorter JA, Paupard MC, *et al.* Status epilepticus-induced alterations in metabotropic glutamate receptor expression in young and adult rats. *J Neurosci* 1997; **17**: 8588–95.

121. Lie AA, Becker A, Behle K, *et al.* Up-regulation of the metabotropic

glutamate receptor mGluR4 in hippocampal neurons with reduced seizure vulnerability. *Ann Neurol* 2000; **47**: 26–35.

122. Brooks-Kayal AR. Rearranging receptors. *Epilepsia* 2005; **46**: 29–38.

123. Staley KJ. Wrong-way chloride transport: is it a treatable cause of some intractable seizures? *Epilepsy Curr* 2006; **6**: 124–7.

124. Dzhala VI, Talos DM, Sdrulla DA, *et al.* NKCC1 transporter facilitates seizures in the developing brain. *Nat Med* 2005; **11**: 1205–13.

125. Haglund MM, Hochman DW. Furosemide and mannitol suppression of epileptic activity in the human brain. *J Neurophysiol* 2005; **94**: 907–18.

126. Scher MS. Neonatal seizures and brain damage. *Pediatr Neurol* 2003; **29**: 381–90.

127. Scher MS. Neonatal seizure classification: a fetal perspective concerning childhood epilepsy. *Epilepsy Res* 2006; **70**: S41–57.

Chapter 44

Nutritional support of the asphyxiated infant

John A. Kerner

Routine nutritional support of the premature infant

Optimal nutritional support is critical in helping to obtain a successful outcome for the ever-increasing number of surviving small premature infants [1]. Although it is paramount to insure that the infant receives an adequate caloric intake, the ability of the very-low-birthweight (VLBW) infant to digest, absorb, and metabolize enteral nutrients is limited. In addition, complications of prematurity, such as respiratory distress, cardiovascular instability, hemorrhagic diatheses, and an immature renal system, create a challenge to the provision of proper nutritional support.

To provide nutrition to the premature infant appropriately, one must have an understanding of the biochemical and physiologic processes that occur during the development of the gastrointestinal tract. By 28 weeks of gestation the anatomic development of the gastrointestinal tract in humans is nearly complete. Yet, as an organ of nutrition, the gut is functionally immature. Details of gastrointestinal tract development have been described previously [2–4], and are summarized in Table 44.1. Further, complications due to the incomplete development of the gastrointestinal tract in the low-birthweight infant have been well delineated by Sunshine (Table 44.2).

Enteral feeding

Gastric feeding: intermittent gavage or continuous infusion

Nasogastric (NG) feeds may be given continuously or intermittently. Intermittent feeding, also known as gavage feeding, is easy to administer, and it is possible to evaluate the gastric emptying time by checking the gastric residual before each meal. The stomach takes less time to empty with human milk than with formula, and when in the prone or lateral position [5–6].

Premature infants are predisposed to develop gastroesophageal (GE) reflux because of their incompetent lower esophageal sphincter, small stomach capacity, and delayed gastric emptying. Hence, to prevent this GE reflux and subsequent risk of aspiration and apnea, it is necessary to feed these infants smaller volumes on a more frequent basis [7]. Also,

gastric distension may interfere with respiratory function [8]. For these reasons premature infants may benefit from continuous NG feeds.

Toce *et al.* demonstrated that infants whose birthweight was between 1000 and 1249 g had better weight gain when fed via continuous NG infusion rather than via gavage feeds [9]. A reduction in stool weight was also reported. Both observations were presumed to be secondary to less stimulation of the gastrocolic reflex, with a resulting longer transit time, allowing for better absorption.

Continuous feeding is not without disadvantages. Nutrients, especially fat, may be lost within the tubing during continuous infusion of breast milk [10]. Preterm formulas with a high mineral content may precipitate and clog the tubing [11]. Further, intermittent feeding may be important in the induction of metabolic and endocrine changes which occur in early postnatal life [12].

Transpyloric feeding

Transpyloric feeding is defined as instilling the nutrients directly into the small intestine. The advantages of this method are minimal gastric distension, lower risk of aspiration, and, at least during the first 10 days of life, potentially greater volume tolerance with less initial weight loss than with NG feeding [13]. Two prospective studies compared continuous NG and transpyloric feeding [14,15], but only one [14] concluded there was an advantage to transpyloric feeding during the first 2–3 weeks of life. Roy *et al.* compared every-2-hour bolus NG feeds versus nasojejunal (NJ) feeds in healthy low-birthweight infants and found no difference in growth or weight gain in the two groups [16]. Since the stomach was bypassed in the NJ group and fat digestion starts in the stomach, more fat malabsorption occurred in the NJ-fed babies. The fat malabsorption may be minimized by duodenal placement of the feeding tube [14].

Further, in two studies, transpyloric feeding was not recommended in infants requiring either ventilatory support via a face mask or nasopharyngeal suctioning [17,18], because of the risk of dislodgement and subsequent aspiration. Lucas evaluated seven randomized trials comparing transpyloric (nasoduodenal or NJ) with intragastric feeding [19]. None of the trials was large or conclusive, but collectively they argue against transpyloric feeding. Lucas stated, "There is no convincing evidence that transpyloric feeding improves

Fetal and Neonatal Brain Injury, 4th edition, ed. David K. Stevenson, William E. Benitz, Philip Sunshine, Susan R. Hintz, and Maurice L. Druzin. Published by Cambridge University Press. © Cambridge University Press 2009.

Table 44.1. Development of the human gastrointestinal tract

Age (weeks)	Crown–rump length (mm)	Stage of development
2.5	1.5	Gut not distinct from yolk sac
3.5	2.5	Foregut and hindgut present
		Yolk sac broadly attached at midgut
		Liver bud present
		Mesenteries forming
4	5.0	Intestine present as a single tube from mouth to cloaca
		Esophagus and stomach distinct
		Liver cords, ducts, and gallbladder forming
		Omental bursa forming
		Pancreatic buds appear as outpouching of gut
5.6	8.0–12.0	Intestine elongates into a loop and duodenum begins to rotate under superior mesenteric artery
		Stomach rotates
		Parotid and submandibular buds appear
		Cloaca elongates and septum forms to divide cloaca
7	17.0	Circular muscle layer present
		Duodenum temporarily occluded
		Intestinal loops herniated into cord
		Villi begin to develop
		Pancreatic anlagen fuse
8	23	Villi lined by single layer of cells
		Small intestine coiling within cord
		Taste buds appear
		Microvilli short, thick, and irregularly spaced
		Lysosomal enzymes detected
		Cloacal membrane which sealed the rectum begins to disappear
9–10	30–40	Auerbach's plexus appears
		Intestine re-enters abdominal cavity
		Crypts of Lieberkühn develop
		Active transport of glucose appears aerobically and anaerobically
		Dipeptidases present
		Microvilli of enterocytes more regular and glycocalyx present
		Mitochondria numerous below microvilli
12	56	Parietal cells present in stomach
		Muscular layers of intestine present
		Alkaline phosphatase and disaccharidases detectable
		Active transport of amino acids present
		Mature taste buds present
		Enterochromaffin cells appear
		Pancreatic islet cells appear
		Bile secretions begin
		Colonic haustra appear
		Coelomic extension into umbilical cord obliterated
		Meconium first detected in ileum
13–14	78–90	Meissner's plexus appears
		Circular folds appear
		Peristalsis detected
		Lysosomes detected ultrastructurally
16	112	Pancreatic lipase and tryptic activity detected
		Lymphopoiesis present
		Peptic activity present
		Swallowing evident – 2–7 mL/24 h
20	160	Peyer's patches present
		Muscularis mucosa present
		Mesenteric attachments complete
		Zymogen granules present and well developed in pancreas (22 weeks)
		Intestine has lost ability to transport glucose anaerobically
24	200	Paneth's cells appear
		Maltase and sucrase and alkaline phosphatase very active
		Ganglion cells detected throughout small and large intestine and in the rectum
		Amylase activity present in intestine
28	240	Enterokinase activity increases
		Esophageal glands present
		Frequency and intensity of duodenal peristaltic contractions increasing
32	270	Lactase activity increases
		Hydrochloric acid found in stomach
34	290–300	Sucking and swallowing become coordinated
		Esophageal peristalsis rapid, non-segmental contraction occurs
		Small intestinal motility becomes coordinated
36–38	320–350	Maturity of gastrointestinal tract achieved

Source: Reproduced with permission from Sunshine [53].

Table 44.2. Complications due to the incomplete development of the gastrointestinal tract in the low-birthweight infant

Incomplete development of motility
  Poor coordination of sucking and swallowing
  Aberrant esophageal motility
  Biphasic esophageal peristalsis
  Decreased or absent lower esophageal sphincter pressure
  Delayed gastric emptying time
  Poorly coordinated motility of the small and large intestine
    Stasis
    Dilation
    Impaired blood supply
    Functional obstruction
Delayed ability to regenerate new epithelial cells
  Decreased rates of proliferation
  Decreased cellular migration rates
  Shallow crypts
  Shortened villi
  Decreased mitotic indices
Inadequate host resistance factors
  Decreased gastric acidity
Decreased concentrations of immunoglobulins in lamina propria and intestinal secretions
  Impaired humoral and cellular response to infection
Inadequate digestion of nutrients
  Decreased digestion of protein
    Decreased activity of enterokinase
    Trypsin activity low prior to 28 weeks
    Decreased concentration of gastric hydrochloric acid and pepsinogen
  Decreased digestion of carbohydrates
    Decreased hydrolysis of lactose
    Decreased ability to transport glucose actively
    Decreased activity of pancreatic amylase
  Decreased digestion of lipids
    Decreased production and reabsorption of bile acids
    Decreased activity of pancreatic lipase
Increased incidence of other problems that may indirectly lead to poor gastrointestinal function
  Hyaline membrane disease
  Intraventricular hemorrhage
  Patent ductus arteriosus
  Hypoxemic–ischemic states

Source: Reproduced with permission from Sunshine [53].

enteral feed tolerance and growth, or reduces aspiration pneumonia" [19].

Polyvinyl chloride tubes were used initially, as they are relatively stiff and easily positioned. However, if left in the duodenum for several days, they harden and may perforate the intestine [20]. Silastic tubes are now commonly used, but they are more flexible and hence difficult to position. They are usually weighted at the tip and placed with the help of gravity. Being more flexible, they can curl back into the stomach. Perforation even with the Silastic tubes has been reported [21].

A change in the microbial flora of the upper intestine of infants fed via transpyloric feeds has been reported. The upper intestine of the normal infant is sterile or contains sparse Gram-positive flora. However, Dellagrammaticus *et al.* have shown that the presence of a tube facilitates colonization with "fecal-type" flora, in which *Streptococcus faecalis* and Gram-negative bacteria predominate [22]. Theoretically, a heavy resident flora of the upper intestine could lead to poorer assimilation of feeds. Conflicting data exist on the relationship of necrotizing enterocolitis (NEC) to transpyloric feeds [17,23]. As detailed later in this chapter, it is not the route of feeding that was responsible in the above studies for the NEC, but rather the increased osmolality of the formula used. In controlled studies, NEC was proven not to be more frequent during transpyloric feeds compared to NG feeds [14,17,24].

The European Society of Paediatric Gastroenterology and Nutrition (ESPGN) issued guidelines for feeding the preterm infant [13].

ESPGN guidelines

Enteral feeding should be introduced as soon as it is safe to do so.

(1) Intermittent gastric tube feeding seems more physiological than transpyloric feeding, and whenever possible should be preferred.

(2) When there are feeding difficulties such as regurgitation, poor gastric emptying, or gastric distension, continuous gastric feeding or even transpyloric feeding may be necessary, as they are useful alternatives either to reduced oral feeding or total parenteral nutrition.

(3) The success of any feeding technique is at least partly the result of the skill of the staff of the unit in following their own practiced routines.

(4) Nursery routines should encourage the mother to play an active role in feeding. This will help her to become confident in the care of her baby [13].

Schanler and colleagues, in an elegant randomized trial in 171 premature infants, showed that bolus tube feeding was associated with significantly less feeding intolerance and greater rate of weight gain than the continuous feeding method [25]. More importantly, his group demonstrated the benefit of early gastrointestinal priming [25].

Gastrointestinal priming is a practice with sound scientific rationale. Also known as "minimal feedings," "gut stimulation," "trophic feedings," or "hypocaloric feedings," this practice attempts to enable the premature infant's intestine to adapt to later advancement of full enteral feedings while preventing the known mucosal atrophy and unphysiologic gut hormone status noted in animals and humans kept NPO [26–28]. Schanler *et al.* were congratulated by Kliegman [29] for their large randomized controlled trial that confirmed the overall safety of gastrointestinal priming (no increased incidence of NEC) while clearly demonstrating the positive effects of this novel feeding practice – better calcium and phosphorus retention, improved feeding tolerance, reduced risk of physiologic jaundice, cholestasis, metabolic bone disease, and glucose intolerance [25]. Kliegman went on to state that "gastrointestinal priming must now become the standard of care for very low birthweight infants" [29]. In Schanler's study the gastrointestinal priming group (prime continuous, prime bolus) received 20 mL/kg per day of milk (either formula or breast milk) from day 4 through day 14 [25].

Early feeding of the preterm infant has been shown to decrease intestinal permeability [30] and increase lactase activity [31]. Trophic feeding has been shown to:

(1) shorten time to regain birthweight
(2) improve feeding tolerance
(3) reduce the duration of phototherapy
(4) reduce duration of parenteral nutrition
(5) lower the incidence of cholestasis
(6) reduce metabolic bone disease
(7) improve gastrointestinal maturation, motility, and hormone responses
(8) improve mineral absorption
(9) enhance enzyme maturation
(10) reduce intestinal permeability
(11) be safe (the practice does not increase the incidence of NEC) [32]

Parenteral feeding

Since sick and premature newborns are often not fed enterally, the alternative is parenteral nutrition (PN). In a review by Moyer-Mileur and Chan, parenteral feeds in VLBW infants requiring assisted ventilation for more than 6 days led to a decrease in the percentage of weight loss from birthweight and a shorter time required for recovery of birthweight than in those fed enterally or by a combination of enteral and parenteral feeds [33]. A delay in enteral feeds increased the tolerance to subsequent enteral feeds in the infants. Tolerance was defined as absence of residuals, abdominal distension, or guaiac-positive, reducing substance-positive stools [33]. Another retrospective study presented inconclusive data regarding the benefits and risks of PN [34].

Limited data exist on the potential benefit of PN in the treatment of preterm infants. A controlled study of peripheral total parenteral nutrition (TPN) composed of casein hydrolysate, dextrose, and soybean emulsion in 40 premature infants with respiratory distress syndrome (RDS) showed that TPN neither favorably altered the clinical course of the syndrome nor worsened an infant's pulmonary status [35]. Among infants weighing less than 1500 g, those who received TPN had a greater survival rate when compared with a control group (71% vs. 37%).

Yu and coworkers performed a controlled trial of TPN on 34 preterm infants with birthweights of less than 1200 g [36].

Infants in the TPN group had a greater mean daily weight gain in the second week of life and regained birthweight sooner than did control infants. Four in the milk-fed control group developed NEC whereas none did in the TPN group. The results of a more recent study conducted by Kerner et al. [37] of 40 infants who weighed less than 1500 g at birth were in agreement with the two mentioned controlled studies [35,36]. No increased risk in using peripheral PN as compared with conventional feeding techniques was found. Also, comparable growth was reported in the two groups.

Fifty-nine infants weighing less than 1500 g were randomly assigned either to a PN regimen via central catheter or to a transpyloric feeding regimen (mother's milk or SMA Gold Cap (Wyeth Laboratories, Philadelphia, USA)) via a Silastic nasoduodenal tube [38]. The authors postulated that some of the problems of enteral feeding in VLBW infants might be overcome if enteral nutrients were delivered beyond the pylorus [39]. The PN group had a higher incidence of bacterial sepsis. Conjugated hyperbilirubinemia occurred only in the PN group. In spite of the observations that 34% (10 of 29) of the infants in the transpyloric group failed to establish full enteral feeding patterns by the end of the first week of life, and therefore had achieved lower protein-energy intake than the PN group, no beneficial effect on growth or mortality was found in the PN group.

The authors concluded that "Parenteral nutrition does not confer any appreciable benefit and because of greater complexity and higher risk of complications should be reserved for those infants in whom enteral nutrition is impossible" [38]. Zlotkin and coworkers disagreed with this conclusion: "Had peripheral-vein feeding been used rather than central venous alimentation, or had nasogastric gavage feeding been used in preference to transpyloric feeding, the morbidity and mortality would have declined and the results comparing TPN with enteral feeds would have been quite different" [40].

A study that remains a model for nutritional support in the VLBW infant was performed by Cashore and associates [41]. They described 23 infants who weighed less than 1500 g in whom peripheral PN was begun on day 2 of life to supplement enteral feedings, thus allowing for adequate nutrition while avoiding overtaxing the immature gastrointestinal tract. These infants regained their birthweight by the age of 8–12 days and achieved growth rates that approximated intrauterine rates of growth. Interestingly, infants weighing less than 1000 g were still not taking all their nutrients enterally by 25 days of age.

Premature infants, especially those who have RDS and are incapable of full oral feeds, often receive PN because of their extremely limited substrate reserve, very rapid growth rate, and perceived susceptibility to irreversible brain damage secondary to malnutrition [40]. A survey of 269 neonatal intensive care units showed that TPN was used exclusively during the first week of life in 80% of infants weighing 1000 g or less at birth [42]. The others received a combination of parenteral and enteral feedings in the first week. Adamkin began PN by 72 hours of age in neonates with a birthweight of less than 1000 g in whom respiratory disease and intestinal hypomotility limited the safety of feedings in the first 1–2 weeks of life [43].

In some nurseries umbilical arterial catheters are used for infusing PN. Few studies exist regarding the safety of this practice. Yu *et al.* studied 34 infants with birthweight < 1200 g and randomly assigned them to TPN via umbilical arterial catheters or enteral feeds [36]. The TPN group had better nitrogen balance, weight gain, less NEC, and unchanged mortality compared with the enterally fed group. No data on catheter-related complications were presented, although bacterial or fungal septicemia did not occur in either group in the study period [36]. Higgs and coworkers described a controlled trial of TPN versus formula feeding by continuous NG drip [44]. The study included 86 infants weighing 500–1500 g. The TPN, including glucose, amino acids, and fat emulsion, was administered by umbilical artery catheter for the first 2 weeks of life. There was no difference in neonatal morbidity or mortality between the two groups. Specifically, there was no difference in septicemia, although four of the 43 TPN babies had "catheter problems," described in the text only as "blockage" of the catheter.

As in the study of Higgs *et al.*, Hall and Rhodes found that morbidity, mortality, and common complications, such as infection and thrombosis, were similar in infants receiving umbilical lines for TPN compared to infants receiving tunneled jugular catheters for TPN [45]. They concluded that TPN by indwelling umbilical catheters presents no greater risk than infusion through tunneled jugular catheters. However, careful analysis of the authors' data raises questions about their conclusions. According to the authors, "Six deaths may have been catheter-related" [45]. Five of those deaths occurred in the umbilical artery catheter group; death resulted from thrombosis of the aorta in one patient, candidal septicemia in two, streptococcal septicemia in one, and enterococcal septicemia in one. One death occurred in the jugular venous catheter group, with right atrial thrombosis, superior vena cava syndrome, and *Staphylococcus epidermidis* on blood culture.

Merritt cautions against the use of umbilical arterial catheters for TPN, as this practice is associated with a high incidence of arterial thrombosis [46]. Coran, a pediatric surgeon, strongly recommends that PN not be given through either umbilical arteries or umbilical veins [47]. PN through umbilical veins causes phlebitis, which may lead to venous thrombosis and portal hypertension. He is especially concerned about infusing PN solutions into an umbilical arterial line, since this practice can lead to thrombosis of the aorta or iliac vessels. Severe damage, such as thrombosis of the aorta, may occur to an artery without being recognized. Only over a period of time will the side effects of umbilical arterial catheter use, such as inappropriate growth of one limb [47], become clinically evident. Even the use of 12.5% dextrose infused through an umbilical arterial line has increased osmolality that has been shown to cause thrombophlebitis [47]. Although the first three studies described earlier all claimed there were no short-term complications, they did not address the problem of long-term complications [48].

Coran stated that if PN is required and peripheral veins are not usable, or if peripheral vein delivery is inadequate to provide necessary calories, he would consider percutaneous subclavian vein catheterization, which he could perform successfully even in a 900 g infant [47]. In a study by Sadig, 52 Broviac catheters were inserted in 40 preterm and 8 term infants [49]. Sixty-nine percent of VLBW infants, and 20% of those weighing more than 1500 g, experienced catheter-associated infections. Seventy-eight percent (14/18) of these infections were successfully treated with antibiotics without catheter removal. The rate of thrombosis was also higher in VLBW infants. A retrospective review compared TPN via umbilical catheters in 48 neonates (birthweight 1.7 ± 0.58 kg) versus administration via central venous catheters in 26 infants (birthweight 2.05 ± 0.89 kg) [50]. There was no difference in infection rate between the two groups when adjustment was made for the number of days of catheter life. Transient hypertension occurred in two (4%) of the umbilical arterial catheter group and in one (3.8%) of the central catheter group. There was one aortic thrombus noted on autopsy in the umbilical arterial catheter group. There was one vegetation on the tricuspid valve in the central catheter group. They concluded that umbilical arterial catheters are a reasonable route for PN solutions.

As nurseries become more comfortable with percutaneous central lines [51,52], hopefully umbilical arterial catheters will be used less frequently to provide nutrition.

Nutritional support of the asphyxiated infant

Asphyxia may cause significant injury to the gastrointestinal tract. This injury may predispose an infant to develop NEC. During acute episodes of shock or hypoxemia the "vital structures," which include the heart, brain, and adrenal glands, are preferentially perfused. Perfusion of the "non-vital" organs, including the skin, muscle, lungs, kidney, and gastrointestinal tract, is decreased significantly. With limited periods of hypoxia, the newborn has some autoregulatory capabilities of maintaining blood flow to the intestine. However, if the period of ischemia is maintained for a prolonged period, perforation and significant mucosal hemorrhage may occur [53]. Coupled with asphyxia, feeding the premature infant heightens the risk for the development of neonatal NEC.

Most centers do not enterally feed an asphyxiated infant for the first 5 days to 2 weeks. This practice is extrapolated from animal data on cellular proliferation and migration. The intestinal mucosa of newborn and suckling rats has a very slow rate of cellular proliferation and migration compared to adult animals [54]. While the turnover of intestinal epithelia in the adult jejunum is 48–72 hours, the rate in the 10-day-old animal is at least twice that long, and in the 2–3-day-old animal it may be even longer [55]. In a study by Sunshine and colleagues in the adult animal, labeled cells reached the tips of the villi within 48 hours [56]. During the same period the labeled cells had migrated only one-eighth to one-fourth of the length of the villi in the suckling animal. There are indications that this same slower rate of turnover of intestinal epithelia exists in the newborn human [57].

Necrotizing enterocolitis

NEC is a well-described and extensively investigated affliction of the high-risk newborn. The etiology of this multifactorial disorder remains elusive, and currently there is no universally accepted theory of pathogenesis [58–61]. Risk factors include prematurity, low birthweight, congenital heart disease, perinatal asphyxia, gastroschisis, and indomethacin exposure [62].

Epidemiology

The incidence varies widely, with some centers reporting rare isolated cases [63] while others report an incidence of 3–5% of all neonatal admissions [64]. Among patients in whom NEC develops, the average birthweight is 1400–1500 g and the mean gestational age is 30–32 weeks [65]. In one study by Stoll and coworkers the overall incidence was 3/1000 live births, but increased to 66/1000 live births for infants less than 1500 g. Similarly, the mortality was 0% for infants greater than 2500 g and increased to 40% for infants less than 1500 g [66]. A recent report described the incidence of NEC as ∼ 1.1/1000 live births, with an in-hospital mortality of 15% [67]. The age at diagnosis ranged from 2 to 44 days and was inversely related to gestational age. All babies > 35 weeks' gestational age were diagnosed by 1 week of age. Stoll *et al.* felt there may be two populations who develop NEC – an early population consisting of term and preterm infants, and a later group of solely preterm babies who are smaller and sicker, who presumably have ongoing insults to their gastrointestinal tracts and are therefore at continued risk to develop the disease. These babies must be closely monitored for the possible development of NEC later in their hospital course [66]. It is important to appreciate that approximately 10% of all NEC cases occur in full-term neonates [58].

There are two distinct patterns of NEC: endemic and epidemic [68]. Superimposed on an endemic rate, epidemics (which refer to cases clustered in location and time) may be observed. No seasonal pattern of occurrence of these epidemics has been demonstrated. Patient characteristics appear to differ during epidemics – they are more mature, with fewer antecedent neonatal illnesses, acquire NEC later, and have been fed for a longer period than those patients who develop NEC during non-epidemic times.

Clinical picture

NEC may assume a broad spectrum of clinical severity. Some infants have little in the way of signs and symptoms, with a benign course, and others have fulminant disease characterized by extensive gangrene, perforation, shock, and death.

The diagnosis of NEC is suspected when two or more typical gastrointestinal signs and symptoms occur simultaneously with non-specific signs [64]. The initial signs and symptoms of 123 consecutive patients are presented in Table 44.3, as found by Walsh and Kliegman in a 9-year study [69]. Not all patients

Table 44.3. Initial signs and symptoms of necrotizing enterocolitis

Signs	Percentage of patients[a]
Abdominal distension	73
Bloody stool	28
Apnea, bradycardia	26
Abdominal tenderness	21
Retained gastric contents	18
Guaiac-positive stool	17
"Septic appearance"	12
Shock	11
Bilious emesis	11
Acidosis	10
Lethargy	9
Diarrhea	6
Cellulitis of abdominal wall	6
Right lower quadrant mass	2

Note:
[a]Total exceeds 100%, as many patients had more than one sign.
Source: Reproduced with permission from Walsh and Kliegman [69].

Table 44.4. Unusual manifestations of necrotizing enterocolitis

10% occur in term infants
10–12% occur in infants who have never been fed
10–15% will not have pneumatosis intestinalis
10–15% will have no blood in stools
10–15% will develop intestinal strictures

Source: Reproduced with permission from Sunshine [53].

will have every symptom, and the signs will vary chronologically in their appearance depending on the severity of the illness (Table 44.4).

Because the initial symptoms of NEC are non-specific and the findings on physical examination may be deceptively benign, radiographic findings are used to support the diagnosis. Radiographic examinations of the abdomen may show non-specific findings of distension, ileus, and ascites [70]. The two diagnostic radiologic signs are pneumatosis intestinalis (intramural intestinal gas) and intrahepatic portal venous gas. One of these is essential to confirm the diagnosis. More severe disease will result in perforation and pneumoperitoneum. However, pneumatosis intestinalis may be subtle and fleeting. It is typically first seen in the ileocecal area but may be seen anywhere from the stomach to rectum. Two patterns are described: a curvilinear intramural radiolucency, probably representing subserosal gas, and a cystic form assuming a foamy or bubbly appearance, probably representing submucosal gas. Gas mixed with stool in the bowel, however, can be difficult to distinguish from pneumatosis intestinalis [66]. Pneumatosis may also be present in other clinical situations – intestinal gangrene secondary to vascular occlusion, Hirschsprung's

Table 44.5. Modified Bell's staging criteria for necrotizing enterocolitis (NEC)

Stage	Systemic signs	Intestinal signs	Radiologic signs	Treatment
IA Suspected NEC	Temperature instability, apnea, bradycardia, lethargy	Elevated pregavage residuals, mild abdominal distension, emesis, guaiac-positive stool	Normal or intestinal dilation, mild ileus	NPO, antibiotics × 3 days pending culture
IB Suspected NEC	Same as above	Bright red blood from rectum	Same as above	Same as above
IIA Definite NEC: mildly ill	Same as above	Same as above, plus absent bowel sounds, ± abdominal tenderness	Intestinal dilation, ileus, pneumatosis intestinalis	NPO, antibiotics × 7–10 days if exam is normal in 24–48 h
IIB Definite NEC: moderately ill	Same as above, plus mild metabolic acidosis, mild thrombocytopenia	Same as above, plus absent bowel sounds, definite abdominal tenderness, ± adominal cellulites or right lower quadrant mass	Same as IIA, plus portal vein gas, ± ascites	NPO, antibiotics × 14 days, NaHCO$_3$ for acidosis
IIIA Advanced NEC: severely ill, bowel intact	Same as IIB, plus hypotension, bradycardia, severe apnea, combined respiratory and metabolic acidosis, disseminated intravascular coagulation, neutropenia	Same as above, plus signs of generalized peritonitis, marked tenderness	Same as IIB, plus definite ascites	Same as above, plus as much as 200 mL/kg fluids, fresh frozen plasma, inotropic agents, ventilation therapy, paracentesis
IIIB Advanced NEC: severely ill, bowel perforated	Same as IIIA, sudden deterioration	Same as IIIA, sudden increased distension	Same as IIB, plus pneumoperitoneum	Same as above, plus surgical intervention

Source: Reproduced with permission from Walsh and Kliegman [69].

disease with enterocolitis, obstruction at the site of bowel atresia, pyloric stenosis, and meconium ileus.

Investigators have developed screening tests for NEC such as breath hydrogen analysis [71,72], urine analysis for D-lactate [73] (produced by enteric flora when fed excess carbohydrate), and, more recently, serum D-lactic acid (a bacterial fermentation product of unabsorbed carbohydrates) levels [74], but these tests have not become routine in clinical monitoring up to the present.

Treatment

Since NEC can manifest within a wide range of severity along a continuum of various stages of bowel disease, the true nature or clinical course that NEC will follow is usually not known until 48 hours of onset.

Bell and associates proposed important clinical staging criteria for NEC, which allowed accurate comparisons of patients with disease of similar severity [75]. Kliegman and associates modified Bell's staging criteria to include systemic, intestinal, and radiographic signs and suggested treatment regimens based on the stages (Table 44.5) [76].

In addition to the recommendations in Table 44.5, a large-bore, double-lumen NG tube should also be placed to decompress the stomach. The length of time the bowel is allowed to "rest" will depend on the progression or lack of progression of the disease and on the philosophy of the institution. PN is recommended in patients with documented NEC during the period of intestinal recovery. When prolonged parenteral feedings are required, a central venous line may need to be placed. PN allows for a slow return to enteral feedings – it is common for this transition to take 1–3 weeks to re-establish full enteral feedings. Infants requiring surgical resection of the bowel will have a more protracted course, especially with extensive

resections, and may develop "short-bowel syndrome." The specifics of such management are described elsewhere [77]. Immediate surgical management of NEC has been reviewed [78–80], and the preferred operation for VLBW infants was recently investigated in a multicenter randomized clinical trial [81]. Moss and colleagues compared the outcomes of primary peritoneal drainage with laparotomy and bowel resection in preterm infants with perforated NEC ($n = 117$, all < 34 weeks' gestation). There were no differences between the two surgeries at 90 days postoperatively; length of hospital stay was also comparable between the two groups [81]. The study suggests that peritoneal drainage is a reasonable alternative to laparotomy [82].

Pathogenesis

There is no universal acceptance of a unifying theory regarding the pathogenesis of NEC. Numerous controlled studies have been performed in order to delineate the neonate at risk. Stoll *et al.* determined that affected infants were quite similar to controls and identified no risk factors [66]. Kliegman *et al.* failed to delineate any important risk factor. They therefore concluded that perinatal problems which precede NEC are equally common to all high-risk infants [76].

A unifying theory must explain the development of NEC in the enterally fed or fasted high-risk neonate and in the healthy term newborn [65]. It seems likely that NEC represents the final response of the immature gastrointestinal tract to one or more unrelated stresses. Because there are many stressful factors, there may be a wide range in the severity of bowel injury, and therefore a continuous spectrum of clinical disease. Perhaps in the mildly affected infant the stresses are not as injurious, and in the severely affected infant multiple stresses act synergistically to produce more severe damage [65].

Enteral feeding

Conflicting opinions exist regarding the relationship of enteral feeding practices and the development of NEC.

It is important to bear in mind that 5–10% of patients who develop NEC have never been fed [58]. Controlled studies comparing feeding techniques in infants with and without NEC fail to consistently support feeding as an important precursor, though controversy certainly persists.

There are numerous ways by which feedings might contribute to the pathogenesis or progression of NEC:

(1) direct mucosal injury by hypertonic feedings

(2) alteration of intestinal flora

(3) structural immaturity of the premature infant's intestine

(4) absence of breast milk's immunologically protective effect in formula-fed infants

(5) the effect of early or large-volume feedings on an alimentary tract compromised by an adverse perinatal event

The pragmatic issues, such as timing of feedings, the rate and volume of feedings, and the osmolality/osmolarity of feedings have been evaluated.

Timing of enteral feeding

There is a definite trend to delay enteral feedings in the sick premature infant. In a survey of 269 neonatal intensive care units by Churella et al. (described previously) most units (80%) gave parenteral feedings during the first week of life to infants weighing < 1000 g at birth [42]. None started enteral feeds alone and 20% used a combination of enteral and parenteral feeds. Sixty-nine percent of those weighing 1001–2399 g received a combination of parenteral and enteral feeds. The first enteral feed was begun at a mean of 7 days after birth for infants < 1000 g birthweight, 5 days after birth for those with a birthweight 1001–1500 g, and 3 days after birth for those infants weighing more than 1500 g [42].

In a prospective study by Eyal et al., delaying feedings in VLBW infants (< 1500 g) from 2–3 days to 2–3 weeks decreased the incidence of NEC from 18% to 3% [83]. It is interesting to note that in those patients (3%) who developed NEC after delayed onset of enteral feeds, the time of the first symptoms ranged from 23 to 60 days, compared to 7–23 days in those infants fed enterally within the first week of life. Hence, those infants in whom enteral feeds are delayed must be observed for a longer period for the development of NEC.

Brown and Sweet felt that NEC was virtually eliminated from their nursery with the initiation of an extremely cautious feeding protocol which fostered late initiation of enteral feeds, slow advancement to reach full feeds 2 weeks after onset of feeds, and prompt discontinuance of feeds when untoward signs suggesting hypoxia, hypoperfusion, or gastrointestinal dysfunction developed (i.e., distension, guaiac-positive stools, or apnea) [63].

On the other hand, Ostertag et al. in a prospective study of 34 low-birthweight infants (< 1500 g) who were fed on day 1 or day 7 did not find any significant increase in the incidence

of NEC: 29% of those enterally fed on day 1 compared to 35% fed enterally on day 7 developed NEC. There were no differences in the perinatal risk factors in the two groups [84]. In a study by Unger and coworkers, delayed initiation of enteral feedings was associated with a decreased incidence of NEC only among male infants with birthweight < 775 g; hence their study did not support elective withholding of enteral feeds in other groups of low-birthweight infants [34].

Rate and volume of enteral feeds

Aggressive feeding practices were found to be associated with NEC by Krousop [85]. In his case material, infants who developed NEC received an average of 43 mL/kg during the initial day of enteral feeds and 72 mL/kg during the second day [85].

Book and associates, in a small prospective study comparing fast and slow feeding rates (increase of 20 vs. 10 mL/day), designed to attain complete enteral feedings at 7 and 14 days respectively, did not find any difference in the incidence of NEC [86]. Goldman, however, in a retrospective uncontrolled study found an increased incidence of NEC when feedings were advanced by large volumes (> 40–60 mL/kg per day) [87]. He also found a higher percentage of disease in infants receiving volumes greater than 150 mL/kg per day. Anderson et al. noted an increased incidence of NEC among those low-birthweight infants fed aggressively – advanced at a rate exceeding 20 mL/kg per day [88].

The mechanism by which excessive feeding predisposes to NEC is uncertain. There may be relative mucosal ischemia due to an imbalance between mucosal blood flow and oxygen extraction due to an excessive load [65]. Alternatively, the already low concentration of lactase in preterm infants may be overwhelmed by the excessive lactose load. The excess lactose is then fermented by the microflora, resulting in H_2 production, initiating NEC [65]. Reducing substances are also a by-product of this bacterial fermentation. Book and coworkers found that 75% of infants who developed NEC had 3–4 plus reducing substances in their stools from 1–4 days prior to clinical manifestations of disease [89].

Walsh and coworkers recommended starting enteral feeds at 1 mL every 1–2 hours and advancing feeds slowly, no greater than 20 mL/kg per day. They successfully fed 1-kg infants who required ventilatory support [65]. However, the infant was continuously monitored for intolerance – increased residuals, distension, guaiac-positive stools, or reducing substances in the stool.

Sweet recommended holding feeds if there were significant residuals in the stomach prior to a feed [90]. If residue persisted, then the bowel was rested for 5–7 days. If abdominal distension developed during feeds, appropriate cultures and radiographs were obtained. Even if they were inconclusive, he would not feed the infant for 1–2 weeks. In his conservative approach, infants who developed sudden episodes of apnea, pallor, bradycardia, or poor skin perfusion were not fed for 1 week or more. They had only one episode of NEC in 5 years out of 300 infants (89 infants weighing < 1000 g and 211 weighing 1000–2500 g). Two recent studies cast doubt on the role of rapid advancement of formula feeding on the increased incidence of NEC [91,92].

Osmolality/Osmolarity of feeds

Both animal studies and clinical data have implicated hypertonic feeds in causing mucosal injury. DeLemos *et al.* produced enterocolitis in goats fed hypertonic formula [93]. Book *et al.* found that feeding infants < 1200 g an elemental formula with an osmolarity of 650 mosmol/L resulted in an 87% incidence of NEC, in comparison to 25% of neonates fed standard cow's-milk-based formula (359 mosmol/L) [94]. Willis *et al.* noted a higher frequency of NEC among infants fed undiluted hypertonic calcium lactate than among those unsupplemented or supplemented with diluted calcium lactate [95]. The American Academy of Pediatrics has recommended that infant feedings have an osmolarity of less than 400 mosmol/L (equivalent to an osmolality of approximately 450 mosmol/kg H_2O) [96].

Hypertonic formulas may be the result of added oral medications. In an excellent review by White and Harkavy, the osmolalities of five oral preparations were studied: theophylline, calcium glubionate, digoxin, phenobarbital, and dexamethasone [97]. The osmolalities of all five were > 3000 mosmol/kg H_2O, and hence they should be given undiluted orally with extreme caution. When mixed with formula, theophylline, calcium glubionate, and digoxin had acceptable osmolalities (< 400 mosmol/kg H_2O), but dexamethasone and phenobarbital elixirs still had osmolalities of approximately 1000 mosmol/kg H_2O, when 3.8 and 1 mL respectively were mixed with 15 mL of formula [97]. Ernst *et al.* showed that 1 mL of Polyvisol added to 30 mL of a standard formula increased the osmolality from 375 to 744 mosmol/kg H_2O [98]. If an intravenous line is required for other reasons, then the intravenous route of drug administration may be preferred over the oral route.

Immunologic considerations

The newborn protects its mucosa by secretory immunoglobulin A (sIgA). sIgA inhibits bacterial adherence to mucosal cells in addition to preventing other toxins and antigenic material from binding to the epithelial cells. However, in term infants sIgA is not demonstrable in intestinal fluids until 1 week of age, and adult values are not reached until 1 month of age [99]. However, nature has its way of protecting the newborn. sIgA-producing plasma cells in the maternal gut are antigenically stimulated and migrate to the breast, where specific antibodies are secreted into the colostrum. Thus the breastfed newborn receives some passive protection against the bacteria he or she is most likely to harbor (i.e., his or her mother's).

The possibility of improving gut defenses has been explored extensively [100]. Eibl and coworkers reported their results using an oral immunoglobulin preparation (73% IgA and 26% IgG) in reducing the incidence of NEC in low-birthweight infants (800–2000 g) [101]. These were infants for whom breast milk was not available. In 88 infants fed the oral IgA–IgG there were no cases of NEC, compared with six cases among the 91 control infants. The IgA–IgG preparation

was made from human serum. In a meta-analysis, the oral administration of IgG or IgG–IgA did not reduce the incidence of definite NEC, suspected NEC, need for surgery, or death from NEC [102].

Benefits of human milk

The possibility that breast milk (containing IgA) offers similar immunoprotective benefit has also been studied. In the non-breastfed premature infant, whose intestine is already immature, there is no protection against bacteria when microbial colonization occurs. Hence, maternal milk has potential importance in protecting the newborn. The work of Barlow *et al.* in rats substantiates the importance of breast milk in preventing NEC [103]. They consistently produced a disease similar to NEC by producing a hypoxic insult in those rats fed artificial formula. All breastfed asphyxiated rats were protected from disease. In the rat model, live milk leukocytes appeared to be prophylactic. They concluded that breast milk induced protective enteric immunity for newborn rats, and it may similarly protect premature infants [103]. However, NEC has been reported in neonates exclusively fed fresh, frozen, or pasteurized human milk [104].

In the past, many nurseries fed premature infants pooled frozen human milk. Kliegman *et al.* found that there was no difference in the incidence of NEC among these infants and those fed commercial formula [105]. The reason for this, despite the theoretical advantages of breast milk, could include the adverse affects of storage on the viability and functional integrity of the cellular components of milk, in addition to the possibility of contamination. In a study by Stevenson *et al.* there was no difference in the intestinal flora of preterm hospitalized infants fed stored frozen breast milk and a proprietary formula. However, all the infants fed breast milk had been treated with parenteral antibiotics [106].

Lucas and Cole reported a large prospective multicenter study of 926 preterm infants formally assigned to their early diet [107]. The results argue strongly for a highly protective effect of human milk on the subsequent development of NEC. In exclusively formula-fed babies, confirmed NEC was 6–10 times more common than in those fed breast milk alone, and three times more common than in those who received formula plus breast milk. Among babies born at more than 30 weeks' gestation, confirmed NEC was rare in those whose diet included human milk; it was 20 times more common in those fed formula only. Pasteurized donor milk seemed to be as protective as raw maternal milk. In formula-fed but not breastfed infants, delayed feeding was associated with a lower frequency of NEC. In babies fed breast milk (alone or with formula) there was a sharp decline in incidence of NEC with length of gestation. Beyond 30 weeks' gestation there was only one confirmed case of NEC among 376 babies receiving human milk. The authors concluded that early introduction of breast milk into the diets of preterm infants could make NEC beyond 30 weeks' gestation a rarity [107].

Schanler *et al.* in a randomized trial confirmed the value of feeding human milk to VLBW infants [25]. In their study, independent of treatment group assignment, those infants receiving the most human milk had a significantly lower incidence of NEC. Further, Schulman *et al.* showed that the feeding of human milk (vs. formula) was associated with decreased intestinal permeability at 28 days of age ($p = 0.02$) [30]. Fresh human milk is composed of numerous immunoprotective factors including neonatal antigen-specific antibodies (IgA, IgM, and IgG), macrophages, lymphocytes, neutrophils, enzymes, lactoferrin, lysozyme, growth factors (e.g., epidermal growth factor, EGF), hormones, oligosaccharides, polyunsaturated fatty acids, nucleotides, and specific glycoproteins. Another potentially beneficial component of human milk that was more recently discovered is platelet-activating factor (PAF) acetyl hydrolase (PAF-AH). This enzyme inhibits the activity of PAF, which is likely to be a significant mediator in the pathophysiologic cascade of NEC [108]. In a recent prospective study of 223 infants, enteral feedings containing at least 50% human milk in the first 14 days of life were associated with a sixfold decrease in the odds of NEC [109].

Ischemia and hypoxia

Ischemia and subsequent damage to the intestinal mucosa have been hypothesized in the pathogenesis of NEC. Investigators developed an ischemic model of NEC in piglets and postulated a "diving reflex." This is a well-documented reflex in marine animals when there is arterial constriction in the vascular beds of the skin, kidney, and gastrointestinal tract in an attempt to preserve cardiac and cerebral blood flow during prolonged diving. Premature infants may respond in a similar manner to repeated episodes of gut ischemia. Factors implicated in the "ischemia–hypoxia" pathogenesis of NEC include prenatal asphyxia, hypotension, hypothermia, umbilical vessel catheterization, patent ductus arteriosus (PDA), polycythemia, and exchange transfusion. Nonetheless, NEC does not develop in the majority of infants with these risk factors [64,66], and NEC has been reported in premature infants with no risk factors [110].

Umbilical vessel catheterization has been widely implicated in the pathogenesis of mucosal ischemia; 80% of infants with umbilical artery catheters have been found to have distinct arterial thrombosis [111]. Plasticizer levels in tissues of neonates with NEC were found to be significantly higher than in those without catheters [112]. A significant increase in portal venous pressure was noted in newborn piglets undergoing exchange transfusion via umbilical venous catheter. The authors concluded that alterations in mucosal vascular pressures produced ischemia secondary to vascular congestion and hemorrhage [113].

The presence of a low umbilical catheter has been reported to increase the risk of NEC, especially if the infant is fed during the period of catheterization. However, a prospective randomized clinical trial did not support this association [114]. Kliegman's own experience reinforces the safety and value of feeding infants as small as 600 g who are on a ventilator while an umbilical catheter is in place [29]. In the study of Schanler *et al.*, there was no association between the use of umbilical catheters, concomitant feeding, and either feeding intolerance or NEC [25].

Role of vitamin E

Premature infants weighing < 1500 g maintained at high serum levels of vitamin E for retinopathy of prematurity (ROP) prophylaxis have been found to have a higher incidence of NEC.

Johnson *et al.* found that premature infants weighing < 1500 g who received prophylactic vitamin E had a higher incidence of NEC and sepsis if maintained at pharmacologic levels (> 3.0 mg/dL or 0.03 mg/mL) for more than 1 week [115]. Hence, they recommended serum vitamin E levels be kept between 1.0 and 3.0 mg/dL. In another study, high serum vitamin E levels (> 3.5 mg/dL) were found in premature infants weighing < 1500 g when receiving the recommended dosage of MVI Pediatric [116]; hence, weekly serum vitamin E is recommended in those infants weighing between 1 and 3 kg. Further, infants with elevated vitamin E levels should have multivitamins held until serum vitamin E levels normalize; infants < 3 kg should receive 2 mL/kg (maximum 5 mL) of MVI Pediatric daily to avoid elevations in serum vitamin E and the increased NEC risk.

The most likely reason for the increased incidence of NEC is that pharmacologic serum vitamin E levels result in a decrease in oxygen-dependent intracellular killing ability, which leads to an increased susceptibility to infection in preterm infants.

Role of infectious agents

Many consider NEC to be an infectious disease, as many infants are colonized with a resistant and invasive organism. These organisms are capable of producing hydrogen gas, which leads to pneumatosis. The most commonly encountered organisms have been *Escherichia coli*, *Klebsiella*, and *Clostridium*, and more recently *Staphylococcus epidermidis* has been implicated in a number of patients [53]. The premature infant has decreased resistance; coupled with the inability to mount an appropriate immune response, these infections can be overwhelming.

Prophylactic use of oral aminoglycosides was initially hailed as a means of either prevention of NEC altogether or prevention of perforation if NEC had already developed. Prospective studies have demonstrated that oral gentamicin does not prevent intestinal perforation or alter the course of the disease. Further, oral aminoglycosides can be absorbed across the damaged intestine and increase serum levels, possibly leading to drug toxicity [65]. In addition, Neu and coworkers showed that in animals who had been asphyxiated the use of gentamicin significantly decreased jejunal lactase levels [117].

Maternal cocaine use

Maternal cocaine use has also been implicated in NEC in infants [80]. Cocaine compromises the uterine blood flow and fetal oxygenation in pregnant ewes, thus potentially impairing fetal gut development [118]. Lopez studied 1284 neonatal intensive care unit admissions and found that 12% of exposed infants and 3% of non-exposed infants developed NEC [119]. In low-birthweight or premature infants, the risk is 2–3 times higher during the first 2 weeks in the exposed babies but rises to five times higher after 2 weeks, particularly in those infants smaller than 1500 g.

Role of corticosteroids

In a large multicenter collaborative trial using antenatal corticosteroids to prevent RDS, a significantly decreased incidence of NEC was noted in infants treated with steroids [120]. Similar results have been shown prospectively in infants treated prenatally, with a trend in reduction of NEC even with postnatal treatment [121]. Additionally, corticosteroids stimulate PAF-AH and inhibit the PAF synthesis pathway [122]. In the study of Schulman et al., antenatal steroid administration was associated with decreased intestinal permeability at 28 days of age ($p = 0.017$) [30]. Corticosteroids are one of the growth factors implicated in the physiologic maturation of the intestinal barrier, and in animal studies they help to mature many components of the microvillous surface and enhance the intestinal barrier to the uptake of antigens [80]. Postnatal glucocorticoids are clearly not the ultimate answer to decrease NEC, since their use is associated with a number of significant adverse effects, including growth retardation, hyperglycemia, hypertension, infections, hypertrophic cardiomyopathy, gastrointestinal bleeding, and intestinal perforation [123].

Newer thoughts on etiology

Enteral feeding, bacterial infection, and mesenteric ischemia appear to play significant roles in the pathogenesis of NEC, but are likely secondary to the basic underlying defects of intestinal barrier immaturity. Contributing to this barrier of young (compared to more mature) intestine may be:

(1) decreased mucus production or immature mucin composition
(2) increased susceptibility to disruption of the epithelial cell layer at the cell membrane and/or the basement membrane level
(3) decreased repair capacity of the epithelial cell layer
(4) decreased tissue antioxidant activity
(5) decreased ability to maintain tissue oxygenation secondary to immature regulation of blood flow and oxygenation
(6) increased susceptibility to inflammatory mediators
(7) dysfunctional immune response
(8) abnormal motility [124]

One – or, more likely, several – of these factors contributing to gut immaturity may then result in mucosal injury that progresses to NEC [125,126].

NEC seems to involve a final common pathway that includes the endogenous production of inflammatory mediators involved in the development of intestinal injury. Endotoxin lipopolysaccharide, PAF, tumor necrosis factor (TNF), and other cytokines together with prostaglandins and leukotrienes are thought to be involved in the final common pathway of NEC pathogenesis [108].

PAF has emerged as a primary mediator of pathogenesis of NEC [127,128]. PAF exerts local paracrine effects, and is rapidly hydrolyzed by PAF-AH. PAF binds to a specific receptor, leading to hypotension, increased vascular permeability, hemoconcentration, lysosomal enzyme release, and platelet and neutrophil aggregation [128]. Gonzalez-Crussi and Hsueh have shown that intra-aortic injection of PAF resulted in experimental bowel necrosis in the adult rat that is similar to NEC [129]. Plasma levels of PAF-AH, the PAF-degrading enzyme, have been shown to be significantly lower in preterm neonates, and PAF levels in stools increase after the initiation of enteral feeding [127].

PAF receptor antagonists or PAF-AH mixed in the formula prevented the development of experimental NEC [127]. The bowel necrosis can be exacerbated by a nitric oxide synthase inhibitor [108].

Epithelial cells of the intestinal mucosa turn over naturally by the removal of some cells via programmed cell death (apoptosis) and by replacement of the dying cells with proliferating cells in the crypts. Abundant apoptosis might lead to a breach in the mucosal barrier, allowing bacterial translocation into the submucosa and triggering an inflammatory cascade. PAF is a potent stimulator of apoptosis in cultured intestinal epithelial cells [129].

Intestinal trefoil factor (ITF) is a cytoprotective peptide secreted by the intestinal goblet cells which has been shown to protect the gut mucosa against damage induced by several injurious agents. In an experimental rat model of NEC, ITF protected against PAF-mediated injury [130]. A proposed schematic of the etiology of NEC is shown in Figure 44.1.

Nitrous oxide is synthesized from arginine and is critical for intestinal barrier function. Inhibition of nitrous oxide synthesis increases intestinal damage. Glutamine and arginine serum levels have both been shown to be significantly lower in premature infants with NEC compared to controls [131].

Salivary EGF has been shown to be decreased in NEC infants compared to controls. There is a question of whether a fall in EGF predicts the onset of NEC. If EGF were low, EGF supplementation could possibly be given [124].

Early colonization of the gut might have an important role in developing susceptibility to NEC. Therefore, the supplementation of infant formula with probiotics might be a feasible prevention strategy to reduce the incidence of NEC in high-risk populations. Bifidobacterial supplementation reduced the incidence of NEC in a neonatal rat model [132]. Supplementation of formula with live bifidobacteria prevented the development of NEC in a quail model [133]. Further work from the laboratory of Butel et al. focused on the contribution of the prebiotic, oligofructose, to the protective role of bifidobacteria [134]. Thus the combination of a probiotic and prebiotic may offer a new therapeutic way of preventing NEC.

Probiotics are live microbial organisms that enhance mucosal IgA responses, increase production of anti-inflammatory cytokines, and normalize gut ecology [135]. Several randomized

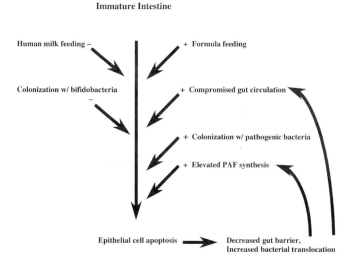

Fig. 44.1. Proposed schematic of the etiology of necrotizing enterocolitis. PAF, platelet-activating factor. – protective effect; + damaging effect. Modified with permission from Caplan and Jilling [127].

prospective studies in human infants (one used Inflor: *Lactobacillus acidophilus* and *Bifidobacterium infantis* [136]) suggest oral probiotics decrease the incidence of NEC, without the development of other infectious complications such as sepsis [136,137]. However, isolated case reports of sepsis following *Lactobacillus* sp. feeding have been described in preterm infants [138]; cases of fungemia following probiotic therapy have been described as well [139]. Data are insufficient at this time to comment on the short- and long-term safety of probiotics. The type of probiotics used, as well as the timing and dosage, are still to be optimized [140]. Therefore, until further studies of efficacy and safety are available, routine use of probiotic therapy in premature infants cannot be recommended [141].

If human milk is not available, altered premature formulas may lower the incidence of NEC. Delipidated formula (formula without fat) has been shown not to alter intestinal permeability, while premature formulas increase intestinal permeability [124]. Carlson *et al.* studied preterm infants fed on experimental formula with egg phospholipids (one or more of which may have enhanced immature intestinal function) in a randomized double-blind clinical study. Those infants fed the experimental formula developed significantly less stage II and stage III NEC compared to controls [142].

Outcome of NEC

In addition to post-NEC strictures, the most common complication is short-bowel syndrome – estimated to be 25% in one review [79]. Since patients with short-bowel syndrome are dependent on PN for varied periods of time, some patients progress to TPN-associated cholestasis, with subsequent cirrhosis and liver failure [79].

Neurodevelopmental outcome has also been studied in babies surviving NEC. Sonntag and colleagues studied 20 of 22 surviving VLBW infants diagnosed with NEC between

1992 and 1996. Severe developmental delay was especially frequent in the NEC group: it was found in 55% of the infants after NEC but only 22.5% of the infants without NEC at 20 months corrected age [143]. In an additional study of 1151 extremely low-birthweight infants, factors significantly associated with increased neurodevelopmental morbidity included chronic lung disease, grades 3–4 intraventricular hemorrhage/periventricular leukomalacia, steroids for chronic lung disease, NEC, and male gender [144].

Prevention of NEC

Given the multitude of known beneficial effects of breast milk for feeding premature infants, administration of fresh breast milk should be given top priority as the most natural and safe way of lowering the risk of NEC [125]. Early gastrointestinal priming with human milk, using the bolus tube-feeding method, "may provide the best advantage for the premature infant" [25].

Since there will continue to be infants for whom breast-milk feeding is not an option, investigation into the ideal nutrient composition for infant formulas and the administration of formula additives should be actively pursued [124]. Premature formulas must be altered to minimize adverse effects on intestinal barrier function. Omega-3 fatty acids and egg phospholipid-containing diets have been used in both animal and human studies [142,145]. These lipids seem to have an anti-inflammatory effect, with reduction of the levels of PAF and leukotrienes in the intestinal mucosa and a significant decrease in the incidence of stage III NEC in less-than-32-week premature infants [80].

In one study, increasing the volume of feedings at a slow versus fast rate was not shown to result in a difference in incidence of NEC [146]. The study was a randomized controlled prospective trial. One hundred and eighty-five preterm infants, < 1500 g, were randomized to receive either "slow" feeding advancement of 15 mL/kg per day or "fast" advancement at 35 mL/kg per day. The authors found no difference in the incidence of NEC between the groups (13% with the slow regimen vs. 9% with the fast regimen). The group randomized to the fast regimen regained their birthweight more rapidly [146]. These unexpected findings suggest that VLBW infants may not require as much caution in their feeding regimens as previously suggested, but few neonatologists currently advance feedings rapidly in preterm infants [127]. Experience dictates a very slow regimen for increases in feeding, beginning early [147,148].

Future therapies potentially beneficial in preventing NEC include:

(1) supplementation of feedings with probiotics (e.g., bifidobacteria) and possibly prebiotics (e.g., oligofructose)

(2) PAF antagonists or recombinant PAF-AH

(3) dietary supplements with growth factors (e.g., EGF, glutamine)

(4) arginine supplementation of the preterm infant's diet – an amino acid essential to intestinal integrity

(5) promotion of intestinal mucus production and addition of mucin to commercially prepared infant formula

(6) antioxidant administration, especially glutathione and vitamin E [124]

A recent clinically oriented study examining multimodal prophylaxis (early trophic feeding with human breast milk, enteral antibiotic, antifungal agent, and probiotics) in a high-risk group has shown a low incidence of NEC, especially when treatment was started within the first 24 hours of life [62,149].

Our knowledge of optimal nutrition in the premature infant is in a continuing state of evolution. Current recommendations for providing nutrition in the asphyxiated premature infant appear below.

Recommendations for nutritional management of asphyxiated infants

Several preventive measures can be proposed for at-risk infants. At-risk infants are those who are suspected to have had an intrauterine or neonatal episode of asphyxia or shock leading to poor bowel perfusion.

Late introduction of feedings

At-risk infants should receive nothing enterally for the first 5 days to 2 weeks of life; they should receive TPN. Enteral feedings are then initiated slowly, but at the first sign of abdominal distension, increasing gastric residuals, regurgitation, guaiac-positive or clinitest-positive (anhydrous Benedict's reagent) stools, enteral feedings should be stopped and not reintroduced for several days to weeks.

Slow advancement of feedings

At the end of 5 days to 2 weeks, or if feedings are to be initiated earlier than stated above (e.g., in tiny newborns on ventilators), one should begin with 1 mL every 1–2 hours and advance slowly to increase the total feedings by no more than 20 mL/kg per day.

Human milk

While early studies suggested that human milk would be protective against NEC, NEC has been described even in infants receiving fresh human milk. However, the immune protection from fresh human milk is thought by many to be very important to the preterm infant, and the large study of 926 preterm infants by Lucas and Cole argues strongly for the protective effects of human milk [107]. The study of Schanler et al. also supported the use of human milk – the greater the quantity of human milk fed, the lower the morbidity [25]. Since human milk may not meet calcium, phosphorus, caloric, and protein needs of low-birthweight infants, it can be supplemented with a human milk fortifier. In our laboratory, we have shown that such supplementation has no adverse effects on key anti-infective factors in human milk [150].

Route of feeding

Intermittent gavage tube feeding appears more physiologic than transpyloric feeding, and, wherever possible, is preferred. Schanler and coworkers confirmed the advantage of such bolus feedings [25]. Enteral nutrition may be the critical element that triggers postnatal gut maturation through release of gut peptide hormones [151]. If the patient has regurgitation, poor gastric emptying, or gastric distension, continuous NG feeding or even transpyloric feeding may be required [13].

Observe for early signs of NEC

Carefully monitor all high-risk infants for any early signs of NEC. These signs may occur up to 60 days of life in infants whose first feed is delayed beyond the first week of life. If the diagnosis of NEC is suspected, feedings are stopped, and the infant receives nutrition by the parenteral route for several days to 2 weeks, depending on the severity of symptoms.

Summary: asphyxia and necrotizing enterocolitis

Asphyxiated infants may have experienced a significant insult to the gut, predisposing them to NEC. Enteral feedings are usually withheld for the first 5 days to 2 weeks after the insult, then advanced slowly. Prolonged bowel rest may arrest gut maturation, but maturation will resume when intraluminal nutrients are reintroduced [152]. Gut atrophy in the chronically parenterally fed infant may lead to increased intestinal permeability to bacteria [153,154].

References

1. Committee on Nutrition. Nutritional needs of low birthweight infants. *Pediatrics* 1985; **75**; 976–86.

2. Grand RJ, Watkins JB, Torti FM. Development of the human gastrointestinal tract. *Gastroenterology* 1976; **70**: 790–810.

3. Lebenthal E, Le PC. Interactions of determinants in the ontogeny of the gastrointestinal tract: a unified concept. *Pediatr Res* 1983; **17**: 19–24.

4. Milla PJ. Development of intestinal structure and function. In Tanner MS, Stocks RJ, eds., *Neonatal Gastroenterology: Contemporary Issues.* Newcastle upon Tyne: Scholium International, 1984: 1–20.

5. Cavell B. Gastric emptying in preterm infants. *Acta Paediatr Scand* 1979; **68**: 725–30.

6. Yu VYH. Effect of body position on gastric emptying in the neonate. *Arch Dis Child* 975; **50**: 500–4.

7. Herbst JJ, Minton SD, Book LS. Gastroesophageal reflux causing respiratory distress and apnea in newborn infants. *J Pediatr* 1979; **95**: 763–8.

8. Pitcher-Wilmott R, Shurack JG, Fox WW. Decreased lung volume after nasogastric feeding of neonates recovering from respiratory distress. *J Pediatr* 1979; **96**: 914–16.

9. Toce SS, Keenan WJ, Homan SM. Enteral feeding in very low-birth-weight infants: a comparison of two nasogastric methods. *Am J Dis Child* 1987; **141**: 439–44.

10. Narayanan I, Singh B, Harvey D. Fat loss during feeding of human milk. *Arch Dis Child* 1984; **59**: 475–7.

11. Moyer L, Chan GM. Clotted feeding tubes with transpyloric feeding of

premature infant formula. *J Pediatr Gastroenterol Nutr* 1982; **1**: 55–7.

12. Lucas A, Bloom SR, Aynsley-Green A. Metabolic and endocrine events at the time of the first feed of human milk in preterm and term infants. *Arch Dis Child* 1978; **53**: 731–6.

13. Bremer HJ, Brooke OG, Orzalesi M, *et al. Nutrition and Feeding of Preterm Infants*. Oxford: Blackwell, 1987: 197–8.

14. Van Caillie M, Powell GK. Nasoduodenal versus nasogastric feeding in the very low birth weight infant. *Pediatrics* 1975; **56**: 1065–72.

15. Whitfield MF. Poor weight gain of the low birthweight infant fed nasojejunally. *Arch Dis Child* 1982; **57**: 597–601.

16. Roy RN, Pollnitz RP, Hamilton JR, *et al.* Impaired assimilation of nasojejunal feeds in healthy low-birth-weight infants. *J Pediatr* 1977; **90**: 431–4.

17. Beddis I, McKenzie S. Transpyloric feeding in the very low birthweight (1500 gm and below) infant. *Arch Dis Child* 1979; **54**: 213–7.

18. Whittfield MF. Transpyloric feeding in infants undergoing intensive care. *Arch Dis Child* 1980; **55**: 571.

19. Lucas A. Enteral nutrition. In Tsang RC, Lucas A, Uauy R, *et al.*, eds., *Nutritional Needs of the Premature Infant*. Baltimore, MD: Williams and Wilkins, 1993: 209–23.

20. Hayhurst EG, Wyman M. Morbidity associated with prolonged use of polyvinyl feeding tubes. *Am J Dis Child* 1975; **129**: 72–4.

21. Rodriguez JP, Guero J, Frias EG, *et al.* Duodenorenal perforation in a neonate by a tube of silicone rubber during transpyloric feeding. *J Pediatr* 1978; **92**: 113–16.

22. Dellagrammaticus HD, Duerden BI, Milner RDG. Upper intestinal bacterial flora during transpyloric feeding. *Arch Dis Child* 1983; **58**: 115–19.

23. Vazquez C, Arroyos A, Valls A. Necrotizing enterocolitis: increased incidence in infants receiving nasoduodenal feeding. *Arch Dis Child* 1980; **55**: 826.

24. Pereira GR, Lemons JA. Controlled study of transpyloric and intermittent gavage feeding in the small preterm infant. *Pediatrics* 1981; **67**: 68–72.

25. Schanler RJ, Schulman RJ, Lau C, *et al.* Feeding strategies for premature infants: randomized trial of gastrointestinal priming and tube-feeding method. *Pediatrics* 1999; **103**: 434–9.

26. Lucas A, Bloom SR, Aynsley-Green A. Gut hormones and "minimal enteral feeding." *Acta Paediatr Scand* 1986; **75**: 719–23.

27. Dunn L, Hulman S, Weiner J, *et al.* Beneficial effects of early hypocaloric enteral feeding on neonatal gastrointestinal function: preliminary report of a randomized trial. *J Pediatr* 1988; **112**: 622–9.

28. Slagle TA, Gross SJ. Effect of early low-volume enteral substrate on subsequent feeding tolerance in very low birth weight infants. *J Pediatr* 1988; **113**: 526–31.

29. Kliegman RM. Experimental validation of neonatal feeding practices. *Pediatrics* 1999; **103**: 492–3.

30. Schulman RJ, Schanler RJ, Lau C, *et al.* Early feeding, antenatal glucocorticoids, and human milk decrease intestinal permeability in preterm infants. *Pediatr Res* 1998; **44**: 519–23.

31. Schulman RJ, Schanler RJ, Laue C, *et al.* Early feeding, feeding tolerance, and lactase activity in premature infants. *J Pediatr* 1998; **133**: 645–9.

32. Schanler RJ. Feeding strategies in premature infants. Presented as a lecture at Advances in Perinatal and Pediatric Nutrition Conference, Stanford University, July 1999. Published in Course Syllabus, 1999: 454–61.

33. Moyer-Mileur L, Chan GM. Nutritional support of very-low-birth-weight infants requiring prolonged assisted ventilation. *Am J Dis Child* 1986; **140**: 929–32.

34. Unger A, Goetzman BW, Chan C, *et al.* Nutritional practices and outcome of extremely premature infants. *Am J Dis Child* 1986; **140**: 1027–33.

35. Gunn T, Reaman G, Outerbridge EW, *et al.* Peripheral total parenteral nutrition for premature infants with the respiratory distress syndrome: a controlled study. *J Pediatr* 1978; **92**: 608–13.

36. Yu VYH, James B, Hendry P, *et al.* Total parenteral nutrition in very low birthweight infants: a controlled trial. *Arch Dis Child* 1979; **54**: 653–61.

37. Kerner JA, Hattner JAT, Trautman MS, *et al.* Postnatal somatic growth in very low birth weight infants on peripheral parenteral nutrition. *J Pediatr Perinat Nutr* 1988; **2**: 27–34.

38. Glass EJ, Hume R, Lang MA, *et al.* Parenteral nutrition compared with transpyloric feeding. *Arch Dis Child* 1984; **59**: 131–5.

39. Dryburgh E. Transpyloric feeding in 49 infants undergoing intensive care. *Arch Dis Child* 1980; **55**: 879–2.

40. Zlotkin SH, Stallings VA, Pencharz PB. Total parenteral nutrition in children. *Pediatr Clin North Am* 1985; **32**: 381–400.

41. Cashore WJ, Sedaghatian MR, Usher RH. Nutritional supplements with intravenously administered lipid, protein hydrolysate, and glucose in small premature infants. *Pediatrics* 1975; **56**: 8–16.

42. Churella HR, Bachhuber BS, MacLean WC. Survey: methods of feeding low-birth-weight infants. *Pediatrics* 1985; **76**: 243–9.

43. Adamkin DA. Nutrition in very very low birth weight infants. *Clin Perinatol* 1986; **13**: 419–43.

44. Higgs SC, Malan AF, Heese H DeV. A comparison of oral feeding and total parenteral nutrition in infants of very low birthweight. *S Afr Med J* 1974; **48**: 2169–73.

45. Hall RT, Rhodes PG. Total parenteral alimentation via indwelling umbilical catheters in the newborn period. *Arch Dis Child* 1976; **51**: 929–34.

46. Merritt RJ. Neonatal nutritional support. *Clin Consult Nutr Support* 1981; **1**: 10.

47. Coran AG. Parenteral nutritional support of the neonate. Tele Session (a group telephone workshop, August 17), Tele Session Corporation, New York, NY, 1981.

48. Kerner JA. The use of umbilical catheters for parenteral nutrition. In Kerner JA, ed., *Manual of Pediatric Parenteral Nutrition*. New York, NY: Wiley, 1983: 303–6.

49. Sadig HF. Broviac catheterization in low birth weight infants: incidence and treatment of associated complications. *Crit Care Med* 1987; **15**: 47–50.

50. Kanarek KS, Kuznicki MB, Blair RC. Infusion of total parenteral nutrition via the umbilical artery. *J Parenter Enteral Nutr* 1991; **15**: 71–4.

51. Nakamura KT, Sato Y, Erenberg A. Evaluation of a percutaneously placed 27-gauge central venous catheter in neonates weighing less than 1200 grams. *J Parenter Enteral Nutr* 1990; **14**: 295–9.

52. Abdulla F, Dietrich KA, Pramanik AK. Percutaneous femoral venous catheterization in preterm neonates. *J Pediatr* 1990; **117**: 788–91.

53. Sunshine P. Fetal gastrointestinal physiology. In Eden RD, Boehm FH,

eds., *Assessment and Care of the Fetus: Physiological, Clinical and Medicolegal Principles.* East Norwalk, CT: Appleton & Lange, 1990: 93–111.

54. Koldovsky O, Sunshine P, Kretchmer N. Cellular migration of intestinal epithelia in suckling and weaned rats. *Nature* 1966; **212**: 1389–90.

55. Herbst JJ, Sunshine P. Postnatal development of the small intestine of the rat. *Pediatr Res* 1969; **3**: 27–33.

56. Sunshine P, Herbst JJ, Koldovsky O, *et al.* Adaptation of the gastrointestinal tract to extrauterine life. *Ann NY Acad Sci* 1971; **176**: 16–29.

57. Herbst JJ, Sunshine P, Kretchmer N. Intestinal malabsorption in infancy and childhood. *Adv Pediatr* 1969; **16**: 11–64.

58. Kliegman RM, Fanaroff AN. Necrotizing enterocolitis. *N Engl J Med* 1984; **310**: 1093–103.

59. Kosloske AM. Pathogenesis and prevention of necrotizing enterocolitis: a hypothesis based on personal observation and a review of the literature. *Pediatrics* 1984; **74**: 1086–92.

60. Neu J. Necrotizing enterocolitis: an update. *Acta Paediatr* 2005; **94**: 100–5.

61. Stevenson DK, Blakely ML. Historical perspectives: necrotizing enterocolitis: an inherited or acquired condition? *NeoReviews* 2006; **7**: e125–34.

62. Lee S, Lee J, Puder M. A.S.P.E.N. Clinical guidelines: complications unique to neonates: necrotizing enterocolitis. *J Parenter Enteral Nutr* (in press).

63. Brown E, Sweet AY. Preventing necrotizing enterocolitis in neonates. *JAMA* 1978; **240**: 2452–4.

64. Frantz ID, L'Heureux P, Engel RR, *et al.* Necrotizing enterocolitis. *J Pediatr* 1975; **56**: 259–63.

65. Walsh MC, Kliegman R, Fanaroff A. Necrotizing enterocolitis: a practitioner's perspective. *Pediatr Rev* 1988; **9**: 219–26.

66. Stoll BJ, Kanto WP, Glass RI, *et al.* Epidemiology of necrotizing enterocolitis: a case control study. *J Pediatr* 1980; **96**: 447–51.

67. Holman RC, Stoll BJ, Curns AT, *et al.* Enterocolitis hospitalizations among neonates in the United States. *Paediatr Perinat Epidemiol* 2006; **20**: 498–506.

68. Moonijian AS, Peckham G, Fox W, *et al.* Necrotizing enterocolitis: endemic vs. epidemic. *Pediatr Res* 1978; **12**: 530.

69. Walsh MC, Kliegman RM. Necrotizing enterocolitis: treatment based on staging criteria. *Pediatr Clin North Am* 1986; **33**: 179–200.

70. Mata AG, Rosenpart RM. Intraobserver variability in the radiographic diagnosis of necrotizing enterocolitis. *Pediatrics* 1980; **66**: 68–71.

71. Kirschner B, Lahr C, Lahr D. Detection of increased breath hydrogen in infants with necrotizing enterocolitis. *Gastroenterology* 1980; **72**: A57/1080.

72. Stevenson DK, Shahin SM, Ostrander CR, *et al.* Breath hydrogen in preterm infants: correlation with changes in bacterial colonization of the gastrointestinal tract. *J Pediatr* 1982; **101**: 607–10.

73. Garcia J, Smith FR, Cucinelli SA. Urinary D-lactate in infants with necrotizing enterocolitis. *J Pediatr* 1984; **104**: 268–70.

74. Rivas Y, Solans C, Spivak W. Serum D-lactic acid level, a new marker for necrotizing enterocolitis. *J Pediatr Gastroenterol Nutr* 2000; **31**: S236.

75. Bell MJ, Ternberg JL, Feigin RD, *et al.* Neonatal necrotizing enterocolitis: therapeutic decisions based upon clinical staging. *Ann Surg* 1978; **187**: 1–7.

76. Kliegman RM, Hack M, Jones P, *et al.* Epidemiologic study of necrotizing enterocolitis among low-birth-weight infants: absence of identifiable risk factors. *J Pediatr* 1982; **100**: 440–4.

77. Kerner JA, Hartman GE, Sunshine P. The medical and surgical management of infants with the short bowel syndrome. *J Perinatol* 1985; **5**: 517–21.

78. Raine PAM. Neonatal necrotizing enterocolitis. In Reed GB, Claireaux AE, Cockburn F, eds. *Diseases of the Fetus and Newborn*, 2nd edn. London: Chapman and Hall, 1995: 1485–91.

79. Dimmitt RA, Moss RL. Clinical management of necrotizing enterocolitis. *NeoReviews* 2001; **2**: e110–17.

80. Israel EJ, Morera C. Necrotizing enterocolitis. In Walker WA, Durie PR, Hamilton JR, *et al.*, eds., *Pediatric Gastrointestinal Disease*, 3rd edn. Ontario: Decker, 2000; 665–76.

81. Moss RL, Dimmit RA, Barnhart DC, *et al.* Laparotomy versus peritoneal drainage for necrotizing enterocolitis and perforation. *N Engl J Med* 2006; **354**: 2225–34.

82. Flake AW. Necrotizing enterocolitis in preterm infants: is laparotomy necessary? *N Engl J Med* 2006; **354**: 2275.

83. Eyal F, Sagi E, Avital A. Necrotizing enterocolitis in the very low birthweight infant: expressed breast milk feeding compared with parenteral feeding. *Arch Dis Child* 1982; **57**: 274–6.

84. Ostertag SG, LaGamma EF, Reisen CE, *et al.* Early enteral feeding does not affect the incidence of necrotizing enterocolitis. *Pediatrics* 1986; **77**: 275–80.

85. Krousop RW. The influences of feeding practices. In Brown EG, Sweet AY, eds., *Necrotizing Enterocolitis.* New York, NY: Grune and Stratton, 1980: 57.

86. Book LS, Herbst JJ, Jung AL. Comparison of fast and slow-feeding rate schedules to the development of necrotizing enterocolitis. *J Pediatr* 1976; **89**: 463–6.

87. Goldman HI. Feeding and necrotizing enterocolitis. *Am J Dis Child* 1980; **134**: 553–5.

88. Anderson DM, Rome ES, Kliegman RM. Relationship of endemic necrotizing enterocolitis to alimentation. *Pediatr Res* 1985; **19**: 331A.

89. Book LS, Herbst JJ, Jung AL. Carbohydrate malabsorption in necrotizing enterocolitis. *Pediatrics* 1976; **57**: 201–4.

90. Sweet AY. Necrotizing enterocolitis: feeding the neonate weighing less than 1500 grams – nutrition and beyond. In Sunshine P, ed., *Report of the 79th Ross Conference on Pediatric Research.* Columbus, OH: Ross Products Division, 1980.

91. Caple J, Armentrout D, Huseby V, *et al.* Randomized controlled trial of slow versus rapid feeding volume advancement in preterm infants. *Pediatrics* 2004; **114**: 1597–600.

92. Kennedy KA, Tyson JE, Chamnanvanikij S. Early versus delayed initiation of progressive enteral feeding for parenterally fed low birth weight or preterm infants. *Cochrane Database Syst Rev* 2000; (2): CD001970.

93. DeLemos RA, Rogers JH, McLaughlin GW. Experimental production of necrotizing enterocolitis in newborn goats. *Pediatr Res* 1974; **8**: 380.

94. Book LS, Herbst JJ, Atherton SO, *et al.* Necrotizing enterocolitis in low-birth-weight infants fed an elemental formula. *J Pediatr* 1975; **87**: 602–5.

95. Willis DM, Chabot J, Radde IC, *et al.* Unsuspected hyperosmolality of oral solutions contributing to necrotizing enterocolitis in very-low-birth-weight infants. *Pediatrics* 1977; **60**: 535–8.

96. AAP Committee on Nutrition. Commentary on breast feeding and infant formulas including proposed standards for formulas. *Pediatrics* 1976; **57**: 278–85.

97. White KC, Harkavy KZ. Hypertonic formula resulting from added oral medications. *Am J Dis Child* 1982; **136**: 931–3.

98. Ernst JA, Williams JM, Glick MR. Osmolality of substances used in the intensive care nursery. *Pediatrics* 1983; **72**: 347–52.

99. Barnard J, Greene H, Cotton R. Necrotizing enterocolitis. In Kretchmer N, Minkowski A, eds., *Nutritional Adaptation of the Gastrointestinal Tract of the Newborn. Nestle Nutrition*, vol. 3. New York, NY: Raven Press, 1983: 103–28.

100. Udall JN. Gastrointestinal host defense and necrotizing enterocolitis. *J Pediatr* 1990; **117**: 33–43.

101. Eibl MM, Wolf HM, Furnkranz H, *et al.* Prevention of necrotizing enterocolitis in low-birth-weight infants by IgA–IgG feeding. *N Engl J Med* 1988; **319**: 1–7.

102. Foster J, Cole M. Oral immunoglobulin for preventing necrotizing enterocolitis in preterm and low-birth-weight neonates. *Cochrane Database Syst Rev* 2004; (1): CD001816.

103. Barlow B, Santulli TV, Heird WC, *et al.* An experimental study of acute neonatal necrotizing enterocolitis: the importance of breast milk. *J Pediatr Surg* 1974; **9**: 587–95.

104. Reisner SH, Garty B. Necrotizing enterocolitis despite breast-feeding. *Lancet* 1977; **ii**: 507.

105. Kliegman RM, Pittard WB, Fanaroff AA. Necrotizing enterocolitis in neonates fed human milk. *J Pediatr* 1979; **95**: 450–3.

106. Stevenson DK, Yang C, Kerner JA, *et al.* Intestinal flora in the second week of life in hospitalized preterm infants fed stored frozen breast milk or a proprietary formula. *Clin Pediatr* 1985; **24**: 338–41.

107. Lucas A, Cole TJ. Breast milk and neonatal necrotising enterocolitis. *Lancet* 1990; **336**: 1519–23.

108. Neu J. Necrotizing enterocolitis: the search for a unifying pathogenic theory leading to prevention. *Pediatr Clin North Am* 1996; **43**: 409–32.

109. Sisk PM, Lovelady CA, Dillard RG, *et al.* Early human milk feeding is associated with a lower risk of necrotizing enterocolitis in very low birth weight infants. *J Perinatol* 2007; **27**: 428–33.

110. Kliegman RM, Fanaroff AA. Neonatal necrotizing enterocolitis: a nine-year experience. Epidemiology and uncommon observations. *Am J Dis Child* 1981; **135**: 603–14.

111. Lehmiller DH, Kanto WF. Relationship of mesenteric thromboembolism, oral feeding and necrotizing enterocolitis. *J Pediatr* 1978; **92**: 96–100.

112. Hillman LS, Goodwin SL, Sherman WR. Identification and measurement of plasticiser in neonatal tissues after umbilical catheters and blood products. *N Engl J Med* 1975; **292**: 381–6.

113. Touloukian RJ, Kadaw A, Spencer RP. The gastrointestinal complications of umbilical venous exchange transfusion: a clinical and experimental study. *Pediatrics* 1973; **51**: 36–42.

114. Davey AM, Wagner CL, Cox C, *et al.* Feeding premature infants while low umbilical artery catheters are in place: a prospective, randomized trial. *J Pediatr* 1994; **124**: 795–9.

115. Johnson L, Bowen FW, Abbasi S, *et al.* Relationship of prolonged pharmacologic serum levels of vitamin E to incidence of sepsis and necrotizing enterocolitis in infants with birth weight 1500 grams or less. *Pediatrics* 1985; **75**: 619–38.

116. Kerner JA, Poole RL, Sunshine P, *et al.* High serum vitamin E levels in premature infants receiving MVI-Pediatric. *J Pediatr Perinat Nutr* 1987; **1**: 75–82.

117. Neu J, Masi M, Stevenson DK, *et al.* Effects of asphyxia and oral gentamicin on intestinal lactase in the suckling rat. *Pediatr Pharmacol* 1981; **1**: 215–20.

118. Czyrko C, Del Pin CA, O'Neill JA, *et al.* Maternal cocaine abuse and necrotizing enterocolitis: outcome and survival. *J Pediatr Surg* 1991; **26**: 414–18.

119. Lopez SL. Time of onset of necrotizing enterocolitis in newborn infants with known prenatal cocaine exposure. *Clin Pediatr* 1995; **34**: 424–9.

120. Bauer CR, Morrison JC, Poole WK, *et al.* A decreased incidence of necrotizing enterocolitis after prenatal glucocorticoid therapy. *Pediatrics* 1984; **73**: 682–8.

121. Halac E, Halac J, Begue EF, *et al.* Prenatal and postnatal corticosteroid therapy to prevent neonatal necrotizing enterocolitis: a controlled trial. *J Pediatr* 1990; **117**: 132–8.

122. Muguruma K, Gray PW, Tjoelker LW, *et al.* The central role of PAF in necrotizing enterocolitis development. *Adv Exp Med Biol* 1997; **407**: 379–82.

123. Thebaud B, Lacaze-Masmonteil T, Watterberg K. Postnatal glucocorticoids in very preterm infants: "the good, the bad, and the ugly." *Pediatrics* 2001; **107**: 413–15.

124. Crissinger KD. Pathogenesis of necrotizing enterocolitis. Workshop presented at the 25th Clinical Congress of A.S.P.E.N. Chicago, IL: Clinical Congress of the American Society for Parenteral and Enteral Nutrition, 2001: 203–4.

125. Crissinger K. Understanding necrotizing enterocolitis: promising directions. *Pathophysiology* 1999; **5**: 247–56.

126. Kliegman R, Walker W, Yolken R. Necrotizing enterocolitis research agenda for a disease of unknown etiology and pathogenesis. *Pediatr Res* 1993; **34**: 701–8.

127. Caplan MS, Jilling T. The pathophysiology of necrotizing enterocolitis. *NeoReviews* 2001; **2**: e103–9.

128. Rabinowitz SS, Dzakpasu P, Piecuch S, *et al.* Platelet-activating factor in infants at risk for necrotizing enterocolitis. *J Pediatr* 2001; **138**: 81–6.

129. Gonzalez-Crussi F, Hsueh W. Experimental model of ischemic bowel necrosis: the role of platelet activating factor and endotoxin. *Am J Pathol* 1983; **112**: 127–35.

130. Chang H, Gonzalez-Crussi F, Hsueh W, *et al.* Prevention of experimental necrotizing enterocolitis with intestinal trefoil factor (ITF). *Gastroenterology* 2000; **118**: A197.

131. Becker RM, Wue G, Galanko JA, *et al.* Reduced serum amino acid concentrations in infants with necrotizing enterocolitis. *J Pediatr* 2000; **137**: 785–93.

132. Caplan MS, Miller-Catchpole R, Kaup S, *et al.* Bifidobacterial supplementation reduces the incidence of necrotizing enterocolitis in a neonatal rat model. *Gastroenterology* 1999; **117**: 577–83.

133. Butel MJ, Roland N, Hilbert A, *et al.* Clostridial pathogenicity in experimental necrotizing enterocolitis in gnotobiotic quails and protective role of bifidobacteria. *J Med Microbiol* 1998; **47**: 391–9.

134. Catala I, Butel MJ, Bensaada M, et al. Oligofructose contributes to the protective role of bifidobacteria in experimental necrotizing enterocolitis in quails. *J Med Microbiol* 1999; **48**: 89–94.

135. Garg P. Necrotizing enterocolitis: newer insights. *J Clin Diagn Res* 2007; **1**: 90–103.

136. Lin HC, Su BH, Chen AC, et al. Oral probiotics reduce the incidence and severity of necrotizing enterocolitis in very low birth weight infants. *Pediatrics* 2005; **115**: 1–4.

137. Bin-Nun A, Bromiker R, Wilschanski M, et al. Oral probiotics prevent necrotizing enterocolitis in very low birth weight neonates. *J Pediatr* 2005; **147**: 192–6.

138. Kunz AN, Noel JM, Fairchok MP. Two cases of *Lactobacillus* bacteremia during probiotic treatment of short gut syndrome. *J Pediatr Gastoenterol Nutr* 2004; **38**: 457–8.

139. Munoz P, Bouza E, Cuenca-Estrella M, et al. *Saccharomyces cerevisiae* fungemia: an emerging infectious disease. *Clin Infect Dis* 2005; **40**: 1625.

140. Barclay AR, Stenson B, Simpson JH, et al. Probiotics for necrotizing enterocolitis: a systematic review. *J Pediatr Gastroenterol Nutr* 2007; **45**: 569–72.

141. Hunter CJ, Upperman JS, Ford HR, et al. Understanding the susceptibility of the premature infant to necrotizing enterocolitis (NEC). *Pediatr Res* 2008; **63**: 117–23.

142. Carlson SE, Montalto MB, Ponder DL, et al. Lower incidence of necrotizing enterocolitis in infants fed a preterm formula with egg phospholipids. *Pediatr Res* 1998; **44**: 491–8.

143. Sonntag J, Grimmer I, Scholz T, et al. Growth and neurodevelopmental outcome of very low birthweight infants with necrotizing enterocolitis. *Acta Paediatr* 2000; **89**: 528–32.

144. Vohr BR, Wright LL, Dusick AM, et al. Neurodevelopmental and functional outcomes of extremely low birthweight infants in the National Institute of Child Health and Human Developmental Neonatal Research Network, 1993–1994. *Pediatrics* 2000; **105**: 1216–26.

145. Akisu M, Baka M, Coker I, et al. Effect of dietary n-3 fatty acids on hypoxia-induced necrotizing enterocolitis in young mice: n-3 fatty acids alter platelet-activating factor and leukotriene B4 production in the intestine. *Biol Neonate* 1998; **74**: 31–8.

146. Rayyis SF, Ambalavanan N, Wright L, et al. Randomized trial of "slow" versus "fast" feed advancements on the incidence of necrotizing enterocolitis in very low birth weight infants. *J Pediatr* 1999; **134**: 293–7.

147. La Gamma E, Browne L. Feeding practices for infants less than 1500 grams at birth and the pathogenesis of necrotizing enterocolitis. *Clin Perinatol* 1994; **21**: 271–306.

148. Brown E, Sweet A. Neonatal necrotizing enterocolitis. *Pediatr Clin North Am* 1982; **29**: 114–70.

149. Schmolzer G, Urlesberger B, Haim M, et al. Multi-modal approach to prophylaxis of necrotizing enterocolitis: a clinical report and review of literature. *Pediatr Surg Int* 2006; **22**: 573–80.

150. Quan R, Yang C, Rubinstein S, et al. The effect of nutritional additives on anti-infective factors in human milk. *Clin Pediatr* 1994; **33**: 325–8.

151. Aynsley-Green A. Metabolic and endocrine interrelation in the human fetus and neonate. *Am J Clin Nutr* 1985; **41**: 399–417.

152. Feng JJ, Kwong LK, Kerner JA, et al. Resumption of intestinal maturation upon reintroduction of intraluminal nutrients: functional and biochemical correlations. *Clin Res* 1987; **35**: 228A.

153. Mascarenhas MR, Kerner JA, Stallings VA. Parenteral and enteral nutrition. In Walker WA, Durie PR, Hamilton JR, et al., eds., *Pediatric Gastrointestinal Disease*, 3rd edn. Ontario: Decker, 2000: 1705–52.

154. Zenk KE, Sills JH, Koeppel RM. *Neonatal Medications and Nutrition: a Comprehensive Guide*, 2nd edn. Santa Rosa, CA: NICU Ink Book, 2000: 527–8.

Early childhood neurodevelopmental outcome of preterm infants

Susan R. Hintz

Epidemiology of preterm birth: framing the issues of sequelae

Preterm birth is a substantial and growing problem for developed nations. In the United States between 1990 and 2004, the proportion of live-born infants delivered preterm (< 37 weeks estimated gestational age, EGA) rose from 10.6% to 12.5%; the proportion delivered very preterm (< 32 weeks EGA) rose from 1.92% to 2.01% [1]. Thus, more than 500 000 preterm infants and 82 000 very preterm infants were born in the United States alone in 2004. With improvements in perinatal and neonatal care and technology over the past decades, survival of preterm infants has improved significantly, particularly among the smallest and most immature subgroups [2]. In the Netherlands, survival to discharge for infants of 22–27 weeks EGA rose from 36.1% to 67.8% between 1983 and 1995 [3]. In two large regional tertiary care centers in Sweden, survival to discharge for live-born infants of 23–25 weeks EGA increased from 55% to 78% from 1992 to 1998 [4]. In the state of Victoria, Australia, survival to discharge among infants of 23–27 weeks EGA increased from 56% in 1991–92 to 72% in 1997; of note in the 1997 birth cohort, survival was 41%, 41%, and 73% for 23-, 24-, and 25-week EGA groups, respectively [5]. For extremely low-birthweight (ELBW) infants overall in Victoria, survival rate increased from 38% in 1985–87, to 56% in 1991–92, to 73% in 1997 [6]. These data may be contrasted with less optimistic reports of relatively recent preterm survival, particularly at the lowest gestational age subgroups [7,8]. However, survival among extremely preterm infants is highly dependent on variables such as approach to intervention or non-intervention [9,10], and regionalization of care [4,5,11,12].

The reported increased survival of extremely preterm infants in the 1990s is linked at least in part with concomitant increased offers of intensive care intervention; survival may be possible even for the most immature infants if support is provided. Yet despite the recognition that survival is achievable – or perhaps because of it – the question has been posed whether the comprehensive costs associated with extremely preterm birth and its sequelae can be justified. Attempts to estimate even the economic consequences of hospitalizations and

services are challenging, and analyses may not be comparable regions; but financial resource utilization is amongst, not surprisingly, significantly greater for preterm than for term children. In a Southern England cohort, adjusted total hospital costs were 443% higher for preterm than term children by 10 years of age [13]. In a statewide Massachusetts cohort, the estimated cost per child for overall early intervention services through age 3 was significantly higher for very preterm infants than for either moderately preterm or full-term infants [14]. Nevertheless, in a regional economic analysis of quality-adjusted survival, Doyle demonstrated that the economic efficiency of neonatal intensive care among ELBW infants to 2 years of age has not declined significantly over two decades, with similar costs per quality-adjusted life-year gained over time [15]. Although important, such economic considerations have little immediate impact for medical providers as they counsel families, or for families as they consider the future for their infants. In these circumstances, discussion around "comprehensive costs" often and appropriately focuses on the potential neurodevelopmental and functional sequelae of preterm birth. For families and other medical decision makers, knowledge of the range of outcomes beyond the neonatal period, and of the clinical and sociodemographic variables associated with adverse outcomes, as well as the limitations of our ability to predict outcomes for an individual child, are critical components in understanding the possible implications and consequences of extremely preterm birth.

Numerous neurodevelopmental outcomes analyses, ranging from small or single-center cohorts to large multisite observational studies, have been published since successful resuscitation of preterm infants became widely achievable. This chapter does not seek to present a comprehensive history of all published neurodevelopmental outcomes studies, but rather we will concentrate on results from larger cohorts and regional population-based studies, presenting more recent data whenever possible. For early childhood outcomes, the attention will be focused on birth cohorts after 1990.

Early childhood neurodevelopmental outcomes

Neurodevelopmental outcome assessments in studies of preterm infants have historically taken place in early childhood (18–30 months of age corrected for prematurity). At this age, a

Fetal and Neonatal Brain Injury, 4th edition, ed. David K. Stevenson, William E. Benitz, Philip Sunshine, Susan R. Hintz, and Maurice L. Druzin. Published by Cambridge University Press. © Cambridge University Press 2009.

battery of exams and tests can be performed, including neurosensory and neurologic exams to assess for blindness, deafness, and cerebral palsy (CP), and standardized cognitive and psychomotor assessments such as the Bayley Scales of Infant Development (BSID). Although these evaluations are important and informative, interpretation and comparison of studies are difficult. Many studies report on outcomes by adverse categories and frequently combine any adverse finding from various aspects of the overall visit to attain an "impaired" or "not impaired" status. The definitions of "adverse" outcomes may not be consistent across studies; indeed, the definitions of the individual components of "impairment" such as CP, blindness, deafness, and developmental delay may also differ across studies. In addition, increasing evidence suggests that assessments into later childhood, adolescence, and adulthood are critically important to understand the true functional and societal outcomes of former preterm infants [16]. Concerns regarding the predictive validity of early childhood cognitive assessment tools, changes in cognitive abilities over time, and an increasing recognition that numerous physical and environmental effects may modify recovery, reinforce the need for later assessments [17–19]. Some neurocognitive, executive function, and behavioral challenges may only be detected at school age. Even recognizing that such learning and attention problems may occur in preterm infants is a critical step to ensuring adequate support and services for families and teachers to help children achieve their best possible outcomes. Nonetheless, a substantial body of literature exists on early childhood neurologic and cognitive outcomes. An understanding of the range of neurodevelopmental outcomes, and the factors associated with adverse outcomes, is critically important both to the medical care team and to the family.

The Victoria Infant Collaborative Study Group (VICS Group)

The Victoria Infant Collaborative Study Group (VICS Group) has reported on several distinct cohorts of preterm infants born 23–27 + 6/7 weeks of gestation in the state of Victoria (Australia). For the purposes of this chapter, we will focus on the most recent published cohorts, born during 1991–1992 ($n = 401$), and 1997 ($n = 208$) [5,20]. Survivors received neurodevelopmental assessment at two years of age corrected for prematurity (1991–92: $n = 219$, 97% of survivors; 1997: $n = 148$, 99% of survivors). Importantly, and different from many other prospective follow-up studies, contemporaneous normal-birthweight (NBW) controls were enrolled and evaluated. Impairments assessed included blindness, deafness, and developmental delay defined as developmental quotient (DQ) on BSID Mental Developmental Index (MDI) 1 SD or more below the mean relative to NBW controls. Neurologic exam for CP was also performed; the authors described "severe" CP as unlikely ever to walk, and "moderate" CP as unable to walk at two years but likely to walk.

Neurodevelopmental outcomes of the VICS cohorts at 2 years of age corrected for prematurity are shown in Table 45.1.

Overall, there were no substantial differences between the two cohorts, with 11–12% diagnosed with CP, and approximately half of children in each of the cohorts with DQ more than 1 SD below the mean of NBW controls. Any neurosensory disability was observed in 45–50% of the preterm cohorts, but also in 20% of the NBW controls. However, moderate to severe disabilities were observed in 21% of the 1991–92 and 27.7% of the 1997 cohort, compared with only 3–4% of the NBW controls. Among only those born at 23–25 + 6/7 weeks' gestation, any neurosensory disability was observed in 58% of the 1991–92 and 56.5% of the 1997 cohort; moderate to severe disabilities were observed in 30% of the 1991–92 and 30.7% of the 1997 cohort. Thus, in these regional analyses, the rates of disability at 2 years among these most premature infants did not change appreciably over the two eras, yet survival increased from 38% in 1991–92 to 58% in 1997. For all ELBW infants in Victoria, moderate to severe neurosensory disabilities were reported in 19% of the 1991–92 and 26% of the 1997 cohorts, while developmental delay was reported in 42% of the 1991–92 and 47% of the 1997 cohort [5,6,11].

The EPICure Study

The EPICure Study is a population-based mortality, morbidity, and neurodevelopmental outcomes study. All infants born at 20–25 + 6/7 weeks' gestation from March through December 1995 were identified in all 276 maternity units in the United Kingdom and Ireland. This cohort is extraordinarily valuable, not least because it is truly population-based, but also because detailed data were collected regarding timing of death from the delivery room through hospitalization [7]. Of 1185 infants born at 22–25 + 6/7 weeks' gestation, 377 (32%) died in the delivery room, 314 survived to discharge. Neurodevelopmental assessment occurred at a median of 30 months of age corrected for prematurity for 283 of the 308 survivors [21,22]. Assessments included a detailed neurologic and functional examination, and administration of the BSID-II MDI and PDI, evaluated with respect to published norms. "Severe disability" was defined as likely to require the child to need assistance to perform daily activities according to neurologic, motor, sensory, and communication domains. Neurologic exam for CP was also performed, classified by limb involvement.

EPICure study 30-month outcomes are shown in Table 45.1 [21]. Approximately 76% of the cohort was free of any neuromotor disability and 66% had no hearing, vision, or communication disability, but only 36% of children were reported to have no developmental disability (BSID-II scores > 85). The proportion of children with disabilities did not appear to differ by gestational age; ≤ 23-week, 24-week, and 25-week groups had 27%, 30%, and 30% moderate to severe developmental disability (BSID MDI or PDI < 70), and 8%, 12%, and 9% were diagnosed with severe neuromotor disability, respectively. However, robust comparisons are difficult, given that patient numbers were quite small, particularly for the ≤ 23 week EGA group. This finding underscores the grave prognosis for survival among the most premature infants in this cohort;

Table 45.1. Early childhood neurodevelopmental outcomes of selected extremely preterm and extremely low-birthweight (ELBW) cohorts

	VICS 1991–92	VICS 1997	EPICure Study	Finnish ELBW	Rainbow 90–91	Rainbow 00–02
Study group description	23–27+6/7 weeks EGA	23–27+6/7 weeks EGA	22–25+6/7 weeks EGA	<1000 g BW, and >22 wk EGA	500–999 g	500–999 g
Birth cohort	1991–1992	1/1/97–12/31/97	March–December 1995	1/1/96–12/31/97	1/1/90–12/31/99	1/1/00–12/31/02
Age at follow-up corrected for prematurity	2 years	2 years	30 months	18 months (neuro) 24 months (BSID)	20 months	20 months
# (% follow-up)	219 (97%)	148 (99%)	283 (92%)	National cohort: 186–207 (89–100%) [a]Regional: 78 (93%)	467 (92%)	152 (92%)
Outcomes						
Blind	2.3%	2.7%	2.5%	0.5%	1%	1%
Deaf/require aids	0.9%	1.4%	1.8%	3.2%	6%	1%
Developmental impairment	DQ[b]≤1SD: 58% 1–2SD: 23% 2–3SD: 11% >3SD: 7.1%	DQ[b]≤1SD: 52% 1–2SD: 24% 2–3SD: 8.8% >3SD: 15%	MDI (n=231), PDI (n=225) 70–84: 34% <70: 30%	MDI mean (SD):Term: 106 (9.6) ELBW: 95 (13) < 85: 22% <70: 1.3%	MDI:<85: 42% <70: 24%	MDI:<85: 43% <70: 21%
Cerebral palsy or motor delay	CP: 11%	CP: 12%	All CP: 18% CP with severe disability: 5.3%	CP: 11% Other motor: 13%	CP: 13%	CP: 5%
Overall disability or impairment	All impairments: 45% Mod-severe: 21%	All impairments: 51% Mod-severe: 28%	Severe developmental, neuromotor, sensory or communication: 23%	All impairments: 58% Severe: 18%	Impaired: 35%	Impaired: 24%

	NRN 95–96 22–26 weeks	NRN 95–96 27–32 weeks	NRN 97–98 22–26 weeks	NRN 97–98 27–32 weeks	NRN 93–96 <25 weeks	NRN 96–99 <25 weeks
Study group description	401–1000 g, 22–26 weeks EGA	401–1000 g, 27–32 weeks EGA	401–1000 g, 22–26 weeks EGA	401–1000 g, 27–32 weeks EGA	501–1000 g, <25 weeks EGA	501–1000 g, <25 weeks EGA
Birth cohort	1/1/95–12/31/96	1/1/95–12/31/96	1/1/97–12/31/98	1/1/97–12/31/98	1/1/93–6/30/96	7/1/96–12/31/99
Age at follow-up corrected for prematurity	18–22 months	18–22 months	18–22 months	18–22 months	18–22 months	18–22 months
# (% follow-up)	716 (84%)	538 (81%)	910 (84%)	512 (82%)	366 (80%)	473 (89%)
Outcomes						
Blind	Unilateral: 2.5% Bilateral: 1.5%	Unilateral: 1.1% Bilateral: 0.4%	Unilateral: 1.6% Bilateral: 1.0%	Unilateral: 0.8% Bilateral: 0.4%	Bilateral: 2.3%	Bilateral: 1.1%
Deaf/require aids	Bilateral: 2.3%	Bilateral: 0.8%	Bilateral: 1.8%	Bilateral: 1.8%	Bilateral: 4.3%	Bilateral: 2.6%
Developmental impairment	MDI<70: 39%	MDI<70: 26%	MDI<70: 37%	MDI<70: 23%	MDI<70: 40%	MDI<70: 47%
Cerebral palsy or motor delay	All CP: 19% Mod-severe CP: 11%	All CP: 11% Mod-severe CP: 7.1%	All CP: 18% Mod-severe CP: 10%	All CP: 11% Mod-severe CP: 6.3%	All CP: 23%	All CP: 21%
Overall disability or impairment	NDI: 47%	NDI: 32%	NDI: 45%	NDI: 28%	NDI: 55%	NDI: 58%

Notes:

BSID, Bayley Scales of Infant Development;

BW, birthweight; CP, cerebral palsy; DQ, developmental quotient;

EGA, estimated gestational age; MDI, BSID Mental Developmental Index;

NDI, neurodevelopmental impairment (see text for definition);

PDI, BSID Psychomotor Developmental Index.

[a] Range of patient numbers for different parts of follow-up exam.

[b] DQ compared with a contemporaneous normal-birthweight control group.

only 18% of $\leq$ 23-week EGA infants admitted alive to a NICU survived to discharge, compared with 48% of 25-week EGA infants.

Finnish National ELBW Cohort

The Finnish ELBW Cohort consists of all ELBW infants of at least 22 weeks' EGA born in Finland from 1/1/1996 to 12/31/1997 [8,23]. Of 529 infants meeting weight and EGA criteria during this time, 351 were live-born, and 211 survived to 40 weeks' gestation equivalent. Three additional patients died in very early childhood. This population included 97% of all Finnish infants born before 27 weeks. Thus the Finnish cohort is overall more mature from the perspective of gestational age than previously discussed cohorts. In addition to obtaining full population-based mortality and in-hospital morbidity data, the cohort was followed at 18 $\pm$ 2 months of age corrected for prematurity for neurologic, hearing, vision, and communication assessments. Cerebral palsy was defined as motor impairment with spastic or dystonic tone, brisk reflexes, positive Babinski's sign, and persistent primitive reflexes. Children were characterized as "normal" if they had no impairments in any of the four assessed areas; "mildly" impaired if they had 1–2 impairments but were not blind, severely hearing-impaired, diagnosed with CP, or had seizures; and "severely" impaired if they had 3–4 impairments or any of the problems excluded in the "mild" category. A regional subcohort of infants born at Helsinki University Hospital ($n = 109$ live-born, $n = 84$ survivors to early childhood) also underwent BSID-II at 24 months of age corrected for prematurity. Healthy, full-term infants, born at Helsinki hospital contemporaneously with the ELBW infants, served as controls (75 of 126 invited controls were entered).

Outcomes are shown in Table 45.1. Normal motor development was reported for 76% (157/207), and normal verbal/communication assessments were reported in 53% (103/195), with 36% demonstrating mild verbal delay and 6% demonstrating severe delay. Ophthalmologic exam was considered completely normal in 77% (151/197), but the majority of those considered "abnormal" had strabismus ($n = 23$) or myopia ($n = 15$); 8% ($n = 14$) of the group required glasses. Although only 22% of the regional subcohort had BSID-II scores < 85 and 1% had scores < 70, this relatively low rate should be viewed with respect to the term control group BSID scores (mean 106, SD 9.6), which are higher than the published population norms. Thus, given that the mean ELBW for the subcohort (95) was a standard deviation below the control mean score, reliance on published norms may underestimate the extent of developmental delay at this time point for this population.

Rainbow Babies ELBW cohorts

Since the late 1970s, Maureen Hack and her colleagues at Rainbow Babies and Children's Hospital, Case Western Reserve University, have undertaken ground-breaking and seminal epidemiologic studies of early childhood, school-age, adolescent, and adult outcomes among VLBW and ELBW infants.

The complete body of work from this group is vast; therefore, for the purposes of this chapter, discussion of early childhood outcomes will focus on the most recent ELBW birth cohorts.

The Rainbow Babies cohorts from the 1990s and 2000–02 consist of all live-born infants with birthweights 500–999 g and without major anomalies born at a single large center in the United States [24–26]. Of 749 ELBW infants born alive in the 1990s, 508 (68%) survived to 20 months; 83 (11%) were not offered assisted ventilation because they were considered non-viable due to immaturity. Of 233 ELBW infants born alive in 2000–02, 165 (71%) survived to 20 months; 26 (11%) were not offered assisted ventilation. Thus it is important to recognize that the Rainbow cohorts are defined by weight, not extreme prematurity, and that a birthweight of less than 500 grams was an exclusion criterion for these studies. The cohorts were followed at 20 months of age corrected for prematurity, and the visit included neurosensory assessment and administration of the BSID MDI and PDI. Cerebral palsy was defined as a moderate to severe persistent disorder of movement and posture. "Major neurologic impairment" was defined as CP, hypotonia, hypertonia, or shunt-dependent hydrocephalus with or without neurologic abnormalities. Overall "neurodevelopmental impairment" was defined as any major neurologic impairment, unilateral or bilateral blindness or deafness (requiring hearing aid), or BSID MDI < 70.

Outcomes for both cohorts are shown in Table 45.1. There were significant differences between the two cohorts on unadjusted analyses, favoring the 2000–02 group [26]. The rate of neurosensory impairment (major neurologic impairment or blindness or deafness) was 23% in the 1990s cohort, but only 9% in the 2000–02 cohort. Adjusting for differences between the cohorts in gestational age only, survival without neurodevelopmental impairment was more likely in the later cohort (OR 1.5, 95% CI 1.1–2.0; absolute observed rates = 41% in the 1990s, 50% in 2000–02). There were also significant increased rates of antenatal steroid use and cesarean section, and decreased rates of postnatal steroid use, sepsis, and severe cranial ultrasonographic abnormality between the cohort periods. After adjusting for these variables, the observed increase in impairment-free survival between the two cohorts was no longer significant, suggesting that the findings could be explained by changes in perinatal and neonatal management. Notably, this apparent improvement in outcomes between the 1990s and 2000–02 is in contrast with analyses by the Rainbow group and others demonstrating increased survival but worse or unchanged neurodevelopmental outcomes between birth cohorts in earlier eras [26–29]. This observation is an encouraging finding when considering the potential outcomes of current and future ELBW and extremely preterm infants.

NICHD Neonatal Research Network Follow-Up Study Group

The National Institute of Child Health and Human Development (NICHD) Neonatal Research Network (NRN) was initiated in 1986 as a multicenter effort in the United States with the main objective of providing a registry of uniformly collected baseline and morbidity and mortality data to provide the basis for planning and implementing clinical trials. The NICHD NRN Follow-up Study Group was later added to provide neurodevelopmental follow-up to ELBW survivors 401–1000 g. Numerous analyses have been published by this Follow-Up group, but for the purposes of this chapter we will focus on neurodevelopmental outcomes of the most recent birth cohorts over a range of gestational ages [29–31].

Membership in the multicenter NRN is through a mechanism of competitive grant application on a 6-year cycle. Participating institutions are major academic tertiary care centers and regional referral centers; thus these patients do not represent a regional or population-based cohort, but likely includes a group of patients at the more critical end of the spectrum of illness. During the period 1993–99, infants from participating centers were eligible for inclusion in the general database if they were < 1500 g, admitted to the institution within 14 days of age. The NRN Follow-Up study database included neurodevelopmental follow-up at 18–22 months of age corrected for prematurity for ELBW survivors (401–1000 g birthweight). Of 2502 ELBW infants born 1/1/93–12/31/94 and cared for at a NRN site, 1586 (63%) survived to discharge (22–25 week: 55%; 27–32 week: 82%). Of 2357 ELBW infants born 1/1/95–12/31/96, 1555 (66%) survived to discharge (22–26 week: 56%; 27–32 week: 87%). Of 2539 ELBW infants born 1/1/97–12/31/98, 1735 (68%) survived to discharge (22–26 week: 61%; 27–32 week: 86%). The cohorts were followed at 18–22 months of age corrected for prematurity, and visits included neurosensory and gross motor functional assessments (GMFCS), and administration of BSID MDI and PDI. Examinations were performed by experienced, certified examiners, who were trained in annual 2-day workshops to assure reliability. Cerebral palsy was defined as a non-progressive central nervous system disorder with abnormal muscle tone in at least one extremity and abnormal control of movement or posture. Moderate to severe CP included children who were non-ambulatory or required assistive devices. Neurodevelopmental impairment (NDI) was defined as MDI or PDI < 70, moderate to severe CP, bilateral blindness, or bilateral deafness requiring amplification.

Outcomes for the 1995–96 and 1997–98 overall ELBW cohorts, stratified by EGA, are shown in Table 45.1 [30]. In the 1993–94 cohort (not shown in the table), moderate to severe CP was diagnosed in 12% and 7.8% of the 22–26-week and 27–32-week groups, respectively. Adjusting for confounding variables in regression analyses, rates of any CP or moderate to severe CP did not change over time, but not surprisingly rates were significantly different between the gestational age groups. In the 1993–94 cohort, MDI < 70 was found in 42% and 30%, and NDI in 50% and 40%, of the 22–26-week and 27–32-week groups, respectively. In regression analyses, a significant decrease in rates of MDI < 70 and NDI over the three eras was noted, but this was primarily explained by differences between rates in the earliest (1993–94) compared

with the second (1995–96) eras. As with the Rainbow cohorts, the NRN group noted significant increases in rates of antenatal steroid use and cesarean section, and decreased rates of postnatal steroid use over the three eras. Although the rates of CP of any severity may be concerning, gross motor function in many of these children may in fact be relatively normal. In separate analyses of GMFCS findings in ELBW survivors born 8/1/95–2/1/98 in the NRN Follow-Up study, many children with CP had normal or mildly delayed gross motor function [31]. The ability to walk 10 steps independently and fluently (GMFCS level 0, normal) or sit with hands free, walk with hands held, and cruise (GMFCS level 1, mildly delayed) was demonstrated by 100% children with spastic monoplegia, 69% of children with hemiplegia, 78% with diplegia, and 38% with triplegia.

The substantial rates of impairment in the lowest EGA range prompted further investigation of outcomes among the most immature infants in the NRN Follow-Up group [29]. Outcomes of infants < 25 weeks EGA born 1993–99 are shown in Table 45.1, stratified by eras (born 1/1/1993–6/30/1996 and 7/1/1996–12/31/1999). Survival to discharge rates were 40% (473/1170) in the first era and 43% (544/1260) in the second era. Despite more aggressive perinatal management, with increased use of antenatal steroids, antenatal antibiotics and cesarean section delivery between the eras, no significant improvements in neurodevelopmental outcomes were observed; in fact, in multivariate analyses, membership in the later birth cohort was associated with significantly greater odds of MDI < 70. However, use of postnatal steroids and rates of bronchopulmonary dysplasia (BPD) were higher in the second era as well, which are factors known to be associated with adverse outcomes in premature infants. Although these variables were included in regression analyses, other aggressive and perhaps untested management strategies may have been applied; such approaches and interventions, and their downstream effects, may have represented unknown variables that could confound analyses. Given the hopeful early neurodevelopmental findings from recent ELBW cohorts [26], analyses of more recent extremely preterm cohorts would be of great interest.

Risk factors associated with neurodevelopmental sequelae

A number of perinatal, neonatal, and sociodemographic variables have been linked with early childhood neurologic and developmental disability in preterm infants (Table 45.2). Outcomes may be influenced by an enormous array of biologic, environmental, and iatrogenic factors. Furthermore, the risk factors themselves may be tightly associated with other variables, and one factor may modify or potentiate the effect of others; therefore, analyses can be complex and challenging to interpret despite the efforts of investigators to consider confounders. Some studies have suggested that little of the variance in outcomes can even be explained by identified major risk factors [32]; thus, unknown or currently unknowable

Table 45.2. Factors reported to be associated with adverse early childhood neurodevelopmental outcomes among ELBW or extremely preterm infants

Cerebral palsy/motor impairment	Developmental/cognitive impairment
Significant brain abnormalities (see text)	Significant brain abnormalities (see text)
No antenatal steroids	Male gender
Early postnatal hospital transfer	Social risk
Male gender	Infection
Infection	Severe necrotizing enterocolitis
Bronchopulmonary dysplasia	Bronchopulmonary dysplasia
Postnatal dexamethasone	Postnatal dexamethasone

factors may be important determinants or modifiers of neurodevelopmental outcomes. Nevertheless, several variables have been consistently recognized to be associated with adverse neuromotor outcomes and overall impairment in early childhood among ELBW and very preterm infants. Risk factors for developmental or cognitive delay are more difficult, in part due to differences among studies with respect to definition of delay, and to social–environmental interactions.

The objectives of neurodevelopmental outcomes studies are not only to provide information to help better predict outcomes, but also to identify factors associated with adverse outcomes that may be modifiable. Recognition of such factors serves as a stimulus for further translational and clinical research, with the hope of uncovering the biologic basis of the connection, and with the ultimate goal of changing care paradigms to improve long-term outcomes for preterm infants.

Brain injury

Cranial ultrasound

Cranial ultrasound (CUS) has been used to image preterm infant brain injury since the late 1970s [33,34]. Given the modality's portability, ease of repeatability, non-invasive technique, and the development of a standardized grading system for intraventricular hemorrhage (IVH) [35], CUS quickly became the neuroimaging standard of care (see also Chapter 24). Although many seem to rely heavily on simply the presence of grade 3 IVH, intraparenchymal hemorrhage (IPH), or cystic PVL to counsel families about the neurodevelopmental outcomes of their preterm infants, the complexity of interpretation and limitations of CUS should give clinicians cause for prudence and careful consideration.

CUS abnormalities and early childhood neurodevelopmental outcomes

Virtually every major study of early childhood neurodevelopmental outcomes among preterm and ELBW infants has confirmed a strong association between major CUS abnormalities and adverse neurodevelopmental outcomes. Definitions of CUS abnormalities as well as specific outcomes differ among studies; however, most consider parenchymal hemorrhage, or

ventricular dilation, or cystic changes, regardless of laterality or extent of the findings, to be severe abnormalities [22,24,29,30]. In some, persistent periventricular echodensity or "flaring" is included [36,37]. This diagnosis may be based on a single CUS, either the "worst" or the "final" imaging study, but a few prospective cohorts, notably that of deVries et al. [37], required serial imaging.

The EPIPAGE study followed 22–32-week EGA infants born in nine French regions during 1997 to 2 years of age [36]. Significant CUS abnormalities were associated with CP; 57% of those with cystic PVL were diagnosed with CP, but only 24% of those with any presumed white-matter injury (WMI) defined as PVL, ventricular dilation, or intraparenchymal hemorrhage or cyst. The EPICure study also found that severe CUS abnormalities were strongly independently associated with CP and severe motor disability [22]. Of importance, when children with motor disability were excluded, severe CUS abnormality was not significantly correlated with BSID MDI score. Hack et al. also found that severe CUS abnormality was significantly associated with neurologic abnormality at 20 months, but not with poor cognitive outcome among patients without significant neurologic impairment [24]. In the National Brain Hemorrhage Study (NBHS) cohort of infants < 2000 g birthweight, parenchymal lesions or ventricular enlargement (PL/VE) on neonatal CUS was independently associated with severe motor disability at 2 years [38]. Although severe cognitive impairment also appeared to be related to PL/VE, this association was not significant after controlling for differences in motor performance. Studies of ELBW and extremely preterm infants from the NICHD NRN have shown grade 3 or 4 intracranial hemorrhage or cystic PVL to be significantly associated with CP and overall neurodevelopmental impairment at 18–22 months [29,30]. These studies also suggested severe CUS abnormalities to be associated with BSID MDI < 70, but patients with severe neuromotor and neurosensory impairment were not excluded from this group; thus cognitive impairment was not assessed separately from motor disability. The EPIPAGE group also reported that severe CUS abnormalities were independently associated with decreasing developmental quotient [39]. In extremely detailed serial CUS studies of patients < 36 weeks in a single center, deVries et al. found that the sensitivity and specificity of major CUS abnormalities for CP at 2 years was an impressive 76% and 95% for patients < 32 weeks EGA. Of importance, among those with major CUS abnormalities who developed CP, approximately 30% were only noted after 28 days. Negative predictive value of major CUS abnormalities for CP was 99%, although positive predictive value was only 48% for < 32-week EGA infants. Major CUS abnormalities were not strongly associated with cognitive delay at 2 years.

Challenges to interpretation

In skilled hands and with meticulous technical attention, much can be seen beyond IVH by CUS. However, CUS is an operator-dependent modality, imaging procedures and views differ among institutions and studies, and there is no uniform approach to serial imaging protocols. For instance, the cerebellum is best seen by US using mastoid fontanel (MF) views, and the trigone and occipital horns of the lateral ventricles are best seen by posterior fontanel (PF) views; however, some still rely solely on the anterior fontanel (AF) views for preterm imaging [40]. Cerebellar hemorrhage may be a more common complication among preterm infants than previously thought, and appears to be associated with long-term neurodevelopmental disabilities [41,42]. Without serial imaging, transient lesions may be missed, including echodense periventricular lesions or collapsing small cystic lesions, both of which may represent evolving WMI [37,43]. Isolated intraparenchymal hemorrhages can be seen by carefully performed CUS; characteristics of the hemorrhage including laterality, midline shift, and extent may be important to predict adverse neurodevelopmental outcomes [44,45]. Nevertheless, studies of ELBW and extremely preterm infants suggest that approximately 30–40% of those with CP or neuromotor impairment in early childhood did not have significant CUS abnormalities [3,24], and normal CUS do not ensure normal neurodevelopmental outcomes [46].

There is little doubt that CUS can be a more valuable predictive diagnostic tool with optimal timing and imaging protocols. But given the inconsistencies in procedures, challenges to interpretation of resulting data, and the extraordinary array of complex variables that influence outcomes, reliance solely on CUS findings – or any single factor – to attempt "perfect prediction" of neurodevelopmental outcome is inappropriate. More detailed measures of the extent of significant parenchymal and WMI seen by neonatal CUS certainly may improve risk assessment for motor and developmental impairment in early childhood [37,44,47], but advanced imaging techniques such as magnetic resonance imaging (MRI) could substantially enhance our capabilities.

Magnetic resonance imaging

Brain MRI has been used more extensively in recent years among preterm infants, both for research and for clinical indications. Availability of MR-compatible infant equipment, monitoring devices, and isolettes [48–50], and recognition that non-sedated imaging is possible and indeed customary in many institutions [51,52], have made MRI a more routine advanced neonatal neuroimaging method. MRI allows for a more comprehensive and detailed picture of the brain, and better delineation of deep structure and cortical injury than CUS. Potentially most important however, MRI provides improved detection of subtle or diffuse WMI [53–55], which appears to be common among preterm infants at term [56,57] and may prove to be critically important to understanding the structure–function relationship of the developing preterm brain and influences on later neuromotor and cognitive outcomes. Advanced MR imaging in preterm infants at near term have shown that even subtle MR-detected WMI is associated with reduced total-brain and gray-matter volumes, reduced cerebellar volume, and reduced basal ganglia and thalamic volume [58–62]; volume reductions which, in turn, are associated with developmental impairment in middle and late childhood among preterm infants [63,64].

MRI findings and early childhood neurodevelopmental outcomes

Increasing numbers of studies have shown that MRI may be an important adjuvant technique to CUS, or superior to CUS, in predicting neurodevelopmental outcome for preterm infants. Among preterm infants with unilateral parenchymal hemorrhage on CUS, abnormal myelination of the posterior limb of the internal capsule (PLIC) on MRI at near term has been reported to be helpful in prognosis of hemiplegia and high-tone motor deficits [65,66]. Notably, although the cerebellum may be seen by appropriate views on CUS, MRI may distinguish important topographic features of cerebellar injury that could help to predict severity of neuromotor and developmental impairment [42]. In preterm infants with inhomogeneous periventricular echodensities on CUS, neonatal MRI may not only clarify the extent and severity of WMI, but predict early childhood MRI injury pattern as well as motor and visual outcomes at 18 months [67,68].

Early studies attempting to compare term-equivalent MRI with CUS predictive capabilities were primarily small, single-center studies, and timing and approach to CUS differed [51,66,68]. However, these studies suggested that MRI may better predict early childhood neuromotor outcome than CUS. The largest study to date was a prospective multicenter effort comparing serial CUS with near-term MRI findings and their association with 2-year outcomes in 167 infants < 30 weeks EGA [52]. This study demonstrated that moderate to severe white-matter abnormalities on near-term MRI were significantly associated with neuromotor delay and cerebral palsy, independent of CUS findings and other risk factors. Increasing WMI severity was also linearly related to worsening BSID MDI scores, but an independent association of moderate to severe WMI with severe cognitive delay was not reached. This study was a substantial and promising step toward distinguishing neuroimaging techniques and injury that can better predict outcomes in this vulnerable population.

Challenges and future directions

Current guidelines do not recommend near-term MRI for routine preterm infant neuroimaging [69]. But recent studies in preterm infants continue to indicate that brain injury or structural abnormalities are better delineated by MRI than by CUS, and emerging evidence suggests that MRI may provide prognostic advantages at least in some situations. Future studies should focus further on identifying specific high-risk groups of preterm infants for which MRI would definitively improve prediction of neurodevelopmental outcomes. But this task will require much larger patient numbers. Of enormous interest is the mechanistic connection between WMI and cognitive delay in preterm infants, supported by studies demonstrating that WMI on near-term MRI is associated with deep gray-matter volume reduction [60,61], and that even mild WMI on MRI in later childhood is associated with lower IQ and total impairment [70]. Quantitative MRI techniques such as diffusion tensor imaging and tractography promise to help clarify this pathway [71].

Antenatal, demographic, and social risk variables

Events and interventions prior to delivery may have significant influences on extremely preterm neurodevelopmental outcomes. Antenatal steroid treatment appears to be protective with respect to adverse early childhood outcomes including CP, PDI < 70, neurologic abnormalities, and motor impairment [22–24,30,70,72]. Antenatal steroids have been shown not only to reduce severity of respiratory distress syndrome and improve survival, but also to protect against IVH [72]. However, analyses indicate that the protective effect of antenatal steroids is independent of severe CUS abnormalities, suggesting an additional mechanism may be at play. Early postnatal hospital transfer (within 24 hours) was identified as a risk factor for CP and severe motor disability by the EPICure study [22]. Although antenatal steroid treatment was less likely among these patients and significant CUS abnormality was more likely, transfer within 24 hours remained a significant risk factor independent of those variables, underscoring the importance of regionalized care for these extremely vulnerable patients [73].

A distinct male disadvantage for death, short-term morbidities, and neurodevelopmental outcomes has been frequently noted for ELBW and extremely preterm infants [21,22,24,30,74]. Male gender has been reported to be an independent risk factor for early childhood cognitive delay, cerebral palsy, and motor impairment. The reasons for this gender-specific vulnerability are obscure, but measurable risk factors and events do not appear to confer differential risk for adverse neurodevelopmental outcomes for boys [74]. Fetal hormonal exposures and genetic influences are important areas for further research.

Measures of social risk have been frequently reported to be associated with significant early childhood cognitive impairment [22,24,29,30,75]. Some investigators have developed cumulative social risk scores based on several variables [24], but many others assess social risk primarily by level of maternal education. Racial or demographic background have also been identified as risk factors for cognitive delay independent of maternal education; racial factors are likely to be markers for reduced socioeconomic circumstances in some cohorts, but not in all [23]. Given that environmental factors may contribute to the effects of social risk on outcome, early developmental intervention and parenting programs may positively modify the adverse influence of social risk [76].

Other major neonatal morbidities associated with adverse outcomes

Preterm infants with bronochopulmonary dysplasia (BPD), usually defined as oxygen requirement at 36 weeks post-conceptional age, have been shown to be at higher risk for all components of neurodevelopmental impairment in early childhood [77–79]. Infants with BPD are more likely to be of lower gestational age and to have other complications such as sepsis and IVH, but in large analyses taking multiple confounders into account, BPD remains an independent risk factor for neuromotor and general cognitive delay. There are a number of postulated explanations for the association of BPD with later neurodevelopmental impairment. In the vulnerable ELBW population, BPD is likely a marker for severity of illness, which is difficult to quantitate in analyses. Approximately 25% of ELBW infants are mechanically ventilated for 40 days or longer [78], and these infants in particular may experience frequent, though short, episodes of hypoxemia. Given the vulnerability of the preterm brain, such desaturation events coupled with other clinical complications may interact to produce neurologic injury during a critical stage of development.

The adverse effects of BPD are challenging to separate from those of postnatal steroids. Although treatment with postnatal steroids, particularly dexamethasone, was studied in an attempt to reduce BPD and thus neurodevelopmental impairment, numerous reports subsequently recognized the independent association of cerebral palsy, neuromotor delay, and developmental and cognitive impairment with postnatal steroid treatment [80]. Steroids may influence neurodevelopmental outcome by inhibition of brain growth [81], perhaps through inhibition of growth factors and facilitation of apoptosis [82]. The American Academy of Pediatrics and the Canadian Paediatric Society do not recommend postnatal steroid treatment for preterm infants to prevent or treat BPD outside randomized controlled trials [83]. However, it should be noted that further analysis by Doyle *et al.* has demonstrated that the adverse effect of postnatal dexamethasone on death or CP is modified by risk of BPD [84]: among infants at very high risk for BPD (> 65%), postnatal dexamethasone actually decreased the risk for death or CP. Furthermore, treatment with other corticosteroids such as hydrocortisone may not adversely affect brain growth and developmental or neurodevelopmental outcome [70,85].

Preterm infants are also at high risk for infection, with more than 50% of ELBW infants treated for at least one episode of culture-proven or clinically suspected sepsis during hospitalization [86]. Both neonatal sepsis and severe necrotizing enterocolitis (NEC) are associated with adverse motor, cognitive, and growth outcomes in early childhood [87,88]. White-matter injury is a key component in the path from infection or NEC to poor neurodevelopmental outcome. The inherent vulnerability of the pre-oligodendroglial cell appears to be central to the sequence of events that place preterm infants at high risk for adverse outcome [56,57]. Factors known to be injurious or directly toxic to developing white matter, such as systemic and cerebral hypoperfusion, ischemia–reperfusion, and cytokine elucidation during a systemic inflammatory response, can be expected during the clinical course of infection or NEC. The potential mechanistic links between WMI and gray-matter volume reduction in the developing preterm infant brain have been discussed earlier; the concept of reduced connectivity will likely prove to be extremely important in explaining the association as research continues.

The premature infant is in a period of dramatic axonal growth and elongation. Both axonal and subplate neuronal injury could result in reduction of important and complex connections during a crucial period in brain development, impairing neuronal differentiation and, subsequently, gray-matter growth [89,90]. In the case of severe NEC requiring surgery, it may be not only that inflammatory responses and perioperative events such as hypotension and hyperventilation are important, but that surgery itself could be a major contributing factor to adverse neurodevelopmental outcomes. Results from the VICS Group revealed that surgery in the neonatal period requiring general anesthesia is associated with adverse neurosensory outcome at 5 years among extremely preterm infants [91]. Animal models have suggested that some anesthetic agents are neurotoxic, associated with apoptosis and injury to the developing brain [92,93].

Because neurodevelopmental outcomes for the complex preterm infant are influenced by multiple factors, some investigators have endeavored to develop scoring systems using several morbidities to improve prediction of outcomes. In results from the Trial of Indomethacin Prophylaxis in Preterm infants, Schmidt et al. developed a scoring method using the presence of BPD, severe retinopathy of prematurity (ROP), and severe brain injury by CUS to predict the combined outcome of death or NDI (CP, cognitive delay, bilateral blindness, or bilateral hearing amplification) at 18 months [94]. Overall, the outcome was observed in 35% of the cohort surviving to 36 weeks postconceptional age (PCA), but among those in which none of the morbidities was present, death or NDI was observed in only 19%, compared with 42% in those with one morbidity, 67% in those with two, and 87% in those with all three. Doyle et al. and the VICS Group also reported on a predictive scoring system for survival free of major sensorineural disability at 5 years of age using presence of PVL, major hemorrhage on CUS, any surgery, exposure to postnatal steroids, or BPD as morbidities [91]. The investigators found that 96% of the group had survived without major disability if none of the neonatal morbidities was present, compared with 83% in those with one, 53% in those with two, and 33% in those with three.

Outcomes in later childhood and beyond

Although a thorough discussion is not within the scope of this chapter, no review of neurodevelopmental outcomes of ELBW and very preterm infants would be complete without noting the critical importance of truly long-term follow-up for these high-risk children to later childhood, adolescence, and beyond [95–97]. Children born extremely preterm or ELBW continue to have motor and cognitive disabilities in childhood, as well as more subtle functional and adaptive impairments. Delineation of some of these problems may not even be reasonably undertaken until 5–8 years of age, and the true impact of these impairments may not be felt until later school age [98]. Follow-up studies at 5–8 years from the Finnish National Cohort [99], EPICure [100], and Rainbow Babies [101] have

shown CP in 13–19%, significant motor skills problems or major disabilities in 20–27%, and moderate to severe cognitive impairment in 20–38%. Families report substantial functional limitations, including emotional delay, trouble understanding or communicating, and need for medication or equipment; needs for special services were significantly greater than for the normal birthweight (NBW) control group. Impairment in academic (32%) and adaptive skills (48%) have also been reported among ELBW children, and are significantly more frequent than in NBW controls [102]. In an ELBW or < 28-week EGA cohort at 8 years ($n = 275$), Anderson et al. reported significant impairment across all tested cognitive and educational abilities compared with NBW controls [103]. Given these concerning findings, it would seem reasonable that long-term follow-up, at least to school age, should be prospectively incorporated into any randomized controlled trial involving preterm infants.

These types of cognitive and educational measures provide important information about the community supports and special services that may be required for children born very preterm and their families. But they do not necessarily present a broader picture of "life outcome" for these children, and therefore may be viewed as overly pessimistic [16]. Assessments of quality of life for former premature infants at adolescence and young adulthood, from the perspective of both the child and the mother, appear to be more positive than earlier maternal assessments even if impairments exist [104]. These findings underscore the importance of recognizing that the larger implications of preterm birth certainly differ among families and children, and may change over time.

Conclusions

Despite advances in perinatal and neonatal management, and improvement in survival, early childhood neurodevelopmental outcomes of extremely preterm and ELBW infants remain guarded. Factors associated with adverse neurodevelopmental outcomes include demographic and socioeconomic variables, but also include numerous neonatal morbidities that may be modifiable. A continued meticulous approach to follow-up to early childhood is needed for these extraordinarily vulnerable infants. But it is also clear that more routine longer-term follow-up to school age and beyond is required to understand the broader implications of extremely low birthweight and very preterm birth, and to evaluate the impact of our interventions during the neonatal period. Crucially, we must improve our recognition and understanding of subtle brain injury associated with adverse outcomes, and the factors associated with such injury. Implementation of more detailed and comprehensive approaches to routine CUS protocols, and expanded use of advanced neuroimaging techniques such as MRI, will certainly assist in this endeavor. A better understanding of the mechanisms and pathways of brain injury and impaired development will inevitably lead us to opportunities for neuroprotective strategies for these extremely high-risk infants.

References

1. Martin JA, Hamilton BE, Sutton PD, et al. Births: final data for 2004. *Natl Vital Stat Rep* 2006; **55** (1). www.cdc.gov/nchs/data/nvsr/nvsr55. Accessed April, 2008.

2. Fanaroff AA, Stoll BJ, Wright LL, et al. Trends in neonatal morbidity and mortality for very low birthweight infants. *Am J Obstet Gynecol* 2007; **196**: 147.e1–8.

3. Anthony S, den Ouden L, Brand R, et al. Changes in perinatal care and survival in very preterm and extremely preterm infants in the Netherlands between 1983–1995. *Eur J Obstet Gyn Reprod Biol* 2004; **112**: 170–7.

4. Serenius F, Ewald U, Farooqui A, et al. Short-term outcome after active perinatal management at 23–25 weeks of gestation: a study from two Swedish tertiary care centres. Part 2: infant survival. *Acta Paediatr* 2004; **93**: 1081–9.

5. Doyle LW, VICS Group. Neonatal intensive care at borderline viability: is it worth it? *Early Hum Dev* 2004; **80**: 103–13.

6. Doyle LW. Evaluation of neonatal intensive care for extremely-low-birth-weight infants. *Semin Fetal Neonatal Med* 2006; **11**: 139–45.

7. Costeloe K, Hennessy E, Gibson AT, et al. The EPICure Study: outcomes to discharge from hospital for infants born at the threshold of viability. *Pediatrics* 2000; **106**: 659–71.

8. Tommiska V, Helnonen K, Lehtonen L, et al. No improvement in outcome of nationwide extremely low birth weight infant populations between 1996–1997 and 1999–2000. *Pediatrics* 2007; **119**: 29–36.

9. Doyle LW, Morley CJ, Halliday J. Prediction of survival for preterm births: data on the quality of survival are needed. *BMJ* 2000; **320**: 648.

10. de Leeuw R, Cuttini M, Nadai M, et al. Treatment choices for extremely preterm infants: an international perspective. *J Pediatr* 2000; **137**: 608–16.

11. Doyle LW for the VICS Group. Changing availability of neonatal intensive care for extremely low birth weight infant in Victoria over two decades. *Med J Aust* 2004; **181**: 136–9.

12. Bode MM, O'Shea TM, Metzguer KR, et al. Perinatal regionalization and neonatal mortality in North Carolina, 1968–1994. *Am J Obstet Gynecol* 2001; **184**: 1302–7.

13. Petrou S. The economic consequence of preterm birth during the first 10 years of life. *BJOG* 2005; **112**: 10–15.

14. Clements KM, Barfield WD, Ayadi MF, et al. Preterm birth-associated cost of early intervention service: an analysis by gestational age. *Pediatrics* 2007; **119**: e866–74.

15. Doyle LW, the VICS Group. Evaluation of neonatal intensive care for extremely low birth weight infants in Victoria over two decades: II. Efficiency. *Pediatrics* 2004; **113**: 510–14.

16. Saigal S, Rosenbaum P. What matters in the long term: reflections on the context of adult outcomes versus detailed measures in childhood. *Semin Fetal Neonatal Med* 2007; **12**: 417–22.

17. Hack M, Taylor HG, Drotar D, et al. Poor predictive validity of the Bayley Scales of Infant Development for cognitive function of extremely low birth weight children at school age. *Pediatrics* 2005; **116**: 333–41.

18. Ment LR, Vohr B, Allan W, et al. Change in cognitive function over time in very low-birth-weight infants. *JAMA* 2003; **289**: 705–11.

19. Kilbride HW, Thurstad K, Daily DK. Preschool outcome of less than 801 gram preterm infants compared with full-term siblings. *Pediatrics* 2004; **13**: 742–7.

20. The Victorian Infant Collaborative Study Group. Outcome at 2 years of children 23–27 weeks' gestation born in Victoria in 1991–92. *J Paediatr Child Health* 1997; **33**: 161–5.

21. Wood NS, Marlow N, Costeloe K, et al. Neurologic and developmental disability after extremely preterm birth. *N Engl J Med* 2000; **343**: 378–84.

22. Wood NS, Costeloe K, Gibson AT, et al. The EPICure study: association and antecedents of neurological and developmental disability at 30 months of age following extremely preterm birth. *Arch Dis Child Fetal Neonatal Ed* 2005; **90**: F134–40.

23. Tommiska V, Heinonen K, Kero P, et al. A national two-year follow-up study of extremely low birthweight infants born in 1996–1997. *Arch Dis Child Fetal Neonatal Ed* 2003; **88**: F29–35.

24. Hack M, Wilson-Costello D, Friedman H, et al. Neurodevelopment and predictors of outcomes of children with birth weights of less than 1000 g 1992–1995.

Arch Pediatr Adolesc Med 2000; **154**: 725–31.

25. Wilson-Costello D, Friedman H, Minich N, et al. Improved survival rates with increased neurodevelopmental disability for extremely low birth weight infants in the 1990s. *Pediatrics* 2005; **115**: 997–1003.

26. Wilson-Costello D, Friedman H, Minich N, et al. Improved neurodevelopmental outcomes for extremely low birth weight infants in 2000–2002. *Pediatrics* 2007; **119**: 37–45.

27. Emsley HCA, Wardle SP, Sims DG, et al. Increased survival and deteriorating developmental outcomes in 23–25 week old gestation infants, 1990–1994 compared with 1984–1989. *Arch Dis Child Fetal Neonatal Ed* 1998; **78**: F99–104.

28. Hintz SR, Poole WK, Fanaroff AA, et al. Changes in mortality and morbidity among infants born at less than 25 weeks during the post-surfactant era. *Arch Dis Child Fetal Neonatal Ed* 2005; **90**: F128–33.

29. Hintz SR, Kendrick DE, Vohr BR, et al. Changes in neurodevelopmental outcomes at 18–22 months corrected age among infants born at less than 25 weeks gestation 1993–1999. *Pediatrics* 2005; **115**: 1645–51.

30. Vohr BR, Wright LL, Poole SK, et al. Neurodevelopmental outcomes of extremely low birth weight infants < 32 weeks' gestation between 1993 and 1998. *Pediatrics* 2005; **116**: 635–43.

31. Vohr BR, Msall ME, Wilson D, et al. Spectrum of gross motor function in extremely low birth weight children with cerebral palsy at 18 months of age. *Pediatrics* 2005; **116**: 123–9.

32. Ambalavanan N, Nelson KG, Alexander G, et al. Prediction of neurologic morbidity in extremely low birth weight infants. *J Perinatol* 2000; **20**: 496–503.

33. Pape KE, Blackwell RJ, Cusick G, et al. Ultrasound detection of brain damage in preterm infants. *Lancet* 1979; **1**: 1261–4.

34. Slovis TL, Kuhn LR. Real-time sonography of the brain through the anterior fontanelle. *AJR Am J Roentgenol* 1981; **136**: 277–86.

35. Papile LA, Burstein J, Burstein R, et al. Incidence and evolution of subependymal and intraventricular hemorrhage: a study of infants with birth weight less than 1500 gm. *J Pediatr* 1978; **92**: 529–34.

36. Ancel PY, Livinec F, Larroque B, *et al.* Cerebral palsy among very preterm children in relation to gestational age and neonatal ultrasound abnormalities: the EPIPAGE Cohort Study. *Pediatrics* 2006; **117**: 828–35.

37. de Vries LS, Van Haastert IC, Rademaker KJ, *et al.* Ultrasound abnormalities preceding cerebral palsy in high-risk preterm infants. *J Pediatr* 2004; **144**: 815–20.

38. Pinto-Martin JA, Whitaker AH, Felman JF, *et al.* Relation of cranial ultrasound abnormalities in low-birthweight infants to motor or cognitive performance at 2, 6, and 9 years. *Develop Med Child Neurol* 1999; **41**: 826–33.

39. Fily A, Pierrat V, Delporte V, *et al.* Factors associated with neurodevelopmental outcome at 2 years after very preterm birth: the population-based Nord-Pas-de-Calais EPIPAGE cohort. *Pediatrics* 2006; **117**: 357–66.

40. DiSalvo DN. A new view of the neonatal brain: clinical utility of supplemental neurologic US imaging windows. *RadioGraphics* 2001; **21**: 943–55.

41. Limperopoulos C, duPlessis AJ. Disorders of cerebellar growth and development. *Curr Opin Pediatr* 2006; **18**: 621–7.

42. Limperopoulos C, Bassan H, Gauvreau K, *et al.* Does cerebellar injury in premature infants contribute to the high prevalence of long-term cognitive, learning and behavioral disability in survivors? *Pediatrics* 2007; **120**: 584–93.

43. Pierrat V, Duquennoy C, van Haastert IC, *et al.* Ultrasound diagnosis and neurodevelopmental outcome of localized and extensive cystic periventricular leucomalacia. *Arch Dis Child Fetal Neonatal Ed* 2001; **84**: F151–56.

44. Bassan H, Benson C, Limperopoulos C, *et al.* Ultrasonographic features and severity scoring of periventricular hemorrhagic infarction in relation to risk factors and outcome. *Pediatrics* 2006; **117**: 2111–18.

45. Bassan H, Limperopoulos C, Visconti K, *et al.* Neurodevelopmental outcome in survivors of periventricular hemorrhagic infarction. *Pediatrics* 2007; **120**: 785–92.

46. Laptook AR, O'Shea RM, Shankaran S, *et al.* Adverse neurodevelopmental outcomes among extremely low birth weight infants with a normal head ultrasound: prevalence and antecedents. *Pediatrics* 2005; **115**: 673–80.

47. Holling EE, Leviton A. Characteristics of cranial US white matter echolucencies that predict disability: a review. *Dev Med Child Neurol* 1999; **41**: 136–9.

48. Rutherford MA. Patient preparation, safety, and hazards in imaging infants and children. In Rutherford MA, ed., *MRI of the Neonatal Brain*. Philadelphia, PA: Saunders, 2002: 3–15.

49. Rutherford MA. Imaging the preterm infant: practical issues. In Rutherford MA, ed. *MRI of the Neonatal Brain*. Philadelphia, PA: Saunders, 2002: 17–21.

50. Bluml S, Friedlich P, Erberich S, *et al.* MR imaging of newborns by using an MR-compatible incubator with integrated radiofrequency coils: initial experience. *Radiology* 2004; **231**: 594–601.

51. Mirmiran M, Barnes PD, Keller K, *et al.* Neonatal brain magnetic resonance imaging before discharge is better than serial cranial ultrasound in predicting cerebral palsy in very low birth weight preterm infants. *Pediatrics* 2004; **114**: 992–8.

52. Woodward LJ, Anderson PJ, Austin NC, *et al.* Neonatal MRI to predict neurodevelopmental outcomes in preterm infants. *N Engl J Med* 2006; **355**: 685–94.

53. Maalouf EF, Duggan PJ, Counsell SJ, *et al.* Comparison of findings on cranial ultrasound and magnetic resonance imaging in preterm infants. *Pediatrics* 2001; **107**: 719–27.

54. Childs AM, Cornette L, Ramenghi LA, *et al.* Magnetic resonance and cranial ultrasound characteristics of periventricular white matter abnormalities in newborn infants. *Clin Radiol* 2001; **56**: 647–55.

55. Miller SP, Cozzio CC, Goldstein RB, *et al.* Comparing the diagnosis of white matter injury in premature newborns with serial MR imaging and transfontanel ultrasonography findings. *AJNR Am J Neuroradiol* 2003; **24**: 1661–9.

56. Volpe JJ. Cerebral white matter injury of the premature infant: more common than you think. *Pediatrics* 2003; **112**: 176–9.

57. Volpe JJ. Encephalopathy of prematurity includes neuronal abnormalities. *Pediatrics* 2005; **116**: 221–5.

58. Dyet LE, Kennea N, Counsell SJ, *et al.* Natural history of brain lesions in extremely preterm infants studied with serial magnetic resonance imaging from birth and neurodevelopmental assessment. *Pediatrics* 2005; **118**: 536–48.

59. Inder TE, Warfield SK, Wang H, *et al.* Abnormal cerebral structure is present at term in premature infants. *Pediatrics* 2005; **115**: 286–94.

60. Inder TE, Huppi PS, Warfield S, *et al.* Periventricular white matter injury in the premature infant is followed by reduced cerebral cortical gray matter volume at term. *Ann Neurol* 1999; **46**: 755–60.

61. Boardman JP, Counsell SJ, Rueckert D, *et al.* Abnormal deep grey matter development following preterm birth detected using deformation-based morphometry. *NeuroImage* 2006; **32**: 70–8.

62. Thompson DK, Warfield SK, Carlin JB, *et al.* Perinatal risk factors altering regional brain structure in the preterm infant. *Brain* 2007; **130**: 667–77.

63. Peterson BS, Vohr B, Staib LH, *et al.* Regional brain volume abnormalities and long-term cognitive outcome in preterm infants. *JAMA* 2000; **284**: 1939–47.

64. Peterson BS, Anderson AW, Ehrenkranz R, *et al.* Regional brain volumes and their later neurodevelopmental correlates in term and preterm infants. *Pediatrics* 2003; **111**: 939–48.

65. de Vries L, Groenendaal F, van Haastert IC, *et al.* Asymmetrical myelination of the posterior limb of the internal capsule in infants with periventricular haemorrhagic infarction: an early predictor of hemiplegia. *Neuropediatrics* 1999; **30**: 314–19.

66. Roelants-van Rijn AM, Groenendaal F, Beek FJA, *et al.* Parenchymal brain injury in the preterm infant: comparison of cranial ultrasound, MRI and neurodevelopmental outcome. *Neuropediatrics* 2001; **32**: 80–9.

67. Sie LTL, van der Knaap MS, van Wezel-Meijler G, *et al.* Early MR features of hypoxic–ischemic brain injury in neonates with periventricular densities on sonograms. *Am J Neuroradiol AJNR* 2000; **21**: 852–61.

68. Sie LTL, Hart AAM, van Hof J, *et al.* Predictive value of neonatal MRI with respect to late MRI findings and clinical outcome: a study in infants with periventricular densities on neonatal ultrasound. *Neuropediatrics* 2005; **36**: 78–89.

69. Ment LR, Bada HS, Barnes P, *et al.* Practice parameter: neuroimaging of the neonate. Report of the Quality Standards Subcommittee of the American Academy of Neurology and the Practice

Committee of the Child Neurology Society. *Neurology* 2002; **58**: 1726–38.

70. Rademaker KJ, Uiterwaal CSPM, Beek FJA, *et al.* Neonatal cranial ultrasound versus MRI and neurodevelopmental outcome at school age in children born preterm. *Arch Dis Child Fetal Neonatal Ed* 2005; **90**: F489–93.

71. Counsell SJ, Dyet L, Larkman DJ, *et al.* Thalamo-cortical connectivity in children born preterm mapped using probabilistic magnetic resonance tractography. *NeuroImage* 2007; **34**: 896–904.

72. O'Shea TM, Doyle LW. Perinatal glucocorticoid therapy and neurodevelopmental outcome: an epidemiologic perspective. *Semin Neonatol* 2001; **6**: 293–307.

73. Vieux R, Fresson J, Hascoet JM, *et al.* Improving perinatal regionalization by predicting neonatal intensive care requirements of preterm infants: an EPIPAGE-based cohort study. *Pediatrics* 2006; **118**: 84–90.

74. Hintz SR, Kendrick DE, Vohr BR, *et al.* Gender differences in neurodevelopmental outcomes among extremely preterm, extremely-low-birthweight infants. *Acta Paediatrica* 2006; **95**: 1239–48.

75. Anderson PJ, Doyle LW. Cognitive and educational deficits in children born extremely preterm. *Semin Perinatol* 2008; **32**: 51–8.

76. Spittle AJ, Orton J, Doyle LW, *et al.* Early developmental intervention programs post hospital discharge to prevent motor and cognitive impairments in preterm infants. *Cochrane Database Syst Rev* 2007; **(2)**: CD005495.

77. Anderson PJ, Doyle LW. Neurodevelopmental outcome of bronchopulmonary dysplasia. *Semin Perinatol* 2006; **30**: 227–32.

78. Walsh MC, Morris BH, Wrage LA, *et al.* Extremely low birth weight neonates with protracted ventilation: mortality and 18-month neurodevelopmental outcomes. *J Pediatr* 2005; **146**: 798–804.

79. Kobaly K, Schlucter M, Minich N, *et al.* Outcomes of extremely low birth weight and extremely low gestational age infants with bronchopulmonary dysplasia: effects of practice changes in 2000–2003. *Pedatrics* 2008; **121**: 73–81.

80. Baud O. Postnatal steroid treatment and brain development. *Arch Dis Child Fetal Neonatal Ed* 2004; **89**: 96–100.

81. Murphy BP, Inder TE, Huppi PS, *et al.* Impaired cerebral cortical gray matter growth after treatment with dexamethasone for neonatal chronic lung disease. *Pediatrics* 2001; **107**: 217–21.

82. Riva MA, Fumagalli F, Racagni G. Opposite regulation of basic fibroblast growth factor and nerve growth factor gene expression in rat cortical astrocytes following dexamethasone administration. *J Neurochem* 1995; **64**: 2526–33.

83. American Academy of Pediatrics, Committee on Fetus and Newborn. Postnatal corticosteroids to treat or prevent chronic lung disease in preterm infants. *Pediatrics* 2002; **109**: 330–8.

84. Doyle LW, Halliday HL, Ehrenkranz RA, *et al.* Impact of postnatal systemic corticosteroids on mortality and cerebral palsy in preterm infants: effect modification by risk for chronic lung disease. *Pediatrics* 2005; **115**: 655–61.

85. Watterberg K. Postnatal steroids for bronchopulmonary dysplasia: where are we now? *J Pediatr* 2007; **150**: 327–8.

86. Adams-Chapman I, Stoll BJ. Neonatal infection and long-term neurodevelopmental outcome in the preterm infant. *Curr Opin Infect Dis* 2006; **19**: 290–7.

87. Stoll BJ, Hansen NI, Adams-Chapman I, *et al.* Neurodevelopmental and growth impairment among extremely low-birth-weight infants with neonatal infection. *JAMA* 2004; **292**: 2357–65.

88. Hintz SR, Kendrick DE, Stoll BJ, *et al.* Neurodevelopmental and growth outcomes of extremely low birth weight infants after necrotizing enterocolitis. *Pediatrics* 2005; **115**: 696–703.

89. Haynes RL, Borenstein NS, DeSilva TM, *et al.* Axonal development in the cerebral white matter of the human fetus and infant. *J Comp Neurol* 2005; **484**: 156–67.

90. McQuillen PS, Sheldon RA, Shatz CJ, *et al.* Selective vulnerability of subplate neurons after early neonatal hypoxia–ischemia. *J Neurosci* 2003; **23**: 3308–15.

91. Doyle LW, VICS Group. Outcome at 5 years of age of children 23 to 27 weeks' gestation: refining the prognosis. *Pediatrics* 2001; **108**: 134–41.

92. Mellon RD, Simone AF, Rappaport BA. Use of anesthetic agents in neonates and young children. *Anesth Analg* 2007; **104**: 509–20.

93. Ikonomidou C, Bosch F, Miksa M, *et al.* Blockade of NMDA receptors and apoptotic neurodegeneration in the developing brain. *Science* 1999; **283**: 70–4.

94. Schmidt B, Asztalos EV, Roberts RS, *et al.* Impact of bronchopulmonary dysplasia, brain injury and severe retinopathy on the outcome of extremely low birth weight infants at 18 months. *JAMA* 2003; **289**: 1124–9.

95. Saigal S, Doyle LW. An overview of mortality and sequelae of preterm birth from infancy to adulthood. *Lancet* 2008; **371**: 261–9.

96. Marlow N. Neurocognitive outcome after very preterm birth. *Arch Dis Child Fetal Neonatal Ed* 2004; **89**: F224–8.

97. Hack M, Flannery DJ, Schluchter M, *et al.* Outcomes in young adulthood for very low birth weight infants. *N Engl J Med* 2002; **346**: 149–57.

98. Saigal S, Hoult LA, Streiner DL, *et al.* School difficulties at adolescence in a regional cohort of children who were extremely low birth weight. *Pediatrics* 2000; **105**: 325–31.

99. Mikkola K, Ritari N, Tommiska V, *et al.* Neurodevelopmental outcome at 5 years of age of a national cohort of extremely low birth weight infants who were born in 1996–1997. *Pediatrics* 2005; **116**: 1391–400.

100. Marlow N, Wolke D, Bracewell M, *et al.* Neurologic and developmental disability at six years of age after extremely preterm birth. *N Engl J Med* 2005; **352**: 9–19.

101. Hack M, Taylor HG, Drotar D, *et al.* Chronic conditions, functional limitations, and special health care needs of school-aged children born with extremely low birth weight in the 1990s. *JAMA* 2005; **294**: 318–25.

102. Taylor HG, Klein N, Drotar D, *et al.* Consequences and risk of < 1000 g birth weight for neuropsychological skills, achievement, and adaptive functioning. *J Dev Behav Pediatr* 2006; **27**: 459–69.

103. Anderson PJ, Doyle LW, VICS Group. Neurobehavioral outcomes of school-age children born extremely low birth weight or very preterm in the 1990s. *JAMA* 2003; **289**: 3264–72.

104. Saigal S, Tyson J. Measurement of quality of life of survivors of neonatal intensive care: critique and implications. *Semin Perinatol* 2008; **32**: 59–66.

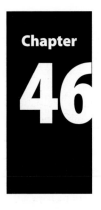

Chapter 46

Cerebral palsy: advances in definition, classification, management, and outcome

Trenna L. Sutcliffe

Overview

Cerebral palsy (CP) is a neurodevelopmental disorder. It begins in early childhood and is a lifelong condition. Core features include abnormal movement and posture due to impairments in coordination and/or muscle tone. CP is not an etiologic diagnosis. Rather, it is a descriptive term based on an individual's clinical picture. Among children diagnosed with CP, there is great heterogeneity with respect to etiology, type of impairment, and severity of impairment. Brain disturbances that lead to CP may occur prenatally, perinatally, or in the young child during brain development and maturation. Although the brain disturbances leading to CP are not progressive, the clinical picture is not static. Clinical features of CP evolve with time, development, learning, motor training, and therapy. The disorder can potentially lead to poor growth of a limb, contractures and poor range of motion, pain secondary to spasticity, inability to complete voluntary movements, neglect of a limb, inability to complete activities of daily living, and poor participation in the community.

CP is the most common cause of physical disability in children. Based on classic definitions for the disorder, 2–3/1000 live births are affected by CP [1]. The prevalence of CP is 77/1000 children for those born less than 28 weeks gestation and 40/1000 in children born between 28 and 31 weeks gestation [2]. The total lifetime costs for those born with CP in the USA in the year 2000 will be $11.5 billion, based on the 2003 dollar value [3]. Lifetime indirect costs, including productivity losses, will be 2–5 times greater than direct costs, emphasizing the tremendous importance of functional participation of persons with CP.

Improved outcome for children with CP, including increased activity and community participation, can occur. However, timely identification and diagnosis, accurate classification, and the development of comprehensive management plans are pivotal in improving long-term outcome. As our knowledge of CP advances, experts in the field are providing consensus statements around these issues to assist clinicians caring for children at risk for or diagnosed with CP.

Definition

CP has been recognized by physicians for more than a century. However, its definition continues to be refined. An English orthopedic surgeon, William Little, initially reported the condition in 1861. He referred to the condition as "cerebral paresis." In 1959 Mac Keith and Polani provided a working definition for the disorder. They described CP as "a persisting but not unchanging disorder of movement and posture, appearing in the early years of life and due to a non-progressive disorder of the brain, the result of interference during its development" [4]. Subsequently Bax revised the definition in 1964 to "a disorder of movement and posture due to a defect or lesion of the immature brain" [5].

The current definition for CP, published in 2007, represents the work of an international committee of experts. The workshop was co-sponsored by the United Cerebral Palsy Research and Educational Foundation in Washington and the Castang Foundation in the UK, with special support provided by the National Institutes of Health/National Institute of Neurological Disorders and Stroke. The definition, based on consensus, states that:

> Cerebral palsy (CP) describes a group of permanent disorders of the development of movement and posture, causing activity limitation, that are attributed to nonprogressive disturbances that occurred in the developing fetal or infant brain. The motor disorders of cerebral palsy are often accompanied by disturbances of sensation, perception, cognition, communication, and behaviour, by epilepsy, and by secondary musculoskeletal problems [6].

The 2007 published definition for CP expands on previously accepted definitions and includes a number of new concepts. It is noted in the revised definition that only individuals who have activity restrictions should be identified as having CP. This concept had not been previously included in earlier definitions and highlights the importance of assessing activity and function (1) in children at risk for CP, prior to making a diagnosis, and (2) in children diagnosed with CP, to inform management plans. This concept is in keeping with the International Classification of Functioning, Disability and Health (ICF), which is the World Health Organization's (WHO) framework for assessing health and disability [7]. This framework emphasizes the assessment and consideration of activity levels and community participation in addition to bodily impairments.

Fetal and Neonatal Brain Injury, 4th edition, ed. David K. Stevenson, William E. Benitz, Philip Sunshine, Susan R. Hintz, and Maurice L. Druzin. Published by Cambridge University Press. © Cambridge University Press 2009.

The revised definition also states that CP results from a non-progressive brain disturbance. This fact distinguishes CP from metabolic disorders or progressive neurologic disorders that may present with motor symptoms in infancy or young childhood. Thus it is important to use a thorough history, as well as ongoing clinical monitoring with serial examinations and neuroimaging, to confirm the diagnosis of CP and exclude progressive disorders. The disturbance occurs to the developing brain and during a time when motor skills are emerging. This distinguishes it from other motor disorders that are due to acquired brain lesions that occur after motor skills have been established. The motor impairments in CP generally manifest clinically in early child development, usually before 18 months of age. Presentation may include delayed or aberrant motor progress. Alternatively, many children who are ultimately diagnosed with CP present with medical issues other than motor delay, such as feeding problems, in early infancy.

The word "disturbance" rather than "lesion" in the current definition is important for our future understanding and interpretation of the disorder. Baxter and Rosenbloom emphasize the significant implications of this word change [8]. The term "brain disturbance" allows for more ambiguity regarding the specific brain pathology and may lead to the inclusion of children previously identified with disorders such as motor dyspraxia or developmental coordination disorder. As a result, the prevalence of CP would increase drastically from what we currently believe it to be. The word "disturbance" emphasizes that CP does not necessarily result from a specific lesion or abnormality in some cases, and that the CP causal pathways are not always fully understood. Fifteen percent of children diagnosed with CP have unexplained etiologies despite neuroimaging and metabolic investigations [9]. Future revisions of the CP definition may continue to use the term "disturbance" as we learn more about the numerous neurobiologic and genetic factors that may ultimately contribute to the CP phenotype.

The inclusion of associated disturbances beyond the motor disorder in the revised definition is also novel. The consideration of associated disturbances is essential for comprehensive assessment and management of children with CP. It emphasizes that, similar to other neurodevelopmental disorders, CP impacts numerous functions in the child. However, the motor impairment remains the primary condition for a disorder to fall under the diagnostic CP umbrella. Associated impairments may result from the same brain disturbance that led to the motor disorder, be secondary to the motor disorder, or result from other disturbances and mechanisms. These disturbances can present at various times throughout childhood, and therefore continual monitoring is indicated.

Classification

A standard system for CP classification has a number of benefits. Firstly, it allows for effective communication among professionals who work with children with CP. Details around type and severity of impairment can be better understood. With respect to research in the field, standardized and detailed classification of study subjects allows for better study comparisons, helps in determining the generalizability of study results, assists in the interpretation of results, and informs policy makers and other professionals of future resource needs. Classification also provides important information to the patient, family, and treating clinician. Long-term outcome and treatment choice may be directed by classification. A comprehensive classification system may also help in monitoring change in a patient over time. Impairments evolve or may be difficult to characterize in young children, and therefore a child's classification may change with time, development, and therapy.

A revised CP classification system has been described, based on consensus among experts at an international workshop [6]. The revised system is more extensive than previously described versions. Previous classification systems focused on the physical distribution of motor impairment alone. The revised classification system provides additional information that may inform comprehensive management plans, provide insight to causation and aid in prognostication. It also subdivides the very heterogeneous group of children diagnosed with CP into classes that are similar in key aspects of the disorder. The key components of the revised classification system include: motor abnormalities, accompanying impairments, anatomical and neuroimaging findings, and causation and timing (Table 46.1).

The classification of motor abnormalities includes information on (1) the type of motor disorder and (2) functional motor abilities. Motor disorder type includes information on increased or decreased muscle tone as well as information on specific movement disorders such as dystonia or ataxia. One should indicate primary versus secondary movement abnormalities. Including information on functional abilities again is in keeping with the WHO's ICF framework. A validated tool to measure activity and function should be considered. Examples of validated tools include the Gross Motor Function Classification System (GMFCS) for gross motor activities and the Manual Ability Classification System (MACS) for fine motor activities [10,11]. Activities such as oromotor function and speech should also be described, although no validated tools are available to measure specific levels of ability.

Data on accompanying impairments may change over time in a given patient. It is important that ongoing monitoring is carried out, to ensure that there are appropriate management plans, which meet patient needs. Accompanying impairments may include epilepsy, abnormal vision or hearing, communication disorders, or cognitive, behavioral, or learning impairments.

It is recommended that information regarding the anatomic distribution of symptoms include a description of involvement without the use of classic terms such as diplegia or hemiplegia. Frequently the clinical picture is not as concrete as these terms lead one to believe, and an appreciation for atypical movement or posture in the "unaffected" limbs is lost. Specific details around muscle tone, function, and/or impairments for each limb, the trunk, and oropharynx should be

Table 46.1. Proposed classification system for cerebral palsy

1. Motor abnormalities	A. Nature of the movement disorder	• Describe tone and movement abnormalities observed on clinical examination (e.g., spasticity, dystonia, ataxia)
	B. Functional motor abilities	• Describe functional limitations due to the motor disorder
		• Include oromotor and speech abilities and limitations
		• List comorbid impairments
2. Accompanying impairments		• Include musculoskeletal impairments that are secondary to the motor disorder (e.g., contractures)
		• Include other impairments that are associated but not directly due to the motor disorder (e.g., seizures, cognitive and learning impairments, hearing and vision impairments)
3. Anatomic and neuroimaging findings	Anatomic findings	• Describe the anatomical distribution of the observed motor abnormalities and functional limitations
		• Refrain from using classic terms such as diplegia or hemiplegia
		• Include all limbs, trunk, and oropharynx
	Neuroimaging findings	• Describe abnormalities observed on brain imaging
		• MRI scan is the preferred mode of brain imaging
4. Causation and timing		• Note the cause and timing of the brain disturbance leading to CP, if known (e.g., postnatal meningitis, brain malformation)

Source: From Rosenbaum *et al.* [6].

described. This information provides a more complete and accurate representation of the patient. Information regarding the neuroanatomic distribution should include specific details of all anomalies documented with imaging. Neuroimaging is recommended by the American Academy of Neurology for all children with CP [12]. Magnetic resonance imaging (MRI) is preferred over computed tomography (CT). Neuroimaging provides data regarding underlying etiology as well as informing research studies that are investigating the concept of CP prevention.

The proposed classification system also includes information regarding the cause and timing of injuries leading to the CP diagnosis. These data may not always be available. When they are available, they may provide insight into prognosis and therapy options as we learn more about the relation between potential neural reorganization and timing of neural injury in children with CP.

Management
General principles
A multidisciplinary team is essential in the management of children with CP. The team may include some combination of the following professionals: developmental pediatrician, neurologist, neurosurgeon, orthopedic surgeon, psychiatrist, physiotherapist, occupational therapist, and speech and language therapist. Additional professionals may be needed for specific issues around feeding, sensory impairments, or other accompanying symptoms that are listed in the revised definition for CP. A multidisciplinary team is frequently needed to adequately address the potential complexity of the movement disorder, symptoms secondary to the movement disorder, and the accompanying impairments. Treatment plans are individualized to the functional needs of each patient, and

the various treatments should be used in a complementary manner.

A comprehensive treatment plan can be created using the WHO's ICF framework. The ICF emphasizes the importance of assessing and promoting a person's activity level and community participation in addition to treating bodily impairments when creating management plans. Quality of life is positively impacted with interventions that not only focus on improving impairments, such as range of motion or muscle tone, but also target a child's ability to complete activities and participate more fully in the community. The ICF framework can help determine therapeutic priorities, as frequently numerous interventions may be considered at any given time.

Treatments to reduce spasticity
Spasticity is an important cause of disability in children with CP. CP is also the most common cause for spasticity in children. Although reducing spasticity is only one component of CP management, this chapter will focus on this aspect of the treatment plan (Table 46.2). Children with CP have improved quality of life when they receive medical management for their motor disorders. This frequently translates into spasticity management. Spasticity is present in more than 80% of individuals with CP, although many children have a mixed clinical picture with components of both spasticity and dystonia.

Numerous advances have been made in the treatment of pediatric spasticity. The treatment of pediatric spasticity is an individualized and potentially complex endeavor. Spasticity may interfere with motor function in some children with CP, but some component of spasticity may be very helpful and essential in other children to maintain posture. Therefore the treating clinician needs to weigh potential benefits and adverse effects of reducing spasticity when creating a treatment plan.

Table 46.2. Treatments to reduce spasticity

Non-pharmacologic treatments	
	Physical and occupational therapy approaches
	Constraint-induced movement therapy
	Electrical stimulation
	Selective dorsal rhizotomy
Pharmacologic treatments	
Oral medications	Baclofen
	Benzodiazepines (valium, clonazepam)
	Dantrolene
	α_2-adrenergic agonists (tizanidine, clonidine)
Locally injected medications	Botulinum toxin injections
	Intrathecal baclofen

Non-pharmacologic treatments

Physical and occupational therapy approaches

Physical therapy (PT) and occupational therapy (OT) are key components of most management plans in pediatric CP. Despite this, there have been few scientifically rigorous studies to demonstrate the benefits of these therapies [13]. Studies that assess the benefits of PT and OT frequently lack objective outcome measures or prospective randomized study designs.

A number of PT and OT approaches and theories are used with children with CP. Long-standing therapies have evolved as the importance of motor-learning principles and dynamic systems theories have been emphasized. Neurodevelopmental treatment (NDT) is a long-standing approach used in pediatric CP. Its focus is to move the child through normal movement patterns. However, despite its extensive history, a thorough review of the intervention showed that there is no strong evidence to support its use [14]. Conductive education, another therapy approach that has been used for decades, aims to teach the child methods to overcome his or her movement difficulties in a structured environment. However, benefits observed with conductive education are similar to those seen with more conventional approaches when they are also provided in an intensive format [15].

Muscle strengthening and resistive exercise programs are also important for children with CP. Children with CP typically have muscle weakness [16]. Research shows that activities such as walking improve when weak muscles are targeted in strengthening programs [17,18].

Constraint-induced movement therapy

Constraint-induced (CI) movement therapy is a promising new intervention for children with CP. CI improves upper extremity function. It is used in children with asymmetric neurologic examinations. The therapy includes restraining the unaffected arm while providing motor training to the affected arm. CI was initially described as restraining the unaffected arm for 90% of waking hours. Subsequently, a number of modified versions of CI have been described. These include but are not limited to casting of the unaffected arm and weekly OT [19], restraint of the unaffected arm for 6 hours per day with intensive therapy [20], or restraint of the unaffected arm for 2 hours per day with parents or teachers providing therapy [21].

Evidence is emerging to support CI as an important component in the management of children with asymmetric CP. Research investigating CI as a rehabilitation tool was initially conducted in adults with stroke [22,23]. A larger multicenter trial of CI in adult stroke patients confirms its benefits [24]. Pediatric CI controlled trials have been done more recently, and these have demonstrated clinical benefits in children with CP [19–21,25]. Observed benefits include increased use of the affected arm, improved quality of skills in the affected arm, and improved use of the affected arm in bimanual tasks. However, the field of pediatric CI is young and requires ongoing investigation to fully understand its clinical and scientific basis.

The underlying mechanism behind CI success is not yet clear. A number of concepts are felt to contribute to CI success in children with CP. The first is "developmental disregard," which describes the phenomenon that children neglect their affected arm to an extent greater than one would expect given the presence of some skills in the limb [26]. Developmental disregard therefore perpetuates the disorder because opportunities to use and provide practice to the affected arm are reduced. CI forces the child to use the affected arm and therefore helps to overcome developmental disregard. The second concept felt to contribute to CI success is reorganization of cortical brain activity. Altered and increased cortical activation for affected arm movements has been demonstrated after pediatric CI [27]. It is believed that these cortical changes may have an important impact on long-term upper extremity function. Ongoing investigations are needed to demonstrate the long-term improvements in children with CP following CI.

CI, as a treatment for pediatric CP, has received significant attention. It therefore has sparked much interest in the concept of increased practice and opportunity as a form of physical intervention for CP. As a consequence, further treatment modalities that borrow from this key concept continue to emerge [28].

Electrical stimulation

Electrical stimulation has been used in children with CP with therapeutic success. There are different forms of the therapy. Neuromuscular electrical stimulation includes stimulation of the muscle through the motor nerve. This form of stimulation results in muscle contraction. It is generally applied transcutaneously but can also be applied percutaneously. Alternatively, threshold electrical stimulation does not result in muscle contraction. It includes electrical stimulation at low intensities and is generally applied for several hours while the child is sleeping at night. Benefits of treatment include increased muscle strength, range of motion, and motor learning. Research shows that neuromuscular electrical stimulation is effective at increasing strength and range of motion in the child with CP [29]. However, further research is needed to determine if electrical stimulation leads to functional gains.

Selective dorsal rhizotomy

Selective dorsal rhizotomy (SDR) is used to treat children with spastic CP involving the lower limbs. It includes the selective disruption of sensory rootlets. The procedural goal is to reduce spasticity while maintaining function. Intraoperative electrophysiological monitoring is frequently used to ensure the preservation of sensation, voluntary muscle control, and bladder function. A meta-analysis of controlled trials demonstrated increased clinical benefit from SDR plus physiotherapy compared with physiotherapy alone [30]. Improved scores on the gross motor function measurement scale (GMFM) have been documented up to 5 years after SDR [31]. Additional benefits include reduced spasticity, increased strength, increased range of motion, and improved function with activities of daily living [31,32]. Children undergoing SDR generally require fewer adjunctive orthopedic procedures and have fewer long-term spinal deformities such as scoliosis. Better preoperative function is associated with increased gains after SDR [33]. Therefore, higher-functioning children should be considered for SDR.

Pharmacologic treatments

Medications are frequently used in the treatment of muscle spasticity in children with CP, generally in an open-trial manner with close monitoring of side effects. The route of delivery may be oral for a generalized effect or local injection for a targeted effect. The decision between these two routes of administration is influenced by the extent of clinical spasticity.

Oral medications

Oral medications are important in the treatment of general spasticity in pediatric CP. These medications include baclofen, benzodiazepines, dantrolene, and α_2-adrenergic agonists. Side effects associated with these medications include weakness and alterations to the central nervous system such as changes in blood pressure or the onset of sedation, ataxia, or dizziness.

Baclofen, a γ-aminobutyric acid (GABA) agonist, binds to $GABA_B$ receptors and reduces the release of excitatory neurotransmitters, working primarily at the level of the spinal cord. It has been used to treat spasticity in CP since 1977. It is used in children with general spasticity to reduce discomfort and allow for better movement to complete activities of daily living or assist in positioning.

Benzodiazepines increase the affinity of GABA to the $GABA_A$ receptor complex and increase GABA-mediated inhibition at the level of the spinal cord as well as supraspinally. They can reduce general spasticity, decrease muscle spasms, and improve overall well-being in children with CP [34,35].

Dantrolene acts at the level of the skeletal muscle and inhibits calcium release from the sarcoplasmic reticulum.

α_2-Adrenergic agonists, such as tizanidine and clonidine, act at the level of the brain and spinal cord. It is believed that they act by hyperpolarizing motor neurons, preventing the release of excitatory amino acids, and facilitating the inhibitory neurotransmitter glycine.

Locally injected medications

Botulinum toxin A (BTX-A) is a neuromuscular blocking agent produced by the bacterium *Clostridium botulinum*. It can transiently weaken a patient's muscles for several months when given intramuscularly. In spasticity management, BTX-A is injected in agonist muscles and its effects are local. Therapeutic goals during BTX-A treatment include improving function, allowing time for the strengthening of antagonist muscles, reducing pain that may be secondary to severe spasticity, and reducing joint deformity. Approval and licensing of BTX-A for pediatric treatment varies from country to country.

BTX-A injections are effective in the management of children with cerebral palsy. BTX-A injections have been used in pediatric CP since the early 1990s, and it is now an established mode of treatment. Seventy-six percent of children with cerebral palsy have functional gains following their first dose of BTX-A [36]. It is used in treating both upper and lower extremities. Injections in both the upper and lower extremities result in decreased tone, increased range of motion, and improved functional abilities [37–41]. Research confirms the safety of BTX-A [42,43]. Current research studies aim to standardize BTX-A treatment approaches and are examining the doses required for optimal outcome as well as injection techniques.

BTX-A treatment is frequently combined with other interventions for optimal results. Similar to other treatments for spasticity, BTX-A injections are rarely given in isolation. Interventions such as physiotherapy, occupational therapy, serial casting, orthoses, and electrical stimulation are frequently employed with BTX-A. However, evidence to demonstrate the added benefit of these combined therapeutic approaches is needed.

Intrathecal baclofen significantly decreases spasticity in both upper and lower extremities in children with CP. Intrathecal administration of baclofen began in the 1980s. Therapeutic goals include reducing contractures, improving positioning and comfort, and providing ease for caregiver tasks in children with generalized spasticity or generalized secondary dystonia.

Intrathecal administration of baclofen has a number of benefits over oral use. It results in higher drug concentrations in the cerebral spinal fluid (CSF) while decreasing the generalized side effects that are observed with oral administration [44]. Baclofen CSF levels are almost undetectable following oral dosing. However, CSF levels of baclofen comparable to serum levels are observed following intrathecal dosing with 1/100 of the oral dose. Pump-specific complications with this treatment approach include CSF leakage, catheter problems (kinks and breaks), catheter infections, and meningitis. Drug administration is done via a subcutaneous pump in the abdomen. A catheter extends from the pump to the intrathecal position.

Indications for intrathecal baclofen include children older than 6 years of age who have severe and generalized spasticity or dystonia. This group of children rarely benefit from oral baclofen treatment. It is recommended that children younger than 4 years of age who have moderate to severe spasticity have an initial trial of oral baclofen before proceeding to intrathecally administered drug [45]. However, there are no size or age limitations for pump insertion. Bolus baclofen dosing via lumbar puncture can be considered to test responsiveness prior to pump implantation.

Outcome

Predicting the long-term outcome of a child diagnosed with CP can be challenging. Outcome is influenced by many factors including but not limited to severity of the motor disorder, social environment, therapeutic interventions, and comorbid conditions. Outcome statistics represent averages from large populations of children diagnosed with CP. Detailed subgroup classification and analyses are not always done in such studies. Therefore data may not always be useful for specific clinical cases because of the tremendous clinical and etiologic heterogeneity within the CP population.

Tools are now being created to assist the clinician in predicting developmental trajectories in children with CP. Examples include the Gross Motor Function Classification System (GMFCS) [10] (Table 46.3) and the Gross Motor Function Measure (GMFM) [46]. Data from the GMFCS and the GMFM, when combined, can provide motor growth curves that describe and predict gross motor function in children with CP [47].

There is an increasing research interest in studying the long-term outcome of children with CP as our knowledge of the disorder advances and novel therapeutic interventions become available. However, classic CP outcome measures may not provide sufficient data. Traditionally, CP outcome studies have measured change in specific body impairments,

such as muscle tone or range of motion. However, a change in impairment status does not necessarily translate into functional benefits or improved quality of life. Increasing emphasis is now being placed on measuring the overall quality of life, health status, and community participation in individuals with CP as we try to document long-term outcome.

Measuring quality of life in children with CP has a number of challenges that are currently being met by researchers in the field. Again the issue of heterogeneity within the CP population impacts the data. This challenge can be met by introducing the recently described CP classification system (Table 46.1) into epidemiologic studies to collect data for specific subgroups. Subgroup data will likely be more useful to clinicians and families. An additional challenge is that many quality-of-life measurement tools are unable to adequately address the vast differences in function seen in children with CP without floor and ceiling effects. Most of these tools were not specifically designed for the CP population. Currently there is significant interest within the field of pediatric CP to create quality-of-life measures that are specific to this population and meet their unique needs.

Despite the challenges mentioned above, outcome data have been collected for children with CP. Most children with CP survive into adulthood. Risk factors for mortality include severely impaired mobility, feeding problems, and intellectual impairment [48,49]. Mortality rates in a Western Australian registry from 1958 to 1994 show rates greater than 1% per annum in the first 5 years of life and then 0.35% for the next 20 years [49]. Mortality rates did not decrease during this time period in this registry. Morbidity studies show that adults with CP have a number of associated medical conditions. Among adult women with CP, seizures occur in 40%, mental retardation in 34%, learning disabilities in 26%, hip and back deformities in 59%, bowel problems in 56%, and urinary problems in 49% [50]. Adults with CP also suffer from unemployment, as only 40% of adults with CP in the United States are employed [51]. These data were produced by studying the CP population without further classification, and are not specific for any one subgroup. Children with comorbid conditions are likely to have more severely involved CP and different long-term outcome than children with less involved CP. This point should be taken into consideration when counseling families.

Advances in the definition and classification of CP will likely contribute to useful outcome data to document our progress with the disorder and the benefits of emerging therapies. The field of CP treatment is moving forward. Our understanding of neural plasticity and motor learning in children with neural injuries is increasing. This information is now being translated into the clinical and therapeutic realms. Knowledge of the underlying mechanisms behind therapies, along with refined disease classification and epidemiologic studies, can help in optimizing treatment choices. The field of CP has come a long way since Dr. Little, and it appears to be at an important point of advancement.

Table 46.3. The Gross Motor Function Classification System (GMFCS) for pediatric cerebral palsy

GMFCS	Description
Level I	Walks without restrictions with limitations in more advanced gross motor skills
Level II	Walks without assistive devices but has limitations in walking outdoors or in the community
Level III	Walks with assistive devices and has limitations walking outdoors or in the community
Level IV	Self-mobility with limitations such that children are transported or use powered mobility devices outdoors or in the community
Level V	Self-mobility is severely limited even with assistive devices

Source: Palisano et al. [10].

References

1. Blair E, Watson L. Epidemiology of cerebral palsy. *Semin Fetal Neonatal Med* 2006; **11**: 117–25.

2. Himmelmann K, Hagberg G, Beckung E, *et al.* The changing panorama of cerebral palsy in Sweden. IX. Prevalence and origin in the birth-year period 1995–1998. *Acta Paediatr* 2005; **94**: 287–94.

3. Honeycutt A, Dunlap L, Chen H, *et al.* Economic costs associated with mental retardation, cerebral palsy, hearing loss, and vision impairment: United States, 2003. *MMWR Morb Mortal Wkly Report* 2004; **53**: 57–9.

4. Mac Keith RC, MacKenzie ICK, Polani PE. The Little Club. Memorandum on terminology and classification of "cerebral palsy." *Cereb Palsy Bull* 1959; **1**: 27–35.

5. Bax MCO. Terminology and classification of cerebral palsy. *Dev Med Child Neurol* 1964; **6**: 295–307.

6. Rosenbaum P, Paneth N, Leviton A, *et al.* A report: the definition and classification of cerebral palsy April 2006. *Dev Med Child Neurol Suppl* 2007; **109**: 8–14.

7. World Health Organization. *International Classification of Functioning, Disability and Health.* Geneva: World Health Organization, 2001.

8. Baxter P, Rosenbloom L. CP or not CP? *Dev Med Child Neurol* 2005; **47**: 507.

9. Carr LJ. Definition and classification of cerebral palsy. *Dev Med Child Neurol* 2005; **47**: 508–10.

10. Palisano R, Rosenbaum P, Walter S, *et al.* Development and reliability of a system to classify gross motor function in children with cerebral palsy. *Dev Med Child Neurol* 1997; **39**: 214–23.

11. Eliasson AC, Krumlinde-Sundholm L, Rosblad B, *et al.* The Manual Ability Classification System (MACS) for children with cerebral palsy: scale development and evidence of validity and reliability. *Dev Med Child Neurol* 2006; **48**: 549–54.

12. Ashwal S, Russman BS, Blasco PA, *et al.* Practice parameter: diagnostic assessment of the child with cerebral palsy. Report of the Quality Standards Subcommittee of the American Academy of Neurology and the Practice Committee of the Child Neurology Society. *Neurology* 2004; **62**: 851–63.

13. Boyd RN, Morris, ME, Graham, HK. Management of upper limb dysfunction in children with cerebral palsy: a systematic review. *Eur J Neurol* 2001; **8**: 150–66.

14. Butler C, Darrah J. Effects of neurodevelopmental treatment (NDT) for cerebral palsy: an AACPDM evidence report. *Dev Med Child Neurol* 2001; **43**: 778–90.

15. Reddihough DS, King J, Coleman G, *et al.* Efficacy of programmes based on Conductive Education for young children with cerebral palsy. *Dev Med Child Neurol* 1998; **40**: 763–70.

16. Wiley ME, Damiano DL. Lower-extremity strength profiles in spastic cerebral palsy. *Dev Med Child Neurol* 1998; **40**: 100–7.

17. Damiano DL, Kelly LE, Vaughan CL. Effects of quadriceps femoris muscle strengthening on crouch gait in children with spastic diplegia. *Phys Ther* 1995; **75**: 658–71.

18. Damiano DL, Abel MF. Functional outcomes of strength training in spastic cerebral palsy. *Arch Phys Med Rehabil* 1998; **79**: 119–25.

19. Willis JK, Morello A, Davie A, *et al.* Forced use treatment of childhood hemiparesis. *Pediatrics* 2002; **110**: 94–6.

20. Gordon AM, Charles J, Wolf SL. Efficacy of constraint-induced movement therapy on involved upper-extremity use in children with hemiplegic cerebral palsy is not age-dependent. *Pediatrics* 2006; **117**: e363–73.

21. Eliasson AC, Krumlinde-Sundholm L, Shaw K, *et al.* Effects of constraint-induced movement therapy in young children with hemiplegic cerebral palsy: an adapted model. *Dev Med Child Neurol* 2005; **47**: 266–75.

22. Taub E, Miller NE, Novack TA, *et al.* Technique to improve chronic motor deficit after stroke. *Arch Phys Med Rehabil* 1993; **74**: 347–54.

23. Wolf SL, Lecraw DE, Barton LA, *et al.* Forced use of hemiplegic upper extremities to reverse the effect of learned nonuse among chronic stroke and head-injured patients. *Exp Neurol* 1989; **104**: 125–32.

24. Wolf SL, Winstein CJ, Miller JP, *et al.* Effect of constraint-induced movement therapy on upper extremity function 3 to 9 months after stroke: the EXCITE randomized clinical trial. *JAMA* 2006; **296**: 2095–104.

25. Taub E, Ramey SL, DeLuca S, *et al.* Efficacy of constraint-induced movement therapy for children with cerebral palsy with asymmetric motor impairment. *Pediatrics* 2004; **113**: 305–12.

26. Deluca SC, Echols K, Law CR, *et al.* Intensive pediatric constraint-induced therapy for children with cerebral palsy: randomized, controlled, crossover trial. *J Child Neurol* 2006; **21**: 931–8.

27. Sutcliffe TL, Gaetz WC, Logan WJ, *et al.* Cortical reorganization after constraint-induced movement therapy in pediatric cerebral palsy. *J Child Neurol* 2007; **22**: 1281–7.

28. Charles J, Gordon AM. Development of hand-arm bimanual intensive training (HABIT) for improving bimanual coordination in children with hemiplegic cerebral palsy. *Dev Med Child Neurol* 2006; **48**: 931–6.

29. Hazelwood ME, Brown JK, Rowe PJ, *et al.* The use of therapeutic electrical stimulation in the treatment of hemiplegic cerebral palsy. *Dev Med Child Neurol* 1994; **36**: 661–73.

30. McLaughlin J, Bjornson K, Temkin N, *et al.* Selective dorsal rhizotomy: meta-analysis of three randomized controlled trials. *Dev Med Child Neurol* 2002; **44**: 17–25.

31. Mittal S, Farmer JP, Al-Atassi B, *et al.* Long-term functional outcome after selective posterior rhizotomy. *J Neurosurg* 2002; **97**: 315–25.

32. Gul SM, Steinbok P, McLeod K. Long-term outcome after selective posterior rhizotomy in children with spastic cerebral palsy. *Pediatr Neurosurg* 1999; **31**: 84–95.

33. Farmer JP, Sabbagh AJ. Selective dorsal rhizotomies in the treatment of spasticity related to cerebral palsy. *Childs Nerv Syst* 2007; **23**: 991–1002.

34. Matthew A, Matthew MC. The efficacy of diazepam in enhancing motor function in children with spastic cerebral palsy. *J Trop Pediatr* 2005; **51**: 109–13.

35. Matthew A, Matthew MC. Bedtime diazepam enhances well-being in children with spastic cerebral palsy. *Pediatr Rehabil* 2005; **8**: 63–6.

36. Linder-Lucht M, Kirschner J, Herrmann J, *et al.* Why do children with cerebral palsy discontinue therapy with botulinum toxin A? *Dev Med Child Neurol* 2006; **48**: 319–20.

37. Fehlings D, Rang M, Glazier J, *et al.* An evaluation of botulinum-A toxin injections to improve upper extremity function in children with hemiplegic

cerebral palsy. *J Pediatr* 2000; **137**: 331–7.

38. Corry IS, Cosgrove AP, Walsh EG, *et al.* Botulinum toxin A in the hemiplegic upper limb: a double-blind trial. *Dev Med Child Neurol* 1997; **39**: 185–93.

39. Baker R, Jasinski M, Maciag-Tymecka I, *et al.* Botulinum toxin treatment of spasticity in diplegic cerebral palsy: a randomized, double-blind, placebo-controlled, dose-ranging study. *Dev Med Child Neurol* 2002; **44**: 666–75.

40. Reddihough DS, King JA, Coleman GJ, *et al.* Functional outcome of botulinum toxin A injections to the lower limbs in cerebral palsy. *Dev Med Child Neurol* 2002; **44**: 820–7.

41. Ubhi T, Bhakta BB, Ives HL, *et al.* Randomised double blind placebo controlled trial of the effect of botulinum toxin on walking in cerebral palsy. *Arch Dis Child* 2000; **83**: 481–7.

42. Naumann MJJ. Safety of botulinum toxin type A: a systematic review and meta-analysis. *Curr Med Res Opin* 2004; **20**: 981–90.

43. Bakheit AM, Severa S, Cosgrove A, *et al.* Safety profile and efficacy of botulinum toxin A (Dysport) in children with muscle spasticity. *Dev Med Child Neurol* 2001; **43**: 234–8.

44. Tilton AH. Injectable neuromuscular blockade in the treatment of spasticity and movement disorders. *J Child Neurol* 2003; **18**: S50–66.

45. Albright AL, Ferson SS. Intrathecal baclofen therapy in children. *Neurosurg Focus* 2006; **21**: e3.

46. Russell DJ, Rosenbaum PL, Cadman DT, *et al.* The gross motor function measure: a means to evaluate the effects of physical therapy. *Dev Med Child Neurol* 1989; **31**: 341–52.

47. Rosenbaum PL, Walter SD, Hanna SE, *et al.* Prognosis for gross motor function in cerebral palsy: creation of motor development curves. *JAMA* 2002; **288**: 1357–63.

48. Strauss DJ, Shavelle RM, Anderson TW. Life expectancy of children with cerebral palsy. *Pediatr Neurol* 1998; **18**: 143–9.

49. Blair E, Watson L, Badawi N, *et al.* Life expectancy among people with cerebral palsy in Western Australia. *Dev Med Child Neurol* 2001; **43**: 508–15.

50. Turk MA, Scandale J, Rosenbaum PF, *et al.* The health of women with cerebral palsy. *Phys Med Rehabil Clin N Am* 2001; **12**: 153–68.

51. Liptak GS, Accardo PJ. Health and social outcomes of children with cerebral palsy. *J Pediatr* 2004; **145**: S36–41.

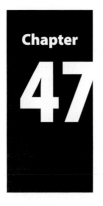

Chapter 47

Long-term impact of neonatal events on speech, language development, and academic achievement

Heidi M. Feldman and Irene M. Loe

Introduction

Language is the medium by which people exchange greetings, requests, thoughts, information, and emotions. As such, language and speech are the foundation of human communication, social interaction, and learning. Children with delays in early language and speech development are at high risk for later disorders in reading, spelling, and writing, academic skills which are highly dependent on language abilities. They are also at risk for general academic underachievement, behavioral disorders, and poor social skills. It is highly important to understand the impact of prematurity, low birthweight (LBW), and associated adverse neonatal events on the early development of language and speech, and also on reading, spelling, writing, and academic achievement.

This chapter begins with a brief summary of developmental milestones in language, speech, and reading as a background to the specific topic. Methods of assessment are described to facilitate understanding of studies to be discussed. The chapter then describes the equivocal results of studies of early language and speech development in children born prematurely. We will demonstrate that delays in language development are usually components of a broader disorder of cognition, sensory abilities, and/or motor skills. The chapter then considers the development of reading, spelling, and writing as language-based skills, as well as overall academic achievement, in children born prematurely. We will demonstrate that problems in reading are also often a component of broader disorders, including cognitive impairments and deficits in executive function. We consider outcomes as a function of potential moderators, including age, gender, and socioeconomic status (SES). Finally, we consider the underlying neural basis for language, speech, and academic achievement in children born prematurely with and without complications. We conclude with directions for future studies.

Language and speech development in typically developing children
Natural history

In typically developing children, language and speech develop slowly in infancy and then rapidly in the toddler–preschool era [1]. Receptive language, or the ability needed to understand language, emerges within the first year of life, beginning with recognition of one's name, the command "no," and verbal requests for routines such as "wave bye-bye." Receptive vocabulary develops before expressive vocabulary and is highly associated with socioeconomic status (SES). Prelinguistic babbling begins at about 6 months of age and true expressive language skill, the ability to produce actual words, emerges early in the second year of life. For most children, expressive vocabulary grows slowly and erratically for several months and then rapidly and consistently beginning between 18 and 24 months of age. Coincident with a surge in vocabulary size is the onset of word combinations or early syntax. At age 2 years, children primarily talk about concrete objects in the here-and-now. By age 3 years, they create short sentences. They show advances in morphology by using morphological markings, such as plural –s and past tense –ed. They show advances in syntax by using grammatical features, such as auxiliary verbs, question markings, and dependent clauses in complex sentences. They begin to discuss past and future. By about age 4–5 years, most typically developing children have mastered the fundamentals of language, including morphology and syntax. They use language for interpersonal conversation and also for narrative discourse, which includes the ability to tell or retell stories or personal events. Progress at school age represents more consistent use of advanced constructions; greater understanding of sentences; growing appreciation for humor, metaphor and non-literal meanings of language; and understanding and discussion of complex or abstract ideas. By age 7 years, most children have mastered all of the speech sounds of the language, including difficult sounds, such as r and l and consonant clusters, such as bl and sp.

Children begin learning to read in kindergarten and first grade. Prereading skills include letter recognition, letter–sound correspondence, and the ability to manipulate the sounds of the language. Reading requires mapping the sounds

Fetal and Neonatal Brain Injury, 4th edition, ed. David K. Stevenson, William E. Benitz, Philip Sunshine, Susan R. Hintz, and Maurice L. Druzin. Published by Cambridge University Press. © Cambridge University Press 2009.

of the language, or phonemes, onto written letters, or graphemes. Many studies have documented that reading is more highly associated with language and speech abilities than with perceptual or performance skills [2]. A child's ability to manipulate the sounds of the language for word play and rhyming is called phonological awareness, and it is highly correlated with skill in reading [3]. Children differ in the ease of reading single words, reading speed, and their ability to understand what they are reading. Difficulty with spelling may be an indication of subtle difficulties with overall reading abilities.

Assessment of language, speech, and reading

It is difficult to assess young children's progress in language and speech development, because they have yet to reliably develop the abilities to sit for extended periods and to cooperate with formal testing. Many research studies and clinical evaluations use parent questionnaires or analysis of language samples in toddlers and preschoolers to circumvent these challenges. Concurrent validity of parent questionnaires is usually good to very good, especially for assessing expressive language skills in children 2 years of age or older [4]. Analysis of language samples is also an excellent though time-consuming approach, especially to assess expressive language skills. As children approach school age, the use of standardized testing is preferable, because the resulting standard score allows the child to be compared to the population of children of that age.

Reading, writing, and spelling are assessed by norm-based assessments, generating a standard score, or curriculum-based assessments, generating a grade- or age-equivalent. Reading disability can be defined in two ways: as a discrepancy between standardized scores on reading achievement tests and measured intelligence tests, or as low achievement in reading abilities regardless of intelligence quotient. Recent literature has favored the latter definition, although federal legislation used discrepancy scores in defining eligibility for special education.

Disorders of language, speech, and reading in the general population

Language delays are common in the preschool era. At kindergarten entry, 6–7.4% of children are estimated to have a language development disorder unrelated to cognitive impairment or other known disorders [5]. Reading disorders are also prevalent, though estimates vary as a function of definition of the disorder. Reading disorders are more likely after early language delays than after typical early language development [6]. Given the high base rates in the population, it is challenging to differentiate idiopathic language, speech, or reading disorders from delays based on prematurity. Two risk factors associated with language, speech, and reading delays in the general population – male gender and low SES – are also risk factors for prematurity and for adverse outcomes following prematurity, again making the attribution of cause very difficult. Language and speech delay are highly likely in children

with sensorineural hearing loss and with cognitive impairments. Virtually all children with severe to profound neural hearing loss have language and speech impairments. Approximately half the children with mild to moderate sensorineural hearing loss have a phonological impairment that adversely affects memory, discrimination, and phonological awareness [7]. In general, children with cognitive impairment have language functioning that is commensurate with their developmental or mental age rather than their chronological age, though the etiology of the cognitive impairment may affect the rate of language learning. Hearing loss and cognitive impairment occur at greater frequency in the aftermath of adverse neonatal events than they do in the general population. For all these reasons, assessments of outcomes of prematurity should include a carefully chosen comparison group.

Language and speech after prematurity
Conflicting results

Studies of the development of language and speech after premature birth vary considerably in their findings and conclusions. We review selected studies in the literature in terms of the age of the children at the time of assessment.

Some studies report that children born prematurely progress normally in terms of language and speech. Reilly and colleagues conducted a large population-based study of children at the very earliest stages of language development, between 8 and 12 months of age. They found that skills at 8 months of age were good predictors of skills at 12 months of age, but multivariate regression models accounted for only about 5% of the variance in the rates of development. In these models, various risk factors were studied, including gender, prematurity, multiple birth, sociodemographic indicators, maternal mental health, vocabulary, and education, non-English-speaking background, and family history of speech–language difficulties. Prematurity did not contribute substantially to the modest variance accounted for in these models [8]. The authors concluded that risk factors explained little variation in early communication trajectories, and therefore that the early developmental course of young infants was more likely to unfold based on biological factors. Eilers and colleagues, also studying the earliest phases of language development, found that the onset of babbling in children born prematurely occurred in line with expectations on the basis of chronological age rather than on the basis of adjusted age, suggesting the importance of exposure to the extrauterine environment in the development of babbling [9]. A study of a Finnish cohort using the Finnish version of a parent-report measure followed a group of prematurely born very-low-birthweight (VLBW) children and full-term controls to age 2 years. They found that the vocabulary size of the groups was similar and the developmental rate was also comparable. The only indication of a difference between the premature and full-term groups was the loss of usual female advantage for language development in the VLBW group and a difference in the composition of the vocabulary across groups, a finding of uncertain significance [10]. Menyuk and colleagues followed a group of prematurely born children (gestational age 27–37 weeks) longitudinally to age 3 years using language samples as the assessment strategy. They found that as a group the preterm children developed more rapidly than peers in terms of vocabulary and grammar [11].

Several studies, by contrast, have found that children born prematurely show delays in multiple aspects of language and speech development. For example, in a New Zealand study of 2-year-old children, extremely preterm children (< 28 weeks GA) scored below very preterm (28–32 weeks GA) and full-term controls on all scales of a parent-report measure, including vocabulary, morphosyntactic complexity, and use of language to discuss the non-here-and-now [12]. Importantly, the differences persisted even after adjusting for substantial socioeconomic differences across the three groups. However, substantial variability was found within each group, such that some children born prematurely outperformed peers born at term.

Vohr and colleagues evaluated language development in LBW infants with respect to gestational age [13]. They compared appropriate-for-gestational-age (AGA) and small-for-gestational-age (SGA) LBW infants to full-term infants at age 3 years. Though only two (5%) of the LBW infants were neurologically abnormal at age 3, the LBW AGA infants continued to lag behind the controls in terms of cognitive and receptive language measures. In this study, socioeconomic factors had a significant effect on the language development of all three groups. Lower gestational age and neurological status at 8 months continued to have a significant effect on language performance at 3 years.

Kilbride and colleagues followed a group of extremely low-birthweight (ELBW) infants who weighed less than 800 grams at birth to age 5 years and compared them to full-term sibling controls [14]. The use of this control group was a creative attempt to control for postnatal macroenvironmental factors and shared genetic backgrounds. Receptive language skills were lower in the preterm group than in the full-term controls. However, other measures, including a well-respected formal measure called the Preschool Language Scale, did not show a group difference.

Others have suggested an association of prematurity and language or speech difficulties using a very different methodology. Among Dutch children referred for speech–language pathology services at age 2–5 years, there was a higher proportion of children born prematurely and LBW than would be expected in the general Dutch population. However, such findings may represent a detection bias rather than a difference in true prevalence [15].

Language and speech after brain injuries

Brain injuries, including intraventricular hemorrhage (IVH) and periventricular hemorrhage (PVH) or periventricular leukomalacia (PVL), have been found to be associated with language and speech outcomes among children born prematurely. Severe grades of IVH, as well as PVH and PVL, are risk factors for adverse neurodevelopmental outcomes, including cognitive impairment and cerebral palsy (CP). Among 3-year-old children, those who had early IVH in association with prematurity and LBW had significantly higher rates of cognitive impairment and CP than children without early IVH and prematurity [16]. Children 5–7 years of age with brain injuries following prematurity had multiple difficulties with narrative discourse, such as shorter productions, more irrelevant talk, a limited ability to differentiate types of narrative discourse, and problems creating integrated discourse. Despite these difficulties, they continued to develop between ages 5 and 7 in these skills [17].

Language abilities tend to correlate highly with cognitive abilities in preterm children with perinatal brain injuries. Language samples of preterm children with PVL at age 2 years found that the size of the lexicon and the amount of verbal output correlated with cognitive abilities, though other measures of language ability did not [18]. In a study that used analysis of language samples as the evaluation method, a comparison of three groups matched on cognitive scores – group 1 with PVL and CP, group 2 with PVL without CP, and group 3 without PVL – found no differences across groups. However, in all three groups substantial correlations of language measures with cognitive scores were observed [17]. Studies of early low-dose indomethacin treatment to decrease both the incidence and severity of IVH in VLBW preterm infants also found that though the treated group had rates of CP comparable to the untreated group, cognitive scores were somewhat better. In this study, language abilities also improved after early indomethacin, and correlated with improved cognitive outcomes [19]. In addition, there were significant gender by treatment effects for boys in reducing IVH, and raising language and cognitive test scores [20]. Additional language and cognitive outcomes from this study are discussed later under the section on moderators of language and speech outcomes.

Academic outcomes after prematurity
Reading and related skills

Numerous follow-up studies of preterm and LBW children document problems with academic achievement in multiple areas, including reading, spelling, and writing skills, as well as mathematics [21–23]. Longitudinal studies document that difficulties begin with prereading skills and persist through adolescence. A longitudinal study in southern Germany evaluated cognitive status and prereading skills in a geographically defined population sample of 6-year-old children who were born at less than 32 weeks' gestation [24]. Compared with term peers, preterm children scored approximately one standard deviation (SD) lower on measures of cognitive and language skills. The rates of major cognitive deficits (> 2 SD below the mean) were 10–35 times higher than in controls. Prereading skills were assessed using adapted measures of phonological awareness, such as rhyming, sound-to-word matching, and number and letter naming tasks. Very preterm children, regardless of whether major neurosensory impairment was excluded, were 3–5 times more likely to score below the 10th percentile in all the prereading tests as well as on measures of speech articulation. Interestingly, a very specific deficit in processing of simultaneous information was found in these very preterm children compared to term controls. When controlling for this simultaneous information processing deficit measured on the German version of the Kaufman Assessment Battery for Children (K-ABC), many of the differences in achievement and language abilities between very preterm children and term controls did not remain [24].

The longitudinal component of this study found stability in reading and other academic problems over time. When the children were again evaluated at the age of 8 years, at the end of Grade 2, control children outperformed VLBW children on standardized reading, spelling, and math tests. The differences in mean reading error and spelling error were approximately three-quarters of a standard deviation [25]. Multiple stepwise regression analyses using sociodemographic variables and measures taken during preschool and kindergarten were conducted to explore the impact on reading, spelling, and math performance at the age of 8 years. Approximately 50% of the variance in reading scores and 41% of the variance in spelling scores were explained by IQ, rhyming skills, and number knowledge. In these models, after accounting for the other factors, prematurity did not significantly contribute to the prediction.

At age 13 years, compared to VLBW children, normal birthweight (NBW) control children showed higher levels of academic achievement, a combined measure reflecting level of educational track within the German school system and performance level within the track. For VLBW/very premature children, IQ had a substantial indirect effect on reading which was mediated by phonological processing assessed at age 6. In addition, IQ differences predicted individual differences in phonological processing, which in turn impacted reading. Throughout the study, there was a correlation of birthweight category and scores. On both phoneme and rhyming tasks, 30% of ELBW children scored below the 5th percentile, compared to 4% of controls. Moreover, 65% of ELBW children fell in the lowest quartile, compared to approximately 45% of VLBW children and 25% of LBW children.

Reading in children with neural injuries

Specific brain injuries also affect reading and spelling outcomes. Downie and colleagues investigated the impact of periventricular brain injury (PVBI) on reading and spelling abilities in the late elementary years [21]. They studied a cohort of preterm children who were born at 23–30 weeks, weighed less than 1000 g, and had received three head ultrasounds during the first 6 weeks of life in order to evaluate for presence and severity of PVBI. Compared with term control children, ELBW children without PVBI performed as well on intelligence (verbal and performance IQ), academic achievement (word attack, word identification, and spelling), cognitive ability tests (auditory working memory), and phonological

processing. ELBW children with mild and severe PVBI received significantly lower scores than either ELBW children without PVBI or children born at term.

In the previously mentioned indomethacin IVH prevention trial, VLBW preterm children with IVH (after receiving either indomethacin or saline) were compared to children without IVH at age 8 years [26]. Children with IVH had significantly lower cognitive (verbal, performance, and full-scale IQ) and achievement scores on the Peabody Individual Achievement Tests–Revised (reading recognition, reading comprehension, and math) compared to children without IVH. In this study both biological and environmental factors (including maternal education and language spoken in the home) were important predictors of outcome. Although grades 3 and 4 IVH had significant negative effects on cognitive scores, they did not contribute to models predicting performance on reading and math achievement tests. Rather, the presence of ventriculomegaly and/or periventricular leukomalacia predicted poor performance on achievement tests [26].

Short-term academic resource use and outcomes

The impact of these cognitive and academic difficulties is accompanied by increased utilization rates of educational resources and supports. In the indomethacin IVH prevention trial, the presence of IVH was associated with significantly increased rates of academic resource support or therapy (62–79%) compared to already high baseline rates in children without IVH (47–49%) at the age of 8 years. Compared to the preterm children without IVH, children with IVH received twice as many individual therapies, were more likely to be in self-contained classrooms, and were more likely to be receiving speech or language therapies. There was no difference in grade repetition among the groups [26].

A population-based cohort study in southern Sweden of extremely preterm (EPT) infants compared to full-term controls at age 10 years found significant differences of approximately 1 SD on tests of cognition and visual–motor integration [27]. The study also found that 38% of the EPT children performed below grade level, and that 30% of EPT children attending mainstream schools received special education [27]. More than half of the EPT children with IQs less than 70 were not previously identified as having mental retardation, and some were not receiving special education. A study of four international population-based cohorts of ELBW survivors (birthweight 500–1000 g) found that school difficulties were serious sequelae of ELBW in all four countries [28]. Although there were some differences among the cohorts on cognitive and achievement measures, more than half of all cohorts required special education assistance and/or repeated a grade.

Long-term outcomes

The cumulative impact of these cognitive and academic difficulties can be substantial. In a longitudinal study of VLBW

(< 1500 g) children born in Cleveland from 1977 to 1979, Hack and colleagues assessed the level of education, cognitive and academic achievement at 20 years of age compared to an NBW control group [29]. They found that fewer VLBW participants had graduated from high school or obtained a general equivalency diploma. Compared to NBW participants, more of the VLBW participants had repeated a grade in school and fewer were enrolled in postsecondary studies. The differences in educational attainment, grade repetition, and current educational program remained significant when excluding the participants with neurosensory impairment or subnormal IQ. On IQ testing and academic achievement subtests, VLBW participants had significantly lower mean scores and higher frequency of subnormal IQ (< 70) and borderline IQ (70–84). The differences in IQ and achievement remained significant after excluding those with neurosensory impairment.

A Canadian cohort aged 22–25 years was found to have more positive outcomes than the Cleveland cohort [30]. In this sample, 82% of the ELBW young adults graduated from high school, compared to 87% of the controls, and a substantial proportion of both groups were pursuing higher education. The Canadian sample was generally of higher SES, and had access to better health care and educational services than did the American counterpart, differences which may contribute to differences in outcomes.

Moderators of language and speech outcomes

Language and speech outcomes of prematurity have been found to vary as a function of the age of assessment. One dramatic example was reported by Ment *et al.* [31]. In this study, a large cohort of infants born weighing 600–1250 g who had participated in the randomized, placebo-controlled trial of indomethacin for IVH prevention were serially evaluated at ages 36, 54, 72, and 96 months, corrected for the degree of prematurity. The study found that the median standard score on the Peabody Picture Vocabulary Test–Revised (PPVT-R) (with a population mean 100, standard deviation 15) increased from 88 at 36 months to 99 at 96 months. Over half of the children gained five points or more in test scores from 3 to 8 years, and improvements in full-scale and verbal IQ scores were also found. Multivariate analyses demonstrated that in addition to age, residence in a two-parent household and higher levels of maternal education were significantly associated with higher PPVT-R scores. Children with early IVH followed by significant brain injury had the lowest PPVT-R scores initially and, unlike the majority of the cohort, they did not demonstrate improvement over time.

Gender is another moderating variable among preterm and VLBW children. In a large multicenter analysis, boys were more likely than girls to have adverse outcomes, including moderate to severe CP and cognitive impairment. In multivariate models including both girls and boys, male gender remained an independent risk factor for cognitive impairment at 22 months of age, even after consideration of other factors.

Boys appear to be not only at higher risk for perinatal and neonatal morbidities, but also at higher constitutive baseline risk for adverse early childhood cognitive and neurologic outcomes [32]. In follow-up studies, boys continue to have worse outcomes than girls. Hack and colleagues reported an interaction between birthweight and gender on an applied problems subtest in academic achievement testing; the difference between preterm boys and controls was greater than the difference between preterm girls and controls [29]. Males also appear to be more vulnerable to brain injuries associated with prematurity, including white-matter injury. The volume of white matter in preterm boys was significantly less than the volume in term boys, whereas the volumes were comparable in girls [33].

Socioeconomic status is highly associated with cognitive and linguistic outcomes in children born prematurely. Low maternal education is an independent risk factor for adverse outcomes in many studies, including those focused on children with brain abnormalities such as ventriculomegaly [34]. The contribution of SES to outcomes for term and preterm infants usually is observed in the toddler years as language is emerging [9]. In children born prematurely, SES is also associated with outcomes beginning in the toddler–preschool years [14]. The magnitude of the SES effect is substantial. Kilbride and colleagues found that the mean scores on cognitive and language measures, but not motor skills, of children with premature delivery in a high-SES family were comparable to the mean for the low-SES full-term children [14]. The effects of low SES have been found in all medical risk categories after premature delivery [35]. SES is not usually considered to exert a direct influence on language, speech, or reading but rather to be a marker for various adverse psychosocial factors, including highly stressful environments, poor access to health and education services, limited verbal input, and poor parenting skills. Interventions that improve the level of parental responsivity also improve social, emotional, and language development, and the VLBW group has been shown to benefit more than the term group from maternal intervention [36].

Language, speech, and reading outcomes in relation to other developmental domains
Language impairments are associated with cognitive and motor functioning

The evidence argues against the development of selective language delays or disorders in the aftermath of preterm delivery. For example, Caravale and colleagues documented that in children with no obvious neurological disorders, problems with receptive vocabulary are accompanied by problems with intelligence, visual perception, visual motor integration, memory, and sustained attention [37]. Severe disabilities including cerebral palsy, cognitive impairment, seizures, hearing impairment, and visual impairment affect 15–25% of the population of children born prematurely. Language and associated skills, such as verbal memory, generally are reduced in children with these disabilities, commensurate with cognitive impairment [38].

The prevalence of specific language impairment (SLI), defined as language abilities significantly below what would be expected on the basis of IQ, is no higher in children born prematurely than in the general population [39]. In a study by Aram et al., differences in the prevalence of SLI between LBW children and controls failed to achieve statistical significance, once children with other disabilities were excluded from the analysis [39]. A higher proportion of preterm than control children had subnormal language abilities, but they were associated with an IQ more than one standard deviation below the mean, hearing impairment, and/or major neurological impairments.

Some studies have even suggested that language and speech skills are less severely affected than cognitive and motor skills after prematurity. Kilbride and colleagues compared a sample of children born prematurely to a comparison group of siblings born at term [14]. Though the groups differed on the intelligence and motor tests, they were not statistically different on expressive language and articulation.

Problems of executive functioning

The relatively poor academic achievement of prematurely born children may relate to deficits beyond cognitive and reading abilities, including problems of executive function. Executive function is an umbrella term referring to multiple complex and interrelated abilities which are used to direct purposeful, goal-oriented behavior. These abilities are used for cognitive, behavioral, emotional, and social functions. They include, but are not limited to, cognitive flexibility, inhibitory control, and the ability to hold information on-line and filter out distraction. Difficulties with executive function are implicated in learning and neurobehavioral disorders, such as attention-deficit/hyperactivity disorder (ADHD). Attention problems are highly associated with reading and learning problems in the population of children born at term, and therefore may contribute to academic difficulties in children born prematurely.

Numerous studies have documented difficulties with executive and other neuropsychological function in children born prematurely from early childhood through adolescence. For example, Caravale and colleagues found problems with sustained attention and memory for location in children aged 3–4 years [37]. A Finnish cohort of ELBW children at age 5 years demonstrated poorer performance compared to Finnish population norms on all domains of the standardized Developmental Neuropsychological Assessment (NEPSY) test, including attention and executive functions, language, sensorimotor function, visuospatial perception, and memory and learning [38]. An Australian study similarly found significant executive dysfunction at age 8 years in an ELBW/very-preterm cohort born during the 1990s compared to NBW peers [40]. A US cohort, also born during the 1990s and evaluated at age 8 years, found similar results [41]. Using a computerized executive function battery, Luciana and colleagues found that compared to age-matched controls, 7- to 9-year-old children born prematurely demonstrated more memory errors on a spatial working memory task, longer planning times on a task of spatial planning and organization, poorer pattern recognition, and shorter spatial memory span [42]. Longitudinal studies document continued impairments in executive function skills of VLBW children into adolescence [43,44].

ADHD

Epidemiologic studies find that the prevalence of ADHD is 4–12% in the general population of 6- to 12-year-olds [45]. The true prevalence of ADHD in children born prematurely is unknown. A retrospective case–control study of clinic-referred children with ADHD found that ADHD cases were three times more likely to have been born LBW than non-ADHD controls [46]. The study accounted for potential family–genetic and environmental confounders, such as prenatal exposure to alcohol and cigarettes, parental ADHD, social class, and family history of comorbid disruptive disorders, indicating that LBW was an independent risk factor for ADHD [46]. In addition, Breslau and colleagues found a 2–3.5-fold increased risk of ADHD among LBW children at age 6 years [47]. At age 11 years, longitudinal follow-up of the same children showed an association between LBW and clinically significant attention problems for children from urban, but not suburban, communities, suggesting an interaction between biologic vulnerability associated with premature birth and environmental risk associated with social disadvantage [48]. Botting and colleagues reported a threefold increase in risk of ADHD at age 12 among a cohort of children with birthweight < 1500 g compared to age-matched classroom controls [49]. A Norwegian study conducted by Indredavik and colleagues found that 25% of their sample of VLBW children had attention problems as adolescents, although only 7% met diagnostic criteria for ADHD [50]. In contrast, a Swedish follow-up study of 10-year-old children born prematurely (< 29 weeks) found rates of general behavior problems of 32%, with 20% meeting DSM-IV criteria for ADHD, compared to rates of 10% and 8%, respectively, in the full-term group [27].

Longitudinal follow-up studies have found an association between parent-reported attention problems, performance on tests of attention, and academic achievement in children born preterm or of low birthweight. In a US study, 7-year-old children with birthweight < 750 g were compared to a matched group of children with birthweight 750–1499 g and term controls on a battery of attention tests [51]. The group < 750 g performed more poorly on measures of vigilance and mental set shifting, but not on a test of visual search. The < 750 g group differed from the comparison groups on only one attention test measuring vigilance after controlling for overall cognitive ability. The 750–1499 g group did not differ from the term group on any measures of attention. Poorer performance on attention tests in this study was associated with higher ratings of attention problems and general behavior problems, lower ratings of social adjustment and school performance, and lower scores on tests of mathematics and written language abilities. After adjusting for influences of SES and general cognitive ability, the attention tests also predicted achievement skills, indicating that such tests serve as meaningful predictors of outcome [51].

A complication in this literature is that parent-reported attention problems do not always align with results of objective testing. A Norwegian study by Elgen and colleagues of a population-based sample of 11-year-old LBW children compared to NBW children showed that mothers reported higher rates of attention problems on the Child Behavior Checklist (CBCL), a standardized behavior questionnaire, in LBW children [52]. The battery of tasks to assess various aspects of attention functions, such as inattention, vigilance, impulsivity, selective attention, and alternating attention, found no specific attention dysfunction in the LBW group compared to the NBW group [52]. Davis and colleagues used a similar method and found that parents reported only 4.4% of VLBW children had attention problem scores in the clinical range, and another 11% had scores in the borderline range [53]. In this study, the LBW children had poorer performance on objective measures of attention than NBW, but their scores did not correlate with parent-rated attention problems [53].

It has been proposed that the attention problems experienced by children born prematurely and of LBW may differ from attention issues in other populations, including those with ADHD defined by strict diagnostic criteria. Fewer comorbid disruptive behavior disorders have been reported in VLBW children than in the population of term children with ADHD [54]. Whereas in otherwise healthy children ADHD is accompanied by a greater predominance of externalizing than internalizing disorders, in children born prematurely attention problems are associated with increased rates of shyness, unassertiveness, withdrawn behavior, anxiety, depression, and social skills deficits [49,55–57].

Neural basis of language, speech, and reading problems in children born prematurely

Hypoxic–ischemic injury

One potential explanation for the developmental delays among prematurely born children could be exposure to periods of sublethal hypoxia and ischemia (HI). Premature infants demonstrate physiologic vulnerability to such HI episodes due to impaired cerebrovascular autoregulation [58]. The typical course of an ill neonate includes clinical episodes of desaturation, apnea, and fluctuations in blood pressure; hence disturbances in cerebral blood flow and lack of autoregulation are implicated in brain injury. Several studies find smaller head circumference in children born prematurely than in children born at term [14], and small head circumference is associated with adverse developmental outcomes [59,60]. Small head circumference may be caused by a loss of cellular elements from HI injury. Though there is evidence of global

reduction of brain volumes among children born prematurely, regional reduction of volumes, particularly of the temporal lobes, has been associated with a decrease in language functioning [61]. Increased gyrification of the temporal lobe, another indication of HI injury, has been associated with poor reading abilities in children born prematurely [62].

It is difficult to reconcile the findings of an association of temporal lobe injuries with language disorders in children born prematurely, given the considerable evidence for cortical plasticity among young children with large lesions in areas of the brain purported to be associated with language skills [18,63]. Children with early left-hemisphere cortical lesions do better on language tasks than do adults with acquired injuries to those same regions, a difference attributed to the plasticity of the central nervous system at young ages [64]. In fact, the ability of the brain to reorganize language skills to the right hemisphere after early left-hemisphere cortical injury has been demonstrated [65,66]. More research is required to determine when neural injuries lead to persistent and severe language disorders, and when recovery and continued development are possible.

White-matter injury

Another possible explanation for poor developmental outcomes after prematurity relates to white-matter damage. Periventricular hemorrhage (PVH) is typically associated with large IVH and appears to result from a venous infarction on the side of the IVH [67] (see Chapter 24). Cystic PVL is characterized by multifocal areas of necrosis deep in the cortical white matter [67]. This most severe of white-matter lesions now affects only 1–4% of infants of birthweight < 1500 g, depending on birthweight category [68].

White-matter damage results from injury to the vulnerable preoligodendroglial cells and to the elongating and developing axons. White-matter damage, as well as injury to the subplate neurons, is thought to result in reduced connectivity and impaired neuronal differentiation. Thinning of the corpus callosum is seen following white-matter injury, particularly in the posterior sections of the corpus callosum [69].

White matter is responsible for rapid communication among brain regions. Though white matter has long been regarded as relevant to motor and visual systems, it had been regarded as irrelevant to higher cerebral function or language because it lacks inherent computational functions. However, recent studies have found that reading ability is highly associated with the integrity of white matter. Using diffusion tensor imaging (DTI) to assess the integrity of white matter, studies have found differences in the left temporal–parietal areas between good and poor readers [70]. Fiber tracking suggests that the site of the difference is within the corona radiata [71]. The location of the differences is difficult to interpret, since these tracts had not previously been thought to contribute to language or reading functions. Further research will be needed to explore these associations in children born prematurely.

Cerebellar injury

Cerebellar hemorrhagic injury may also be associated with developmental disorders in language, speech, and reading in children born prematurely [72]. Traditionally, the cerebellum was thought to be involved in motor activities and coordination. However, the cerebellum has now been implicated in cognitive, language, and reading tasks, though its precise function is not clear. Reduced right anterior cerebellar volumes have been found in anatomic studies of poor readers [73]. Cerebellar damage may often be part of an extensive pattern of injuries after prematurity or found as an isolated lesion. Infants with isolated cerebellar hemorrhagic injury had lower expressive language, receptive language, and cognitive scores than full-term controls [72]. Children with both parenchymal and cerebellar damage fared no worse than those with isolated cerebellar injury [72].

Neural organization

Functional neural organization may differ in children born prematurely in comparison to full-term controls, even in the absence of frank neural damage. Functional imaging studies demonstrate patterns of neural activation in response to specific exposures or specific neuropsychological processes. Ment and colleagues conducted an fMRI study of phonologic and semantic processing of language using preterm and term children aged 12 years [74]. Their paradigm asked participants to listen passively to a meaningful story or randomly presented combinations of speech elements from that story. The pattern of brain activity in the semantic processing task (the meaningful story) in preterm children resembled the pattern of brain activity in the phonologic processing task (the disconnected sounds) in term controls. Children with low verbal IQ scores and poor language comprehension were more likely than the others to show this pattern during scanning. These findings suggest that prematurity alters aspects of language processing. However, a potential problem with the interpretation is that the children born prematurely may have been processing the input differently. The authors attempted to rule out this possibility by asking comprehension questions at the end of the semantic task. However, participants may have been able to answer the questions correctly based on their familiarity with the story rather than their on-line processing during the scan. Functional imaging has enormous promise for contributing to our understanding of language, speech, reading, executive functioning, and related areas in the aftermath of prematurity.

Clinical implications

In summary, language and speech may be delayed or disordered in the aftermath of prematurity, LBW, and associated adverse complications. The evidence suggests that such delays are not isolated or specific but rather part of a complex of other developmental problems. In addition, sociodemographic variables are associated with language and speech disorders; for instance, these disorders are more prevalent in boys than in girls, and in children of low socioeconomic status than in children from the middle class. Language and speech should be a central component of the comprehensive evaluation of children born prematurely. Children with early delays in language and speech should be referred for early intervention or speech and language services. Speech and language therapy has been shown to be generally effective at improving outcomes for children with language and speech disorders [75].

Problems of reading, spelling, writing, and academic achievement are also highly prevalent in the aftermath of prematurity. Academic problems are also associated with other developmental problems, including cognitive impairment and deficits in executive function. These academic problems are also more common among boys and children of low socioeconomic status. Given the enormous importance of academic achievement, follow-up of children born prematurely should continue until their literacy and executive function skills can be accurately evaluated. Prematurity must be conceptualized as a chronic condition for many children. Systematic long-term follow-up with a strong emphasis on functional assessment may be required through adolescence to adulthood.

Directions for future research

Learning more about the neural basis of developmental disorders after prematurity is essential. Such information may explain the developmental disorders that follow prematurity. Such information may also allow neonatologists and colleagues to improve clinical care in the newborn period to reduce these injuries. Studies on the effectiveness of neural protection require clinical trials with adequate long-term follow-up to evaluate improvements in outcomes at least until school age.

We must also investigate educational and behavioral interventions that can improve outcomes in children born prematurely. At the present time, infant specialists, speech/language therapists, and educators generally intervene with children who have delays on the basis of developmental levels, not on the basis of etiology or pathophysiology. We need to consider whether specialized instructional methods for children born prematurely or children with specific neural injuries would allow more rapid gains than interventions based on generalized approaches. Furthermore, we must evaluate interventions for school-age children with reading and attentional problems in the aftermath of prematurity and associated neural injuries. We must determine whether children born prematurely benefit to the same degree as full-term children from pharmacological and behavioral management treatments for ADHD.

Finally, continued long-term follow-up of children born prematurely is important to document the outcomes of medical management in the newborn period, and education and therapy throughout childhood. Such studies must consider functional outcomes in multiple domains, including learning, communication, socialization and interpersonal relationships, educational attainment, and success in major life areas. Such follow-up should utilize a systematic and comprehensive approach, such as the International Classification of Functioning, Disability, and Health [76]. As we uncover more information about the long-term outcomes of such children, we can further refine our treatment and management strategies.

References

1. Feldman HM. Evaluation and management of language and speech disorders in preschool children. *Pediatr Rev* 2005; **26**: 131–42.

2. Rayner K, Foorman BR, Perfetti CA, *et al.* How psychological science informs the teaching of reading. *Psychol Sci* 2001; **2**: 31–74.

3. Wagner RK, Torgesen JK. The nature of phonological processing and its causal role in the acquisition of reading skills. *Psychol Bull* 1987; **101**: 192–212.

4. Feldman HM, Dollaghan CA, Campbell TF, *et al.* Measurement properties of the MacArthur communicative development inventories at ages one and two years. *Child Dev* 2000; **71**: 310–22.

5. Law J, Boyle J, Harris F, *et al.* Prevalence and natural history of primary speech and language delay: findings from a systematic review of the literature. *Int J Lang Commun Disord* 2000; **35**: 165–88.

6. Scarborough HS, ed. *Developmental Relationships Between Language and Reading: Reconciling a Beautiful Hypothesis with Some Ugly Facts.* Mahwah, NJ: Lawrence Erlbaum Associates, 2005.

7. Briscoe J, Bishop DV, Norbury CF, *et al.* Phonological processing, language, and literacy: a comparison of children with mild-to-moderate sensorineural hearing loss and those with specific language impairment. *J Child Psychol Psychiatry* 2001; **42**: 329–40.

8. Reilly S, Eadie P, Bavin EL, *et al.* Growth of infant communication between 8 and 12 months: a population study. *J Paediatr Child Health* 2006; **42**: 764–70.

9. Eilers RE, Oller D, Levine S, *et al.* The role of prematurity and socioeconomic status in the onset of canonical babbling in infants. *Infant Behav Dev* 1993; **16**: 297–315.

10. Stolt S, Klippi A, Launonen K, *et al.* Size and composition of the lexicon in prematurely born very-low-birth-weight and full-term Finnish children at two years of age. *J Child Lang* 2007; **34**: 283–310.

11. Menyuk P, Liebergott J, Schultz M. *Early Language Development in Full-term and Premature Infants.* Hillsdale, NJ: Lawrence Erlbaum Associates, 1995.

12. Foster-Cohen S, Edgin JO, Champion PR, *et al.* Early delayed language development in very preterm infants: evidence from the MacArthur-Bates CDI. *J Child Lang* 2007; **34**: 655–75.

13. Vohr BR, Garcia-Coll C, Oh W. Language and neurodevelopmental outcome of low-birthweight infants at three years. *Dev Med Child Neurol* 1989; **31**: 582–90.

14. Kilbride HW, Thorstad K, Daily DK. Preschool outcome of less than 801-gram preterm infants compared with full-term siblings. *Pediatrics* 2004; **113**: 742–7.

15. Keegstra AL, Knijff WA, Post WJ, *et al.* Children with language problems in a speech and hearing clinic: background variables and extent of language problems. *Int J Pediatr Otorhinolaryngol* 2007; **71**: 815–21.

16. Vohr B, Allan WC, Scott DT, *et al.* Early-onset intraventricular hemorrhage in preterm neonates: incidence of neurodevelopmental handicap. *Semin Perinatol* 1999; **23**: 212–17.

17. Hemphill L, Feldman HM, Camp L, *et al.* Developmental changes in narrative and non-narrative discourse in children with and without brain injury. *J Commun Disord* 1994; **27**: 107–33.

18. Feldman HM, Evans JL, Brown RE, *et al.* Early language and communicative abilities of children with periventricular leukomalacia. *Am J Ment Retard* 1992; **97**: 222–34.

19. Ment LR, Vohr B, Allan W, *et al.* Outcome of children in the indomethacin intraventricular hemorrhage prevention trial. *Pediatrics* 2000; **105**: 485–91.

20. Ment LR, Vohr BR, Makuch RW, *et al.* Prevention of intraventricular hemorrhage by indomethacin in male preterm infants. *J Pediatr* 2004; **145**: 832–4.

21. Downie AL, Frisk V, Jakobson LS. The impact of periventricular brain injury on reading and spelling abilities in the late elementary and adolescent years. *Child Neuropsychol* 2005; **11**: 479–95.

22. Aylward GP. Neurodevelopmental outcomes of infants born prematurely. *J Dev Behav Pediatr* 2005; **26**: 427–40.

23. Aylward GP. Cognitive and neuropsychological outcomes: more than IQ scores. *Ment Retard Dev Disabil Res Rev* 2002; **8**: 234–40.

24. Wolke D, Meyer R. Cognitive status, language attainment, and prereading skills of 6-year-old very preterm children and their peers: the Bavarian Longitudinal Study. *Dev Med Child Neurol* 1999; **41**: 94–109.

25. Schneider W, Wolke D, Schlagmuller M, *et al.* Pathways to school achievement in very preterm and full term children. *Eur J Psychol Educ* 2004; **19**: 385–406.

26. Vohr BR, Allan WC, Westerveld M, *et al.* School-age outcomes of very low birth weight infants in the indomethacin intraventricular hemorrhage prevention trial. *Pediatrics* 2003; **111**: e340–6.

27. Stjernqvist K, Svenningsen NW, Stjernqvist K, *et al.* Ten-year follow-up of children born before 29 gestational weeks: health, cognitive development, behaviour and school achievement. *Acta Paediatr* 1999; **88**: 557–62.

28. Saigal S, den Ouden L, Wolke D, *et al.* School-age outcomes in children who were extremely low birth weight from four international population-based cohorts. *Pediatrics* 2003; **112**: 943–50.

29. Hack M, Flannery DJ, Schluchter M, *et al.* Outcomes in young adulthood for very-low-birth-weight infants. *N Eng J Med* 2002; **346**: 149–57.

30. Saigal S, Stoskopf B, Streiner D, *et al.* Transition of extremely low-birth-weight infants from adolescence to young adulthood: comparison with normal birth-weight controls. *JAMA* 2006; **295**: 667–75.

31. Ment LR, Vohr B, Allan W, *et al.* Change in cognitive function over time in very low-birth-weight infants. *JAMA* 2003; **289**: 705–11.

32. Hintz SR, Kendrick DE, Vohr BR, *et al.* Gender differences in neurodevelopmental outcomes among extremely preterm, extremely-low-birthweight infants. *Acta Paediatr* 2006; **95**: 1239–48.

33. Reiss AL, Kesler SR, Vohr B, *et al.* Sex differences in cerebral volumes of 8-year-olds born preterm. *J Pediatr* 2004; **145**: 242–9.

34. Ment LR, Vohr B, Allan W, *et al.* The etiology and outcome of cerebral ventriculomegaly at term in very low birth weight preterm infants. *Pediatrics* 1999; **104**: 243–8.

35. Landry SH, Smith KE, Swank PR. Environmental effects on language development in normal and high-risk child populations. *Semin Pediatr Neurol* 2002; **9**: 192–200.

36. Landry SH, Smith KE, Swank PR. Responsive parenting: establishing early foundations for social, communication, and independent problem-solving skills. *Dev Psychol* 2006; **42**: 627–42.

37. Caravale B, Tozzi C, Albino G, *et al.* Cognitive development in low risk preterm infants at 3–4 years of life. *Arch Dis Child Fetal Neonatal Ed* 2005; **90**: F474–9.

38. Mikkola K, Ritari N, Tommiska V, *et al.* Neurodevelopmental outcome at 5 years of age of a national cohort of extremely low birth weight infants who were born in 1996–1997. *Pediatrics* 2005; **116**: 1391–400.

39. Aram DM, Hack M, Hawkins S, *et al.* Very-low-birthweight children and speech and language development. *J Speech Hear Res* 1991; **34**: 1169–79.

40. Anderson PJ, Doyle LW, Victorian Infant Collaborative Study Group. Executive functioning in school-aged children who were born very preterm or with extremely low birth weight in the 1990s. *Pediatrics* 2004; **114**: 50–7.

41. Taylor HG, Klein N, Drotar D, *et al.* Consequences and risks of <1000-g birth weight for neuropsychological skills, achievement, and adaptive functioning. *J Dev Behav Pediatr* 2006; **27**: 459–69.

42. Luciana M, Lindeke L, Georgieff M, *et al.* Neurobehavioral evidence for working-memory deficits in school-aged children with histories of prematurity. *Dev Med Child Neurol* 1999; **41**: 521–33.

43. Taylor HG, Minich N, Bangert B, *et al.* Long-term neuropsychological outcomes of very low birth weight: associations with early risks for periventricular brain insults. *J Int Neuropsychol Soc* 2004; **10**: 987–1004.

44. Taylor HG, Minich NM, Klein N, *et al.* Longitudinal outcomes of very low birth weight: neuropsychological findings. *J Int Neuropsychol Soc* 2004; **10**: 149–63.

45. Brown RT, Freeman WS, Perrin JM, *et al.* Prevalence and assessment of attention-deficit/hyperactivity disorder in primary care settings. *Pediatrics* 2001; **107**: E43.

46. Mick E, Biederman J, Prince J, *et al.* Impact of low birth weight on attention-deficit hyperactivity disorder. *J Dev Behav Pediatr* 2002; **23**: 16–22.

47. Breslau N, Brown GG, DelDotto JE, *et al.* Psychiatric sequelae of low birth weight at 6 years of age. *J Abnorm Child Psychol* 1996; **24**: 385–400.

48. Breslau N, Chilcoat HD. Psychiatric sequelae of low birth weight at 11 years of age. *Biol Psychiatry* 2000; **47**: 1005–11.

49. Botting N, Powls A, Cooke RW, *et al.* Attention deficit hyperactivity disorders and other psychiatric outcomes in very low birthweight children at 12 years. *J Child Psychol Psychiatry* 1997; **38**: 931–41.

50. Indredavik MS, Vik T, Heyerdahl S, *et al.* Psychiatric symptoms and disorders in adolescents with low birth weight. *Arch Dis Child Fetal Neonatal Ed* 2004; **89**: F445–50.

51. Taylor H, Hack M, Klein NK. Attention deficits in children with <750 gm birth weight. *Child Neuropsychol* 1998; **4**: 21–34.

52. Elgen I, Lundervold AJ, Sommerfelt K, *et al.* Aspects of inattention in low birth weight children. *Pediatr Neurol* 2004; **30**: 92–8.

53. Davis DW, Burns B, Snyder E, *et al.* Attention problems in very low birth weight preschoolers: are new screening measures needed for this special population? *J Child Adolesc Psychiatr Nurs* 2007; **20**: 74–85.

54. Szatmari P, Saigal S, Rosenbaum P, *et al.* Psychiatric disorders at five years among children with birthweights less than 1000 g: a regional perspective. *Dev Med Child Neurol* 1990; **32**: 954–62.

55. Hack M, Youngstrom EA, Cartar L, *et al.* Behavioral outcomes and evidence of psychopathology among very low birth weight infants at age 20 years. *Pediatrics* 2004; **114**: 932–40.

56. Weindrich D, Jennen-Steinmetz C, Laucht M, *et al.* Late sequelae of low birthweight: mediators of poor school performance at 11 years. *Dev Med Child Neurol* 2003; **45**: 463–9.

57. Anderson P, Doyle LW, Callanan C, *et al.* Neurobehavioral outcomes of school-age children born extremely low birth weight or very preterm in the 1990s. *JAMA* 2003; **289**: 3264–72.

58. Back SA. Perinatal white matter injury: the changing spectrum of pathology and emerging insights into pathogenetic mechanisms. *Ment Retard Dev Disabil Res Rev* 2006; **12**: 129–40.

59. Peterson J, Taylor HG, Minich N, *et al.* Subnormal head circumference in very low birth weight children: neonatal correlates and school-age consequences. *Early Hum Dev* 2006; **82**: 325–34.

60. Hack M, Breslau N, Weissman B, *et al.* Effect of very low birth weight and subnormal head size on cognitive abilities at school age. *N Eng J Med* 1991; **325**: 231–7.

61. Kesler SR, Ment LR, Vohr B, *et al.* Volumetric analysis of regional cerebral development in preterm children. *Pediatr Neurol* 2004; **31**: 318–25.

62. Kesler SR, Vohr B, Schneider KC, *et al.* Increased temporal lobe gyrification in preterm children. *Neuropsychologia* 2006; **44**: 445–53.

63. Feldman HM, Janosky JE, Scher MS, *et al.* Language abilities following prematurity, periventricular brain injury, and cerebral palsy. *J Commun Disord* 1994; **27**: 71–90.

64. Bates E, Reilly J, Wulfeck B, *et al.* Differential effects of unilateral lesions on language production in children and adults. *Brain Lang* 2001; **79**: 223–65.

65. Booth JR, MacWhinney B, Thulborn KR, *et al.* Developmental and lesion effects in brain activation during sentence comprehension and mental rotation. *Dev Neuropsychol* 2000; **18**: 139–69.

66. Booth JR, Macwhinney B, Thulborn KR, *et al.* Functional organization of activation patterns in children: whole brain fMRI imaging during three different cognitive tasks. *Prog Neuropsychopharmacol Biol Psychiatry* 1999; **23**: 669–82.

67. Volpe JJ. *Neurology of the Newborn*, 4th edn. Philadelphia, PA: Saunders, 2001.

68. Fanaroff AA, Stoll BJ, Wright LL, *et al.* Trends in neonatal morbidity and mortality for very low birthweight infants. *Am J Obstet Gynecol* 2007; **196**: 147.e1–8.

69. Nosarti C, Rushe TM, Woodruff PWR, *et al.* Corpus callosum size and very preterm birth: relationship to neuropsychological outcome. *Brain* 2004; **127**: 2080–9.

70. Deutsch GK, Dougherty RF, Bammer R, *et al.* Children's reading performance is correlated with white matter structure measured by tensor imaging. *Cortex* 2005; **41**: 354–63.

71. Ben-Shachar M, Dougherty RF, Wandell BA. White matter pathways in reading. *Curr Opin Neurobiol* 2007; **17**: 258–70.

72. Limperopoulos C, Bassan H, Gauvreau K, *et al.* Does cerebellar injury in premature infants contribute to the high prevalence of long-term cognitive, learning, and behavioral disability in survivors? *Pediatrics* 2007; **120**: 584–93.

73. Leonard C, Eckert M, Given B, *et al.* Individual differences in anatomy predict reading and oral language impairments in children. *Brain* 2006; **129**: 3329–42.

74. Ment LR, Peterson BS, Vohr B, *et al.* Cortical recruitment patterns in children born prematurely compared with control subjects during a passive listening functional magnetic resonance imaging task. *J Pediatr* 2006; **149**: 490–8.

75. Law J, Garrett Z, Nye C. Speech and language therapy interventions for children with primary speech and language delay or disorder. *Cochrane Database Syst Rev* 2007; (**3**): CD004110.

76. World Health Organization. *The International Classification of Functioning, Disability and Health.* Geneva: WHO, 2001.

Neurocognitive outcomes of term infants with perinatal asphyxia

Steven P. Miller and Bea Latal

Introduction

Neonatal brain injuries represent a group of common yet heterogeneous disorders, which result in long-term neurodevelopmental deficits. A significant proportion is related to hypoxic–ischemic brain injury, either diffuse or focal (e.g., stroke). Neonatal brain injury is recognized clinically by a characteristic encephalopathy that evolves over days in the newborn period [1]. This clinical syndrome includes a lack of alertness, poor tone, abnormal reflex function, poor feeding, compromised respiratory status, and seizures [2]. Neonatal encephalopathy occurs in 1–6/1000 live term births, and is a major cause of neurodevelopmental disability [1]. Up to 20% of affected infants die during the newborn period, and another 25% sustain permanent deficits of motor and also cognitive function [3,4]. Functional motor deficits are often described as cerebral palsy, a non-progressive disorder of motor function or posture originating in early life. Cognitive deficits include mental retardation or learning disabilities, and impaired executive functions, language skills, or social ability. Other forms of neonatal brain injury, particularly in the term newborn, such as stroke, have an incidence as high as 1/4000 live births [5]. More than 95% of infants with neonatal stroke survive to adulthood, and many have some form of motor or cognitive disability.

Thus, neurocognitive deficits that follow neonatal encephalopathy are serious problems that frequently result in lifelong disability with serious impact for the child, family, and society. In addition, even if neurocognitive deficits are mild, they affect academic achievement and quality of life. Despite the prevalence of these deficits, predicting the long-term outcome of newborns with encephalopathy in the earliest days of life remains a considerable challenge. However, recent advances in newborn brain imaging have yielded important insights into expected patterns of neurocognitive outcomes. Understanding the full spectrum of neurocognitive outcome following neonatal encephalopathy is critical to applying and evaluating emerging strategies, such as hypothermia, to protect the neonatal brain from injury [6–8]. An understanding of the neurocognitive outcomes following neonatal encephalopathy

needs to consider the etiology of the brain injury, the timing of this injury, and the selective vulnerability of the neonatal brain to injury. These factors lead to characteristic patterns of brain injury in neonatal encephalopathy that are each associated with different profiles of neurocognitive deficits.

This chapter will focus on describing the brain injuries leading to neurocognitive deficits following neonatal encephalopathy, including the etiology and timing of brain injury in this condition, as well as the most commonly observed patterns of brain injury. The spectrum of neurocognitive abnormalities following neonatal encephalopathy will be discussed, and the profile of abnormalities associated with each of the main patterns of brain injury will be described. A case study will be used to highlight a typical profile of neurocognitive outcomes.

Brain injuries leading to neurocognitive deficits following neonatal encephalopathy
Etiology of neonatal encephalopathy

Neonatal encephalopathy is a heterogeneous condition with multiple etiologies. It is increasingly clear that most neonatal brain injury is metabolic, whether from transient ischemia–reperfusion or from inherited defects in metabolic pathways resulting in energy failure. Hypoxic–ischemic encephalopathy (HIE) accounts for a substantial fraction of neonatal brain injury, yet many cases of neonatal encephalopathy have no documented hypoxic–ischemic insult [1,9]. Other causes of neonatal encephalopathy include metabolic abnormalities such as acute bilirubin encephalopathy, hypoglycemia and inborn errors of metabolism, infections, trauma, and malformations of cerebral development. As many etiologies of neonatal encephalopathy have specific therapies, and the underlying cause of the encephalopathy is an important determinant of neurocognitive outcome, a critical part of clinical management is to determine the underlying etiology.

Timing of brain injury in neonatal encephalopathy

Recent studies are beginning to elucidate the antenatal, perinatal, and postnatal factors that underlie the vulnerability of the newborn brain, as well as the mechanisms that contribute to resilience and recovery. There is continuing controversy as to whether neonatal encephalopathy from hypoxia–ischemia

Fetal and Neonatal Brain Injury, 4th edition, ed. David K. Stevenson, William E. Benitz, Philip Sunshine, Susan R. Hintz, and Maurice L. Druzin. Published by Cambridge University Press. © Cambridge University Press 2009.

is primarily related to insults sustained in the antepartum or intrapartum period. Careful epidemiological studies suggested that neonatal encephalopathy is primarily related to antenatal risk factors (events well before birth), and that intrapartum factors (events at or near birth) account for a minority of cases [10,11]. In a prior study of risk factors for neonatal encephalopathy, 69% of cases had antepartum risk factors such as maternal hypothyroidism, pre-eclampsia, or chorioamnionitis, 5% had only intrapartum risks such cord prolapse or abruptio placentae, and 24% had both antepartum and intrapartum risks [10]. In recent years, magnetic resonance imaging (MRI) has emerged as a valuable tool for determining the timing and etiology of neonatal brain injury. In prospective studies using MRI in the first days of life, it is increasingly apparent that most term newborns with encephalopathy presumed secondary to hypoxia–ischemia have an acquired brain injury at or near the time of birth that progresses over several days [12,13]. In one prospective cohort of neonatal encephalopathy, more than 90% of affected newborns had evidence of perinatally acquired insults on MRI, with a very low rate of long-standing antenatal brain injury [12]. The imaging findings of acquired brain injury in these studies include brain swelling, loss of gray–white matter differentiation, abnormal signal intensities in the deep gray nuclei or posterior limb of the internal capsule, or an acutely developing region of infarction. The use of diffusion-weighted MRI has also greatly improved our ability to assess the onset of brain lesions in term newborns with encephalopathy. The reduction in free water diffusion in areas of brain injury, reflected in decreased average diffusivity or decreased apparent diffusion coefficients on diffusion-weighted imaging, evolves over the first days of life and normalizes over the second week following acute brain injury in the term newborn [14,15].

Taken together, it is possible that antenatal factors may lead to greater susceptibility to perinatal problems in some, while in others an acute sentinel is documented as a single perinatal event. These data suggest that because the brain injury is recent, it may be amenable to postnatal interventions, such as hypothermia, in the first days of life. With the increasing application of therapeutic hypothermia in newborns with moderate to severe encephalopathy, it is expected that the neurocognitive sequelae outlined below will change over the next 5–10 years. The recent brain imaging data also indicate the urgent need to discover the mechanistic link between antenatal risk factors and brain injury that occurs near the time of birth, so that new prevention strategies for encephalopathy can be implemented to further improve neurocognitive outcomes.

As the etiology of a newborn's encephalopathy, and its treatment, are key determinants of the expected neurodevelopmental outcome, this chapter will focus on acquired neonatal brain injury presumed secondary to hypoxia–ischemia. For the purpose of this chapter, the term "neonatal encephalopathy" is used instead of "perinatal asphyxia," as hypoxic–ischemic insults may not be documented, even when other causes of encephalopathy are excluded.

Selective vulnerability in the neonatal brain

Neonatal brain injury involves a complex set of interrelated biochemical and molecular pathways including oxidative stress, excitotoxicity, inflammation, and genetic effects, as addressed elsewhere in this volume (see Chapters 1 and 2). Underlying these mechanisms is a selective vulnerability of specific cell types at specific developmental stages. Together, these factors underlie the regional vulnerability of the developing brain in the human newborn, including the characteristic patterns of injury and resultant neurodevelopmental outcomes.

Patterns of brain injury in neonatal encephalopathy

Advanced neuroimaging techniques, such as MRI, can now be applied in the human newborn to better understand the heterogeneity of brain injury associated with neonatal encephalopathy. The typical patterns of brain injury in neonatal encephalopathy are each associated with different patterns of neurodevelopmental outcomes. In a primate model of term neonatal brain injury, the specific regional distribution of injury was associated with different durations and severities of ischemia: partial asphyxia caused cerebral white-matter injury, while acute and profound asphyxia produced selective injury to the basal ganglia and thalamus [16,17]. As changes on MRI correspond closely to histopathological changes found on postmortem examination [18–21], MRI can be applied in vivo to better understand the heterogeneity of brain injury associated with neonatal encephalopathy. A comparable regional vulnerability is observed in the brain of term newborns following hypoxia–ischemia, resulting in two major patterns of injury detectable by MRI: (1) a *watershed-predominant* pattern involving the white matter, particularly in the vascular watershed, extending to cortical gray matter when severe, and (2) a *basal-nuclei-predominant* pattern involving the deep gray nuclei, perirolandic cortex, and hippocampus, extending to the total cortex when severe [1,22–25]. These patterns reflect the predominant regions of injury, with frequent overlap in affected newborns. Involvement of the hippocampus has been linked to specific neurocognitive deficits later in childhood [26]. As expected from the primate models, newborns with basal nuclei patterns of injury have the most intensive need for resuscitation and the most severe clinical encephalopathy. Focal infarctions of the brain, either arterial or venous, are an additional but under-recognized pattern of injury in the term newborn, occasionally occurring in the setting of neonatal encephalopathy [12,27]. Consistent with observations of childhood stroke, many newborns with stroke have multiple risk factors for brain injury, including intrapartum complications [28].

Spectrum of neurocognitive abnormalities following neonatal encephalopathy

The neurocognitive outcome following neonatal encephalopathy is variable and may include deficits of neuromotor, neurosensory, and cognitive functions. Cognitive deficits may result from the cerebral cortical injury that frequently accompanies basal nuclei injury. In contrast, the watershed pattern of injury is most commonly associated with cognitive impairments that are not accompanied by major motor deficits [25]. The clinical correlate of the basal nuclei pattern of injury in the neonatal period is a severe encephalopathy, while the watershed pattern more frequently manifests as a more moderate encephalopathy. While both patterns may be accompanied by neonatal seizures, these are seen in almost 90% of those with the basal nuclei pattern and closer to half of those in whom watershed injury predominates [25]. The cognitive deficits associated with watershed injury may not be apparent in early infancy and often need more prolonged follow-up for detection. It should be stressed that abnormal outcome following neonatal encephalopathy is not limited to cerebral palsy and often requires follow-up beyond 1 year of age to be detected [25]. Postnatal factors such as socioeconomic status also have important effects on neurodevelopmental outcome following brain injury in the term newborn [29].

The American College of Obstetricians and Gynecologists task force on neonatal encephalopathy and cerebral palsy concluded that an acute intrapartum event could result only in cerebral palsy of the spastic quadriplegic or dyskinetic type, and could not account for cognitive deficits alone [30]. Our clinical experience and recently reviewed data suggest that the outcome of neonatal encephalopathy includes cognitive deficits as a prominent feature, even in the absence of cerebral palsy, and that this is associated with the watershed pattern of injury and white-matter damage [25,29,31]. A number of studies examining the long-term outcomes of children with neonatal encephalopathy or children with risk factors for hypoxia–ischemia have described isolated cognitive deficits in the absence of functional motor deficits [26,29,32–36]. In this era of increasing medical litigation, it is critical to stress that these studies address the outcomes of critically ill newborns with overt encephalopathy, rather than children identified later in life on the basis of isolated cognitive impairments. In addition to these clinical reports, experimental studies using a variety of large and small animal models demonstrate the selective vulnerability of the developing brain to hypoxia-ischemia. In the immature brain exposed to hypoxia–ischemia, injury predominates in the hippocampus, striatum, and parasagittal cortex [23]. The resulting hypoxic–ischemic injury often causes impairments in memory, learning, and spatial orientation, frequently in the absence of gross motor deficits [31]. The learning and behavior abnormalities may not be evident early in life but may only become apparent in adolescence. These studies highlight the need for a better understanding of the early brain lesions that underlie long-term neurodevelopmental impairments in this population. In addition, it is mandatory to assess the full spectrum of specific neurocognitive outcomes following neonatal encephalopathy, which include the following domains: (1) neuromotor (cerebral palsy and other motor abnormalities), (2) neurosensory (vision and hearing), (3) epilepsy, (4) cognitive abilities (general, memory, executive function, language), (5) behavior, and (6) quality of life.

Specific neurocognitive outcomes following neonatal encephalopathy

Compared to the extensive literature on outcomes of other populations at risk for neurodevelomental impairment such as children born preterm, the body of literature is remarkably small for term-born survivors of neonatal encephalopathy. Previous publications on long-term outcome described children who suffered from "asphyxia" defined by abnormal biochemical or clinical markers (pH, base excess, Apgar, intrauterine distress with bradycardia, abnormal cardiotocogram), but in whom the neurologic impairment after birth was not a defining criterion [37,38]. It is thus difficult to compare outcomes in these studies to those from studies using the severity of neonatal encephalopathy as a defining criterion [34,39,40]. The current definition of hypoxic–ischemic encephalopathy mandates clinical signs of neonatal encephalopathy in the absence of other etiologies. While recent *imaging* studies support the assumption that once other causes of neonatal encephalopathy are excluded, such as genetic syndromes or congenital infections, the remaining cases are primarily related to hypoxia–ischemia, few of the *outcome* studies rigorously document intrapartum asphyxia (according to ACOG guidelines) in all subjects. Overall, studies of outcome following neonatal encephalopathy presumed secondary to hypoxic–ischemic injury have focused on mortality, neurologic disability, and, to a much lesser extent, cognition.

In addition to the major motor and cognitive disabilities that can be diagnosed in early childhood, a complete assessment of neurocognitive outcomes needs to consider domains that are more readily assessed as children develop to school age: learning (including writing, reading, and math), executive functions, behavior, and social competence. Impairments in these domains are often only detected with the increased demands of school and peer groups. Neurocognitive or intellectual abnormalities are increasingly recognized as important long-term sequelae, even in the absence of major motor impairments [31]. Intellectual abilities and in particular executive functions such as planning, organization, flexibility, and attention play an increasingly important role in today's society. In addition, specific dysfunctions such as attention-deficit/hyperactivity disorder, developmental coordination disorder, autism spectrum disorder, or specific language impairment may follow neonatal brain injury, either in isolation or more often in conjunction with each other [41].

"Quality of life," an individual's subjective perception of physical and psychological health, is an important aspect of outcome that is only beginning to be probed following neonatal brain injury. Thus the assessment of long-term neurocognitive outcomes needs to consider the child's function in a variety of environments – family, school, employment, and society.

Many studies on neurocognitive sequelae after neonatal encephalopathy report outcomes at an early age [33,42]. Early cognitive testing has limited predictive value for later functioning, in part because early developmental testing relies on cognitive concepts that differ from those later intellectual assessments where memory, executive function, language and visuomotor functions are specifically tested. Thus early prognosis of later cognitive functioning is difficult, and may be impacted by a host of other factors such as genetic and environmental, in particular socioeconomic, factors [29,40]. Very few studies report long-term outcome into adolescence or young adulthood [40,43–45]. These studies, however, usually did not perform detailed neonatal brain imaging, limiting our ability to link long-term outcomes with patterns of injury in the newborn. Knowledge on long-term outcome of these children is crucial not only for parental counseling but also for tailoring follow-up services and appropriate therapies, and for advising teachers and therapists, caring for these children.

Neuromotor outcome

Cerebral palsy
In survivors of HIE, cerebral palsy or severe disability ranges from 13% to about 36% [1,25,32–34,36,44,46], but strongly depends on the severity of encephalopathy. Survivors of a severe neonatal encephalopathy face a high risk of cerebral palsy. In one study, all surviving children after severe encephalopathy had a severe disability [36]. A more recent study reported that 42% of children with severe encephalopathy were diagnosed with cerebral palsy at age 7 years [34]. At school age, spastic quadriparesis is the most common severe neurologic disability, although athetoid or spastic hemiparesis may also occur. Other disabilities often co-occur with cerebral palsy, including sensorineural hearing loss, cortical blindness, and learning difficulties [34].

Motor function in the absence of cerebral palsy
Few studies have examined motor functioning in the absence of cerebral palsy in children with neonatal encephalopathy. Their results indicate that motor problems in the absence of cerebral palsy may occur, and may also occur in children after mild neonatal encephalopathy. Parents reported an increased rate of minor motor impairments and fine motor problems for school-age children with low Apgar scores and signs of neonatal encephalopathy (seizures, feeding difficulties, and/or ventilator treatment) [35]. The presence of a neonatal encephalopathy seems to be a critical risk factor for impaired motor skills. In a cohort with mild intrapartum fetal asphyxia, but without neonatal neurological signs in the majority, no differences in gross and fine motor performance were seen at 7 years of age (assessed by the Bruinicks–Oseretsky Test of Motor Proficiency and the Motor Accuracy Test) [47]. A recent study examined motor performance using a standardized motor test (Movement Assessment Battery for Children) in 61 9- to 10-year-old children with neonatal encephalopathy but without cerebral palsy and related motor performance to corpus callosum size on MRI. Definitely abnormal motor performance ($\leq$ 5th percentile) was more frequently diagnosed in children with moderate, but importantly also in children with

mild encephalopathy (37.5% and 29% respectively) [48]. Similar findings were reported for 5- to 6-year-old children: 23.5% of children with neonatal encephalopathy without cerebral palsy were diagnosed with minor neurological dysfunction and/or perceptual–motor difficulties [32].

Neurosensory outcome

Vision
Impaired visual function after neonatal encephalopathy can be due to (1) "cortical visual impairment," resulting from injury in the posterior visual pathway, including the primary visual cortex [49], or (2) injury in other central nervous system structures (e.g., optic radiation, basal ganglia, or thalamus) [50] that may then affect acuity, visual fields, or stereopsis. Severe visual impairment or blindness occurs in 11–25% of children after severe or moderate encephalopathy, most often in association with neurological disability [51,52]. Abnormalities can be detected in the first years after birth and are related to the extent of cerebral injury on MRI, in particular to basal ganglia involvement [50]. Visual abnormalities persist to school age and are highly related to early visual abnormalities [53].

Hearing
Children with neonatal encephalopathy are at increased risk for sensorineural hearing loss [36,51]. Hearing loss may be associated with neurological disabilities, but not necessarily [1,52,54]. The pathophysiology of sensorineural hearing loss after HIE is not fully understood; it may be due to selective injury to brainstem and dorsal cochlear nuclei [1,55]. It appears that hearing loss is not associated with gentamycin treatment or familial deafness [54]. While there is no increase in parentally reported hearing impairments in children with low Apgar scores and signs of encephalopathy [35], survivors of moderate encephalopathy without cerebral palsy are at substantial risk of hearing loss, with up to 18% affected, by parental report [44].

Epilepsy
Post-neonatal epilepsy frequently occurs after moderate or severe neonatal encephalopathy, affecting 20–50% of survivors [56,57]. Two recent studies reported a significantly lower incidence of epilepsy, 9.4%, in infants who were treated for both clinical and subclinical seizures in the neonatal period [58,59]. The occurrence of post-neonatal seizures is strongly related to the diagnosis of cerebral palsy and developmental delay [59].

Cognitive ability

General
A limited number of studies have presented results on cognitive abilities. Overall, cognitive functions may also be impaired in the absence of cerebral palsy or major disability [34,36]. Overall, 30–50% of children with moderate (grade 2) HIE have mental deficits at follow-up [60]. Marlow et al. demonstrated that intellectual performance in children with severe encephalopathy without cerebral palsy is significantly poorer than in

controls, with a mean difference of 11 IQ points [34]. Another study including children after aEEG detected neonatal seizures (moderate and severe encephalopathy) showed that 11% of children with moderate encephalopathy manifested global delay in the absence of cerebral palsy at 5 years of age [59]. Robertson and Finer found that 42% of non-disabled children (that is, in the absence of cerebral palsy, mental retardation, severe neurosensory deficits, or seizure disorders) in the moderate encephalopathy group were delayed on school-readiness tests [61].

In addition to generally diminished intellectual performance, children in the moderate encephalopathy group were more likely to have problems in reading, spelling, and arithmetic compared to those with mild encephalopathy or controls at 8 years of age [36]. No difference was found between mildly encephalopathic newborns and controls [36]. A large study by Moster and colleagues from Norway compared children with low Apgar scores (0–3) and signs of neonatal encephalopathy to those with normal Apgar scores and no neonatal signs. Neurodevelopmental and behavioral outcomes were assessed by parental questionnaire. Children with major neurological disabilities were excluded. The authors found that children with low Apgar scores and signs of neonatal encephalopathy had a sevenfold increased risk of need for extra resources in kindergarten and a threefold increased risk of intervention at school. They also were judged by their parents to perform below average in reading, writing, spelling, and mathematics [35].

It appears that the proportion of children with cognitive deficits may rise with increasing age of follow-up and increasing intellectual demands: a study examining 28 children at age 15–19 years detected definitive cognitive dysfunctions in 71% of the children [44]. These dysfunctions are coupled with educational problems, which may continue into adulthood, leading to a higher unemployment rate and a lower proportion of survivors obtaining a university degree [43].

Memory and executive functions

Little information is available on specific neurocognitive deficits after neonatal encephalopathy. However, short- and long-term memory problems, in particular auditory memory, are prevalent in survivors of moderate or severe neonatal encephalopathy. A study by Lindström et al. showed that 64% of parents of children with moderate encephalopathy reported short-term memory problems and problems with time perception, interfering with the child's daily life [44]. Deficits in short- and long-term memory may not be detected following a mild encephalopathy [47]. However, Robertson and Finer showed that cognitive function of children after moderate encephalopathy was particularly affected in areas of auditory memory, attention, and short-term recall. They also demonstrated for children after mild encephalopathy that visual attention for letters and objects (assessed by the Detroit Tests of Learning Aptitude) was significantly diminished compared to a neonatal and peer comparison group [40]. Marlow and colleagues confirmed these findings in a cohort of 65 children at 7 years of age, 50 of whom were free of motor

disability. Although childhood survivors of moderate neonatal encephalopathy had similar overall IQ scores compared to control children, specific cognitive impairments were detected: language and auditory memory (narrative memory, sentence repetition) on a standardized neuropsychological assessment scale (NEPSY) [34].

Language

Language development may also be impaired after neonatal encephalopathy [54]. Children following moderate encephalopathy are reported to have more problems in speaking and listening, reading and spelling compared to those with mild encephalopathy or controls [34,36]. Similar results were reported at school age for children with low Apgar scores and signs of neonatal encephalopathy compared to children with normal Apgar scores and no neonatal encephalopathy [35].

Behavior

Childhood survivors of neonatal encephalopathy without motor disability are at increased risk for behavioral problems such as hyperactivity and emotional problems [34]. Children with low Apgar scores (0–3) and signs of neonatal encephalopathy were more likely to manifest behavioral problems such as aggressivity, passivity, and anxiety as assessed by parental questionnaire using the Yale Children's Inventory Scale [35]. They were also almost four times more likely to need follow-up by a special resource center for children with educational or behavioral problems [35]. However, from this study it is unknown if these behavioral outcomes differed in individuals with mild or moderate encephalopathy. Other studies suggest that behavioral differences are not detected at 8 years of age in survivors of perinatal asphyxia (defined by an umbilical artery base deficit greater than 12 mmol/L) with only mild or no encephalopathy [47]. It is increasingly clear that behavioral problems following a moderate encephalopathy may persist into late adolescence. Comparing adolescents after moderate neonatal encephalopathy to a sibling comparison group, significant differences are seen on the Conners scale ($p < 0.003$), on the inattention subscale of the ADHD Rating Scale IV ($p < 0.006$), and on the Asperger Syndrome Screening Questionnaire [44].

Quality of life

Quality of life is a multidimensional construct integrating an individual's subjective perceptions of physical, social, emotional, and cognitive functioning [62]. Quality of life can be assessed by means of self- or proxy-reports. No study has been published on long-term quality of life of children after neonatal encephalopathy using instruments that reflect the above-mentioned construct. One study examined social interaction using standardized questionnaires (Conners 10-item scale, Asperger Syndrome Screening Questionnaire) [44]. Difficulties making friends or interacting with peers were reported more frequently for teenage children with moderate neonatal encephalopathy compared to their siblings [44]. In a study of family stress and function in 7-year-old children after mild neonatal encephalopathy no difference in the number of major life events (e.g., divorce, loss of job, etc.) was found between affected children and controls [47]. This finding is not unexpected, since major life events have been associated only with major child disabilities, but not with minor neuro-cognitive problems.

Patterns of brain injury in relation to neurocognitive outcomes

The severity of clinical encephalopathy in the first days of life is an important predictor of neurodevelopmental outcome [2,30]. Children with mild encephalopathy do not appear to have an increased risk of neurocognitive sequelae compared to normal children [40,63], even when selected motor functions, short- and long-term memory, and behavior are tested [47]. At the other end of the spectrum, the majority of children with severe encephalopathy die, and the remainder suffer from severe disabilities such as cerebral palsy, mental retardation, or epilepsy [36]. Determining the outcome of moderate encephalopathy is more difficult, as the spectrum of neuro-cognitive disability is broad. In this context, neonatal brain imaging, with MRI in particular, is emerging as a powerful tool to accurately predict neurocognitive outcomes.

While it is accepted that the risk of an abnormal neuro-developmental outcome increases with the severity of brain injury detected by MRI, the pattern of injury also conveys important prognostic information regarding the *pattern* of neurodevelopmental outcomes [25,64]. Abnormal signal intensity in the posterior limb of the internal capsule on MRI, and injury predominantly in the basal ganglia and thalamus, are associated with severely impaired motor and cognitive outcomes [25,65]. In fact, the pattern of brain injury on MRI is even more predictive of neurodevelopmental outcome than is the *severity* of brain lesions, and is often associated with specific profiles (or patterns) of neurocognitive impairments [12,25].

The basal-nuclei-predominant and watershed-predomin-ant patterns of injury are associated with impairments in different developmental domains. Both the basal-nuclei-predominant pattern and abnormal signal intensity in the posterior limb of the internal capsule on MRI have been associated with severely impaired motor and cognitive out-comes [25,64–66]. As the basal-nuclei-predominant pattern of injury is frequently accompanied by cerebral cortical and white-matter injury in a watershed distribution [25], and with cerebellar injury [67,68], cognitive deficits with this pattern of injury may result from damage to areas outside the deep gray nuclei themselves. In contrast, newborns with the watershed pattern have predominantly cognitive impairments, which often occur without functional motor deficits [25].

It is important to recognize that the detection of cognitive deficits in survivors of neonatal encephalopathy, with or with-out co-existing motor deficits, may be delayed beyond the first year of life. In one cohort, cognitive deficits associated with the watershed pattern of injury were detected at 30 months, but were largely under-recognized at 12 months of age [29]. Additionally, term newborns with encephalopathy and an abnormal MRI are more likely to have neurological impair-ments such as minor perceptual–motor difficulties at 5 years of age, even in the absence of gross motor deficits or differences in IQ [32]. Newborns with the watershed-predominant pattern of injury on neonatal MRI in the setting of an overt neonatal encephalopathy appear to be at highest risk of long-term cogni-tive deficits in the absence of overt motor signs. It is also important to note that some survivors of neonatal encephal-opathy with persistent white-matter damage on follow-up MRI at 2 years of age still have normal outcomes at this time point [69]. The child's postnatal environment, including socio-economic conditions and access to rehabilitative services, will also directly impact the presentation and severity of abnormal neurocognitive outcomes, especially at later time points [29]. It is at these later time points in childhood that some of the specific neurocognitive deficits described above, such as impaired executive functions, may be most readily examined.

Advanced quantitative brain imaging techniques, such as MR spectroscopy and diffusion tensor imaging, can now be applied to measure subtle brain injuries, such as white-matter injuries, and determine their association with long-term neurocognitive outcomes [29,70,71]. For example, in a recent case series using advanced volumetric techniques, five survivors of neonatal encephalopathy examined between 8 and 14 years of age with delayed recall, in the setting of intact semantic memory and motor function, were found to have bilateral hippocampal atrophy on MRI [26].

Conclusions

Childhood survivors of neonatal encephalopathy are at risk of a broad spectrum of neurocognitive and behavioral–social deficits. With sophisticated and detailed measures of cognition there appears to be an association between specific cognitive deficits, such as language and memory deficits, with the sever-ity of neonatal encephalopathy and the pattern of brain injury. This recognition allows physicians and caregivers an oppor-tunity to optimally care for infants following neonatal enceph-alopathy by identifying those who may benefit most from rehabilitative services and early intervention, to maximize educational and social function and thus independent func-tion throughout development. In this era of potential therapies for neonatal brain injury, including hypothermia, we need a better understanding of the full spectrum of motor *and* cognitive outcomes of survivors of neonatal encephalopathy. Studies into the mechanisms that contribute to resilience and recovery from neonatal brain injury offer further promise to prevent neurocognitive deficits following neonatal encephal-opathy. In addition, a better understanding of the postnatal factors impacting neurocognitive outcomes, including envir-onmental and social influences, will ultimately lead to better interventions to improve the outcome of affected newborns.

Case study

Baby Girl M was born to a healthy 31-year-old primigravid mother, after an uneventful pregnancy at 40 weeks' gestation. Before delivery, the mother noted decreased fetal movements. Because of an abnormal fetal heart tracing and meconium-stained amniotic fluid an emergent cesarean section was performed. The Apgar scores were 1 and 5 at 1 and 5 minutes respectively; the arterial cord pH was 6.98. The birthweight was 3130 g, length was 50 cm and head circumference was 35 cm (all 50th–90th percentile). The newborn required positive-pressure ventilation for a few minutes before breathing spontaneously. Multifocal clonic seizures were noted clinically at 12 hours of life and treated with phenobarbital. The child was neurologically abnormal on the first day of life, with poor spontaneous movements, hypotonia, a high-pitched cry, and decreased suck and gag reflex. These abnormalities persisted until discharge on day 17 of life, when the child manifested limited responsiveness to visual and auditory stimuli, marked truncal hypotonia with hyperextension of the lower extremities, poor spontaneous movements of the extremities, and exaggerated muscle stretch reflexes. MRI of the brain on the fourth day of life revealed moderate watershed injury accompanied by mild signal abnormalities in the basal ganglia and thalamus.

The child was serially examined until 12.5 years of age with attention to the domains outlined in Table 48.1. By 2 years of age a mild cerebral palsy (level 1 on the gross motor function classification system for cerebral palsy, GMFCS [72]) was evident, with significant cognitive delay (MDI = 70), in the setting of microcephaly (head circumference below the 3rd percentile). At 5 years of age generalized tonic–clonic seizures occurred and were treated with valproate.

At 6 years of age the child manifested an intellectual deficit with an IQ of 75 as assessed by the Kaufman Assessment Battery for Children [73]. Working memory (visual and auditory) was particularly affected. Language performance was even more delayed than the overall cognitive functional level; a dysarthria accompanying her mild cerebral palsy was also noted. Motor functioning was impaired, classified as level 1 on the GMFCS. She received speech and language therapy, occupational and physical therapy, and she went to a special kindergarten.

Table 48.1. Proposed follow-up template for survivors of neonatal encephalopathy. Examination ages and intervals are suggestions and may be increased if clinically necessary. For each developmental domain, *options* for standardized examination tools are listed; they can be replaced by other standardized tests. The choice of appropriate assessment tools for specific cognitive testing should be discussed with a neuropsychologist.

Age	Domain	Assessment tool
3 months	Neurology	Standardized neurological examination including clinical assessment of hearing and vision
9–12 months	Neurology	Standardized neurological examination; for cerebral palsy: gross motor function classification system [72]
	Cognition	Bayley Scales of Infant Development III – Cognitive or equivalent [74]
	Motor	Bayley Scales of Infant Development III – Motor or Alberta Infant Motor Scale [74,75]
2–3 years	Neurology	Standardized neurological examination; for cerebral palsy: gross motor function classification system [72]
	Cognition	Bayley Scales of Infant Development III – Cognitive or equivalent [74]
	Motor	Bayley Scales of Infant Development III – Motor or equivalent [74]
	Behavior/social	Bayley Scales of Infant Development III – Adaptive Behavior; *optional:* screening for autism (e.g., childhood autism checklist) [76]
	Specific	Language: Bayley Scales of Infant Development III – Language [74], or other, e.g., the clinical linguistic and auditory milestone scale in infancy [77]
4–6 years	Neurology	Standardized neurological examination; for cerebral palsy: gross motor function classification system [72]; acuity and hearing
	Cognition	Wechsler Preschool and Primary Scale of Intelligence 3rd edn. [78] or Kaufman-ABC [73]
	Motor	Standardized motor test: Movement-ABC II [79], Bruinicks-Oseretsky Test of Motor Proficiency [80], or Zurich Neuromotor Assessment [81]
	Behavior/Social	Screening for behavioral abnormalities, e.g., strength and difficulties questionnaire [82]
	Specific	Language (standardized test or questionnaire)
10–12 years	Neurology	Standardized neurological examination; for cerebral palsy: gross motor function classification system [72]; acuity and hearing
	Cognition	Wechsler Intelligence Scale for Children, 4th edn. [83] or Kaufman-ABC [73]
	Motor	Standardized motor test: Movement-ABC II [79], Bruinicks–Oseretsky Test of Motor Proficiency [80], or Zurich Neuromotor Assessment [81]
	Behavior/	Screening for behavioral abnormalities, e.g., strength and difficulties questionnaire [82]; Youth Self Report [84]; quality of life [85,86]
	Quality of life	
	Specific	Testing of specific intellectual functions: reading, writing, working memory, executive function, using standardized tests

From 6 until 12 years of age, she continued in a special-education school and received the same therapies. At 12 years of age the motor impairment was evident on standardized testing (Zurich Neuromotor Assessment) and intellectual functioning further decreased compared to 6 years of age with an IQ of 62 on the Wechsler Intelligence Scale for Children–revised version [83]. Her behavior was normal and she was a happy and contented girl with a good quality of life according to her parents. Her special interests were animals and flowers.

References

1. Volpe JJ. *Neurology of the Newborn*, 4th edn. Philadelphia, PA: Saunders, 2001.

2. Miller SP, Latal B, Clark H, *et al.* Clinical signs predict 30-month neurodevelopmental outcome after neonatal encephalopathy. *Am J Obstet Gynecol* 2004; **190**: 93–9.

3. Vannucci RC, Perlman JM. Interventions for perinatal hypoxic–ischemic encephalopathy. *Pediatrics* 1997; **100**: 1004–14.

4. Finer NN, Robertson CM, Richards RT, *et al.* Hypoxic–ischemic encephalopathy in term neonates: perinatal factors and outcome. *J Pediatr* 1981; **98**: 112–17.

5. Nelson KB, Lynch JK. Stroke in newborn infants. *Lancet Neurol* 2004; **3**: 150–8.

6. Gluckman PD, Wyatt JS, Azzopardi D, *et al.* Selective head cooling with mild systemic hypothermia to improve neurodevelopmental outcome following neonatal encephalopathy: the CoolCap study. *Pediatr Res* 2004; **55**: 582A.

7. Inder TE, Hunt RW, Morley CJ, *et al.* Systemic hypothermia selectively protects the cortex in term hypoxic–ischemic encephalopathy. *Pediatr Res* 2004; **55**: 583A.

8. Shankaran S, Laptook AR, Ehrenkranz RA, *et al.* Whole-body hypothermia for neonates with hypoxic–ischemic encephalopathy. *N Eng J Med* 2005; **353**: 1574–84.

9. Ferriero DM. Neonatal brain injury. *N Eng J Med* 2004; **351**: 1985–95.

10. Badawi N, Kurinczuk JJ, Keogh JM, *et al.* Intrapartum risk factors for newborn encephalopathy: the Western Australian case–control study. *BMJ* 1998; **317**: 1554–8.

11. Badawi N, Kurinczuk JJ, Keogh JM, *et al.* Antepartum risk factors for newborn encephalopathy: the Western Australian case-control study. *BMJ* 1998; **317**: 1549–53.

12. Cowan F, Rutherford M, Groenendaal F, *et al.* Origin and timing of brain lesions in term infants with neonatal encephalopathy. *Lancet* 2003; **361**: 736–42.

13. Chau V, Poskitt KJ, Sargent MA, *et al.* Comparison of computer tomography and magnetic resonance imaging scans on the third day of life in term newborns with neonatal encephalopathy. *Pediatrics* 2009; **123**: 319–26.

14. Barkovich AJ, Miller SP, Bartha A, *et al.* MR imaging, MR spectroscopy, and diffusion tensor imaging of sequential studies in neonates with encephalopathy. *AJNR Am J Neuroradiology* 2006; **27**: 533–47.

15. McKinstry RC, Miller JH, Snyder AZ, *et al.* A prospective, longitudinal diffusion tensor imaging study of brain injury in newborns. *Neurology* 2002; **59**: 824–33.

16. Myers RE. Four patterns of perinatal brain damage and their conditions of occurrence in primates. *Adv Neurol* 1975; **10**: 223–34.

17. Myers RE. Two patterns of perinatal brain damage and their conditions of occurrence. *Am J Obstet Gynecol* 1972; **112**: 246–76.

18. Childs AM, Cornette L, Ramenghi LA, *et al.* Magnetic resonance and cranial ultrasound characteristics of periventricular white matter abnormalities in newborn infants. *Clin Radiol* 2001; **56**: 647–55.

19. Felderhoff-Mueser U, Rutherford MA, Squier WV, *et al.* Relationship between MR imaging and histopathologic findings of the brain in extremely sick preterm infants. *AJNR Am J Neuroradiol* 1999; **20**: 1349–57.

20. Hope PL, Gould SJ, Howard S, *et al.* Precision of ultrasound diagnosis of pathologically verified lesions in the brains of very preterm infants. *Dev Med Child Neurol* 1988; **30**: 457–71.

21. Schouman-Claeys E, Henry-Feugeas MC, Roset F, *et al.* Periventricular leukomalacia: correlation between MR imaging and autopsy findings during the first 2 months of life. *Radiology* 1993; **189**: 59–64.

22. Barkovich AJ, Hajnal BL, Vigneron D, *et al.* Prediction of neuromotor outcome in perinatal asphyxia: evaluation of MR scoring systems. *AJNR Am J Neuroradiol* 1998; **19**: 143–9.

23. McQuillen PS, Ferriero DM. Selective vulnerability in the developing central nervous system. *Pediatr Neurol* 2004; **30**: 227–35.

24. Sie LT, van der Knaap MS, Oosting J, *et al.* MR patterns of hypoxic–ischemic brain damage after prenatal, perinatal or postnatal asphyxia. *Neuropediatrics* 2000; **31**: 128–36.

25. Miller SP, Ramaswamy V, Michelson D, *et al.* Patterns of brain injury in term neonatal encephalopathy. *J Pediatr* 2005; **146**: 453–60.

26. Gadian DG, Aicardi J, Watkins KE, *et al.* Developmental amnesia associated with early hypoxic–ischaemic injury. *Brain* 2000; **123**: 499–507.

27. Ramaswamy V, Miller SP, Barkovich AJ, *et al.* Perinatal stroke in term infants with neonatal encephalopathy. *Neurology* 2004; **62**: 2088–91.

28. Lee J, Croen LA, Backstrand KH, *et al.* Maternal and infant characteristics associated with perinatal arterial stroke in the infant. *JAMA* 2005; **293**: 723–9.

29. Miller SP, Newton N, Ferriero DM, *et al.* Predictors of 30-month outcome after perinatal depression: role of proton MRS and socioeconomic factors. *Pediatr Res* 2002; **52**: 71–7.

30. American College of Obstetricians and Gynecologists. Neonatal encephalopathy and cerebral palsy: executive summary. *Obstet Gynecol* 2004; **103**: 780–1.

31. Gonzalez FF, Miller SP. Does perinatal asphyxia impair cognitive function without cerebral palsy? *Arch Dis Child Fetal Neonatal Ed* 2006; **91**: F454–9.

32. Barnett A, Mercuri E, Rutherford M, *et al.* Neurological and perceptual–motor outcome at 5–6 years of age in children with neonatal encephalopathy: relationship with neonatal brain MRI. *Neuropediatrics* 2002; **33**: 242–8.

33. Dixon G, Badawi N, Kurinczuk JJ, *et al.* Early developmental outcomes after newborn encephalopathy. *Pediatrics* 2002; **109**: 26–33.

34. Marlow N, Rose AS, Rands CE, *et al.* Neuropsychological and educational problems at school age associated with

neonatal encephalopathy. *Arch Dis Child Fetal Neonatal Ed* 2005; **90**: F380–7.

35. Moster D, Lie RT, Markestad T. Joint association of Apgar scores and early neonatal symptoms with minor disabilities at school age. *Arch Dis Child Fetal Neonatal Ed* 2002; **86**: F16–21.

36. Robertson CM, Finer NN, Grace MG. School performance of survivors of neonatal encephalopathy associated with birth asphyxia at term. *J Pediatr* 1989; **114**: 753–60.

37. Goodwin TM, Belai I, Hernandez P, *et al.* Asphyxial complications in the term newborn with severe umbilical acidemia. *Am J Obstet Gynecol* 1992; **167**: 1506–12.

38. Nelson KB, Ellenberg JH. Apgar scores as predictors of chronic neurologic disability. *Pediatrics* 1981; **68**: 36–44.

39. Sarnat HB, Sarnat MS. Neonatal encephalopathy following fetal distress: a clinical and electroencephalographic study. *Arch Neurol* 1976; **33**: 696–705.

40. Robertson CM, Finer NN. Long-term follow-up of term neonates with perinatal asphyxia. *Clin Perinatol* 1993; **20**: 483–500.

41. van Handel M, Swaab H, de Vries LS, *et al.* Long-term cognitive and behavioral consequences of neonatal encephalopathy following perinatal asphyxia: a review. *Eur J Pediatr* 2007; **166**: 645–54.

42. van Schie PE, Becher JG, Dallmeijer AJ, *et al.* Motor outcome at the age of one after perinatal hypoxic–ischemic encephalopathy. *Neuropediatrics* 2007; **38**: 71–7.

43. Kjellmer I, Beijer E, Carlsson G, *et al.* Follow-up into young adulthood after cardiopulmonary resuscitation in term and near-term newborn infants. I. Educational achievements and social adjustment. *Acta Paediatr* 2002; **91**: 1212–17.

44. Lindström K, Lagerroos P, Gillberg C, *et al.* Teenage outcome after being born at term with moderate neonatal encephalopathy. *Pediatr Neurol* 2006; **35**: 268–74.

45. Viggedal G, Lundalv E, Carlsson G, *et al.* Follow-up into young adulthood after cardiopulmonary resuscitation in term and near-term newborn infants. II. Neuropsychological consequences. *Acta Paediatr* 2002; **91**: 1218–26.

46. Badawi N, Felix JF, Kurinczuk JJ, *et al.* Cerebral palsy following term newborn encephalopathy: a population-based

study. *Dev Med Child Neurol* 2005; **47**: 293–8.

47. Handley-Derry M, Low JA, Burke SO, *et al.* Intrapartum fetal asphyxia and the occurrence of minor deficits in 4- to 8-year-old children. *Dev Med Child Neurol* 1997; **39**: 508–14.

48. van Kooij B, van Handel M, Uiterwaal C, *et al.* Corpus callosum size in relation to motor performance in 9- to 10-year-old children with neonatal encephalopathy. *Pediatr Res* 2008; **63**: 1–6.

49. Van Hof-van Duin J, Mohn G. Visual defects in children after cerebral hypoxia. *Behav Brain Res* 1984; **14**: 147–55.

50. Mercuri E, Atkinson J, Braddick O, *et al.* Basal ganglia damage and impaired visual function in the newborn infant. *Arch Dis Child Fetal Neonatal Ed* 1997; **77**: F111–14.

51. Robertson C, Finer N. Term infants with hypoxic–ischemic encephalopathy: outcome at 3.5 years. *Dev Med Child Neurol* 1985; **27**: 473–84.

52. Shankaran S, Woldt E, Koepke T, *et al.* Acute neonatal morbidity and long-term central nervous system sequelae of perinatal asphyxia in term infants. *Early Hum Dev* 1991; **25**: 135–48.

53. Mercuri E, Anker S, Guzzetta A, *et al.* Visual function at school age in children with neonatal encephalopathy and low Apgar scores. *Arch Dis Child Fetal Neonatal Ed* 2004; **89**: F258–62.

54. D'Souza SW, McCartney E, Nolan M, *et al.* Hearing, speech, and language in survivors of severe perinatal asphyxia. *Arch Dis Child* 1981; **56**: 245–52.

55. Roland EH, Hill A, Norman MG, *et al.* Selective brainstem injury in an asphyxiated newborn. *Ann Neurol* 1988; **23**: 89–92.

56. Brunquell PJ, Glennon CM, DiMario FJ, *et al.* Prediction of outcome based on clinical seizure type in newborn infants. *J Pediatr* 2002; **140**: 707–12.

57. Clancy RR, Legido A. Postnatal epilepsy after EEG-confirmed neonatal seizures. *Epilepsia* 1991; **32**: 69–76.

58. Hellstrom-Westas L, Blennow G, Lindroth M, *et al.* Low risk of seizure recurrence after early withdrawal of antiepileptic treatment in the neonatal period. *Arch Dis Child Fetal Neonatal Ed* 1995; **72**: F97–101.

59. Toet MC, Groenendaal F, Osredkar D, *et al.* Postneonatal epilepsy following amplitude-integrated EEG-detected

neonatal seizures. *Pediatr Neurol* 2005; **32**: 241–7.

60. Dilenge ME, Majnemer A, Shevell MI. Long-term developmental outcome of asphyxiated term neonates. *J Child Neurol* 2001; **16**: 781–92.

61. Robertson CM, Finer NN. Educational readiness of survivors of neonatal encephalopathy associated with birth asphyxia at term. *J Dev Behav Pediatr* 1988; **9**: 298–306.

62. Koot HM. The study of quality of life: concepts and methods. In Koot HM, Wallander JL, eds., *Quality of Life in Child and Adolescent Illness.* Hove: Bunner-Routledge, 2001.

63. Thornberg E, Thiringer K, Odeback A, *et al.* Birth asphyxia: incidence, clinical course and outcome in a Swedish population. *Acta Paediatr* 1995; **84**: 927–32.

64. Roland EH, Poskitt K, Rodriguez E, *et al.* Perinatal hypoxic–ischemic thalamic injury: clinical features and neuroimaging. *Ann Neurol* 1998; **44**: 161–6.

65. Rutherford MA, Pennock JM, Counsell SJ, *et al.* Abnormal magnetic resonance signal in the internal capsule predicts poor neurodevelopmental outcome in infants with hypoxic–ischemic encephalopathy. *Pediatrics* 1998; **102**: 323–8.

66. Krageloh-Mann I, Helber A, Mader I, *et al.* Bilateral lesions of thalamus and basal ganglia: origin and outcome. *Dev Med Child Neurol* 2002; **44**: 477–84.

67. Le Strange E, Saeed N, Cowan FM, *et al.* MR imaging quantification of cerebellar growth following hypoxic-ischemic injury to the neonatal brain. *AJNR Am J Neuroradiol* 2004; **25**: 463–8.

68. Sargent MA, Poskitt KJ, Roland EH, *et al.* Cerebellar vermian atrophy after neonatal hypoxic-ischemic encephalopathy. *AJNR Am J Neuroradiol* 2004; **25**: 1008–15.

69. Rutherford M, Pennock J, Schwieso J, *et al.* Hypoxic–ischaemic encephalopathy: early and late magnetic resonance imaging findings in relation to outcome. *Arch Dis Child Fetal Neonatal Ed* 1996; **75**: F145–51.

70. Nagy Z, Lindstrom K, Westerberg H, *et al.* Diffusion tensor imaging on teenagers, born at term with moderate hypoxic–ischemic encephalopathy. *Pediatr Res* 2005; **58**: 936–40.

71. Rutherford M, Counsell S, Allsop J, *et al.* Diffusion-weighted magnetic resonance imaging in term perinatal brain injury:

583

a comparison with site of lesion and time from birth. *Pediatrics* 2004; **114**: 1004–14.

72. Palisano R, Rosenbaum P, Walter S, *et al.* Development and reliability of a system to classify gross motor function in children with cerebral palsy. *Dev Med Child Neurol* 1997; **39**: 214–23.

73. Kaufman A, Kaufman N. *Kaufman Assessment Battery for Children (K-ABC).* Circle Pines, MN: American Guidance Service, 1983.

74. Bayley N. *Bayley Scales of Infant Development*, 3rd edn. San Antonio, TX: Psychological Corporation, 2005.

75. Piper M, Darrah J. *Alberta Infant Motor Scale: Motor Assessment of the Developing Infant.* Philadelphia, PA: Saunders, 1994.

76. Baron-Cohen S, Allen J, Gillberg C. Can autism be detected at 18 months? The needle, the haystack, and the CHAT. *Br J Psychiatry* 1992; **161**: 839–43.

77. Wachtel RC, Shapiro BK, Palmer FB, *et al.* CAT/CLAMS: a tool for the pediatric evaluation of infants and young children with developmental delay. Clinical Adaptive Test/Clinical Linguistic and Auditory Milestone Scale. *Clin Pediatr* 1994; **33**: 410–15.

78. Wechsler D. *Wechsler Preschool and Primary Scale of Intelligence*, 3rd edn. New York, NY: Psychological Corporation, 2002.

79. Henderson S, Sugden D. *Movement Assessment Battery for Children*, 2nd edn. Sidcup: Harcourt Brace Jovanovich, 2007.

80. Bruininks R. *Bruininks–Oseretsky Test of Motor Proficiency.* Circle Pines, MN: American Guidance Service, 1978.

81. Largo RH, Fischer JE, Rousson V. Neuromotor development from kindergarten age to adolescence: developmental course and variability. *Swiss Med Wkly* 2003; **133**: 193–9.

82. Goodman R, Ford T, Simmons H, *et al.* Using the Strengths and Difficulties Questionnaire (SDQ) to screen for child psychiatric disorders in a community sample. *Br J Psychiatry* 2000; **177**: 534–9.

83. Wechsler D. *Wechsler Intelligence Scale for Children*, 4th edn. New York, NY: Psychological Corporation, 2003.

84. Achenbach T. *Manual for the Youth Self Report and 1991 Profile.* Burlington, VT: University of Vermont, 1991.

85. Fekkes M, Theunissen NC, Brugman E, *et al.* Development and psychometric evaluation of the TAPQOL: a health-related quality of life instrument for 1–5-year-old children. *Qual Life Res* 2000; **9**: 961–72.

86. Robitail S, Simeoni MC, Erhart M, *et al.* Validation of the European proxy KIDSCREEN-52 pilot test health-related quality of life questionnaire: first results. *J Adolesc Health* 2006; **39**: 596 e1–10.

Chapter 49

Appropriateness of intensive care application

William E. Benitz, David K. Stevenson, and Ernlé W. D. Young

Introduction

Ethical questions in medicine revolve around three core topics: what needs to be decided, on what basis, and by whom. These matters are not unique to the perinatal period, nor to patients with brain injury, but both of those circumstances may have ethical implications in the decision-making process, and in combination they raise questions that are unique. Because these situations touch so many critical aspects of human existence – birth, death, personhood, parenthood, etc. – it is not surprising that ethical matters related to the perinatal period have garnered a disproportionate amount of attention in the public discourses on medical ethics, nor that brain integrity lies at the core of so many of the contentious cases. The philosophical underpinnings of medical ethics have been reviewed exhaustively in many other venues, so this discussion will focus on aspects that are unique to or uniquely framed by brain injury or dysfunction in the perinatal period.

What is to be decided?

In the lay literature, ethical dilemmas are often framed as "life-or-death" decisions, with the implication that death or survival are options to be freely selected by patients, family members, or care providers, and that the ultimate outcome is within their control. In reality, that is rarely the case. In the case of a patient whose vital signs are rapidly failing despite full application of intensive care measures, this fact is obvious and there is no (or at most a very short-lived) ethical problem. Ethical problems arise when there is no detectable brain function (including spontaneous respiratory effort) but otherwise stable vital signs, when brain function is severely impaired but vital signs are sustained without aggressive medical interventions, when there is no realistic prospect for recovery from a life-threatening illness (independent of neurological condition), when the anticipated future quality of life is so dismal as to be outweighed by the burdens of life-sustaining medical measures, or when medical interventions for other conditions pose risks to neurological integrity or may result in prolonged survival with substantial neurological impairments due to associated or coincident neurological injuries. In all of these

situations, the questions confronted can be reduced to two items: the objective of medical intervention and the methods to be applied to achieve that objective. In the United States, and other societies in which active euthanasia is not overtly practiced, these choices do not translate directly to decisions about life or death.

In general, the "default" objective of medical care, and neonatal intensive care in particular, is restoration of patients to health, at least to the extent that they are able to leave the hospital and resume (or in the case of an infant, assume) their role in society. This is almost always assumed to be the goal of medical care at the time that an infant is admitted to a neonatal intensive care unit. For the infant, this means becoming a member of a family, with the ability to recognize, interact with, and experience family members. For most, it also implies a capacity for developmental progression, with acquisition of new behaviors, such as language, locomotion, and self-care. In the rare circumstances in which the severity of known neurological disorder – anencephaly or intractable seizures in an infant with trisomy 18, for example – makes it clear that these expectations cannot be met, the goal of restoration to health is not realistic, and identification of alternative objectives becomes mandatory. The consequences of failure to do so are exemplified by the case of "Baby K" [1]. This anencephalic child was born at Fairfax Hospital in Falls Church, Virginia, on 13 October 1992. Nationally, the standard of care for anencephalic infants requires only the provision of comfort measures: nutrition, hydration, warmth, human companionship, and being allowed to die peacefully. When they experience respiratory distress, they are not offered mechanical ventilation. In this case, however, the child's mother, believing that "all life should be protected" [2], wanted her child to have cardiopulmonary resuscitation and mechanical ventilation when she had trouble breathing. Despite the fact that "the hospital and physician concluded that such treatment was medically and ethically inappropriate" [1], leading to a protracted litigation further discussed below, Baby K was intubated and supported with mechanical ventilation. She was eventually weaned from the ventilator and discharged to a nursing home. In this instance, the national standard of care that warrants withholding of aggressive treatment – at the outset – was circumvented. This was, at least in part, a consequence of asynchrony between the goals of Baby K's physicians (based on their recognition that she could not be

Fetal and Neonatal Brain Injury, 4th edition, ed. David K. Stevenson, William E. Benitz, Philip Sunshine, Susan R. Hintz, and Maurice L. Druzin. Published by Cambridge University Press. © Cambridge University Press 2009.

restored to health and social function) and her mother (who either denied that assessment or was satisfied with more limited results). From her perspective, merely prolonging life – an alternative goal for her medical care – appears to have been appropriate.

The objective of restoration to health may also be deemed unrealistic when medical conditions, independent of coincident neurological disease, are incompatible with survival without ongoing intensive care measures, such as mechanical ventilation, continuous drug infusions to support the circulation, or dialysis. The extreme difficulty of reaching consensus in these situations is demonstrated by Ryan Nguyen [3], who was born "six weeks before his due date, asphyxiated, and with barely a heart beat." The initial resuscitation attempt was successful, but weeks later the infant's physicians at Sacred Heart Medical Center in Spokane, Washington, when confronted with Ryan's multiple medical problems, including "kidney failure, bowel obstructions, and brain damage," decided that aggressive medical treatments "would only prolong his suffering and that he would never survive infancy. They suggested that his life support be withdrawn." Clearly, they had concluded that the continued application of intensive care technology was inappropriate, for two reasons: even with intensive care, the child would not survive beyond infancy, and applying the technology was cruel, since the burdens imposed by treatment would be disproportionately massive relative to any possible benefits. Other medical experts (from the Children's Hospital and Medical Center in Seattle) concurred with this assessment by the child's neonatologists at Sacred Heart Medical Center. This suggests that the initial recommendation to forgo further intensive care was not impulsive or arbitrary but was carefully considered and had the unequivocal support of colleagues in the field. However, even as one group of physicians was attempting (for what seemed to them good reason) to say no to the continued application of intensive care, another group was willing to say yes. Neonatologists "at a medical center in Portland, Oregon [Legacy Emmanuel Children's Hospital], reading about the baby in a newspaper, said they were willing to treat him and that he was likely to survive. Almost immediately, Ryan was transferred to their care." The parents' wishes, reinforced by their pro-life lawyer and a court order requiring continued hemodialysis for the infant's kidney failure (obtained before the baby's transfer from Spokane to Portland) prevailed over the professional judgment (and integrity) of the original perinatal team and their consultants. Five months after admission to the Portland hospital, Ryan was discharged home and was reported to be doing well. In this case, the conclusion that recovery to the point of survival without intensive care was impossible may have been incorrect (in retrospect). Nonetheless, a key difference between Ryan's physicians at Sacred Heart and Emmanuel lies in the different goals for his care: minimizing suffering in the first instance and restoration to health in the second. His parents' unwillingness to adopt the goals recommended by his doctors in Spokane lay at the heart of the ensuing conflict.

These cases frame the choices of objectives for intensive care: restoration of health, minimizing suffering, and prolonging life. When there is consensus that the first of these is not achievable, either of the latter may be ethically appropriate, depending upon specific circumstances. These objectives are not mutually exclusive; the desire to prolong life may be tempered by respect for the burden imposed on the patient by life-sustaining interventions, for example. If consensus on the objectives of medical care can be achieved, conflicts and ethical problems related to the second group of decisions – how best to care for the patient in question – often dissolve. The necessity for careful attention to those choices does not.

The objective of restoration of health – supported by realistic expectations of success among the medical team – typically will dictate choices driven by medical expertise rather than by family members' desires. That is not to say that the choices confronted are devoid of ethical or moral dimensions. This is exemplified by the circumstance of the extremely low-birthweight infant with an intraparenchymal cerebral hemorrhage and necrotizing enterocolitis with extensive bowel infarction. For this infant, the probability of survival is low and that for significant neurodevelopmental impairment is high [4]. For some families, this prospect is sufficiently unpalatable to lead to choice of an alternative objective of care (minimal suffering), based upon both the immediate suffering endured during intensive care and long-term suffering related to complications of short-bowel syndrome and sequelae of a major neurological injury. For others, the potential for survival and hope for a better-than-expected neurodevelopmental outcome may be the basis for continuation of aggressive intensive care. Such choices clearly are contingent upon the values brought to the situation by each family.

Evolving medical technologies have created new challenges for parents and practitioners, who now must consider the neurodevelopmental implications of interventions primarily designed to address non-neurological conditions. For example, technical advances over the last two decades have made palliative and curative neonatal heart surgeries possible, substantially increasing the number of newborns being treated surgically for congenital heart disease (CHD). Babies with previously lethal cardiac anomalies can now be palliated or even cured of their heart disease, leaving them with repairs (sometimes incomplete), and potentially a legion of other associated neurologic and physical injuries, defects, or limitations. The relationship between congenital heart disease and cerebral injuries is complex and multifaceted. The same pathological processes may lead to disturbances of early fetal development of both heart and brain. This may arise in well-described genetic disorders, such as the DiGeorge/velocardiofacial syndrome (VCFS) or Down syndrome, or with congenital infections such as rubella, but congenital heart disease is also associated with developmental brain malformation in ways that appear to be independent of discrete syndromes. Whether this association is a consequence of shared antecedents, a reflection of altered intrauterine hemodynamics, or both, in different instances is unknown. There is certainly great potential for cerebral injury as a complication of congenital heart disease in the perinatal period, from severe hypoxemia (in transposition of the great vessels with intact septum and a restrictive foramen ovale, for example), reduced cerebral perfusion (in left-heart obstructive lesions, in particular), and from paradoxical emboli or cerebral abscesses (associated with intracardiac right-to-left shunts). These events can occur before, during, or after interventional catheterizations or heart surgery. The complex relationship between cardiac surgery (including the potential cerebral sequelae of intraoperative cardiopulmonary bypass) and the brain is discussed in Chapter 38. In short, some brain abnormalities are inherited in association with congenital heart disease, and others are acquired in association with it, sometimes in the process of diagnosis or treatment.

Whatever the mechanisms of injury, the decision makers for these vulnerable patients have to decide between impending death of the child, if intervention is not undertaken, and substantial risks for brain dysfunction (intrinsic or acquired) and often-lifelong disabilities because of other physical and functional incapacities. Late sequelae of hypoplastic left heart repairs, for example, include intractable seizures, neurodevelopmental delays, failure to thrive, and diminished exercise tolerance [5–8]. These decisions are not easy, and there is no universal right answer as to whether cardiac surgery should be undertaken in lethal complex CHD, such as hypoplastic left heart syndrome (HLHS). Moreover, the decisions are made more difficult because conditions like HLHS are not uniform. They vary across a developmental spectrum of structural cardiac malformations and are associated with a variety of concomitant conditions. For these immediately lethal anomalies, a choice to do nothing beyond comfort care remains understandable, but willingness to recommend non-intervention varies enormously between physicians in different specialties (with neonatologists much more likely to support non-intervention than intensivists, cardiologists, or surgeons) [9]. For less likely lethal anomalies which have protracted natural histories leading to later disability or death, the choice to do nothing seems less acceptable, because it would entail prolonged suffering and possibly avoidable death. For these conditions, for which it is possible to correct the defect and prevent protracted disability or death, discussions to restrict intervention seem less defensible morally. What is not ethical is the assumption that just because a lethal condition is technically amenable to palliation a surgical procedure must be undertaken. The fullest context of the patient, including co-existence of any other anomalies or developmental disabilities, is also relevant, and might render the palliation or even curative surgery futile or produce only a prolongation of suffering.

Recent clinical trials that have provided evidence that hypothermia ameliorates the neurodevelopmental impairments that follow acute intrapartum asphyxial events raise the possibility of a new kind of ethical challenge [10–12]. This is the first intervention with demonstrated efficacy for improving outcomes for infants who have sustained hypoxic–ischemic insults, requiring treatment of approximately six infants to produce one additional neurologically intact survivor. This treatment is quite tempting for families and medical professionals confronted with an infant with low Apgar scores, metabolic acidosis documented at or soon after birth, and behavioral or electroencephalographic evidence of cerebral dysfunction. At this writing, however, it is premature to recommend this treatment without qualification. While the data seem convincing, it is not clear whether the perceived benefits are real or only artifacts of palliation bias. The criteria for selection of the best candidates for treatment have not been identified, and the most severely injured infants may benefit least. Fortunately, these early reports suggest that the risk of survival with severe neurological debilitation is not increased by induced hypothermia. As these and other treatments evolve, parents and physicians will have to balance the promise of benefit against potential, and as yet unknown, adverse consequences.

If there is agreement that the goal is to minimize suffering, it may be easy to reach a decision to discontinue mechanical ventilation, remove the endotracheal and nasogastric tubes, and use opioid analgesics liberally but judiciously. Most importantly, agreement on this goal allows attention to be refocused on palliative care. The fact that the "life-or-death" decision about survival of the infant is not entirely within the control of the family or medical team should not lead to a nihilistic conclusion that the situation is completely out of control. On the contrary, decisions about the timing or manner of discontinuation of presumably life-sustaining treatments (e.g., mechanical ventilation) may facilitate the presence of parents or those who provide their social supports and permit the infant the benefit of comfort measures. For a neonate, these include being clean, dry, warm, pain-free, not hungry (if feeding is medically feasible), human companionship, and relief from the indignities of continued invasive medical interventions. The latter does not equate to "withdrawal of care," however. This language, which has been a part of the ethical literature in neonatology for many years [13], is best discarded, as it implies and creates reasonable fears of abandonment of the patient by the medical care team. Even if all medical measures are discontinued, the team should continue to provide emotional support for the family and attention to the continuing needs of the infant. In many instances, this may include medical measures that enhance comfort, as well as management of pain or other distressing symptoms, such as gentle suctioning of the oropharynx for a baby who cannot swallow oral secretions. Such medical interventions should be chosen or adapted carefully to minimize noxious effects. For pain relief, sublingual administration of fentanyl is preferable to subcutaneous injections of morphine. Providing family members – grieving parents, in particular – an opportunity to hold and comfort their dying baby, in a quiet and private setting, with the support of others of their choosing (family, friends, clergy, social workers, or other members of the medical team) has become a routine but extremely important part of this process. For infants whose demise can be anticipated to fall hours or days after elimination of aggressive medical interventions, or whose anticipated rapid demise fails to materialize, the support of the medical team may be extended to allow the family to escape from confinement in a hospital room, to the hospital chapel, garden, or other more pleasant location. The recent expansion of hospice programs to encompass dying neonates now enables discharge of such infants home or to a hospice facility, with all necessary services to maintain comfort and support the family. The medical team must be familiar with all of these options to advise the family and guide their choices.

The patient for whom the objective is simply prolongation of life may be the most problematic, as neither the purpose of that choice nor the measures used for that purpose are always obvious. In some instances, this may be only a short-term objective, with a clear intent to continue intensive care measures only for a defined period – until family members can come to support the parents or perhaps until a religious ritual is completed. The potential for conflict is much greater when the goal is open-ended. Many instances of conflict between care providers and family members hinge on unspoken but critical differences in expectations that follow from imprecise communication on this issue: frustration, anger, and rejection on the part of care providers who mistake a request for life-prolonging care for a demand for rescue of an unsalvageable patient, or similar responses by family members who mis-apprehend acquiescence to such a request for tacit affirmation of their unreasonable hopes for recovery. We will return to this problem in the discussion of futility later in this chapter. Nonetheless, explicit articulation of this aim will facilitate more appropriate decisions about the details of the medical care provided. Fundamentally, this becomes the technical problem of identifying and applying measures that maintain vital signs, physiological homeostasis, consciousness, or what-ever signs of "life" are deemed confirmatory that life is, in fact, being sustained. (Problems related to disagreements on this matter are addressed below.) In this context, however, appli-cation of medical interventions may differ from the way in which the same measures might be incorporated into care of a patient for whom recovery is expected. For instance, worries about the impact of tracheostomy on speech acquisition might be irrelevant for an infant who is not expected to survive beyond a year (even with life-prolonging intensive care) or for one with profound cranial nerve deficits (Moebius syn-drome) not compatible with acquisition of speech. In general, slowly accruing adverse effects, such as development of opiate dependence and tachyphylaxis or oxygen-associated lung injury, may be more acceptable to enhance comfort in the short term in this setting than might be the case if recovery to discharge from intensive care or from the hospital were the goal.

What is the basis for ethical decisions?

It is not the conclusion of the decision-making process that makes a decision ethical or not, but rather the process by which it is reached, and, to some extent, the rationale for the ultimate decision. For example, a recommendation to discontinue hospital care for a handicapped infant precipitated by exhaustion of his insurance coverage would likely be viewed as driven by the physician's self-interest (or greed) and, therefore, unethical. On the other hand, a similar decision, leading to exactly the same outcome, but reached jointly with the family after consideration of the infant's intractable pain and dependence upon invasive medical procedures, would not raise ethical concerns. What, then, are the requirements for a process to be seen as ethical? Although there are some broad principles that can be invoked as generic answers to this question, their application will often depend upon the specific situation at hand. Rather than attempt to cover all of those possibilities, we will focus on a few circumstances that high-light problems specific to brain injury in the perinatal period.

Establishment of the concept of brain death has simplified management of patients who are unresponsive, without signs of cortical or brainstem function. When it can be established that there has been irreversible cessation of brain function, most would argue that discontinuation of intensive care is not only permissible, but mandatory. Despite an ongoing debate about whether such individuals are actually dead or the label is merely a "convenient semantic construct" [14], this concept has proven helpful, perhaps by allowing family members to recognize that their beloved relative is no longer present, despite persisting signs of physiological functioning of other organs (particularly the heart). Criteria for recognition of brain death, defined as irreversible cessation of brain function, initially developed for adults, have been adapted for applica-tion in children [15], but diagnosis of brain death in newborn infants is fraught with both false-positive and false-negative conclusions [16], particularly in the first 7 days after injury [15]. Even advocates for the feasibility of diagnosing brain death recognize special requirements, involving use of com-binations of observations and longer periods of observation, in these patients [17]. For this reason, it is rarely possible to invoke this concept in support of withdrawal of intensive care measures in neonates.

There are situations, though, in which the medical care providers believe that there is virtually no chance that an infant will survive, even with continuation of intensive care. The key word here is "virtually." The second usage of "virtually" in the Oxford English Dictionary (second edition) is: "In effect, though not formally or explicitly; practically, to all intents, as good as." While it may seldom be possible to assert, with absolute certainty, that an infant has no chance of sur-viving, even with continued intensive care, it may be said that the probability of surviving is so low as to make death prac-tically, or to all intents, or as good as, certain. Although, in theory, probability can approach but never be synonymous with certainty, in practice the effect or result of causal factors with an extremely high level of probability may be almost always the same as certainty. Hence, use of the term "virtually" no chance of surviving – even with intensive care.

In practice, determination that there is virtually no possi-bility of survival almost always depends upon synthesis of numerous clinical data elements, not all of which are necessarily related to neurological assessments. A determination that a given outcome is virtually certain has to be based on empirical data, not subjective belief or bias alone. This is why physicians may find themselves at odds with nurses in the intensive care nursery. Nurses, at the bedside for 24 hours a day, 7 days a week, tend to intuit sooner than physicians (who attend their tiny patients more episodically) that an infant is or is not "going to make it." Physicians have to be persuaded of this by empirical evidence: not only the evidence the particular infant is providing, but also its corroboration by similar findings by their peers in similar circumstances as documented in the medical literature. This is how a "national standard of care" comes to be developed, on the basis of repeated and consistent empirical clinical findings. Stahlman has argued that:

> The decision to withhold or withdraw life-sustaining treatment can be justified only if one has a set of medical (not social or emotional) circumstances whose outcomes can be predicted with accuracy. This accuracy has been significantly increased by certain types of modern technology, and by long-term follow-up studies on medical and behavioral outcomes of a wide variety of neonatal conditions, including extreme prematurity, chronic lung disease, and many congenital abnormalities [18].

Where these findings, in the case of a given neonatal patient with specific medical complications or conditions, suggest that survival is unprecedented – the application of neonatal intensive care technology notwithstanding – a physician may, with confidence and in good conscience, recommend that aggressive treatments be withdrawn. The use of the phrase "virtually no chance of survival," with the implication that the recommendation is based on probability rather than absolute certainty, may prompt a few parents to refuse the recommendation and to insist on continued aggressive treatments. Statistical probability applies to groups and has little to say about discrete individuals. Even odds of winning as low as one in several million do not deter multitudes of people from buying lottery tickets. Nevertheless, most reasonable people accept the fact that a prognosis of "virtually" no chance of survival is to all intents indistinguishable from one where there is "absolutely" no chance at all.

In the Nguyen case, not all the physicians consulted agreed that little Ryan had virtually no prospect of surviving his multiple medical problems [3]. There was also no generally agreed-upon standard of care for babies in his condition. Although, as the case of Baby K brings home, having a national standard of care is not an infallible means of limiting aggressive treatments considered inappropriate, it is more often true that the lack of a medical consensus is commonly the reason why doing this is difficult and, at times, impossible. The challenge to academic neonatal medicine, in particular, is to establish national standards of care for patients in more and more categories. One of the positive benefits of managed care and its emphases on cost-effectiveness, outcome assessment, and evidence-based medicine is that it is driving research of this kind. Without the backing of a community standard

or, even better, a national standard of care, the individual neonatologist who is convinced that an infant has virtually no chance of surviving even with continued aggressive treatments, and who accordingly recommends their withdrawal, is out on a limb, and very much at the mercy of the whims and wants of parents or family members.

The approach to these conundrums has often been framed in terms of futility, since the care providers typically see continuation of intensive care measures as pointless. Unless those measures fail to maintain the presence of vital signs (such as when CPR does not restore a heart beat or where vasopressors fail to maintain blood pressure), however, family members may perceive the situation differently. As Moseley and colleagues have pointed out, if an intervention is truly futile, "it will generally be provided for only a short period of time before it fails" [19]. From this perspective, it is apparent that futility is largely in the eye of the beholder, as family members may rightly apprehend that intensive care measures that have not yet failed *are* demonstrably effective in maintaining signs of life in their baby. In effect, then, the only way to determine whether an intervention is futile is to try it out and see if it works. Consequently, it may not be helpful to inform a desperate parent that a requested intervention is futile or pointless. On the other hand, it would be an abrogation of the physician's moral responsibility to acquiesce to requests for interventions that are not medically plausible (i.e., can reasonably be expected to alter some relevant aspect of physiology or pathology in that particular patient). Asking a physician to rub an untested herbal mixture on the child's brow in order to get rid of the brain damage does not fall within the boundaries of a treatment with proven medical efficacy. And asking the physician to keep the child alive for the sole purpose of allowing God to perform a miracle is, from a physiological standpoint, to prolong the dying process. While the principle of non-maleficence prohibits the medical team from providing care that would actually be harmful, it may nonetheless be acceptable to permit or even facilitate activities of a non-medical nature – rites or ceremonies of religious or cultural significance, for example – as long as the risk of harm is absent or minimal, even though those measures are, from a medical perspective, futile.

Morreim has pointed out that the so-called futility debate "turns on intractable conflicts of deeply held beliefs about the value of life" [20]. On one hand are the "vitalists," who believe that all life is fully, even infinitely, valuable, regardless of its quality. On the other are those whom Morreim describes as "qualitists" (for want of a better term), "who believe that there are some conditions under which a life is no longer of value to the person who has it – that such a person would be better off, or at least not worse off, dead." Central to this controversy is the fact that vitalists conflate the meanings of "human life" and "personal life," while qualitists insist on distinguishing the two concepts. Those in the latter camp do not regard the terms "human life" and "personal life" as synonymous, and attempt to emphasize what to them seems to be an important distinction: we are *human* by virtue of our membership of the human species (by having human DNA), but we are *persons* only as we have actual or potential capacities for sentience (being able to experience pain or pleasure), responding to external and internal stimuli, relating to our environments and to one another, and for being, at least in some slight measure, self-determining moral agents. These capacities, so far as we can tell, depend entirely on neocortical function. For qualitists, if neocortical function is absent, we are not persons, though we continue to be human beings. On the other hand, vitalists equate human life with personal life. This fosters the view that a fertilized egg, a fetus, a severely neurologically impaired neonate, or – at the other end of the life cycle – a permanently vegetative adult, simply by being a member of the human species, are all persons. Persons are sacred; their right to life is inviolable. Therefore, except in the case of those with afflictions incompatible with survival, everything that can be done technologically must be done to ensure their survival. Withholding and withdrawing life-sustaining treatments are not seen as moral options; indeed, the implication of this position is that it is mandatory to continue all treatments until the patient has died.

The ramifications of the vitalist view are evident in the public discussion of the matter of 8-week-old twins joined at the pelvis in Great Britain. Unless surgically separated, both were expected to die; if separated, one would die and the other might survive. An appeals court in London ruled, over the opposition of the babies' parents, that they must be separated. Writing in the *New York Times* [21], Sirico remarked, "Here, as in the case of abortion, one simple principle applies: There is no justification for deliberately destroying innocent life. In this case, the court has turned its back on a tenet that the West has stood by: Life, no matter how limited, should be protected." It comes as no surprise to the reader to learn that Sirico is a Roman Catholic priest. He exemplifies the vitalist position perfectly.

The two views of what constitutes personal life may be further described, respectively, as passive and active. The vitalist view is passive: personhood is acquired simply by virtue of being a member of the human species. The qualitist sees it differently: we become persons, not merely by being endowed with human genes, but by becoming actively involved in reacting and responding to stimuli within our various environments, forming relationships, and, eventually, making choices. Dworkin refers to this as the "investment" each of us has made, is making, and will continue to make to become the persons we are [22]. If these kinds of activity are preempted because the neocortex is either absent or has been destroyed, personhood either is not or is no longer possible. For example, Dworkin writes:

> The life of a single human organism commands respect and protection, then, . . . because of the complex creative investment it represents and because of our wonder at the divine or evolutionary processes that produce new lives from old ones, at the processes of nation and community and language through which a human being will come to absorb and continue hundreds of generations of

cultures and forms of life and value, and, finally, when mental life has begun and flourishes, at the process of internal personal creation and judgment by which a person will make and remake himself, a mysterious, inescapable process in which we all participate, and which is therefore the most powerful and inevitable source of empathy and communion we have with every other creature who faces the same frightening challenge [22].

The vitalists gained the upper hand during the "Baby Doe" era. The Federal Rehabilitation Act of 1973 was invoked to warn healthcare providers that to withhold services from handicapped infants (the term then in vogue) that ordinarily would be provided to others would constitute a violation that could render their institutions ineligible for federal financial assistance. In order to implement the threat of action under the Rehabilitation Act, the Department of Health and Human Services issued an "interim rule" in March 1983; the final rules were promulgated in January 1984. These regulations (named for "Baby Doe", from whom life-sustaining treatments had been withheld in 1982 at the request of the parents, against the advice of their pediatrician and the hospital) [23] expressly excluded "quality of life" from the decisional process in the intensive care nursery [24]. These rules were eventually struck down by the Supreme Court, but their legacy endures in the Federal Child Abuse Amendments of 1984 and, more significantly, in the Americans With Disabilities Act of 1990. The Americans With Disabilities Act expands the Rehabilitation Act in several respects. As Greely points out, "Perhaps most importantly, it includes physicians along with other healthcare providers as 'public accommodations' under the Act who, subject to a few limitations, have to make services available regardless of a patient's disability" [25].

Despite these developments, there is a widespread consensus among adults that supports the qualitist position. Although some, like the husband of Helga Wanglie, who refused to allow discontinuation of assisted ventilation despite her permanent vegetative state, do make other choices [26], many – if not most – of us would not want biological existence extended mechanically (in our own case) when personal life, as we understand it, is no longer possible. The fear that this could happen as a result of physicians mindlessly subscribing to the technological imperative gave impetus to the so-called "right to die" movement; so-called because, strictly speaking, death is not so much a right as a destiny. What the term "right to die" means is the right to die with some measure of control, dignity, and humanity. This right is now recognized and may be expressed in legally binding advance directives, such as the Durable Power of Attorney for Health Care or California's Advance Health Care Directive (or its equivalent in other states), which allow competent adults to specify, beforehand, that they desire life-sustaining treatments to be withheld or withdrawn when these will merely maintain biological existence in the absence of qualities they deem necessary for a personal life. These legal provisions are of little help when the patient is an infant, however. What they do provide to those responsible for decision making for infants with severe neurological injuries is the legal and moral authority to decide, on their behalf, to discontinue medical measures, including those that are potentially life-sustaining, when there is consensus that those measures are no longer appropriate.

These are the broad lines of the debate between the two camps. As Morreim observes: "At every juncture, each side's argument presupposes as true its distinctive view about the value of fetal [or neonatal] life" [20]. The debate hinges on deeply held beliefs, and the values to which they give rise. These may not be amenable to rational persuasion. They may have to be accepted as givens by which people in both groups live and for which, if necessary, they might be prepared to fight and die. Consequently, neither futility nor the concept of personhood has led to consensus positions that help resolve disagreements about requests for aggressive interventions for neurologically compromised infants.

Parallel arguments about parental demands for *withholding* interventions, however, have been more productive, and – fortuitously – the results are more generally applicable, independent of the direction of the parent–physician disagreement. While the focus of this public debate has often been more on *who* should decide (as discussed below) than on *why* or *how*, the conversation has produced a reasonable consensus that the basis of ethical decisions for patients who cannot speak for themselves, and children in particular, should be the *best interests* of the patient. This concept was implicit in the assertion in the 1924 Geneva Declaration of the Rights of the Child that "mankind owes the child the best that it has to give" [27] and was made explicit in the 1959 United Nations Declaration of the Rights of the Child in the statement that "In all actions concerning children, whether undertaken by public or private social welfare institutions, courts of law, administrative authorities or legislative bodies, the best interests of the child shall be a primary consideration" [28]. By 1983, this principle had been incorporated into consensus statements issued both by a Presidential Commission and by the American Academy of Pediatrics [29,30]. What remained, then, was to work out what is meant by "best interests" and how they might be determined.

Most would agree that the best interests of the patient would lie in selection of medical and other care measures that offer the greatest potential for benefit and the least prospect of harm, but every attempt to help entails some risk of harm. Every intervention, however safe and efficacious it may be in the majority of cases, will sometimes prove neither safe nor effective. Vaccination provides a good example of this. While millions of children benefit from being vaccinated, there are rare exceptions – children who develop damaging and sometimes lethal reactions to the vaccines. Therefore, between the two cardinal biomedical ethical principles of non-maleficence (requiring that, above all else, the physician do no harm) and beneficence (mandating the attempt to benefit or to help the patient) there is the moral notion of proportionality. The challenge for those responsible for care of an infant with brain injury is therefore to find the optimal balance between beneficial and noxious consequences of care.

For the most part in neonatal medicine, the risk or probability of harm is outweighed by the prospect of benefiting the patient. However, there may come a time in the aggressive treatment of some patients when the balance shifts. Harms, mostly iatrogenic in nature, may begin to outweigh the help that is being afforded, becoming disproportionately burdensome relative to meager benefits. At this juncture it is not merely ethically permissible to stop treating the infant aggressively, it is obligatory. To continue on an aggressive course that is doing more harm than good is cruel. This is morally as well as medically reprehensible, as it violates the principle of non-maleficence.

But how are harms to be defined? The infant has no language, except body language, with which to communicate. In a neonate with a neurological injury, even these tenuous signals may be attenuated. The assessment of harms and benefits, of necessity, must be made by those caring for the infant rather than by the patient him- or herself. Adult observers will rely on both subjective and objective indicators of harm, and these may be in conflict with one another. Nurses are commonly the first to protest that an infant is being harmed rather than helped by aggressive treatments, claiming that their tiny patients are "being tortured." Physicians, on the other hand, may dismiss these assertions as overly subjective, as emotional rather than empirical deductions, because they see objective signs of improvement in the data being provided by their patients. While acknowledging the unfortunate side effects of their treatments, they may continue to insist that these are more than outweighed by the actual and hoped-for benefits [31]. This is particularly likely to happen when clinicians are also investigators, and have enrolled their patients in clinical trials. In a recent study, Catlin and Stevenson found that "despite awareness of the high morbidity and mortality, 96% of the physicians [interviewed] offered resuscitation to all ELBW neonates in the delivery room. The main factors affecting their decisions were 'the role of physician;' having been 'trained to save lives;' the belief that 'if called, I resuscitate;' the inability to determine gestational age; requests from parents to 'do everything;' and the need to move from a 'chaotic' delivery room to a controlled neonatal intensive care unit" [31].

How can these opposing points of view be reconciled in the best interests of the patient being treated? One criticism of the claim that infants are not being harmed because there are objective signs of improvement is that those making this claim are looking at isolated trees, but not at the forest as a whole. The infant's renal function may be somewhat improved, or her lungs may appear marginally better, or the intracranial bleed may seem slowly to be resolving, but the patient may not be getting better at all. Treatments may have effects without necessarily providing benefits. The tendency to focus on isolated organ systems rather than the whole person can blind even the most objective observer to the fact that, overall, less good than harm is being done. The role of the nurse as advocate for a holistic view of the patient may be to teach physicians, who are generally more oriented to an objective perspective, how to observe the subtle nuances of the infant's body language over time. This body language may eloquently proclaim the disproportionality of harms to benefits. The same may be true for parents who visit their child infrequently and continue unrealistically to insist, despite all evidence to the contrary, that the child is getting better and that aggressive treatments cannot be forgone. Requiring these parents to spend uninterrupted time at their child's bedside is often the most effective way of breaking through their denial, and winning their agreement that the time has come to switch from a curative to a palliative course. Conversely, parents who are able to spend substantial time at the bedside are often better able to recognize and describe the signs of suffering exhibited by their own baby.

The necessity for involvement of multiple members of the nursing staff to provide round-the-clock care for a neonatal patient provides a valuable safeguard against an overly subjective assessment of an infant's distress. If not one nurse, but *every* nurse, who spends a shift of 8 or 12 hours with a patient agrees that, on balance, the infant is being harmed rather than helped, this admittedly subjective point of view becomes powerfully compelling. Those who dispute it on the basis of the objective data being monitored have to be challenged to spend as much time at the infant's bedside as those who claim that the moment has arrived when shifting from an aggressive to a more palliative course is warranted. Besides, the subjective view may correlate well with the aggregate data, if not with the indications for particular organ systems.

Determination of "best interests" must also balance immediate and short-term benefits against long-term harm and vice versa. Short-term pain during recovery from surgery to repair a bowel atresia may be easily justified by long-term, pain-free survival, but the immediate benefit of prolongation of life with palliative surgery for complex congenital heart disease may not outweigh the later burdens of survival with major neurological impairments from coincident brain injuries. Evaluation of the long-term impacts of survival with severe neurosensory and developmental impairments, often compounded by significant ongoing medical problems, is especially difficult. The views of medical professionals, parents, and (later on) the affected infants in this regard may be quite disparate. This disparity is evident in the observation that self-reported health-related quality of life is not related to birthweight or presence of disability among extremely low-birthweight survivors followed up at 21–25 years of age [32]. It was stated more poignantly by a young man in his early twenties, blind from retinopathy of prematurity and dependent on a wheelchair for ambulation but attending college, who inquired of a panel discussing strategies for "avoiding bad outcomes" (i.e., withholding of intensive care), "Am I a bad outcome?" The answer to this question is not self-evident. Because it is laden with value judgments, different observers can be expected to reach different conclusions.

The key to discerning the infant's best interest, and to implementing the moral notion of proportionality in the trade-off between harms and benefits, is teamwork. As Stevenson and Young stated:

> The fact that there is a treatment team, rather than a solitary treating physician, can be a useful check and balance against overly subjective interpretations – one way or the other. In this respect, many heads (and hearts) are better than one. When a consensus begins to emerge among all who are participating in the care of an infant that the harms of continued treatment (or nontreatment) are outweighed by the benefits, then it becomes difficult for any one member of the group to make claims to the contrary; increasingly persuasive arguments in support of such claims will be necessary [33].

Continuous involvement of the parents in these processes, as advocated by the AAP [30,34], will provide the greatest opportunity for successful resolution.

It is generally assumed that the interests of the child can be and should be determined independently of the interests of the other members of the family. Hardwig has argued that there is a "presumption of equality" between the patient and the family which requires that the interests of both, whether they be medical or non-medical, must have equal consideration [35]. And Blustein has observed that "to treat the patient in the family appropriately, the physician must be cognizant of the patient in the family" [36]. These comments by Hardwig and Blustein suggest that the interests of the child and of the parents should not be viewed in isolation from one another. The 1983 American Academy of Pediatrics statement on treatment of critically ill newborns emphasized the limitations of this view, however:

> While the needs and interests of parents, as well as of the larger society, are proper concerns of the pediatrician, his or her primary moral and legal obligation is to the child-patient. Withholding or withdrawing life-sustaining treatment is justified only if such a course serves the interests of the patient. When the infant's prospects are for a life dominated by suffering, the concerns of the family may play a larger role. Treatment should not be withheld for the primary purpose of improving the psychological or social well being of others, no matter how poignant those needs may be [30].

The revised (2007) AAP statement on non-initiation or withdrawal of intensive care for high-risk newborns essentially reiterates this position:

> The physician's role is to present the treatment options to the parents and provide guidance as needed. The parents' role is to participate actively in the decision-making process. Decisions to continue, limit, or stop intensive care must be based only on the best interest of the infant . . . the physician's first responsibility is to the patient. The physician is not obligated to provide inappropriate treatment or to withhold beneficial treatment at the request of the parents. Treatment that is harmful, of no benefit, or futile and merely prolonging dying should be considered inappropriate. The physician must ensure that the chosen treatment, in his or her best medical judgment, is consistent with the best interest of the infant [34].

These comments are tempered, in the more recent statement, by recognition that such decisions often cannot be made totally independent of parental wishes and values, however:

> There may be cases . . . in which the prognosis is uncertain but likely to be very poor and survival may be associated with a diminished quality of life for the child; in these cases, parental desires should determine the treatment approach . . . The physician . . . must be sensitive to the parents' concerns and desires, which are often based on a complex combination of values and influences derived from their cultural, religious, educational, social, and ethnic backgrounds [34].

When parental interests do appear to be clearly contrary to the medical needs of the child, responsibility for the care of the child may be taken away from the parent. However, this cannot be done with a fetus. In past years, the clinical status of the fetus could only be determined indirectly by examining the pregnant woman. This produced a single-patient model in which the benefits and burdens of care were identical for both the fetus and its mother. This unitary model has yielded to one in which the woman and fetus can be viewed as separate individuals with distinct medical needs. The shift from a unitary to a dyadic concept occurred for two reasons, one political and the other medical. The political reason was the effect of the discourse employed by the anti-abortion movement, which, in response to the US Supreme Court decision in *Roe* v. *Wade*, promulgated the view that the fetus is a person with a right to life from the moment of conception. The medical reason was improvement in medical diagnostic capabilities. The array of diagnostic tools that have become available has helped, as Fasouliotis and Schenker observed, "penetrate the opaque environment and reveal the fetus to clinical observation in all its anatomical, physiological, and biochemical particularity" [37].

The goals of the obstetrician are to promote the health of both the pregnant woman and the developing fetus. In most instances, these objectives are consonant, as the well-being of the fetus is dependent on the health of the mother. There are circumstances in which they may diverge, however, such as when maternal inattention to her own health compromises fetal health or when concerns about fetal integrity lead to consideration of invasive procedures, such as cesarean delivery or fetal (and therefore, necessarily, maternal) surgery, which have health risks but few or no health benefits for the mother. If the mother chooses to accept those risks for the benefit of her fetus, or if the benefits for the fetus are minimal, hypothetical, or unknown, there may be no conflict of any consequence. When the mother is unable or unwilling to consent to procedures intended to benefit her fetus (such as emergency cesarean section to rescue a fetus experiencing an acute hypoxic–ischemic event), or is requesting interventions that may benefit herself but compromise the fetus (such as elective induction of labor before term, which might alleviate her of the burdens of continuation of pregnancy but expose the fetus to complications of prematurity), maternal and fetal interests do come into conflict. Is there any approach that can morally justify an action in favor of the fetus that is incompatible with the woman's interests or needs, or conversely? One approach, claiming that the fetus's right to life trumps all needs or desires of the pregnant woman except her own right to life, justifies overriding the autonomy of the woman in order to take care of the fetus. Another denies that the fetus has any rights at all, focusing on the medical problems of the woman whatever the attendant cost to the fetus. The critical issue is whether coercive measures can justifiably be used to compel maternal interventions for fetal benefit [38]. Because treating a woman against her will would be an exception to the legal rule against battery and a violation of the moral rules of autonomy and bodily integrity, and would destroy the pregnant woman's ability to trust the physician, there is now consensus that there is no ethical basis for such coercion. But this does not mean that the pregnant woman is entirely free of obligation. As Nelson and Milliken observed,

> Persuasive arguments can be made that a pregnant woman not intending to have an abortion has an ethical obligation to accept reasonable nonexperimental medical treatment and to behave otherwise in a manner that will benefit and not harm her fetus . . . Nevertheless it is quite another matter to transfer this obligation into a legal duty by enforcing it with the coercive power of the law [38].

What has been suggested is that treatment of the pregnant woman and of the fetus as separate beings does not, in case of a conflict, call for coercive measures being brought to bear against the woman. The costs of such tactics outweigh the benefits. In these situations, the only recourse for the physician may be to pursue persuasion.

Who decides?

In countries like Sweden, where the provision of medical care is the responsibility of the state, and where savings in one area can effectively be allocated to provide needed services elsewhere, the government, acting on the advice of experts in the field and after paying attention to lobbyists (parents and people with disabilities), may ultimately decide when providing neonatal intensive care is inappropriate. The ethical foundation of these decisions is the principle of *distributive justice*, which calls for the fair distribution of medical resources among potential recipients. In such societies, the question at hand then becomes the extent, if any, to which treatment of brain-damaged infants can be justified, given the competing claims for treatment of other patients.

In the best of all possible worlds, we would not experience pain, suffering, or debilitation, and therefore would not have to expend our wealth on health care. In the second-best world, we would always receive the best of care for all of our medical needs. As Hume, the eighteenth-century philosopher observed, "If nature supplied abundantly all our wants and desires . . . the jealousy of interest, which justice supposes, could no longer have a place" [39]. Thus, in this world, we would utilize an economy of abundance in which the way medical resources are distributed would be irrelevant. But, in our own real world, we must employ an economy of scarcity in which the patterns of distribution are of importance, not only from the standpoint of economic efficiency but also from the standpoint of fairness or distributive justice.

In an economy of scarcity, there are two general sorts of decisions that are called for: macro allocation and micro allocation. In the USA, macro allocation decisions are made by the Federal Government for medical research, for medical schools and hospitals, for Medicare and Medicaid, and by state agencies, health organizations, private foundations, and insurance companies. These are the product of two important questions: (1) How much of our economic resources should be allotted for health care, with the more specific issue being the relative importance of such care in comparison to other social goods, such as education, housing, law enforcement, and food programs? (2) How should what is allotted be distributed to specific undertakings such as research, crisis care, and technological innovation? Micro allocation decisions, or rationing, are made by doctors and hospitals when there is a scarcity of resources relative to demand. Our concern will be with the issue of rationing as it applies to brain-damaged infants. This will require us to ask whether the resources expended in the treatment of these infants satisfy the principle of distributive justice.

When we deal with problems of allocation, we are concerned to know what portion of the economic pie is to be designated for health care. When we deal with problems of medical rationing, we are concerned to know what portion of the allocated portion of the economic pie is to be designated for different parts of the healthcare system. One approach is to recognize that since almost all people want to live, and since almost all parents want their children to survive, the rationing of resource should be based on a lottery [40]. This offers each patient in the lottery an equal chance to win or to lose. But there is a limiting condition in its use. Let us suppose that allocations have allowed us to identify those patients for whom insufficient resources are available and who are therefore legitimate participants in the lottery. Once the lottery is run and appropriate distributions have been made, we are in no position to know what distribution should be made to the next new patient.

The second approach is to measure the outcome of our monetary investments in health care against the costs involved in these investments. This allows us to compare the relative efficiencies of different treatments. For instance, when we compare extremely low-birthweight infants in the NICU with elderly patients in the ICU, we find clear evidence that expenditures for treatment of the infant population are much more cost-effective than for the adult population [41].

Other results based on quality-adjusted life year (QALY) assessments indicate that care for low-birthweight infants is "significantly more cost effective than . . . coronary artery bypass surgery, treatment for severe hypertension, or routine Pap smears for women aged 20 to 74" [42]. The population that was studied by Cutler and Meara included brain-damaged infants. This suggests that the cost efficiency of treating hypoxic children is similar to that of treating low-birthweight infants. But this evidence must be treated with caution, since not all hypoxic infants are of low birthweight.

In the USA, which does not have a centralized system and where there is no effective mechanism for transferring savings achieved in one sector to another where an infusion of resources could be of obvious benefit, authority for deciding when intensive care is inappropriate and for what reasons is more diffuse. The experts may line up on one side of the issue, to find themselves opposed by parents or other experts, on the other, with the state remaining neutral. At the present time, infants enter the NICU on a first come first served basis, limited only by the availability of staff and beds. In those instances in which the infant is discovered to have malformations such as anencephaly or pulmonary hypoplasia, or genetic conditions such as epidermolysis bullosa, or an injury such as chronic lung disease or liver failure, parents will often consent to the withdrawal of life support. The studies mentioned above appear to support the conclusion that continued treatment of infants surviving hypoxic insults is cost-efficient. Given this result, the burden of proof falls on those who would deny that the treatment of hypoxic infants is cost-efficient. In societies that have not chosen to prohibit medical interventions for brain-injured neonates as a matter of resource allocation, decisions about initiation and continuation or discontinuation of such measures fall to the parents and treating physicians, and there inevitably are times when the parents and medical professionals cannot agree upon the best course of action. The case of Baby K reminds us how it may be almost impossible to say no, and how little help is provided by appeal to the principle of distributive justice.

When dealing with competent adult patients, the answer to the question of "who decides" is determined by the moral principles of autonomy, self-determination, and bodily integrity. It is obvious that the newborn infant is unable to exercise autonomy on his or her own behalf, so it must fall to another party to do so. In the early days of neonatal intensive care, difficult decisions about care of infants – particularly those related to end-of-life care or withholding of potentially life-sustaining measures – were mostly left up to the baby's parents, who were considered to be acting as the baby's *surrogate*. The deference of the medical profession to parental wishes to withhold treatment is evident in the 1963 "Johns Hopkins case," in which surgical repair of duodenal atresia in a 33-week-gestation premature infant with trisomy 21 was not undertaken when the parents declined to consent to the surgery [43]. The baby died of starvation 15 days later. By report, "the physicians acquiesced to this decision, even though allowing the baby to starve to death created great consternation among the staff" [44]. This case, and undoubtedly others like it, received little public attention until the 1971 release of a documentary film [45], based on this and at least one similar case [43], that publicly raised questions about the appropriateness of such decisions and, in doing so, provided much of the impetus for development of the field of biomedical ethics. Despite the negative public reaction to the non-treatment decision [46], physicians continued to defer to parents' requests for non-intervention, with 80% of pediatricians responding to a 1977 survey indicating that they thought parents should have the right to refuse consent for surgery for an infant with trisomy 21 and duodenal atresia [47]. Another 1977 survey of pediatric surgeons and pediatricians indicated that more than 90% of the surgeons and more than 80% of the pediatricians would acquiesce to parental refusal to consent to surgery in this circumstance [48]. These attitudes embodied the idea that parents should be universally entitled to make medical decisions on behalf of their children, and particularly those too young to speak for themselves. Although infants are incapable of defining for themselves an acceptable (or unacceptable) quality of life, it seems not unreasonable to allow their parents a degree of freedom to do this for them. After all, parents are at liberty to impart their values to their children in virtually every other aspect of their lives. If infants either lack or are likely not to have those capacities (for responsiveness to stimuli, for relationships, and for self-determination) that their parents believe necessary for the attainment of personhood, it is arguably their right to forgo the artificial support systems that will not restore these capacities but merely prolong biological existence.

After the much-publicized and controversial case of Baby Doe in 1982 [23], a public consensus began to emerge that unlimited deference to parental wishes might not be appropriate. In that case, the parents refused surgery to repair esophageal atresia in their newborn son, who also had trisomy 21. Triggered by disagreement from the family's pediatrician, the hospital went to court, unsuccessfully seeking an order to override the parents' right to make this decision and to compel performance of the surgery. While this court decision seemed to be a victory for advocates for complete parental autonomy, the ensuing controversy drew the attention of President Reagan, who ordered promulgation of the ill-fated "Baby Doe rules" discussed previously. Although these rules did not survive the scrutiny of the Supreme Court, they did create a precedent for denial of parental pre-eminence, and subsequent public discussion of the matter seems to have assumed that parental choices no longer had primacy. The 1983 AAP policy statement on treatment of critically ill newborns [30], issued to voice strong opposition to the Baby Doe regulations, advocated delegation of responsibility for such decisions to institutional review committees, suggesting that "parents should be involved" "at each step of [the] review."

In the 1992 case of Baby K, however, the child's mother, believing that "all life should be protected" [2], wanted her anencephalic child to have cardiopulmonary resuscitation and mechanical ventilation when she had trouble breathing. The hospital filed a declaratory judgment action to determine its obligations to provide this kind of emergency medical treatment to Baby K, "since the hospital and physician concluded that such treatment was medically and ethically inappropriate" [1]. A panel of the Fourth Circuit Court of Appeals ruled, by a margin of two to one, "that federal patient anti-dumping law, EMTALA [Emergency Treatment and Active Labor Act of 1986], required that all patients with emergency conditions be treated and stabilized, even when the medical standard was not to treat." The hospital argued against application of the statutory language of EMTALA, but the court rejected all arguments. Legal analysts were dismayed. Barry Furrow, professor at the Widener University School of Law in Wilmington, Delaware, wrote:

> The court's focus on stabilization under the Act, in the case of an anencephalic newborn, misses the point of the Act. Since Baby K is not a case of "patient dumping" for economic reasons, and the standard of care is generally accepted as to non-treatment, this is a better case for a judicial interpretation of the statute that is not stubbornly literal, but rather attentive to both medical practice and the congressional intent in passing EMTALA [49].

Although Baby K was eventually weaned from the ventilator and discharged to a nursing home, she required readmission on several occasions. Baby K, aka Stephanie Harrell, died at 2 years of age, after her sixth return to the emergency department at Fairfax Hospital for resuscitation because of respiratory distress. While the case of Baby Doe led to limitations on parental autonomy in making decisions on behalf of infants with neurological disabilities, the case of Baby K exemplifies the limitations of the resulting diffusion of responsibility among parents, medical professionals, ethics committees, and public entities.

Indeed, neither this diffusion of authority nor its redelegation to ethics committees has eliminated conflicts between family members and care providers. Even when a consensus of treating physicians and the medical team in general is supported by an ethics committee review, families may cling to hope and refuse withdrawal of medical interventions, as demonstrated by the recent Gonzales case in Texas [50]. Emilio Gonzales was an incapacitated, deaf, blind 17-month-old with Leigh syndrome who spent 5 months on life support in a pediatric intensive care unit. After determination by his physicians that his condition was hopeless, his physicians exercised the process defined by the Texas Advanced Directives Act, also known as the Texas Futile Care Law. Under this 1999 law [51]:

(1) The physician's refusal to comply with the patient's or surrogate's request for treatment must be reviewed by a hospital-appointed medical or ethics committee in which the attending physician does not participate.

(2) The family must be given 48 hours' notice and be invited to participate in the consultation process.

(3) The ethics-consultation committee must provide a written report detailing its findings to the family and must include this report in the medical record.

(4) If the ethics-consultation process fails to resolve the dispute, the hospital, working with the family, must make reasonable efforts to transfer the patient's care to another physician or institution willing to provide the treatment requested by the family.

(5) If after 10 days (measured from the time the family receives the written summary from the ethics-consultation committee) no such provider can be found, the hospital and physician may unilaterally withhold or withdraw therapy that has been determined to be futile.

(6) The patient or surrogate may request a court-ordered time extension, which should be granted only if the judge

determines that there is a reasonable likelihood of finding a willing provider of the disputed treatment.

(7) If the family does not seek an extension or the judge fails to grant one, futile treatment may be unilaterally withdrawn by the treatment team with immunity from civil and criminal prosecution.

(Similar laws have been enacted in California, Virginia, and other states.) After obtaining review by the ethics committee and approaching 31 other institutions, all of which declined to accept a transfer for further care, the treating physicians and hospital were prepared to discontinue care after the required 10-day waiting period. Emilio's mother sought and obtained an injunction to extend that deadline. Emilio died while still receiving intensive care before the court issued its final ruling, so the legal status of this law remains ambiguous. The court's willingness to delay withdrawal of care suggests that the judicial system remains reluctant to override the wishes of families. As Truog has pointed out, "the law's effectiveness for achieving closure . . . relies on a due process approach that is more illusory that real and that risks becoming a rubber-stamp mechanism for systematically overriding families' requests for care that seem unreasonable to the clinicians involved" [52]. It should not be surprising that families may mistrust a process (review by a hospital-appointed ethics committee) that almost always agrees with the treating physicians' assessment of futility, as demonstrated by the report of affirmation of that position in 43 of 47 cases reported from another Texas hospital [53]. It should be apparent that this approach, though well intended and thoughtfully designed, fails to bring resolution to these dilemmas. Truog has summarized this well in his conclusion that "Rather than jeopardize the respect we hold for diversity and minority viewpoints, . . . we should seek to enhance our capacity to tolerate the choices of others, even when we believe they are wrong" [52].

Implementing the recommendation that parents be regarded as the principal decision makers regarding forgoing potentially life-sustaining care for their infants will require a high degree of unanimity among all the nursery staff that, in a given case, an infant's capacities for personal life are so profoundly diminished that the parents' request to forgo life-sustaining treatment is appropriate and ought to be respected. In the absence of unanimity there could be repercussions, both for the attending neonatologists and for the institution, not only in terms of litigation but also, and this is of perhaps greater concern, unwanted media attention and the adverse publicity that can be associated with it. These practical considerations may in the end prevail over the moral and medical judgment of the physicians and, hence, the parents. It is generally assumed that the interests of the child can and should be determined independently of the interests of the other members of the family who normally serve as its surrogates. This is a questionable assumption, particularly for a mother or father suddenly confronted with the birth of a neurologically damaged child. Given the shock and stress that ensues, in which parents have to absorb the technical information about the conditions of their child and also their often dizzying roles as caretakers, asking the parent for a dispassionate assessment of the interests of the child may not be a reasonable request [54,55]. But there does not appear to be a better alternative.

So what is the state of affairs at this point in time? We can decide which medical interventions to apply or withhold, but decisions about life and death are out of our hands. Decisions should be based upon the "best interests" of the patient, but these are value-laden, often difficult to determine, and sometimes the subject of intense disagreement. Arguments based on the moral principles of distributive justice, autonomy, surrogacy, and substituted judgment have failed to produce consensus on who should have final authority for decisions when conflicts cannot be resolved, and attempts to diffuse this responsibility through constructs like infant care review committees have not succeeded in eliminating intractable disagreements. The courts have shown some willingness to compel medical treatments against parental wishes, but not to the extent of mandating maternal interventions for fetal benefit, nor have they formally condoned cessation of intensive care against parental wishes, despite legislation in several states providing legal mechanisms for doing so. As these issues remain unresolved, the de facto authority for decision making continues to rest with parents, unless there is compelling evidence that their choice to withhold treatment is contrary to the best interests of the infant.

Nearly 2500 years ago, Hippocrates (ca. 460–370 BCE) said, "Life is short; art is long; opportunity fugitive; judgment difficult. It is the duty of the physician not only to do that which immediately belongs to him, but likewise to secure the cooperation of the sick, of those who are in attendance, and of all external agents" [56]. It has been hard to improve upon that advice.

References

1. In the matter of baby K. In: *LEXIS*, US App. 4th Cir., 1994.

2. Greenhouse L. Court order to treat baby with partial brain prompts debate on costs and ethics. *New York Times* 1994 February 20; Sect. 20.

3. Kolata G. Battle over a baby's future raises hard ethical issues. *New York Times* 1994 December 27; Sect. A1.

4. Hintz SR, Kendrick DE, Stoll BJ, *et al*. Neurodevelopmental and growth outcomes of extremely low birth weight infants after necrotizing enterocolitis. *Pediatrics* 2005; **115**: 696–703.

5. Cirak B, Wang P, Avellino AM. Implications of a neurosurgical intervention in a patient with a surgically repaired hypoplastic left heart syndrome. *Pediatr Neurosurg* 2007; **43**: 488–91.

6. Tabbutt S, Nord AS, Jarvik GP, *et al*. Neurodevelopmental outcomes after staged palliation for hypoplastic left heart syndrome. *Pediatrics* 2008; **121**: 476–83.

7. Davis D, Davis S, Cotman K, *et al*. Feeding difficulties and growth delay in children with hypoplastic left heart syndrome versus D-transposition of the great arteries. *Pediatr Cardiol* 2008; **29**: 328–33.

8. Schultz AH, Wernovsky G. Late outcomes in patients with surgically treated congenital heart disease. *Semin Thorac Cardiovasc Surg Pediatr Card Surg Annu* 2005: 145–56.

9. Kon AA, Ackerson L, Lo B. How pediatricians counsel parents when no "best-choice" management exists: lessons to be learned from hypoplastic left heart syndrome. *Arch Pediatr Adolesc Med* 2004; **158**: 436–41.

10. Eicher DJ, Wagner CL, Katikaneni LP, *et al.* Moderate hypothermia in neonatal encephalopathy: efficacy outcomes. *Pediatr Neurol* 2005; **32**: 11–17.

11. Gluckman PD, Wyatt JS, Azzopardi D, *et al.* Selective head cooling with mild systemic hypothermia after neonatal encephalopathy: multicentre randomised trial. *Lancet* 2005; **365**: 663–70.

12. Shankaran S, Laptook AR, Ehrenkranz RA, *et al.* Whole-body hypothermia for neonates with hypoxic–ischemic encephalopathy. *N Engl J Med* 2005; **353**: 1574–84.

13. Whitelaw A. Death as an option in neonatal intensive care. *Lancet* 1986; **2**: 328–31.

14. Isaacs D. Brain death. *J Paediatr Child Health* 2003; **39**: 224–5.

15. American Academy of Pediatrics Task Force on Brain Death in Children. Guidelines for the determination of brain death in children. *Pediatrics* 1987; **80**: 298–300.

16. Volpe JJ. Brain death determination in the newborn. *Pediatrics* 1987; **80**: 293–7.

17. Ashwal S. Brain death in the newborn: current perspectives. *Clin Perinatol* 1997; **24**: 859–82.

18. Stahlman M. Withholding and withdrawing therapy and actively hastening death. In Goldworth A, Silverman W, Stevenson DK, *et al.*, eds., *Ethics and Perinatology*. New York, NY: Oxford University Press, 1995: 162–71.

19. Moseley KL, Silveira MJ, Goold SD. Futility in evolution. *Clin Geriatr Med* 2005; **21**: 211–22, x.

20. Morreim EH. Profoundly diminished life: the casualties of coercion. *Hastings Cent Rep* 1994; **24**: 33–42.

21. Sirico RA. An unjust sacrifice. *New York Times* 2000 September 28; Sect. A31.

22. Dworkin R. *Life's Dominion: an Argument About Abortion, Euthanasia, and Individual Freedom*. New York, NY: Alfred A. Knopf, 1993.

23. Wallis C. The stormy legacy of Baby Doe. *Time* 1983 September 26.

24. Stevenson DK, Ariagno RL, Kutner JS, *et al.* The "Baby Doe" rule. *JAMA* 1986; **255**: 1909–12.

25. Greely HT. Baby Doe and beyond: the past and future of government regulations in the United States. In Goldworth A, Silverman W, Stevenson DK, *et al.*, eds., *Ethics and Perinatology*. New York, NY: Oxford University Press, 1995: 296–306.

26. Capron AM. In re Helga Wanglie. *Hastings Cent Rep* 1991; **21**: 26–8.

27. League of Nations. Geneva Declaration of the Rights of the Child of 1924, adopted September 26, 1924. *League of Nations OJ* 1924; Spec. Supp. 21: 43.

28. United Nations. Declaration of the Rights of the Child, proclaimed by General Assembly resolution 1386 (XIV) of 20 November 1959.

29. President's Commission for the Study of Ethical Problems in Medicine and Biomedical and Behavioral Research. *Deciding to Forgo Life-Sustaining Treatment*. Washington, DC: US Government Printing Office, 1983.

30. American Academy of Pediatrics Committee on Bioethics. Treatment of critically ill newborns. *Pediatrics* 1983; **72**: 565–6.

31. Catlin AJ, Stevenson DK. Physicians' neonatal resuscitation of extremely low-birth-weight preterm infants. *Image J Nurs Sch* 1999; **31**: 269–75.

32. Saigal S, Stoskopf B, Pinelli J, *et al.* Self-perceived health-related quality of life of former extremely low birth weight infants at young adulthood. *Pediatrics* 2006; **118**: 1140–8.

33. Stevenson DK, Young EWD. Introduction: a thematic overview. In Goldworth A, Silverman W, Stevenson DK, *et al.*, eds., *Ethics and Perinatology*. New York, NY: Oxford University Press, 1995: 6.

34. American Academy of Pediatrics Committee on Fetus and Newborn. Noninitiation or withdrawal of intensive care for high-risk newborns. *Pediatrics* 2007; **119**: 401–3.

35. Hardwig J. What about the family? *Hastings Cent Rep* 1990; **20**: 5–10.

36. Blustein J. The family in medical decision making. *Hastings Cent Rep* 1993; **23**: 6–13.

37. Fasouliotis SJ, Schenker JG. Maternal–fetal conflict. *Eur J Obstet Gynecol Reprod Biol* 2000; **89**: 101–7.

38. Nelson LJ, Milliken N. Compelled medical treatment of pregnant women: life, liberty, and law in conflict. *JAMA* 1988; **259**: 1060–6.

39. Hume D. *Treatise of Human Nature*. Oxford: Clarendon Press, 1888.

40. Harris J. What is the good of health care? *Bioethics* 1996; **10**: 269–91.

41. Meadow W, Lantos JD, Mokalla M, *et al.* Distributive justice across generations: epidemiology of ICU care for the very young and the very old. *Clin Perinatol* 1996; **23**: 597–608.

42. Cutler DM, Meara E. The technology of birth: is it worth it? *Forum Health Econ Policy* 2000; **3**: Article 3.

43. Antommaria AM. "Who should survive?: one of the choices on our conscience": mental retardation and the history of contemporary bioethics. *Kennedy Inst Ethics J* 2006; **16**: 205–24.

44. Robertson JA. Involuntary euthanasia of defective newborns: a legal analysis. *Stanford Law Review* 1975; **27**: 213–69.

45. *Who Should Survive? One of the Choices on Our Conscience*. [Film]. Joseph P. Kennedy Jr. Foundation, distributor, 1971.

46. McGehan F. Hopkins was wrong to let infant die in '63 case, symposium decides. *Baltimore Sun* 1971 October 17; Sect. 20, 16.

47. Todres ID, Krane D, Howell MC, *et al.* Pediatricians' attitudes affecting decision-making in defective newborns. *Pediatrics* 1977; **60**: 197–201.

48. Shaw A, Randolph JG, Manard B. Ethical issues in pediatric surgery: a national survey of pediatricians and pediatric surgeons. *Pediatrics* 1977; **60**: 588–99.

49. Furrow BR. Baby K: a legal and ethical viewpoint. *ASMLE Briefings* 1994 (10): 1, 5.

50. Moreno S. Case puts Texas futile-treatment law under a microscope. *Washington Post* 2007 April 11.

51. Texas Futile Care Law. *Texas Health & Safety Code*. 1999: Chapter 166, Section 46.

52. Truog RD. Tackling medical futility in Texas. *N Engl J Med* 2007; **357**: 1–3.

53. Fine RL, Mayo TW. Resolution of futility by due process: early experience with the Texas Advance Directives Act. *Ann Intern Med* 2003; **138**: 743–6.

54. Hackler JC, Hiller FC. Family consent to orders not resuscitate: reconsidering hospital policy. *JAMA* 1990; **264**: 1281–3.

55. Rhoden NK. Litigating life and death. *Harv Law Rev* 1988; **102**: 375–446.

56. Coar T. *The Aphorisms of Hippocrates*. London: Valpy, 1882.

Chapter 50

Medicolegal issues in perinatal brain injury

David Sheuerman

Introduction

Perinatal hypoxic-ischemic brain injury is an important and often troublesome medicolegal problem for practicing physicians. Brain injury to infants occurring during the perinatal period is probably the most common cause of severe long-term neurological deficit in patients, and consequently the incentive for legal action is high.

Although vast advances in care have taken place during the past several decades in the practice of perinatal medicine, the incidence of brain injury and its sequelae has not seen a significant decline. Litigation involving these types of injuries has remained a constant over many years despite endeavors in education of both physicians and patients, and improvements in care. This chapter will attempt to explore and explain the manner in which legal principles are applied to complex medical issues in the medicolegal examination of perinatal brain injury. The rules of law in this chapter refer either to California law or to general medical negligence principles in the USA.

The term "medical malpractice," often misused and frequently misunderstood, refers to any professional act or omission to act that encompasses or represents an unreasonable lack of knowledge, care, or skill in carrying out one's professional duties. As used herein the term "malpractice" is synonymous with "negligence."

Although there are a number of legal theories which may be brought against a physician for allegedly fault-worthy conduct in perinatal or other medical contexts, the vast majority of such legal actions are based on allegations that a physician or other practitioner was negligent – that is, that he or she did not perform in a reasonable manner as compared to other practitioners of similar standing acting under the same or similar circumstances.

Duty

The first element of the theory of negligence as malpractice is establishing that a duty was created by the practitioner–patient relationship. In certain instances, whether such a "duty" has been created is a contested legal issue. Such circumstances might include where an informal communication which might be construed as a consultation takes place, or where a physician volunteers to help in an emergency situation. Once a sufficient relationship has been established, the practitioner has a duty to possess and utilize that degree of knowledge, care, and skill exercised by a reasonable and prudent physician under the same or similar circumstances. A physician owes the patient a duty to act in a manner consistent with the standards established by his or her profession, commonly referred to as the "standard of care."

There is no clear or precise definition of the duty of a particular physician under each factual scenario. Thus, because most medical malpractice cases, especially those in the perinatal area, are highly technical, the standard of care is defined by witnesses who profess to carry special medical qualifications and who are asked to provide guidance to the judge or jury. In general, the finder of fact is instructed to base its decision solely on the opinions of such experts in deciding whether the physician in question acted with ordinary prudence [1] (Box 50.1). Instructions are also given to the jury on physician duty [2] (Box 50.2).

Breach of duty

The second element of a cause of action for medical malpractice is proof, only more likely than not, that the physician did not comply with the duty described above. It is thus alleged that the physician breached his or her duty by failing to act within the applicable standard of care. This is obviously a vigorously contested issue in each medicolegal case, with a variety of criteria to be examined in supporting the plaintiff or the defense case, mostly surrounding the opinions of the various experts. In the perinatal arena, consensus statements and guidelines such as those published by the American College of Obstetricians and Gynecologists (ACOG) and the American Academy of Pediatrics (AAP) are frequently utilized to clarify the standard of care in the community. Of course, it is not possible for any consensus statement or clinical practice guideline to encompass or anticipate each clinical scenario or to speak to the important aspect of physician judgment employed in each case. The jury is instructed by the court to utilize a specific framework in evaluating whether the physician deviated from the standard of care [3] (Box 50.3).

Physicians asked to consult on a given case and to render their opinion whether the practitioner(s) met the standard of

Fetal and Neonatal Brain Injury, 4th edition, ed. David K. Stevenson, William E. Benitz, Philip Sunshine, Susan R. Hintz, and Maurice L. Druzin. Published by Cambridge University Press. © Cambridge University Press 2009.

Box 50.1 Medical negligence: standard of care determined by expert testimony

You must determine the standard of professional learning, skill, and care required of the defendant only from the opinions of the physicians (including the defendant) who have testified as expert witnesses as to such standard.

You should consider each such opinion and should weigh the qualifications of the witness and the reasons given for his or her opinion. Give each opinion the weight to which you deem it entitled.

(You must resolve any conflict in the testimony of the witnesses by weighing each of the opinions expressed against the others, taking into consideration the reasons given for the opinion, the facts relied upon by the witness, and the relative credibility, special knowledge, skill, experience, training, and education of the witness.)

Source: California BAJI 6.30 [1]

Box 50.2 Duration of physician's responsibility

Once a physician has undertaken to treat a patient, the employment and duty as a physician to the patient continues until the physician withdraws from the case after giving the patient notice and a reasonable time to employ another doctor, or until the condition of the patient is such that the physician's services are no longer reasonably required.

A physician may limit his or her obligation to a patient by undertaking to treat the patient only for a certain ailment of injury or only at a certain time or place. If the employment is so limited, the physician is not required to treat the patient for any other ailment or injury or at any other time or place.

Source: California BAJI 6.05 [2]

Box 50.3 Duty of physician

A physician performing professional services for a patient owes that patient the following duties of care:
(1) The duty to have that degree of learning and skill ordinarily possessed by reputable physicians, practicing in the same or a similar locality and under similar circumstances.
(2) The duty to use the care and skill ordinarily exercised in like cases by reputable members of the profession practicing in the same or a similar locality under similar circumstances.
(3) The duty to use reasonable diligence and his/her best judgment in the exercise of skill and the application of learning.
A failure to perform any one of these duties is negligence.

Medical perfection not required

A physician is not necessarily negligent because he or she errs in judgment or because his or her efforts prove unsuccessful. The physician is negligent if the error in judgment or lack of success is due to a failure to perform any of the duties as defined in these instructions.

Source: California BAJI 6.00.1, 6.02 [3]

Box 50.4 Alternative methods of diagnosis or treatment

Where there is more than one recognized method of diagnosis or treatment, and no one of them is used exclusively and uniformly by all practitioners of good standing, under the same or similar circumstances, a physician is not negligent if, in exercising his or her best judgment, he or she selects one of the approved methods, which later turns out to be a wrong selection, or one not favored by certain other practitioners.

Source: California BAJI 6.03 [4]

---

from the treatment the consultant believes he or she would have given, the standard must have been breached. This is clearly an incorrect application of the law, which provides that different methods may be employed by different practitioners and, where no uniformity of opinion exists, the physician is not negligent merely because he or she chooses a method different from or not favored by other physicians [4] (Box 50.4).

A generally accurate description by a testifying expert witness is "a physician must use the care a reasonable physician might employ in the same or similar circumstances." An error in judgment does not constitute negligence. Intentionally, and by necessity, the legal definition of the "standard" to be met is vague. The author proposes that if one may logically surmise that the practitioner has demonstrated adequate knowledge to apply the necessary skills and has utilized that knowledge in a logical manner in an attempt to achieve the desired result, the physician has met the standard of care, regardless of the outcome of the treatment.

Causation

The third element that must be proved by the plaintiff, again by a preponderance of the evidence, is that the act or omission said to be negligent by the physician was a cause of the resulting injury. The closeness of this connection is described as "legal" or "proximate" cause. In the law, the concept of causation differs markedly from the concept of etiology in medicine. The law requires only that a particular act or omission be a "substantial factor," and not necessarily the major or most immediate cause of the injury, as a physician would apply the term to describe the etiology of an injury.

Physicians involved in the legal process, whether as defendants, retained experts, or treating physicians, often confuse (or allow themselves to be confused) when they are being cross-examined regarding their opinions on causation. Plaintiffs' burden of proof to show something did or did not happen by a "preponderance" of the evidence requires only that the "likelihood" of the occurrence or non-occurrence is greater than 50%. Thus, words such as "probably" or "likely" have critical meaning in the legal forum. Physicians are to be cautioned that use of these words in an answer (or a response linked to a question containing these words) constitutes a medical opinion which may make or break the legal case. The jury receives instruction on causation [5] (Box 50.5).

Causation is a critical element in the evaluation of most perinatal brain-injury cases. Numerous criteria are evaluated in an attempt to prove the likelihood or lack of causation in

care commonly apply very different standards in the application of the "standard of care" to a given set of facts and circumstances. Many consultants are misled into believing that if the practitioner in question acted in a manner which deviated

Box 50.5 Cause: substantial factor test

The law defines cause in its own particular way. A cause of injury, damage, loss, or harm is something that is a substantial factor in bringing about an injury, damage, loss, or harm.

There may be more than one cause of an injury. When negligent or wrongful conduct of two or more persons contributes concurrently as (a) cause(s) of an injury, the conduct of each is a cause of the injury regardless of the extent to which each contributes to the injury. A cause is concurrent if it was operative at the moment of injury and acted with another cause to produce the injury. It is no defense that the negligent or wrongful conduct of a person not joined as a party was also a cause of the injury.

Source: California BAJI 3.76, 3.77 [5]

the perinatal period, including epidemiology, indicators of intrauterine injury, evaluation of fetal heart-monitor tracings, consideration of alternative causes of brain injury to those occurring in the perinatal period, correlation of clinical findings and timing of the hypoxic–ischemic event by use of Apgar scores, blood gases, brain imaging, placental pathology, hematologic markers such as nucleated red blood cells [6], and the like.

Damages

The fourth element of the medical malpractice lawsuit is plaintiffs' proof of the nature and extent of damages. During the perinatal brain-injury case, damages may include a wide range of financial, physical, and emotional injury to the patient.

General or non-economic damages are awarded for pain and suffering, mental anguish, grief, and emotional conditions which are thought to flow inevitably from the injury caused by the defendant as a natural and foreseeable consequence of the injury.

"Special" or "economic" damages in the perinatal brain-injury case are presented by a team of experts on each side, which has grown into a cottage industry, often thought by the defense to represent extreme departures from reason. The plaintiffs' bar, on the other hand, argue that defense experts are hired to unreasonably reduce just compensation for legitimate injuries. Economic damages in a severe perinatal injury case will generally include:

- Healthcare services, often including those of a pediatrician, internist, dentist, podiatrist, nutritionist, vision specialist, occupational and physical therapist, speech therapist, psychological services, behavioral intervention, therapeutic recreation, lab, emergency room, case manager, financial manager, and acute hospitalization.

- Medical supplies, including medications, bowel and bladder supplies, gastrostomy supplies, respiratory supplies and equipment, medical equipment including wheelchair, orthotics, mechanical bedding, bedside equipment and supplies.

- Diagnostic testing, chest, hips, spine, and other x-rays, neurodiagnostic studies such as magnetic resonance imaging/computed tomography of the head, electroencephalograms, and various laboratory work are claimed as intermittent needs.

- Attendant care, often alleged to be necessary around the clock, can, alone, easily generate damages of several hundred thousand dollars per year for life. The level of care required is a frequently contested issue, often involving millions of dollars, depending on whether the jury finds care should be provided by a trained attendant, a licensed vocational nurse, or a registered nurse.

- Home modifications, such as access ramps, widened hallways, lowered cabinets, and specialized bathroom facilities are commonly prescribed.

In many cases, such lifetime damages are funded by the purchase of an annuity, generally at a small fraction of the expenses projected by the plaintiffs. An exemplar of such damages can be found as part of a typical life care plan (Box 50.6).

Documentation

No discussion of medicolegal issues in any area of medicine can ignore the critical importance of careful and accurate charting. One must recognize that the practitioner's primary responsibility is to provide quality care to the patient, even if that endeavor detracts from accurate charting. The ability to time precisely particular events or to record all "significant" information is highly dependent on clinical circumstances. However, when trying to defend one's actions years after an event has taken place, failure to record, as recommended by obstetric and nursing organizations, makes it far more likely that a lay jury will infer a negative event is represented by lack of documentation. Often the issue in a perinatal case brought years after the event involves when the status of the fetus was compromised. Long time periods of undocumented fetal heart rates often simply reflect long periods of fetal well-being. Plaintiffs will argue, perhaps supported by suboptimal blood gases or low Apgar scores, that the lack of documentation reflects lack of adequate monitoring. Both ACOG and NAACOG (the organization for obstetric, gynecologic, and neonatal nurses) have published standards requiring specific frequency of recording as well as specifying the characteristics required to be noted. For instance, ACOG provides that auscultated fetal heart rates should be recorded in the chart after each observation [7]. The practitioner must recognize that the events of labor, delivery, or neonatal care often are not even examined by lawyers or consulting experts until several years after the events. Substandard record keeping alone, where the actual care was adequate, has led to many malpractice suits.

Terminology matters

Accurate and consistent use of terms (or the reverse) is often the difference between the filing or the successful prosecution of cases alleging substandard perinatal care. The term "fetal distress" is most commonly misapplied in medical charts to the reaction of the fetus to the stress of labor, and the term's indiscriminate use can lead to confusion or worse.

ACOG has stated, "Terms such as asphyxia, hypoxia, and fetal distress should not be applied to continued electronic fetal monitoring or auscultations" [8].

Box 50.6 Exemplar: future medical needs, neonatal brain injury

I. Future medical care
A. *Physicians*
   1. Internist: four times a year over life expectancy after age 18.
   2. Pediatrician: 4–6 times a year until age 18.
   3. Other (neurologist, ophthalmologist, immunologist, gastroenterologist, hematologist, pulmonologist, rehabilitation medicine, orthopedist, etc.): 10–12 visits per year over the patient's life expectancy.
B. *Ancillary medical care*
   1. Dentist: cleaning 3–4 times per year. Currently, seeing a special pediatric "special needs" dentist. Because of oral tactile defensiveness, as patient ages, will likely need examination and cleaning under anesthesia.
   2. Podiatrist 1–2 times per year over the patient's life expectancy.
   3. Nutritionist: two times per year over the patient's life expectancy.
   4. Low-vision specialist: one time per year until age 18.
C. *Counseling*
   1. Individual counseling for mother six times per year over the patient's life expectancy.
   2. Family counseling for parents as a couple six times per year over the patient's life expectancy.
   3. Sibling (5-year-old brother) four times per month for 3 months, then one time per month until age 18.
D. *Behavioral intervention*
   1. A behavioral specialist to assist with a program of environmental and behavioral modification to extinguish negative self-mutilating behavior and the behavior of kicking, pinching, and biting others. Initial intervention at 6–12 sessions for the first 6 months, supervised by a psychologist. Thereafter, two visits per year over the patient's life expectancy.

II. Diagnostic testing
A. *Routine blood chemistry*
   1. Complete blood count: six times per year on average over the patient's life expectancy, exclusive of inpatient lab.
   2. Sequential multiple analyzer count (SMAC) 20: two times per year over the patient's life expectancy.
   3. Valproic acid levels: two times per year over the patient's life expectancy.
   4. Immunoglobulin G levels.

III. Neurodiagnostic studies
A. *Magnetic resonance imaging/computed tomography head scans*
   4–6 more times over the patient's life expectancy.
B. *Electroencephalogram*
   4–6 more times over the patient's life expectancy.

IV. Radiologic studies
A. *Chest x-ray*
   2–4 per year over the patient's life expectancy. Based on this track record thus far, this is a conservative estimate.
B. *Joint x-ray/spine x-ray*
   Approximately 1–2 per year over the patient's life expectancy to follow scoliosis; rule out fractures/dislocation secondary to anticipated falls.

V. Gastrointestinal studies
A. *Upper gastrointestinal endoscopy*
   4–6 per year over the patient's life expectancy for recurrent obstruction, gastrointestinal bleeding, and vomiting.

VI. Rehabilitation therapy
A. *Physical therapy*
   One time per week until age 18. Then four times per year over the patient's life expectancy to re-evaluate lower-extremity range of motion, mobility status, and equipment.
B. *Occupational therapy*
   Two times per week until age 18. Thereafter, four times a year to re-evaluate equipment, upper-extremity range of motion, and self-care potential.
C. *Speech therapy*
   One time per week until age 18. Thereafter, re-evaluations are appropriate once every 3–5 years.
D. *Therapeutic recreation*
   One time per year over the patient's life expectancy, to assist with the selection of developmentally appropriate recreational activities.

VII. Equipment
A. *Feeding supplies*
   1. Gastrostomy tubes (Mic Key buttons with adapters for both J-tube site and separate G-tube site). Buttons are changed every 3–4 months.
   2. Feeding bags with tubing.
   3. Intravenous pole.

Box 50.6 (*cont.*)

    4. Feeding pump.

    5. Syringe.

    6. 2 × 2 dressings for both G-tube and J-tube sites.

    7. Stockinette (wrapped around abdomen to secure G-tube and J-tube dressings).

  B. *Incontinence supplies*

    1. Diaper wipes.

    2. Diapers (approximately eight per day).

    3. A&D ointment.

    4. Gloves.

    5. Bactroban ointment.

  C. *Respirator equipment*

    1. Suction machines, portable.

    2. Yangauer suction handle.

    3. Pulse oximeter.

    4. Pulmoaide.

  D. *Mobility aids*

    1. Wheelchair: pediatric manual Quickie wheelchair with head rest, lateral trunk and lateral thigh supports, hip abduction wedge, detachable foot rests, anti-tip bars, heavy-duty wheels, back support with lumbar insert, chest and lap belts, handles on back for parents to push chair.

    2. Bilateral ambulatory foot orthotics: will require a new pair every 12 months until age 18. Thereafter, replace every 2–3 years.

  E. *Equipment*

    1. Hospital bed.

    2. Bath equipment: shower chair and hand-held shower hose will be needed after age 8–10 years. Currently, parents lift him in and out of bathtub.

  F. *Safety equipment*

    1. Restraint jacket to use in any bad conditions (traveling).

    2. Helmet.

    3. Vail bed enclosure.

    4. Bilateral arm splints to hold elbows in extension to prevent self-mutilation.

    5. Other: Porto-Cath, implanted. Change? How often?

VIII. Medications

  A. *See attached.*

  In addition, is frequently on antibiotics several times per year. These include Keflex, Septra, etc., per J-tube, and Rocephin, intramuscularly as an outpatient.

IX. Tube feeding

  A. *Vivonex* via J-tube at 65 ml/hx24H/day.

Practitioners have been cautioned by ACOG against indiscriminate use of the term "fetal distress." Instead, the term "non-reassuring fetal status" is recommended [9].

Another term used with consistent imprecision is "perinatal asphyxia." According to ACOG, "long usage prevents its abandonment" [10]. The current AAP and ACOG guidelines state that "asphyxia" should be reserved to describe neonates with all the following conditions:

(1) acidemia, pH below 7.0 on arterial cord blood

(2) Apgar score of 0–3 for longer than 5 minutes

(3) objective neonatal neurological signs and symptoms (seizures, coma, hypotonia, etc.)

(4) multisystem organ dysfunction (cardiovascular, gastrointestinal, hematologic, pulmonary, or renal) [11]

It should be noted, effective in 1998, the International Classification of Diseases (ICD) dropped "all inclusion terms" for "fetal distress" except metabolic acidemia.

Similarly, the term "hypoxic–ischemic encephalopathy" (HIE) is frequently applied indiscriminately by perinatal providers as it occurs with other such "diagnoses." Once the term is applied to the patient by one practitioner it is commonly repeated in subsequent chart entries by others, without appropriate consideration of whether the neonate displaying neurological depression actually had evidence antepartum or intrapartum of events likely to compromise oxygen supply to the fetus. Once the term is used in the chart (and frequently buttressed by multiple entries simply parroting it) it is extremely difficult for the defense team to demonstrate to a jury of lay people that the infant's depression is more likely a result of perinatal ischemic stroke, congenital metabolic condition, infectious etiologies, or placental vasculopathies. Litigation experience shows that, once discovery ensues, comparison of records of the neonate's siblings can uncover similar developmental delays, demonstrating a likely genetic cause of the original neurological compromise and subsequent delay. However, because these causes are often difficult to prove, the diagnosis of HIE is often applied by default. A more complete review of the factors to be considered in the "cause and effect" analysis of perinatal depression can be found in Chapter 1.

Authorities, including Nelson, have advocated that when encephalopathy and/or later cerebral palsy occurs in a term or near-term infant without the obvious antecedent asphyxial events, a diagnosis of neonatal encephalopathy (NE) is the appropriate term [12]. This appears to be a preferred approach from both the therapeutic and the medicolegal perspective.

The absence of subsequent markers of HIE, including positive findings on magnetic resonance imaging, should also be noted as significant in the diagnostic process and accompanying documentation.

Case study: obstetrics/labor and delivery

In a case alleging negligent care by two obstetricians, the hospital nursing staff, and the anesthesiologist, the minor plaintiff brought this action for severe brain injury following uterine rupture.

The mother of the baby was a 25-year-old gravida 3 para 1 with a relatively uncomplicated prenatal course admitted to the subject hospital for induction at 40 4/7 weeks' gestational age due to a low amniotic fluid index. The patient had no known risk factors for the eventual complication, a uterine rupture. She had previously delivered a 3500+ g infant by uncomplicated vaginal delivery.

The patient was in the hospital for induction for approximately 12 hours on the day prior to delivery. During that time she received oxytocin augmentation, which was discontinued around midnight to allow her to rest overnight. On the following day, the obstetricians began a trial of misoprostol for induction. After approximately 7 hours of relatively normal, albeit slow progress of labor (there was dispute whether the fetal monitors reflected fetal well-being and whether there was evidence of hyperstimulation), the mother requested her labor epidural. She testified, as compared with her previous pregnancy, that she felt delivery was imminent.

The external fetal monitor belt was removed for placement of the epidural. A few minutes after the epidural was in, the mother reported a tearing sensation and severe pain, which the experienced nursing staff interpreted as labor pain. The fetal monitoring Doppler was being reattached; however, the nurses had not obtained a fetal heart beat since attempting to replace the external fetal monitor belt following the epidural. The next 6–8 minutes passed as the nursing staff attempted to obtain a fetal heart rate, without success. The obstetrician was called, arrived within 5 minutes, and delivered the baby from the abdomen by cesarean section within 20 minutes of her arrival.

Allegations against prenatal obstetrician

Plaintiff alleged the prenatal care was negligent in that the position of the baby at 29 weeks was confirmed as transverse and that no accurate testing regarding presentation was done thereafter until the uterine rupture occurred. Plaintiff complained the obstetricians did not assess the position of the fetus sonographically on several visits leading up to the delivery and

failed to document that the fetus was in vertex position throughout the period of induction at the hospital.

Plaintiff complained various drugs were used to promote cervical ripening and dilation without any descent of the fetus and without dilation in the mother. Plaintiff claimed these drugs, rather than promoting ripening, induced hypercontractility. Plaintiff alleged the prenatal obstetrician was negligent in failing to confirm a vertex presentation during the last few prenatal visits. That obstetrician testified he most probably conducted a Leopold's maneuver to determine fetal presentation, given the mother's excessive weight gain and the fact that the first baby was nearly macrosomic. However, that obstetrician failed to document in the medical record that he had performed a Leopold's maneuver, nor did he document fetal presentation. Plaintiff alleged, had the examination been performed, it would have likely diagnosed a transverse lie requiring cesarean rather than vaginal delivery.

Plaintiff further claimed that the patient was not adequately informed concerning the risks and benefits of oxytocin under the circumstances of having a low amniotic fluid index, and that the obstetricians further failed to explain the risks involved in the use of misoprostol.

Allegations against labor obstetrician

Plaintiff complained the obstetrician managing the labor and delivery was negligent in failing to consider the potential for uteroplacental insufficiency, and thereby discontinue the use of misoprostol; failing to confirm fetal presentation before ordering the use of misoprostol; and failing to observe the patient adequately to "insure" normal fetal heart rate and uterine contraction patterns in a patient laboring under misoprostol induction. Plaintiff alleged the mother of baby was hyperstimulated, and that according to misoprostol protocols the patient's dosage should have been reduced or discontinued.

Allegations against anesthesiologist

Plaintiff claimed the anesthesiologist was negligent in ignoring complaints of severe pain at the time the epidural was administered despite two preceding doses of narcotic medications without relief; plaintiff alleged removal of the fetal monitor during epidural administration was negligent in the face of "abnormalities" present on the fetal heart-rate monitor and with contractions occurring every 1–2 minutes.

Plaintiff contended it was the responsibility of the anesthesiologist practicing in the labor and delivery department to know the status of both mother and fetus and to be "sure" that both were stable at all times. Plaintiff complained of the anesthesiologist that he made no inquiries of the status of the fetus and that he prematurely left the patient's room shortly after giving the epidural. Plaintiff alleged the standard of care required the anesthesiologist to remain in the room for 15–20 minutes following epidural administration. Had he done so, plaintiff alleged, he would have been aware of the report by the mother of baby that she felt a rip or tearing pain and that this would have alerted him to the occurrence of a uterine rupture. Plaintiff complained that when the nurse, following the epidural, was unable to obtain a fetal heart rate, the anesthesiologist should have immediately contacted the obstetrician rather than allowing the nursing staff to evaluate the reasons for loss of fetal heart rate.

Allegations against hospital (nursing staff)

Plaintiff alleged the hospital nursing staff failed to determine fetal position on vaginal exams, failed to contact the obstetrician to report decelerations in the absence of uterine contraction, failed to detect hyperstimulation, failed to administer terbutaline to reduce the frequency of contractions, failed to evaluate the patient's complaints of pain described as hallmarks of uterine rupture, and delayed contacting the obstetrician once the fetal heart tones were found to be undetectable.

The prenatal obstetrician defended his actions by arguing that he did in fact determine this fetus was in a vertex presentation based on the fact that he had written in his record the location of the fetal heart rate and had performed an abdominal examination. An ultrasound examination was done shortly before admission for the primary purpose of determining the amniotic fluid volume. He argued that he certainly would not have scheduled the patient for an induced labor had there been a transverse lie at the time of his examination. He testified he utilized four methods to determine the vertex presentation on his final prenatal visit: (1) location of the fetal heart rate in the lower quadrant; (2) palpating the fetal back through the abdominal wall; (3) vaginal examination with palpation of vertex; (4) ultrasound confirmation of vertex presentation. However, only heart-sound location was documented.

He testified that misoprostol is a synthetic prostaglandin E_1 analog which can be administered intravaginally or orally for cervical ripening and induction; it had been studied in randomized clinical trials, and had been found to be an effective agent for induction of labor. Reports of uterine rupture in use of misoprostol had occurred, he argued, only in patients with prior cesarean section.

The labor and delivery obstetrician argued that she most likely did discuss the risks of induction with the patient despite the fact that she had made no note of such. She also argued that fetal presentation was vertex at the time of her initial evaluation although, again, she did not make a note of that. She argued that the fetal heart rate and contraction patterns were adequate and reassuring. She saw no evidence of hyperstimulation. She argued that she was paged stat and that she arrived in 5 minutes' time. The baby was delivered within 20 minutes of her arrival.

The anesthesiologist defended his case by responding to the plaintiff's contention that he should have "questioned the indication for the epidural" by pointing to the mother's own testimony that she did feel as though she was in labor at the time of the epidural and had compared this labor to her previous delivery. He argued that the nursing staff, far more experienced in managing labor than he, also felt the patient was in labor.

The anesthesiologist responded to the plaintiff's criticism that the fetal heart monitor should not have been moved during epidural administration by pointing to the fact that there is no standard or guideline requiring such monitoring in the face of many hours of a reassuring heart-rate pattern. He argued that it would be substandard either not to remove or to move the fetal monitor strap to place the epidural and such would violate the sterile field. The nursing staff would then have been free to position the Doppler on the patient's abdomen during placement of the epidural if that was felt to be warranted.

The anesthesiologist argued that he did not prematurely exit the patient's bedside and that his chart reflected he recorded the patient's blood pressures every 5 minutes from the time he first saw her until the time of delivery. Thus, he argued, the plaintiff's testimony that he left the room and did not return was due to faulty memory.

The anesthesiologist responded to the allegation that he had failed to contact an obstetrician under emergency circumstances by arguing that the nurses were making constant attempts to locate the fetal heart rate and that the normal interaction between the obstetrician and the staff is that the notification to obtain an obstetrician for a problem is made by the nurses, not the anesthesiologist. He argued it is not the role of the anesthesiologist to assume the tasks of the labor and delivery nurses, whose roles are carefully coordinated, with certain responsibilities assigned to them.

Discussion

This case points out several common areas in which plaintiffs may make allegations of substandard care. First, failure to adequately document fetal presentation by the obstetricians left them open to claims that the baby was inappropriate for induction despite the logical inference that trained obstetrical personnel, including physicians and nurses, would not induce a patient for vaginal delivery in a transverse lie. In fact, the prenatal obstetrician would not have even been in the case had he documented fetal position. The physicians' and nurses' failure to document their informed-consent discussions or even the fact that such discussions took place with the patient left them open for criticism that they had not advised the patient as to the risks of induction with a low amniotic fluid index. Informed consent should always be documented. In many jurisdictions, the jury is instructed that a failure to give informed consent may subject the physician to liability for any injury caused by the treatment, even if the treatment itself is provided appropriately [13] (Box 50.7).

Serious questions arose in this case as to the time of the uterine rupture and the ability of the team to respond to this catastrophic event. The defendants argued that the baby and the placenta were both extruded into the abdomen at the time of the rupture. Thus, regardless of whether the baby had a heart rate at that time, the rupture of the placenta resulted in complete and total asphyxia of the child from the point of rupture. Utilizing the mother's testimony and the chart to establish this timing, it became difficult to conceive of a scenario where this child could have been delivered without having suffered severe brain damage unless an obstetrician was present at the time of the rupture.

Box 50.7 Duty of disclosure

It is the duty of the physician to disclose to the patient all material information to enable the patient to make an informed decision regarding the proposed treatment.

Material information is information which the physician knows or should know would be regarded as significant by a reasonable person in the patient's position when deciding to accept or reject a recommended medical procedure. To be material a fact must also be one which is not commonly appreciated.

When a procedure inherently involves a known risk of death or serious bodily harm it is the physician's duty to disclose to the patient the possibility of such outcome and to explain in lay terms the complications that might possibly occur.

Even though the patient has consented to a proposed treatment or operation, the failure of the physician to inform the patient as stated in this instruction before obtaining such consent is negligence and renders the physician subject to liability for *any* injury caused by the treatment if a reasonably prudent person in the patient's position would not have consented to the treatment if he or she had been adequately informed of all the significant perils. (Italics added)

Source: California BAJI 6.11 [13]

Demonstrating their awareness of this weakness in their case, the plaintiffs were highly motivated to find flaws in the prenatal care and in the early labor pattern to circumvent the causation defense which became operative at the time of rupture. Thus the plaintiff was motivated to focus less on the delay in diagnosis after the rupture had occurred. This was an area that was problematic for the defense where substantial delays took place between the time of the apparent rupture and notification to the obstetrician.

This case also illustrates how allegations of negligence may shift in focus if, for instance, at a particular time, causation cannot be proven to be linked with a particular act or mission. Here, it was likely that the infant suffered severe irreparable brain damage within 8–10 minutes of the rupture, making a therapeutic response to the event virtually impossible. Delay in notification to the obstetrician was thus less significant. The focus of the case therefore shifted to the weaker negligence arguments, such as the allegation that a 29-week prenatal ultrasound showing the baby was transverse indicated the baby was transverse at the time of induction.

The case against the hospital and the anesthesiologist settled before trial with approximately 80% of the payment coming from the hospital. The case went to trial against the two obstetricians. There was a finding of negligence by the jury, who also concluded that this negligence (by the prenatal obstetrician) was not a cause of injury to the child. The resulting judgment was for the physicians.

Case study: obstetric discharge/pediatric follow-up

This action was brought by a 5-year-old child with severe athetoid cerebral palsy from bilirubin encephalopathy which developed between 3 and 5 days after birth. Plaintiff alleged "early discharge" resulted in missed hyperbilirubinemia.

Plaintiff was delivered with Apgars of 9/9 at approximately 36 weeks' gestational age (a few days short of the AAP definition of "term"). The child was observed for approximately 32 hours in the hospital without any indication of jaundice. During that time, the child voided and stooled normally, had normal feeding habits, normal laboratory values, including hematocrit and hemoglobin levels, had frequent normal vital signs, normal skin color, normal activity, and normal tone. A cephalohematoma of unspecified size was noted.

Mother and child were discharged by the obstetrician with instructions to the mother to observe for color, feeding, activity, sleep, voiding, stools, and signs of illness. The mother was shown a videotape with similar instructions, which included a section on jaundice. At the time of discharge the mother was instructed to return to the pediatrician's office in "1–2 days."

The medical records and the mother's deposition testimony reflect that the child did well at home until approximately 3 days following discharge. The medical records and the mother's testimony also reflected the child exhibited symptoms of opisthotonos, the hallmark of bilirubin encephalopathy, on the third evening following discharge. The testimony demonstrated the mother had not returned to the pediatrician's office during that 1- to 2-day period as instructed at the time of discharge.

The records indicated the mother called the pediatrician's office for the first time 4 days post-discharge. The child was seen by the pediatrician at approximately midday on the fifth day of life. The pediatrician charted a relatively benign newborn exam, except that the child was jaundiced to the mid-abdomen. The pediatrician sent the patient to the hospital laboratory for a bilirubin level, which came back in approximately 2.5 hours, revealing a bilirubin level of 32 mg/dL. In light of the relatively benign physical examination, the pediatrician elected to order a retest stat to determine if there was lab error. The entire process between the completion of the pediatrician's first exam and the completion of the second blood test was approximately 4 hours. When the retest came back at the same level, the parents were sent immediately to the nearest neonatal intensive care unit. In the meantime, the pediatrician called the neonatologist at the neonatal intensive care unit for the purpose of preparing the staff for accepting the child for treatment. The neonatologist in charge ordered blood from the blood bank and began preparations for treatment. Because of the time required to obtain the blood, the transfusion did not take place for approximately an additional 4 hours.

Allegations against obstetrician

Plaintiff's experts alleged the obstetrician had violated the standard of care in the "early" discharge because the patient was at increased risk for potential elevated concentration of free ("toxic") bilirubin due to (1) prematurity, (2) cephalohematoma, (3) breastfeeding, (4) mother's receipt of oxytocin during labor, and (5) Asian ancestry. Plaintiff also alleged the obstetrician deviated from the standard of care in failing to educate the mother "vigorously" regarding her need to watch for jaundice, contending that the baby had a 50% increased risk of hyperbilirubinemia at the time of discharge. Plaintiff relied heavily on ACOG and AAP literature advocating against "early discharge."

Allegations against pediatrician

Plaintiff alleged the pediatrician was negligent because he failed to: (1) obtain a complete history of symptoms in a baby at "very high risk" for hyperbilirubinemia, and therefore did not conduct the appropriate physical examination; (2) did not order the initial bilirubin test stat; (3) did not inform the lab to phone with the results of the bilirubin in the initial order; and (4) that he reordered the bilirubin test after receiving the result of 32 mg/dL, without having the mother stay at the hospital to receive the results.

The plaintiff's attorney retained two experts on the subject of hyperbilirubinemia. One, a nationally recognized expert in the pathophysiology of hyperbilirubinemia, with extensive writings on the subject, was called to express opinions only on causation. This physician gave testimony which contradicted much of the causation testimony of the second plaintiff expert. The defense argued that had the mother followed the obstetrician's instructions to return the baby to the pediatrician in 1–2 days, the treatment would have been available. Plaintiff expert 1 admitted that had this child been treated with the standard therapies in the 3 days following discharge, she would have had no great injury whatsoever. Plaintiff expert 1 also acknowledged that, based on the serum bilirubin lab values taken at the time of the first test, the child's level had either peaked or was on its way down when the pediatrician first examined the child. This expert further admitted that if the child was truly exhibiting opisthotonic movements, characterized by back-arching on the previous evening, this would be an indication of bilirubin brain toxicity even before the pediatrician saw the child.

Plaintiff expert 2, a retired physician, clearly was an advocate for the plaintiff. Causation was strenuously contested throughout the cross-examination of this expert. Plaintiff expert 2 refused to acknowledge that the back-arching movements witnessed by the parents before the child was seen at the pediatrician's office were characteristic of opisthotonos. This expert claimed that most, or all, of the brain damage would have been avoided and/or reversed if treatment had been initiated by the pediatrician on the first visit. Plaintiff expert 2 produced a self-generated "table" of neonatal signs of bilirubin-induced neurological dysfunction progressing to kernicterus, purporting to correlate clinical signs in three stages, with those stages being (1) reversible, (2) partially reversible, and (3) irreversible. This table was not the product of any controlled studies, nor had it been submitted for publication. Both plaintiff experts admitted that bilirubin encephalopathy does occur at levels over 20%. Expert 1, along with the

---

Box 50.8 Patient's duty to follow instructions

A patient has a duty to follow all reasonable and proper advice and instructions regarding care, activities, and treatment given by such patient's doctor.

A doctor is not liable for any injury resulting *solely* from the negligent failure of the patient to follow such advice and instructions.

However, if the negligence of the doctor is a cause of injury to the patient, the contributory negligence of the patient, if any, in not following such advice and instructions does not bar recovery by the patient against the doctor, but the total amount to which the patient would otherwise be entitled shall be reduced in proportion to the negligence attributable to the patient. (Italics added)

Source: California BAJI 6.28 [14]

---

defense experts, testified that the bilirubin level had peaked or was on the way down at the time the mother presented the child to the pediatrician's office. Thus, the bilirubin level on the morning before the child arrived at the pediatrician's office was approximately 30 mg/dL. Bilirubin toxicity to the brain cells, it was acknowledged, may occur even before clinical symptoms are present. Following the expert depositions, the plaintiff dismissed the case and refiled it in a different jurisdiction before the running of the statute of limitations. Plaintiff's expert 1 was not to be called in the refiled case. Thereafter, the case was settled for a small fraction of the proffered damages.

Discussion

The defense had legitimate fears of how the jury might react to specialty society (e.g., ACOG, AAP) guidelines advocating against early discharge. While the practitioners here sought to balance the discharge with early pediatric follow-up, deviations from such guidelines can be devastating at trial.

The hospital staff had documented (twice) the discharge instructions to the mother, to return the child to the pediatrician's office in 1–2 days. Moreover, they had the mother sign the discharge instructions, acknowledging receipt and understanding. That follow-up instructions were given is frequently denied by plaintiffs. Signed instructions are a valuable and effective way to rebut such denials. However, the doctor is protected from liability only for injury resulting solely from the negligent failure of the patient to follow instructions [14] (Box 50.8).

This case illustrates the enormous impact a thorough analysis of the causation elements of the case may have on the ultimate result. Objective evidence utilizing the natural progression of the bilirubin levels led to a strong conclusion that the child's encephalopathy had occurred before the visit to the pediatrician's office. This strong causation defense again caused the plaintiffs to focus arguments against the obstetrician, which may not have been made otherwise. The fact of the serious contradictory testimony between the two plaintiff experts also weighed heavily on the ultimate outcome of the case.

References

1. California BAJI (Book of Approved Jury Instructions), 6.30.

2. California BAJI (Book of Approved Jury Instructions), 6.05.

3. California BAJI (Book of Approved Jury Instructions), 6.00.1, 6.02.

4. California BAJI (Book of Approved Jury Instructions), 6.03.

5. California BAJI (Book of Approved Jury Instructions), 3.76, 3.77.

6. Altshuler G. Placental insights into neurodevelopmental and other childhood diseases. *Semin Pediatr Neurol* 1995; **2**: 90–9.

7. ACOG Technical Bulletin. Fetal heart rate patterns: monitoring, interpretation, and management. No. 207, July 1995 (replaces No. 132, September 1989). *Int J Gynaecol Obstet* 1995; **51**: 65–74.

8. American College of Obstetricians and Gynecologists. *Intrapartum Fetal Heart Rate Monitoring.* Technical bulletin 132. Washington, DC: American College of Obstetricians and Gynecologists, 1989.

9. American College of Obstetricians and Gynecologists. *The Intrauterine Device.* Technical bulletin 104. Washington, DC: American College of Obstetricians and Gynecologists, 1987.

10. American College of Obstetricians and Gynecologists. *Fetal and Neonatal Neurologic Injury.* Technical bulletin 163. Washington, DC: American College of Obstetricians and Gynecologists, 1992.

11. American Academy of Pediatrics, American College of Obstetricians and Gynecologists. Relationship between perinatal factors and neurologic outcome. In Poland RL, Freeman RK, eds., *Guidelines for Perinatal Care*, 3rd edn. Elk Grove Village, IL: AAP, 1992: 221–4.

12. Nelson KB. Is it HIE? And why that matters. *Acta Paediatr* 2007; **96**: 1113–14.

13. California BAJI (Book of Approved Jury Instructions). 6.11 (revised), Duty of disclosure.

14. California BAJI (Book of Approved Jury Instructions). 6.28, Duty of patient.

Index